TEXTBOOK OF SURGERY

FOR MEDICAL STUDENTS AND DOCTORS

TEXTBOOK OF SURGERY

for medical students and doctors

By

Ijaz Ahsan

FRCS (Ed), FCPS (Pak),
FRCPS (Glas), FCS (Lanka)
Formerly
Professor of Surgery and Principal, King Edward Medical College, Lahore;
Dean, Postgraduate Medical Institute, Lahore;
Principal, Allama Iqbal Medical College, Lahore;
Dean, Faculty of Medicine and Dentistry, University of Lahore,
President, College of Physicians and Surgeons Pakistan,
Karachi, Pakistan.

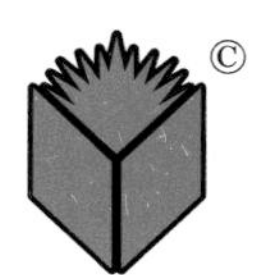

Paramount Books (Pvt.) Ltd.
Karachi | Lahore | Islamabad | Hyderabad | Faisalabad | Peshawar | Abbottabad |

Textbook of Surgery

by

Ijaz Ahsan

First Edition 1991
Second Edition 1997
Third Edition 2015

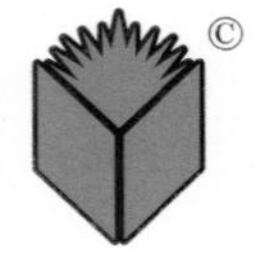

Paramount Books (Pvt.) Ltd.

152/O, Block-2, P.E.C.H.S., Karachi-75400. Tel: 34310030
Fax: 34553772, E-mail: info@paramountbooks.com.pk
Website: www.paramountbooks.com.pk

ISBN: 978-969-637-076-5
Printed in Pakistan

CONTENTS

To
Yousaf, Mariam, Mudassar,
Daaniyal and Faiz,
wishing them the best

FOREWORD

It was a privilege to be asked to write a foreword to this superb text, but beyond this, it was a pleasure to be able to read the book itself. It would be no exaggeration to say that this is a superb book, designed as an entry point into the broad field of surgery, and thus indispensable for medical students, to nurses who are developing their careers in the area of surgery, and to junior surgical residents in training.

The charm and appeal of the book lies in its simplicity, directness, accuracy and completeness. In distinction to much more sophisticated volumes which have been written to cover this field, sometimes in five separate volumes, the scope is broad but the text is limited. Thus one can read it quickly, easily, with pleasure and with satisfaction.

In a text directed towards this particular audience, one should not criticize the lack of depth, in as much as the complexity of surgical pathophysiology today is such that one could spend endless pages probing deeper and deeper into the molecular biology of each of the systems discussed. In addition, the complexity of surgical technique is such that one would hardly be expected to pursue it with any degree of effectiveness, but again, this is hardly what one looks for as an entry point into the field. I might comment in passing on the illustrations, which would be fascinating for a young student entering the surgical world.

Obviously, this book is only a preface to a career, and the young men must clearly pursue each of the areas which are covered with a wide brush, in much more depth and precision than is available in these pages. One could not, however, ask or expect this to be done at this level of simplicity, and with the objectives that the author had in mind, it would have been very unwise to extend the length of this volume to pursue any of the areas in further depth. All in all, I seldom encounter a text which would be more satisfactory for an individual entering into this extraordinarily broad and complicated field which we refer to, in the most general terms, as surgery. With this group in mind, I would certainly recommend this text wholeheartedly, and encourage everyone to use this as the initial step into a marvellously complex and increasingly satisfying career.

William V. McDermott Jr., M.D.
David W. and David Cheever Professor of Surgery,
Harvard Medical School, Boston, Massachusetts, USA

PREFACE

A textbook for an undergraduate medical student should contain only that much which he needs, and no more. Before writing a single word in such a book, one must think many times: does the student actually need it? And if it is decided that he does, it should be explained in as easy a language as possible. This is the student's first exposure to the subject. Make it pleasant, and he will follow the subject to the ends of the earth; make it difficult and he will never go near it again. Such is the book I tried to write. The success of the previous editions has encouraged me to continue with the same policy.

Most medical students will not become surgeons; they will become general practitioners or pursue specialties other than surgery. This book should give them a sufficient understanding of surgical illnesses and their management. On the other hand, those students who take up surgery as a career will have all the time in the world to learn the ropes.

At the same time, dental and nursing students and postgraduates, and surgical residents, will find the book useful for an understanding of the principles and practice of surgery. Again, doctors from non-surgical specialties could keep this book on their shelf for reference in respect of surgical illnesses.

To conclude, the author is hopeful that every reader will find in the book what he is looking for. This will be adequate compensation for his efforts, and those of the contributors.

Ijaz Ahsan

ACKNOWLEDGEMENTS

My teachers of surgery Professors Amiruddin, Riyaz Qadeer and Sardar Ali Sheikh set me on the road leading to the production of this book. I am grateful to my colleagues, each eminent in his own field, for their valuable contributions in updating the book; their names appear in the List of Contributors. I am also indebted to Professor Ziaul Meraj and Drs. Saeed Ahmed and Jamil Sarfraz for a number of clinical photographs and images. I am indebted to Professors Anwaar A. Khan and Salman Waris for some up-to-date information about GI endoscopy and urology respectively. I am obliged to Professor Rashid Lateef Khan, whose insistence made me embark on this project. The publisher represented by Zainul Abedin, Asfiya Aziz, Nasser Gaba, Dilshad Alam and Bushra Ahmed were most courteous and helpful throughout.

CONTRIBUTORS

The author is greatly indebted to the following colleagues for help in updating the book for the present third edition:

Abdul Majid Chaudhary

FRCS (Ed), FRCS (Glas), FCPS (Pak), MHPE (Holland), FCS (SL)
President, SAARC Surgical Care Society,
Principal and Chairman Department of Surgery,
Lahore Medical and Dental College, Lahore, Pakistan

ENDOCRINES

Amjad Mehboob

MBBS, FCPS (Medicine)

Fellow in Infectious Diseases, Shaukat Khanum Memorial Cancer Hospital and Research Centre, Lahore, Pakistan

INFECTIOUS DISEASES

Aun Raza

MBBS, FCPS (Medicine)

Fellow in Infectious Diseases, Shaukat Khanum

Memorial Cancer Hospital, and Research Centre Lahore, Pakistan

INFECTIOUS DISEASES

Arshad Taqi

FCPS (Anesthesiology)

Professor of Anesthesiology, Rashid Latif Medical

College, Lahore, Pakistan

ANESTHESIA

Ather Saeed Kazmi

MBBS, MRCP, FRCR

Consultant Clinical Oncologist, Shaukat Khanum Memorial Cancer Hospital and Research Centre, Lahore, Pakistan

ONCOLOGY

Dilawaiz Nadeem

FRCS (Edin), FRCS (Glas), MCH

Orth (Dundee), MD Paeds Ortho (Dundee), FRCS Trauma and Ortho (Ed)

Diplomate Intercollegiate Board in Orthopedic Surgery (UK)

Professor of Orthopedic Surgery, Services Institute of

Medical Sciences, Lahore, Pakistan

ORTHOPEDICS

Faisal Sultan

MBBS, FRCP (Edin), FCPS (Pak)

Diplomate American Board of Internal Medicine (Infectious diseases)

Consultant Physician, Shaukat Khanum Memorial

Cancer Hospital and Research Centre, Lahore, Pakistan

INFECTIOUS DISEASES

Farid Ahmed Khan

FRCS (Edin), FCPS (Plastic Surgery)

Chairman and Professor of Plastic Surgery, King Edward Medical University, Lahore, Pakistan

PLASTIC SURGERY

Ijaz Hussain Shah

FCPS (Plastic Surgery)

Senior Registrar Plastic Surgery, Mayo Hospital,

Lahore, Pakistan

PLASTIC SURGERY

Jamil Sarfraz

MD

Diplomate, American Boards of Internal Medicine,

Diagnostic Radiology and Nuclear Medicine.

Director of Radiology, Kane Community Hospital,

Affiliate of University of Pittsburgh Medical Center,

Kane, Pennsylvania, USA

IMAGING

Kamran Chima

Diplomate, American Boards of Internal Medicine, Pulmonary Disease and Critical Care Medicine

Professor of Pulmonology and Critical Care,
Services Institute of Medical Sciences, Lahore, Pakistan

PULMONARY MEDICINE and CRITICAL CARE

Khalid Durrani

MBBS, FRCS (Edin)

Professor of Surgery, University College of Medicine, University of Lahore, Lahore, Pakistan

G.I.TRACT

Khurram Mir

FRCS (Edinburgh), Masters in Medical Sciences (Glasgow), FRCS Urology (Edin), Fellow of the European Board of Urology

Consultant Urologist, Shaukat Khanum Memorial Cancer Hospital and Research Centre, Lahore, Pakistan

UROLOGY

Mohammad Asim Yusaf

MBBS, FRCP (Edin)

Consultant Gastroenterologist and Medical Director, Shaukat Khanum Memorial Cancer Hospital and Research Centre, Lahore, Pakistan

STOMACH AND DUODENUM

Mohammad Zia-ul-Miraj Ahmad

MBBS, FRCS (Edin), Dipl. Paeds. Surg. (London), DCH (Glasgow), DU (London) Professor of Pediatric Urology, Children's Hospital and The Institute of Child Health, Lahore

PEDIATRIC SURGERY AND PEDS UROLOGY

Parvez Raja

FRCS (Edin)

Professor of Cardiac Surgery,

Faisalabad Institute of Cardiology, Faisalabad, Pakistan

CARDIAC SURGERY

Saad bin Anis

MBBS

Postgraduate Resident in Surgery, Allama Iqbal

Medical College, Lahore, Pakistan

PRINCIPLES

Saeed Ahmed

FRCS, FRACS

Consultant Pediatric Urologist, Adelaide Children's Hospital, Adelaide, Australia; King Faisal Specialist Hospital, Riyadh, Saudi Arabia

PEDIATRIC UROLOGY IMAGES

Salman A. Shah

MD, FACS, Diplomate, American Boards of

Surgery and Thoracic Surgery

Assistant Professor of Pediatric Cardiac Surgery, Children's Hospital, Lahore, Pakistan

PEDIATRIC CARDIAC SURGERY

Samir Qazi

BDS, MPhil, FFDRCS

Associate Professor of Oral and Maxillofacial Surgery, CMH Lahore Medical College, Institute of Dentistry, Lahore, Pakistan

ORAL AND MAXILLOFACIAL SURGERY

Tariq Salahuddin

FRCS, FCPS

Professor of Neurosurgery, Ameeruddin Medical

College, Post Graduate Medical Institution, Lahore Pakistan

NEUROSURGERY

Zahid Niaz

MBBS, FCPS (Pak), FRCS (gow)

Professor of Surgery, Allama Iqbal Medical College, Lahore, Pakistan

PRINCIPLES

Part I

PRINCIPLES

Chapter

1 INTRODUCTION

Surgery has been practiced from time immemorial. The earliest examples of surgical work included the care of wounds, the drainage of abscesses and the splinting of fractures. Modern surgical practice has come a long way from those early days. Before a student embarks upon a detailed study of the subject, he should have a general idea of what surgery is all about, and what is its scope. At the same time he should be knowledgeable about the way in which, over the centuries, surgery has evolved to attain its present state of refinement and advancement.

THE SCOPE OF SURGERY

Surgery can be defined as that branch of medicine which treats diseases and injuries by manual or operative methods. Let us see what this means in actual practice.

If a viscus is diseased, it may be *removed* by operation, for example an appendix which is inflamed, or a testis which is the seat of a cancer.

If an organ is irreversibly diseased but is vital for life, e.g. the heart or the liver, it may be *removed and replaced* by another, taken from a living donor or a fresh cadaver (transplantation).

If a bone is broken, its ends are brought into alignment and held together, either in a fiber-glass cast or by internal fixation by a nail, until they unite to each other.

Many internal organs are in the form of *hollow tubes*, e.g. intestines, arteries, veins, ureters, bile ducts, etc. If such a tube gets blocked, the contained fluid, e.g. blood, urine or bile, accumulates and stagnates in the tube, producing harmful effects on the person's health. Such a tube needs to be *unblocked*, and an important part of any surgeon's work consists of unblocking such tubes. In this sense surgeons are plumbers, or in other words biological engineers.

There are many methods of dealing with such a block in a tube:

- The *material* blocking the tube may be *removed* by slitting open the tube. For example, a polyp in the small intestine, or deposits of cholesterol in an artery, may be removed through an incision in the wall of the intestine or artery.
- In other cases, the narrowing may be eliminated by shifting a *flap* of the wall of the tube across the narrow area to widen it, as at the pelviureteric junction in a case of hydronephrosis.
- If the blockage is due to excessive hypertrophy of a sphincter, it may be dealt with by *dividing the sphincter,* as in infantile pyloric stenosis.
- If the block cannot be eliminated by one of the above methods, the blocked segment of the tube may be *removed* and the continuity of the tube restored, as in the case of the intestine or an artery:
  - In the case of the intestine, the ends are simply brought together and joined to each other.
  - Unlike the intestine which has a mesentery, arteries are firmly adherent to the bed on which they lie. Thus with an artery, the ends normally cannot be mobilized and brought together; therefore, the gap is usually filled either by a segment of a vein, or by a tube made of synthetic material.
- If the tube can neither be unblocked nor removed, the block may be *bypassed*. For example, in a case of inoperable carcinoma of the cecum, the ileum may be joined to the transverse colon, bypassing the obstruction.

The job of a surgeon consists of finding out the cause of the patient's symptoms, i.e. the nature of his illness, and using the appropriate operation or other mode of treatment to remedy the defect. For this he must first possess knowledge of the natural history of different surgical conditions. At the same time, he must be familiar with the different methods of examination and investigation to extract the maximum information from the patient for arriving at the correct diagnosis. Next, he must know which operation or other method of treatment suits his patient the best, and should be able to employ it. Finally, if a complication arises during the postoperative course, he should be able to deal with it.

But that is not all. The surgeon should not be a mere robot carrying out the above-mentioned functions to perfection. He should above all be a compassionate human being, pleasant and smiling. Most patients are afraid of surgical operations. If the practitioner of the art is seen by them to be friendly, their fear of the operation is considerably reduced, which makes it easier for them to withstand what they expect to be an ordeal. In cases with incurable illnesses, the surgeon must utter words of encouragement, and must never let the patient feel he has been forsaken by his medical attendants.

The reader should remember that on becoming a surgeon he is going to have the privilege, but also the responsibility, of working on the most precious asset of an individual, namely his health and life, and that the patient's welfare should always be his first and foremost concern. He will be judged by how well he discharges this responsibility. Surgery offers a fascinating, although a demanding career. The author feels privileged in welcoming newcomers into this field.

THE EVOLUTION OF SURGERY

Surgery is as old as mankind itself. Human skulls in which circular fragments have been removed as if by a trephine have been found dating back to the Stone Age. Such operations were performed for headache and for epilepsy in order to allow the egress of evil spirits! However, apart from the splinting of fractures and the drainage of abscesses, not much of consequence was achieved in the ancient world. One of the reasons for the slow development of surgery was the severe punishments reserved for surgeons in the case of failure. For example, under the code of Hammurabi in western Asia about 4,000 years ago, if the patient died after operation, the surgeon's hands were cut off!

Even from those far-off times, examples of accurate recording are occasionally found. From the Egypt of 5,000 years ago, the Edwin Smith Papyrus describes a series of 48 cases of trauma, listed from the head downwards, and enumerated in order of increasing severity of injury, which is indeed startling for a paper written so far in the past. The value of fixation in the treatment of fractures was appreciated, and splints were made from linen bandages impregnated with resin.

In ancient times it was believed that illnesses were due to the wrath of capricious and merciless gods. The single greatest achievement in the history of medicine was the negation of this belief, as well as the exclusion of demons, spirits and sin as the cause of disease. Only after this was done could a true cause and effect relationship be sought for and established. It should be remembered that in backward countries and societies these beliefs are still held by some.

Darius I of Persia established at Sais around 500 B.C. what seems to have been the first school of medicine. Students were selected "from among the sons of men of consequence, no sons of the poor were among them".

The god of Greek medicine was Aesculapius. During the 5th century B.C., numerous temples of health were erected to him. The priests treated patients with a combination of mysticism, burnt offerings and baths. The best known pupil from one of these schools was Hippocrates. He was distinguished by his straightforward observations and logical deductions. He clearly recognized the principle of traction in the reduction of fractures and dislocations. He classified physicians into the ordinary practitioners, those of a higher class, and the intelligent ones. In those days the surgeon was usually to be found in the first category.

An opportunity for the development of physicians of the second category arose with the founding of a medical school by Alexander's successor Ptolemy Soter at Alexandria in the 4th century B.C. Scholars and books were brought here from Greece and from the whole world. Dissections of the human body were started and normal body functions studied. The pulse was counted and the flow of blood through arteries and veins noted. The lens was removed for the treatment of cataract. The library became a fabulous institution, containing 700,000 papyrus rolls; when it was destroyed by the invading armies of Julius Caesar, civilization received a very severe blow.

Some of the achievements in medicine have been preserved for us by the writings of Celsus and Galen. The former's treatise *De Medicina* is a remarkable document. The last two of eight books concern surgery. The cardinal signs of inflammation are stressed, the treatment of fistulas, the drainage of abscesses, use of the ligature, and debridement of wounds is described. The removal of bladder stones is detailed.

The Romans possessed a strong antipathy to the medicine of a foreign people. For centuries the contributions of Hippocrates and the Alexandrian school were held in contempt. In its place they preferred to adhere to mysticism, and were without physicians for 600 years until after the conquests by Pompey in the first century B.C., many Greek physicians began to migrate to Rome.

The development of medicine over the next 1500 years was to be colored by the work of Galen. Apart from numerous anatomical dissections, he studied function. He called attention to the fact that injury to the spinal cord between the first and second cervical vertebrae produced instant death, between the third and fourth respiratory paralysis, while below the sixth the muscles of the thoracic cage were paralyzed and there was chiefly diaphragmatic respiration.

The millennium following upon the death of Galen was quite unproductive, for two main reasons. Firstly, the authority of Galen was so great that none could challenge it for many centuries after his death, and this led to intellectual stagnation. Secondly, the Christian Church took hold in the Mediterranean area, and the concept of cure by prayer and miracle was strengthened. It was believed that disease was caused by sin. Therapy was thus directed to the soul and not the body. There was an edict against dissection of the human body. At the same time the body was not to be mutilated, and therefore the making of an incision was condemned. Under such a situation, surgery could not develop, and in fact rapidly declined in Christian lands.

Fortunately the intellectual leadership, which now moved eastward to the Islamic world, carried with it the Greek achievements which were translated into Arabic, preserved and modified.

The prominent names among the Muslims are those of Rhazes (860 to 932 A.D.) and Avicenna (980 to 1037 A.D.). One whole book in the former's *Continens* is devoted to surgery. The writings of these two dominated European medicine for a long time.

In 1092 the Pope decreed that monks were not to wear beards. A barber was therefore employed in most monasteries. It was also the custom for monks to be bled at intervals, and naturally it was the barber who performed this function also. These barber-surgeons soon started performing minor surgical procedures, first inside the monastery, but later in society in general.

In 1163 the Council of Tours declared that 'the Church abhorreth bloodshed'. Now, most educational institutions were operated by the Church, and had to respect this ban. Therefore by default surgery had to be practiced by uneducated and often unethical craftsmen —the barber and the lithotomist.

From then onwards, and through the middle ages and renaissance, translations of Arabic medical books into Latin filled a gap and accelerated the development of European medicine.

During the sixteenth century, impressive advances were made in the study of both the structure and function of the human body. Vesalius concentrated on anatomy. Inspired by the depiction of the human form by artists of the caliber of Raphael and Michaelangelo, he hired artists of the first rank to illustrate his dissections. William Harvey was impressed with the demonstration by Fabricius of one-way valves in veins, and deduced the system of circulation of the blood.

During the seventeenth century Malpighi in Italy demonstrated, under a microscope, capillaries and capillary circulation, the layers of the skin, nerve pathways in the spinal cord, and the glomeruli of the kidneys. It was also shown that blood contained a solid component, the red cells. Boyle showed that air was necessary for an animal to sustain life, and that the lungs provided this function. His assistant Hooke gave the concept of the cell, and study of cells of different organs elucidated the intricate details of microscopic anatomy.

The eighteenth century witnessed the performance of operations on the abdomen, including colostomy. John Hunter made important contributions in experimental surgery, including the implantation of lead pellets into the shaft of long bones of puppies to demonstrate that longitudinal growth took place at the epiphysis. His pupil Abernathy demonstrated the regeneration of peripheral nerves following neurectomy and suture.

In America, surgery hardly existed until after the revolution. The first medical school in America was started in Philadelphia in 1761. William Shippen, the first professor of surgery, had studied with Hunter in London. In Boston, John Warren, also a surgeon, played an important part in the founding of the Harvard Medical School. Because of its late beginnings, surgery in America was saved from the turmoil of being involved with barbers, of being controlled by the church, and of having to contend with overbearing physicians. At first, American surgery represented a transfer from European centers; later it assumed a character of its own.

The discovery of anesthesia during the nineteenth century was a quantum leap forwards. Both ether and chloroform were first used in the 1840's. Surgical operations could now take place in a calm and quiet atmosphere, and the surgeon could proceed in an unhurried manner. Before this time, the surgeon had to employ strong men to restrain the patient on the operation table, and it is obvious that only the simplest procedures had been possible under those circumstances. It is not a mere coincidence that a very large number of complicated and extensive operative procedures were first carried out during the succeeding half of the same century; anesthesia had made the job of the surgeon much easier. Thus we notice Kocher with his thyroidectomy, Halsted and his radical mastectomy, Langenbech with his cholecystectomy, and Billroth and Polya with their respective gastrectomies, all within the span of a few decades. By achieving these 'firsts' due to the availability of anesthesia, the surgeons of that generation assured their place in history, and appear larger-than-life even today.

From that time onwards, the speed of scientific progress picked up considerably, so much so that more advancements have been made during the twentieth century than in the previous fifty centuries combined. Removal of the lung for cancer, and removal and substitution of the esophagus by the stomach have become routine procedures.

Since the Second World War, developments in the field of surgery have proceeded with mind-boggling speed. Operations like replacement of the heart, liver or kidneys, which could not even be imagined a few decades ago, are commonplace. Whereas previously, surgery consisted mainly of ablative procedures, advances in surgery are more and more being made in the field of reconstruction, whether in the case of the urethra in cases of stricture, the rectum in congenital anomalies, the thumb in cases of loss due to trauma, or the mandible after its excision for malignant disease. At the same time, plastic surgeons are constantly inventing newer and better methods of correction of defects due to congenital anomalies and loss of tissues.

Finally, with the emergence of large numbers of independent states around the globe, medical schools in their dozens and hundreds have come up in these countries. With the numbers of physicians multiplying with geometric progression, specialization and super-specialization is the order of the day. More and more medical schools in these countries are achieving a reputation and status unimaginable a few decades ago. Often only a year or two elapses between the introduction of a new technique in the advanced countries and its adoption in the developing countries. In this environment of intense international competition, the future of surgery is assured worldwide.

Chapter

2 WOUNDS

This is one of the most important chapters in this book, because all his life a surgeon has to take care of wounds. Most of these he has made himself. Whether he operates upon the stomach or the kidney, the hand or the foot, a wound inevitably results. Again, he has to look after wounds sustained at home, in the factory, in traffic accidents, and due to assault by different weapons. He should thus have a very clear understanding of the process of wound healing to be able to take good care of the thousands of wounds he will come across during his surgical career.

Historical note

In ancient times wounds were taken care of gently. The principles were: removal of foreign bodies, suturing, and covering with clean materials. However, in the fourteenth century, with the increasing use of gunpowder and the frequency of bullet wounds, aggressive methods of wound care were employed. Boiling oil and hot cautery replaced simple washing. Cleanliness was forgotten. This attitude produced disastrous results. The mortality rate after amputation of the thigh ranged from 80 to 100%, mostly due to sepsis.

In the sixteenth century, during a particular battle the supply of oil was exhausted and Ambrose Pare, the surgeon, had to treat amputation wounds without boiling oil. To his surprise, these wounds healed rapidly without the normally expected complications.

From this beginning the era of gentle wound care evolved. John Hunter and others showed that minimizing tissue injury produced rapid healing. Most technical advances in wound care since then have been based on this concept of minimum interference. Finally, the late nineteenth century witnessed the discovery of bacteria and the introduction of aseptic surgical techniques to keep micro-organisms away from wounds. This inaugurated the modern era of wound management.

THE PROCESS OF HEALING

The inflammatory response

Inflammation, followed by repair, commences as soon as a wound is inflicted, and goes through the following stages:

- Injury causes hemorrhage from damaged vessels. *Platelets* derived from the hemorrhage release clotting factors to produce fibrin, which is hemostatic and also forms a mesh for the migration of inflammatory cells and fibroblasts. Platelets are also the first cells to produce several essential cytokines which modulate most of the subsequent events in wound healing.
- Within a few hours white blood cells accumulate in the wound. At first the predominant cell is the *polymorphonuclear leucocyte*. These cells die, lyse, and release acid hydrolases.
- Soon the proportion of *monocytes* increases. These cells continue their activity of clearing the debris for several weeks. It is of interest to note that wound healing proceeds normally in the absence of both polymorphs and lymphocytes. In contrast to this, monocytes must be present for normal production of fibroblasts, and for invasion of the space by them. It should be remembered that while inflammatory cells regulate connective tissue matrix repair, the messengers of repair are the cytokines, which in the past were called 'growth factors'.
- *Fibroplasia*. It is at this stage of wound healing that *fibroblasts* make their appearance, and soon they start laying down collagen fibers. Most of these fibroblasts are derived from the local mesenchymal cells.
- As the fibroblasts and capillaries advance into an area, the previously laid *fibrin strands* get dissolved by the enzyme plasminogen activator produced by the endothelial cells of the capillaries. If large amounts of fibrin, blood clot or dead tissue are present, they constitute a physical barrier against fibroblast penetration. It is only after the macrophages have

removed all this matter that fibroblasts can come in and start laying down *collagen fibers*.

- *Maturation.* When the fibroblasts, with the help of nutrients brought by the capillaries, have laid down collagen, they themselves are no longer required. Both fibroblasts and capillaries now get greatly reduced in number. The wound now matures by type-III collagen fibers being replaced by type-I fibers, which become realigned along the lines of tension.
- *Contraction.* Finally the wound contracts due to the activity of *myofibroblasts*. The resulting tissue, the *scar*, has decreased vascularity and the collagen fibers are aligned along the lines of tension.

Components of healing

Three separate mechanisms are involved in all healing processes:

Epithelialization

This is the process whereby keratinocytes migrate and divide to re-surface loss of skin or mucosa. This activity ceases when epithelial contact is re-established with adjacent epithelial cells. It proceeds most rapidly in a moist, highly oxygenated environment.

Contraction

This is the process which leads to spontaneous closure of full-thickness skin wounds. It is the form of migration that involves the whole thickness of the skin and subcutaneous tissues. It therefore proceeds most readily in areas where the skin is loose such as the back of the neck. It is due to forces exerted by specialized fibroblasts which contain contractile elements in their cytoplasm and are called myofibroblasts. It is the same process that leads to constriction of tubular organs such as the common bile duct or esophagus after injury. It is a physiological process and must be distinguished from the pathological process of scar contracture or cicatrization which produces distortion and limitation of movement.

Table 2.1 Components of extracellular matrix

Component	Function
Collagen	Strength, support and structure for all tissues
Elastin	Allows tissues to expand and contract
Fibronectin	Mediates cell adhesion
Proteoglycans	Store moisture, absorb shock
Hyaluronic acid	Provides fluid environment for cell movement

Connective tissue formation

This is the process whereby fibroblasts are recruited to the site of injury and produce a new connective tissue matrix. It is the mechanism by which the main body of the wound is united, and the strength of a wound following surgery depends upon it. The cross-linked collagen in the connective tissue provides strength and integrity to all the tissues. The major components of the extracellular matrix and their functions are given in (Table 2.1).

Cytokines in wound healing

A cytokine is a soluble molecule produced by a cell to induce a biological effect elsewhere. It acts as a messenger at its destination. The effect varies according to the cytokine and the cell, but typically these molecules signal certain cells to activate, divide, or home in on a particular site in the body. Some examples of cytokines are given in (Table 2.2).

Types of wounds

Wounds are of two types — closed and open wounds.

CLOSED WOUNDS

Healing by first intention

When a surgeon incises the skin cleanly with a sharp knife and then sutures the wound neatly, co-apting the wound edges accurately, there is very little dead tissue or extraneous matter in the wound, which, therefore, heals very promptly. Repair in this manner is called healing by first intention. The duration and intensity of this inflammatory response depends upon the amount of local tissue damage. In the usual clean incision acute inflammation subsides within a few days. While dead material is being removed from the deeper areas the epidermis at the wound edges begins to thicken within a few hours of injury. If the wound has been sutured carefully, the edges are closely coapted to each other. Epithelial cells migrate across the defect and within 48 hours the entire wound surface is epithelialized, many layers of cells being produced. At the same time, the superficial layers become keratinized, as in the normal skin.

If the wound is a badly lacerated one, or has been made by the surgeon without using fine and gentle technique, extensive tissue injury may be present, which may prolong the inflammatory response for many weeks, or even months. The presence of foreign bodies or bacteria also prolongs the time taken for healing.

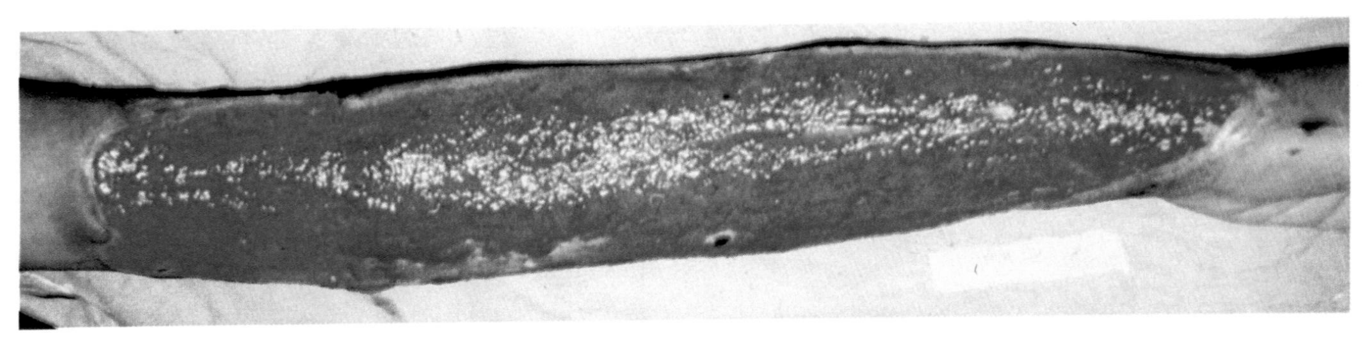

Fig.2.1 Full-thickness skin loss arm, The area is nicely granulating. At the lowermost margin a thin layer of light pink skin is growing upwards. The area is fit to receive split-skin grafts. The rounded ends of looped capillaries produce the granulations which give the tissue its name. To show appearance of granulation tissue.

Table 2.2 Some cytokines that promote wound healing

Cytokine	Source	Function
Platelet-derived growth factor (PGDF)	Platelets, macrophages, endothelial cells and smooth muscle cells	Fibroblast proliferation; chemotaxis;collagen metabolism; macrophages; angiogenesis
Tumor necrosis factor (TNF)	Macrophages, mast cells, T-lymphocytes, other tissues and cells	Fibroblast proliferation; ditto plus collegenase, neutrophil chemotaxis
Epidermal growth factor (EGF)	Platelets, saliva, urine, milk, plasma	Fibroblast and epithelial cell proliferation; granulation tissue formation

OPEN WOUNDS

Healing by second intention

The basic morphological and chemical processes operating in open wounds are the same as in incised and sutured wounds. However, the clinical problem presented is entirely different. Contraction takes place which distorts the wound, and epithelialization over the wound becomes a problem, especially if skin has been lost. The natural healing of an open wound is called *healing by second intention* or by granulation.

Open wounds without skin loss

Granulation tissue

If an incised wound is allowed to remain open it begins the healing process normally. An inflammatory exudate collects on the surface. Marginal epithelial cells mobilize, divide and migrate down the edges under the exudate. Injured venules branch and form capillary networks, and fibroblasts invade the injured area. The surface of such a wound is granular due to the looped ends of the advancing capillaries. This appearance has given it the name of *granulation tissue* (Fig.2.1).

Delayed primary closure

If the wound is heavily contaminated it is best left open for a few days. During this period the number of bacteria on the wound becomes greatly reduced, and the wound can be closed. This *delayed primary suture* can prevent infection from developing in contaminated wounds.

Open wounds with skin loss

If an area of skin has been lost and the wound is left alone, it is closed by the process of contraction. The wound contracts by stretching the surrounding skin, *not by production of new skin.* In regions which are away from joints and where the skin is loose, wound contraction produces minimal deformity. However, where mobility is important, e.g. the fingers, contraction resulting even from a small wound produces serious functional impairment.

Avoiding contraction

Contraction can best be eliminated or minimized *by immediately replacing the missing skin.* Full thickness grafts or flaps work best in this respect; partial thickness grafts are less effective, because they themselves contract down to some extent. But if the areas of skin loss are large, they represent the only practical method available for replacing the loss.

In areas where the tissues are fixed and there is little excess of skin (e.g. over the skull or lower leg), even maximal contraction cannot close a large defect. Sufficient skin simply cannot be pulled into the wound. The wound remains uncovered as an open ulcer, and has to be treated by a skin graft.

Open wounds are covered by a plasma protein exudate, which becomes dry and also contains dead cells. This is called a *scab.* In the case of burns the denatured collagen of the dermis may remain in place. This is called an *eschar.* In either case granulation and epithelialization occur beneath the surface of the scab or eschar.

Epithelialization

Epithelial cells can migrate up to 2.5cm from the wound edge to close a defect. However, defects which are too large cannot be covered by this process. In such a case the wound becomes a chronic open ulcer. Adequate coverage by skin grafts can prevent this disastrous complication.

The stimulus for epithelial repair is unknown. The loss of contact between cells undoubtedly plays a part. When an area is denuded of epithelium, the marginal cells divide and migrate across the area. This activity ceases when contact is re-established with adjacent epithelial cells.

The normal epidermis is very firmly attached to the underlying dermis by a strong basement membrane which has an undulating surface for a more secure cation union. The hair follicles and sweat glands also provide a strong epidermal-dermal junction. On the other hand, the junction of epithelium with scar tissue is quite weak and flimsy. Even minor shearing forces produce epithelial separation and loss. At the same time, whereas normal skin is quite thick, having many layers of cells and squames, the epithelium covering scar tissue is usually much thinner. For both the above-mentioned reasons, epithelialized scar tissue is not as strong as normal skin, and remains a poor substitute for skin.

Phases of healing

Healing passes through three stages:

Lag phase

During the first few days nothing seems to be happening in the wound, and therefore this has been called the *lag phase.* It should better be called the preparation phase, because during this period the metabolites required for repair are being collected at the site.

Fibroplasia

During the next few weeks the cells and capillaries proliferate. Neutrophils and macrophages are prominent, and fibroblasts lay down collagen in increasing amounts. In an open wound this fibrocellular tissue is called granulation tissue, because its surface is granular due to the looped ends of advancing capillaries. This is the phase of proliferation or fibroplasia.

Maturation

After a few weeks these activities slow down. Fibroblasts and capillaries are now fewer in number, but strength progressively increases. This third phase is called the *maturation* or *differentiation* phase, and lasts many months.

TIDY AND UNTIDY WOUNDS

Rank and Wakefield's classification of wounds into tidy and untidy is the most suitable for a clear understanding of wounds. The salient features of the two are as follows:

Tidy wounds

These are usually single, are inflicted by sharp weapons, and contain no devitalized tissue. Fractures are unusual in this type of wounds, while tendons, arteries and nerves may be cut. These wounds include surgical incisions, glass cuts, knife wounds etc.; if they are simply closed, they are expected to undergo primary healing.

Untidy wounds

These result from crushing, tearing, avulsion etc. and contain devitalized tissues. They are often multiple and irregular. Tendons, arteries and nerves, if injured, are crushed, not cut. Fractures are common and often with multiple fragments (Fig.2.2).

Such wounds must not be closed primarily, as the result could be wound dehiscence, infection and delayed healing. At worst it may end up in gas gangrene or death.

Wound excision

The correct management of untidy wounds is wound excision, i.e. excision of all devitalized tissue to create a tidy wound; the wound may then be closed if desired, or closed after a few days by *delayed primary closure.*

Factors influencing wound healing

General factors

Age

Healing proceeds more rapidly in a younger patient, provided he is well nourished. This increased vigor of repair may explain why hypertrophic scars and keloids are more common in the young.

The strength of scars

Because of formation of fibrous tissue, with the passage of time wounds become stronger. At two days, bursting strength in an incised rat skin wound is about 100gm per linear centimeter. When collagen fibers appear on the third day, bursting strength increases rapidly, and by three weeks has reached over 1 Kg per linear centimeter. It should be noted that gain in strength does not stop here. Skin wounds continue to gain strength rapidly for about four months, and then more slowly for one year. However, normal elasticity, which is important in some tissue functions, is lost in scars.

The role of collagen fibers

Most of the strength of scars comes from the collagen fibers they contain. Scars gain strength in three ways:

- The number of collagen fibers increases.
- The strength of individual fibers increases.
- The irregularly arranged collagen fibers are replaced by fibers which are oriented more effectively.

Scar remodeling

The appearance of a scar changes over a period of many months. This process is called *scar maturation.* The red, firm scar becomes pale and soft, and is no longer adherent to the underlying structures.

With scar formation all injured tissues get bound together in a single unit by strong collagen fibers. This has different effects at various sites. In abdominal incisions it does not matter if the peritoneum, muscles, fascia and skin are welded into one unit. However, in many situations such a result is unsatisfactory. For example if a wound of a finger involves skin, tendon and bone, all injured components are quickly united by scar. The scar becomes strong, but active movements become impossible and the finger becomes stiff, resulting in a major disability.

Abnormal collagen metabolism

Production

In a normally maturing scar, collagen is at the same time being synthesized and lysed. This balance may be disturbed in different situations:

- In keloids and hypertrophic scars, there is excessive synthesis and diminished lysis of collagen.
- In scurvy the synthesis of collagen fails due to lack of vitamin C and the wound breaks down, because in the meantime lysis is continuing normally.

Arrangement

In uninjured skin, collagen fibers are arranged in well-organized bundles. In sutured wounds, they lie in a haphazard manner, later coalescing to form irregular masses. However, the normal architecture is never restored.

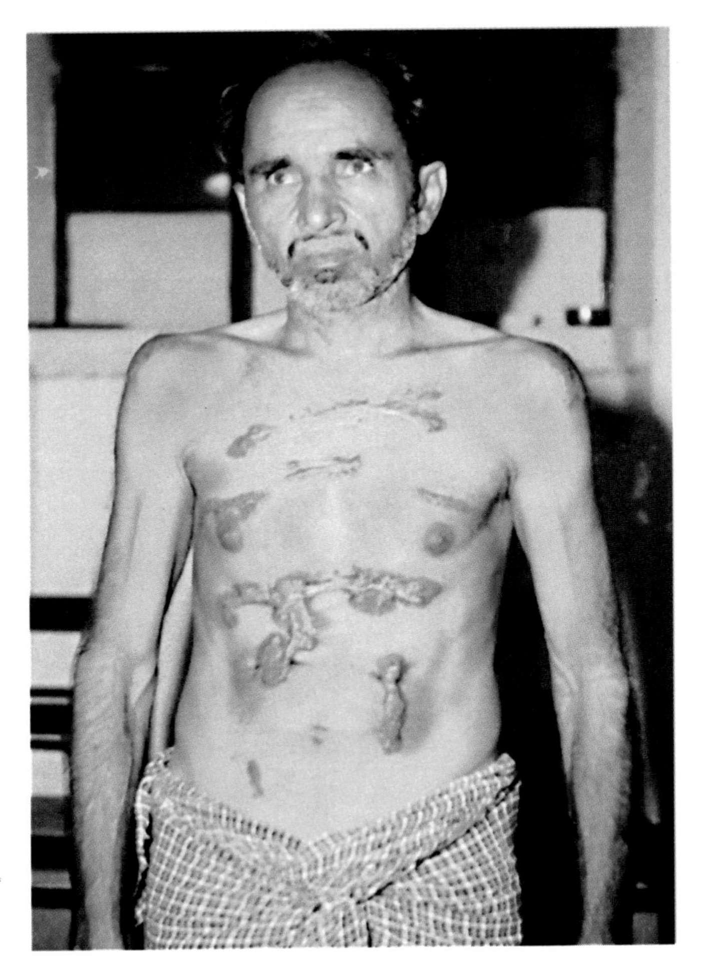

Fig.2.3 Multiple keloids over chest and abdomen

HYPERTROPHIC SCARS AND KELOIDS

Keloids and hypertrophic scars are both abnormal healing processes that occur after trauma or surgery. However, hypertrophic scars remain within the boundaries of the original wound and regress with the passage of time. By contrast, keloids extend beyond the boundaries of the original wound and do not regress. They usually recur after excision unless additional therapy is given. Keloids are normally pink in their early stages, but become hyperpigmented later. They are most common among persons from the black African races, and occur less often in light-skinned people. The most common sites of occurrence include the sternum and shoulder. (Fig.2.3). Keloids contain a significant number of mast cells and have abnormally high histamine content. As a result, these patients often suffer severe itching.

In both keloids and hypertrophic scars there is overabundant production as well as decreased degradation of collagen. This is probably because of an excess of growth factors. Keloid cells produce increased amounts of cytokines, e.g. the transforming growth factor (TGF-b). If antibodies to TGF-b are placed in guinea pig wounds at the time of closure, the wounds heal without any scars. This suggests that in the future, inhibition of this growth factor may play a significant role in the clinical control of keloids and hypertrophic scars.

Treatment

At the present time the treatment of keloids and hypertrophic scars is not satisfactory:

- For severe itching, an oral *antihistamine* is often helpful.
- *Triamcinolone* may be injected into the keloid or hypertrophic scar. The adult dose consists of 2ml of a solution containing 40mg/ml, injected every 6 weeks to avoid systemic effects. The itching and pain are often relieved. The treatment also makes the lesion softer and smaller, and may be the only therapy required for small lesions. Complications include local atrophy of the skin and subcutaneous tissues, which may be severe.
- *Surgical* treatment should be carried out only after careful consideration, because whereas a hypertrophic scar will usually regress without operation, a keloid tends to recur after excision. The patient should be made aware of the high risk of recurrence. Triamcinolone may be used in conjunction with surgery, being injected into the wound margins at the time of closure after excision.
- The pattern of formation of new collagen in a wound is abnormal. While the fibers are being formed, their molecules get cross-linked and thus irreversibly fixed. If this cross-linking could be delayed, a more normal pattern of collagen would have time to develop. β-aminoproprionitrile and penicillamine have shown promise in this respect. Finally, compression has also been of benefit in some cases.

Radiation therapy produces very equivocal results. There have been no long-term follow-ups reported, and the late development of skin cancer after radiation constitutes a potential hazard.

THE CARE OF WOUNDS

This is a very important part of a surgeon's work, and good care of wounds pays rich dividends. If an operation wound heals promptly, a satisfied patient goes home within a few days; if the wound gets septic the matter may linger on for months, causing much distress, financial loss and frustration. During the past two decades wound healing has attracted considerable attention:

- The mechanisms of repair are being defined at a *biochemical* and *molecular* level, and advances in molecular biology are helping the development of new drugs to enhance wound healing.
- The *economic* loss imposed by chronic wounds is being realized.
- *Reconstructive techniques* have improved with the advent of musculocutaneous flaps and microvascular free-tissue transfers.

And yet, in this age of advanced technology, in actual practice wounds are often badly managed. First of all, aseptic technique is not strictly adhered to. It is no use our discussing the properties of the latest and most expensive antibiotic in eradicating infection, if we are not first willing to take elementary aseptic precautions.

The *after-care* of wounds should be carried out meticulously:

- A separate set of instruments should be used for each dressing.
- The number of visitors to wards should be restricted; they bring in bacteria.
- Septic cases should be properly isolated.
- The care of perineal wounds resulting after operations on anal fistulae should not be handed over to the most junior member of the surgical team without supervision.
- In the tropical countries ceiling fans should be switched off while dressing wounds, in order to minimize the chances of cross-infection.

Antiseptics

Antiseptics are chemicals which are capable of killing free-living organisms. Unfortunately, many also have a corrosive action, and leave stains. At the same time only a few kill spores. Thus in this respect they are inferior to steam sterilization or the hot air oven. The common antiseptics employed in surgical practice include the following:

For the skin

Alcohol

This is the cheapest and best chemical available for the routine cleansing of the skin around wounds, and allows removal of grease, dirt, etc. It is used in the form of methylated spirit; the methyl alcohol is added to make it poisonous, so that it cannot be misused by being drunk as an intoxicant.

Ether

Ethyl ether is a strong solvent of fats. A gauze swab soaked in ether solution removes particularly sticky grease, dirt, dried up discharge and marks of adhesive plaster in a most efficient manner. This solvent property of ether is not widely appreciated; *it should be available on every dressing trolley for this purpose.*

Povidone iodine solution

Povidone iodine has completely displaced tincture of iodine, which consisted of alcohol with the addition of 2 % iodine. With the latter, cases of sensitivity to iodine were numerous. When combined with povidone, iodine is free of this toxicity. Its antiseptic effect, when applied and left on an area of skin, is considerable. Because of its bland nature, it can also be applied to wounds.

Cetavlon

Cetavlon, diluted 1 in 40 or 1 in 100, is a mild antiseptic as well as detergent. It is used for cleansing wounds during dressings.

Chlorhexidine

Chlorhexidine is a soapy solution and is widely used by surgeons for washing their hands and forearms during scrubbing up.

For the wound

Sodium hypochlorite

This solution looks and smells like lime water. The wound is lightly packed with gauze soaked in this liquid. It clears up dirty wounds, helping greatly in the removal of sloughs. It comes under the label of Eusol.

Hydrogen peroxide

This solution produces a foam of oxygen and is useful in wounds infected with anaerobic organisms.

Mercurochrome

This solution is applied to a wound for its continuing effect, and is probably useful. However, it stains the wound red, and it becomes difficult to judge whether this is due to inflammation or to the color of the solution. It is therefore no longer popular.

Acriflavine

Acriflavine has similar properties but again, because it colors everything yellow, has lost its popularity.

For instruments

Pure phenol and cresol

These are very strong antiseptics and are suitable for immersion of sharp instruments for sterilization.

Glutaraldehyde 2%

This solution is effective, and is gentle to delicate instruments like cystoscopes. Spores require 10 hours of immersion for destruction.

CARE OF DIFFERENT KINDS OF WOUNDS

Surgical wounds

Most clean and sutured operation wounds require very little care:

- Because they have been made under aseptic conditions, infection is not a problem.
- Because a minimum of trauma has been inflicted by using a sharp knife and gentle dissection, there is not much debris to be removed.
- Because absolute hemostasis has been achieved, there is no hematoma.
- Because the wound margins and edges have been accurately brought together, there is no dead space where serum could collect and become infected.

All that is required in most cases is a *dry gauze dressing,* especially for the first day or two, until the wound becomes sealed off by coagulated serum.

Cotton-wool gauze is the best material for this purpose. It conceals the wound from view, protects it from dust, flies and knocks, and gently splints it. It soaks up any slight discharge, but very importantly, it allows free evaporation of sweat, and prevents the accumulation of moisture. Only if a complication e.g. hematoma or infection arises does the treatment have to vary from this simple routine.

Incised wounds

Incised wounds are inflicted by pieces of glass or by knives. In these wounds damage to the tissues is minimal. They may be closed by primary suture. Divided tendons, nerves and major vessels should be repaired at the same time. Penetrating wounds can damage important structures. This is the reason for the rule that all stab wounds of the abdomen must be explored.

Lacerated wounds

These commonly follow road traffic accidents. They are often contaminated with dirt and organic matter. If crushed and dead muscle is present, the risk of infection is increased. *Dead tissue must be removed thoroughly.* After this some of these wounds can be sutured primarily. However, the stitches should be applied loosely, in order to avoid tension and not allow any excessive exudate to collect.

Many lacerated wounds are so contaminated that after debridement they are best left open, being closed about a week later by the method of *delayed primary suture.* Repair of tendons and nerves is usually postponed for 4 to 6 weeks in these irregular wounds.

Crushed wounds

These commonly occur in severe industrial or road traffic accidents. *The main danger is from dead tissue,* all of which must be removed. At the same time, marked inflammatory edema occurs in the injured tissues. If such a wound is sutured, tissue tension increases further and may cause more necrosis. All tension must be relieved by longitudinal incisions into the deep fascia. After this the wound must be left open.

Open wounds

Open wounds require much more detailed care, and for much longer, than closed wounds. The dressing should be such which will not adhere to the granulation tissue, otherwise each time it is removed this tissue is damaged. Gauze impregnated with Vaseline is commonly used. The amount of Vaseline should not be excessive, otherwise it prevents the serum or other discharge from escaping into the overlying cotton wool. The cotton wool is held in place by a gauze bandage.

Avoid sealing a wound

It is very bad practice to seal a dressing overlying a septic wound with adhesive plaster. In fact by sealing even a clean sutured wound with adhesive plaster one creates a humid environment by preventing evaporation of perspiration from that portion of the skin. This excessive humidity can encourage infection. Therefore, even clean sutured wounds should not be sealed by adhesive plaster.

Sitz baths

Especially when on the limbs, open wounds may be treated by warm sitz baths. Normal saline is the most physiological fluid for this purpose. It can easily be prepared by adding two teaspoonfuls (9–10gm) of table salt to every liter of water. This method is usefully employed in perineal wounds. The patient is asked to sit in a basin of warm normal saline once or twice a day for a few minutes. This causes both irrigation and fomentation, and expedites wound healing.

The value of fomentation

Before the advent of antibiotics, hot fomentation was the only available method of management of inflammation and infection, and it was very useful. Nowadays an excessive amount of reliance is placed on antibiotics. They are sometimes used even when there is no infection but only inflammation, following trauma. Certainly, antibiotics have a place in the treatment of infection, but fomentation has an action complementary to that of antibiotics.

Hot fomentation causes marked vasodilatation, so that many times more blood circulates through the inflamed tissues. Not only does this blood bring in more oxygen and nutrients, it also helps to promptly remove the waste products of inflammation, so that they do not accumulate in the tissues and produce deleterious effects. In short, the vasodilatation produced by fomentation greatly accelerates the process of inflammation and repair, resulting in earlier wound healing; therefore, fomentation should be employed more often. Even if antibiotics are employed, fomentation does no harm. The vasodilatation produced by fomentation allows larger quantities of antibiotics to be brought into the inflamed tissues, with beneficial effects.

Treatment of edematous granulations

An infected wound often shows pale, edematous granulations. These can be made more firm and pink by extracting fluid from them. For this purpose:

Magnesium sulphate glycerine paste is very useful. Because it is strongly hypertonic, it extracts fluid due to its very high osmotic pressure. The hypertonicity also destroys bacteria. This paste should never be used on a fresh wound, because at that time the ends of severed nerves in the tissue are exposed, and mag. sulph. paste would cause intense pain. However, in a few days the nerve ends have been covered by a layer of granulations. Although the paste can cause the patient some discomfort this is short-lived, as it quickly becomes diluted. Improvement in the condition of the wound is usually very rapid.

Silver nitrate. If a small area of the wound shows excessive granulations, a 10 to 15% *solution of silver nitrate* can be applied. The caustic effect makes the granulations more firm. Alternatively, the surface of the wound may be touched by a crystal of silver nitrate. This has a very good astringent effect.

If a silver nitrate crystal is used, care should be taken to remove it after touching the wound surface with it, as otherwise it can cause a burn. For the same reason silver nitrate powder should not be used, as it can spill over and cause a burn. To minimize the pain resulting from touching with silver nitrate, xylocaine jelly may be applied to the wound surface a few minutes in advance of the treatment.

Eusol. If sloughs are present in the wound, Eusol solution (a transparent solution containing sodium hypochlorite) can be used to help them separate. Gauze dipped in Eusol is used to dress the wound.

The importance of rest

For prompt healing of the wound it is extremely important to give rest to the injured part. This is especially important for wounds overlying joints, e.g. elbow or knee. Each movement of a joint stretches the wound and tears and damages the delicate granulation tissue which is being gradually built up by the microscopic processes of repair. Because movement of every joint takes place many times a day, the granulation tissue never gets an opportunity for uninterrupted healing, and the wound may become a chronic ulcer. Rest to the part, by bed rest or by splinting the limb, helps the same wound heal within a few weeks. In such a wound any number of antibiotics cannot achieve what simple rest can.

In the *upper limb,* rest can be provided quite simply by placing the limb in a sling. In the *lower limb*, the patient cannot hop around with one leg in a sling; so bed rest has to be enforced. Neglect of such a precaution leads to greatly delayed healing in the wounds resulting from even straightforward minor operations on the feet. This can best be explained to the patient by reminding him that if he were to walk about, he would be placing the weight of the whole body on the wounded part hundreds of times a day.

In the case of *abdominal operations,* if the only consideration was prompt wound healing one would advise absolute bed rest. However, this type of rest produces its own problems. Immobility after a major abdominal operation can result in hypostatic pneumonia. It can also produce deep vein thrombosis, which may lead to pulmonary embolism and death. Therefore one has to work out a compromise between the requirements of the wound and of general care of the patient. Early gentle but not excessive mobilization of the patient is advised, followed by gradual return to activity over a period of a few weeks.

BANDAGES AND DRESSINGS

A firm bandage applied properly over a pad of cotton-wool benefits a wound in many ways:

- By exerting firm and even pressure on the wound it discourages excessive edema formation, collection of serum and the formation of a hematoma.
- If the wound is near a joint the bandage, by splinting the part, discourages movement and reduces the resultant pain.
- The cotton wool serves to absorb any discharge that may come out from the wound.

Every medical student should be taught to apply a well-fitting bandage to any part of the body, because on occasion a medical graduate may have to apply such a dressing.

The importance of cotton wool as a dressing material

For thousands of years cotton wool has served as the best material for the dressing of wounds:

- The important feature of cotton is its absorbent property. Unlike silk or nylon, it soaks up a large volume of fluid. Thus, it removes the fluid from immediate contact with the surface of the wound, where it would have caused maceration of the tissues.
- At the same time, being freely water-miscible, it allows fluids to seep through it and evaporate, producing a dry environment, in which bacteria cannot grow.

Role of different parts of a dressing

The surgeon must have a clear concept of the purpose of each of the different components of a dressing:

- If the wound is a *clean sutured incision,* commonly a small amount of sterilized gauze is placed to cover the wound, and is held in place by adhesive plaster. The gauze:
    - o Serves to conceal the wound from view.
    - o It absorbs any small quantity of serum that may seep through the wound.
    - o If the environment is unhygienic it prevents dust and flies settling on the wound.
- If the wound is *clean and dry* but needs some support and splintage, the gauze is covered by pads of cotton wool, and the whole is held in place by a bandage. The bandage is applied firmly, and helps exert *gentle* pressure on the wound, which reduces the tendency to edema formation and minimizes the pain. The cotton wool helps to distribute the pressure of the bandage evenly and makes the dressing more comfortable.
- If the wound is an *open* one, the gauze may adhere to the granulation tissue and make the change of dressing a painful experience. Therefore a layer of Vaseline gauze is applied to the wound surface first, followed by dry gauze, cotton wool and bandage. Here the cotton serves a dual purpose:

Table 2.3 Wound dressings

Class	Composition	Properties	Indicated in wounds with
Films	Semiocclusive polyurethane	Provides moist environment	Nil or minimal exudates
Impregnates	Fine mesh gauzes with antibacterials	Does not adhere, promotes epithelialization	Moderate exudate
Calcium alginate	Fibers of calcium alginate	Highly absorbent, facilitates moist healing	Much exudate
Foams	Polyurethane film coated, absorbent	Absorbs fluid, debrides, vapor permeable	Much discharge, sloughs
Hydrocolloids	Hydrophilic colloid	Absorbs fluid, promotes granulation, epithelialization	Partial thickness wounds, pressure ulcers

- It helps distribute the pressure of the bandage evenly.
- It soaks up any discharge of serum, pus or blood etc.

If the discharge from a wound soaks the dressing, it is important to change the dressing promptly, otherwise the skin exposed to the discharge becomes macerated and irritated. At the same time, the moist external surface of the dressing allows the spread of the infection to the patient's bedclothes and thence further afield. This is the reason for the frequent change of dressings in discharging wounds, otherwise in clean incised and sutured wounds the dressing can be left in place for some days.

Modern dressings

During the last few decades, many new 'active' dressings have become available; some of them with their constituents are listed in (Table 2.3).

Silastic foam

A good material for use as dressing for the deeper wounds is silastic foam. Two solutions are provided. These are mixed and poured into the wound. The silastic foam which forms quickly sets to produce a sponge, which conforms to the contours of the wound and provides an exact fit. It can be removed from the wound, washed and used again. It is inert and non-adherent.

Chapter

3 TRAUMA

Trauma is defined as damage inflicted upon the body by an external force. About two centuries ago trauma was rarely a cause of death or serious disability. There were very few roads, and the horse-driven carriages of those days were slow. The arrival first of the railways and then of automobiles and aircraft changed all that. Today travelers move at speeds unimaginable in those days, and when a collision takes place the injuries inflicted on the body are proportionately severe. At the same time the number of automobiles has increased to millions. It is therefore not surprising that trauma counts as one of the major killers today. In order to understand how to look after a patient who has undergone a surgical operation or other kind of trauma, one must be familiar with the manner in which his body normally responds to injury, i.e. the changes which occur in the post-traumatic state, and how they are produced.

After major trauma the body responds in a well-organized manner to the injury, conserving fluids, providing energy, if necessary at the cost of the body cell mass, etc. In this chapter we will discuss first the body's metabolic response to trauma, and then the management of trauma.

Metabolic response to trauma

CIRCULATORY FLUID VOLUME

One of the most important effects of trauma is a loss of circulating body fluids. Before discussing the effects of such a loss it is necessary to consider why it is important to maintain a normal blood volume, and to see how it is maintained during health.

Importance of maintenance of normal blood volume

In order to sustain life and health it is essential that oxygen and nutrients be supplied to the cells of the different organs, and that waste products be carried away from them. These two processes require perfusion of a sufficient amount of blood through the capillaries passing adjacent to the different cells. This perfusion in turn depends upon an adequate cardiac output, which is maintained by a sufficient blood volume and venous return. Therefore, for normal function of the cells of the different organs it is important that blood volume be maintained within normal limits.

Trauma lowers the blood volume

This is brought about in two ways:

- From direct loss of blood.
- From loss of fluid in the form of an exudate.

This fluid is sequestrated in the injured organ, so that a *'third space'* is formed. The result is that it is no longer available for exchange, and if a large quantity of fluid is thus lost, hypovolemia ensues.

Response to reduced blood volume

When the blood volume falls, the stimulation of the baroreceptors is reduced. Therefore the *nervous system is no longer inhibited to the same extent* as before. This loss of inhibition has the following important effects:

- There is *increased sympathetic activity*. The adrenal medulla secretes more adrenaline and noradrenaline which constrict the arteries except those of the heart and brain. This helps in restoring the blood pressure to normal.
- The *kidney secretes more renin*, which leads to the formation of angiotensin. The latter is a peptide having vasoactive properties. It constricts the

arterioles and veins, thus reducing the vascular bed. It also constricts the renal arterioles, causing the kidney to conserve water and salt. In this manner it leads to an increase in the body fluid volume, which helps in raising the arterial blood pressure.

- The secretion of *ACTH and ADH* from the anterior and posterior pituitary is reflexly increased.

In this way a decrease in blood volume causes a compensatory build-up of body fluids as well as an increase in blood pressure, thereby compensating for the original deficit and restoring the internal environment to normal.

Biphasic response

The metabolic response to trauma manifests itself as a biphasic response, consisting of the ebb and flow phases.

Ebb phase

The ebb phase begins immediately after injury and is accompanied by decreased intravascular volume, hypotension, decreased cardiac output, poor tissue perfusion, lactic acidosis, hypothermia and hemodynamic instability. Loss of intravascular volume is an important factor in its development. However, the initial fall in cardiac output takes place before major loss of vascular volume, and is produced by neurohumoral mechanisms including histamine, activated complement factors, oxidants and prostanoids. Metabolic expenditure at this time shows a hypometabolic state, with a decrease in oxygen consumption.

Flow phase

If successful resuscitation takes place, the flow phase of the physiological response to trauma sets in. Cardiac output is restored to normal and later rises to more than twice the resting state for uninjured individuals.

The accompanying *hypermetabolic response* is characterized by:

- A large increase in metabolic expenditure.
- Increased heat elimination.
- Erosion of body cell mass.
- Weight loss.

The magnitude of this response is proportional to the size of the injury. The patient remains hypermetabolic as long as wound healing continues; this persists as long as the wound is hyperemic and immature and only declines to normal values when the wound is fully mature.

Acidosis

In low flow states and in cardiovascular collapse, large quantities of lactic acid accumulate and acidosis results. *This acidosis is the result of the hypoperfusion and anaerobic metabolism, and it interferes further with cellular function.* It has profound effects on the cardiovascular system:

- It reduces myocardial contractility.
- It decreases the response of the myocardium and peripheral vessels to catecholamines.
- It predisposes the heart to the development of arrhythmias.

If compensatory mechanisms are blocked or the change occurs too rapidly, death may result.

CENTRAL NERVOUS SYSTEM AND ENDOCRINE CHANGES

The main stimuli which activate the endocrine response to injury are *hypovolemia and pain*. The hormonal response is diffuse, including increased release of:

- Adrenaline and noradrenaline.
- ACTH.
- Hydrocortisone.
- Antidiuretic hormone.
- Renin.
- Aldosterone.
- Growth hormone.
- Glucagon.

The hypothalamus controls these responses. The afferent pathways are shared to a considerable extent. The result of this sharing is that the neuroendocrine response to injury is well-coordinated.

HORMONES TAKING PART IN THE NEUROENDOCRINE RESPONSE

A large number of hormones take part in the response to trauma:

Adrenaline and noradrenaline

These are both secreted in response to trauma. *The secretion of these two hormones is the most basic of all post-traumatic hormonal responses.* This is so firstly because they are stimulated by all forms of trauma and stress. Secondly, they produce widespread effects on the circulation, on metabolism, and on the activity of other hormones:

- They increase the cardiac output and raise the blood pressure.
- They produce vasoconstriction in the skin, gastrointestinal tract, kidneys etc. to conserve blood for the essential organs, namely the heart and brain.

- Adrenaline stimulates glycogenolysis and lipolysis and inhibits the release of insulin. The increased secretion usually lasts only a day or so, unless the injury is a severe and persisting one.

If, however, because of continuing trauma, or because of the mistake of over-administration of these hormones by the surgeon, their levels remain high for a prolonged period, their effects on the body are harmful due to two reasons:

- The energy stores (e.g. glycogen stores in the liver) become exhausted.
- *Prolonged peripheral vasoconstriction produces ischemia of cellular tissues.* Thus:
    - o Ischemic damage *of* the kidney produces oliguria or anuria.
    - o In the stomach it results in acute gastric erosions, leading to hematemesis and/or melena.

Hydrocortisone

Injury leads to an increased secretion of ACTH and therefore of hydrocortisone. In the presence of significant hypovolemia ACTH secretion will persist until blood volume is restored.

In patients who have been on steroids for a long time the adrenal cortex undergoes atrophy. If they are not given steroids during an operation they may sometimes die because of failure of hydrocortisone release from an adrenal rendered inactive by atrophy. Thus hydrocortisone is necessary for the normal response to trauma, and it is very important to ask for a history of corticosteroid administration during the preoperative work-up of the patient.

Antidiuretic hormone (ADH)

In most cases of trauma there is an increased secretion of ADH from the posterior pituitary due to afferent stimuli acting on the hypothalamus. Hypovolemia also stimulates ADH release. This hormone acts on the distal tubule to increase water reabsorption. In the presence of ADH, if water is given without salt, sodium gets diluted and hyponatremia results. If administration is continued, water intoxication may result, which produces disorientation, or even coma.

Renin

In most cases of trauma there is increased secretion of renin by the cells of the juxtaglomerular apparatus of the renal afferent arterioles. Renin secretion is increased by:

- Sympathetic stimulation of the juxtaglomerular apparatus.
- Lowered renal arterial pressure.
- Decreased delivery of sodium to the distal tubules.

Renin:

- Converts angiotensinogen to angiotensin I.
- The latter is converted by an enzyme to angiotensin II.
- Angiotensin II:
    - o Stimulates the adrenal cortex to secrete aldosterone.
    - o It also increases the secretion of antidiuretic hormone and of ACTH from the pituitary.

Aldosterone

This hormone acts on the distal nephron to increase reabsorption of sodium in exchange for potassium and hydrogen. *This effect is critical for life. It is the main mechanism by which the kidney can excrete the potassium and acid which builds up in severe trauma, and thus prevent a dangerous degree of hyperkalemia and acidosis, which could be fatal.*

Growth hormone

The growth hormone causes lipolysis; further, it antagonizes insulin and has pro-inflammatory effects.

Glucagon

This is a diabetogenic hormone produced by the alpha cells of the pancreatic islets. Secretion is increased by hypoglycemia and by sympathetic stimulation acting on the alpha cell. The main result of glucagon secretion in trauma is an *increase in blood glucose.* This is brought about by stimulation of glycogenolysis, gluconeogenesis and lipolysis.

Insulin

It may be noted that secretion of insulin is never increased in response to trauma. In fact in the immediate post-traumatic period there is a relatively diabetic glucose tolerance curve, due to increased levels of adrenaline, ACTH, cortisol and glucagon, and reduced levels of insulin.

METABOLIC CHANGES AFTER TRAUMA

After a severe injury there is marked tissue wasting and weight loss. This is due partly to semi-starvation and partly to the greatly increased catabolism following injury. *After injury the basic fact which stands out is that the body cell mass is sacrificed, while the extracellular volume is preserved.*

Body cell mass

When cells are destroyed the products of cellular lysis are released into the extracellular fluid. Some of these compounds are converted into glucose and burned for energy. Most of the nitrogen is excreted in the urine as urea.

Skeletal muscle is the worst sufferer

The tissue most affected is skeletal muscle. This is shown by the visible and rapid decrease in bulk of the palpable muscles. The caloric requirements are increased to 5,000–6,000 per day. Relative starvation is the rule, and is the cause of the negative nitrogen balance. This release of the products of cellular protoplasm to the extracellular fluid, and their excretion, produces the following effects:

- A negative nitrogen balance.
- The loss of intracellular electrolytes (particularly potassium, phosphate and sulphate) into the extracellular fluid and thence to the urine via the kidneys.

Little effect on viscera

Whereas skeletal muscle mass is rapidly reduced, this catabolism of the post-traumatic state does not have much impact on the cell mass of *visceral* organs such as brain, heart, lungs, kidneys, gastrointestinal tract and liver. At the same time, even muscle recovers completely without any residual weakness. This suggests that each muscle cell is maintained intact in spite of severe reduction in its protoplasm.

Transient loss of tissues

Medium grade injury in the adult causes a loss of approximately 1kg of wet lean muscle. At the same time body fat is lost. There is no evidence that this transient drain on muscle cells and fat after injury has any harmful effects on the healing of wounds and fractures, or the later achievement of a positive nitrogen balance.

Prolonged starvation

On the other hand *prolonged* starvation, either before or after injury, has clearly adverse effects upon all aspects of wound healing and bodily function, and is favorably affected by increased nutritional intake.

The importance of protein

It must be remembered that body protein is not designed primarily as a source of fuel, but performs other important functions in the form of enzymes, plasma proteins, structural protein, cardiac and skeletal muscle etc. During starvation the body attempts to conserve protein by burning fat instead.

The need for alimentation

In short-term starvation the body is able to replenish protein at a rate equal to its degradation. However, with prolonged fasting in the presence of marked catabolism due to trauma, endogenous plasma proteins are burned. In this situation the liver cannot synthesize albumin at a rate equal to its loss. Therefore it becomes necessary to replace plasma proteins from exogenous sources. *Thus it is very important to administer amino acids, albumin or plasma to surgical patients who are in a catabolic state and unable to eat.* This is necessary not only to replace the plasma protein which has been lost externally or into the third space, but also that which is burned as fuel.

However, it is now realized that the hyperalimentation often provided during recent decades in such cases is itself a metabolic stress, and that therefore nutritional support should be provided to a more moderate extent.

Extracellular fluid volume

While the body cell mass is being reduced by lysis of protoplasm, the body devotes several active mechanisms to the conservation of extracellular fluid, and thus to the maintenance of plasma and blood volume.

Firstly, the level of sodium in the urine, sweat and saliva falls, preserving this ion.

The importance of sodium. The question might be asked: why is it so important to conserve sodium? The answer is that the *total osmolality* of extracellular fluid (and therefore its total volume) is largely determined by the sodium content. Sodium is the *water-holding* ion of the extracellular fluid.

After injury a mechanism for conservation of fluid comes into play. There is a sharp restriction in the excretion of free water (antidiuresis). This is shown by a rising urine osmolality due to reabsorption of water in the distal tubules. In spite of the fact that it contains a reduced amount of sodium, the *osmolality of the urine is high.* This is due to the raised concentrations of the waste products of cellular lysis, namely phosphate, potassium and urea.

Large water loads should therefore not be given to the postoperative patient. He is more apt to retain this water than the normal person. After injury patients are more easily swamped with sodium and water loads than in the normal state.

The plasma *protein* level falls due to dilution. This produces a tendency towards tissue edema, especially of the lungs and brain.

Cardiovascular function

High cardiac output

In the post-traumatic patient or after a low-flow state, elevated cardiac output is usual. This is due to two factors:

- The effect of catecholamines, which stimulate the heart.
- The shift of the oxyhemoglobin dissociation curve to the left. The oxyhemoglobin does not give up its oxygen to the tissues easily. Therefore in order to supply sufficient oxygen to the tissues an increased cardiac output is required.

In heart disease

In persons with heart disease who cannot support a high cardiac output, the following undesirable effects can result:

- *Cardiac* arrhythmias and congestive cardiac failure.
- Peripheral *tissue* anoxia with lactic acidosis.
- *Organ* failure (brain or kidneys).

Renal function

Post-surgical renal damage

Any significant reduction of blood volume produces renal vasoconstriction with hypoperfusion of the kidneys. When glomerular filtration rate falls below 20ml per minute the kidney becomes very vulnerable to nephrotic damage from porphyrin pigments, drugs or chemical poisons. It is this combination of factors which results in post-traumatic renal insufficiency.

When there is decreased perfusion pressure at the afferent arteriole of the glomerulus, the juxtaglomerular apparatus interprets it as volume deficiency, and stimulates the production of renin, angiotensin and aldosterone. The result is a rise in blood pressure, retention of sodium and an alkalotic trend.

If hydration and an osmotic load (in the form of mannitol, glucose or salts) are maintained, the result is well-filled renal tubules and high glomerular filtration rates. This is how adequate hydration and solute loading protect the kidney.

Gastrointestinal tract

Reduced gut function

After severe injury anywhere in the body both absorption and motility of the gastrointestinal tract are reduced. If the injury involves the peritoneal cavity this reduction in gastrointestinal function is much more severe and prolonged. If efforts are made to feed the patient at this time the result is abdominal distension, severe peristaltic abdominal pain, and vomiting. It is in such a situation that special diets are particularly useful.

Special diets

The slow infusion of a *hydrolyzed diet* into the small bowel (e.g. through a feeding jejunal tube), may be well absorbed and provide satisfactory nutrition in the post-traumatic patient, even though peristalsis is slow and the patient unable to hydrolyze and absorb a full protein-starch diet. When the total surface of available gastrointestinal tract is inadequate, e.g. after massive resection of small bowel, the use of diets containing the basic elements of food, e.g. amino acids, glucose, etc. *('elemental diets')* helps convalescence greatly, as these diets do not have to be digested before absorption.

Lungs

A variety of mechanisms can damage the lungs after trauma. They may arrive at the lungs by the airway, by the bloodstream, or by direct trauma:

- **Airway.**
  - Aspiration of gastric contents.
  - Inhalation of smoke chronically (heavy smoking) or acutely (burns).
  - Prolonged mechanical ventilation.
  - Prolonged immobilization in one posture, allowing secretions to collect and become infected.
- **Blood stream.**
  - Fluid overload with osmotic dilution and pulmonary edema.
  - Multiple small platelet emboli from the area of trauma.
  - Micro-organisms from peripheral infection.
  - Vasoactive substances affecting pulmonary circulation: serotonins, catecholamines, and the kinins.
  - Microemboli of transfused blood.
- **Direct trauma to chest and lungs.**
  - Unstable rib cage, e.g. crushed chest.
  - Prolonged open chest with collapsed or underperfused lung tissue.

When the combined effect of these different factors is great, post-traumatic pulmonary insufficiency results. The most common conditions predisposing to pulmonary insufficiency are a history of heavy smoking, chronic asthma, emphysema and bronchiectasis.

Brain

When arteriosclerosis is present, as in older people, cerebral function is very sensitive to poor perfusion. The left-shifted oxyhemoglobin dissociation curve of alkalosis further reduces cerebral function. The symptoms produced by cerebral dysfunction are: disorientation, hallucination, extreme restlessness and coma.

Hypocarbia and alkalosis reduce cerebral function by producing cerebral vasoconstriction, and may lead to loss of consciousness. *This is a very bad sign in a surgical patient.* The brain needs an adequate supply of well-oxygenated blood with normal levels of glucose.

COMPONENTS OF ACUTE INJURY

Acute trauma commonly has three components: the local tissue wound, the volume reduction produced, and the catabolic state induced by the injury.

The tissue wound

Every wound initiates catabolism, and a continuously open wound inhibits anabolism. It fills up with a coagulum of albumin, globulin and mucopolysaccharides. This is changed to procollagen, and with the invasion of fibroblasts collagen is formed and tensile strength is gradually resumed.

Interestingly, this early and most significant phase of wound healing is completed during the period of negative nitrogen balance. Restoration of nitrogen anabolism is not necessary for wound healing. However, it is important for regaining muscular strength and vigor. The only substance required from outside the body for wound healing is ascorbic acid. Even here, deprivation of this substance for up to a month has no effect on wound healing if the patient has normal stores to begin with.

Hematomas in the tissue are a common result of injury or surgical operation. The blood undergoes hemolysis, and presents the kidney with a load of porphyrin pigments to excrete. If kidney function is impaired, these pigments (hemoglobin, methemoglobin or myoglobin) can be nephrotoxic.

In the body's economy the wound has a high priority in its demand on building materials. Even in emaciated patients with advanced cancer undergoing palliative surgery one commonly finds strong healing and a firmly cicatrized wound. Conversely wound dehiscence, in which there is almost complete absence of fibroplasia, is as likely to occur in the previously healthy person as in the nutritionally depleted patient.

Burns

Burns provide an example of wounds that cannot be closed for many weeks or months; they are chronically colonized and infected. As long as a burn or other wound remains open, it inhibits protein anabolism and the resumption of growth. The patient remains ill and in negative nigrogen balance. As soon as the wound is healed or grafted the nitrogen balance becomes positive even on a low intake of calories and nitrogen, either by mouth or by the intravenous route.

Volume reduction, hypoperfusion and the low flow state

The confusion between injury and shock causes a great deal of difficulty. It is better to avoid the term shock altogether. It is preferable to use the terms 'volume reduction' and 'low flow state'.

Volume reduction

The term volume reduction means any reduction in the *effective* circulating volume of the blood. This may be due firstly to simple hemorrhage. Secondly, it may be the result of acute desalting water loss, as in vomiting, diarrhea, pancreatic fistula, intestinal obstruction etc.

Low flow state

The low flow state is defined as a situation in which hypoperfusion of tissues passes the boundaries of physiological compensation *with disordered metabolism of all tissue cells as a result of anoxia. In other words* volume reduction, if severe and prolonged, leads to a low flow state.

Cellular deterioration

The key to differentiation between volume reduction and a low flow state lies in the occurrence of *cellular deterioration.* This can be measured in many ways:

- By the deterioration of *function* of specific organs e.g. brain and kidney, whose function is obvious clinically.
- By the accumulation in the blood of those electrolytes which are normally present *intracellularly,* and their excretion in the urine.
- By the temperature and pulse rate.
- By the raised blood levels of catecholamines.
- By the production of prolonged severe tissue acidosis.

The presence of the above indicators of a low flow state indicates the existence of a *very critical situation.*

Catabolic state

The catabolism occurring after trauma shows a number of differences from simple starvation:

- In simple starvation the maximum rate of nitrogen loss is 5 to 7gm of nitrogen per 70kg per day; in posttraumatic catabolism this figure lies in the range of 15 to 25gm.
- In starvation the blood *sugar* level falls and remains low; after severe trauma it rises.
- The blood *urea* nitrogen level falls in starvation but rises after major injury.

- In starvation urinary excretion of *creatinine* is very gradually reduced as the body cell mass falls; after severe injury it rises sharply.

In spite of these clear differences, starvation contributes an important component to post-traumatic metabolism, especially when it is continued for more than a few days after injury or operation.

Management

Predigested foods and balanced intravenous feeding mixtures are important in damping out the starvation component in the post-traumatic period. This is especially important in chronically ill patients with intestinal diseases, wounds, burns or chronic sepsis.

PHASES OF CONVALESCENCE

Four phases of convalescence are commonly recognized:

Acute injury phase

The patient has a rapid pulse with elevated cardiac output. He feels ill, desires to sleep, requires analgesics, does not wish to be disturbed, and wishes to remain immobile. *If the operation is smoothly performed with a minimum of tissue trauma and body fluids are restored to normal, both pain and the endocrine response to injury are minimized.* Body temperature is usually elevated after injury. Excellence of surgical and anesthetic technique reduces this fever to a minimum. In two to five days this phase draws to a close. The patient looks brighter, the pulse rate and temperature are reduced, and he enters the turning point phase. Catecholamine responses have ceased.

Minimum access surgery, by greatly reducing the amount of tissues dissected, has made it possible to minimize the endocrine response to surgery.

Turning point phase

In this phase peristalsis returns, flatus is expelled, appetite improves, and diuresis occurs. The patient desires to see visitors and to 'return to living'. Food is assimilated easily as in simple starvation. Muscle protein synthesis occurs rapidly. The young woman again applies her lipstick and powder.

Anabolic phase

There is increasing strength, appetite, and food intake, normal absorption and a positive nitrogen balance. Most patients are returned home. Both growth hormone and insulin are active, restoring nitrogen compounds to the synthesis of actin and myosin in muscle.

Fat gain phase

When nitrogen balance returns to zero balance (indicating that muscle mass has been restored) the patient continues to gain weight and remains in positive caloric balance. Nearly all of this additional weight is due to the deposition of fat.

In conclusion, it will be seen that the body responds to trauma by a series of well-coordinated changes. A breakdown occurs only if a compensatory mechanism is overstretched.

Complications

Most surgical *complications* inhibit normal nitrogen anabolism. The most common of these include:

- Prolonged wound sepsis.
- Unhealed wounds.
- Septic fractures.
- Intestinal fistulae.

The condition of such a patient does not improve. He remains hospitalized or is discharged home to remain in bed.

As stated above, positive nitrogen balance is not required for the healing of the wound. However, it is essential for gain in strength and for the social rehabilitation of the patient.

Management of trauma

GENERAL CONSIDERATIONS IN TRAUMA

Even today a number of the patients who reach hospital die of surgically remediable causes. This percentage can be reduced by providing the necessary facilities as well as trained manpower.

Facilities

The facilities for undertaking the care of victims of trauma at the site of the accident, at the hospital, and at a specialized trauma center, should include the following:

Ambulances

Well-equipped ambulances with staff trained in the care of trauma victims.

Emergency rooms in hospitals

Emergency rooms in hospitals each provided with a ***'trauma area'*** equipped for emergency resuscitation. This room should contain such items as overhead operating lights, oxygen, cardiac monitors and a defibrillator.

A cabinet in the room should contain the following items:

- Laryngoscopes with different-sized blades.
- Endotracheal tubes of different sizes.
- Tracheostomy tray.
- Closed chest drainage tray and different-sized tubes.
- Venesection tray.
- Central venous catheters.
- Syringes for abdominal paracentesis.
- Pericardiocentesis and peritoneal lavage catheters.
- Intravenous fluids with tubing.

The cabinet shelves should have clearly visible labels under each tray or set of instruments. The trays should be kept in this trauma room and not in central supply, as a delay of even a few minutes may prove fatal in the very urgent case.

Trauma system and trauma centers

Within a city or province, a Trauma System provides for rapid transport of victims of major trauma to specified hospitals (called Trauma Centers), because they have concentrated resources and expertise to treat severely injured patients immediately and effectively. The integration of pre-hospital care, rapid transport and immediate surgical treatment within a trauma system *reduces preventable deaths* from this cause from nearly 25% to about 5%.

Priority by type of injury

There are three groups of patients according to the urgency of the case:

- *Injuries immediately threatening life,* by interfering with vital physiological functions, e.g. obstruction of an airway or excessive bleeding from a wound. The primary treatment is to establish an airway and control the bleeding. Such a patient may require operation e.g. laparotomy or thoracotomy within a few minutes, for occluding major vessels to control massive internal bleeding.
- *Injuries* posing *no immediate threat to life.* These include patients with either blunt trauma or gunshot or stab wounds to the chest or abdomen, but where the vital signs are stable. Most patients with trauma belong to this category. They usually require surgical procedures within 1 or 2 hours. X-rays may be obtained to determine the course of the missile and the extent of the possible associated injuries, such as fractures. *A doctor must be constantly in attendance,* because such a patient may develop shock (e.g. from internal hemorrhage) at any moment; if this happens he must be taken to the operating room immediately.
- *Injuries producing occult damage*. These are patients in whom the exact nature of the damage is not apparent. Surgical exploration may be delayed for hours or days, as with delayed rupture of the spleen.

DETAILS OF MANAGEMENT OF TRAUMA

Advanced trauma life support

Advanced Trauma Life Support (ATLS) protocols have improved the management of trauma. There are two types of injured patients being brought to emergency departments:

- Patients with serious and *life-threatening* injuries.
- Patients with significant injuries requiring early treatment but *not threatening life*.

The basic philosophy of ATLS includes:

- Primary survey with simultaneous resuscitation.
- Identification and treatment of life-threatening injuries.
- Secondary survey which proceeds to identify the other serious injuries.
- Definitive care of the injured patient with a multidisciplinary approach.

Triage

When large numbers of casualties suddenly result, it is important to separate those who are critically ill and require immediate attention from the rest. Triage [*Triage* Fr.: sorting out] is an important concept in modern-day health care systems. It focuses on:

- Identification of those immediately at risk of loss of life.
- Then moving to the management of urgent cases and prioritizing those into clinically stable but seriously ill, and into the most appropriate order of evacuation.
- Identifying the most appropriate receiving clinical unit.

In multiple trauma, two types of situations requiring triage are seen:

- *Multiple casualties.*

Here the number and severity of injuries do not exceed the ability of the facility to render care. Priority is given to life-threatening injuries followed by those with poly-trauma.

- *Mass casualties.*

The number and the severity of the injuries exceed the capabilities and facilities available to the staff. In this situation, those with the greatest chance of survival and the least expenditure of time, equipment and supplies are priorities. This situation may be faced in volcanic eruptions, thunderstorms, rail accidents and bomb blasts.

Simple triage (at the site)

Simple triage is usually used at the site of a mass casualty incident, in order to sort patients into:

- Those who need critical attention and immediate transport to the hospital.
- Those with less serious injuries.

This step can be started before transport becomes available. The categorization of patients based on the severity of their injuries can be aided by the use of printed triage tags.

Advanced triage (at the hospital)

At the hospital, doctors decide:

- Which patients need to be operated upon immediately.
- Which can wait for a few hours.
- The most appropriate clinical unit to receive each patient.

Injury severity score (ISS)

A good trauma scoring system for the individual patient is the Injury Severity Score. This assigns a score from 0 to 75 based on severity of injury to six regions:

- Head and neck.
- Face.
- Chest.
- Abdomen.
- Extremities.
- External.

Each region is scored from 0 to 5 (from uninjured to critically injured), the figures being summed up to create the ISS.

Trimodal pattern of death

A trimodal pattern is seen in deaths from trauma. There are three peaks:

- *Immediate* deaths which include 50% of all deaths, and it is not possible to prevent them. These are usually cases of massive head injury and major cardiovascular events.
- *Early* deaths, within the first few hours, often from trauma to the trunk-'torso trauma'. These account for 30% of deaths.
- *Late* deaths, accounting for 20% of mortality. These usually result from sepsis and multiple organ failure and, are influenced by inadequate early resuscitation and care.

The 'Golden hour'

This has led to the concept of the 'golden hour' to describe the urgent need for treatment of trauma victims within the first hour of injury for best results. Modern-day emergency services are based on this principle.

Multidisciplinary team approach

A multidisciplinary team is constituted before the arrival of multiple or mass casualties. This comprises of general surgeon, orthopedic surgeon, neurosurgeon, vascular surgeon, physician, radiologist and a team of residents.

It is mandatory to identify a *team leader* who will plan and command the whole scene and his role should be to pass the orders and communicate with the team members rather than providing the hands-on care himself.

A *spokesperson* of the team should also be appointed who will communicate with the outside world, family and the media, and use the media to mobilize the heath-care facilities from the other hospitals.

Preparation

Pre-hospital phase

Good communication is needed between the emergency room team and the emergency services, so that the team can be mobilized well before the patients arrive in the emergency.

In-hospital phase

Resuscitation area

A separate resuscitation area is allocated where all the life-saving equipment should be available in functional status. The fluids to be administered should also be available, *warmed to the appropriate temperature.* Laboratory and x-ray facilities should be arranged in this area.

MIST protocol

The patients should be examined according to the **MIST** protocol:

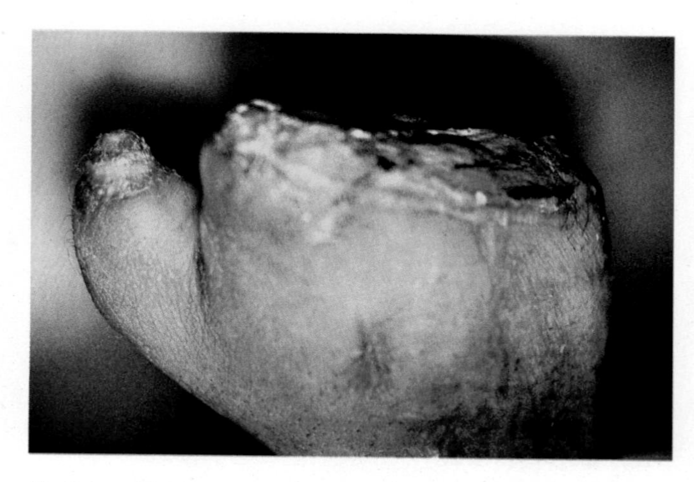

Fig.3.1 Traumatic amputation due to right hand getting sliced by by the blade of a fodder-cutting machine. The cut surface has been skin grafted. The proximal phalanx of the thumb has been exposed, and will require coverage by a tubed pedicle flap.

- **M**echanism of injury.
- **I**njuries identified, including information on injuries to other casualties involved in the same event.
- (vital) **S**igns at the scene.
- (any) **T**reatment administered.

PRIMARY SURVEY AND RESUSCITATION

This includes early triage, and several scoring systems have been devised to assess the initial trauma and outcome of the patients. Examples of such scores include:

- Injury Severity Score (ISS).
- Mangled Extremity Severity Score (MESS).
- Glasgow Coma Scale (GCS) etc.

The Primary Survey is based on the **ABCDE** of trauma care:

A. Airway maintenance with control of cervical spine.

B. Breathing with ventilation.

C. Circulation with control of hemorrhage.

D. Disability and neurological status.

E. Exposure: completely undressing the patient. Environmental control.

Airway with control of cervical spine

Every unconscious multiple trauma patient, and one with an injury above the clavicle, must be presumed to be having a cervical spine injury until proved otherwise. Therefore the cervical spine is immobilized and attention paid to the airway.

All foreign bodies/materials are cleared off from the airway, and blood and other liquids in the pharynx are cleared with the help of a sucker.

Oral, facial and maxillary trauma and fractures, and laryngeal edema, are identified.

Breathing with ventilation

100% oxygen is administered and ventilation assessed by the adequate function of the lungs, chest wall and diaphragm. Engorgement of neck veins, deviation of trachea, asymmetry of the chest wall, hyper-resonance (pneumothorax), dullness on percussion (hemothorax) and any sucking wound on the chest should be identified immediately.

Actions

- A three-dimensional dressing is applied to a sucking chest wound.
- In a case of tension pneumothorax, a wide bore needle is passed two centimeter below the mid-clavicular line in the 2nd intercostal space.
- In the emergency room tube thoracotomy is done as a life-saving procedure.
- In cases of oropharyngeal trauma an endotracheal tube is passed or a tracheostomy done to deliver the oxygen.

Circulation with control of hemorrhage

Blood loss can be assessed by observing an altered level of consciousness, which is an indication of significant blood loss to such an extent that the cerebral circulation has been affected. Similarly, pallor along with cold clammy peripheral skin is a sign of massive blood loss. A thready, irregular and rapid pulse is a sign of shock and needs urgent fluid replacement.

Disability

A complete neurological examination is carried out with evaluation of sensory and motor function and size of pupil. The other causes of altered consciousness like alcohol intake, hypoglycemia and drug abuse should also be assessed.

The *neurological status* of the patient is assessed at the same time. A Glasgow Coma Scale score of 8 or less will need definite airway protection by the passage of an airway, as follows:

Oral airway

By fingers below and behind the mandible, the chin is lifted and the jaw thrust forwards *(chin-lift and jaw-thrust maneuvers).* This is followed by the passage of an oral airway. Special attention is paid to pediatric patients.

Exposure

The patient is completely undressed and the front, back and the perineal area examined for any missed injuries. The *environment is controlled to prevent heat loss and hypothermia.*

Adjuncts to the primary survey

- Two short wide-bore cannulas, size 16 or 14, are passed into peripheral veins. They provide fluid rapidly, and are thus better than central venous lines with their long, thin catheters.
- ECG, x-rays of the chest, pelvis and cervical spine (lateral view) are obtained.
- Blood sugar is checked and full blood count, urea, electrolytes, toxicology, clotting screen and cross-matching is ordered.
- A urinary catheter and a nasogastric tube are passed.

SECONDARY SURVEY

This starts once the primary survey is complete and the patient has been resuscitated. The aim of the secondary survey is to identify all the injuries and to do a complete physical examination. The AMPLE mnemonic is helpful:

A. **Al**lergy.

M. **M**edication including tetanus prophylaxis.

P. **P**ast medical history.

L. **L**ast meal.

E **E**vents of the incident.

Complete physical examination

Each region of the body is examined to document the details of injuries in a systematic way:

Head and face

Oral, facial, maxillary, mandible, ocular, nose, zygoma fractures are documented. Any nasal or ear discharge or bleed, and signs of basal skull fracture, are noted.

Neck

Engorged and distended neck veins are seen. The cervical spine is palpated anteriorly and posteriorly; it is stabilized with a hard cervical collar until injury to the cervical spine is ruled out by x-rays.

Chest

The chest is re-evaluated for rib fractures, flail chest, diaphragmatic injury, cardiac tamponade, sternal fractures and distant heart sounds.

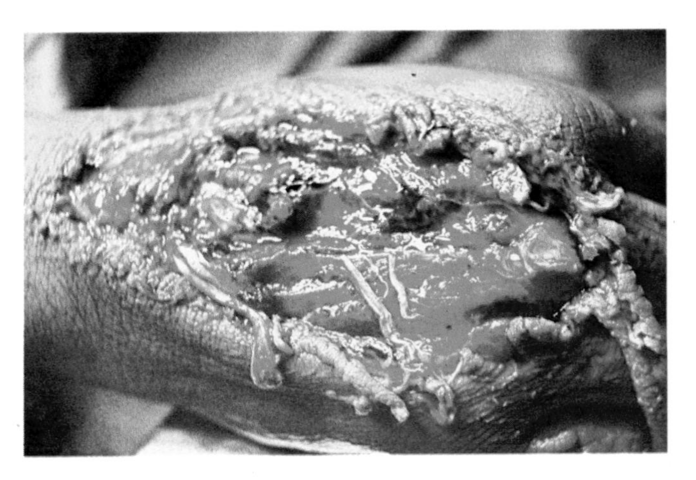

Fig.3.2 Back of hand severely traumatized by a crushing injury, with loss of skin, irregular skin margins, torn tendons, crushed muscles and much exudate.

Neurological

The Glasgow Coma Scale is evaluated after every 15 minutes; any sign of deterioration is documented and urgent help from a neurosurgeon sought. The sensory and motor examination is carried out and any deficit noted; a spinal surgeon is involved in the management.

Abdomen and pelvis

The abdomen is palpated for tenderness and any distension is looked for. Any bruise in the right and left hypochondrium is looked for, and a high level of suspicion is observed for liver or splenic trauma. Bowel sounds are heard, the genitalia are properly examined, and a digital rectal examination carried out. Stability of the pelvis is assessed by applying pressure on both anterior superior iliac spines. Tenderness on iliac spines, greater trochanters and symphysis pubis is noted to rule out any pelvic trauma.

Extremities

Long bone fractures are associated with massive hemorrhage. The limbs are examined for obvious swelling, deformity, abnormal movement, crepitus and loss of movement at the joints. The neurovascular status of the limbs is documented. Special attention is given for the compartment syndrome. Hands are often badly injured (Fig.3.1 and 2)

Log roll

Once the anterior examination is complete, a 'log roll' is done (the patient rolled over like a log), by three persons. The posterior part of the body especially spine is assessed for any missed injuries. Inspection, palpation and percussion are carried out.

Regular re-evaluation

Once the whole examination is completed, it is mandatory to continue the monitoring of the patient. Pulse oximetry, oxygen inhalation and urine output, at the rate of 1ml per kg per hour in adults, are monitored.

Analgesia

This is a very important part of the initial management, as pain and anxiety can produce changes in vital signs. Generally an intravenous dose of opiate is given judiciously, so that the respiratory function is not compromised at the same time.

Documentation and legal considerations

It is very important to keep a meticulous record. The time must also be noted from arrival to step-wise intervention. Informed consent must be obtained if possible, otherwise in life-threatening conditions, it can be obtained retrospectively. Forensic material like clothing and bullets etc. must be properly saved for the police. Blood samples for alcohol and drugs must also be sent and documented.

Definitive care and transfer

The airway must be properly secured and life-saving procedures like tracheostomy, tube thoracotomy and emergency splenectomy must be done before transferring the patient. An experienced anesthesiologist should accompany the patient.

PHASES OF TRAUMA CARE

Complete trauma care should consist of five phases: pre-hospital phase, resuscitation, operation, intensive care and rehabilitation.

Pre-hospital phase

As mentioned above, pre-hospital care helps most in patients belonging to the second group listed above, who can be saved if medical care is provided early. Pre-hospital care can be divided into basic life support and advanced life support.

Basic life support

Basic life support includes the following skills, in which all pre-hospital personnel, e.g. ambulance drivers, should be adequately trained. *This can save lives:*

- *Extrication,* i.e. removing the victim from the site of the accident while providing immobilization of the spine and extremities to prevent further injury.
- *Spinal protection,* including strapping the patient to a back board and immobilizing the head with sandbags and tape.
- *Immobilization* of the extremities with splints: this prevents further damage to vessels, nerves and soft tissues and reduces the extent of hemorrhage around the fracture.
- *Control* of external *bleeding:* this can be achieved by firm pressure over the wound.
- Cardiopulmonary *resuscitation* if required. An adequate airway must be ensured and ventilation provided first, because without it cardiac massage is of no use.

Advanced life support

Airway

A patient who answers when questioned has an adequate airway and can be assumed to be able to protect that airway from aspiration. On the other hand a patient who is unconscious whether due to head injury or hypovolemia is at risk for aspiration, and requires control of the airway. In comatose patients an endotracheal tube should be passed. This protects the patient from aspiration. It also enables gas exchange to be controlled. Further, the patient can be hyperventilated to control intracranial pressure.

Circulation

The *blood pressure* is assessed by palpation. If the radial pulse cannot be palpated, the arterial pressure is probably less than 80mm Hg. *Peripheral perfusion* is estimated by evaluating the time required for capillary refilling. Delayed capillary filling (determined by compressing the capillary bed and watching for filling in less than two seconds) is a good clinical indicator of shock. If a patient has peripheral evidence of hypoperfusion and a blood pressure less than 90mm Hg, he has lost 20–40% of blood volume, i.e. in the adult about 1–2 liters.

Short wide-bore catheters should be inserted into peripheral veins and isotonic crystalloid solution i.e. Ringer's lactate administered. Hemorrhage should be arrested by direct pressure and fractures splinted before or during transport.

Brain. In severe head injury a patent airway must be established and hyperventilation initiated as first line therapy and mainstay of treatment. In addition, circulating volume must be restored, to maintain cerebral perfusion pressure.

Resuscitation

Primary survey

At the hospital, a primary survey is carried out to identify life-threatening conditions and management is begun immediately:

Airway

The *airway* is reassessed and cleared of blood, vomit and foreign body. The lungs are auscultated to assess the adequacy of ventilation. If this is inadequate (i.e. respiratory distress or respiratory rate greater than 35), the patient should be ventilated by a bag valve device (e.g. Ambu bag) connected to a mask until definitive airway control can be obtained with an endotracheal tube. Injuries which can compromise ventilation and perfusion, and require definitive airway management, include:

- Open pneumothorax.
- Tension pneumothorax.
- Massive hemothorax.
- Massively crushed chest.

Hemodynamic status

This is next assessed; useful indicators of the same include:

- Blood pressure.
- Pulse.
- Skin perfusion.
- Urine output.
- Mental status.
- Central venous pressure.

A rough estimate can be made on the basis of the first three. A 15–20% blood volume loss will cause a drop in the blood pressure; with a loss of 30% the blood pressure will be in the range of 60–80mm Hg. With a 40% loss it will be less than 50mm Hg. The pulse rate will be raised and the skin pale and cool.

Fluid loss is rapidly replaced by Ringer's lactate, given through at least two short large-bore intravenous catheters:

- If less than 15% of blood has been lost, 1 to 2 liters of Ringer's lactate raise the blood pressure to normal levels.
- If 2 liters of Ringer's lactate fail to restore blood pressure or peripheral perfusion, blood must be given.
- If the patient is in severe hypotension, transfusion with uncrossmatched blood (type O, Rh negative) may have to be carried out.
- Exsanguinating hemorrhage should be controlled by direct pressure on the wounds.

Splinting of fractures reduces blood loss at the fracture site.

Neurological examination

A brief *neurological* examination utilizing the components of the Glasgow Coma Scale and the size of the pupil completes the primary survey. If the Glasgow Coma Score is 8 or less, aggressive brain resuscitation should be carried out.

Secondary survey

After life-threatening conditions have been dealt with, a thorough history of the accident is taken and a complete examination of the patient carried out from head to toe, in order not to overlook any injury. The *skull* is palpated for hematomas, the eyes for pupillary reactions, and the ears for hemorrhage. The *mouth* is examined for retropharyngeal hematomas and retained foreign bodies. The *neck* is evaluated for venous distension or tracheal deviation (indicating increased intrathoracic pressure) and cervical fractures. *Cranial nerve* function is determined.

Inspection of the *chest* identifies sucking chest wounds and the paradoxical movements of a flail chest. Palpation reveals the crepitus or tenderness of probable fractures. The chest is auscultated at the apex for pneumothorax and at the base for hemothorax. Distant heart sounds with distended neck veins indicate cardiac tamponade.

The *abdomen* is inspected for bruises and hematomas, palpated for tenderness, percussed for free fluid e.g. blood, and auscultated for absence of bowel sounds. *All these clinical methods can be used even where no ultrasound or CT scan is immediately available.*

Pain over the pubis or iliac crest, pelvic instability or perineal hematomas suggests pelvic fractures.

The *extremities* should be assessed for tenderness, bruising, crepitus, skin integrity and the presence of peripheral pulses and neurological deficit.

Evaluation for *vascular* injury should include examination of the neck, supraclavicular spaces, groins and all extremities for large expanding hematomas.

Neurological examination should include motor and sensory evaluation, as well as re-evaluation of the patient's level of consciousness, pupillary size and Glasgow Coma Score.

Where to resuscitate

Most patients are best resuscitated in an emergency room. However, a few should be taken straight to the operating theatre. These include all patients:

- In cardiac arrest.
- With uncontrollable external hemorrhage.

- With massive soft tissue injuries, e.g. traumatic amputation, massive degloving injuries.
- With penetrating trauma to the chest who remain hypotensive in spite of pre-hospital resuscitative efforts.
- With hemodynamic instability in spite of peripheral volume administration.

Rapid volume resuscitation and open chest cardiac massage can be rewarding in patients with cardiac arrest who have at least one vital sign present, i.e.:

- A palpable pulse.
- Evidence of cardiac activity.
- Respiratory excursion.

Operation

Hemorrhage is arrested, devitalized tissue removed, injured soft tissues repaired and fractures stabilized. In the case of major multiple system injury, simultaneous operations by two or three teams may be necessary. *The importance of early and expeditious operation in trauma patients cannot be over-emphasized.*

Intensive care

Patients who have suffered severe injury require a period of intense observation and care. This may entail simple observation of vital signs in a high-risk patient or may necessitate mechanical support of ventilation and circulation. Particular attention is paid to:

- Cardiopulmonary function.
- Fluid and electrolyte balance.
- Coagulation parameters.

It is common to add the following:

- Invasive monitoring of left and right ventricular function.
- Intracranial pressure.
- Arterial and venous pressures.

Such monitoring allows for early recognition of problems and early institution of treatment.

Rehabilitation

Rehabilitation is the process by which biological and psychosocial functions are restored to the level which existed before the injury. It requires cooperation between members of a team including a surgeon, an occupational therapist, a physiotherapist and a social worker. Throughout this difficult period the patient should receive words of encouragement and support from all members of the medical team.

COMPLICATIONS OF TRAUMA

Complications may arise in the management of major trauma due to overlooked injuries, infection, and respiratory failure.

Overlooked injuries

All trauma patients, regardless of outward appearance, should be examined from head to foot. Further, they should be examined serially to assess the effects of resuscitation. This includes continuous evaluation of:

- Ventilation.
- Circulation.
- Level of consciousness.

Failure to improve should prompt immediate re-evaluation. Similarly, a decreasing level of consciousness may suggest a severe closed head injury that was not previously suspected. Many injuries fail to manifest any signs or symptoms and may lead to disastrous consequences if overlooked. These occult injuries usually occur in association with other more easily detectable injuries.

Immunosuppression and infection

Major trauma, whether operative, blunt or penetrating, is accompanied by some degree of immunological compromise, so that the chances of infection are increased. At the same time, the chances of sepsis in a trauma victim are greater:

- The more severe the injury.
- The greater the number of organs injured.
- The larger the number of units of blood administered.
- The longer the operative procedure.
- The more severe and prolonged the state of shock.
- In the very young and the very old.
- In patients with a poor nutritional status.
- In patients on steroids and certain antibiotics.
- After the use of certain anesthetic agents as halothane, cyclopropane, ether and nitrous oxide.

The best indicators of the immunosuppressed state include decreased *T-cells* with decreased *helper cells* and increased *suppressor cells,* a pattern which is sustained until the risk of infection recedes. Of equal importance are the *immunosuppressive peptides* which are generated by injury within half an hour. Their presence can similarly be correlated with risk of infection.

Post-traumatic respiratory failure

Acute respiratory failure is a common complication after major trauma, and may be produced by:

- Respiratory obstruction:
  - Aspiration/foreign body.
  - Head injury with failure to protect the airway.
  - Expanding neck hematoma.
  - Burns.
- Ventilatory failure:
  - CNS injury producing flaccid paralysis.
  - Spinal cord injury:
    - Between C2 and C3 (phrenic paralysis).
    - Between T5 and T10 (intercostal paralysis).
  - Diaphragmatic rupture.
  - Severe flail chest.
  - Severe malnutrition.
  - Gas exchange derangements (ARDS).
- Neurogenic.

ABDOMINAL TRAUMA

Abdominal trauma is seen in a large number of persons injured in automobile accidents. The spleen, liver, kidneys and bowel are the most frequently injured abdominal organs. Early diagnosis facilitates optimal management. Sometimes the patient is unconscious because of associated head injury, shock or alcoholism. Chest injuries and fractures may further complicate the diagnostic problems. The index of suspicion should be high even in cases of supposedly minor abdominal trauma if diagnostic errors are to be avoided.

Clinical manifestations

One should find out how the patient got injured, as this helps in assessing the likelihood of abdominal injury. *In spite of the large number of modern diagnostic aids available, a careful and detailed history and physical examination are the most helpful measures for detecting intra-abdominal injury.*

Apart from the abdomen the entire patient must be examined thoroughly because of the high incidence of associated trauma. Abdominal pain and tenderness are the most reliable of all physical findings. *Abdominal rigidity indicates intraperitoneal injury and is an indication for exploratory laparotomy.*

If the blood pressure falls to low levels this suggests *internal hemorrhage.* If the systolic blood pressure has fallen below 70mm Hg due to hemorrhage, up to 30 to 40% of blood volume has probably been lost. A liter of Ringer's lactate solution should be infused within 15 to 20 minutes while blood is being grouped and cross matched. If after coming up, the blood pressure again falls to hypotensive levels, blood transfusion must be immediately started and the abdomen explored. Other subtle signs of internal hemorrhage include:

- Moderate tachycardia.
- Narrowing of the pulse pressure.
- Cold hands and feet.
- Rapid breathing.

Investigations

If *hemoglobin* and *hematocrit* are determined very soon after injury or hemorrhage they will be normal, as enough time has not elapsed for hemodilution; at a later stage both levels will be lowered.

The *serum amylase* may be raised if the pancreas has been injured.

Blood gas determinations should be carried out repeatedly in all patients with multiple injuries, especially those with chronic pulmonary disease, chest injuries or possible aspiration of gastric contents.

X-rays are not of much help in abdominal trauma for detecting injuries to the soft tissues, except for gas under the diaphragm in a perforated stomach or duodenum. In internal hemorrhage the density in the region may be increased, and fluid accumulation between bowel loops may be shown up.

Peritoneal tap and lavage

Blunt trauma to the abdomen may produce severe intraperitoneal injury with minimum physical signs. In suspected cases a *peritoneal tap* with a needle may be carried out in both flanks. A positive abdominal tap is correct in about 95% of cases. However, a negative tap does not rule out intra-abdominal injury and should be followed by peritoneal lavage or CT scan. If signs of peritoneal irritation are present urgent laparotomy should be carried out whether or not the abdominal tap or lavage are positive.

CT scan

In retroperitoneal injuries physical signs may be few and peritoneal lavage unreliable. In such cases CT scan has a definite place. However, patients with unstable vital signs should not be candidates for a CT scan because the scanning takes time. Finally, continued clinical evaluation is essential even if the CT scan is negative.

Effect of lengthy operations

If a lengthy operation is carried out for trauma during which large quantities of blood are lost, the patient's condition can deteriorate during the procedure due to the following reasons:

- Evaporation from the extensive surfaces of the intestines can lead to *hypothermia* from excessive heat loss.
- The citrate contained in the large quantities of blood transfused can cause *acidosis*.
- Dilution of blood and hypothermia can result in defective coagulation (*coagulopathy*).

The above conditions, especially when they occur together, can be dangerous.

Procedure for a patient in extremis

In such a situation, sometimes the best course to follow consists of immediate termination of the laparotomy. Further, if the intestines are so distended that the abdomen cannot be closed without embarrassing the respiration, the skin alone may be closed, leaving the muscular abdominal wall open. The patient should now be taken to the intensive care unit, where his metabolic derangements can be corrected over a couple of days. He is then returned to the operation theatre and the procedure completed.

PEDIATRIC TRAUMA

Trauma is one of the leading causes of death in children. The initial management of trauma is the same according to the ATLS protocol i.e. ABCDE followed by the primary and secondary survey. The physiological reserve of a child is much less than that of an adult; therefore, once the condition of the child deteriorates, recovery is more difficult. Most of the children die of head injury and respiratory distress. Compared to the body volume, the surface area, which is responsible for heat loss, is greater in children; so care must be taken to protect the patient from hypothermia.

Airway and cervical spine control

Control of the airway is the first priority, as children die of airway obstruction rather than cardiopulmonary arrest. In children the tongue is short, oropharynx is straight and epiglottis is flabby, so jaw thrust can be used but not chin lift. Before clearing the airway the child is pre-oxygenated, and only then the secretions are removed. An airway should not be used except in dire situations. Only uncuffed endotracheal tubes are used. The vagal response is strong in children; therefore premedication is done with atropine to reduce the secretions before intubation. Nasopharyngeal tubes are not used in children. Care of the cervical spine is the same as in adults.

Breathing and ventilation

The respiratory rate must be constantly monitored as hypoventilation can lead to respiratory acidosis which can prove fatal. Otherwise the care is the same as for adults.

Circulation and hemorrhage

Tachycardia is the earliest sign of shock in children. The vital signs must be monitored aggressively in children. Cold clammy peripheries, mottled skin and reduced pulse pressure must be noted as signs of shock. If intravenous access is not obtained after two attempts, the intra-osseous route should be used; the diaphyseal tibia is the ideal route. Urine output at the rate of 2ml per kg per hour should be expected.

Disability

Death due to head injury is more common in children due to diffuse axonal injury. The GCS should be monitored constantly.

Exposure

It is similar to the adult patient but care must be observed regarding hypothermia which can be prevented by the use of blankets, proper wrapping and instituting warm fluids.

Pediatric secondary survey

This is based on similar protocols as observed for the adult patient. Care must be given to detect duodenal and pancreatic trauma, small bowel and bladder injury and injury to the lumbar spine.

Chapter

4 BURNS, GRAFTS AND FLAPS

BURNS

A burn constitutes one of the commonest types of emergency received in any hospital. It affects the patient not only physically but also psychologically with devastating effects, and may result in chronic disability. Age is no barrier, ranging from babies to elderly people. The problem is present in both the developed and under-developed world. Burn injuries represent a diverse and varied challenge to medical and paramedical staff.

In 1945, the concept was introduced that major burns were best cared for in a 'burn centre'. This resulted in rapid improvement in survival and a reduction of morbidity of burned patients. Further, it led to the emergence of regional specialty treatment centers in other disciplines also.

CAUSES OF BURNS

Burns may be caused by heat, electricity, chemicals and friction.

Frequency of different types of burns

Burns of different types occur with the following frequency:

- Flame 55%
- Scalds 40%
- Chemical and electrical burns 5%

Thermal injuries

These injuries can be divided into the following types:

Scalds

The common mechanisms are spilling hot drinks or liquids, or being exposed to hot bathing water. Scalds tend to cause superficial to superficial dermal burns. About 70 % of burns in children are scalds.

Flame burns

Flame burns comprise 50% of adult burns. They are often associated with inhalational injury and other concomitant trauma. Flame burns tend to be deep dermal or full thickness.

Contact burns

Touching a very hot object may result in this type of burn, and these are commonly seen in people with epilepsy or those who use alcohol or drugs. They are also seen in elderly people after loss of consciousness.

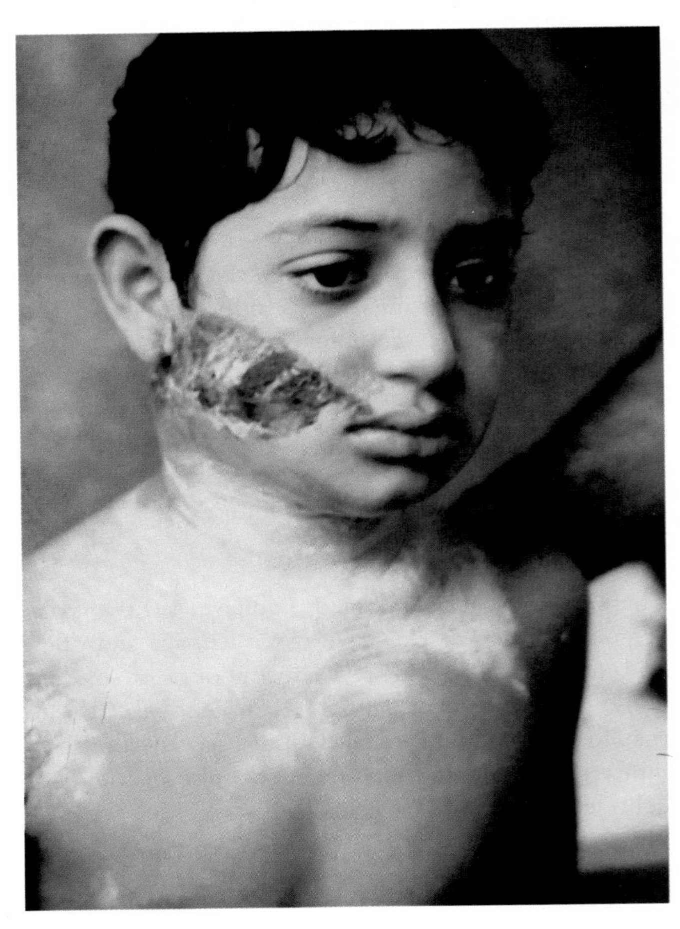

Fig.4.1 Friction burn. Superficial partial-thickness burn face sustained when the patient's cheek was rubbed along a metalled road.

Burns from brief contact with very hot substances are usually due to industrial accidents. Contact burns tend to be deep dermal or full thickness.

Deaths from oil stoves

In some underdeveloped countries, young women cooking the family meal over kerosene oil stoves sometimes die from severe burns. The mother-in-law is often blamed; at other times it is thought that the stove bursts. The truth is otherwise.

The mother-in-law does not kill, as suggested by the fact that over one-third of the young girls dying are unmarried. The stove does not burst; in a study carried out in the author's clinical unit not a single piece of metal from a stove was recovered from any young girl's body. At the same time, our researchers recovered the suspected stoves; none of them had burst.

The real cause is carelessness in the use of these rather imperfectly made stoves. A set of instructions, on the lines of the following, broadcast on the radio and TV helped considerably reduce the incidence of these tragic accidents:

Do not pour kerosene oil into a lighted stove; do not carry a lighted stove; do not wear synthetic clothes: if you have to, wear a cotton apron over them, etc. etc.

Electrical injuries

An electric current travels through the body from one point to another, creating "entry" and "exit" points. The tissue between these two points can be damaged by the electrical energy. The amount of heat generated, and hence the level of tissue damage, is proportional to the voltage, which is therefore the main determinant of the degree of tissue damage. These electrical injuries can be divided into high and low voltage injuries:

High voltage injuries

These injuries occur when the voltage is 1,000 volts or greater. There is extensive tissue damage and often limb loss. There is usually a large amount of soft and bony tissue necrosis. Muscle damage gives rise to rhabdomyolysis, and renal failure may occur. This injury pattern needs more aggressive resuscitation and debridement than other burns.

Contact with voltage greater than 70,000 volts is invariably fatal.

Low voltage injuries

These are those injuries that occur due to voltage less than 1,000 volts

"Flash" injuries

These can occur when there has been an arc of current from a high tension voltage source. The heat from this arc can cause superficial flash burns to exposed body parts, typically the face and hands. However, clothing can also be set alight, giving rise to deeper burns. No current actually passes through the victim's body.

Chemical injuries

Chemical injuries are usually a result of industrial accidents, but may also occur with household chemical products. These burns tend to be deep, as the corrosive agent continues to cause coagulation necrosis until completely removed.

Alkalies

Alkalies tend to penetrate deeper and cause worse burns than acids. Cement is a common cause of alkali burns.

Acids

In acid burns hydrofluoric acid, widely used for glass etching and in the manufacture of circuit boards, is one of the more common culprits. It causes a continuing, penetrating injury, and must be neutralised with calcium gluconate, either applied topically in a gel or injected into the affected tissues.

Friction

Friction can also occasionally result in a burn (Fig.4.1).

Incidence of burns by age

Burns occur at different ages with the following frequency:

- 1–4 years old 20%.
- 5–14 years old 10%.
- 15–64 years old 60%.
- > 65 years old 10%.

THE BODY'S RESPONSE TO A BURN

Burn injuries result in both local and systemic responses:

Local response

The three zones of a burn were described by Jackson in 1947:

Zone of coagulation

This occurs in the centre, at the point of maximum damage. In this zone, coagulation of the proteins results in irreversible loss of tissue.

Zone of stasis

In the surrounding zone of stasis perfusion is decreased, but the tissue can still be saved. The effort should be to improve perfusion and prevent the injury becoming irreversible.

Zone of hyperemia

In the outermost zone perfusion is increased due to vasodilatation. Such a situation recovers unless there is severe sepsis or prolonged hypoperfusion.

If tissue is lost, the wound becomes deeper as well as wider.

Systemic response

The release of cytokines and other inflammatory mediators at the site of injury has a systemic effect once the burn reaches 30% of total body surface area.

Cardiovascular changes

Capillary permeability is increased, leading to loss of intravascular proteins and fluids into the interstitial compartment. Peripheral and splanchnic vasoconstriction occurs. Myocardial contractility is decreased, possibly due to release of tumor necrosis factor. These changes, coupled with fluid loss from the burn wound, result in systemic hypotension and end-organ hypo-perfusion.

Respiratory changes

In a patient with a major burn the function of the lung can be impaired by the following factors:

- An unyielding leathery eschar may be present around the thorax, which limits respiratory excursions and hinders ventilation.
- The large volumes of salt-containing solutions infused may lead to considerable weight gain, making the chest wall heavy and hard to move.
- Toxaemia affecting the gut may produce reflex ileus which elevates the diaphragm, further reducing the vital capacity.
- An inhalation burn may result in gross edema of the respiratory passages.
- Smoke particles provoke an allergic reaction, producing alveolitis and pneumonia.

All the above factors combine to produce coughing which predisposes the patient to the development of collapse of the lung, bronchopneumonia and other pulmonary complications.

The kidneys

In cases with very extensive burns, renal damage sometimes occurs. The events leading to a harmful effect on the kidney occur in the following sequence:

- In response to the trauma and hypovolemia of the major burn the posterior pituitary releases antidiuretic hormone and the adrenals release aldosterone, so both water and salt are maximally reabsorbed from the tubules. Thus a greatly reduced volume of concentrated urine with a small amount of sodium is passed.
- The injured cells in the burned area release myoglobin and hemoglobin besides other waste products.
- If an adequate glomerular filtration rate is not maintained, or if renal ischemia occurs due to severe hypotension, these waste products cannot be effectively removed, and acute tubular necrosis occurs. This is the basis of the renal failure which was previously a common event in burn shock.
- If volume losses are replaced by similar fluid, renal blood flow is maintained, a good urinary output (30–50ml/hr in an adult) is ensured, and damage to the kidney is prevented.

The gut

Stress ulceration

This often occurs in a major burn. This can take one of two forms:

- *Curling's ulcer.* This is the acute duodenal ulcer which can occur in any extensive burn and is called a Curling's ulcer.
- *Acute gastric erosions.* Acute gastric erosions can occur due to the stress associated with a major burn. These are multiple tiny erosions in the gastric mucosa, and are found in the fundus and body of the stomach.

Either of these two forms of ulceration present with hematemesis and melena, which may be massive. Their incidence after major burns can be reduced by the prophylactic use of proton pump inhibitors.

Reflex ileus

This may occur due to intestinal paralysis probably from the toxins of bacteria infecting the burn. This delays the onset of oral feeding. At the same time the resulting abdominal distension splints the diaphragm, impairs ventilation, especially in the lower lobes of the lungs, and predisposes the patient to the development of respiratory infections.

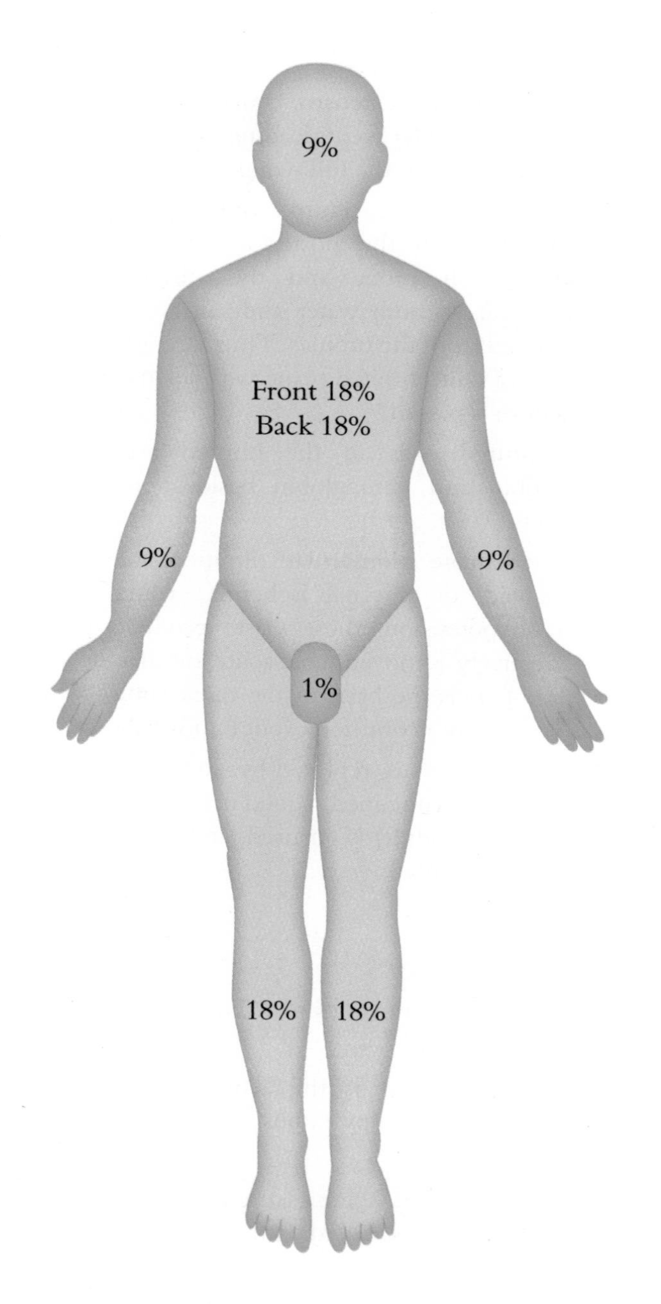

Fig.4.2 Wallace's Rule of Nine

Metabolism

In a major burn, due to loss of the skin barrier over a large area of the body surface, fluid losses from evaporation are greatly increased. The resultant cooling causes shivering, leading to a markedly elevated metabolic rate and much loss of energy. This hyper-metabolic state leads to severe catabolism and rapid loss of weight. It can be corrected by early closure of the burn wound by skin grafts and increasing the enteral feeding in the patient. Therefore nasogastric tube feeding should be started promptly in all patients with burn greater than 15% total body surface area. In this way fluids and nutrients are provided to the patient through the most physiological route.

Immunity

As a major burn is a very extensive wound, it produces deficiencies in both cellular and humoral defences. There is lymphocytopenia, with delayed rejection of allograft skin. The level of immunoglobins is depressed, as is the inflammatory response. *This reduced immunity predisposes the patient to septic complications* both locally in the burn wound and at distant sites, as explained later.

EVALUATION

The severity of a burn depends upon the following factors:

- The age of the patient.
- The extent of the burn.
- The depth of the burn.
- The actual site involved.
- Whether an inhalation burn has also occurred.
- The presence of coexisting disease states.

The age of the patient is important; burns in persons below the age of 3 years and over 60 years have more serious consequences for the patient than at other ages.

The extent of the burn is recorded in terms of percentage of body surface area burned. A burn diagram should be used, the exact location and extent of the burn being drawn on the body diagram.

Wallace's Rule of Nine

An estimate can be made in adults by using the Wallace's Rule of Nine (Table 4.1). What this formula loses in accuracy it more than gains by ease of committing to memory. Further, if for example, the whole of the front of an arm is not burnt, the area can be considered as a fraction of 9%, estimated, and recorded (Fig.4.2).

Lund and Browder chart

This chart, if used correctly, is the most accurate method. It compensates for the variation in body shape with age and therefore can give an accurate assessment of the burnt area in children.

However for the undergraduate and a general duty doctor, the simplicity and ease of application of the Rule of Nine makes it a great deal more attractive.

Table 4.1 Wallace's Rule of Nine

Head and neck	9%
Right upper limb	9%
Left upper limb	9%
Front of chest and abdomen	18%
Back of chest and abdomen	18%
Right lower limb	18%
Left lower limb	18%
Genitals	1%
Total	100%

Depth of a burn

The depth of a burn is difficult to estimate. Generally, scalds tend to be superficial, and chemical and electrical burns are deep. Redness of the skin and thin water blisters generally occur in superficial burns, and thick blisters and leathery eschar in deep burns, but appearances may be deceptive. Sensation is not as helpful for estimating the depth of a burn as was once thought. In deep burns pinprick sensation is absent, but it can also be absent in burns of moderate depth.

However, for the initial treatment of burns it is only necessary to separate those injuries which are clearly superficial and will heal rapidly from those which are deeper and will require hospitalization and specialized care. Accurate differentiation between superficial and deep burns becomes possible by the second week after the burn.

During the first few days, the extent of the burn is more important than its depth, for estimating fluid requirements and directing care. Later, when the question of skin grafting arises, burn depth assumes more significance.

Site of burn

Burns of the face and neck, hands, feet and perineum pose special problems in their reconstruction and rehabilitation.

Inhalation injury

A common cause of instability and increased morbidity in burn patients is severe inhalation injury producing extensive damage to the airways with pending obstruction, and this should be detected during the primary survey. Burnt nasal hair, conjunctivitis, hoarseness, bronchitis and carbon particles in the sputum should raise suspicion of inhalation injury.

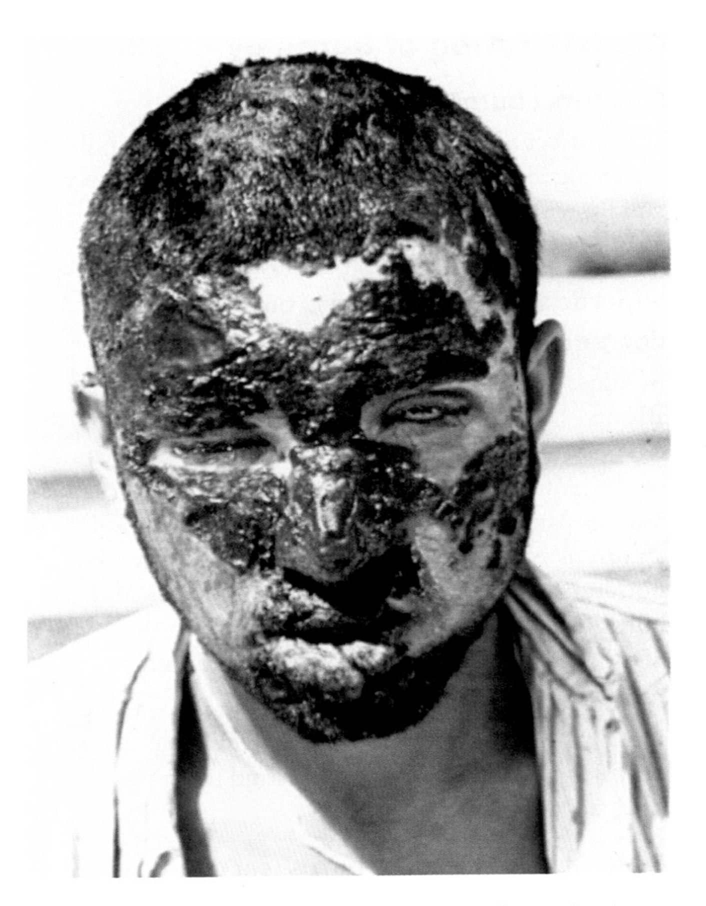

Fig.4.3 Healing partial thickness burns face. The burnt layers of the skin are in the form of scabs which are dry and are falling off.

Associated injuries and diseases

A secondary survey should detect associated injuries such as head injuries, fractures, etc. Coexisting disease, whether cardiovascular, respiratory, renal or metabolic, can complicate the care of a burned patient and increase the mortality. On the other hand epilepsy and alcohol or drug abuse tends to predispose patients to burns.

Laboratory studies

These should include blood count, electrolytes, biochemistry profile and blood gases, as well as carboxyhemoglobin concentration if indicated.

Criteria for admission

After evaluating the patient, the following types of patients should be considered for admission:

- Suspected airway burn.
- Where intravenous fluids or surgery may be required.
- Significant burns of hands or face.
- Poor social or psychiatric background.

Classification of burns by depth

Epidermal burns (first-degree)

These affect only the epidermis and are due to sunburn. Blistering may occur but is not common. Healing occurs rapidly, within a week, by regeneration from undamaged keratinocytes within skin adnexa.

Superficial partial thickness burns (second-degree)

In these burns epidermis and part of the dermis is affected (Fig.4.3). The characteristic features in this type of burn are the blisters which form on the surface of the skin; the exposed superficial nerves make these injuries painful and exquisitely sensitive to stimuli, even a current of air. Since the basal layers of the skin are not destroyed, regeneration occurs promptly and these burns usually heal spontaneously in two or three weeks without infection. The rate of regeneration depends on the density of the skin adnexa.

If a burn has not healed by two weeks, the depth has probably been assessed incorrectly and referral should be made to a burns unit.

Deep partial thickness burns (second-degree)

These burns are more severe, with many areas of marginally viable tissue. They show a decreased sensitivity to stimuli, e.g. pinprick. They can be defined as burns that take longer than three weeks to heal; this prolonged healing often results in hypertrophic scar formation. The skin only survives and heals under the most optimal conditions; otherwise it gets converted into a full-thickness burn. Only after 10 to 14 days can it be predicted accurately whether excision and skin grafting would give results better than natural healing.

Full thickness burns (third-degree)

In these burns all regenerative elements have been destroyed, and healing only occurs from the edges and is associated with considerable contraction. All such injuries should therefore be excised and grafted unless they are less than 1cm in diameter in an area where function would not be compromised.

Fourth-degree burns

These burns involve injury to subcutaneous tissues, such as fat, fascia, muscle or bone. After a burn is sustained edema, decreased blood supply or bacterial invasion may further injure or destroy cells that have survived the initial thermal insult.

TREATMENT OF BURNS

Emergency treatment

First aid

The aims of first aid should be to stop the burning process, cool the burn, provide pain relief, and cover the burn.

Stopping the burning process

The heat source should be removed. Flames should be doused with water or smothered with a blanket or by rolling the victim on the ground. Rescuers should take care to avoid burn injury to themselves. Clothing can retain heat, even in a scald burn, and should be removed as soon as possible. Adherent material, such as nylon clothing, should be left on.

Cooling the burn

Active cooling removes heat and prevents progression of the burn. This is effective if performed within 20 minutes of the injury. Immersion or irrigation with running tepid water (15°C) should be continued for up to 20 minutes. This also removes noxious agents and reduces pain, and may reduce edema by stabilising mast cells and histamine release. Iced water should not be used as intense vasoconstriction can cause burn progression. Cooling large areas of skin can lead to hypothermia, especially in children. Chemical burns should be irrigated with copious amounts of water.

Analgesia

Exposed nerve endings will cause pain. Cooling and simply covering the exposed burn will reduce the pain. Opioids may be required initially to control pain, but once first aid measures have been effective non-steroidal anti-inflammatory drugs such as ibuprofen taken orally will suffice.

Covering the burn

Dressings should cover the burn area and keep the patient warm. Polyvinyl chloride film ('cling' film) is an ideal first aid cover. Hand burns can be covered with a clear plastic bag so as not to restrict mobility. Use of topical creams should be avoided at this stage as these may interfere with subsequent assessment of the burn.

Primary survey

The initial management of a severely burnt patient is similar to that of any trauma patient. A modified "advanced trauma life support" primary survey (ABCDEF) is performed, with particular emphasis on assessment of the airway and breathing. The burn injury must not distract from this sequential assessment, otherwise serious associated injuries may be missed.

A—Airway with cervical spine control

An assessment must be made as to whether the airway is compromised or is at risk of compromise. The cervical spine should be protected unless it is definitely not injured. Inhalation of hot gases will result in a burn above the vocal cords. This burn will become edematous over the following hours, especially after fluid resuscitation has begun. This means that an airway that is patent on arrival at hospital may occlude after admission. This can be a particular problem in small children. If there is any concern about the patency of the airway then intubation is the safest policy.

B—Breathing

All burn patients should receive 100% oxygen through a humidified non-rebreathing mask on presentation. Breathing problems are considered to be those that affect the respiratory system below the vocal cords. There are several ways that a burn injury can compromise respiration:

- Mechanical restriction of breathing.
- Blast injury.
- Smoke inhalation.
- Carboxyhemoglobin.

C—Circulation

Intravenous access should be established with two large bore cannulas. This is an opportunity to take blood for checking full blood count, urea and electrolytes, blood group, and clotting screen. Peripheral circulation must be checked. Any deep or full thickness circumferential extremity burn can act as a tourniquet, especially once edema develops after fluid resuscitation. This may not occur until some hours after the burn. If there is any suspicion of decreased perfusion due to circumferential burn, the tissue must be released with *escharotomies*, i.e. longitudinal incisions through the full thickness of skin of the trunk or a limb.

D—Neurological disability

All patients should be assessed for responsiveness with the Glasgow coma scale; they may be confused because of hypoxia or hypovolemia.

E—Exposure

Complete exposure of the patient is done to assess the burn and also the associated injuries, if there are any.

F—Fluid resuscitation

The resuscitation regimen should be determined and begun. This is based on the estimation of the burn area. A urinary catheter is mandatory in all adults with injuries covering > 20% of total body surface area, to monitor urine output.

Analgesia

Superficial burns can be extremely painful. All patients with large burns should receive intravenous morphine at a dose appropriate to body weight. This should be titrated against pain and respiratory depression.

Investigations

The nature of the investigations required will vary with the type of burn.

Secondary survey

At the end of the primary survey and the start of emergency management, a secondary survey should be performed. This is a head to toe examination to look for any concomitant injuries.

Dressing the wound

Once the surface area and depth of a burn have been estimated, the burn wound should be washed and any loose skin removed.

Definitive treatment

Definitive management of the patient with a major burn resolves itself into the following steps:

- Fluid replacement.
- Monitoring.
- Nutritional care.
- Care of the burn wound.
- Rehabilitation.

FLUID REPLACEMENT

All the fluid formulas are only guidelines, and their success relies on adjusting the amount of resuscitation fluid against monitored physiological parameters. The main aim of resuscitation is to maintain tissue perfusion to the zone of stasis and so prevent the burn deepening. This is not easy, as too little fluid will cause hypoperfusion whereas too much will lead to edema that will cause tissue hypoxia.

The greatest amount of fluid loss in burn patients is in the first 24 hours after injury. For the first eight to 12 hours, there is a general shift of fluid from the intravascular to interstitial fluid compartments. This means that any fluid given during this time will rapidly leave the intravascular compartment.

Colloids have no advantage over crystalloids in maintaining circulatory volume. Fast fluid boluses probably have little benefit, as a rapid rise in intravascular hydrostatic pressure will just drive more fluid out of the circulation. However, much protein is lost through the burn wound, so there is a need to replace this oncotic loss.

Volume of fluid

The greater the body weight and the more extensive the burn, the larger the volume of fluid required for replacement of the losses.

First 24 hours

If, as recommended above, *buffered salt solution,* i.e. Ringer's lactate, is used during the first 24 hours, 4ml of the solution is required for every one per cent of body surface burnt per kilogram body weight during the 24 hours. Thus the volume is:

4ml/kg body weight/% body surface area burnt

However, if *colloid* is used, less than half the above amount is required and only 1.5 to 2ml per kg per one per cent body surface burnt is given in the 24 hours. Thus the volume administered is:

1.5 to 2ml/kg body weight/% body burnt

Examples of colloid solutions include human plasma protein fraction, human albumin 4.5%, or a synthetic plasma expander like Dextran 110.

Speed of administration

Whichever of the above two types of fluids, i.e. salt solution or colloid, is chosen for administration, 1/2 of it is given in the first 8 hours, 1/4 in the second 8 hours, and the remaining 1/4 in the third 8 hours. This is because the loss of fluid is greatest in the first 8 hours, and slows down later.

Urine output

In major burns the urine output should be closely monitored, as it indicates whether replacement of fluid has been adequate or not. An output of 30–70ml of urine per hour is required. If this much urine is passed, it indicates that the fluid losses are being satisfactorily replaced, and that sufficient fluid is being provided to help excrete the increased quantities of waste products resulting from the raised level of catabolism due to the major burn.

Second 24 hours

During the second 24 hours after the burn approximately half the above amounts will be required, as the losses of fluids from the burn are gradually decreasing in amount.

Fluid replacement in children

Small-sized objects have a larger surface area per kg of weight. Children are smaller in size than adults, therefore this rule applies to them also, i.e. compared to their weight, their surface area is greater. Now, the larger the surface area the greater the fluid loss per kg, and a similarly large volume of fluid is required for replacement.

In actual practice it works out like this: when Ringer' lactate solution is used, instead of the 4ml/kg body weight/1 % body burnt recommended above for adults, 5ml is used. Similarly, when colloid is used, instead of the 1.5 to 2ml/kg body weight/1 % body burnt, 2.5ml is used. Except from this difference in the volumes used, fluid replacement in children is carried out on the same lines as in adults.

However, it should be remembered that even if a clinician follows a particular formula very carefully, he cannot be sure that the fluid and electrolyte requirements have been correctly met. It is only by repeated clinical observation that one can be certain in this respect. The patient with a major burn should have his fluid requirements evaluated and the necessary adjustments made, not on a daily but an hourly basis.

Indicators of adequate fluid replacement

The parameters to watch, in assessing the adequacy of the circulation, are the following:

- The patient should be mentally alert.
- The pulse rate should be below 120/min.
- The urine volume should be at least 30ml/hr in the adult and 1.2ml/kg/hr in the child.
- If a central venous line has been passed, the central venous pressure should be between 6 and 8cm of water.
- The hematocrit value should be less than 60%.
- High tension electrical injuries, because of their depth, require substantially more fluid (up to 9ml × (burn area) × (body weight) in the first 24 hours) and a higher urine output (1.5–2ml/kg/hour).
- Inhalational injuries also require more fluid.

Investigations at intervals of four to six hours are mandatory for monitoring a patient's resuscitation status. These include packed cell volume, plasma sodium, base excess, and lactate. Burns units use different resuscitation formulas.

Escharotomies

A circumferential deep dermal or full thickness burn is inelastic and on an extremity will not stretch. Fluid resuscitation leads to the development of burn wound edema and swelling of the tissue beneath this inelastic burnt tissue. Tissue pressures rise and can impair peripheral circulation.

Circumferential chest burns can also cause problems by limiting chest excursion and impairing ventilation. Both of these situations require escharotomy, i.e. division of the burn eschar. Only the burnt skin is divided, not any underlying fascia, differentiating this procedure from a fasciotomy.

Incisions are made along the mid lateral or medial aspects of the limbs, avoiding any underlying structures. For the chest, longitudinal incisions are made down each mid-axillary line to the subcostal region. The lines are joined up by an incision running parallel to the subcostal margin (chevron incision). This creates a mobile breastplate that moves with ventilation.

Escharotomies are best done with electro-cautery, as they tend to bleed. Although they are an urgent procedure, escharotomies are best done in an operating theatre by experienced staff.

MONITORING

All major burn victims require cardiac monitoring, preferably with periodic arterial blood gas determinations, at least during the first 24 hours after the burn is sustained.

NUTRITIONAL CARE

In every major injury, including any extensive burn, the metabolic rate is greatly increased, with a marked catabolic response, so that there is weight loss, a negative nitrogen balance, and retarded wound healing. During the catabolic phase the levels of the catabolic hormones (glucagon and catecholamine) in the plasma are elevated, whereas the level of the anabolic hormone (insulin) is lowered.

Protein catabolism does not proceed uniformly in all tissues; muscle protein is sacrificed to save the structural and functional integrity of vital organs such as the heart and liver, so muscle wasting is a marked feature. The negative nitrogen balance can be corrected if a sufficient caloric and nitrogen intake is provided (about 20 grams of nitrogen per square meter of body surface per day). If this is not done, the patient becomes severely malnourished.

If fat is omitted from the enteral and parenteral solutions, essential fatty acid deficiency may develop after prolonged nutritional therapy. The patient develops dermatitis, thrombocytopenia, impaired wound healing and loss of hair. This can be prevented by weekly parenteral administration of a litre of lipid emulsion.

Water-soluble vitamins (B complex and C) are depleted rapidly, and 250 to 500mg vitamin C should be administered daily. The fat-soluble vitamins (A, D, E and K) are depleted more slowly, and need replacement only after prolonged parenteral feeding.

Frequent determinations of calcium, magnesium and phosphorus levels should be carried out, apart from electrolytes. Finally, zinc is an important co-factor in wound healing, and periodic measurements of zinc, copper, manganese and chromium provide guidelines for replacement.

Consequences of malnutrition

Inadequate nutritional replacement produces the following serious consequences:

- Profound weight loss.
- Decreased immunological response.
- Decreased leucocyte function, and therefore reduced host resistance.
- Impaired wound healing.
- Superior mesenteric artery syndrome. In the emaciated supine patient the acute angle between the aorta and the superior mesenteric artery is further reduced so that the third part of the duodenum is compressed between these two structures. This leads to anorexia, nausea and vomiting, and results in poor food intake and further malnutrition.
- In the bedridden supine patient most of the energy utilized is spent on maintaining normal respiratory function. When the energy available becomes insufficient even for this activity, ineffective respiratory effort causes *atelectasis,* and lung infection by opportunistic pathogens supervenes. The most common cause of death in these patients is pulmonary sepsis.

Although the effects of severe malnutrition have been described above in the case of a major burn, *a similar situation arises in a major injury of any type*, especially one complicated by infection.

Remedial measures for malnutrition

The consequences of severe malnutrition can be minimized by paying attention to the following aspects of patient care:

- *Control of heat loss.* In major burns, a great deal of heat is lost due to evaporation from the extensive burn surfaces. If the patient is treated without dressings, radiation also plays a part in heat loss. As a response to this heat loss, the metabolic rate is greatly increased in order to maintain the body temperature, but this leads to rapid loss of weight. This hypermetabolic state can be controlled by insulative occlusive dressings. If the patient is being treated without dressings, electric heaters may be used to keep the environmental temperature at 31° C.

- *Pain.* Apprehension and *pain* potentiate the release of catecholamine; they are controlled by analgesics and tranquilizers.
- *Infection.* This is prevented by isolation, careful nursing and the judicious use of antibiotics.
- *Early closure.* The burn wound is *closed early,* as this step alone greatly reduces the catabolic state.
- *Provision of calories.* However, the most important aspect of the nutritional management of the burn patient is the provision of an *adequate number of exogenous calories* and nitrogen. Extensive tissue breakdown in major burns results in protein catabolism. Nitrogen is produced, and appears in the urine as urea. If nutritional support is not provided, protein catabolism is further increased in order to provide energy. This results in a decrease in lean body mass and loss of weight. With small burns this weight loss is minor, e.g. about 5% of body weight for a 10% burn. However, if nutritional support is not provided in cases of burns exceeding 40% of body surface, up to 30% of body weight can be lost, leading to severe malnutrition.
- *Route of administration.* Whenever possible the gastrointestinal tract should be used for providing nutrition; this is not only the best method but also very much cheaper. Parenteral nutrition should be reserved only for those patients where the gut cannot be employed. Complete homogenized diets are well tolerated by the patient with a major burn. On the other hand, partially digested diets have a high osmolality, and may cause diarrhea and dehydration.

Advantages of enteral feeding

The advantages of enteral feeding are many:

- Enteral nutrients maintain the integrity of the digestive tract and minimize the chances of bacterial translocation from the gut, which could result in the sepsis syndrome.
- An oral diet preserves the gut mucosa and the output of enzymes by it. Oral feeding stimulates the elaboration of trophic hormones, e.g. gastrin.
- Enterally administered calories stimulate release of insulin, which promotes anabolism.

Additional measures

- ***Temperature.*** Low environmental temperatures increase the metabolic expenditure and lead to loss of weight. This tendency can be eliminated by keeping the ambient temperature at 31° C, i.e. four degrees higher than the neutral temperature for normal subjects.
- ***Pain*** on dressing and other procedures increases metabolic expenditure. This can be reduced by analgesics and sedation.
- ***Physical exercise*** promotes preservation of muscle bulk, and supervised physical therapy should be provided to all patients requiring prolonged hospitalization from any cause.
- ***Closure.*** Expeditious wound closure is the most effective measure for minimizing the loss of energy from the wound.

CARE OF THE BURN WOUND

The aims of the local treatment of the burn are three:

- Avoidance of further damage to cells already injured.
- Prevention of infection.
- Early closure of the burn wound.

In a small burn wound, full-thickness excision and grafting can be carried out if necessary. However, in the more extensive burns this is not possible, because as the area to be excised increases, the available donor sites decrease. As large scale excision cannot be carried out the wound has to be supported while the reversibly injured cells heal. This demands protection from bacterial invasion.

Protection from infection

The skin is not sterile. It contains many bacteria in the hair follicles and sweat glands. The surgeon's aim is to prevent an increase in these exogenous bacteria to levels sufficient to cause burn wound sepsis.

Historical evolution

Historically, the local care of burns has evolved through three stages:

Occlusive dressings

Classically, burns were treated locally by occlusive dressings. After cleansing and debridement an inner layer of gauze impregnated with petroleum jelly etc. was covered by a layer of absorptive cotton wool and held in place by a gauze bandage. This dressing remained intact until exudate soaked through it, or odour, pain or fever made inspection of the wound necessary. The

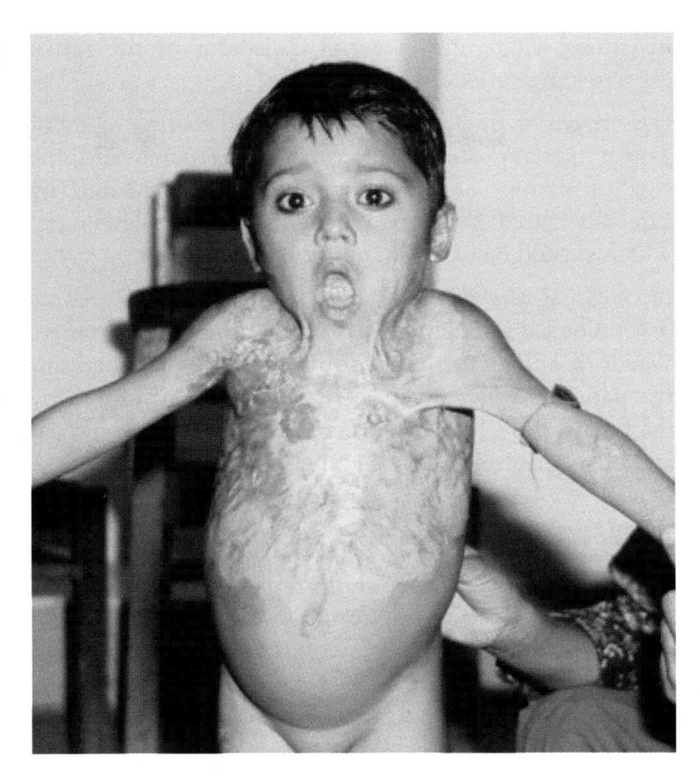

Fig.4.3 (a) Post-burn contracture front of neck and left shoulder

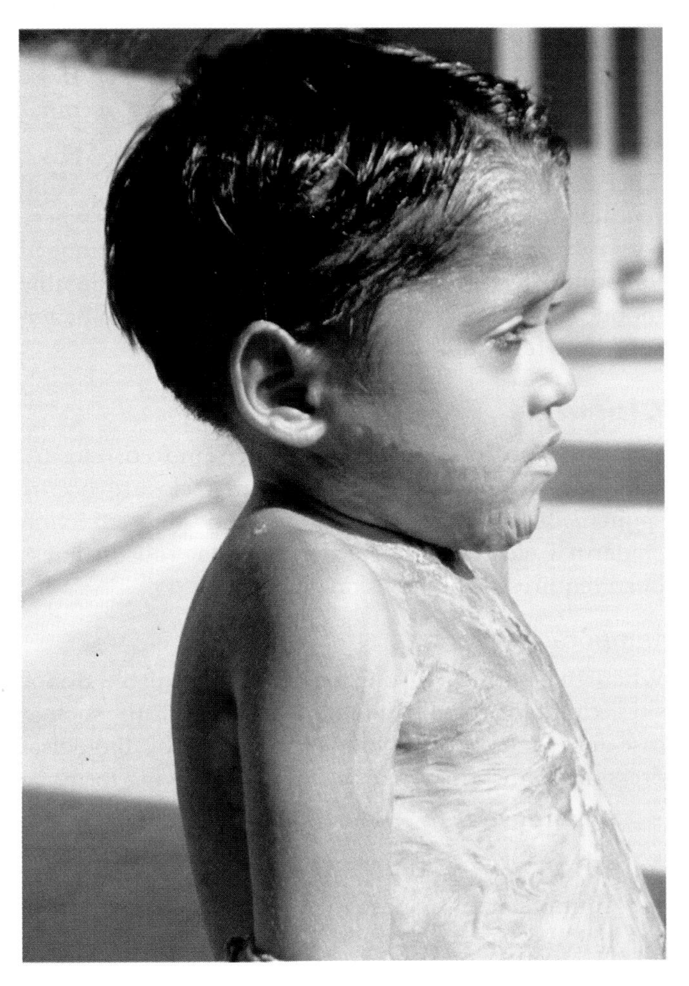

Fig.4.3 (b) After excision of contractures

idea behind these dressings was to protect the wound from bacteria, which were supposed to come from the environment.

In due course it was shown that normal skin contains up to 10 organisms/gm. of tissue (in the hair follicles and sweat glands as mentioned above). It was thus realized that not only was the main threat from within the skin, but also that occlusive dressings, by providing a warm and moist environment, actually encourage the multiplication of bacteria and pave the way for invasive infection.

Exposure treatment

To overcome this problem exposure treatment was introduced. In this method a dry eschar forms over the burn wound and acts as a physiological dressing. This prevents the access of exogenous bacteria.

However, even this exposure treatment has its limitations. As with occlusive dressings, the only organisms from which the patient is protected are the exogenous bacteria, and these are not the major offenders. At the same time the drying up of the injured cells damages them further and burn wounds treated by exposure become deeper.

Semi-open technique

Because of dissatisfaction with both open and closed methods the semi-open technique was evolved. In this method an ointment or solution containing a chemotherapeutic agent is applied to the wound surface. The three most commonly used agents are the following:

- Silver sulphadiazine cream.
- Silver nitrate solution.
- Mefenide acetate.
- Cerium nitrate also boosts cell-mediated immunity.

This is the only method by which the multiplication of endogenous bacteria can be prevented. The effectiveness of these agents can be monitored by quantitative analysis of biopsies taken from the burn wound.

Debridement

In a partial thickness burn some of the cells in the superficial layers of the skin are dead. As they separate from the deeper layers of viable cells they need to be trimmed away. This debridement is best carried out daily by the patient soaking in a tub of warm normal saline, which can be easily prepared by making a 1% solution of common salt (1% NaCl, or 10 gram/litre, is very close to 0.9%, which is isotonic saline). The eschar becomes softened and can be gently cut away.

The method is relatively painless and helps avoid repeated sessions of anesthesia. In those countries where bath tubs are not common, a series of showers arranged longitudinally over a specially designed sterilisable mobile stretcher is an excellent, and perhaps even better, substitute for a tub bath.

Closure

Once the necrotic tissue has been removed, closure can follow. In partial thickness burns closure occurs spontaneously by regeneration from the surviving epidermal elements in the dermis. The full-thickness burn requires closure by skin grafts.

Temporary coverings

When the burn is very extensive, the available donor sites cannot provide enough skin grafts. In such a case temporary closure can be achieved by biological dressings, which may take one of the following forms:

- Skin from other persons (homograft).
- Skin from animals (heterograft).
- Amniotic membranes.
- Synthetic dressings, e.g. nylon mesh with a collagen peptide coating.

These dressing are only temporary, and permanent closure with the patient's own skin (autografts) remains the goal of treatment. When skin grafting large areas priority should be given to the face, the neck, and the various flexion creases of the body.

Adjunct procedures

Physical therapy

If a burn destroys skin over the flexor aspect of a joint, skin grafting must be carried out as early as possible. As soon as the grafts have taken, movements at the joint should be encouraged, and carried out daily. For about six months splints must be worn at night to maintain anti-contracture postures during sleep.

REHABILITATION

Rehabilitation should start the moment a burn is sustained. From the beginning burned limbs are elevated and exercised to minimize the edema and reduce the need for escharotomy. The burn team should include a play therapist, who encourages children to take part in games where they are not conscious of the active exercises they are performing.

Hypertrophic scarring. This is a very troublesome sequel of a burn. Certain patients are prone to severe hypertrophic scar formation. Scar hypertrophy can be reduced by carefully fitted pressure garments over healed scars, which should be worn for about 6 months.

Psychological rehabilitation. Apart from physical measures psychological rehabilitation is of the utmost importance. Words of encouragement should be spoken throughout the patient's convalescence. If the face is disfigured by the burns, skilful plastic surgery helps greatly in physical as well as psychological rehabilitation (Fig.4.4).

COMPLICATIONS OF BURNS

The most important complications are burn wound sepsis, distant septic complications, the smoke inhalation syndrome, complications involving the gastrointestinal tract, and contractures. Marjolin's ulcer is a squamous cell carcinoma which occurs as malignant degeneration in longstanding chronic ulcers in burn scars.

Burn wound sepsis

The most important cause of death after massive burns is burn wound sepsis, when microorganisms invade subeschar tissue and bacteremia results. The burnt skin being avascular, systemic antibiotics cannot affect bacterial growth. Moreover, host resistance is very low due to reduction in the amounts of complement and gammaglobulins available, and impairment of the activity of neutrophils and monocytes. If local antibiotics are not used, rapid bacterial colonization can occur.

Creams

Until now local antibiotic creams have been applied to the surface of the burn. These have reduced the incidence of bacterial colonization of the subeschar tissue considerably, but still not sufficiently often.

Subeschar infusion

If wound biopsy shows the presence of over 10^4 organisms per gram of tissue it means that bacteria have escaped control. In such cases antibiotic solutions have recently been infused deep to the eschar. The entire daily dose, usually of carbenicillin, is dissolved in normal saline and distributed under the eschar. This practice has considerably improved the outlook in Pseudomonas septicemia, which used to be uniformly fatal. Cultures of wound, sputum, urine and blood should be obtained from all patients of major burns twice a week. The same organisms are likely to be involved in later life-threatening

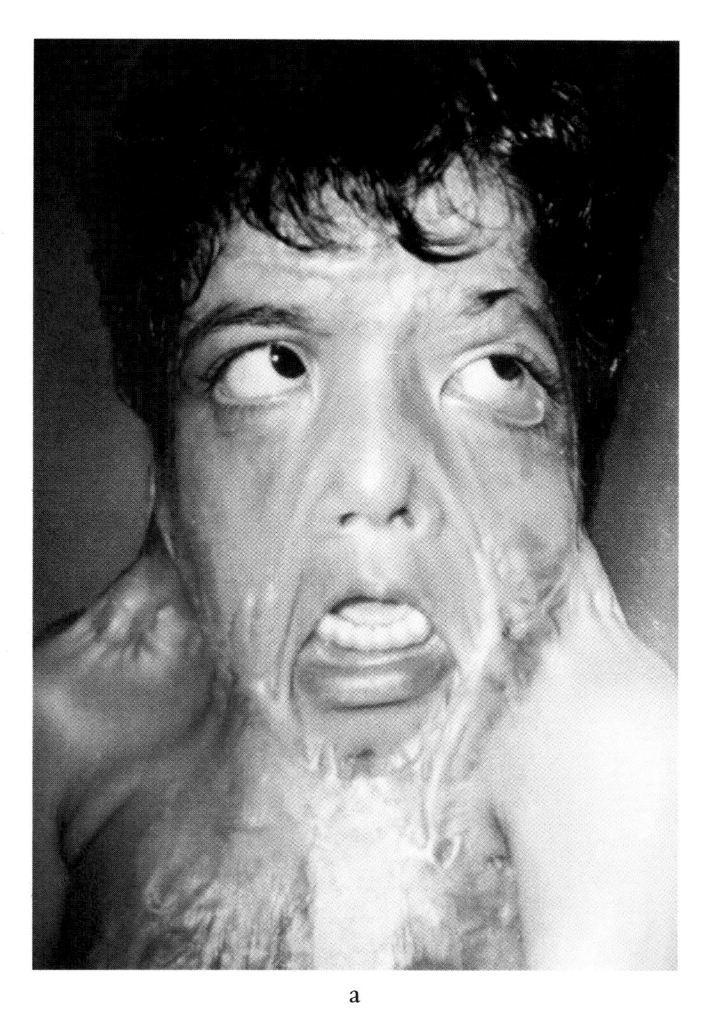

a

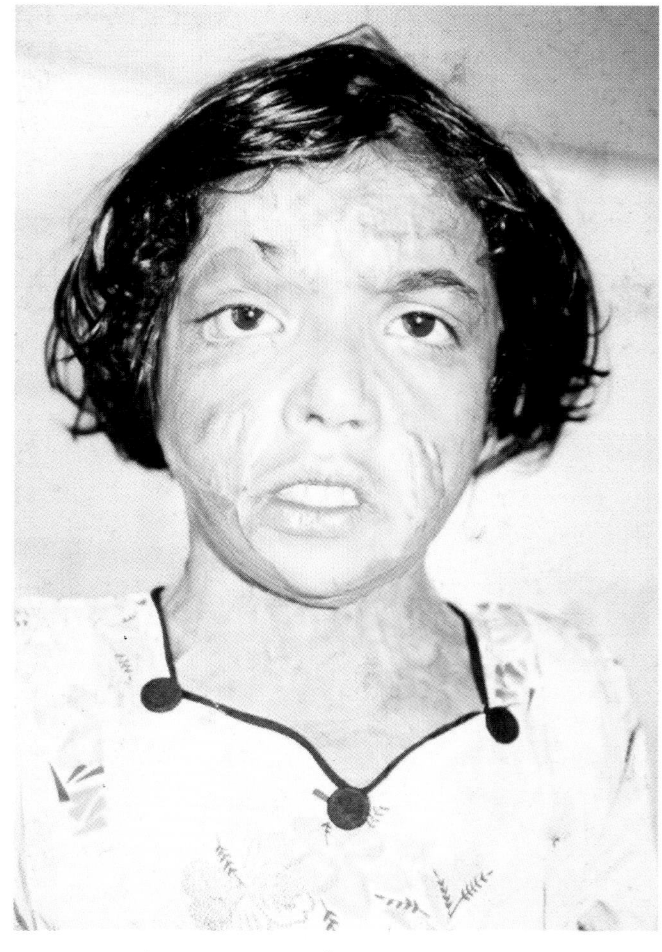

b

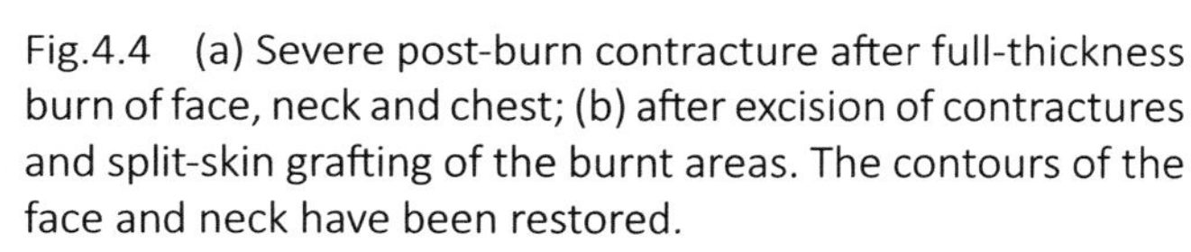

Fig.4.4 (a) Severe post-burn contracture after full-thickness burn of face, neck and chest; (b) after excision of contractures and split-skin grafting of the burnt areas. The contours of the face and neck have been restored.

infections, and selection of antibiotics is made easier by reviewing these earlier reports.

Stimulation of immune mechanisms

Recently, monoclonal antibodies have been produced against endotoxin, and they have improved the survival of patients with gram-negative bacteremia and shock.

The future

It is likely that monoclonal antibodies to cytokines will shortly prove to be effective for treating patients with life-threatening infections.

Control of infection

The following measures should be taken in this connection:

- Patients with major burns should be isolated in single rooms, which should be closed for decontamination regularly. The rooms should be ventilated with non-recirculating air exchange systems.
- Each room should be provided with its own wash-basin, and the personnel of the burns unit should wash their hands each time before handling the patient or carrying out any procedure. Chlorhexidine gluconate is probably the most effective cleaning agent for reducing the incidence of nosocomial infections.
- Patients should not return from convalescent floors to visit patients in the critical care burns unit, as they are sometimes carriers of serious nosocomial infections.

Distant sepsis

In patients with extensive burns the resistance of the host is reduced, therefore distant septic complications

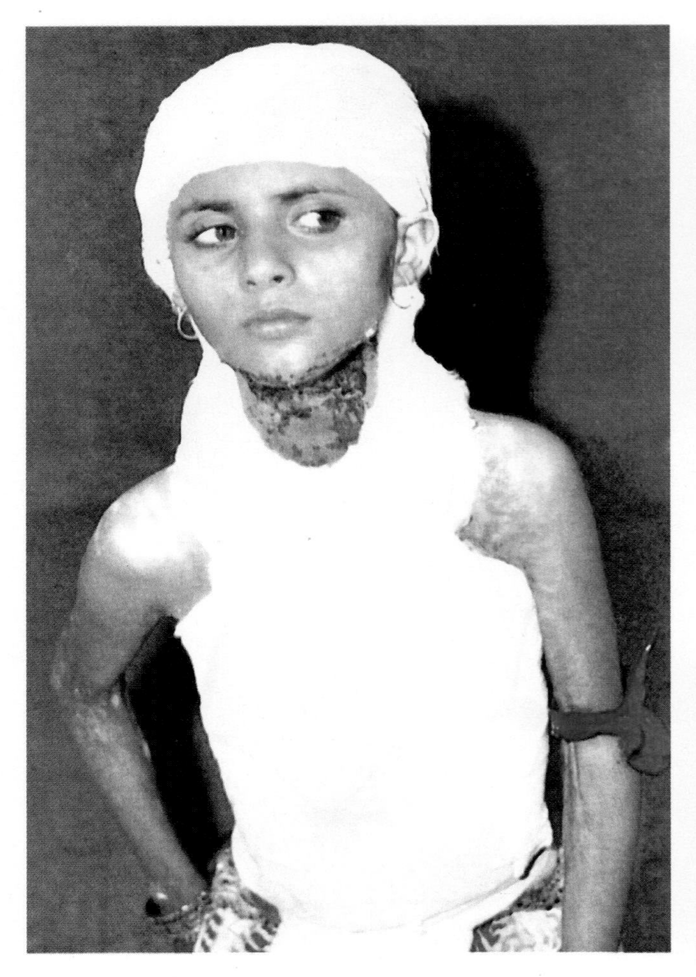

Fig.4.5 Minerva jacket for split-skin grafts applied after excision of burn contracture front of neck, to prevent recurrence of contracture.

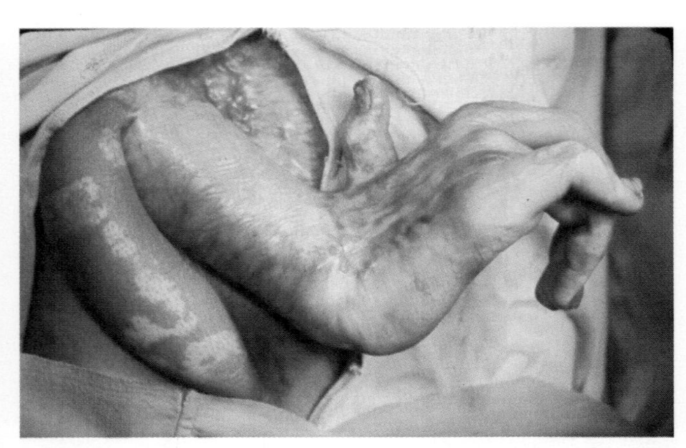

Fig.4.6 (a) Severe post-burn contracture dorsum of forearm and hand. Tubed pedicle flap from abdominal wall was attached to forearm a few weeks ago, and is ready to be spread out on the raw area after excision of the contracture.

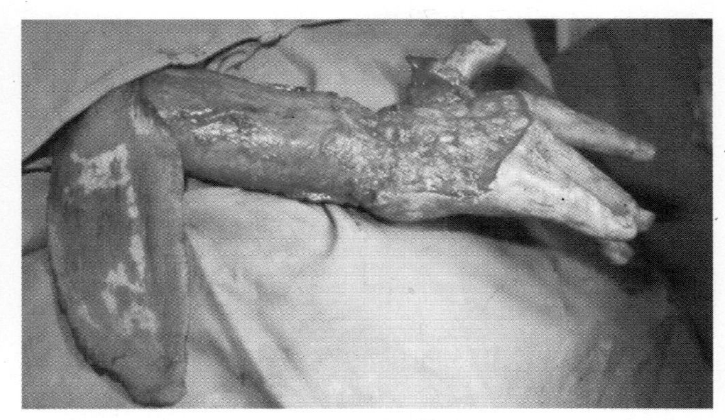

Fig.4.6 (b) The contracture has been removed, relieving the hyperextension at the wrist. Tubed pedicled flap opened out to spread it over the area.

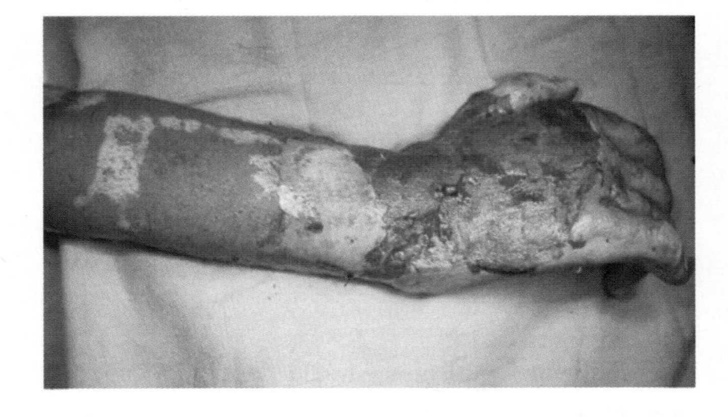

Fig.4.6 (c) The flap has taken. The contracture has been relieved.

are common. The usual sites of such complications are the lungs, the veins, and the urinary tract.

Bronchopneumonia

This is the most common complicating infection in cases of severe burns. Air infected with organisms from the burn is probably inhaled, because sputum cultures show the same organisms as have colonized the burn.

Suppurative thrombophlebitis

This occurs quite commonly in cases with massive burns. It usually follows prolonged venous cannulation. Local physical signs e.g. calf tenderness and edema may be absent, so detection is difficult. The patient may present with bacteremia of unknown origin, when blood cultures often yield staphylococci. The diagnosis may be confirmed by surgical exploration of all peripheral veins which have been cannulated. If pus is found, the entire offending vein or veins must be excised, otherwise fatal septicemia could result.

Urinary tract infections

Most patients with major burns require indwelling urinary catheters to guide fluid administration during resuscitation. Such catheters should be removed as early as possible, as with increasing duration of catheter placement the likelihood of infection increases, so that after 7 to 10 days most patients will have positive urine cultures. The causative organisms are usually the same as in the burn wound.

Smoke inhalation syndrome

If smoke is inhaled in sufficient quantities, progressive bronchospasm can develop within 24 hours, with expiratory wheezes, tachypnea and respiratory failure. Bronchopneumonia often develops due to bacterial growth distal to the occluding plugs of mucus. X-ray changes are seen only 72 hours after the injury.

Treatment

This includes rapid fluid resuscitation, performance of escharotomies over the chest, and monitoring of respiratory function. Humidified air and oxygen should be provided as required. If respiratory failure threatens, an endotracheal tube should be passed and mechanical ventilation carried out. Antibiotics are given parentally. The routine use of steroids should be avoided, as they result in higher morbidity and mortality.

Gastrointestinal complications

These include Curling's ulcer, acute cholecystitis, acute pancreatitis, and superior mesenteric artery syndrome.

Curling's ulcer

(Stress ulceration of the stomach and duodenum)

Mucosal erosions are seen in over three-fourths of patients with burns of over 35% of the body surface, and one-fifth of these progress to frank gastric or duodenal ulcers. Keeping the pH above 5, H_2 blockers have proved effective in preventing these lesions.

Acute pancreatitis

This is seen in one-third of the patients in critical care burns units. Treatment consists of supportive measures, nasogastric suction and parenteral nutrition.

Acute cholecystitis

This may be seen from time to time, either due to hematogenous spread from a primary focus in the septic patient, or in patients with marked dehydration, ileus or pancreatitis. Physical examination is difficult and ultrasound or CT examination should be employed. Once the diagnosis is made, cholecystectomy is indicated to avoid perforation of the gallbladder. In an unstable critically ill patient tube cholecystostomy may be carried out.

Superior mesenteric artery syndrome

This has been described above as one of the manifestations of advanced malnutrition.

Contractures

If a large area of skin is burned near a flexion crease and is left untreated, the fibrous tissue formed during healing pulls the surrounding skin inwards to produce a contracture which bends and fixes the neighbouring joint towards it and produces a contracture (Figs.4.3 to 4.6).

Marjolin's ulcer

Marjolin noted that chronic ulcers in old burn scars often resulted in malignant degeneration, commonly in the form of a squamous cell carcinoma but occasionally as a basal cell carcinoma. Therefore, malignant degeneration should be suspected in any healed burn scar which exhibits chronic breakdown. If biopsy shows malignancy, wide excision should be carried out. If cancer is not present, an unstable burn scar should be excised and resurfaced.

Skin grafts

Introduction

If an area of skin is lost in such a way that it cannot be closed primarily, the defect has to be filled in by skin brought from the outside in the form of a graft. If this is not done, two problems arise:

- The raw area takes a very long time to heal, with infection and a purulent discharge continuing in the meantime.
- Especially if the area of skin loss lies over a joint, a contracture results. This produces an unsightly deformity, and at the same time limits joint motion, sometimes resulting in considerable disability. It can also cause cosmetic issues, especially over the face and the hands.

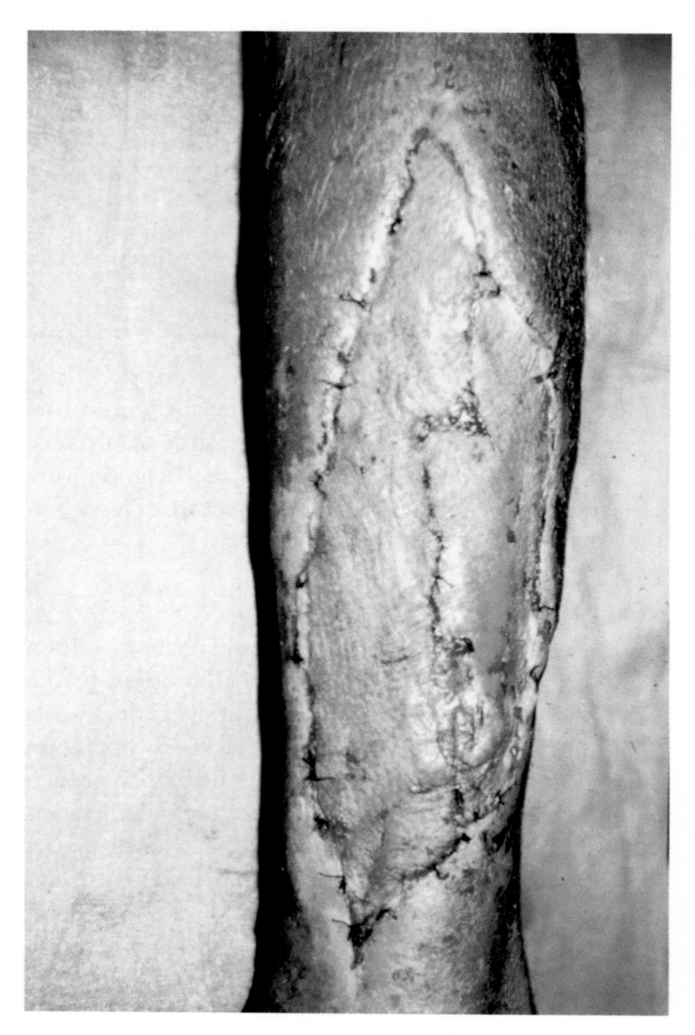

Fig.4.7 Split skin grafts over a burnt area have been followed by a 100% take. A few stitches remain to be removed.

The skin defect can be filled either by skin grafts or flaps.

- A skin graft is a segment of skin which has been totally separated from its normal bed (donor site) and is transferred to a new area (recipient site).
- A skin flap is a segment of skin and subcutaneous tissue which is transferred from its original position to another site while maintaining its own blood supply through a 'pedicle' or, (as in a 'free flap'), the pedicle is anastomosed with blood vessels at the recipient site.

Sources of grafts

- An *autograft* is a graft transplanted from one area to another in the same individual.
- A *homograft* (or/allograft) is transplanted from one individual to another in the same species.
- A *heterograft* (or xenograft) is transplanted from one individual to another of a different species.

Thickness of grafts

On the basis of thickness, skin grafts are divided into two types:

- Partial thickness (split skin) grafts (Fig.4.7)
- Full thickness grafts.

Partial-thickness grafts

These are commonly taken from the outer side of the thigh. They may be cut thin, medium or thick.

The thicker grafts have the following characteristics:

- They look better.
- They contract less.
- However, their chances of survival are less than those of the thinner grafts, because they have more cells to be nourished before a blood supply is established.

When partial-thickness grafts are taken, the deeper layers of skin are left behind, and the donor area heals spontaneously within about a fortnight. Therefore even very large skin defects can be covered by this method, and partial-thickness grafting is the standard method for resurfacing extensive burns.

Full-thickness grafts

These grafts give the best color match, the most padding, and the least contraction. However, they can survive only over very vascular recipient sites. Further, the donor sites cannot heal spontaneously, because the whole thickness of skin has been removed. Therefore only relatively small-sized grafts can be taken, so that the resultant skin defect can be dealt with by primary closure. For example, if a small skin tumor is removed from the face and a skin defect results, an elliptical segment of skin can be taken from the retroauricular or supraclavicular regions to repair it (Fig 5, chapter 50).

Composite grafts

A composite graft is a graft containing more than one tissue detached from its original site and applied to the recipient site, from where it takes its nourishment.

Example. Due to trauma, or after removal of a small skin tumor, there may be loss of an ala of the nose. The ideal tissue for replacement of the defect is a piece of cartilage covered on both sides with skin. This can be obtained by excising a triangular segment from the middle of the margin of the pinna. This contains two layers of skin with cartilage in between. The defect in the helix can be closed by direct suture using fine suture materials. Such a transplant is an example of a composite graft.

'Take of a graft'

The success of skin grafting, or 'take', depends on the ability of the graft to receive nutrients and, subsequently, on vascular ingrowth from the recipient bed.

The phases of revascularization

Skin graft revascularization, or 'take', occurs in three phases:

Serum imbibition

The first phase involves a process which lasts for 24 to 48 hours, and in which the graft imbibes serum. Absorption of nutrients into the graft occurs by capillary action from the recipient bed. This prevents the graft from drying up and also provides some nutrition. Initially, a fibrin layer forms when the graft is placed on the recipient bed, binding the graft to the bed.

Inosculation

[*inosculate*: to unite tubes; to make continuous]

The second phase is an inosculatory phase in which recipient and donor end capillaries are aligned for joining up. At the end of 48 hours, a fine vascular network is established in the fibrin layer between the graft and its recipient bed. Capillary buds from the blood vessels in the recipient bed make contact with the graft vessels.

Revascularization

In the third phase, these "kissing" capillaries open up to each other, the graft is revascularized and becomes pink.

To optimize the take of a skin graft, the recipient site must be prepared. Skin grafts require a bed with adequate blood supply; they do not take on exposed bone, cartilage, or tendon.

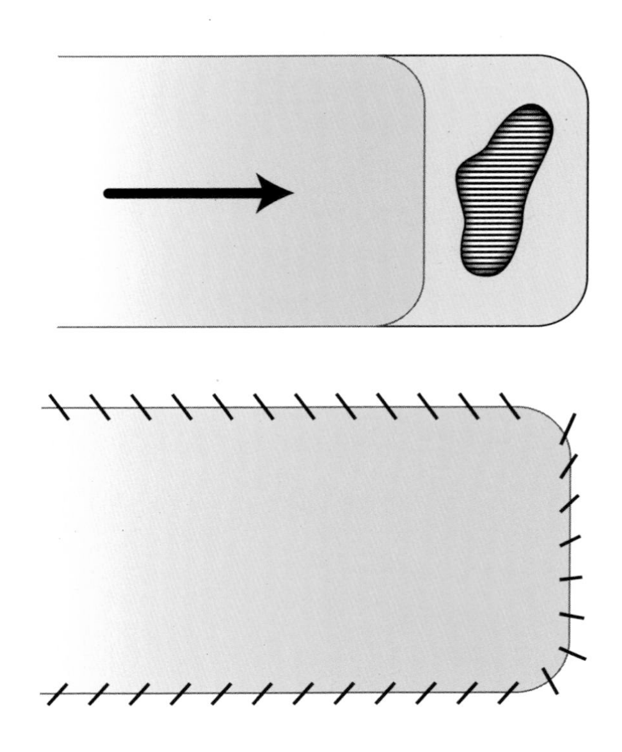

Fig.4.8 Advancement flap. A quadrangular area is excised around the lesion. The skin flap on the left advances to the right to fill the defect.

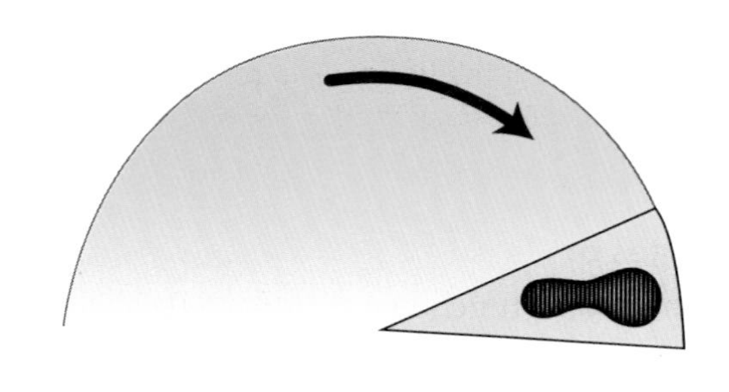

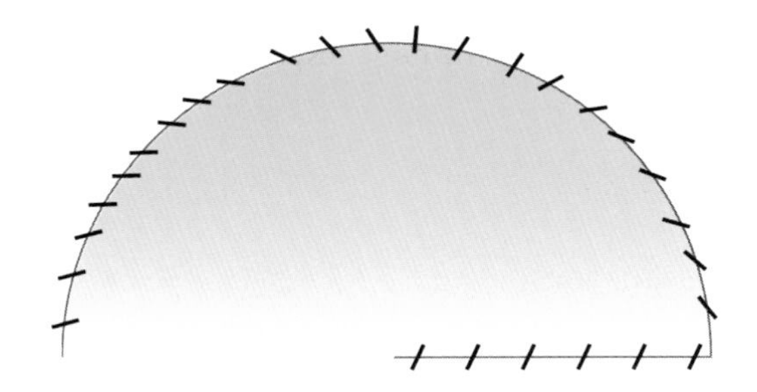

Fig.4.9 Rotation flap. After excision of the sectoral area around the lesion, the large semi-circular flap stretches and rotates into the defect.

Skin flaps

As mentioned above, a skin flap is a segment of skin and subcutaneous tissue which is transferred from its original position to another site while maintaining its own blood supply through a 'pedicle' or, (as in a 'free flap'), the pedicle is anastomosed with blood vessels at the recipient site.

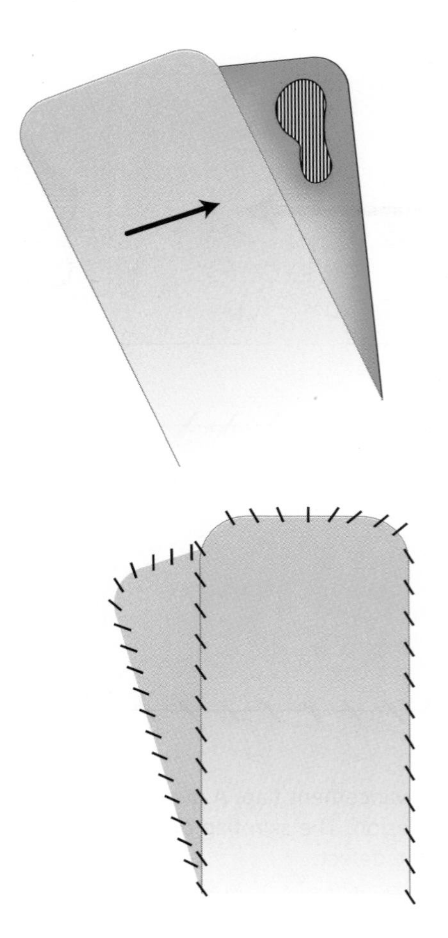

Fig.4.10 Transposition flap. After excision of a triangular area around the lesion, a large quadrangular area of skin moves sideways to fill the defect. The resulting raw area on the left has been split-skin grafted.

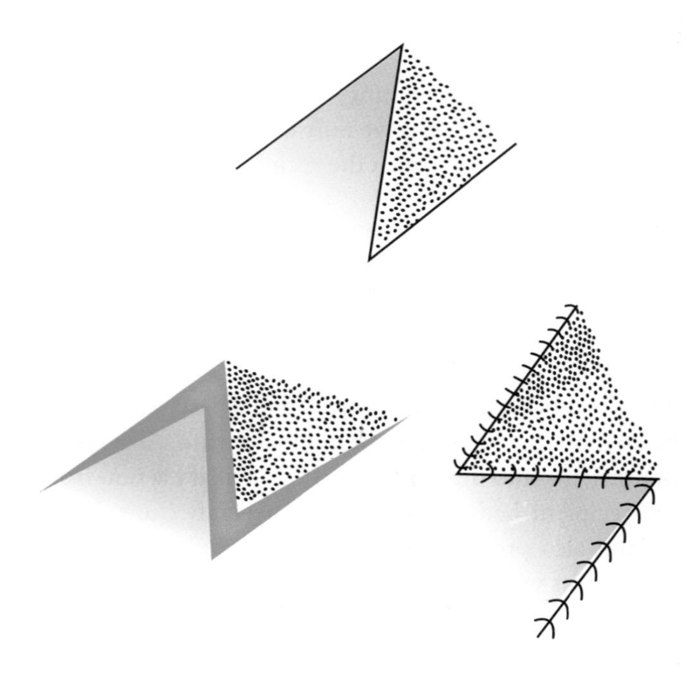

Fig.4.11 Z-plasty. a. A Z-shaped line is marked on the skin in such a manner that the line requiring lengthening becomes the middle limb of the Z. b. Incisions have been made along the lines marked out. c. The shaded triangle has been rotated to the left, the unshaded to the right; the distance between the extreme ends of the Z has been increased.

Advantages of flaps

The cosmetic and functional results of flaps are better than those of skin grafts:

- The original colour and texture of the skin is maintained.
- Hair growth, sweating and sensation are at least partly preserved.
- The flaps are more durable, especially over.
- pressure points.

Indications for uses of flaps

Reconstruction by a flap may be required in any of the following situations:

- If the recipient area lacks the vascularity required to support a skin graft.
- If padding is required over a bony prominence.
- If further surgery will be required beneath the reconstructed area.

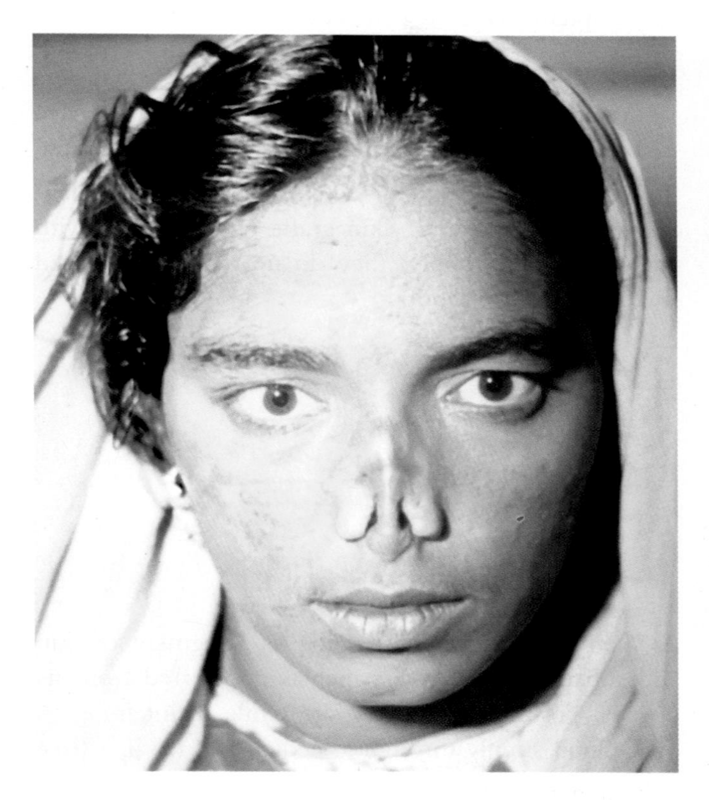

Fig.4.12 Nose cut for alleged adultery

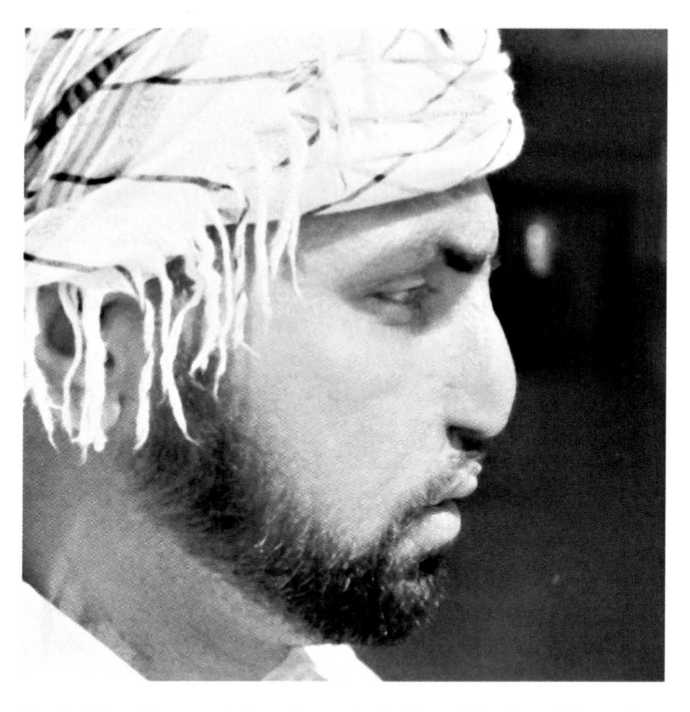

Fig.4.13 Nose cut for alleged adultery. Final position after forehead flap rhinoplasty. The patient was able to go back to his job as a school teacher.

- If a good aesthetic result will be achieved by a skin flap.

Causes of failure of skin flaps

If a skin flap fails it is commonly due to an error of technique. Some examples follow:

- Suturing a flap under tension may cause necrosis by interfering with the venous or arterial flow.
- Pressure on the flap by a tight constricting dressing may similarly compromise the circulation.
- If hemostasis is imperfect, a hematoma may form and cause considerable damage to the flap.
- Infection is not common, but can severely damage a flap when it does occur. In flaps with a poor blood supply the organisms are mostly anaerobic. With well-vascularized flaps, infection is usually due to the beta-hemolytic streptococcus.

Classification of skin flaps

Skin flaps may be classified as follows:

- Arterial pattern flaps.
- Random pattern flaps:
    - o Local flaps:

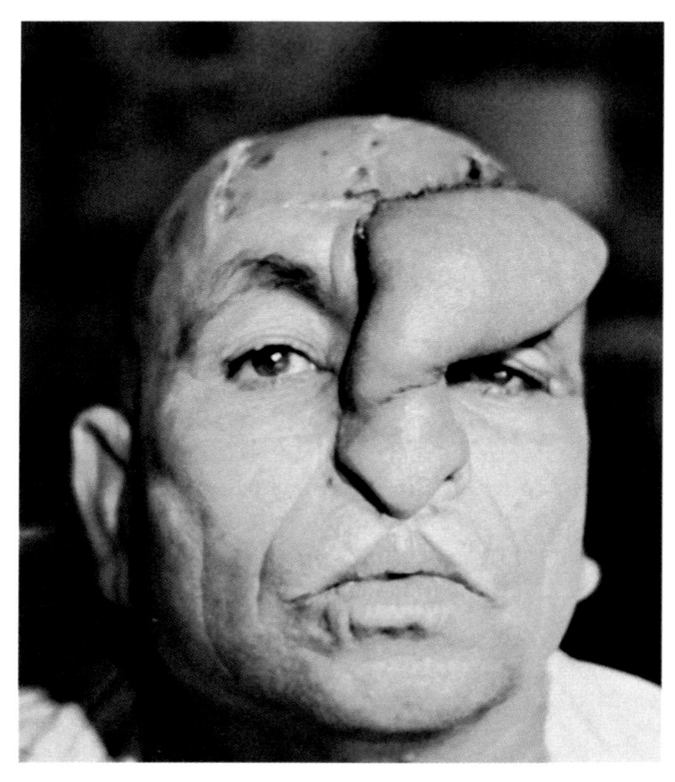

Fig.4.14 (a) Nose cut for alleged adultery. Scalping flap from anterior part of scalp attached to nose. Partial thickness grafts on raw area of scalp have taken.

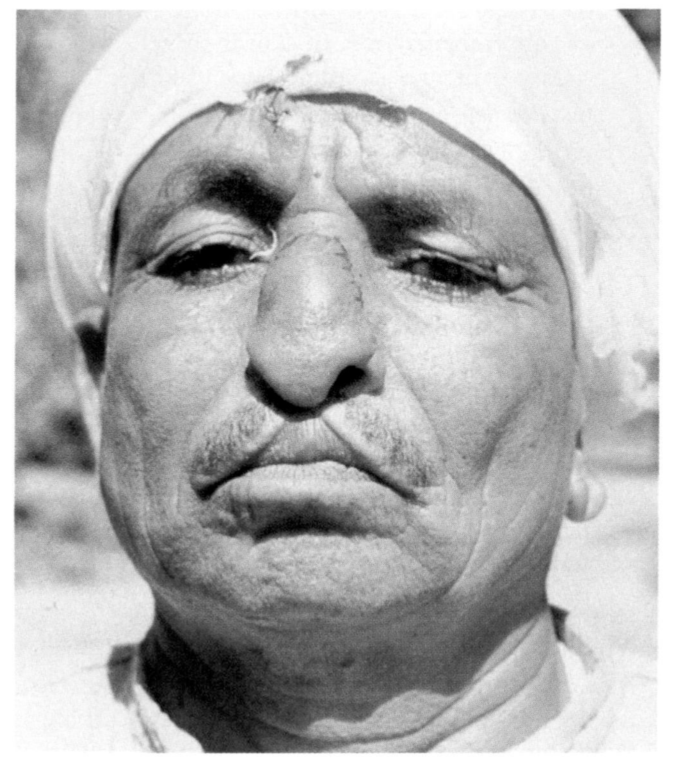

Fig.4.14 (b) Final position. The pedicle has been divided and the basal part of the flap returned to the scalp.

        - Advancement flap.
        - Rotation flap.
        - Transposition flap.
        - Z-plasty.
    - Flaps from a distance, e.g. tubed pedicle flap.
- Myocutaneous flaps.
- Free flaps.

Arterial pattern flaps

An arterial pattern flap carries with it a cutaneous artery which enters its base and runs longitudinally within the flap. Such a flap can be fairly long because of its feeding artery. One example is the long flap of the forehead containing the anterior branch of the temporal artery, the *'scalping' flap* (Figs. 4.13 and 14), used for a nose cut for alleged adultery (Fig.4.12).

Random pattern flaps

These flaps lack an anatomically recognized artery. Therefore there are strict limitations on their length, which should usually not be more than twice their width, otherwise blood supply in the distal part may be insufficient, leading to necrosis of that part. These flaps may take the following forms:

- *Local flaps.*
    - *Advancement flaps*: In this variety of local flap a quadrangular area of skin is stretched forwards to cover an adjacent defect (Fig.4.8).
    - *Rotation flaps*. Here, a semicircular segment of skin rotates and stretches to fill a defect (Fig.4.9).
    - *Transposition flaps*. In this type, a quadrangular piece of skin hinges laterally to resurface an adjoining area (Fig.4.10, 16).
    - *Z-plasty*. In this technique two triangular skin flaps are interchanged in position to gain length along a scar at the expense of adjacent tissues. This method enables a surgeon to lengthen a contracted scar or to treat a web contracture (Fig.4.11).
- *Flaps from a distance.* Examples of such flaps include an arm flap which is brought directly to the nose. When a flap is brought over a distance e.g. from the abdominal wall to the hand, its pedicle is usually 'tubed'. It is therefore called a tubed pedicle flap (Fig.4.6).

Myocutaneous flaps

At many sites in the body, a muscle can be elevated with its longitudinal segmental blood supply, carrying its overlying skin with it. Such a flap is called a myocutaneous flap. It helps not only in providing good full-thickness skin for resurfacing a defect, but also in filling irregular defects of body contour. An example of such a flap is the use of the latissimus dorsi muscle during the operation of mammoplasty following a mastectomy for breast cancer.

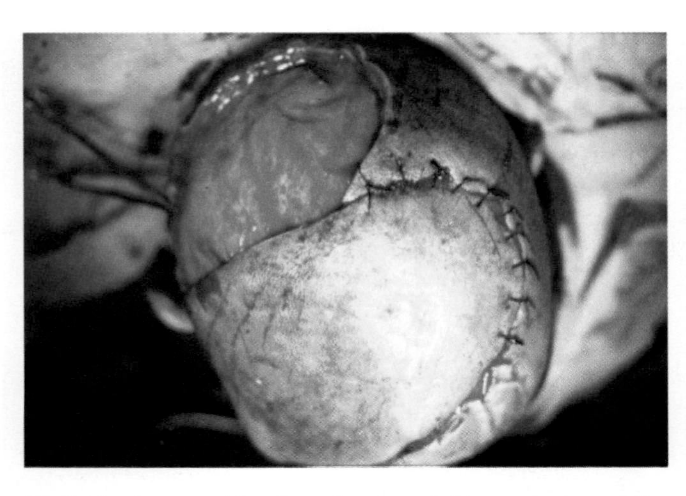

Fig.4.15 Transposition flap. An area of skin on the top of the skull had been lost in a burn. A transposition flap has been brought forwards from behind and stitched in place, to shift hair-bearing area to front of scalp. The raw area left behind was split-skin grafted during the same operation.

Free flaps

The use of extremely fine instruments and suture materials, with the help of magnification *(microvascular techniques)*, has enabled anastomoses of arteries and veins of less than 1mm diameter to be carried out satisfactorily. This has allowed free-flap transfers, the vessels of the graft being anastomosed to the vessels of the recipient site, with high success rates. Because a specially tailored composite mass of tissues can be transported to a distant site in just one step, these techniques have quite a wide applicability.

Microvascular operations need very lengthy operating sessions. However, sometimes they represent the only solution to a complicated reconstructive problem.

Reconstructive ladder

This is a term used to describe levels of increasingly complex surgical management of wounds. To select a method of treatment, the surgeon should first consider employing the lowest rung of the ladder, and then move upwards until a suitable technique is arrived at:

Rung 1: Healing by secondary intention.

Rung 2: Primary closure.

Rung 3: Delayed primary closure.

Rung 4: Split thickness skin graft.

Rung 5: Full thickness skin graft.

Rung 6: Random flap.

Rung 7: Arterial pattern flap.

Rung 8: Free microvascular flaps flap.

Chapter 5 SHOCK

In order to live and function every cell in the body requires that oxygen and nutrients be supplied to it, and waste products be carried away from it. Both these processes depend upon an adequate circulation of blood. Any serious interference with circulation therefore causes disordered function of all the cells in the body.

The term 'shock' has been used for two centuries to describe a progressive but gradual collapse of vital organ function after injury or surgery. Up to the 1960s shock was defined as 'decreased blood flow to vital organs'. However, during the 1970s it was found that in shock due to sepsis a high cardiac output and low peripheral resistance is present. Therefore the old definition of shock as decreased blood flow to vital organs is not valid. Shock should be defined as a state of inadequate tissue perfusion.

CLASSIFICATION OF SHOCK

Shock can be classified into five types based on the underlying cause: hypovolemic, cardiogenic, obstructive, distributive and endocrine, the last being seen only occasionally (Table 5.1).

In the first two types of shock, the problem is a falling cardiac output, which may be due to insufficient blood volume (hypovolemic shock). or inefficient working of the heart as a pump (cardiogenic shock). Obstructive shock is due to obstruction of the blood flow outside the heart.

The next three types can be grouped together as *distributive circulatory failure* i.e. a condition in which, although the cardiac function is normal or above normal, the tissues are under-perfused because of peripheral pooling of blood.

MONITORING THE PATIENT IN SHOCK

Nine primary measurements are useful in the initial assessment and follow-up of patients in shock (Table 5.2).

Table 5.1 Classification of shock

Type	Examples
Hypovolemic	Hemorrhage
	Burns
	Vomiting, diarrhea
Cardiogenic	Myocardial infarction
	Arrhythmias
	Cardiac surgery
	Pulmonary embolism
Obstructive	Cardiac tamponade
	Tension pneumothorax
	Pulmonary embolism
	Aortic stenosis
Distributive	Septic shock
	Neurogenic shock
	Anaphylactic shock
Endocrine	Hypo-and hyperthyroidism
	Adrenal insufficiency

Table 5.2 Hemodynamic and metabolic parameters in shock.

S.No.	Measurements	Average normal values
1	Arterial blood pressure	120/80mm Hg
2	Pulse rate	70 per minute
3	Central venous pressure	5 ±2cm H2O
4	Cardiac output	5.8 liters/min
5	Arterial PO2 tension	85–100mm Hg
6	Arterial PCO2	40mm Hg
7	Hemoglobin concentration	14 ±1gm/100ml
8	Urine flow	50ml/hour
9	Arterial blood lactate	5–8mg/100ml

Pulse and blood pressure

A rapid pulse and low blood pressure are cardinal signs of shock and should be carefully monitored in all seriously ill patients. Decreased blood pressure is always significant, but the pressure may be normal or nearly normal until marked depletion of vascular volume occurs. This happens because hypovolemia results in severe vasoconstriction, which reduces the capacity of the vascular bed. In such a situation the cardiac output may be low and yet the blood pressure may be maintained. In spite of these limitations, however, the level of blood pressure is a useful guide.

Pulse pressure, i.e. the difference between systolic and diastolic pressures, is related to cardiac output and normally is about 40mm Hg. If this decreases to 20, then even if systolic pressure is normal, blood flow is probably inadequate. On the other hand if the pulse pressure is near 40mm Hg, flow is likely to be adequate even though the systolic pressure is only 80 or 90mm Hg. Thus, one should be interested in finding out not only whether the systolic pressure is maintained, but also whether *pulse* pressure is adequate.

Continuous monitoring of the pulse is used in recovery rooms for seriously ill patients and for all patients after general anesthesia. It is useful to have warning devices that alert one if any arrhythmia arises.

Central venous pressure (CVP)

During critical illness the central venous pressure is an important guide to the adequacy of the circulation. The CVP reflects the volume of blood returning to the heart and the ability of both the right and left ventricles to propel it. It is therefore a good guide, during volume replacement, about the quantity of fluids to be administered. If the CVP is low, it means more fluid is required; if high, it shows that fluid should be restricted.

The ultimate aim of the circulatory system is to maintain a good cardiac output, to enable oxygen and nutrients to be carried to the different organs and tissues and for waste products to be carried away from them. Thus if cardiac output can be determined, we have the most direct evidence of the adequacy of the circulation.

Arterial blood gases and pH

An arterial oxygen tension (PaO_2) of between 85 and 100mm Hg is normal, depending upon the age of the patient. A tension below 60mm Hg indicates a marginal respiratory reserve, and an increased concentration of oxygen in the inspired air is required. The main causes of a reduced PO_2 in the arterial blood are the following:

- *Hypoventilation.*
- *Impaired diffusion.* This occurs in some disease states where the blood gas barrier is thickened. The hypoxemia resulting from this cause can be corrected by administering higher concentrations of oxygen to the patient.
- *Shunt.* This occurs when some blood reaches the arterial system without passing through ventilated portions of the lung. Examples include cases of Fallot's tetralogy. Also, a consolidated pneumonic lobe contains a perfused but completely unventilated area of lung, and acts as a shunt.

Most patients suffering from shock or sepsis hyperventilate. This has two harmful effects:

- The strenuous muscular exercise involved in hyperventilation causes exhaustion.
- The alkalosis resulting from hyperventilation shifts the oxyhemoglobin dissociation curve to the left. Thus hemoglobin does not easily give up its oxygen, and the supply of oxygen to the tissues suffers.

Hemoglobin concentration

Hemoglobin concentration is of fundamental importance in oxygen transport to the tissues. If the oxygen content of the inspired air is increased to 100%, this raises hemoglobin saturation only from 97 to 100%. On the other hand even moderate changes in hemoglobin concentration or cardiac output have a strong influence on oxygen transport. If hemoglobin concentration falls from 15gm/dl to 10gm/dl, the oxygen carrying capacity of blood is reduced by one third. If at the same time cardiac output falls to half (from 6 to 3 liters per minute) oxygen consumption will fall very markedly, from 300 to as little as 100ml per minute, which is a serious matter.

Urine flow

In hypovolemic shock cardiac output falls, renal vessels constrict, and renal blood flow diminishes. *In all patients under treatment for shock the urine flow should be measured every hour.* This should be at least 30ml per hour in an adult. However, in sepsis and trauma there is an increased osmolar load due to increased breakdown of cellular proteins; therefore a urine volume of at least 1,000ml per 24 hours is required.

Acute renal failure usually occurs as follows:

- A period of decreased rate of urine flow sets the stage for renal injury.
- Obstruction of tubules may result from precipitation of casts from concentrated urine.

Arterial blood lactate level

In shock the perfusion of tissues with blood is inadequate, and this produces a decreased tissue pO_2. The result is that the breakdown of glucose is partially arrested at the anaerobic phase, with accumulation of lactate and other ions. The raised level of lactate in the arterial blood can be estimated, *and is an indicator of the severity of shock.*

Tissue perfusion

In the past, parameters like pulse rate, blood pressure and urine output were employed for assessing the presence and severity of shock. However, all these parameters monitor the 'vital' organs whose circulation is maintained till the advanced stages of shock, while the intestine and the muscles may be underperfused, with coagulation and inflammation proceeding apace, and where reperfusion could injure these organs and produce multiple organ dysfunction.

Occult hypoperfusion

When vital signs are normal but the gut and muscles are underperfused, the condition is called occult hypoperfusion, and is manifested only by:

- Lactic acidosis.
- Reduced mixed venous oxygen saturation.

These two tests should therefore be carried out. If the situation persists for more than 12 hours, the mortality rate rises two to three times.

Mixed venous oxygen saturation

The percentage saturation of oxygen in the venous return, collected by a central line placed in the right atrium, indicates the oxygen delivery and extraction by the tissues. Normal venous oxygen saturation levels are 50 – 70 %. Levels below 50 % indicate insufficient delivery of oxygen and increased extraction by the cells, which is seen in hypovolemic and cardiogenic shock.

In contrast in septic shock, venous saturation is greater than 70% due to *disordered utilization of oxygen by the cells*. If in septic shock the venous saturation is below 70%, then the patient is not only in septic, but also in cardiogenic or hypovolemic shock, which should be dealt with by inotropes and fluids respectively.

Monitoring regional tissue perfusion

Modalities of monitoring regional tissue perfusion include:

- Near-infrared spectroscopy for pulse oximetry.
- Muscle tissue oxygen probe. Near-infrared light penetrates into *tissues* relatively well. The amount of light reflected back to the *probe* varies with the *oxygen* saturation of the tissues.
- Sublingual capnometry (for CO_2).

HYPOVOLEMIC SHOCK

This is the commonest type of shock and is caused by insufficient circulating blood volume. Its causes include:

- Hemorrhage (internal and/or external).
- Loss of fluid from the circulation due to:
  - Burns.
  - Vomiting and diarrhea (the commonest causes in children).
  - Excess urine loss due to:
    - Diabetic ketoacidosis.
    - Diabetes insipidus.

The patient has a low blood pressure (below 90mm Hg), rapid pulse (above 100), a low central venous pressure (below 3cm H_2O, and a low urine output (under 20ml per hour), with high urinary osmolality. There is usually a dramatic response to rapid volume replacement. The hematocrit is a guide to the type of fluid required. In hypovolemic shock due to pancreatitis the hematocrit may be as high as 60, due to loss of fluid leading to hemoconcentration. Plasma and physiological saline i.e. Ringer's lactate solution should be given. This has two effects:

- It restores the blood volume.
- It reduces the hematocrit and therefore the viscosity to normal.

The less viscous blood passes through the capillaries more easily, so that the cardiac output, urine flow and blood pressure are all increased. At the same time the pulse rate falls towards normal.

On the other hand the patient in shock with a bleeding duodenal ulcer who has a very low hematocrit, e.g. 20, will require blood.

The peripheral vessels are severely constricted in hypovolemic shock. This is best dealt with by volume replacement. Vasodilator drugs should not be used, because the little blood that is available will be pooled in the dilated vessels, reducing the venous return and cardiac output even further.

Response to hypovolemia

The response of the body to hypovolemia may be considered under three headings, namely cardiovascular, endocrine and metabolic responses.

Cardiovascular responses

A fall in blood pressure acts through the stretch receptors in the carotid sinus and the aortic arch. The sympathetic nervous system is reflexly stimulated. This increases the peripheral resistance by arteriolar constriction, and raises the cardiac output by increasing the rate and force of cardiac contraction. At the same time the *effective* blood volume is increased by enhanced vasomotor tone in the veins, which squeezes blood from the large venous reservoirs into the great veins. Thus blood is diverted from the extremities, bowel and kidneys to more vital areas of the heart and brain, the vessels of which constrict little even under intense sympathetic stimulation. When capillary pressure falls there is a net movement of extracellular fluid into the capillary, restoring plasma volume. This is seen after moderate blood loss (up to 1500ml).

Endocrine responses

Catecholamines

An acute reduction of blood volume stimulates the production of *epinephrine* and *norepinephrine* from the adrenal medulla and nerve endings. Some other conditions simulating release of these hormones include acidosis, sepsis and prolonged low-flow states. These catecholamines increase the rate and force of cardiac contraction and dilate the arteries in the myocardium and skeletal muscles. At the same time they constrict the arteries in the skin, kidneys and viscera. They also stimulate the production of glucagon and inhibit the production and peripheral action of insulin.

Antidiuretic hormone and aldosterone

Hypotension results in increased firing by baroreceptors, which causes increased secretion of *antidiuretic hormone* by the posterior pituitary. This hormone helps restore plasma volume by retention of water. Diminished renal blood flow activates the renin-angiotensin system, which promotes the elaboration of *aldosterone*; this hormone also helps preserve plasma volume by retention of salt.

Maximal cardiovascular and endocrine responses occur when the effective circulating volume has been decreased by 30 to 40%. Further reduction in the circulating volume cannot be adequately handled by compensatory mechanisms, and shock follows.

Metabolic responses

In the shock state catecholamines enhance glycogen and protein breakdown but are ineffective in stimulating the breakdown of fats (lipolysis). With the decreased availability of fat as fuel, the body becomes dependent on the oxidation of carbohydrate reserves, and increased formation and deamination of amino acids are characteristic of the shock state. In shock the rate of urea production is elevated, indicating faster protein breakdown. Skeletal muscle is the major tissue supplying amino acids as fuel.

Viscosity

When flow rates are slow as in shock, the viscosity of normal blood in small vessels can itself be a factor impairing tissue perfusion. Anything that decreases the hematocrit and fibrinogen concentration will decrease viscosity and improve perfusion. For this purpose low molecular weight dextran can be used, but equally effective are those fluids that simply decrease hematocrit and fibrinogen concentration, e.g. saline or Ringer's lactate.

Treatment of hypovolemic shock

The nine parameters listed in (Table 5.2) should be measured at the outset, and the response to therapy observed. Two peripheral lines are employed, using short wide-bore cannulas of size 14 or 16, for rapid fluid administration. If prompt infusion of the appropriate fluids restores the parameters to normal the problem is under good initial control. A central venous line is not required, but may be used subsequently for monitoring the central venous pressure.

Failure to achieve hemodynamic and metabolic stability promptly is dangerous. The chronic low-flow state promotes vital organ failure of the kidneys, liver and heart. In the hypovolemia of trauma crystalloids must be used in addition to blood. There are two reasons for this:

- Fluid is lost into the injured or operated area, which must be replaced.
- It is desirable to reduce the hematocrit and fibrinogen concentration in small vessels to decrease viscosity and promote flow in the vessels. In the low-flow state better oxygen transport is achieved if the blood is less viscous, e.g. with a hematocrit of 30% rather than 50%.

Blood pressure

Arterial pressure is a guide to therapy. The blood volume must be reduced by 15 to 25% before systolic pressure falls below 80 to 90mm Hg. If a patient is alert, has a normal ECG, and a urine flow of 50ml per hour, the systolic pressure is probably adequate even if it is only 80mm Hg.

Pulse pressure

The pulse pressure is helpful as a guide to volume replacement. In shock a higher diastolic pressure is usually seen due to severe arteriolar vasoconstriction. Thus a blood pressure of 80/40mm Hg is preferable to one of 120/100.

Composition of fluid

The best fluid to start on all patients in shock or with trauma is *Ringer's lactate.* Equally effective is 5% glucose in normal saline with 2 ampoules (90 meq) of sodium bicarbonate added to each liter to buffer the solution to pH 7.4. The reason why Ringer's lactate is best is that it closely resembles tissue fluid in composition. During trauma tissue fluid is lost and therefore Ringer's lactate is its best replacement. Recent work has shown, however, that it is the volume and speed of replacement that determines outcome more than the type of fluid. Further, that a liter of a hypertonic solution is desirable as the initial infusion because, apart from providing fluid, it draws fluid from the tissues into the vessels.

If hypovolemic shock is due to hemorrhage, transfusion of *blood* is carried out, using the appropriate number of units of blood. When massive transfusion is required, blood should always be warmed. At the same time clotting factors should be replaced continuously. In conditions in which there is excessive loss of plasma proteins, as in acute pancreatitis, peritonitis or burns, the use of plasma, or electrolyte solutions to which albumin has been added, is of great value.

The difficulty of achieving a balance between under-transfusion and over-transfusion should not be underestimated, even with all monitoring facilities. It should be remembered that prolonged hypoperfusion carries the risk of organ tissue damage, whereas if supervision is close, fluid overload can be reversed with diuretics or hemofiltration.

Ventilation

All patients in shock should receive oxygen by mask. Respiratory failure may require further measures, e.g. ventilation.

Diuretics

If hypovolemia has been corrected but oliguria (a urine flow of less than 20ml per hour) persists, the use of diuretics should be considered. Urine output should be monitored hourly with an indwelling catheter.

Mannitol

The diuretic in common use in hypovolemic shock is mannitol. This is an osmotic diuretic. It produces diuresis because it is filtered by the glomerulus but not reabsorbed by the renal tubules, thus obligating the excretion of water. At the same time its administration results in an increase in intravascular volume. Therefore, if a diuretic has to be used in a patient recovering from hypovolemic shock, it should be mannitol. It is given as 25gm in 250ml of 5% glucose in water over a period of 25 minutes. If there is a good response the dose may be repeated.

Vasodilators

If pre-load and contractility have been optimized but cardiac output still remains inadequate, reduction of ventricular after-load may be useful. This is achieved by the use of vasodilators.

Sodium nitroprusside acts directly on arterioles and to some extent veins. It produces a fall in the peripheral resistance and venous return, thus reducing ventricular pre-load.

Nitroglycerine acts directly and causes predominant venous dilatation, thus reducing pre-load. It also reduces after-load by relaxing arteriolar smooth muscle.

Hydralazine given by i.v. bolus in a dose of 10–20mg may be used to reduce after-load.

Acid-base correction

The best way to correct metabolic acidosis in shock is by restoring adequate tissue perfusion, by fully restoring the circulating volume. However, sodium bicarbonate may be required in addition. The dose may be roughly determined by the following method:

- Multiply the body weight (in kg) by 0.2, to obtain the volume of extracellular fluid.
- Now find out the deficit of sodium bicarbonate in each liter. This value is obtained by subtracting the level in the patient's serum from the normal level, (i.e. 27 meq/l minus the value of sodium bicarbonate in meq/l in the patient's serum).
- Now multiply the deficit in meq/l with the number of liters in the extracellular fluid. In other words multiply 1. with 2. Thus:

Dosage of sodium bicarbonate required, in meq = 0.2 x body weight x (27 minus sod. bicarb.in meq in the patient's serum).

In low-flow states the ability to buffer the acidity in banked blood is reduced, so when rapid massive transfusions are required, an ampoule (45 meq) of sodium bicarbonate should be given with every two units of blood.

CARDIOGENIC SHOCK

Cardiogenic shock is caused by the failure of the heart to pump effectively. This can be due to:

- Myocardial infarction, due to damage to the heart muscle.
- Dysrhythmias.
- Cardiomyopathy/myocarditis.
- Congestive heart failure.
- Cardiac valve problems.

The blood lactic acid level is raised.

The important hemodynamic abnormalities in cardiogenic shock include:

- Low systolic blood pressure (80mm Hg or less).
- Low cardiac output (2.0 liters per minute per square meter).
- Normal or raised peripheral vascular resistance.

Clinical features

The initial clinical evaluation of cardiogenic circulatory failure should determine the nature of the failure, the underlying cause and the severity of the problem. A full clinical history should be taken and physical examination carried out to detect ischemic, valvular or congenital heart disease, or hypertension.

Investigations

An *ECG* will identify acute myocardial infarction, left ventricular hypertrophy, heart block or arrhythmias.

Chest x-ray is required for the assessment of heart size, pulmonary markings and pleural effusion.

If pulmonary edema or cardiogenic shock is present, treatment should begin immediately. If there is less urgency, an *echocardiogram* provides information about the size, thickness and performance of the heart.

Treatment

The treatment of cardiogenic shock consists of the following:

- Improvement of *myocardial contractility* by inotropic drugs. (e.g. dopamine 0.5 to 5mg/kg/min).
- The reduction of cardiac *preload* by diuretics. (e.g. furosemide 10 to 100mg intravenously).
- The reduction of *afterload* by vasodilators. (e.g. sodium nitroprusside infusion of 10 to 15mg/min, increasing by 10mg/min every 5 to 15 minutes).

The success or failure of therapy should be measured against clear endpoints, such as doubling of cardiac output, or a 25% reduction in pulmonary artery occlusion pressure.

Monitoring

The ECG, arterial pressure, cardiac output, and pulmonary artery occlusion pressure should be monitored throughout the period of therapy. An arterial catheter is essential for monitoring patients receiving vasodilator or inotropic therapy, particularly when the blood pressure is labile.

OBSTRUCTIVE SHOCK

Obstructive shock is due to obstruction of blood flow outside of the heart. Examples include:

- *Cardiac tamponade*, in which venous return is impaired:
    - o In *pericardial effusion,* due to excess fluid in the pericardium.
    - o In *constrictive pericarditis*, due to a hardened and shrunken pericardium.
- *Tension pneumothorax*; through increased intrathoracic pressure, venous return being impaired.
- *Pulmonary embolism*, due to a thromboembolic incident in the blood vessels of the lungs, hinders venous return.
- *Aortic stenosis* hinders circulation by obstructing the ventricular outflow tract.

DISTRIBUTIVE CIRCULATORY FAILURE

The next three forms of shock, namely septic, neurogenic and anaphylactic shock, can be grouped together under the heading of 'distributive circulatory failure.' In each of these types, the pre-capillary smooth muscle sphincters in the skin and splanchnic circulation undergo relaxation, resulting in a marked increase in the capacity of the vascular bed in these organs. Diversion of blood supply to these non-essential organs results in insufficient oxygen delivery to the vital organs, and shock results.

SEPTIC SHOCK

This is the most common cause of distributive shock, and is caused by an overwhelming systemic infection resulting in vasodilation and leading to hypotension. Common conditions resulting in septic shock include peritonitis and major burns. Septic shock can be caused by:

- Gram negative bacteria such as *Escherichia coli*, Proteus species and *Klebsiella pneumoniae* which release an endotoxin which produces adverse biochemical and immunologic effects which are harmful to the body.
- Gram-positive cocci, such as pneumococci and streptococci, Gram-positive bacteria, and certain fungi.

In septic shock the cardiac output is adequate but blood is distributed improperly to different parts of the body. This is due mainly to excessive vasodilatation in the peripheral vascular system, including the skin and splanchnic bed. This is brought about as follows: with the lysis of white cells, mediators like cytokines are liberated in the form of a cascade. These produce relaxation of pre-capillary sphincters in the skin and splanchnic circulation, diverting blood supply to non-essential organs, and resulting in insufficient oxygen delivery to the vital organs.

Sepsis syndrome

The sepsis syndrome, and associated multiple organ dysfunction syndrome, is the most common cause of death in patients in critical care units. The cardiac function is normal while the peripheral vascular resistance is low, therefore the cardiac output is high. But in spite of this the filling pressures are low (high output failure). At a later stage, cardiac output along with the function of other organ systems may be greatly impaired. Those patients who do not generate high cardiac outputs in the face of a septic insult have a poor prognosis.

The patient is commonly over 45 years of age, and the genitourinary and gastrointestinal tracts are the most common sites of invasion. Several factors predispose to sepsis. These include:

- Diabetes mellitus.
- Steroid therapy.
- Immunosuppressive therapy.
- Indwelling urinary or intravenous catheters.
- Excessive use of antibiotics.
- Cancer chemotherapy.
- Radiation therapy.

Clinical features

There is a hyperdynamic circulation. This is manifested by a high cardiac output, warm and dry extremities and a raised central venous pressure. As mentioned above, this is probably in an effort to supply oxygen to the deficient cells. However, in spite of this there is profound hypotension and oliguria.

Hyperventilation is especially valuable as an early sign of septic shock. After operation hyperventilation may be due to:

- Pneumonia.
- Atelectasis.
- Pulmonary embolism.
- Myocardial infarction.

But it can also be due to septic shock.

The clinical features of sepsis syndrome include the following:

- Fever > 38.5°C or < 36°C.
- Tachycardia >100/min.
- Tachypnea > 20/min.
- Hypotension< 90mm Hg systolic BP.
- Evidence of localized septic focus.

Manifestations of end-organ failure

These include:

- Metabolic acidosis, pH < 7.2.
- Arterial hypoxemia PO_2 < 10kPa.
- Increased plasma lactate.
- Oliguria < 0.5ml/kg/hour for 1 hour.
- Coagulation defect:
    - Prothrombin level 1.5 times control.
    - PTT 1.5 times control.
    - Thrombocytopenia < 80000/cu mm.
- Acute deterioration in mental status.
- Any other sign of organ system failure.

Sepsis syndrome is the pathophysiological response to systemic infection or endotoxemia. It can be produced by a wide range of organisms including Gram-positive and Gram-negative bacteria, protozoa, viruses, and fungi. In a significant number of cases an infective organism is never isolated. Endotoxemia, though not invariable, is usually present in severe sepsis syndrome with multiple organ dysfunction syndrome, and is associated with a poor prognosis.

Multiple organ dysfunction syndrome (MODS)

The intestine contains very large numbers of bacteria in its lumen, and in the normal state of health its mucous membrane acts as a barrier between these bacteria and the host circulation and tissues. Food within the lumen of the gut is the most important stimulus for mucosal growth.

When, as in cases on intravenous alimentation (usually in patients under critical care), enteral feedings are impossible or inadequate, the intestinal mucosa may atrophy. In such cases bacteria can pass across the mucosal barrier and enter the tissues and the circulation.

The presence of micro-organisms and their toxins triggers an immunological and inflammatory cascade. Complement is activated and a number of host-derived mediators released, including tumor necrosis factor, interleukins, and myocardial depressant factor.

These and other mediators are responsible for vasodilatation, hypotension, and multiple organ dysfunction syndrome (MODS). This process is more likely to take place in inflammatory bowel disease and in obstructive jaundice, where endotoxin can spill over into the circulation.

Early warning signs

These include:

- Mental status changes.
- Increased respiratory rate, pulse, temperature and white blood count.

Later:

- Hypoxia.
- Hypocarbia, and.
- X-ray findings of ARDS make their appearance.

Once this happens, the associated mortality escalates. Increasing encephalopathy accompanies progressive respiratory failure. The onset of renal failure, usually due to acute tubular necrosis, increases the mortality rate greatly. Upper gastrointestinal bleeding, bacteremia, and severe malnutrition are seen.

As the number of failing organ systems increases, the associated mortality rises. Once four organ systems are involved, the mortality is virtually 100 percent. In the final stages coagulopathies and wound breakdown develop along with hepatic failure, most patients dying of hepatic and oliguric renal failure.

Summation of effects of humoral mediators

How do so many different organ systems fail together? It is probable that MODS is a summation of the effects of a large number of different humoral mediators, which are all triggered by uncontrolled infection:

- Prostaglandins, kinins, serotonin and histamine mediate vasodilatation.
- Corticosteroids and norepinephrine cause hypermetabolism.
- Oxygen free radicals produce membrane damage.
- Tumor necrosis factor causes tissue injury and shock.
- Interleukin-1 produces protein breakdown and fever.
- Thyroid and growth hormones produce acute catabolism.
- Complement is responsible for damage to the microcirculation.

Bacterial translocation

Many patients succumbing to MODS show no evidence of a septic focus anywhere in the body. In these it is felt that the microorganisms enter the circulation by migrating across the gut mucosal barrier, begin the septic cascade and perpetuate MODS. This transmigration of living bacteria or their endotoxins has been shown to occur in a number of conditions including hemorrhagic shock, burns, malnutrition, sepsis and jaundice.

Diagnosis

The presence of multiple organ dysfunction syndrome is clinically obvious, diagnostic criteria being as below. The greater the number of organ systems involved, the worse the prognosis:

Circulatory failure

Pulse <40/min.

Mean b.p. <50mm Hg.

Ventricular tachycardia or fibrillation.

Respiratory failure

Respiratory rate >40/min.

$Paco_2$ >50mm Hg.

PaO_2 <60mm Hg.

Hematological failure

White cell count < 1,000/cu mm.

Platelets< 20,000/cu mm.

Hematocrit < 20%

Evidence of disseminated intravascular coagulation.

Neurological

Glasgow coma score < 6

Seizures.

Gastrointestinal failure

Ileus.

Hemorrhage.

Acute renal failure

Urine output < 400ml/24 hours.

Hepatic failure

Coagulation defects.

Rising hepatic enzymes.

Rising alkaline phosphatase.

Management

Prevention

Treatment of septic shock is properly based on *prevention of the septic conditions leading to it*. Antibiotic therapy has not reduced the incidence of infection with complicating sepsis. Further, *prolonged antibiotic therapy permits the development of antibiotic resistant strains of Gram-negative bacteria* and their invasion of the bloodstream. If a prophylactic antibiotic is used, as in a patient undergoing elective surgery on the gastrointestinal tract, it should be started before the operation or not given at all. It has been shown conclusively that if an antibiotic is started after the operation it is quite ineffective in preventing infection.

The antibiotic should preferably be administered intravenously with induction of anesthesia. In lengthy operations, when blood loss is excessive, and when contamination has occurred, antibiotics may be repeated 4-hourly during surgery. There is no evidence that prolonged courses of prophylactic antibiotics given after surgery reduce the incidence of infection, and they can encourage the development of antibiotic resistance.

Catheters

Intravenous, intra-arterial and urinary catheters are frequent sources of infection and sepsis. *They should be used sparingly, and removed as soon as possible.*

Treatment

Early recognition of septic shock is important, and *hyperventilation is a particularly valuable warning sign.* Management aims at organ system support where required, suppression or amelioration of the toxic effects of the septic process, and identification and eradication of the septic focus.

Organ system support

Some forms of organ system support, such as mechanical ventilation and hemofiltration, are readily available. Others, such as the support of the brain, circulation and gastrointestinal tract, have to be approached indirectly by trying to attain supranormal levels of oxygen delivery.

Appropriate antibiotics are selected, but these will prove ineffective unless surgical drainage of the focus of infection is undertaken.

Antibiotics

These have to be given intravenously because if administered orally or intramuscularly they would not be absorbed due to inadequate tissue perfusion. Treatment is usually started with one of the aminoglycosides (gentamycin or kanamycin), but when culture and sensitivity tests are available, a less toxic but effective drug should be substituted. If the infection is by gram-positive cocci, a synthetic penicillin is used. In anaerobic infections bacteroides are frequently seen. A commonly used combination consists of 10 million units of penicillin, 4mg per Kg per day of gentamycin and 500mg 8 hourly of metronidazole. If gram-positive bacilli are present they are most likely clostridia, and penicillin only is required.

Hemodynamics

A higher than normal cardiac output is required. This may require administration of blood, saline, isoproterenol or all three.

Drainage of abscesses

Patients in whom a septic focus is drained have a very much better prognosis than those where this is not done.

Corticosteroids

This therapy is not of proven value; however it is widely used. Large doses are used (50–150mg per kg of hydrocortisone in a single bolus). The benefits are stated to be three-fold: firstly, the function of the lungs and the kidneys is improved. Secondly, steroids stabilize cellular and subcellular membranes. Thirdly, they stabilize the membranous portion of the microcirculation.

Immunotherapy

Many attempts have been made to interrupt the inflammatory cascade of sepsis. Recently, antibodies against the lipopolysaccharide part of endotoxin have been used in cases of Gram-negative sepsis, with significant reduction in overall mortality, particularly in those presenting in shock. Such immunotherapy may, in time, become the standard treatment for sepsis.

'Selective decontamination' of the gut

This has been attempted, in patients with major trauma or granulocytopenia and those receiving liver transplants, by the use of nonabsorbable antibiotics selected to decrease enteric flora. Combinations of these antibiotics include oral polymyxin, amphotericin and gentamicin with a systemic β-lactam like ceftazidime. A decrease in the incidence of nosocomial lung infections has been reported, although mortality has not been affected.

Both *selective decontamination* and *early enteral feeding* hold out hope for the future.

Some definitions

- **Systemic inflammatory response syndrome** (SIRS)

  The presence of two or more of the following:

  - Abnormal body temperature.
  - Abnormal heart rate.
  - Abnormal blood gas.
  - Abnormal white blood cell count.

- **Sepsis**

SIRS in response to an infectious process.

- **Severe sepsis**

Sepsis with sepsis-induced organ dysfunction or tissue hypoperfusion manifesting as:

  - o Hypotension
  - o Elevated lactate, or
  - o Decreased urine output.

- **Septic shock**

Severe sepsis plus persistently low blood pressure despite the administration of intravenous fluids.

NEUROGENIC SHOCK

Neurogenic shock is a type of shock which follows serious interference with the balance of vasodilator and vasoconstrictor influences to both arterioles and venules. It is seen in clinical syncope, as with sudden exposure to unpleasant events such as the sight of blood, the hearing of bad tidings, or the sudden onset of severe pain. It is also seen in paralysis of vasomotor influences, as in high spinal anesthesia.

The clinical picture in neurogenic shock is different from that seen in hypovolemic shock. Although the blood pressure can be very low, the pulse rate is usually slower than normal, and the skin is warm. Not only is the cardiac output reduced but also the resistance of the arterioles and the tone of the veins is diminished. The blood volume is normal. However, as the reservoir capacity of both arterioles and venules is greatly increased, there is a decreased venous return leading to a reduction in the cardiac output.

Treatment

If neurogenic shock is not corrected, the blood flow to the kidneys is reduced and damage to the brain results as well. Subsequently, all the harmful effects of hypovolemic shock appear.

Fortunately the treatment is simple. Shock in high spinal anesthesia can be treated by a vasopressor such as ephedrine or phenylephrine, which increases cardiac output and at the same time produces peripheral vasoconstriction.

In mild cases of neurogenic shock such as fainting, simply removing the stimulus or relieving pain will be adequate treatment, so that the vasoconstrictor nerves can regain the ability to maintain the normal resistance of arterioles and venules. At the same time, *the patient should immediately be placed in a recumbent position* to facilitate venous return and increase cardiac output.

In cases of *spinal cord transection* there may be a great deal of loss of blood and extracellular fluid into the area of injury. It may be difficult to decide about the relative need for fluid replacement and vasopressor drugs. Central venous pressure measurements are of great help in such a situation. It is better to slightly overexpand the volume than to give an excessive amount of vasopressors.

ANAPHYLACTIC SHOCK

Anaphylaxis is defined as an unusual or exaggerated reaction to a foreign protein or other substance. The antigen combines with IgE on the mast cells, releasing large amounts of histamine and slow release substance-anaphylaxis (SRS-A). These chemicals produce bronchospasm, laryngeal edema and respiratory distress. Due to the resulting massive vasodilatation and hypoxia, the patient ends up in hypotension and shock. The drug most often responsible for anaphylactic shock is penicillin. Other agents include dextrans and serum injections. The mortality is around 10%.

Treatment

The aims of treatment in severe allergic reactions are three:

- To correct arterial hypoxemia.
- To restore intravascular fluid volume.
- To inhibit further release of chemical mediators.

The administration of antigen is stopped. An adequate airway is ensured and oxygen is added to the inspired air. Adrenaline is given intravenously, intramuscularly or via the endotracheal tube: 4–8mg i.v. for hypotension, 0.5ml of 1:1000 (0.5mg) for cardiovascular collapse.

Fluids are given in sufficient quantity, both crystalloids and colloids. If there is bronchospasm, adrenaline or aminophylline are used. In cases with pulmonary edema positive pressure ventilation is provided. For inotropic action adrenaline or noradrenalin may be used in a dose of 2–4mg/minute. Acidosis may need to be corrected. It should be remembered that steroids provide no benefit in the acute phase, and antihistamines are useful only in angioneurotic edema.

ENDOCRINE SHOCK

This may have elements of hypovolemic, cardiogenic and distributive shock. It is based on endocrine disturbances such as:

- *Hypothyroidism*, due to reduced cardiac output.
- *Thyrotoxicosis,* due to a reversible cardiomyopathy.
- *Acute adrenal insufficiency*, usually the result of discontinuing corticosteroid treatment without tapering the dosage.
- *Relative adrenal insufficiency* in critically ill patients, where hormone levels are insufficient to meet the higher demands.

Chapter

6 HEMORRHAGE AND TRANSFUSION

Hemorrhage

Hemorrhage is normally a serious matter, and its control is one of the important duties of a surgeon. He should be able to detect the source of the bleeding and should know how to stop it.

Source of the hemorrhage

Hemorrhage may occur from an artery, from a vein, or from capillaries:

- If an *artery* is bleeding the blood is bright red and comes in spurts, in time with the pulse. If the bleeding continues for a long time, and especially if replacement of blood loss has been carried out with electrolyte solutions, the blood may be quite watery.
- If the blood is coming from a *vein* it is dark red, and flows steadily without spurts. The beginner might imagine that bleeding from veins ought to pose a lesser problem than hemorrhage from the high-pressure arteries. However, such is not always the case. Hemorrhage from large, and especially deep-seated, veins can tax the ingenuity of the most experienced surgeon, and therefore should not be taken lightly.
- *Capillary* hemorrhage is bright red, and may be quite a rapid ooze. In certain blood disorders it may continue for many hours, and the blood loss can become quite serious.

Hemorrhage from a wound

When a wound is sustained, either due to operation or trauma, hemorrhage may take place either immediately, after a few hours, or after a few days. Depending upon the time at which it occurs, it is classified as follows:

Primary hemorrhage

Primary hemorrhage is that which takes place at the time of the injury or operation.

Reactionary hemorrhage

This usually occurs within a few hours, and is most commonly due to slipping of a ligature or dislodgement of a clot or after the increase in blood pressure after resuscitation.

Secondary hemorrhage

This occurs usually after one to two weeks due to sloughing off of the vessel wall due to infection or pressure necrosis. Other causes of erosion of the arterial wall include pressure from a drainage tube or fragment of a bone, and infiltration by a cancer. There may be 'warning hemorrhages' in the form of bright red stains on the dressing, followed by a sudden severe hemorrhage.

Secondary hemorrhage is especially common after anorectal operations. This is due to the presence of a certain degree of infection along with moisture which causes maceration of the tissues. Hemorrhoidectomy wounds are especially prone to this complication, because they involve division and ligation of the arteries supplying the piles.

External and internal hemorrhage

Alternatively, hemorrhage can be classified as external and internal hemorrhage.

External hemorrhage

This takes place onto an external surface of the body, for example when the femoral artery is cut across. The quantity of blood lost is easy to estimate, as it is all visible.

Internal hemorrhage

This is invisible or concealed hemorrhage, as in the case of:

- Rupture of the spleen.
- Ruptured ectopic gestation.
- Fracture of the femur.

Concealed and revealed hemorrhage

In certain cases concealed hemorrhage can become revealed, as in hematemesis or melena from a peptic ulcer, or hematuria following blunt trauma to the kidney.

Clinical features of hemorrhage

When external bleeding takes place it is visible. Apart from this, the signs and symptoms of blood loss are as follows: there is increasing pallor and a rising pulse rate. The patient is restless, and in advanced cases there are deep sighing respirations, a condition which is called *air hunger*. The skin is cold and moist, the veins are empty, and there is thirst.

The *pulse* and *blood pressure* should be recorded every 15 or 30 minutes. When they stabilize, they can be recorded every 2 to 4 hours. The blood pressure is normal at first, and falls only after a good deal of blood has been lost. Therefore, even if the blood pressure is normal, it is possible that severe hypovolemia may be present. In such a situation the blood pressure is being maintained by shutting off large parts of the vascular bed by vasoconstriction in the non-essential organs. Any further loss of blood volume can lead to sudden collapse and even death.

Warm hands and feet

It is therefore important to *palpate the hands and feet to see if they are warm or cold*. If they are warm, it means there is no vasoconstriction, and implies that the blood volume is sufficient. On the other hand cold extremities indicate serious hypovolemia.

Classification according to blood loss

With respect to the volume of blood lost, hemorrhage can be classified as follows:

- *Class I* Hemorrhage: loss of less than 15% of total blood volume; this produces very little effect on pulse or blood pressure, as when a person donates a bottle of blood.
- *Class II* Hemorrhage: loss of 15 to 30%; produces tachycardia and decreased pulse pressure.
- *Class III* Hemorrhage: loss of 30 to 40%, with tachycardia, tachypnea, hypotension, oliguria and impaired mental status.
- *Class IV* Hemorrhage: loss of greater than 40%, with tachypnea, tachycardia, hypotension, oliguria, depressed Glasgow Coma Scale (GCS).

The lethal triad

Also called the 'trauma triad of death', this is a combination of hypothermia, acidosis and coagulopathy in cases of severe trauma, that produces a vicious cycle, resulting in a significant increase in the mortality rate.

It arises as follows: the volume depletion of major hemorrhage causes hypoperfusion. The resulting hypoxemia results in anaerobic glycolysis and raised serum lactate levels i.e. metabolic *acidosis*. Resuscitation with cool fluids and tissue exposure at operation causes *hypothermia*. At low temperatures clotting factors are inactive. The resulting *coagulopathy* leads to further hemorrhage, completing the vicious circle.

Replacement of blood loss

Blood loss of up to 20% of total blood volume should be replaced with crystalloid solutions; 20 to 50% loss with crystalloids and red blood cell concentrates; and loss greater than 50% with crystalloids, red blood cells and albumin or plasma.

ESTIMATING THE SIZE OF A HEMORRHAGE

Before the blood lost during a hemorrhage is replaced, the clinician should arrive at a rough estimate of the amount of blood loss. In a severe hemorrhage, the hemoglobin level, hematocrit, central venous pressure, cardiac output and urine output are all reduced, and the extent of their fall can give some idea of the amount of blood lost.

Hemoglobin level

Immediately after hemorrhage, there is no change in the hemoglobin level. However, within a few hours the blood is diluted by the movement of extracellular fluid into the blood vessels, and the hemoglobin level falls.

Packed cell volume or hematocrit

As in the case of hemoglobin, the packed cell volume also falls due to hemodilution.

Central venous pressure (CVP)

If the blood volume is low the veins are not well filled, and the hydrostatic pressure in the major veins (central venous pressure) is low. Conversely, if the blood volume is excessively high, the CVP is raised. The normal lower and upper levels of CVP, measured at the level of the midaxillary line, are 4 and 10cm of water respectively. If measured at the sternal angle the readings are 3 to 4cm lower.

For the purpose of measurement of the CVP, an intravenous catheter is passed either into the internal jugular vein in the neck, or into the subclavian vein through the infraclavicular route. A chest x-ray is taken to ensure that its tip is lying at the lower end of the superior vena cava or in the upper third of the right atrium. A saline manometer is connected to the catheter through a 3-way stopcock.

If the CVP is low the venous return should be supplemented by intravenous infusion; if it is high the amount of fluid given should be restricted. Single measurements of CVP are in fact less useful than serial measurements. At the same time, the response of the CVP to a fluid challenge (a rapid infusion of 100 to 200ml) is a good indicator of circulatory status and right ventricular function.

It is better to measure the CVP with an electronic pressure transducer. Not only are the readings more accurate, they are available continuously. Transducers show readings in mms Hg (1mm Hg = 1.36cm H_2O).

Cardiac output

In hypovolemia it is particularly important to restore and maintain a good cardiac output. Before a commonly used method of estimating cardiac output is described, a few points may be mentioned:

- Cardiac output is the product of the pulse rate and stroke volume (cardiac output = pulse rate x stroke volume).
- Pulse rate is easy to measure, stroke volume is not; it requires elaborate equipment.
- Pulse pressure (systolic minus diastolic pressure) is easy to estimate, and is a good measure of stroke volume.
- Thus if the pulse rate and pulse pressure are known, a rough estimate of cardiac output can be arrived at.

Simple method of estimating cardiac output

If the pulse rate and pulse pressure are measured and both are found to be reduced, the cardiac output must be low. This should alert the clinician so that he can take remedial action. In a situation where even a blood pressure apparatus is not available, the pulse pressure can be roughly estimated by feeling the pulse. If the pulse pressure is low, the pulse is 'thready' or of 'low volume'. *If the pulse is not only slow but also thready, it means the cardiac output is low.*

Urine

The urine output is a good indicator of renal blood flow, which is determined by the cardiac output. Therefore, the amount of urine passed should be carefully monitored in every case of severe hemorrhage. The level in the urine bag should be read every hour and the urine output recorded, which should be above 25–30ml per hour at the very least.

Measurement of blood loss

It is not always easy to estimate the exact amount of blood lost during trauma or operation. However, a few guidelines may be of some help.

If *blood clot* is found around the site of injury it is helpful to remember that clot which is of the size of a closed fist is about 500ml in volume.

In a *fracture* of the tibia if a moderate degree of swelling is present, 500 to 1,500ml of blood may have been extravasated into the muscles. In a fracture of the femur as much as two liters of blood may be lost into the tissues.

Weighing the swabs

Perhaps the best method of estimating blood loss during operations is to weigh the swabs used to mop up the blood, and to deduct their preoperative weight from this weight. A delicate weighing scale is required for this purpose, but it is much better than pure guesswork. In extensive operations such as partial gastrectomy, the figure obtained this way should be multiplied by one and a half, and for even more extensive operations like abdominoperineal resection of the rectum, by 2.

The aim of familiarization with the amount of blood lost during operation can also be achieved in a different manner. Drapes can be arranged as in an operation, known volumes of blood, e.g. from 10ml to 200ml, spilt onto the drapes, and the size and disposition of the bloodstains noted. This can help estimate the amount of blood as it is actually lost during an operation.

THE TREATMENT OF HEMORRHAGE

The treatment of hemorrhage resolves itself into two parts:

- The arrest of bleeding (*hemostasis*). This is discussed in the next part of this chapter.
- The replacement of the blood lost. This is carried out by *blood transfusion* or by infusion of plasma substitutes. This subject is discussed in the third and last of part of this chapter.

Hemostasis

Hemostasis is defined as the arrest of hemorrhage, either by the physiological processes of vasoconstriction and coagulation, or by surgical means.

PHYSIOLOGICAL METHODS OF HEMOSTASIS

The process of hemostasis begins immediately after injury. It is a complex process that prevents or terminates blood loss, provides a fibrin network for tissue repair, and ultimately removes the fibrin when it is no longer required. On the other hand endothelial cells 'do their best' to keep the vessels open by preventing clotting:

- They inactivate adenosine diphosphate, thus interfering with platelet recruitment.
- They provide an environment in which thrombin is inactivated.
- They release thrombomodulin that downmodulates the coagulation process.

Steps of hemostasis

Four major events take part in the process of hemostasis, both simultaneously and consecutively. They are: vascular constriction, platelet plug formation, fibrin formation and fibrinolysis.

Vasoconstriction

Vasoconstriction is the initial vascular response to injury. It is dependent on local contraction of smooth muscle that provides a reflex response to various stimuli including sympathetic nerve stimulation and circulating nonepinephrine. A powerful constrictor of smooth muscle, thromboxane, is also released by platelets. Serotonin, bradykinin and fibrinopeptides are also capable of contracting smooth muscle.

Mechanical factors play an important part in the arrest of hemorrhage. Of these, two are particularly important: the manner of division of the artery and the size of the cavity into which bleeding is taking place.

Manner of division of the artery

If a medium-sized artery is cut right across it can retract very well. At the same time it can contract down fully, so that hemostasis can take place. On the other hand if the same artery is incompletely divided the elastic fibers and smooth muscle in its wall contract, and the lateral tear in the artery tends to gape open and enlarge in size. Thus blood continues to flow, resulting in severe hemorrhage. Therefore, a lateral tear is far more dangerous than a complete transection.

Size of the cavity

The size of the cavity into which bleeding takes place is important in hemostasis. If bleeding takes place into a cavity which is *small* in size, it quickly fills up until it can accommodate no more blood, and hemorrhage stops. On the other hand bleeding into one of the *major* body cavities namely the pleural or peritoneal cavities is dangerous, because:

- Very large quantities of blood can be accommodated in those spaces without tamponade, so that arrest of bleeding does not take place.
- At the same time in the case of the pleural cavity the accumulating blood reduces the vital capacity and interferes with ventilation.

Finally, when there is low perivascular pressure, as with the muscle atrophy of old age, in prolonged steroid therapy, and in the Ehlers-Danlos syndrome (defective conversion of procollagen to collagen), bleeding tends to be more persistent.

Function of platelets

Platelets are 2-micron fragments of megakaryocytes, numbering 150,000 to 400,000 per cu mm in the circulating blood, with a life span of 7 to 9 days. They play a very central role in coagulation and hemostasis. Normally they do not adhere to each other or to the vessel wall. However, when a vessel is disrupted, platelets form a plug which stops bleeding. Injury to the intima exposes subendothelial collagen to which platelets adhere within a few seconds. This requires von Willebrand factor, a protein that is lacking in patients with von Willebrand's disease. The platelets then develop pseudopodial processes and also initiate a release reaction that recruits other platelets from the circulating blood. As a result a loose platelet aggregate forms, sealing the disrupted blood vessel.

Platelets provide coagulation factors to most steps of the coagulation cascade:

- When platelets come across damaged tissues with their exposed collagen, they aggregate and release *thromboxane A2* and *serotonin*, which promote the contraction of divided vessels and the further aggregation of platelets.
- Platelet factor 3 promotes coagulation by providing phospholipid to several stages of the coagulation process such as the activation of factors X and II.
- They also provide platelet factor 4, platelet-derived growth factor and adenosine diphosphate (ADP), which help in compaction of the platelets and the formation of an amorphous plug.
- Platelet factor 4 also inhibits heparin.
- Finally, the lipoprotein surface provided by the platelets catalyses the conversion of prothrombin into thrombin.

The mass of fused platelets forms a plug in the damaged vessel. The platelet plug contracts, reinforcing the

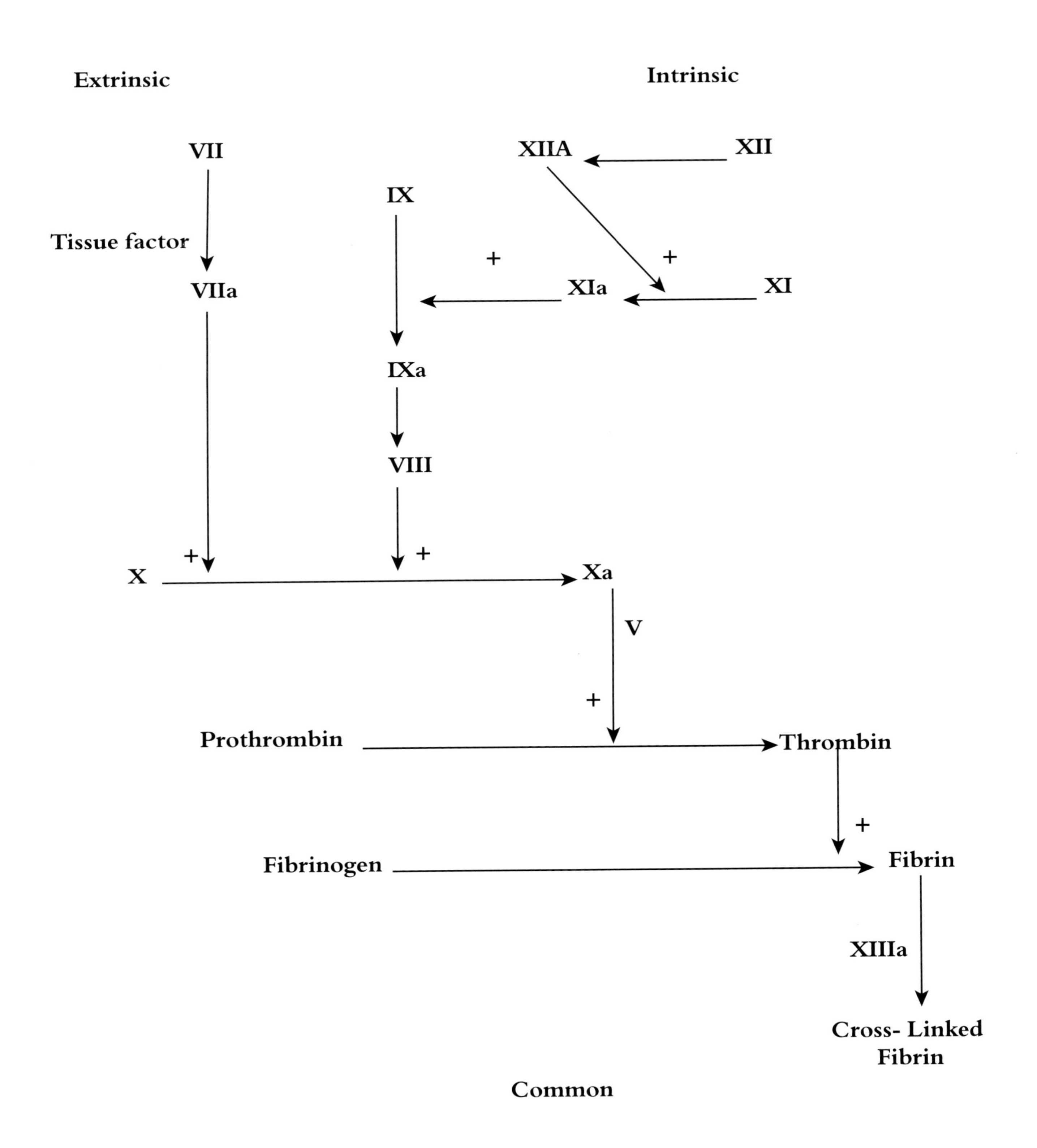

Fig.6.1 Schematic version of the coagulation system

contraction of the vessel. At the same time thrombin, which itself is a product of coagulation, helps the aggregation and fusion of platelets. Finally, platelets also play a role in fibrinolysis by releasing an inhibitor of plasminogen activation.

Fibrin formation (coagulation)

The next important step in the process of hemostasis is the formation of a fibrin clot. Before this can take place a series of reactions occurs, involving about a dozen different coagulation factors acting one after the other.

Initiating pathways

There are two initiating pathways, the intrinsic and the extrinsic:

- The intrinsic pathway involves components *normally present* in the blood, and comes into play in intact blood vessels.
- The extrinsic pathway is initiated by *tissue proteins*; this happens when a vessel is damaged and blood spills into the tissues or onto the exterior.

At every step of each of the pathways there is an increase in effect, so that the whole acts as an amplification system. The series of steps is shown in schematic form in (Fig.6.1).

Fibrinolysis

If fibrin was formed in excess, or in areas where it was not necessary, it would have disastrous results. An efficient system for dissolving excessively formed clot is therefore required.

Fibrinolysin

This is provided by fibrinolysin, also called plasmin. This is a strong proteolytic enzyme that breaks down fibrin into much smaller soluble fragments, thus dissolving *excessive* amounts of clot. It is derived from a precursor plasma protein (plasminogen). Fibrinolysis is initiated at the same time as the clotting mechanism under the influence of circulating kinases, tissue activators, and kallikrein present in many organs including vascular endothelium.

SURGICAL METHODS OF HEMOSTASIS

At the site of the accident

In a first-aid situation away from hospital, the following methods may be employed for controlling hemorrhage:

Packing

The wound may be packed with gauze or with any clothing material available. This is held in place by a bandage applied firmly. Unfortunately, nonprofessionals are often not aware of the fact that this simple step can save lives.

Tourniquets

The cord-like Samway's tourniquet can be used to stop bleeding from a limb. However, there are many disadvantages associated with its use:

- There is no way of regulating the pressure, so that very excessive pressure may be applied.
- The pressure is applied through a narrow rubber cord i.e. it is not distributed over a wide area, so that its harmful effect is further increased. The result is that damage to nerves and traumatic spasm of the arteries can occur.

B.P. cuff

The cuff of a blood pressure apparatus is free from both these defects. The pressure can be controlled to be just a little higher than the systolic pressure. Further, this pressure is distributed over the much wider area of the broad sphygmomanometer cuff. For these reasons damage to nerves or arteries is much less common with its use.

If a tourniquet is not tied tightly enough, it may occlude only the veins and not the arteries, and may encourage bleeding instead of stopping it. If a tourniquet is forgotten after being applied and is not removed, disastrous consequences may result, including gangrene requiring amputation of the limb.

Various expedients have been employed to avoid such a major tragedy. For example:

- The letter "T" may be written on the patient's forehead.
- Alternatively, the tourniquet may be attached to the operating table, so that the patient cannot be lifted off the table and onto the trolley without releasing it.

A tourniquet should not be left on for longer than about 45 minutes. If it has to be employed for a longer period, it should be released for a few minutes at the expiry of this period, and then reapplied.

At the hospital

The following methods may be employed to arrest bleeding:

- The most common method is to grip the bleeding point in the jaws of an artery forceps. The blood vessel is now *ligated* by catgut etc. If it is a small vessel it can also be sealed off by diathermy.

- *Artery supplying a viscus.*

In the case of an artery supplying a viscus, there are many methods of dealing with it:

- o The bleeding viscus may be *excised*, as in splenectomy.
- o The artery supplying the bleeding viscus may be *ligated*. For example, in a case of persistent profuse hematuria after prostatectomy, (Fig.6.2), or when an inoperable cancer of the uterine cervix continues to bleed furiously, the *internal iliac arteries* may be ligated on both sides, and the bleeding usually stops.
- o If bleeding is occurring into the lumen of a hollow viscus, *endoscopy* may be carried out and the bleeding point dealt with. Two examples follow:
  - ▪ In bleeding from esophageal varices, band ligation of the varices is carried out; this procedure has replaced injection of a sclerosing agent.
  - ▪ In the case of a bleeding artery in the base of a peptic ulcer, *diathermy or laser* coagulation of the bleeding point is carried out.
- o *Therapeutic embolization*. If the lumen of a bleeding artery could be filled with small artificial emboli, it would get occluded and the bleeding would stop. This is the basis of this method. A Seldinger catheter is passed up into the aorta, usually from the femoral artery. This catheter has a fine angulated tip, which is positioned into the origin of the concerned visceral artery. Artificial emboli consisting of blood clot or plastic microspheres are injected into the bleeding artery. This usually helps control the bleeding. Examples of the use of this technique include embolization of the following arteries:
  - ▪ The gastroduodenal artery, to treat a bleeding duodenal ulcer.
  - ▪ The hepatic artery, to relieve the pain of a cancer of the liver, by causing it to shrink in size due to reduced blood supply.
  - ▪ The renal artery, to arrest persistent hemorrhage from an inoperable tumor of the kidney.

Because it is a relatively minor procedure, therapeutic embolization is specially indicated in cases of advanced malignancies for palliation.

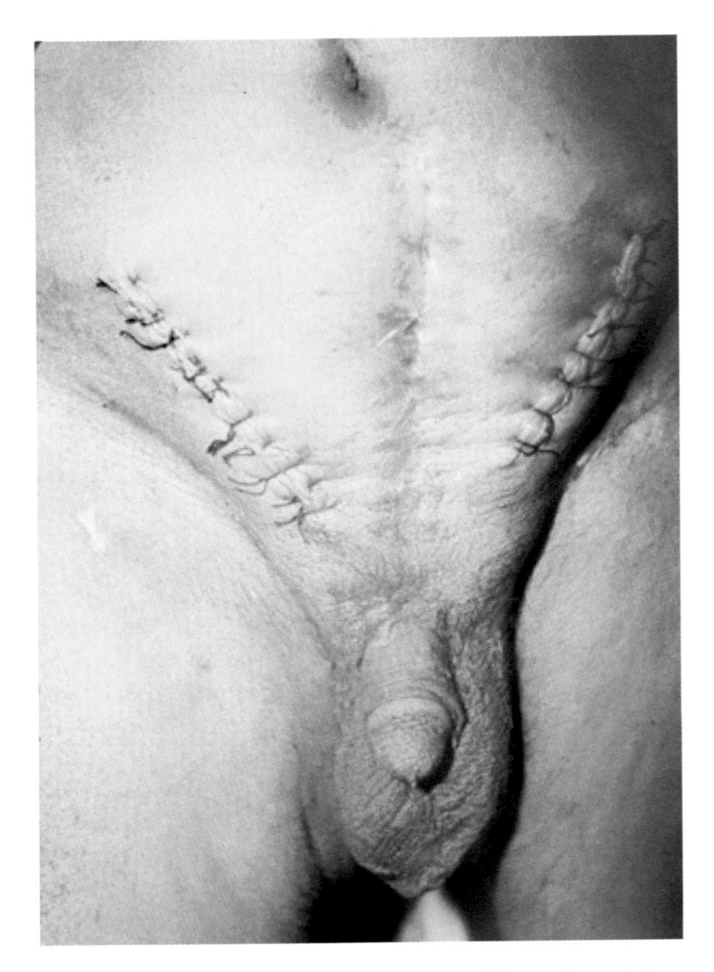

Fig..6.2 After suprapubic prostatectomy (through a midline incision), the patient developed uncontrollable hemorrhage. This was treated by bilateral internal iliac artery ligation, after which the bleeding completely stopped.

ABNORMALITIES OF COAGULATION

Congenital disorders of coagulation

Hemophilia

The most common congenital abnormality of hemostasis is hemophilia A. It arises due to lack of factor VIII activity. This is a sex-linked inherited disorder in which males exhibit the disease and females act as carriers. The condition can also occur without any family history, suggesting that spontaneous mutation can also occur.

The main problem is bleeding, both spontaneous and after even slight trauma. The most common surgical problems are orthopedic. Repeated hemorrhages occur into joints, leading to severe disabilities. At the same time, spontaneous retroperitoneal bleeding may occur, causing severe abdominal pain, tenderness and paralytic ileus. The clues to diagnosis are:

- A falling hematocrit value.
- Laboratory evidence of poor control of the disorder.
- Other evidence of spontaneous bleeding.

Death usually results from hemorrhage into the central nervous system.

Treatment

The treatment of hemophilia aims at maintaining factor VIII levels by repeated infusions to prevent spontaneous bleeding. If operation is to be carried out or active bleeding is occurring, higher levels of factor VIII are maintained. However, it is generally better to tide the patient over without operation. It should be mentioned that preparations of factor VIII are very expensive.

Hemophilia B (Christmas disease)

This is a congenital deficiency of factor IX. It is less common than hemophilia A, and the clinical manifestations are usually milder. Patients with the severe form of the disease require substitution therapy to prevent spontaneous bleeding. Even those with minor disease require substitution therapy whenever major or minor surgery is performed. During severe hemorrhage, treatment should aim to achieve plasma factor IX levels of 20 to 50 percent of normal for about five days, and then at 10 to 20 percent of normal for another 10 days. When an operation is required, plasma levels of 50 to 70 percent of normal should be achieved.

Acquired disorders of coagulation

Platelet abnormalities

Thrombocytopenia

Thrombocytopenia is the most common abnormality of hemostasis that results in bleeding in the surgical patient. It may be due to:

- Massive blood loss with replacement by stored blood.
- Leukemia, uremia or cytotoxic therapy: the number of megakaryocytes in the marrow is generally reduced.
- Idiopathic thrombocytopenic purpura (ITP), systemic lupus erythematosus (SLE), the secondary hypersplenism and splenomegaly of sarcoid, Gaucher's disease, lymphoma and portal hypertension. The marrow shows a normal number of megakaryocytes.

Thrombocytopenia is often accompanied by impaired platelet function. A variety of drugs also interfere with platelet function. These include aspirin, ibuprofen, indomethacin, lignocaine and penicillins.

In general 60,000 platelets per cu mm are adequate for normal hemostasis. If an elective operation is planned, a count greater than 50,000 per cu mm requires no specific therapy. Occasionally, thrombocytopenia may be seen due to vitamin B_{12} or folic acid deficiency, after total gastrectomy or in cases of severe intestinal malabsorption. Supplying the appropriate nutrient corrects the thrombocytopenia in a few days. If the patient has ITP or SLE and a low count, steroids generally help to raise it to more normal levels.

In massive blood transfusion, prophylactic administration of platelets is not recommended. However if required, 4 to 8 platelet packs raise the circulating platelet count sufficiently. If the patient is refractory to standard platelet transfusions, human leucocyte antigen-compatible platelets have proved effective.

Liver disease

Liver disease has multifarious effects on coagulation:

- All the prothrombin-related factors are produced solely in the liver (factors II, VIII, IX and X), and all may be depleted if the liver is diseased.
- Factor V is manufactured only in the liver and does not store well in banked blood. Deficiency of this factor is often the major clinical defect.
- Factor I (fibrinogen) is also produced only in the liver. However, dangerously impaired synthesis seems to occur only in the advanced stages of liver disease.
- The liver produces antiplasmins and removes circulating products of fibrinolysis. Thus, in serious liver disease fibrinolysis escapes control and becomes excessive, producing bleeding.
- The indirect effects of liver disease add to the problem. Destruction of liver tissue produces fibrosis around portal tracts and results in portal hypertension. This causes enlargement of the spleen with excessive destruction of platelets, which produces thrombocytopenia. Portal hypertension also produces esophageal varices which can bleed. If the cirrhosis is due to alcoholism there may also be gastritis or duodenal ulcer, either of which can also bleed.

Thus it will be seen that due to a combination of all the above factors, in advanced liver disease there is a marked tendency to bleed.

Drugs

Perhaps the most common cause of acquired coagulation disorders today are drugs, and a history of intake of such drugs should be carefully elicited in all cases of bleeding disorders.

Aspirin causes impairment of the function of all platelets circulating at the time of exposure, and should be stopped for six days before an elective operation. Similarly, antitumor agents impair the production of platelets.

Anticoagulants

Spontaneous bleeding may be a complication of anticoagulant treatment with either heparin or the vitamin K antagonists (warfarin-like drugs), and can result in a rectus sheath hematoma simulating appendicitis. The incidence of bleeding complications with heparin is reduced with a continuous infusion technique, regulating the partial thromboplastin time.

Certain surgical procedures should not be carried out in the presence of anticoagulation:

- Prostate surgery, because of the additional problem of local fibrinolysis.
- Blind needle aspirations.

If a patient on heparin requires an emergency operation, heparin should be discontinued; the operation can then be carried out safely after a few hours. If more rapid reversal is required, 1mg of protamine sulphate for every 100 units of the last dose of heparin is effective.

Disseminated intravascular coagulation (DIC)

Normally, coagulation is initiated locally as a reaction to local vascular injury. On the other hand in disseminated intravascular coagulation there is an explosive activation of the coagulation cascade throughout the vascular tree. Interestingly, this results not in vascular occlusion but a bleeding tendency. This is because the initial thrombus formed undergoes rapid lysis. Further cycles of coagulation and instantaneous lysis result in the depletion of coagulation factors including fibrinogen, and consumption of platelets. The principal causes of DIC include:

- Severe infections.
- Shock.
- Severe burns.
- Snake bite.
- ABO incompatible transfusion.
- Malignant disease (metastatic carcinoma, leukemia).
- Obstetric disorders:
  - Eclampsia.
  - Amniotic fluid embolism.
  - Retained dead fetus.
- Intravascular hemolysis (e.g. after systemic absorption of hypotonic fluids during transurethral prostatectomy.

Most cases of DIC are triggered by *sepsis*, particularly that due to Gram –ve organisms. Malignant disease, especially in the presence of multiple metastases, is also an important cause.

Clinical features

There is widespread bruising and extensive purpura, with persistent oozing of blood from surgical wounds and venepuncture sites. Epistaxis is common. There may be signs of vascular occlusion in the distal parts of the limbs.

Laboratory tests

In fulminant cases, the blood is incoagulable:

- Both the *cephalin kaolin clotting time* and *prothrombin time* are greatly prolonged, but are corrected by adding normal plasma to the patient's plasma.
- The *thrombin time* is also prolonged.
- The *fibrinogen level* is below 1.0 g/l (normal 2–4 g/l).
- *Fibrinogen degradation test* levels in the blood are very high, reflecting hyperfibrinolysis.
- The *platelet count* is reduced.

Treatment

The underlying cause must be identified; its treatment removes the stimulus for further consumption of coagulation factors.

- *Fresh frozen plasma* should be infused, being a good source of coagulation factors, including fibrinogen.
- *Cryoprecipitate* is a concentrate of fibrinogen, so that volume overload is avoided. This should also be given, as well as *platelet concentrates*.
- Patients often need *blood* in addition to plasma products.

Inhibitors of fibrinolysis, e.g. tranexamic acid are useless and may precipitate thrombosis. Low-dose heparin is also not widely advocated any longer.

Investigation of bleeding disorders

A carefully taken history and physical examination help in determining the following:

- Whether there is a generalized hemostatic defect. This may be suggested by bleeding from multiple sites, spontaneous bleeding and bleeding into the skin.
- Whether the defect is inherited or acquired. A family history of a bleeding disorder should be sought. Severe inherited defects become apparent in infancy, while mild inherited defects come to light only later, for example after surgery, childbirth or trauma.

- Whether the bleeding suggests a coagulation defect or a vascular/platelet defect.
    - Coagulation disorders are typically associated with hemarthroses and muscle hematomas.
    - Vascular/platelet bleeding is characterized by easy bruising and spontaneous bleeding from small vessels. The bleeding is mainly into the skin and from mucous membranes, often from the nose.

Laboratory tests for disorders of coagulation

the common tests utilized are the following:

- *Whole blood clotting time* measures the intrinsic coagulation system, but is insensitive and variable.
- The *one-stage prothrombin time (PT)* reflects the extrinsic clotting system i.e. factors II, V, VII and X, but is most sensitive to deficiencies of factor VII. Therefore it is the standard method for monitoring patients receiving vitamin K antagonists.
- The *activated partial thromboplastin time (APTT)* also measures the intrinsic clotting mechanism; unlike the whole-blood clotting time the results are very reproducible and fairly sensitive. It is sensitive to factors VIII, IX, XI and XII, as well as the factors normally detected by the one-stage prothrombin time. It is useful for screening hemophiliacs, for assessing coagulation in patients with liver disease before surgery, for regulating the dose of heparin, etc.

Tests of fibrinolysis

- *Fibrin degradation products* can be measured by immunological methods.
- The *euglobulin clot lysis time* is a rapid and sensitive test of fibrinolysis.

Platelets

- The *platelet count* can be measured. However, a great deal depends upon the functional state of the platelets.
- One of the best tests of platelet *function* is a carefully performed *bleeding time*.

Tests for *provoked petechiae* are less sensitive and less reproducible.

Importance of the history

To conclude, it must be emphasized that in the care of the bleeding patient the various laboratory tests are less important than: Careful history-taking and clinical examination, past history of bleeding and response to trauma, recent history of ingestion of drugs, knowledge of the functional state of the liver, and an enquiry for the presence of malignancy, dead tissue, uncontrolled infection and areas of poor perfusion. To order laboratory tests or to commence treatment without thorough investigation into these factors is like putting the cart before the horse.

A questionnaire can be designed to ask about:

- Prolonged bleeding after biting the tongue or after dental extraction.
- Bleeding problems after minor and major operations.
- Bruising without injury.
- Excessive menstrual bleeding.
- Aspirin taken during the preceding week.

The further course to be followed depends on the results of the tests.

- If the history is negative: if the operation is minor, no tests are required. In the case of a major operation, platelet count, blood smear and PTT should be carried out.
- If the history suggests defective hemostasis and the operation is major: bleeding time and APTT should be carried out in addition to the above tests.

Excessive bleeding after operation

Excessive bleeding during or shortly after operation may occur due to:

- *Ineffective local hemostasis*. Excessive bleeding at operation without bleeding from other sites suggests inadequate local surgical control of hemorrhage. However, operations on the prostate, pancreas and liver may be followed by excessive bleeding even after careful hemostasis, because operative trauma may activate plasminogen and cause fibrinolysis on the raw areas. Interruption of plasminogen activation by administration of epsilon aminocaproic acid for a day or two usually proves effective for hemostasis.
- An *undetected hemostatic defect* or consumption coagulopathy.
- A *hemolytic transfusion reaction* in a patient under anesthesia may manifest itself by diffuse bleeding in a previously dry operative field. The hemolysed red cells release adenosine diphosphate which causes platelet aggregation, the platelet aggregates being swept away by the blood.
- During *biliary tract surgery* in cirrhotic patients, diffuse bleeding may occur due to portal hypertension and coagulopathy. Vasopressin is used intravenously to reduce the portal hypertension, while epsilon aminocaproic acid (EACA) can be employed to control the increased fibrinolysis.

Blood transfusion

Blood transfusion can be a life-saving procedure. However, it can also be followed by serious reactions due to incompatibility and otherwise. Therefore, blood should be transfused only when really indicated, and stringent precautions should be taken before and during the transfusion. This is all the more important because of the rising incidence of AIDS and hepatitis along with intravenous drug abuse.

INDICATIONS FOR BLOOD TRANSFUSION

The important indications for blood transfusion include the following:

- Following *hemorrhage*, which may be due to:
  - Trauma with severe blood loss.
  - Bleeding from pathological lesions, e.g. from the gastrointestinal tract.
  - Major operative procedures with extensive dissection, in which a fair amount of blood is lost.
- After *extensive burns*, where a good deal of blood is destroyed in the burnt skin.
- *Before operation*, in a case of chronic anemia, where surgery is indicated urgently and there is insufficient time for iron therapy. However, this indication is now questioned, and the teaching that a hemoglobin value of less than 10 g/dl mandates preoperative blood transfusion is challenged. The cardiac output does not rise until the hemoglobin value falls to 7 g/dl. According to this view, even patients with a hemoglobin value below this figure in whom significant bleeding during operation is not expected are not considered candidates for preoperative transfusion.
- *Postoperatively*, in a patient where severe anemia has resulted from an infection.
- In a patient with a *bleeding disorder*, e.g. hemophilia or thrombocytopenia, either to prevent hemorrhage or to arrest it.

Which blood component to transfuse?

It is normally preferable to transfuse only the component or product required by the patient rather than whole blood. Not only is this the most effective way of using donor blood which is a scarce resource, it also reduces the risk of complications from transfusion of unnecessary components of the blood.

Whole blood should be reserved for acute blood loss; even here packed cells or red cell concentrates plus crystalloid or colloid solutions are acceptable alternatives.

Fresh frozen plasma

This contains most of the *coagulation factors* in concentrations approaching those in normal plasma. It is a very good source of coagulation components, but quite large volumes are required for clinical effect. It has an important role in the following conditions:

- In patients with multiple coagulation defects resulting from hepatic insufficiency.
- In disseminated intravascular coagulation.
- Where labile clotting factors have been depleted by the transfusion of very large volumes of old stored blood.

Cryoprecipitate (cold precipitate)

This was developed when it was found that a cold precipitate of plasma was rich in antihemophilic globulin (AHG) i.e. Factor VIII. It also contains von Willebrand factor along with some fibrinogen. It is no longer used for the treatment of hemophilia and von Willebrand's disease because of the greater risk of virus transmission compared to virus-inactivated coagulation factor concentrates.

Factor VIII and IX concentrates

These are freeze-dried preparations obtained from large pools of plasma. They are used in hemophilia and von Willebrand's disease.

Washed red cell concentrates

These are useful in patients who have severe recurrent urticarial or anaphylactic reactions.

Platelet concentrates

These can be stored for up to five days at 22°C. They are used to treat bleeding in patients with severe thrombocytopenia.

Albumin

4.5% and 20% solutions are available. They are inappropriate fluids for acute volume replacement or in shock. They are indicated in acute severe hypoalbuminemia, the 20% solution being particularly useful in patients with nephrotic syndrome or liver disease who are fluid-overloaded and resistant to diuretics.

Immunoglobulins

These are used in hypogammaglobulinemia to prevent infections.

Recycled blood

Because of the fear of AIDS as well as hepatitis, cardiac surgeons have started using recycled blood. During an operation where a considerable quantity of blood is inevitably lost, a suction machine sucks up the blood from the cavity the surgeon is working in. The blood is passed through a highly efficient filter and allowed to flow right back into a vein.

Advantages

- The system is quite safe.
- At the same time, because it is fresh, recycled blood has superior oxygen carrying and clotting qualities than banked blood once the heparin has been neutralized.
- Another advantage of recycling is that one can use an almost indefinite amount of blood.

The same technique can be usefully employed in other branches of surgery.

PLASMA AND BLOOD SUBSTITUTES

Plasma substitutes

If massive bleeding has occurred or is taking place, the lost blood must be replaced promptly. If blood is not available immediately, at least the normal blood volume must be re-established immediately. Volume replacement can be carried out using one of a number of plasma substitutes available:

Dextrans

These are polysaccharides of different molecular weight. In the concentrations used, their osmotic pressure is the same as that of plasma. They induce rouleaux formation of the red blood cells and therefore interfere with blood grouping and cross-matching, so the blood sample for these tests must be taken before dextran is infused.

Low molecular weight dextran (40,000)

This restores blood volume promptly, but its action is of brief duration because the kidney rapidly excretes the small molecules. It prevents sludging of red cells in small vessels. In the kidney this action prevents the renal shutdown which can occur in cases of severe hypotension.

High molecular weight dextrans (70,000 and 1,10,000)

These are retained in the circulation for a longer time, so their action is more prolonged. However, they are associated with a higher incidence of allergic reactions.

Gelatin

Gelatin has a molecular weight of 30,000 and is used as a 4% solution, and up to a liter can be infused.

Blood substitutes

The future

Natural hemoglobin when outside the red blood corpuscles breaks up into its two subunits, hem and globin. These are small molecules, which leak into the urine and damage the kidneys. Free hemoglobin therefore cannot be used for transfusion into patients.

Artificial blood

Recently, researchers have been able to grow large quantities of subunits a and b of human hemoglobin in the gut bacteria Escherichia coli. The subunits are next linked together to produce hemoglobin. These workers have been able to join the subunits in such a manner that they cannot split from each other when free in the blood, and therefore this hemoglobin can be administered to the patient without fear of hemoglobinuria.

As hemoglobin can be manufactured on a large scale by E. coli, it appears that such hemoglobin will be available commercially in the near future, and will for the first time provide an oxygen-carrying blood substitute in abundant quantities to be used during wars and natural calamities. This preparation will have the advantage of being completely free of all infectious agents like the AIDS and hepatitis viruses. Besides, this kind of hemoglobin-based artificial blood requires no typing or cross-matching. It will therefore be a very great advance in the subject of blood transfusion.

COMPLICATIONS OF BLOOD TRANSFUSION

Although the availability of blood transfusions has greatly advanced the frontiers of surgery, it must be remembered that a number of serious complications can follow after blood transfusions, including the following:

Incompatibility

The ABO blood groups are of very basic importance in every case of blood transfusion. Let us see how a transfusion reaction develops. The ABO antigens are two, A and B. Each person carries in his red cells either one (A or B), or both (AB), or none (O). If he carries the antigen A, his blood does not have any anti-A antibodies.

Now, many plants have both A and B antigens, and every human being gets exposed to them. So this person who belongs to group A develops anti-B antibodies at an early age. These antibodies are powerful hemolysins. Therefore, if he now receives blood of the B or AB groups, severe intravascular hemolysis is produced, which often results in disseminated intravascular coagulation and renal failure. Up to 10% of these cases end up in mortality.

At the same time, if a very large quantity of plasma containing anti-A or anti-B antibodies is infused into a recipient whose red cells contain A or B, hemolysis will occur, but usually will be less severe.

Misidentification

This is the commonest cause of transfusion reactions. Although ABO incompatibility can and does occur from time to time, the irony of the situation lies in the fact that the majority of transfusion reactions occur from simple misidentification; either the patient or the blood is incorrectly identified, or the blood sample sent for cross-matching is wrongly labeled. The unnecessary deaths from some of these wrongly labeled units of blood can be prevented by being careful, and by strict adherence to a routine for proper identification.

Rh antigens

A person either carries the Rh antigen in his red blood cells and is therefore Rh +ve, or he does not carry such antigen, and is Rh-ve. If a patient is receiving blood for the first time, no untoward reaction takes place even if the recipient is Rh-ve and the donor Rh +ve.

However, with repeated transfusions of Rh +ve blood into an Rh-ve person, anti-Rh antibodies develop in the plasma of the recipient, and can cause a reaction. Thus Rh antigens are important only in Rh-ve persons, and then only if they have either been transfused previously with Rh +ve blood, or have been pregnant with an Rh +ve fetus.

Morbidity and mortality

If a full unit of incompatible blood has been given, the mortality and morbidity rate is high. In about 20% of patients an acute hemorrhagic diathesis is seen with a fall in platelet count, increase in fibrinolytic activity, and consumption of coagulation factors due to disseminated intravascular coagulation.

O-negative blood

If blood is required in a dire emergency which allows no time for grouping and cross matching, O Rh-ve blood should be used.

Laboratory findings

These include hemoglobinuria with a free hemoglobin level of over 5mg/dl, and evidence of antigen incompatibility of donor and recipient blood. A bladder catheter shows the dark color and low volume of urine. A positive Coomb's test shows transfused cells coated with patient autoantibody.

Treatment

- The transfusion is stopped.
- A sample of the recipient's blood is taken and sent to the blood bank with the suspected unit of blood.
- The serum bilirubin is determined.
- A Foley catheter is passed and the hourly urine output recorded.
- Mannitol or furosemide plus sodium bicarbonate are given intravenously.
- Dialysis is sometimes required.
- During recovery, losses of sodium and potassium due to the diuresis may require replacement.

Other transfusion reactions

- *Pyrexial reactions.*

The patient develops fever with rigors. The most common cause of these reactions is the presence of impurities in the donor apparatus. These reactions were very common in the past when red rubber tubings were repeatedly used in transfusion sets. Their incidence was minimized by the introduction of plastic disposable transfusion sets.

- *Allergic reactions.*

The patient develops an urticarial rash and tachycardia; rarely, acute anaphylaxis may occur. This is the result of an allergic reaction to plasma products in the donor blood. The transfusion should be stopped and an antihistaminic drug administered, e.g. chlorpheniramine, 10mg.

Infections

Three common types of infection can occur in the recipient:

- *Bacterial infection.*

This usually occurs if the donor blood is left in a warm room for some hours before being transfused, as any bacteria in the blood can multiply their numbers. Septicemia and even death can result.

- *Hepatitis.*

A common and serious complication of blood transfusion is the transmission of the virus of serum hepatitis. Severe hepatitis arises about three months after the transfusion. The causative organism is the hepatitis B or hepatitis C virus (HBV or HCV). The advanced countries have a low incidence of HBV, which is widespread in the developing countries. HCV was identified as recently as 1988, and in countries where blood was not tested for HCV markers, was responsible for the great majority of cases of post-transfusion hepatitis. However, since the introduction of screening for HCV in donor blood, this incidence has fallen to only 4%. All donors should be asked if they have suffered from jaundice in the past, and should be tested for hepatitis B and C antigen. However, the test is not sensitive enough to eliminate all possibility of the disease.

- *Thrombophlebitis.*

This may occur in a vein into which the transfusion has been given, and usually results from a lack of observation of aseptic precautions. If suppuration develops, wide incision and drainage, or even excision of the vein, must be carried out for prompt relief from the infection.

Congestive cardiac failure

Congestive cardiac failure can occur if blood is transfused too rapidly specially in the elderly, or when there is cardiovascular insufficiency. If blood has to be transfused in a case of anemia, it is better to give packed red cells; at the same time the transfusion should be given slowly, over a period of many hours.

Air embolism

Air may be sucked into an open vein at the end of the transfusion. If a drip chamber is used which contains a plastic float that plugs the exit when the fluid falls to a low level, this complication is prevented. Collapsible bags for blood and intravenous fluids are also relatively safe, unless they have been punctured by a needle for adding some drug to the infusate.

Coagulation defects

These may arise as follows:

- *Stored blood* is low in platelets, factor V and factors VIII. Therefore, if large volumes of stored blood are used these factors may get diluted and hemorrhage can occur.
- *Disseminated intravascular coagulation (DIC):* This commonly follows ABO incompatibility. When coagulation takes place in the blood vessels the various coagulation factors namely fibrinogen, factor II, V, VIII and platelets, get used up, so that hemorrhage results. For the treatment of DIC these factors have to be replaced.

Massive transfusion

This is defined as replacement of more than 1 blood volume in 24 hours or > 50% of blood volume in 4 hours. It occurs in settings like severe trauma, ruptured aortic aneurysm, and in surgical and obstetric complications. The mortality is high, due to hypotension, hypothermia, coagulopathy, acidosis, citrate toxicity, shock, and the underlying disease.

In treatment, the aim should be to maintain the values of different parameters given below at the levels indicated:

- Temperature $>35\ ^0C$
- pH >7.2
- Ionised calcium >1.1mmol/L
- Platelets $>50\text{x}10^9$/L
- PT/APTT <1.5x of normal
- Fibrinogen >1g/L

Chapter

7 FLUIDS AND ELECTROLYTES

If the cells of the body are to function efficiently, their internal environment, i.e. composition of the extracellular and intracellular fluids, must remain constant. For this, it is necessary that water and different electrolytes used up in the various metabolic processes be replaced in like amounts. In the normal healthy person this takes place by ingestion of appropriate quantities of water and food as dictated by thirst and appetite, both of which are extremely elegant mechanisms for regulation of the internal environment; we are not sufficiently cognizant of their accuracy because we take them for granted.

Where oral intake is not possible for one reason or the other, the same must be provided by an alternative route, commonly intravenously. For this purpose one must know the normal amounts of fluids and salts ingested and excreted every day. At the same time in many surgical illnesses, as well as after operations, excessive quantities of water and salts are lost. In such situations we must know how to assess the amounts lost, in order to replace them accurately. It will thus be seen that fluid and electrolyte management is a very important part of the care of surgical patients.

NORMAL EXCHANGE OF FLUIDS AND ELECTROLYTES

A healthy 70kg adult consumes on an average about 2,500ml of water per day. About 1,500ml of this is water taken as such by mouth. The rest is water extracted from solid food or gained as *water of oxidation*. The salt (sodium chloride) intake of this average adult is about 5gm per day.

How to replace the water and salt?

Let us now see how the above-noted basal amounts of water and salt can be replaced intravenously, if it is so desired.

If one was to replace all the 2,500ml as plain water, one will need to make it isotonic, because if plain water was given intravenously in such a quantity it would cause intense hemolysis, being severely hypotonic, and would kill the recipient. In clinical practice water is made isotonic by adding 5% glucose to it, this being the amount of glucose which makes it exactly isotonic with plasma. An added bonus in using glucose is the fact that glucose is quickly metabolized, providing some ready energy, leaving behind just water. Thus, electrolytically speaking a 5% aqueous solution of glucose is simply water. In other words if one gives 2,500ml of 5% glucose in water, one is really giving 2,500ml of plain water.

Now, how does one add 5gm of sodium chloride to this 2,500ml of water? In clinical practice the most common method by which this is done is by replacing 500ml of 5% glucose by the same volume of normal saline. This gives 500 x 0.9/100 = 4.5gm of salt, which is fairly close to the 5gm of salt required.

To sum up, then, the normal basal requirement of water and salt is made good by administering 2,000ml of 5% glucose and 500ml of normal saline. This is also called the *maintenance requirement*. Another method of giving the same quantities of water and salt is to administer 2,500ml of l/5th normal saline. *This maintenance requirement never varies*, i.e. in a 70kg adult it is 2,500ml of water, with 5gm of salt.

Method of calculation in a patient

When calculating the fluid needs of any particular patient:

- This *maintenance* requirement is first noted down.
- To this are added any losses due to *operation or fever*.
- Finally, any losses from the *gastrointestinal tract*, due to vomiting, nasogastric aspiration, diarrhea or discharge from an intestinal fistula, are recorded and added to the total.

We shall see in detail, in due course, how the abnormal losses are assessed in different situations. However, *the concept of maintenance requirement has been introduced at this stage for the sake of clarity*, so that the full requirements can later be built up on this basic value.

Incidentally, every clinician should have a sip or two of 5% glucose, and of normal saline, to see how they taste. In fact if he tasted some of the other intravenously administered nutrients as well, he would come to no harm.

CLASSIFICATION OF BODY FLUID CHANGES

Disorders of fluid balance may be of three types, namely disturbances of volume, concentration and composition. For ease of understanding, the three types are discussed in turn. However, it should be noted that in any patient more than one type of change is commonly present.

Volume changes

The most common fluid disorder in the surgical patient is reduction in the volume of the extracellular fluid. *Remember that the fluid lost is not water alone; both water and electrolytes are lost,* in approximately the same proportion as that in which they exist in the extracellular fluid.

Volume deficit

Volume deficit may be produced by two different kinds of processes:

- Fluid is actually lost from the body; in surgical practice this commonly occurs when *gastrointestinal fluid* is lost due to:
  - Vomiting.
  - Gastroduodenal suction, after operation or in cases of intestinal obstruction.
  - Diarrhea.
  - Drainage from a fistula, usually intestinal.
- No fluid is actually lost from the body. *However, fluid is lost from the blood vessels and is 'sequestrated' into the tissue spaces or body cavities.* Examples of such losses of fluids include the following conditions:
  - *Soft tissue injuries and infections,* fluid being lost into the injured tissues.
  - *Peritonitis,* fluid being lost into the peritoneal cavity.
  - *Intestinal obstruction,* large volumes of fluid collecting in the lumen of the intestine.
  - *Burns,* great quantities of fluid being trapped in the edematous burn wound.

Clinical features

The symptoms and signs of volume deficit are manifested by the different organ systems as follows:

CNS.	Sleepiness, apathy, anorexia.
Cardiovascular.	Tachycardia, collapsing pulse, collapsed veins, hypotension.
Tissue signs.	Decreased skin turgor.
Metabolism.	Reduction in body temperature.

Volume excess

In surgical practice this happens commonly when too much fluid is given intravenously. At the same time, volume overload can take place in renal failure, due to the inability of the kidneys to excrete a normal volume of water. The signs are those of circulatory overload, e.g. distended neck veins, crepitations at the lung bases, and edema of the feet. In the elderly patient congestive cardiac failure with pulmonary edema may develop rather quickly even with a moderate volume excess.

Our forensic colleagues tell us how frequently, at postmortem examinations, they find lungs overloaded with fluid in patients dying after stab or bullet wounds. We should therefore be careful not to overinfuse our patients.

Concentration changes

If the serum *sodium* level becomes very low or very high, it can be diagnosed by clinical examination. However, one should not allow the situation to reach that stage. Serum electrolyte determinations should be carried out repeatedly, so that minor deviations from the normal are detected and corrected promptly. Disorders of sodium concentration include hyponatremia and hypernatremia.

Hyponatremia

When the serum sodium level is low the osmolality of the extracellular fluid falls. This causes water to move into the cells to restore osmolality. In the brain increased intracellular water causes raised intracranial pressure, with muscle twitchings or even convulsions.

Hypernatremia

In this condition CNS signs occur in the form of restlessness and weakness. In severe cases the patient is delirious and behaves like a maniac.

Mixed volume and concentration changes

The most common example is seen in volume and concentration changes in a patient who is losing large volumes of gastrointestinal fluids but continues to drink plain water. The result is an extracellular deficit with hyponatremia. This can also occur if, after operation gastrointestinal losses are replaced by only 5% glucose in water. On the other hand, if a patient with oliguric renal failure is given an excess of water, the result is raised extracellular volume and hyponatremia.

The importance of kidney function

Normally functioning kidneys minimize these changes. The result is that some of our mistakes in fluid administration are compensated and masked. However, when a patient is in oliguric renal failure, he is especially prone to develop these fluid disorders. In these patients, therefore, fluid management must be extremely precise.

'Functional' renal failure

It should be remembered that when a patient has a significant deficit of volume, even if he has normal kidneys his glomerular filtration rate (GFR) is reduced. Thus the patient is in a state of 'functional' renal failure, because with a low GFR the kidneys' ability of maintaining fluid hemostasis is lost. Fortunately, these changes are reversible with early correction of the extracellular fluid volume deficit.

Composition changes

The most common change of composition involves an excess or deficit of hydrogen ions, i.e. acidosis or alkalosis. The other important changes of composition include excess or deficit of potassium, calcium and magnesium.

ACID-BASE BALANCE

In different disease states either acidosis or alkalosis may occur. Either of these may be due to a disorder of respiration or metabolism.

Respiratory acidosis

This condition occurs when alveolar ventilation is decreased, so that $C0_2$ is retained. Examples of these conditions include the following:

- Airway obstruction.
- Pneumonia.
- Pleural effusion.
- Hypoventilation due to the pain of upper abdominal incisions.
- Abdominal distension from paralytic ileus limiting diaphragmatic movements.

These factors may operate singly or in combination. The problem can be particularly serious in the patient with chronic lung disease, because in such a patient pre-existing respiratory acidosis may be made worse in the postoperative period. After operation restlessness, hypertension and tachycardia are commonly due to pain. However, it must be remembered that *they can also be due to inadequate ventilation with a raised* $PaCO_2$ which can be dangerous if it remains undetected and uncorrected.

Prevention

Strict attention to tracheo-bronchial hygiene during the postoperative period is an important preventive measure, especially in patients with chronic lung disease:

- Deep breathing and coughing are taught before, and supervised after, operation.
- Humidified air is inhaled to prevent hardening of secretions.
- Oversedation is avoided, as it depresses respiration.

Management

Whenever possible the underlying defect should be corrected. At the same time, steps must be taken to ensure adequate ventilation. Occasionally, an endotracheal tube may have to be passed and the patient placed on a ventilator.

Respiratory alkalosis

After operation the patient may hyperventilate. The most common factors leading to such hyperventilation include apprehension and pain. Occasionally the cause may be hypoxia, and rarely nervous system injury.

Complications of respiratory alkalosis

Severe respiratory alkalosis can produce the following complications:

- *Hypokalemia,* producing ventricular arrhythmia and fibrillation.
- Shift of the oxyhemoglobin dissociation curve to the left. Thus hemoglobin cannot easily unload oxygen at the tissue level, and hypoxia may result.
- The level of ionized *calcium* may be significantly depressed, and tetany and convulsions may result.

Treatment is directed towards preventing the condition by the proper use of mechanical ventilators and by correcting pre-existing potassium deficits.

Metabolic acidosis

This condition results when:

- Fixed acids are either produced in excess or retained in the body. Some examples follow:
    - o In diabetic acidosis (due to excess production).
    - o In lactic acidosis (due to excess production).
    - o In azotemia (due to retention).
- Bicarbonate base is lost from the body, e.g. in:

- o Diarrhea.
- o Small bowel fistula.
- o Renal insufficiency, with inability to reabsorb bicarbonate.

Compensation initially occurs by an increase in the rate and depth of ventilation, which washes out $C0_2$.

Common causes of metabolic acidosis

The conditions commonly resulting in metabolic acidosis include the following:

- One of the very important functions of the kidney is the *regulation of pH*, by the excretion of nitrogenous waste products and acid metabolites, and the resorption of bicarbonate. If *renal damage* occurs and these regulatory functions are lost, metabolic acidosis develops rapidly and may be difficult to control.
- However, metabolic acidosis can occur even in a patient with normal kidneys. This happens when more chloride is given than the kidneys can handle. *The typical patient is one who has suffered excessive losses of alkaline gastrointestinal fluids* (biliary, pancreatic, small bowel secretions). He has been on intravenous fluids for many days, having been given mostly isotonic sodium chloride solution. Because these solutions have only chloride and no bicarbonate they will not correct the pH change. The use of a balanced salt solution, such as lactated Ringer's solution, is required.
- Another common cause of severe metabolic acidosis in surgical patients is *acute circulatory failure*. In this condition inadequate perfusion of the tissues results in tissue hypoxia. Due to the inadequate supply of oxygen, carbohydrates cannot be broken down to CO_2 and H_2O. Anaerobic glycolysis leads to formation of lactic acid.
- Finally, acute *hemorrhagic shock also* produces a profound drop in pH due to lactic acidosis. Attempts to raise the blood pressure with vasopressors simply worsen the situation. Similarly, efforts to correct the acidosis by infusing large quantities of sodium bicarbonate, without restoring the blood flow, are futile. The indiscriminate use of sodium bicarbonate during resuscitation of patients in hypovolemic shock should be discouraged because:
  - o A mild metabolic alkalosis is common following resuscitation, partly due to the alkalinizing effect of blood transfusions and the administration of lactated Ringer's solution.
  - o After restoration of hepatic blood flow the lactate in lactated Ringer's solution and the citrate in the transfused blood are metabolized and bicarbonate is formed.

Once adequate tissue perfusion is restored, the lactic acid that had accumulated during the shock episode is rapidly cleared.

If excessive quantities of sodium bicarbonate are administered at the same time, severe metabolic alkalosis can result. An alkaline pH is highly undesirable, because it shifts the oxyhemoglobin dissociation curve to the left. Hemoglobin does not readily give up its oxygen, and oxygen unloading at the tissue level suffers.

On the other hand if volume replacement is carried out promptly, adequate tissue perfusion and therefore oxygenation is restored. The lactic acid is quickly metabolized and the pH returns to normal. This volume replacement should not be carried out using blood alone, but blood and lactated Ringer's solution should be used together. In this way the pH returns to normal more promptly. In fact the recent tendency is to use more Ringer's lactate than blood.

Anion gap

Routine electrolyte estimations determine the levels of the cations sodium and potassium, and the anions chloride and bicarbonate. The total of the former exceeds that of the latter. This is due to the presence of organic anions which are not normally measured. The difference is called the anion gap.

The anion gap is a useful tool in the management of acid-base disorders. Its value is found by subtracting the sum of the chloride and bicarbonate from the serum sodium concentration. The unmeasured anions that account for the 'gap' are sulphate, phosphate, lactate, and other organic anions.

Significance of anion gap

If the acidosis is due to loss of bicarbonate (e.g. diarrhea) or gain of chloride (e.g. administration of ammonium chloride), the anion gap will be normal. On the other hand if the acidosis is due to increased production of an organic acid (e.g. lactic acid in circulatory shock) or the retention of sulphuric or phosphoric acid (**e.g.** in renal failure), the concentration of these *unmeasured* anions (i.e. the anion gap) will be increased.

Causes of anion gap

- The most common cause of an elevated anion gap is *shock* or inadequate tissue perfusion from any cause, resulting in accumulation of large quantities of lactic acid.
- *Diabetic ketosis* and *starvation* cause elevation of the anion gap by formation of ketoacids.

- *Renal failure* produces the same effect by the retention of sulphuric or phosphoric acids.

Metabolic alkalosis

Metabolic alkalosis results from loss of fixed acid, e.g. during the vomiting of pyloric stenosis, or due to gain of base bicarbonate. It is aggravated by any pre-existing potassium depletion. Compensation is primarily by renal mechanisms, because respiratory compensation is generally of a minor degree.

Most patients with metabolic alkalosis have some hypokalemia. When cellular potassium is depleted sodium and hydrogen enter the cell. This produces an intracellular acidosis and extracellular alkalosis. The dangers of metabolic alkalosis are the same as those described under respiratory alkalosis, namely hypoxia, hypokalemia and tetany.

In *pyloric stenosis* persistent vomiting or gastric suction produces a hypochloremic, hypokalemic metabolic alkalosis. Proper management requires replacement of the extracellular fluid volume deficit with isotonic sodium chloride solution, along with replacement of potassium. Volume restitution should be started first and a good urine output obtained before potassium is administered, otherwise dangerous hyperkalemia could result. Temporary control of the alkalosis with this method is usually successful, but control of the underlying cause should be achieved as soon as possible.

Potassium abnormalities

Potassium is the major cation of intracellular water, 98% of the potassium in the body being located within the cells at a concentration of approximately 150 meq/liter. Disorders of potassium concentration include hypokalemia and hyperkalemia.

Hypokalemia

The more common problem in surgical patients is hypokalemia which may occur due to one or more of the following causes:

- Loss of gastrointestinal fluids by diarrhea, intestinal fistula, etc.
- Prolonged administration of potassium-free parenteral fluids (because in the meantime obligatory renal loss of potassium continues).
- Parenteral hyperalimentation with inadequate potassium replacement.
- Excessive renal excretion of potassium.

Potassium plays an important role in the regulation of the acid-base balance. The physical signs of potassium deficit are produced by the failure of contractility of skeletal, smooth and cardiac muscle. There is muscular weakness, progressing to flaccid paralysis. Abdominal distension occurs due to paralytic ileus. The ECG shows flattening of T waves and depression of ST segments.

Treatment

Treatment of hypokalemia firstly involves prevention. While replacing gastrointestinal losses, potassium should also be replaced. It should be remembered that while treating hypokalemia, *potassium should not be given directly into a vein,* as the sudden rise of potassium concentration in the blood can cause cardiac arrest. Instead, potassium is added to the intravenous fluids and given as a drip. No more than 40 meq should be added to a liter of intravenous fluid, and the rate of administration should not exceed 40 meq per hour.

Hyperkalemia

The most common cause of hyperkalemia is chronic renal failure. After severe injury or surgical operation, and also in a catabolic state from any cause, a large number of cells are broken down and a significant amount of intracellular potassium released into the extracellular space. Similarly, potassium also moves out of the cells in acidosis. *However, the serum potassium level rises markedly only if the kidneys fail to excrete the excess potassium, in oliguric or anuric renal failure.*

The *clinical signs* of hyperkalemia are manifested in the cardiovascular and gastrointestinal (GI) systems.

The GI symptoms include nausea, vomiting, intestinal colic and diarrhea.

The cardiovascular signs are first seen on the ECG: peaked T waves, widened QRS complexes, and depressed ST segments. At higher levels of potassium the T waves disappear, and heart block and diastolic cardiac arrest develop.

Treatment

Treatment of hyperkalemia includes the following measures:

- Exogenously administered potassium is withheld.
- The following measures are taken to reduce the potassium level in the blood:
    - 50ml of 50% glucose solution is given intravenously along with insulin. The glucose stimulates the synthesis of glycogen, resulting in an uptake of potassium and reducing its level in the serum.
    - 50–150 meq of sodium lactate or bicarbonate are given intravenously. This raises the pH and shifts potassium into the cells.

- o 10% calcium gluconate is given in a dose of 10–30ml in a liter of intravenous fluid as an infusion. It helps counteract the effects of hyperkalemia on the myocardium.
- o The underlying cause of hyperkalemia is corrected if possible.

Calcium abnormalities

The total amount of calcium in the body is about 1,000gms in the average adult, most of which is found in the bones. The normal daily intake of calcium is 1 to 3gm. Most of this is excreted via the gastrointestinal tract, and about 200mg is excreted in the urine per day. The normal serum calcium level is 8.5 to 10.5mg/dl (2.2–2.6mmol/1). About half of this is non-ionized, and bound to protein and other substances in the plasma. The other half is ionized, and is responsible for neuromuscular stability. Disturbances of calcium metabolism are not a problem in the uncomplicated postoperative patient, and therefore administration of calcium is not required in such cases.

Hypocalcemia

The common *causes* of hypocalcemia include acute pancreatitis, chronic renal failure, hypoparathyroidism, and massive soft tissue infections (necrotizing fasciitis).

The *symptoms* of hypocalcemia (serum level less than 8mg/dl i.e. 2mmol/1) are numbness and tingling of the circumoral region, fingers and toes. The signs are muscle cramps, tetany with carpopedal spasm, convulsions, and prolongation of the Q-T interval on ECG.

Treatment consists of correction of the underlying cause alongwith repletion of the deficit. Acute symptoms can be relieved by intravenous calcium gluconate. Patients requiring prolonged replacement may be given calcium lactate by mouth. Routine administration of calcium during massive blood transfusions is probably not required. Only those patients who are receiving blood as rapidly as 100ml per minute require calcium administration; in other cases dangerous levels of hypercalcemia can result.

Hypercalcemia

The two main *causes* of hypercalcemia are cancer with bony metastases, and hyperparathyroidism. The former is most common in a patient with metastatic breast cancer who is receiving estrogen therapy.

Treatment

This is urgent. Measures to lower the serum calcium level are instituted immediately. The extracellular fluid volume is depleted in these cases; the deficit is rapidly made good, and this immediately lowers the serum calcium level by dilution.

The treatment of hypercalcemia in the patient with metastatic cancer is that of prevention. If the serum calcium level is raised the patient is placed on a low-calcium diet, and measures are taken to ensure adequate hydration.

Magnesium abnormalities

Magnesium deficiency occurs infrequently. Plasma magnesium concentration ranges between 1.5 and 2.5meq/l (0.7–1.1mmol/1). Most of the magnesium is excreted in the feces, and the remainder in the urine.

Magnesium deficiency

Magnesium deficiency occurs in:

- Starvation.
- Malabsorption syndrome.
- After very long-continued losses of gastro-intestinal fluids.
- After the use of intravenous fluids with magnesium-free solutions.
- Acute pancreatitis.
- Diabetic acidosis.
- Late stages of a major burn.

The magnesium ion is essential for the proper functioning of most enzyme systems. Thus depletion is characterized by *neuromuscular* and *central nervous system hyperactivity.* The symptoms are similar to those of calcium deficiency, including muscle tremors and tetany, progressing to delirium and convulsions in severe cases.

The diagnosis of magnesium deficiency cannot be made without awareness of the syndrome. *In the surgical patient who exhibits disturbed neuromuscular or cerebral activity in the postoperative period, magnesium deficiency must be kept in mind.* This is especially so if he has had long-continued dysfunction of the gastrointestinal tract and has been maintained on magnesium-free intravenous fluids. Cases of small gut fistulas of many weeks' duration provide most of the examples.

Treatment is by parenteral administration of magnesium sulphate or chloride. If renal function is normal 80 meq of magnesium sulphate are given over 6–8 hours. The pulse, blood pressure, respiration and ECG are monitored for signs of magnesium toxicity, which can cause cardiac arrest. Calcium chloride or gluconate should be available to counteract any adverse effects of a rapidly rising magnesium level.

Magnesium excess

Causes

- *The most common cause of hypermagnesemia (as of hyperkalemia) is severe renal insufficiency,* when the magnesium which is liberated during the normal processes of metabolism cannot be excreted.
- Magnesium excess is seen in *massive trauma* because large numbers of body cells are damaged, and the magnesium contained inside them is liberated into the extracellular fluid.
- Magnesium also moves out of the cells in *acidosis*.

Acute symptoms may be controlled by the slow intravenous administration of 5 to 10 meq of calcium chloride or gluconate. If elevated levels persist, peritoneal dialysis or hemodialysis is required.

NATURE AND QUANTITIES OF I.V. FLUIDS

Fluid requirements for metabolism

As stated before, an average adult consumes about 2,500ml of water daily. About 1,500ml water is taken by mouth, the rest being either extracted from solid food or gained as water of oxidation. The daily water losses include 800 to 1,500ml as urine, 600 to 900 as insensible loss, and 250ml in stools.

Even if a person is deprived of access to water he must still excrete a minimum of 500 to 800ml of urine per day in order to excrete the products of catabolism, in addition to the mandatory insensible loss through the skin and lungs. This insensible loss is increased by hypermetabolism, hyperventilation and fever. The loss due to fever amounts to about 250ml per degree centigrade of fever per day.

Nature of fluids lost during illness

Losses of extracellular fluid into the area of the operation or wound are isotonic. Gastrointestinal losses are usually isotonic or slightly hypotonic. Replacement of both these type of losses should be by isotonic salt solutions.

The solution most suitable for this purpose is *Lactated Ringer's solution*. Its composition is very similar to that of extracellular fluid. It contains 130 meq sodium balanced by 109 meq chloride and 28 meq lactate. This fluid has minimum effects on body fluid composition and pH even when infused in large quantities. *Normal saline contains too much chloride for routine use*. In Ringer's lactate this excess chloride is replaced by lactate, which has a very useful buffering action.

Table 7.1 Electrolyte content of parenteral fluids in mEq/l.

Solution	Cations					Anions	
	Na	K	Ca	Mg	NH_4	Cl	HCO_3
Extracellular fluid	142	4	5	3	0. 3	103	27
Lactated Ringer's	130	4	3			109	28*
0.9% sodium chloride	154					154	
M/6 sodium lactate	167*					167	

*Present as lactate, which is converted into bicarbonate

Constituents of available I.V. fluids

In the advanced countries the clinician describes the patient's clinical parameters as well as serum electrolyte values to the pharmacist, who prepares an appropriate mixture of fluids and electrolytes and sends it to the ward to be administered to the patient. Elsewhere in the world, however, the clinician has to fend for himself.

Before we discuss the replacement of the fluids lost due to illness, we should be conversant with the composition of the different fluids which are commercially available (Table 7.1):

5% glucose in water

This solution contains no electrolytes, and therefore electrolytically speaking, this is plain water. As explained before, the purpose of the 5% glucose is to render the fluid exactly isotonic with plasma, so that there is no hemolysis on its administration. At the same time, the glucose provides instantly available energy. This fluid is used where plain water is required.

Lactated ringer's solution

This is very similar, though not identical to, Hartmann's solution. As can be seen in (Table 7.1), it closely approximates the composition of tissue fluid. Therefore when tissue fluid is lost during operations, whether on the surface or into the 'third space', lactated Ringer's solution constitutes the appropriate replacement. At the same time this is a more physiological solution than normal saline, which contains much more chloride than tissue fluid. In Ringer's lactate, some of this chloride is replaced by lactate, which acts as a useful buffer to neutralize the excess acid produced in infections, trauma etc.

0.9% saline

('Normal' saline) If excessive vomiting has taken place with resultant loss of chloride, this is a more suitable fluid than Ringer's lactate.

l/6th molar and molar lactate

These solutions are used to buffer excess acid produced in cases of metabolic acidosis, e.g. in diabetes, extensive trauma and fulminant infections. If the acidosis is severe, full-strength i.e. molar lactate is used; if more moderate, l/6th molar lactate.

Which fluid to use?

Isotonic sodium chloride contains 154 meq of sodium and 154 meq of chloride per liter. The high concentration of chloride is a load on the kidneys that cannot be rapidly excreted. Thus dilutional acidosis may result. However, this solution is ideal where there is a deficit of extracellular fluid volume with hyponatremia, hypochloremia and metabolic alkalosis, as in *pyloric stenosis*.

On the other hand if volume deficit is present with metabolic acidosis, as in diabetes, *M/6 sodium lactate* may be given. The lactate is converted into bicarbonate and helps correct the acidosis.

If hyponatremia is so *severe* as to produce symptoms, the choice of fluid would again depend upon the accompanying acid-base derangement:

- If *acidosis* is present *molar sodium lactate* is used.
- In the case of *alkalosis 3% sodium chloride* may be employed.

When the pH has returned to normal the remainder of the volume deficit can be corrected by a balanced salt solution like *Ringer's lactate.*

ADMINISTRATION OF FLUIDS

Preoperative fluids

Correction of volume changes

The most frequent abnormalities noted in the surgical patient are changes in the volume of extracellular fluid, especially depletion. This may result from:

- External losses.
- Internal redistribution.

The 'third space'

As explained in detail earlier, internal redistribution is also called loss into a *'third space.'* Examples are seen in:

- Extensive burns.
- Crush injuries.
- Generalized peritonitis. Many liters may be lost into the peritoneal cavity.
- Inflammation or strangulation of the bowel. Swelling of the bowel and secretion of fluid into the lumen of the obstructed gut cause great losses.
- Massive infections of the subcutaneous tissues cause similar deficits.

Estimation of deficit

Exact measurement of these losses is impossible and unnecessary. An estimate of the deficit can be made from the severity of the clinical signs:

- Mild deficit represents a loss of approximately 4% of body weight.
- Moderate loss is about 7% of body weight.
- Severe loss equals about 10% of body weight.

In a 70kg man this would amount to 3, 5 and 7 liters respectively.

It should be remembered that when such a loss of extracellular fluid volume occurs rapidly, cardiovascular signs e.g. tachycardia and hypotension predominate, while the tissue signs are minimal or absent.

Fluid replacement should be started, and changed according to the response of the patient noted on frequent clinical observation. Successful resuscitation is indicated by:

- Reversal of the signs of volume deficit.
- Stabilization of the pulse and blood pressure.
- A urine volume of 30 to 50ml per hour.

It should be noted that in certain situations a high urinary output may be misleading. For example:

- The excessive administration of glucose may produce an osmotic diuresis.
- An osmotic agent like mannitol produces urine at the expense of vascular volume.
- Acute renal damage from shock and injury may impair the ability of the tubules to concentrate the urine, so that a large volume of dilute urine is produced.

When pure extracellular fluid volume loss has taken place, the use of a balanced salt solution such as lactated Ringer's is indicated.

Correction of concentration changes

The nature of the fluid required depends upon the type of disorder:

Severe hyponatremia

5% sodium chloride solution or molar sodium lactate is used, depending on the patient's acid-base status: chloride in cases with alkalosis, lactate for acidosis.

The sodium deficit can be estimated as follows:

- First estimate the deficit per liter by deducting the patient's serum sodium level from the normal sodium level.
- Then estimate the quantity of total body water in liters.
- Finally multiply the deficit per liter by the number of liters to obtain the total deficit.

Example

If a young adult female weighing 60kg has a serum sodium of 125 meq/1, the total deficit is calculated as follows:

In females, body water constitutes 50% of body weight.

Thus total body water = 60 x 0.5 = 30 liters.

Now the deficit per liter = 140 – 125 = 15 meq.

So the total deficit = 30 x 15 = 450 meq.

Half this calculated deficit is administered by intravenous infusion. Further correction is facilitated when renal function is restored by correcting the volume deficit.

Mild hyponatremia

In the presence of metabolic alkalosis, isotonic sodium chloride is used.

To correct acidosis, M/6 sodium lactate is employed.

When the pH change has been corrected, the remainder of the volume deficit can be repaired with lactated Ringer's solution.

Hyponatremia with volume excess

This is treated simply by restriction of water. As the excess water is excreted the serum sodium level rises to normal.

Severe hypernatremia with a volume deficit

5% glucose in water may be infused slowly until symptoms are relieved; as it is infused the volume deficit is made good, and at the same time the raised serum sodium level drops to normal due to dilution.

Correction of composition changes

Correction of a *potassium* deficit should be started only after an adequate urine output is obtained. Potassium chloride is available in 20 meq and 40 meq ampoules for addition to intravenous fluids. More than 40 meq should not be added to a liter of intravenous fluid. Potassium must never be given by direct injection, but by infusion.

Calcium and magnesium are rarely needed during preoperative preparation, except in acute pancreatitis, chronic starvation and massive subcutaneous infections.

Prolonged periods of fluid restriction, and the use of laxatives and enemas for preparation of bowel, may cause an acute loss of extracellular fluid. *Such losses should be recognized and corrected* to prevent complications during the operation.

Intraoperative fluids

If preoperative replacement of extracellular fluid volume has been incomplete, hypotension may develop during induction of anesthesia. *This should be prevented by replacing abnormal losses of fluids and electrolytes before operation.*

At the beginning of the 20th century it was discovered that after surgical operations changes occurred in urine output, blood volume and fluid and electrolyte composition. In the following 25 years saline solutions were given to patients undergoing operation, often in excessive amounts. Investigations carried out in the 1930s indicated that after surgical operations water and saline should be withheld, because most of the administered fluid is retained. Later work showed that proper management lies somewhere between the above two extremes. Some useful guidelines regarding fluid replacement during operations are as follows:

- Blood should be replaced as it is lost.
- Replacement of extracellular fluid should begin during the operative procedure. Balanced salt solution should be given during operation at the rate of 0.5 to 1 liter per hour. The maximum should not exceed 2 to 3 liters during a four-hour major abdominal procedure.

Postoperative fluids

The first day

Immediately after operation extracellular fluid may continue to be lost into the site of injury or operation. Several liters of extracellular fluid may be slowly deposited in such areas within a day or so after injury. This may produce circulatory instability. Postoperative hypotension and tachycardia require prompt investigation and proper therapy. The following parameters must be monitored carefully:

- Pulse rate and volume.
- Blood pressure.

- Skin warmth and color, and body temperature.
- Hourly urine output.

Circulatory instability is most often caused by underestimated losses of fluids. Careful monitoring will show oliguria in addition to the rapid pulse and low blood pressure. An additional 500–1,000ml of isotonic salt solution often resolves the problem. No potassium should be given during the first 24 hours unless a definite potassium deficit exists.

Later postoperative period

The problem is simply one of accurate measurement and replacement of all losses. This means the replacement of both the measurable losses which are mostly gastrointestinal, and the insensible losses.

Gastrointestinal losses are isotonic or slightly hypotonic, and are replaced by an isotonic salt solution. The amount of potassium required for replacement is 40 meq. daily for renal excretion of potassium, in addition to about 20 meq per liter for replacement of gastrointestinal losses if present.

The *insensible loss* is usually relatively constant, between 600 and 900ml daily. This may be increased by hypermetabolism, hyperventilation and fever to a maximum of about 1,500ml daily. It is replaced by 5% glucose in water.

Finally, in the *febrile* patient, sweating seldom exceeds 250ml per degree centigrade of fever per day, and should be replaced by 1/4 normal saline.

FLUID NEEDS IN NEWBORNS AND INFANTS

Before going into the details of fluid needs in the newborn, the following background must be kept in mind. In nature, whenever a female mammal gives birth, not only is the mother exhausted but the infant animal is also unable to look after itself properly. Therefore nature stuffs extra fluid and salt in the neonate to last it a few days. Similar is the case with the human being. When a baby is born it looks bloated due to extra salt and water. During the first few days the baby loses weight, and it should be remembered that most of this weight loss occurs due to excretion of the surplus salt and water. The stable position is arrived at in about a week's time.

As the infant grows older, through the months and years, his weight increases at a greater rate than his surface area. Fluid requirements depend greatly on the area of the surface from which fluid losses take place. As the surface area becomes relatively less with growth, the fluid requirements *per kilogram* gradually get reduced.

With this background it is easy to understand the water and salt requirements during infancy, if these have to be given intravenously.

Water requirements

First week

- On the day of birth the baby requires only about 60ml perkg per 24 hours.
- In two days, this figure rises to 80ml.
- It peaks at the age of one week at 100ml/kg/24 hours.

Later

After this the fluid needs gradually decline during childhood, as follows:

- Below a weight of 10kg the requirement remains at 100ml/kg/day.
- Between 10 and 20kg body weight, it is reduced to about 80ml/kg/day.
- Above 20kg body weight, it is reduced to about 60ml/kg/day.

All the above information can be expressed in an easy-to-remember formula (Table 7.2).

> *Note:* The formula consists of average figures, but what it loses in accuracy it more than gains by its ease of being committed to memory.

Table 7.2 Fluid volume requirements of an infant (in ml/kg/24 hours)

Age			Body weight	
0–2 days	3–7 days	7 days and > (<10kg)	10–20kg	>20kg
60	80	100	80	60

Salt requirements

How much *salt* should be added to this water? During the first one week the baby's body contains so much excess salt that he needs no more salt. Therefore, 5% glucose in water may be given. But the liver is immature and needs more glucose. So in fact 10% glucose in water is ordered. After one week the baby should be given the same proportion of salt as the older infant or adult, i.e. 1/5th normal saline. To sum up, the basal fluid requirements of the baby work out to be those given in (Table 7.3).

ASSESSING FLUID LOSS AT OPERATIONS

The composition of the fluid

The fluid lost at operation is tissue fluid. This is closely mimicked by Ringer's lactate solution. Therefore, apart from any blood given for blood loss, the entire fluid given after operation is commonly replaced by Ringer's lactate solution.

The amount to be replaced

A simple guideline for estimating third-space replacements after major abdominal surgery is as follows:

For each quadrant of the abdomen either affected by the disease process or involved in surgical dissection, one fourth of the maintenance volume of fluid will be required as additional increment for volume replacement of third-space shifts. As mentioned above, the fluid will not be hypotonic solution but

Ringer's lactate, preferably with 5% glucose. For example, if the maintenance volume for a patient was 2,000ml, for a one-quadrant dissection 500ml Ringer's lactate solution will be added.

Examples in a 10kg infant

- Procedure: *Appendectomy* (1 quadrant).

  Maintenance fluid: 10 x 100 = 1,000ml of ¼ normal saline.

  Operation losses: ¼ x 1,000 = 250ml of Ringer's lactate solution.
- Procedure: *Right hemicolectomy* for irreducible intussusception (2 quadrants).

  Maintenance fluid: 10 x 100 = 1,000ml of ¼ normal saline.

  Operation losses: 2 x ¼ x 1,000 = 500ml of Ringer's lactate solution.
- Procedure: *Malrotation* (4 quadrants)

  Maintenance fluid: 10 x 100 = 1,000ml of 1/4 normal saline.

  Operation losses: 4 x 1/4 x 1,000 = 1,000ml of Ringer's lactate solution.

When calculating for an operation on an area other than the abdomen, the procedure should be assessed as equivalent to an abdominal operation affecting one, two, or more quadrants, and the fluid needs determined accordingly.

Table 7.3 Basal fluid requirements of an infant

Age/weight	Volume of fluid/kg/24 hours
0–2days	60ml of 10% glucose in water
3–7 days	80ml of 10% glucose in water
7 days+ (but less than 10kg body weight)	100ml of 1/5 normal saline
10–20kg body weight	80ml of 1/5 normal saline
>20kg body weight	60ml of 1/5 normal saline

CALCULATING AN ACTUAL PATIENT'S REQUIREMENTS

A useful method of calculating the fluid needs of a patient over a 24-hour period is to prepare a proforma as in (Table 7.4).

The various losses which commonly require replacement include maintenance requirements, operation losses (into the 'third space'), gastrointestinal losses (e.g. vomiting, diarrhea or losses from fistulae), losses due to fever, and last but not least, summer losses in tropical countries:

- The basal *maintenance* requirements never vary, and as explained at the beginning of this chapter, in the case of a 70kg man amount to about 2,500ml of l/5th normal saline.
- *Operation losses* depend upon the severity of the

Table 7.4 Proforma for calculating a patient's requirements

	Glucose 5% in 1/5 normal saline	Ringer's lactate solution	Other, e.g. blood, molar lactate etc./ (where indicated)
Maintenance volume			
Operation losses			
G.I. losses			
Losses due to fever			
Summer losses			
Totals			

operation. As explained above, a simple guideline for assessing third-space losses after major surgery is as follows:

For each quadrant of the abdomen either affected by the acute illness or involved in surgical dissection, a quarter of the maintenance volume of fluid will be required as an additional increment for volume replacement of third-space shifts. This fluid is preferably Ringer's lactate, as it closely resembles the extra-cellular fluid which is lost.

- *Gastrointestinal losses* also approximate Ringer's lactate in composition, except that during vomiting more acid is lost, and during diarrhea there is a greater loss of potassium.
- As mentioned above, in a 70kg man each degree centigrade of *fever* increases the water loss by about 250ml per day. This fluid is probably about one fifth normal saline.
- Similarly, due to acclimatization and salt conservation, *summer losses* are also probably about one-fifth normal saline.

Example

Let us take the example of a 70kg man who undergoes appendectomy in a tropical country during the month of May. He is running a temperature of 39°C.

The requirements can be worked out as follows:

- Maintenance needs: 2500ml glucose 5% in l/5th normal saline.
- Operation losses: 2500 x 1/4 = 625ml (Hartmann's)(as 1 quadrant is dissected in appendectomy).
- G.I. losses: Nil.
- Fever losses: 500ml (1/4 normal saline). (2 x 250ml)
- Summer losses: 1,000ml (1/4 normal saline).

(approx.)

Entering these data in a chart like (Table 7.4) is a useful method of ensuring that all the different types of losses are not only considered, but also their volumes are calculated and added to make up the total volume of fluid to be infused.

INTRAVENOUS ALIMENTATION

If fluids have to be administered intravenously for a prolonged period of time, water and electrolytes are not sufficient. Nutrients must also be given, otherwise the body's own tissues are burnt, and the patient starts losing weight rapidly. Each of the major types of nutrients must be given for optimal effect. Carbohydrates are utilized for ready energy, and proteins as replacement for wear and tear of cells and for synthesizing enzymes and hormones. Fats are given not only to serve as energy stores, but also for providing the essential fatty acids.

The nutrient fluids commonly available include the following:

- *Glucose,* 10% and 25% solutions.
- *Amino acid solutions.* Usually these contain a 5% solution of the different essential amino acids in 10% sucrose.
- *Fat emulsions.* These come in two concentrations, 10% and 20%.

When nutrients are given parenterally, there is an optimal ratio between their quantities which is desirable. This is necessary in order to ensure the correct number of protein and non-protein calories, as well as enough fats for essential fatty acids.

A suitable proportion of these fluids for most cases requiring parenteral nutrition is as follows:

10% glucose solution	4 parts.
Amino acid solution	3 parts.
Fat emulsion	1 part.

It may be mentioned that such a solution is likely to contain insufficient quantities of the different electrolytes, namely sodium, potassium, and chloride, and these have to be topped up appropriately. Most of the above-mentioned solutions can be given through the peripheral veins, which is very convenient. However, if 25% glucose solution or 20% fat emulsion have to be employed, the infusion has to be given through one of the central veins.

Central venous lines

When fluids have to be given intravenously, they are normally administered through one of the peripheral veins, commonly in an arm or a leg. However, in two types of situations it is preferable to use one of the central veins, commonly either the subclavian or the internal jugular veins:

- *Intravenous alimentation.* The hyperalimentation fluids, e.g. 25% glucose, are markedly hyperosmolar, and can cause thrombophlebitis if given into a peripheral vein. In the great veins the rapid flow of blood quickly dilutes the fluid, so that it cannot damage the intima of the vein. Therefore these concentrated fluids are best given into the great veins, i.e. the venae cavae. Hoever, recently there as been a move away from hyperalimentation .

- *Conditions of hemodynamic instability.* If the patient is not hemodynamically stable, as in hypovolaemia or hypervolaemia, it is important to know the level of pressure in the central veins (central venous pressure) so that the correct volume of fluids can be infused.

Water manometer

For this purpose, a water manometer is constructed as follows:

A needle is passed into the subclavian or internal jugular vein, and through the needle a catheter is passed into the vein and advanced so that its tip lies in the superior vena cava. The catheter is now connected to the intravenous drip tubing through a 3-way stopcock. To the side-arm of the stopcock is attached a tubing which is fixed in a vertical position, with a measuring tape fixed along its side (Fig.7.1). The intravenous fluid is allowed to flow into the vertically fixed tubing, and to fill it up. The zero level of the measuring tape is kept at the level of the manubrium sterni. When the lever of the stopcock is rotated so that the central veins are in communication with the vertically fixed tubing, the height of the fluid column in the tubing indicates the central venous pressure.

The normal level of central venous pressure recorded at the sternal angle varies between 1 and 7cm of water. If the pressure is low, the venous return should be supplemented by intravenous infusion; if excessively high, intravenous diuretics may be required.

Electronic transducers

Electronic transducers can be connected to the central venous tubing, and give more accurate *and continuous* readings.

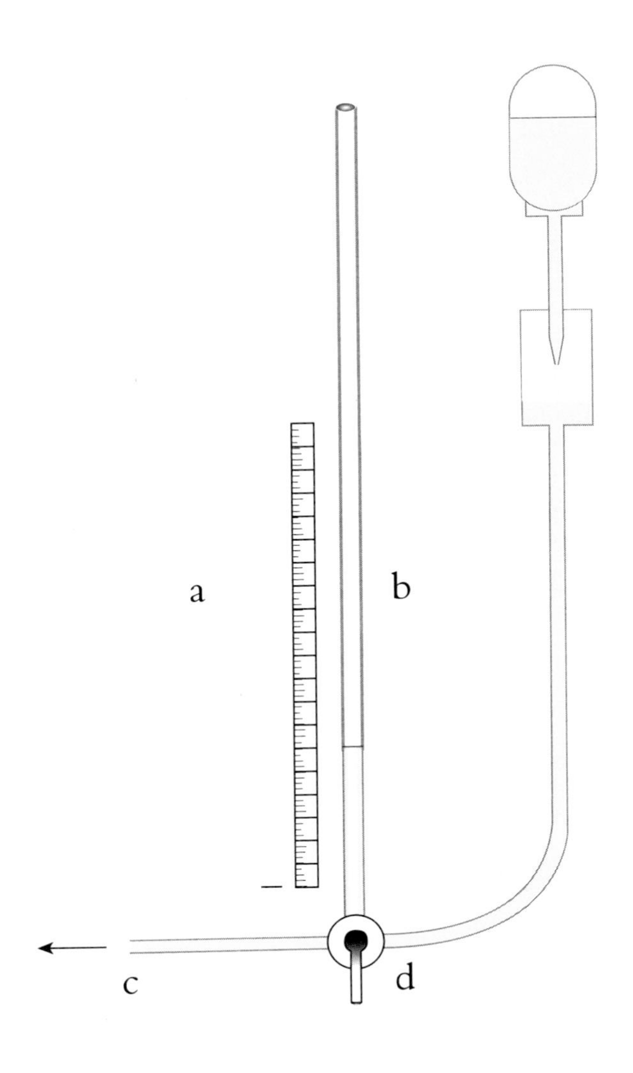

Fig.7.1 Water manometer for measuring central venous pressure. a. ruler, b. water column, c. tubing leading to patient, d. 3-way stopcock

Chapter

8 PREOPERATIVE PREPARATION

Before a patient can be subjected to the stress of anesthesia and surgery, an assessment must be made of his suitability for surgery. It should be remembered that when a person takes exercise, the oxygen demand of his body increases. He gets exhausted early if the exercise is too hard or he is not in good health. Similarly, due to the stress of surgery, the oxygen demands of the body increase, and the patient gets exhausted if the surgery is extensive or he is not keeping good health.

Changes produced by stress

The stress of surgery produces a number of physiological changes:

- *Metabolic changes.* There is an increase in the metabolism, which is dependent on the extent of the surgery. This results in an increased oxygen demand, which increases the burden on the cardiorespiratory system.
- *Endocrine changes.* The levels of stress hormones including catecholamines, steroids and antidiuretic hormone rise. The result is hyperglycemia, catabolism, and fluid and salt retention.
- *Surgical bleeding* results in activation of the hemostatic system. This system may become uncontrolled and increase the risk of arterial and venous thrombosis.

PREOPERATIVE ASSESSMENT

The *objectives* of preoperative assessment of the patient are the following:

- To assess the ability of the patient to withstand the stress of surgery and the resultant physiological changes.
- To optimise the patient for surgery; this may require modification of his lifestyle, and changes in the treatment he is receiving for concurrent medical diseases.
- To formulate an anesthetic plan and discuss it with the patient.
- To get an informed consent for surgery and anesthesia.

Preoperative assessment has several *components:*

- A history is obtained.
- A complete physical examination is carried out.
- Laboratory and imaging investigations that can help in the management of the patient are requested.

History

History includes history of present illness, past history and family history.

History of present illness

This includes the reason the patient is undergoing surgery, the events leading to this condition and any associated ongoing medical illnesses.

Past history

This deals with any medical illnesses in the past. In case of chronic medical conditions like diabetes mellitus and hypertension a complete history of the course of the disease including duration, treatment and end-organ effects, and current state of control should be obtained. History of previous anesthetic exposures is very important.

A history of allergy to foods, drugs and latex is important as these events become very difficult to manage during anesthesia.

Family history

This is similarly important. Genetic disorders like malignant hyperthermia and pseudocholinesterase deficiency run in families and a history of a problem during anesthesia in a family member may require further workup and modification of anesthetic technique.

Physical examination

Physical examination is carried out in a systematic manner:

Table 8.1. Physical activities described in METS

ACTIVITY	METS
Sleeping	0.9
Walking @ 4 miles/hour	4.5
Jogging or running	>6.0
Swimming (fast)	7.0
Squash	12.0

General physical examination

This includes height and weight measurement, and looking for the presence of edema, pallor, jaundice or cyanosis. Obese patients are at high risk of complications; they should be identified for detailed systemic examination. The pulse should be checked for rate and rhythm; blood pressure should be checked in both arms, preferably with the patient lying down and standing up.

Examination of the airway

This is essential for all patients requiring anesthesia. Signs of a difficult airway include:

- Receding chin.
- Thick neck, prominent incisors, large tongue.
- Restricted neck movements at the atlanto-occipital joint.

Systematic examination

This should include a detailed examination of the CVS and respiratory systems, looking for signs of obstructive or restrictive airway disease, heart failure or cardiac murmurs. The carotid arteries should be auscultated for a bruit.

Neurological injuries may occur during anesthesia. Any pre-existing neurological impairment should be identified and documented before surgery.

Laboratory investigations

There is no place for routine investigations for all patients; they increase the cost of surgery and cause unnecessary delay. Laboratory tests should be ordered in the light of the history and physical examination. Certain tests are, however, routinely recommended in some population groups:

- Hemoglobin in all children, and in women of menstruating age.
- Renal function in all elderly, hypertensive and diabetic patients.
- ECG in all patients above 65 years, and in patients with longstanding diabetes or hypertension.
- The value of a routine x-ray chest is doubtful; it should be ordered if the history and clinical examination suggests its need.
- Some centres suggest routine screening for Hepatitis B and C, keeping in view the prevalence of the disease in the population to protect the medical staff. It is more rational to treat all patients as potential carriers and take universal precautions to avoid contamination.

Assessment of physical activity

The level of routine physical activity is a good indicator of the general health of the patient. If someone gives a history of ischemic heart disease but jogs for 30 minutes without any symptoms, there is reason to believe that the disease is stable and does not need further testing before surgery. Similarly a 70 year old who walks in the park at a brisk pace for one hour every day is healthier than a 50 year old who gets breathless after walking for 15 minutes.

METS

Exercise capacity is described in terms of metabolic equivalents (MET). One MET is equal to the amount of energy expenditure of an average resting adult, who consumes 250ml of oxygen per minute. The intensity of the physical activity is measured in multiples of one MET. (Table 8.1) gives the relationship between routine daily physical activities and METs.

Predicting the risk

Clinicians would like to know the risk to the patient before taking him to surgery. One such association between the condition of the patient and the risk of complications of surgery is suggested by the American Society of Anesthesiologitsts, which classifies patients into 5 categories according to the presence of systemic disease and its effect on physical activity (Table 8.2). It has been shown that the risk of complications increases manifold as the patient moves from ASA class 1 to 5. Further, the risk is doubled in case of emergency surgery.

Who should perform the preoperative evaluation?

An anesthetist is generally considered to be the most suitable person to perform pre-anesthetic evaluation. Due to busy operating room schedules they are not always available in the outpatient department when patients are being scheduled for surgery. It is therefore important that surgeons should look for concurrent medical illness and arrange for the patient to be seen by the anesthetist before scheduling the operation. This will prevent the operations from being postponed on the day of surgery. The anesthetist will, after a thorough history and clinical examination, order necessary investigations, and ask for a specialist consultation if required.

Standard questions

A few standard questions can help identify the patients requiring a more detailed assessment:

- Do you suffer from *diabetes, or blood pressure*?
- Have you felt *chest pain* or discomfort in the past?
- How much can you *walk* without getting tired or breathless?
- Have you *seen a doctor* or a healthcare provider for any symptoms that have been distressing you in the recent past?
- Are you taking any *medicines* that your doctor told you to take continuously?
- Have you been *anesthetised* in the past? Was the anesthesia uneventful?
- Do you have *allergy* to any drug or food item? How severe was the allergic response when *it occurred?*
- *Do you smoke*? Since when and how many cigarettes every day?
- Do you *drink* alcohol or take any illicit substance?

An important issue is when to seek consultation from other specialties. Physicians often write comments like "fit for anesthesia and surgery". They should keep in mind that only the surgeon and anesthetist can decide about the patient's fitness for anesthesia. Others should suggest management of the patients in their area of expertise, and in the end inform whether the patient's medical condition is optimized or they need more time to make it better.

Table 8.2. The ASA physical status classification

1.	Healthy person.
2.	Mild systemic disease.
3.	Severe systemic disease.
4.	Severe systemic disease that is a constant threat to life.
5.	A moribund person who is not expected to survive without the operation.

Note: If the surgery is an emergency, the physical status number is followed by an 'E', for example '3E'.

COMMON MEDICAL CONDITIONS AND THEIR EFFECTS ON ANESTHESIA AND SURGERY

These include the following:

Anemia

Whatever the underlying cause of anemia, it compromises the oxygen carrying capacity of the blood. Surgery involves blood loss, which may aggravate the anemia when the loss is significant.

Cardiac disease

Many patients above 40 years of age present with ischemic heart disease. The patient may give a history of angina or myocardial infarction. These patients are at risk of myocardial infarction, serious arrhythmias or heart failure in the perioperative period. The risk depends on the severity of the disease and the type of surgery.

The American Heart Association has determined the risk predictors for cardiac patients undergoing non-cardiac surgery:

- ***Major risk predictors.*** Unstable angina, recent myocardial infarction, major arrhythmias and heart failure.
- ***Clinical risk predictors.*** History of heart disease, compensated or prior heart failure, cerebrovascular disease, diabetes mellitus, and renal insufficiency.
- ***Type of surgery:***
    - o *High risk.* Major vascular surgery.
    - o *Intermediate risk.* Carotid endarterectomy; orthopedic surgery; prostate surgery; intraperitoneal and intrathoracic surgery; head and neck.
    - o *Low risk.* Endoscopic procedures; eye; breast surgery; superficial procedures.

Patients who have undergone coronary interventions like angioplasty and stenting or coronary artery bypass grafting in the past and are receiving prophylactic antiplatelet therapy, have an increased risk of bleeding during surgery. Withdrawing these agents increases the risk of coronary thrombosis. These drugs need to be stopped for at least 7 days before surgery, in consultation with the cardiologist.

Pulmonary diseases

Chronic obstructive pulmonary disease, infections of the respiratory tract and bronchial asthma are common medical problems. They compromise the patient's ability to cough or take deep breaths, which increases the risk of postoperative pneumonia. Restrictive lung diseases are less common but these patients can go into respiratory failure if they have a poor reserve. These patients should be carefully assessed. Pulmonary function tests can give very useful information; they should be requested when the disease is significant. Preoperative preparation should include:

- Control of active infection.
- Chest physiotherapy and removal of secretions.
- Incentive spirometry (a simple device that helps increase the inspiratory effort).

Diabetes mellitus

With the incidence of diabetes on the rise, a large number of patients presenting for surgery are likely to be diabetics. Management of diabetic patients presents many challenges to the anesthetist. The patients suffer from long-term end-organ complications and control of the blood sugar may be impaired due to the stress of surgery.

Long-term complications of diabetes include:

- Nephropathy.
- Autonomic and sensory neuropathy.
- Ischemic heart disease.
- Cardiomyopathy.

The result in advanced cases is ischemic heart disease, heart failure, and chronic renal failure. Patients with diabetic autonomic neuropathy may experience severe hypotension during anesthesia.

The patients have to fast in preparation for surgery; oral hypoglycemic agents are withdrawn and replaced with insulin in most cases. Stress of surgery changes the metabolic balance of the body. These patients may go into hypoglycemia, hyperglycemia or diabetic ketoacidosis.

These complications can be prevented by careful preoperative preparation and good diabetic control during the perioperative period.

Hypertension

This is defined as a blood pressure of more than 140/90 on 2 or more occasions. Hypertensives are at a high risk of developing ischemic heart disease, heart failure, cerebrovascular accidents and renal dysfunction. Serious blood pressure swings are seen during anesthesia in poorly controlled hypertensive patients. It is desirable that patients undergoing surgery should have their blood pressure controlled before surgery unless the operation is an emergency where blood pressure control is continued during surgery.

Renal dysfunction

Patients with diabetes mellitus or hypertension, and the elderly, have varying degrees of renal dysfunction, and the risk of postoperative renal failure is increased by:

- Excessive blood loss and hypotension during anesthesia.
- Nephrotoxic drugs like non-steroidal anti-inflammatory analgesics and aminoglycoside antibiotics.
- Contrast media used for imaging.

Serum creatinine gives a good estimate of renal function; it should be checked in all diabetic and hypertensives, and in patients above 65 years of age.

Liver disease

Patients may present with acute hepatitis or cirrhosis leading to liver failure. Liver disease increases the risk of bleeding during surgery, interferes with drug metabolism, alters the fluid and electrolyte balance. Anesthesia and surgery on the other hand can cause liver injury particularly when hepatic blood flow is compromised during surgery. Anesthesia in the patient with liver failure is associated with high mortality. Raised aminotransferases are strongly suggestive of liver injury; a rise of more than twice normal requires consultation with a hepatologist. Serum albumin, bilirubin and prothrombin time are indicators of synthetic and metabolic functions of the liver.

Neurological and muscular disorders

Neuromuscular disorders, both congenital and acquired, can affect the course of anesthesia. Whereas the effect of non-depolarizing muscle relaxants is exaggerated in patients with myopathies, giving succinylcholine to these patients can cause cardiac arrest due to massive potassium release. Similar effect is seen in patients with poliomyelitis, motor neurone disease and paraplegias. It is important to identify these conditions preoperatively to avoid life-threatening situations.

Patients with neurological conditions like Parkinsonism and epilepsy sometimes receive medication that may adversely interact with anesthetic agents. Withdrawal of drug therapy can aggravate the medical condition. These patients need to be carefully evaluated and prepared before surgery. A neurology consultation may be required to change the drug regime.

PREOPERATIVE PREPARATION

Surgery is scheduled once it is agreed that the benefit of surgery is more than any risk due to extensive surgery or the patient's medical condition. Preparation for surgery requires a systematic approach:

- Discuss the risks and benefits of anesthesia and surgery and get an informed consent.
- Give clear instructions to the patient about preoperative fasting.
- Patients with medical illnesses are taking drugs that interact with the anesthetic agents or otherwise have an adverse effect on the course of anesthesia and surgery. Withdrawal of these medicines on the other hand can lead to exacerbation of the medical condition. They should be given precise instructions on whether to continue or stop these drugs. Current evidence suggests as follows:
    - *Oral hypoglycemics* should be stopped before surgery. These are substituted with plain insulin on a sliding scale for procedures that require more than 12 hours fast.
    - *Antihypertensive drugs* are continued on the day of surgery. Some institutions stop ACE inhibitors on the morning of surgery because there is some evidence that they may cause hypotension during anesthesia.
    - *Statins, nitrates and beta blockers* should be continued in patients with ischemic heart disease in the perioperative period.
    - *Tricyclic antidepressants and monoamine oxidase inhibitors* have a potential to cause serious drug interactions with some of the drugs used during anesthesia. Antidepressants have a long half-life and their withdrawal can cause serious depression. These drugs should be continued and their interactions should be kept in mind while planning the anesthetic.
    - Patients receiving *anticoagulant or antiplatelet drugs* pose a unique challenge. These drugs need to be discontinued to avoid excessive bleeding. Antiplatelet drugs like aspirin and clopidogril should be stopped seven days before surgery; risk of coronary thrombosis must be kept in mind while doing so. Oral anticoagulant *warfarin* should be stopped at least five days before surgery and prothromin time should be monitored in case of patients on long-term anticoagulation.
    - *Low molecular weight heparins* (LMWH) are frequently used for prevention of deep vein thrombosis; they are continued in the perioperative period unless there is a surgical contraindication. They are omitted on the morning of surgery and started again when the surgeon feels comfortable after the procedure. It is recommended that spinal or epidural block should be given 12 hours after the last dose of LMWH.

Preoperative preparation and boils

In elective operations make sure there is no septic focus anywhere in the body, even such innocuous lesions as boils. If present, they must be treated first before scheduling the operation. Otherwise, with the resistance of the patient lowered due to the trauma of surgery, infection may metastasize to other parts of the body including the surgical wound, with serious consequences for the patient.

Preoperative fasting

The following instructions for fasting are given to all patients to prevent vomiting or regurgitation of the food during anesthesia:

- Have a light meal six hours before anesthesia.
- Clear fluids may be continued upto three hours before anesthesia.
- For children, mother's milk can be continued until four hours before operation, but one should wait for six hours before anesthesia if the child is fed formula or cow's milk.

It may be mentioned that these recommendations are not valid if gastric emptying is delayed due to any reason or the patient has gastric reflux. In this case the duration of the fast should be prolonged.

To conclude, the detection of any factors that can result in disturbances of metabolism, and corrective action concerning them, considerably reduces the risks of anesthesia and surgery.

Chapter

9 ANESTHESIA

Surgical procedures can only be performed well if the patient feels no pain and the surgeon has a free access to the surgical field during the procedure. The anesthesiologist provides these conditions to the surgeon by using one of the two techniques: general anesthesia and regional anesthesia.

GENERAL ANESTHESIA

General anesthesia is defined as the induction of a state of unconsciousness with the absence of pain sensation over the entire body, through the administration of anesthetic drugs.

There are three components of general anesthesia:

- Amnesia. The patient remains unconscious during the procedure and has no recall of the events afterwards.
- Analgesia. The patient feels no pain during the procedure. However, a painful stimulus will cause increase in heart rate and blood pressure even in an anesthetised patient.
- Muscle relaxation. The muscle tone is abolished to give free access to the surgeon.

Properties of a good anesthetic agent

These include:

- Analgesia and muscle relaxation during the surgical procedure.
- Rapid elimination of the drug from the brain allowing rapid recovery from anesthesia.
- No interaction with other drugs and agents.
- Absence of side effects.

Combinations of drugs

None of the available drugs fulfills all these criteria; therefore the anesthetists use combinations of drugs to achieve their goals. Intravenous or inhalational anesthetic agents are used to induce and maintain amnesia; analgesia is provided with systemic analgesics or neuronal blockade. Muscle relaxants are not required in every case; they are used when needed to provide muscular relaxation. They paralyse the respiratory muscles also; therefore these patients need positive-pressure ventilation with a ventilator.

INTRAVENOUS ANESTHETIC AGENTS

These induce a rapid and smooth sleep. They are short acting, the affect of a single dose lasting about 3–5 minutes. They are commonly used for induction of anesthesia; maintenance with these drugs would require repeated boluses or a continuous infusion. Currently available intravenous anesthetic agents include the following:

Propofol

This is an alkylphenol, which is prepared in a lipid emulsion. It induces sleep rapidly with a dose of 1.5–3.0mg/kg.The duration of effect is 3–5 minutes. There is a risk of severe hypotension with these doses, particularly in patients who are hemodynamically compromised.

Propofol does not have an analgesic effect. It has the advantage that it can be given as intermittent boluses on continuous infusion without the risk of delayed recovery. It is very effectively used in the technique called *total intravenous anesthesia* as a sole agent for induction and maintenance of anesthesia.

Ketamine

This is the only anesthetic available that has analgesic properties. A dose of 3–5mg/kg induces sleep in less than one minute, the effect lasting for 10–15 minutes. It is a strong analgesic in a dose of 0.2–0.5mg/kg. Muscle tone is maintained, therefore there are less chances of airway obstruction. It can also be given in repeated doses or as a continuous infusion. These characteristics make it a useful drug for battlefield conditions. However, its use by untrained people has caused many deaths, and it should be used only when people who are trained in the management of the airway are monitoring the patient. Side-effects include increased salivary secretions and hallucinations.

Benzodiazepines

These are normally used as sedatives; they can be used for induction of anesthesia at higher doses. *Midazolam* is the drug of choice due to its short recovery time and strong amnesic effect. It is commonly used to reduce the requirement of other anesthetic agents in hemodynamically compromised patients.

Dexmedetomidine

This is a highly selective α_2 blocker that is used for sedation in the ICU. It can also be used for preoperative sedation to reduce the requirement of anesthetic agents and prevent a rise in the blood pressure and heart rate on laryngoscopy and intubation. It can cause a significant fall in blood pressure. It is expensive and currently not available in most of the developing countries.

INHALATION ANESTHESIA

In this technique small amounts of anesthetic agents are added to the inspired gases, resulting in loss of consciousness. Currently available agents are volatile liquids that are added to the inspired air.

Nitrous oxide

This is a gas which has some anesthetic properties; it is used to provide analgesia and reduce the requirement of anesthetic agents.

Anesthesia machine

The technique requires a special delivery apparatus commonly known as an anesthesia machine. The components of the anesthesia machine include:

- *Cylinders* containing compressed oxygen, nitrous oxide and air stored under high pressure. They are mounted on the machine or kept in a dedicated area outside the operating room and delivered to the machine through a system of pipes (central supply of gases).
- *Regulators* deliver these gases to the machine at a working pressure.
- *Flowmeters* control the flow and ratio of gas mixture, which passes through the vaporizer.
- *Vaporizers* control the amount of anesthetic agent added to the gas mixture.
- The *delivery system* conveys a controlled mixture of gases to the patient.

This system must ensure a minimum concentration of oxygen in inspired air and get rid of exhaled carbon dioxide from the expired air.

Inhalation anesthetic agents

Halogenated hydrocarbons

Currently available agents, with the exception of nitrous oxide, are halogenated hydrocarbons. *They cause anesthesia but do not possess analgesic properties.* When the agent is added to a gas mixture its concentration in the alveoli rises; the level in the brain rises simultaneously, causing anesthesia. They are largely removed from the body through the lungs; only a small percentage is metabolized in the liver.

Other effects

Other effects of these agents include cardiac depression, vasodilatation and bronchial dilatation. Cardiac depression is counteracted by reflex sympathetic stimulation.

Difference between agents

The difference between individual agents is due to the speed of onset and termination of anesthesia. This varies with the solubility of the agent in the blood. The more soluble agents have more rapid onset of anesthesia and recovery.

The common agents

These include:

Halothane

This is the oldest of this group. It has the slowest onset and recovery profile among this group. A pleasant smell makes it suitable for inhalation induction in children. There is less sympathetic stimulation leading to bradycardia, hypotension and arrhythmias. It is an economical agent, which is very useful in trained hands but it has recently fallen out of favor in the affluent countries.

Isoflurane

This has an irritant smell; induction and recovery times are faster than halothane. It causes vasodilatation and reflex tachycardia in clinical concentrations. Cerebral and splanchnic blood flows are maintained which makes it a useful agent in neuroanesthesia and patients with compromised liver function.

Sevoflurane

This has a sweet smell, a rapid induction and recovery profile. It causes vasodilatation and reflex tachycardia. It is the agent of choice for induction of anesthesia in children.

Desflurane

This has the fastest induction and recovery times. Hemodynamic effects are favorable. High cost and need for special vaporizers have prevented its widespread use.

MUSCLE RELAXANTS AND REVERSAL AGENTS

Muscle relaxants

Muscle relaxation is required during anesthesia to facilitate endotracheal intubation and provide good exposure for surgery. Muscle relaxants reduce the need for anesthetic agents but they should not be used as substitutes for anesthesia because a paralyzed patient may be awake yet unable to move. *It must be emphasized that these drugs cause paralysis of respiratory muscles; ventilation should be supported in all patients receiving muscle relaxants.*

These drug act on the acetylcholine receptors situated on the neuromuscular junction. They are classified into two groups according to their effect on acetylcholine receptors:

- ***Depolarizing muscle relaxants***. The drug binds to the acetylcholine receptors and causes membrane depolarization resulting in uncoordinated muscle contraction (seen as fasciculation). This is followed by a period of paralysis.

  Succinylcholine. This is the only drug available for clinical use in this group. It has a rapid onset of effect and brief duration of action. The onset of effect is within 60–90 seconds and the effect lasts 3–5 minutes; this makes it the drug of choice when rapid intubation is required.

  In patients with burns and conditions associated with muscle wasting, muscle fasciculations may increase intracranial pressure and cause release of large amounts of potassium, leading to life-threatening hyperkalemia.

- ***Non-depolarizing muscle relaxants***. These drugs are competitive antagonists on acetylcholine receptors. Their onset of effect is slower and duration of effect longer than succinylcholine. The drugs are classified according to their chemical structure or duration of effect:
  - ***Aminosteroids***. These include:
    - *Vecuronium*; this has minimal effects on cardiovascular or respiratory systems.
    - *Rocuronium*; this has the most rapid onset among all non-depolarizing agents.
    - *Pancuronium*.
  - ***Benzylisoquinolines***. These include *atracurium* and *cis-atracurium*.

Their metabolism is independent of the liver and kidney, which makes them ideal for use in patients with renal or hepatic failure

Reversal agents

The effect of non-depolarizing agents can be reversed by administering an anticholinesterase, which increases the amount of acetylcholine at the neuromuscular junction.

Neostigmine is one such drug, which is given in combination with atropine or glycopyrrolate for this purpose.

Recently, *sugamadex* has been introduced for rapid reversal of the effect of rocuronium by forming a bond and removing them from their site of action.

COMPLICATIONS OF GENERAL ANESTHESIA

Airway obstruction

The pharynx is a soft and collapsible structure. During anesthesia the tongue falls back against the posterior pharyngeal wall and muscles of the palate lose their tone, resulting in airway obstruction. Airway obstruction was the most common cause of mortality during the early days of anesthesia. Different techniques and equipment have developed over a period of time to ensure a patent airway during anesthesia.

Aspiration of gastric contents

If the acidic gastric contents are regurgitated during anesthesia, they can enter the airway since the airway's protective reflexes are diminished. This results in severe lung injury depending on the volume and acidity of gastric contents.

Gastric contents are increased in:

- Intestinal obstruction.
- Pregnancy.
- Morbid obesity.
- Patients who had a recent meal.
- Gastroesophageal reflux disease; this increases the risk of regurgitation.

The following measures are recommended in all patients at increased risk of aspiration:

- *Proton pump inhibitors.*
- *Prokinetic agents* like metachlopramide are used to promote gastric emptying.
- The airway is protected with an *endotracheal tube.*

Hemodynamic changes

Factors contributing to these changes include:

- Cardiac depressant and vasodilator effects of anesthetic agents.
- Blood loss and fluid shifts during surgery.
- Pain.
- Stimulation of autonomic nervous system. Tachycardia, bradycardia, hypotension and hypertension are all dangerous. Patients with cardiac disease or those undergoing significant blood loss will require *continuous monitoring* and tight control of blood pressure.

Hypothermia

A fall in body temperature below 35^{0}C during surgery increases the risk of wound infections and cardiac arrhythmias; it causes postoperative shivering and increased oxygen demand. Body temperature is maintained during anesthesia by measures like covering the patient and avoiding cold infusions. Active warming is sometimes required, particularly in children.

Hypoxia

Failure of oxygen delivery from the anesthesia machine was a common cause of death during anesthesia in earlier days. Safety features have been incorporated in recent models to prevent delivery of hypoxic mixture of gases.

REGIONAL ANESTHESIA

Local anesthetics block nerve transmission by blocking voltage-gated sodium channels. Nerve fibers are enclosed in sheaths, which form a barrier to drug penetration; the drug should reach the nerve membrane in sufficient quantity to block impulse transmission. Concentration of the drug required to block individual fibres depends on the diameter of the nerve fibres. Smaller fibres carrying pain sensations are blocked more easily than large motor fibers.

Local anesthetics

These are classified according to their chemical structure:

- *Amide linked* drugs are metabolized by the liver.
- *Ester linked* drugs are metabolized by plasma cholinesterases.

Names of commercially available local anesthetics belonging to each group are shown in (Table 9.1).

Supplements to local anesthetics

- *Adrenaline* is used to prolong the effect of local anesthetics.
- *Opioids* are commonly used in the spinal and epidural spaces to reduce the need for local anesthetics and prolong their side-effects.
- Tramadol, Clonidine and Ketamine have also been employed to increase the duration of analgesia.

TECHNIQUES OF REGIONAL ANESTHESIA

These include the following:

- *Nerve* blocks.
- *Plexus* blocks e.g. brachial plexus, cervical plexus, lumbar or sacral plexus.
- *Central neuraxial* blocks e.g. spinal or epidural anesthesia.

Nerve and plexus blocks

These require a sound knowledge of anatomy. Nerves are identified by:

- Eliciting paraesthesias when the needle touches the nerve.
- Using electrical stimulation and ultrasound guidance.

Central neuraxial blocks

These involve blocking impulse transmission in the spinal cord or spinal nerves. The techniques used are:

- *Spinal anesthesia.* These drugs are injected into the cerebrospinal fluid (CSF). A small amount of local anesthetic will block a large area of the body.
- *Epidural anesthesia.* These drugs are injected into the epidural space. A large volume of drug is required to block multiple spinal segments. The catheter may be left in the space for intermittent injections or continuous infusion.
- *Combined spinal and epidural anesthesia.* The epidural space is approached with a wide-bore needle; a spinal needle is passed through it to inject local anesthetic into the CSF. The spinal needle is withdrawn and a catheter is passed into the epidural space for subsequent injections.

Complications and side-effects of central neuraxial blocks

- *Hypotension.* Blockade of sympathetic nerves results in vasodilatation and fall in blood pressure. The degree of hypotension depends on the number of spinal segments blocked. Hypotension may become severe and life-threatening if not treated with vasopressors and intravenous fluids. These techniques should be avoided in patients with limited cardiac reserve.

- *Total spinal anesthesia.* Inadvertent injection of a large dose of local anesthetic into the subarachnoid space will result in paralysis of respiratory muscles and extreme hemodynamic instability requiring cardio-respiratory support till the block wears off.
- *Post-dural-puncture headache.* Puncture of the dura mater leads to leakage of CSF. If this leak is significant the patient will develop severe headache, which is aggravated on standing. Headache occurs in 0.2–25% of all the patients receiving spinal anesthesia; it is more common and severe with large-bore cutting spinal needles. Management consists of rest, analgesics and plenty of fluids; injection of patient's fresh blood in the epidural space "epidural blood patch" can seal the leak; this is considered to be a definitive treatment of this kind of headache.
- *Backache.* This is a distressing problem that is the most frequent cause of the patient's refusal to receive repeated spinal or epidural anesthesia. It is more common with epidural than spinal technique for unknown reasons.
- *Neurological injury.* This is uncommon, but the results can be devastating for the patient. The causes include direct needle trauma, chemical injury and accidental injection of a neurotoxic agent. *Only preservative-free drugs should be used for neuraxial anesthesia, since most of the preservatives are neurotoxic.*

Local anesthetics can cause neurological injury; continuous intrathecal 5% lignocaine caused injury to the sacral nerves in a number of cases.

- *Local anesthetic toxicity.* Most common causes of such toxicity are over-dosage and inadvertent intravascular injection. The affected systems are CNS and CVS and clinical features depend on the serum levels of the drug. An early symptom is tinnitus or circumoral numbness; light headedness may lead to convulsions and coma, and respiratory arrest will follow in severe cases. CVS signs include arrhythmias and cardiac arrest. Bupivacaine toxicity causes cardiac arrest that is difficult to reverse. Maximum dose of local anesthetic should not be exceeded and injection should be made with frequent aspirations to prevent intravascular injection.

Monitoring during anesthesia

It is important that patients should be continuously monitored during anesthesia. Blood pressure and heart rate can rapidly change.

Table 9.1 Amide linked and ester linked local anesthetics

Amide linked	Ester linked
Lignocaine	Benzocaine
Bupivacaine	Procaine
Levobupivacaine	Chloroprocaine

The patients are commonly paralyzed and artificially ventilated:

- They may become disconnected from the ventilator.
- Oxygen supply may drop. There may be sudden blood loss.

Anesthesia should be administered by a trained anesthetist. It is generally agreed that display of the following parameters is mandatory during anesthesia:

- Concentration of oxygen in inspired gases.
- Heart rate and rhythm.
- Blood pressure.
- Body temperature.

A typical monitor used during anesthesia provides continuous display of these parameters:

- ECG monitor that gives a continuous display of 3-lead ECG.
- Pulse oximeter that shows oxygen saturation and waveform of arterial pulsation.
- Non-invasive blood pressure monitor that gives intermittent BP readings.
- Capnograph that shows a tracing of CO_2 throughout the respiratory cycle.
- Nasopharyngeal and surface temperature.

Airway management during anesthesia

This is the most important skill learned in anesthesia, since airway obstruction is one of the most common causes of anesthetic accidents:

- The airway can be secured by simple maneuvers like jaw thrust, chin-lift and extension at the atlanto-occipital joint.
- An *endotracheal tube* is passed through the nose or mouth into the trachea. It provides a patent airway and a seal for positive-pressure ventilation, and prevents the pharyngeal contents from soiling

the airways. The seal is provided with the help of an inflatable cuff on the tracheal end. The tube is placed into the trachea under direct vision using a *laryngoscope*.

- *Supraglottic devices* are sometimes used instead of the endotracheal tube. They consist of a breathing tube attached to a cup or inflatable cuff that forms a seal over the larynx:
  - o A *laryngal mask airway* is the most commonly used supraglottic device.
  - o An *Intersurgical i-Gel airway* has been introduced recently; it contains a channel for passing an orogastric tube.

Recovery from anesthesia

Anesthetic agents are stopped when the surgeon has completed the operation. Inhalation anesthetics are washed off mostly through the lungs; the effect of muscle relaxants and intravenous agents also wears off. Patients resume spontaneous breathing once they are awake and the effect of paralysis is finished. Reversal agents are given for any residual muscle paralysis. Airways are suctioned clear of any secretions. The airway device is removed once the patient is sufficiently awake.

Recovery from anesthesia is a dangerous period. Common problems at the time of recovery include:

- *Airway obstruction.* The airway may be obstructed if the patient is not fully awake or incompletely recovered from muscle paralysis.
- *Laryngospasm* can occur due to airway irritation; this will completely occlude the airway leading to severe hypoxia.
- *Hypoxia.* Hypoventilation and alveolar collapse are common during the immediate postoperative period. Supplemental oxygen should be given to all postoperative patients.
- *Agitation.* This is a common problem. The patient may be difficult to control, sometimes pulling out his IV line.

Causes of agitation

These include:

- Pain.
- Residual effect of anesthetic agents.
- Hypoxia.
- Confusion.
- *Hemodynamic instability.* Changes in blood pressure and heart rate are common. This can be dangerous in case of patients with heart disease.

All postoperative patients should be shifted to a designated postoperative area and monitoring should be continued till they are fully recovered from the effects of anesthesia

Chapter

10 CRITICAL CARE

When a patient is very ill and may die, his condition is referred to as critical. Such a patient has usually developed failure of one or more of the physiological systems. The assessment and management of the disturbed physiology in such a case is defined as critical care. The failure of each system is considered separately for ease of understanding. However, these failures often coexist. Patients dying in a critical care unit often develop what is called 'multiple organ dysfunction syndrome'. In the progression from single to multiple organ dysfunction syndrome, systemic or localized infection often plays a very important part and greatly decreases the chances of survival.

The critical (or 'intensive') care unit is an integral part of a modern acute hospital, providing an environment for the observation and treatment of the severely ill patient. Many large hospitals are able to support separate medical, surgical, neurosurgical and respiratory units, while in smaller institutions a single multidisciplinary unit serves the needs of several specialties.

The critical care clinician must be able to sustain the physiological equilibrium of the patient by pharmacological and mechanical means. This requires constant surveillance, anticipation of adverse events and aggressive and prompt intervention when necessary. The nurse occupies a key position in the provision of critical care, and a 'one to one' nurse to patient ratio is highly desirable.

A major component of critical care is counselling and support for the relatives of the patient. This job should not be delegated to the junior medical or nursing staff but should be undertaken by the seniormost member of the surgical team.

MONITORING

Critical illness is normally severe. Many systems are affected, and changes in the different physiological variables take place rapidly. Traditional clinical evaluation cannot always be relied upon in critically ill patients, as major changes may occur which are not accompanied by obvious clinical findings. Therefore it is necessary to employ sensitive equipment to measure ('monitor') these parameters continuously, or at least frequently. The different parameters repeatedly measured in the critical care unit relate to the hemodynamic, respiratory, renal, neurologic, metabolic and temperature regulating functions.

Hemodynamic monitoring

The hemodynamic state of the critically ill patient can be accurately assessed by measurement of the following parameters:

ECG

This provides continuous information about heart rate and rhythm, and rapidly shows up any arrhythmias.

Arterial catheterization

This is indicated whenever there is a need for continuous monitoring of blood pressure and/or frequent sampling for blood gases.

Blood pressure

Medical conditions in which precise and continuous blood pressure data are necessary include:

- Shock from any cause.
- Use of potent vasoactive drugs.
- High levels of respiratory support.
- High-risk patients undergoing extensive operations.
- Controlled hypotensive anesthesia.

The systolic, diastolic and mean arterial pressures can be continuously displayed.

Blood gases

Regularly repeated analysis of blood gas tensions and pH is necessary in any acute illness with cardiovascular or respiratory dysfunction:

- The *radial* artery is the most commonly used site

for arterial catheterization because of its superficial location and because of the dual blood supply to the hand.

- The *femoral artery* can also be used. Major advantages include its superficial location and large size. Disadvantages include the difficulty of maintaining a clean dressing in the presence of draining abdominal wounds, and the presence of arteriosclerotic disease in the older patients.

Problems associated with arterial catheterization include:

- Failure to cannulate.
- Hematoma formation.
- Disconnection from the monitoring system with bleeding.
- Infections at the catheter site; these are usually seen when a catheter is left in place for longer than 4 days.

Central venous catheterization

The most common indications for central venous catheterization are:

- To secure access for fluid therapy, drug infusions or parenteral nutrition.
- For central venous pressure monitoring.

Central venous pressure (CVP) is, by definition, the pressure in the right atrium. It is raised in the following conditions:

- If the venous return is high.
- If the venous tone is increased.
- If the intrapericardial or intrathoracic pressure is high.
- If the right ventricle is not functioning properly.

A low level of CVP may be the result of:

- Hypovolaemia.
- Reduction of venous tone.
- A combination of both of these.

When monitoring CVP the catheter should be attached to a pressure transducer[1] for electronic measurement rather than to a water manometer; the latter is less reliable as it cannot respond to the full range of pressure variations.

Central venous cannulation

A radiopaque catheter is passed from a subclavian, internal jugular or antecubital vein into the right atrium. This should be done under full aseptic precautions. The head side of the table is lowered. This helps avoid air embolism. It also increases the venous return, which distends the veins and makes puncture of the vein easier. The actual method of insertion of the catheter differs according to the vein chosen for cannulation:

Subclavian vein. A 20-gauge needle on a syringe is inserted at a point below the midpoint of the clavicle and directed towards the tip of a finger in the suprasternal notch. When blood is aspirated freely a guide wire is inserted through the needle. The needle is withdrawn leaving the guide wire inside the vein. After dilating the track by passing a dilator over the wire, a catheter is passed over the wire into the subclavian vein. The guide wire is removed leaving the cannula in place.

Internal jugular vein. A line is drawn between the mastoid process and the sternoclavicular joint. The carotid artery is palpated on this line; the internal jugular vein lies immediately lateral to the artery at the mid-point of this line. A 7-cm needle on a syringe is inserted caudally into the internal jugular vein. The syringe is removed and the soft end of a Seldinger wire is passed through the needle into the vein. The needle is removed over the wire, and the catheter is passed over the wire into the vein after dilating the tract with a dilator. The wire is removed. The catheter is sutured into position and covered with a transparent, sterile self-adherent dressing.

Fluid should be infused only if blood can be easily withdrawn. The position of the catheter tip must be checked by a chest x-ray; it should be located at the lower border of the superior vena cava or the upper third of the right atrium. The CVP should be measured continuously using a pressure transducer. If such a facility is not available, a fluid manometer is used, when readings can be taken only intermittently. The mid-axillary line in the fourth intercostal space is commonly used as the zero level, as it lies at the level of the right atrium. Alternatively, the sternal angle can be used for this purpose. Marked from the midaxillary line, the normal range of CVP is 3 to 7mm Hg (0.4 to 1.0 kPa).

Complications

Complications of central venous cannulation include the following:

- Damage to adjacent structures, e.g. pleura in the case of puncture of the subclavian vein, with resulting pneumothorax or hemothorax.
- Line sepsis due to introduction of infecting organisms through the catheter, especially if care is not taken to ensure a sterile field at the time of central venous line insertion.
- Air embolism: this is a constant threat, so infusion systems should be well sealed and examined frequently.

1 Transducer: a device that converts one form of energy into another, in this case pressure into an electrical signal.

Pulmonary artery catheterization

In this method a balloon-tipped catheter is advanced to the right atrium. The balloon is inflated and the catheter with the inflated balloon moves with blood flow through the right ventricle and pulmonary artery into one of its small branches. The balloon wedges into a small branch and then flow of blood in the distal segment of the pulmonary artery is interrupted. Now, a stagnant system in which no forward flow is present has the same pressure at its proximal as at its distal end, i.e. in this case the left atrium. Therefore the *pulmonary artery occlusion pressure (PAOP)* is a reliable index of the left atrial pressure. This in turn is roughly the same as left ventricular pressure at the end of diastole, and indicates the state of function of the left ventricle. Thus pulmonary artery occlusion pressure is a good indicator of the state of function of the heart.

Low levels of PAOP are found in hypovolemia. High levels are seen in hypervolemia or with a failing left ventricle.

Cardiac output

The cardiac output can be estimated using the *thermodilution* technique. A known volume of fluid at a known temperature (colder than the body) is injected through the proximal port of the pulmonary artery catheter. The fall in temperature is registered downstream by a thermistor[1] located 4cm from the catheter tip. The more generous the blood flow, i.e. cardiac output, the more the cold fluid is diluted and the less the fall in temperature. Applying an appropriate formula, the cardiac output can be calculated.

Complications of pulmonary artery catheterization include:

- Arrhythmias.
- Coiling, looping or knotting of the catheter in the right ventricle.
- Pneumothorax may be seen as with CV-line insertion.

Respiratory monitoring

The critically ill patient may be unable to maintain a level of ventilation sufficient for adequate gas exchange. In such a situation ventilation may have to be carried out artificially by a ventilator. Monitoring ventilation and gas exchange is thus of particular importance in:

- Deciding if ventilation is required.
- Assessing response to therapy.
- Making optimum use of the ventilator.
- Deciding if a weaning trial is indicated.

Respiratory rate

This should be measured in every patient. The normal respiratory rate is 12–16 per min in a normal healthy adult and higher in children. The respiratory rate increases in:

- Pain.
- Anxiety.
- Fever.
- Sepsis.
- Shock.
- Acidosis (diabetic ketoacidosis, uremia, septicemia, induced lactic acidosis).

The rate may be slow in:

- A patient on opiate narcotics.
- Excessive sedation.
- Brain injury.
- A patient who is exhausted and gasping and needs to be put on mechanical ventilation.

Tidal volume

This is the volume of air moved in or out of the lungs in any single breath. If the tidal volume is depressed the patient may have difficulty in both oxygenation and ventilation. In weaning patients from a ventilator rapid shallow breathing indicates that weaning is likely to fail. Tidal volume can be measured at the bedside using a hand-held spirometer (Wright respirometer).

Vital capacity

This is defined as the maximal expiration following a maximal inspiration. The vital capacity is reduced in:

- Diseases involving the respiratory muscles.
- Obstruction to ventilation.
- Patients who fail to cooperate fully.

It can be readily measured at the bedside in a manner similar to the one used for tidal volume.

Expiratory peak flow

This is measured by a peak flow meter and helps in the management of patients with airway obstruction due to asthma. This is a relatively inexpensive piece of equipment which *should be in regular use in every surgical unit.*

Blood gases and pH

Arterial blood samples are assayed for partial pressures of oxygen and carbon dioxide (PO_2 and PCO_2), pH, base

1 Thermistor: a thermometer whose impedance varies with the ambient temperature, and which can measure extremely small changes in temperature.

deficit, etc. At the same time, arterial oxygen saturation can be measured percutaneously by a sensor applied as a clip onto a digit. The device measures the absorbance of light transmitted through well-perfused tissue, such as the finger or ear.

However, it should be remembered that if the blood supply to the skin is reduced, the sensitivity of this device is reduced. This device measures pulsatile signals which can be impaired by:

- Peripheral vasoconstriction.
- Hypoperfusion and hypotension.
- Peripheral vascular disease.

Mixed venous blood oxygen saturation can be measured by determining arterial blood gases (ABGs) in a sample of mixed venous blood taken from the pulmonary artery catheter. Oximetric catheters are also available which display mixed venous oxygen saturation continuously.

Mixed venous oxygen saturation indicates how much oxygen has been extracted by the peripheral tissues, with lower levels of mixed venous oxygen saturation when hypoxic tissues extract more oxygen. It is desirable to improve the mixed oxygen saturation close to normal (normal venous oxygen saturation 75%). Central venous oxygen approximates the true mixed venous oxygen saturation and can be used instead.

Renal monitoring

The reasons for monitoring renal function are three:

- The kidney serves as a monitor of the adequacy of tissue perfusion.
- If acute parenchymal renal failure threatens, monitoring of the renal function helps guide therapy.
- If renal function is impaired, the doses of certain drugs have to be reduced proportionately to the degree of renal failure to avoid toxicity, and renal function monitoring helps indicate the degree of reduction required.

Blood urea

Blood urea nitrogen (BUN) has often been used to estimate renal function. However, BUN is affected by glomerular filtration rate and urea production. The latter may vary considerably from time to time. Therefore, BUN is an unreliable monitor of renal function.

Serum creatinine

The value of serum creatinine far exceeds that of blood urea nitorgen (BUN). In contrast to BUN concentration, plasma creatinine levels are not influenced by protein metabolism or rate of fluid flow through the renal tubules. If glomerular filtration rate is reduced by 50%, the plasma creatinine will double, assuming that creatinine production remains constant.

Neurological monitoring

Several methods have been used to evaluate brain function and the effects of therapy; these include the Glasgow coma scale, intracranial pressure monitoring and electrophysiological monitoring.

Glasgow coma scale (score)

This scale was initially developed to help predict outcome after head injury. It is now also commonly used as an objective means of measuring the level of consciousness (Table 1, Chapter 44).

Intracranial pressure monitoring

This is important, because it allows calculation of *cerebral perfusion pressure*, which is defined as the difference between the mean arterial pressure and the intracranial pressure (ICP). ICP values above 40mm Hg represent dangerous and life-threatening levels of intracranial hypertension. The most common indication for ICP monitoring is head injury, in which monitoring is indicated if the Glasgow coma score after resuscitation is 7 or below. ICP monitoring is also recommended in cases of subarachnoid hemorrhage and hydrocephalus and after craniotomy. The ICP may be monitored by the use of one of the following types of equipment:

- A catheter passed into a ventricle and connected to a transducer.
- A 'subarachnoid bolt' which is screwed through the skull and into the subarachnoid space.
- Fiber-optic catheters carrying transducers at their tips, which can be placed into the subarachnoid space, cerebral parenchyma or ventricles.

The major risk of ICP monitoring is infection. The catheter or bolt should be removed as early as possible, because if monitoring is employed for less than 3 days, the infection rate should be minimal.

Electrophysiological monitoring

The electroencephalogram (EEG) reflects electrical activity recorded on the surface of the scalp. Intraoperative EEG recording has been used for monitoring the adequacy of cerebral perfusion during:

- Carotid endarterectomy.
- Cerebrovascular surgery.
- Open heart surgery.
- Induced hypotension for a variety of surgical procedures.

Metabolic monitoring

During recovery from surgery and trauma if artificial feeding has to be carried out, the simple everyday function of ingestion of food becomes complicated, involving metabolic balance studies and mathematics, with the potential for serious side effects.

The stress of illness, fever, etc. can increase the expenditure of energy, for example by 25% in multiple trauma patients and 50% in cases of extensive burns. However, even an increase of 50% results in a need for less than 3000 kcal in a patient weighing 70kg. *It is being increasingly realized that excessive calorie administration may be harmful.* Carbohydrates given in excess are turned into fat; the liver may develop fatty infiltration resulting in hepatic dysfunction. Thus, too many calories are as harmful as too few. A patient's calory requirements can be determined by indirect calorimetry.

Indirect calorimetry

Oxygen consumption and carbon dioxide production by the patient are measured, and requirements of calories are derived from these figures. Methods of determination of oxygen consumption include the following:

- The Fick equation, which calculates *oxygen consumption* from the product of the cardiac output and the arterial-venous oxygen content difference.
- Douglas bag collection of expired gases.
- Commercially available computerized indirect calorimeters.

The benefits of metabolic monitoring include the following:

- The increased calorie requirements resulting from the illness, with its accelerated metabolism, can be measured.
- Patients with hypometabolism or hypermetabolic states can be identified.
- As the caloric requirements vary widely, metabolic monitoring is more desirable than administering quantities by rote or formula.

Commercially available indirect calorimeters can now measure oxygen consumption and carbon dioxide production, and can help more precise prescription of nutritional therapy.

C-reactive proteins

During the acute phase of different inflammatory conditions a number of proteins are produced. The most clinically important of these 'acute phase proteins' is the C-reactive protein. It is synthesized exclusively in the liver and its value rises within six hours of an acute event. Its level in the plasma increases:

- With temperature (being triggered by IL-1).
- In inflammatory conditions.
- After trauma.

Advantages

- It follows the clinical state of the patient much more rapidly than the ESR.
- Is not affected by the level of hemoglobin.
- It is easily and quickly measured using an automated immunoassay.

It is being increasingly used in place of the ESR, which has traditionally been used to monitor the progress of inflammatory and degenerative conditions. However, determination of C-reactive protein requires more sophisticated equipment and is more expensive.

Temperature monitoring

Temperature is normally taken in the mouth, rectum or axilla. The temperature in these peripheral parts of the body is often influenced by such factors as mouth breathing, temperature of the environment, etc. Therefore it is recommended that core temperatures be taken in the critically ill patient. Core temperature is measured:

- By a thermistor wire directly against the tympanic membrane,
- A thermistor probe into the esophagus or deep into the rectum.

Other devices are commercially available for measuring bedside core temperature in ICU patients:

- Pulmonary artery thermistor catheters.
- Urinary bladder thermistor probes.
- Auditory canal probes.

Pulmonary artery blood temperature

This is increasingly used as a reliable indicator of core temperature, although the need for a catheter is an obvious disadvantage of this method.

Urinary bladder catheters have the advantage of giving both exact measurements of urine output and continuous readings of core temperature.

CARDIOPULMONARY RESUSCITATION (CPR)

From the standpoint of the general duty doctor, the most important part of this chapter is this section, dealing with resuscitation of the patient from cardio-respiratory arrest. Cardiac arrest can take place at any time and any place. Therefore every member of the medical and nursing staff should be thoroughly trained in the procedure of resuscitation. At the same time *the necessary equipment for dealing with this emergency should be available in all hospital departments and emergency services.*

Causes of cardiac arrest

The common causes leading to cardiac arrest include:

5 H's:

- **H**ypoxia.
- **H**ypovolemia.
- **H**ypothermia.
- **H**ydrogen ion (Acidosis).
- **H**ypokalemia/**H**yperkalemia.

5 T's:

- **T**hrombosis (Pulmonary).
- **T**ension Pneumothorax.
- **T**amponade (Cardiac).
- **T**oxins.
- **T**hrombosis (Cardiac).

Types of cardiac arrest

Absence of a circulation may be produced by:

- *Circulatory obstruction*. A massive pulmonary embolism or air embolism may block the path of the circulating blood. It should be remembered that as little as 50ml of air carelessly introduced at venesection can kill a patient.
- *Asystole*. Absence of systole indicates severe depression of the myocardium. The heart beat first becomes slow and feeble and finally stops. The myocardium is dilated, toneless and cyanosed.
- *Ventricular fibrillation*. This usually occurs when the heart is irritable, either from trauma or manipulation during operation, or due to drugs. A fibrillating heart is less depressed and more likely to recover than a heart where asystole has set in.

MANAGMENT OF CARDIAC ARREST

Prevention

It is better to prevent cardiac arrest than to treat it.

- For a start *every surgical operation should be carried out under an ECG, a blood pressure monitor and a pulse oximeter.* It is far better to detect any disorder at the stage of a simple arrhythmia than to allow it to develop into fibrillation or asystole due to lack of monitoring. All patients under intensive care are normally constantly monitored.
- Secondly, *great care should be exercised while administering different drugs intravenously. The sudden influx of almost any drug into the circulation can produce a severe arrhythmia*; therefore intravenous injections should be given very slowly and after being diluted. Some agents, for example potassium ions, cannot safely be given through a syringe or into the drip tubing; these should be added to the contents of the drip bottle, for slow infusion.

Recognition

If cardiac arrest takes place and the circulation remains suspended for more than 8 to 10 minutes, permanent brain damage is the nearly certain consequence, and recovery highly unlikely. Because only a few minutes are available in which to reverse the situation, it is essential that cardiac arrest be recognized immediately. Recognition of the cardiac arrest is based on three signs:

- Absent response.
- Absent or gasping respiration.
- Absent major pulses.

Absent major (carotid) pulse is the most important sign. If the carotid pulse cannot be felt, cardiac arrest must be assumed and immediate cardiopulmonary resuscitation corrective action taken. It must be emphasized that *the ECG alone is of no value for the diagnosis of cardiac arrest because* electrical activity can continue on the ECG without effective cardiac contractions (*pulseless electrical activity*).

The main value of the ECG or rhythm analysis after cardiac arrest lies in its ability to detect ventricular fibrillations/tachycardia (pulseless), in which case defibrillation is required. Ventilation is best carried out in such a situation by mask to mouth or, if a mask is not available, mouth to mouth insufflation of lungs initially, and later by an Ambu bag and endotracheal tube, subject to availability.

Treatment

Treatment can be divided into three phases:

A. Immediate measures (basic life support, BLS)

The person immediately available should follow the BLS protocol for the cardiopulmonary resuscitation of the victim, as follows:

- Check for responsiveness and for chest movements (Minimum for five seconds but no more than 10 seconds).
- Activate the emergency response system and call for a defibrillator.

- Check for carotid pulse (min for 5 seconds but no more than 10 seconds).

If no pulse is detected, immediately start chest compression over the left lower half of sternum.

- Push Hard (2cm) and Fast (100/min).
- Allow complete chest recoil in between compressions. Allow a minimum of interruptions (less than 10 seconds).
- Maintain the airway patency by Head tilt/Chin lift maneuver and give two effective breaths after every 30 compressions (30: 2).

  Note:

  - o Seal of mouth or mask should be tight so that there is no air leak.
  - o Give breath over one second.
  - o Check for the chest rise after each breath.
  - o If two rescuers are available, they should change their position after every 2 minutes or 5 cycles of CPR (30:2) to avoid fatigue.
- As soon as an AED (Automated Electrical Defibrillator) arrives, analyze the rhythm and, if required, deliver the shock within 45 seconds of the arrival of the AED:

  Note:

  - o Avoid contact with the patient while analyzing and delivering the shock.
  - o Immediately resume the CPR for 2 minutes or 5 cycles, after delivering the shock.
  - o Re-analyze the rhythm after 2 minutes or 5 cycles of continuous CPR, and not before.

B. Definitive management (Advanced cardiac life support, ACLS)

Electrocardiographic monitoring (cardiac monitor/ECG strip) should be started as soon as possible. It immediately allows us to determine which of the following types of cardiac arrest is present:

- Aystole/pulseless electrical activity.
- Ventricular tachycardia (pulseless).
- Ventricular fibrillation.

At the same time, any signs of recovery appear first on the ECG.

Further action

This now depends upon the type of rhythm shown by the ECG:

- *Defibrillation.* If ventricular tachycardia (pulseless) or ventricular fibrillation is present, the cardiac defibrillator is used and external defibrillation attempted immediately, as follows:
  - o Energy used: 360 J (if monophasic) or 200 J (if biphasic).

    Establish I/V access, if not available yet.
  - o Resume CPR immediately after delivering the shock, and reassess the rhythm only after 5 cycles or 2 minutes (of CPR).
  - o If rhythm is again shockable, defibrillate with the same energy. Also push first bolus of 1mg adrenaline (repeat every 3 to 5 mins). Consider advanced airway (LMA/ETT etc).
  - o If shock is again advised after two minutes of CPR, give amiodarone (300mg bolus then 150mg bolus) after the shock.
- If *Asystole/pulseless electrical activity* is present:
  - o Continue good quality CPR (as described previously) with 1mg adrenaline (repeat every 3 to 5 mins); alternatively, vasopressin 40 units I/V can replace first or second dose of adrenaline.
  - o Reassess rhythm after every 2 mins or 5 cycles of CPR, and not before.
  - o Consider advanced airway (LMA/ETT [1]etc).

Note:

- o If breaths are being delivered through an advanced airway (ETT/LMA), the rate should not be greater than 10 to 12 breaths/minutes.
- o During BLS/ACLS, consider the causes of cardiac arrest (5H's/5 T's, given above) in order to provide prompt and specific remediation as soon as possible.
- o If end-tidal CO_2 ($EtCO_2$) is less than 10mm Hg or diastolic BP less than 20mm Hg, you need to improve the quality or adequacy of CPR.

C. Later treatment (return of spontaneous circulation, ROSC)

When rhythm and blood pressure are restored the patient is still watched very closely, because another episode of cardiac arrest can occur. The following steps should be considered:

- SpO_2 should be maintained around 94%.
- Consider maintaining advanced airway (LMA/ETT) with ($EtCO_2$) monitoring, if not done before.

1 LMA: Laryngeal mask airway.

ETT: Endotracheal tube.

- Give I/V bolus of crystalloids (normal saline or Ringer's Lactate).
- Provide inotropic cardiac support as required (dopamine, nor-adrenaline).
- If ACS is suspected on 12-lead ECG, alert call should be sent to CCU/Cardiac catheterization lab.
- If return of consciousness is delayed, induced total body hypothermia down to 32°C may help reduce the extent of cerebral damage.

Open cardiac massage

The chest is opened through the fifth left intercostal space. The wound does not bleed because there is no circulation. If a rib-spreader is available both hands can be passed into the chest, the pericardium widely opened, and cardiac massage carried out very efficiently between the two hands. Without a rib spreader only one hand can be introduced into the chest and massage is less effective. Massage should be carried out with the flat of the hand so as not to damage the myocardium. The rate should be 50 to 60 compressions per minute. The purpose of the massage is to:

- Improve the tone of the heart muscle.
- Increase the coronary flow.
- Ensure a supply of oxygenated blood to the brain.

The arrested heart is toneless, distended and blue. After massage it should become smaller and more firm and pink. After the tone has returned, an effort should be made to get it to beat normally.

A toneless heart has a tendency to distend with blood returning from the body. This should be prevented by effective massage, otherwise irreversible damage can occur. The routine use of bicarbonate is discouraged because of cerebral edema, and bicarbonate is given only if indicated, i.e pH <7.2.

Summary

In order to put the whole subject of cardio-respiratory resuscitation in a nutshell and to commit it to memory, the student need only remember the first four letters in the alphabet as follows:

A for **A**irway.

B for **B**reathing.

C for **C**ardiac massage/**C**ompressions.

D for **D**rugs/**D**efibrillation/**D**ifferential Diagnosis

Remember, the earlier you start the CPR with correct sequence and timing, the better will be the outcome.

INFECTION IN THE CRITICAL CARE UNIT (CCU)

Nosocomial infection in the CCU

A nosocomial infection is that which develops at least 48 hours after admission to hospital (Latin: *nosocomium,* a hospital). It affects 15 to 40% of critical care unit (CCU) patients and contributes to approximately 70% of late deaths in such units.

Definitions

Colonization is the presence of a pathogenic organism on two or more occasions.

Infection is the presence of many pathogenic organisms, with leucocytes and the clinical signs of inflammation.

Sepsis (SIRS) is a syndrome comprising inflammation (fever and leucocytosis) and organ system failure; a micro-organism may or may not be identified. This is better known as SIRS i.e. Systemic Inflammatory Response Syndrome.

Predisposing factors

The incidence of nosocomial infection depends upon:

- Length of stay in the CCU.
- Number of invasive procedures.
- Nature of the underlying illness.
- Mode of presentation.

After 24 hours about 10% of patients are colonized, while more than 90% can be colonized after 2 weeks. These factors are to some extent interdependent; the longer a patient stays in the unit the more procedures are likely to be performed.

The role of catheters

The passage of different catheters and tubes increases the chances of developing nosocomial infection:

- Endotracheal intubation and mechanical ventilation carries a 20 to 60 % incidence of pneumonia.
- Up to 30% of patients with urinary catheters develop urinary tract infections.
- Up to 15% of infections occur in vascular lines, and rules regarding the insertion and management of arterial and venous lines need to be strictly enforced.

Factors associated with an increased incidence of vascular catheter infections include:

- Infusion of hypertonic solutions.
- Frequent disconnection of infusion lines.
- Length of time the catheter remains in place.

Moral: Except for tunnelled feeding lines and those required for hemodialysis, no vascular lines should remain in position for more than five days.

Prevention of infection

Control of infection requires strict adoption of preventive measures, early recognition of infection, and application of disciplined antibiotic policies. Insistence on the following precautions pays rich dividends:

- Hand washing.
- Disinfection.
- Isolation procedures.
- Strict control of antibiotic prophylaxis and therapy.

Sites sampled

The usual sites sampled in the microbiological survey of an infected patient include:

- Wounds and discharge sites.
- Lungs and airways.
- Blood.
- Urine.
- Invasive lines.
- CSF.
- Other aspirates.

Nosocomial pneumonia

Overall, nosocomial pneumonia occurs in about 1% of hospital patients, but in critical care units the incidence may reach 5 to 25%. Such pneumonias may be responsible for up to a quarter of critical care deaths. The factors which predispose towards nosocomial pneumonia in critical care patients are the following:

- Advanced age.
- Obesity.
- Cigarette smoking.
- Diabetes mellitus.
- Chronic heart, lung or kidney disease.
- Malignant disease.
- Low Glasgow coma score.
- Endotracheal intubation.
- Oropharyngeal colonization with Gram-negative organisms.
- Gastric colonization in ileus and reduced gastric acidity.

For diagnosis of nosocomial pneumonia, the purely clinical criteria of fever, leucocytosis, purulent sputum and new or progressive infiltrates on chest x-rays are not specific enough to use in the critically ill. Fever and leucocytosis may be due to a variety of infectious or even non-infectious conditions.

Bronchoalveolar lavage and quantitative cultures

A better diagnostic criterion consists of quantitative cultures of material obtained by a protected specimen brush and broncho-alveolar lavage. Significant infection is indicated by the presence of more than 10^3 colony forming units in 1ml of lavage fluid. The number of infections increases from 10 % at 10 days to over 25% at 30 days. Bronchoalveolar lavage offers the advantage that Gram staining of a centrifuged deposit of the fluid obtained may provide an immediate indication of pneumonia: if more than 25% of white cells in the deposit contain intracellular organisms it is highly likely that the patient has pneumonia.

Bronchial lavage

At the same time, blind bronchial lavage with an undirected catheter is almost as sensitive and specific as fibreoptically-guided bronchoalveolar lavage.

Prevention

Measures to this end include:

- Sheathed suction catheters which allow a single catheter to be used for 24 hours without repeated disconnection of the circuit.
- Humidification using heat/moisture exchange filters also serve as microbiological filters.
- Prevention of stress ulcers with the use of a cytoprotective agent like sucralfate, rather than antacids and H2-blockers; the latter increase the gastric pH and may encourage bacterial colonization of the gastric secretions.
- Change of posture every few hours to discourage the development of dependent lung collapse.

Management

All ventilated critical care patients who are considered to have nosocomial pneumonia should undergo fibreoptic bronchoscopy for bronchial lavage. Alternatively, lavage should be carried out through a non-directed catheter passed as far into a lobar bronchus as possible. If on cytological examination more than 25% of white cells contain organisms, empirical therapy should be commenced, based on the results of Gram staining.

The most popular antibiotic regimen for nosocomial pneumonia consists of an aminoglycoside and an antipseudomonal β-lactam. This may be combined with vancomycin to cover methicillin-resistant staph aureus.

Infection in the immunocompromised patient

The most common causes of immunocompromise are:

- Malignancy.
- Chemotherapy.
- Corticosteroid treatment.
- Splenectomy.
- Immunosuppression after transplantation.
- Acquired immune deficiency syndrome (AIDS).

Immunocompromise can take the form of failure of phagocytosis, defective cell-mediated immunity, and defective antibody-mediated immunity.

Treatment

Attempts to reduce infection using isolation procedures have failed. As the *risk of infection is related to the number of interventions*, invasive procedures should be limited to essential diagnostic interventions. The oropharynx and sinuses should be checked daily. The appearance of new infiltrates on chest x-rays indicates an opportunistic pneumonia until proved otherwise. Unfortunately, prophylactic antibiotics are very often associated with the development of bacterial resistance.

Confirmed infection requires immediate and effective treatment. A combination of a third generation cephalosporin with an aminoglycoside and a penicillinase-resistant penicillin (oxacillin or nafcillin) eliminates most of the likely organisms. Finally, persistent fever in the face of adequate antibiotic therapy should raise the suspicion of fungal infection.

CYTOKINES IN SEPSIS

A major breakthrough in the understanding of sepsis has occurred in the last decade with advances in molecular biology. The substances which are produced in severe inflammation and cause host autoinjury and death have been identified, and are called cytokines (cyto = cell; kinesis = motion). A cytokine is a soluble molecule produced by a cell to induce a biological effect elsewhere; it acts as a messenger at its destination. The effect varies according to the cytokine and the cell, but typically these molecules signal certain cells to activate, divide, or home in on a particular site in the body.

The most important cytokines in the mediation of lethal sepsis are:

- Tumor necrosis factor.
- Interleukin-1.

They are synthesized not only by monocytes/macrophages, but by other cells including neutrophils, lymphocytes and endothelial cells.

Tumor necrosis factor (TNF)

This plays a key role in critical illness:

- Administration of TNF to laboratory animals induces all the host alterations associated with severe infection.
- In patients with overwhelming infection there is a close relationship between circulating TNF levels and death.
- In animals given a lethal dose of live Gram-negative organisms, if monoclonal antibodies effective against TNF are administered, a fatal outcome is prevented. This shows that in lethal Gram-negative infection it may be *substances produced by the host* (in this case TNF), and not bacterial poisons by themselves, that cause death.

Interleukin-1 (IL-1)

This exists in a and b forms, the latter being the more important. Administration of interleukin-1b to animals and human beings results in all the responses seen in acute infection. Stimuli for IL-1 release include all inflammatory, infectious and immunological processes.

Actions

- IL-1 acts on the CNS, inducing fever by stimulating local release of prostaglandins in the anterior hypothalamus, and inducing anorexia by direct action on the satiety center.
- It also multiplies the effects of TNF a *hundredfold*.

The lethality of acute infection is due to TNF and IL-1b acting synergistically and causing hypotension, tissue injury and death in animals subjected to experimental sepsis.

Synergy between cytokines—the 'cytokine cascade'

During health, the synthesis of TNF is strongly repressed. It is *only when cells are triggered by endotoxins* and other stimuli that they elaborate TNF. The result depends upon the amounts of TNF produced:

- *Low* levels of endotoxemia trigger TNF production. Fever occurs but without lethal responses like hypotension or coagulopathy.
- If the levels of TNF are *high* enough for secondary synthesis of interleukin-1b, lethal responses can take place and result in death. The induction of a cytokine cascade represents an inappropriately severe

response to an inflammatory stimulus, and leads to death through:

- o Hypothermia.
- o Coagulopathy.
- o Visceral hypoperfusion and reperfusion injury.
- o Lactic acidosis.
- o Myocardial depression.
- o Peripheral vasodilatation, or the capillary leak syndrome.

All of these alterations may be induced by TNF or interleukin-1b.

Blocking the cytokine cascade

The mortality in severe surgical sepsis is constant at 50 to 70%. It is not likely that better antibiotics or hemodynamic support will reduce it. Theoretically, *modification of the cytokine cascade could reduce the death rate*:

- If the endotoxin-induced generation of cytokines could be inhibited.
- If cytokine receptors could be inhibited.
- If effective monoclonal *antibodies* against cytokines (TNF and interleukin-1b) could be developed. This is a promising approach, as these antibodies may be more applicable in severe inflammatory states rather than just those initiated by endotoxin. In animals they have been found to be most effective when given prophylactically.

After severe inflammatory or infective episodes the host releases not only large amounts of potentially lethal cytokines but also antidotes to these cytokines. Lethal effects of cytokines are seen when the antidotes are exhausted, leading to unopposed cytokine activity. Blocking the activity of either TNF or interleukin-1 could theoretically prevent the full consequences of the disease.

Acute inflammation in a localized focus of infection is an 'ally' of the host. On the other hand, intravascular activation of the same mechanism behaves as a 'foe', causing the entire body to behave like a massive wound, with intravascular mediator activation, capillary leak and often lethal consequences. Unfortunately none of the drugs which has been used in randomized control trials, such as antibodies against lipid A or coagulation proteins, has shown any benefit in humans with septic shock.

ACUTE RESPIRATORY DISTRESS SYNDROME

Disordered exchange of gases in the lungs often follows shock and trauma, and is the most common cause of respiratory failure. In 1967 Ashbaugh described acute respiratory distress in twelve patients without underlying lung disease. This 'acute respiratory distress syndrome' (ARDS) may develop in a variety of clinical situations, of which *severe sepsis is the most important*. Apart from this, ARDS can occur as a non-specific reaction to a wide variety of insults including:

- Shock (especially septic shock).
- Trauma.
- Burns.
- Fat embolism.
- Cardiopulmonary bypass.
- Amniotic fluid embolism.
- Aspiration pneumonia.

Pathogenesis

In patients with trauma and sepsis, *endotoxemia activates complement and other components of the immune-inflammatory cascade;* this causes leucocytes to be sequestered in pulmonary capillaries. The sequestered leucocytes release proteases, cytokines, and toxic superoxide radicals, which injure endothelial cells.

Pathophysiology

ARDS is the earliest manifestation of a generalized inflammatory response and *is often followed by the development of a multiple organ dysfunction syndrome*. Severe infection or large areas of devitalized tissue can trigger a massive inflammatory response. Although beneficial when directed against local areas of infection or necrotic tissue, *dissemination of this response can produce widespread tissue damage*. The pulmonary epithelium is damaged, reducing surfactant production and lowering the threshold for alveolar flooding, thus leading ultimately to *non-cardiac pulmonary edema* which is a cardinal feature of ARDS. The pathological changes result in:

- Reduced functional residual capacity.
- Increased venous admixture (shunt).
- Reduced lung compliance.
- Hypoxemia which is refractory to treatment.

Obstruction of the pulmonary circulation results from:

- Vascular compression by interstitial edema as well as edema of the vessel wall.
- Constriction of the pulmonary vessels by:
  - o Increased autonomic nervous activity.
  - o Hypoxic vasoconstriction.
  - o Circulating substances such as catecholamines,

5-hydroxytryptamine, thromboxane, fibrinogen degradation products (FDPs), complement and activated leucocytes.

Presentation

The recognition of acute respiratory dysfunction is not difficult:

- The patient has acute respiratory distress and requires an increasing concentration of oxygen in the inspired air (greater than 0.5) to maintain a partial pressure of arterial oxygen (PaO_2) of more than 50mm Hg.
- Chest x-rays show extensive lung infiltrates.
- During mechanical ventilation the lungs are stiff and require high inflation pressures.
- Cardiogenic pulmonary edema should be excluded by measuring pulmonary artery wedge pressure.
- A bed side echocardiogram can exclude left ventricular or valvular dysfunction.

Management

There is no specific treatment for ARDS except to remove or suppress the injurious agent, and to support the patient until lung function returns. The clinician should anticipate its development by remaining aware of the precipitating causes. An aggressive approach to the management of these underlying disease processes may help prevent progression to respiratory failure.

The aim of *respiratory support* is to achieve adequate oxygen supply without impeding cardiac output. To ensure delivery of sufficient oxygen, the hemoglobin concentration should be maintained at 11 g/100ml of blood. Further, respiratory support in this condition is based on:

- Oxygen.
- Intermittent positive pressure ventilation.
- Positive end-expiratory pressure (PEEP).

However, it should be noted that excessive positive end-expiratory pressure results in damage to the alveoli (barotrauma).

Tissue hypoxia

The clinician should be alert to the signs of tissue hypoxia, such as:

- Metabolic acidosis.
- Mental obtundation.
- Cardiac arrhythmias.

If such signs are not present it is reasonable to assume that oxygen delivery is adequate.

Indications for mechanical ventilation

These fall into two categories:

- Inadequate alveolar *ventilation* with increasing pCO_2.
- Inadequate *gas exchange* with increasing alveolar-arterial oxygen gradient and arterial hypoxemia; the clinician should anticipate problems before they arise.

Lung collapse

Because the patient is often nursed for prolonged periods in the supine position, extensive collapse of the dependent parts of the lungs is common. Oxygenation is greatly improved by:

- Sitting the patient as upright as possible.
- Rolling him from side to side once every few hours.

Supportive care improves the outcome and includes:

- Back care.
- Stress ulcer prophylaxis with sucralfate.
- DVT prophylaxis.

Circulatory support

Fluid administration should be regulated to ensure adequate cardiac output without aggravating the pulmonary edema. Measurement of pulmonary capillary wedge pressure provides a more reliable assessment of the filling status of the patient than determination of central venous pressure, but has its own complications.

Prognosis

If multiple organ support is maintained, the chances of recovery are improved. Even after positive pressure ventilation for weeks a good functional recovery is possible. Although better monitoring and better ventilators are available today, the patients in intensive care units are older and sicker with mutliorgan dysfunction. Therefore mortality from ARDS remains 40–50%.

Chapter

11 SURGERY AND DIABETES

Diabetes mellitus is a very common condition, affecting upto 10% of the population. It is of considerable importance for the surgeon for the following reasons:

- Diabetes is a major metabolic defect of carbohydrate, protein and fat metabolism, and special management is required during a surgical procedure.
- It can cause infection, vascular disease and neuropathy. If any of these conditions already exists, diabetes can aggravate it.
- Surgical infection aggravates the diabetic state, so that the requirements of insulin are increased.
- Hypoglycemia must be considered as a possible cause whenever an unconscious patient is brought for treatment.
- The perioperative mortality rate in diabetics is much higher than in the general population, being around 8%; most deaths occur due to diseases associated with diabetes, including atherosclerosis, nephropathy, hypertension, ischemic heart disease and infection (63% of diabetics have cardiovascular disease, 44% have peripheral vascular disease, and 24% suffer from cerebrovascular disease). Also, many patients suffer from autonomic and peripheral neuropathies, which may lead to postural hypotension or cardiac arrest.

Diagnosis

The diagnosis of diabetes is made on the basis of a fasting venous blood glucose level above 140mg/dl (7.8mmol/l) and an abnormal glucose tolerance test, i.e. blood glucose above 200mg/dl (11.0mmol/l) two hours after ingestion of 75 g of glucose.

SURGICAL COMPLICATIONS OF DIABETES

The complications of diabetes which are of special concern to the surgeon include neuropathy, infection, and angiopathy; and specially in the case of the foot they lead to the clinical conditions of ulcer and gangrene.

Peripheral neuropathy

Peripheral neuropathy leads to the development of ulcers on the sole of the foot as follows:

- Loss of *sensory* nerve supply leads to anesthesia, so that repeated minor trauma remains undetected and uncared for, predisposing to the development of an ulcer.
- Loss of *motor* nerve supply results in muscle atrophy leading to the development of foot deformities. The pressure distribution on the sole of the foot becomes abnormal, with increased weight-bearing on the metatarsal heads. This leads first to the degeneration of the fat pads underlying the metatarsal heads, and later to the development of an actual ulcer.

Infection

Infection predisposes the part to the development of gangrene. It does so by producing hypoxia of the tissues, by increasing the demand for oxygen while reducing its supply:

- The *increased demand* for oxygen results from the raised metabolic rate in the tissues due to the infection.
- The *reduced supply* of oxygen results from vascular insufficiency, which itself is produced as follows:
    - o Inflammatory edema increases tissue tension and compresses the blood vessels.

Table 11.1 Basic features of diabetic foot

	Neuropathy	Ischemia
Presentation	Paraesthesias	Claudication
	Numbness	Rest pain
	Pain	
Lesions	Ulcers	Ulcers
	Abscess	Gangrene
	Digital gangrene	

- o If gas-producing organisms are responsible for the infection, the pressure of the gas adds greatly to the tissue tension.
- o Bacterial toxins produce thrombosis, which leads to occlusion of small vessels.

Angiopathy

- In patients suffering from diabetes, *atherosclerosis* develops at a much earlier age than in the general population.
- At the same time a *microangiopathy* occurs in the small blood vessels of diabetics; thickening of the basement membrane reduces the lumen of these vessels so that the flow of blood through them is diminished.

Ulcer and gangrene

In the development of an ulcer on the sole of the foot the major role is played by neuropathy, although infection and angiopathy also contribute their share. On the other hand, in the development of gangrene all three of the above-named factors make significant contributions (Fig.11.1).

THE DIABETIC FOOT

The foot, being farthest away from the heart, has a modest blood supply at the best of times. In old age atherosclerosis further reduces the circulation to the foot. If diabetes supervenes, microangiopathy and neuropathy greatly increase the chances of onset of gangrene. The widespread belief that diabetic arterial disease is primarily localized to the small vessels is erroneous. Although diabetics develop a microangiopathy, the primary pathology is of typical large-vessel atherosclerosis.

Investigations

Doppler pressure determination in the toes accurately determines arterial insufficiency. Arterial disease is unlikely when the ratio between the pressure in the toe and in the brachial artery (toe-brachial pressure ratio) exceeds 0.70.

Arteriography may be required to exclude the possibility of reconstructible arterial disease of the infrapopliteal or tibial vessels.

Management

- In every diabetic patient the peripheral pulses, the condition of the skin of the foot, and sensations in the foot should be carefully tested. If the circulation is *normal* and there is no neuropathy, the patient should be instructed in the meticulous care of his feet, and the feet checked periodically for the early onset of ischemic changes.
- If the circulation is even slightly *impaired* as indicated by the pulses, the sensations, or by the trophic changes, *urgent measures* should be undertaken to prevent damage to the skin which might lead to ulceration and gangrene. The most important precaution is the wearing of well-fitting shoes. The feet are protected from damage done by tight fitting shoes, and corns and callosities can be prevented from developing. In countries with a warm climate where open sandals can be worn, specially in summer, this is not such a problem.

Instructions to the patient

The surgeon should explain to the patient that even minor ulcerations could get complicated, and lead to possible loss of the whole limb. However, it is no use just telling the patient to take good care of his feet, because he will not know what to do.

A detailed set of written instructions should be given to him, on the following lines:

- o Inspect feet daily for blisters and cuts, specially between the toes.
- o Wash the feet daily, dry carefully.
- o If feet are cold at night, wear socks; *do not use hot water bottles.*
- o Use properly fitted shoes, avoid pointed shoes, start wearing new shoes gradually.
- o Don't walk barefooted.
- o Cut nails straight across.
- o Don't cut corns yourself; get professional help. See your doctor regularly and have your feet examined.

One of the reasons for including the above list of instructions in this book is to serve as a model. Whenever a patient is suffering from a condition where some of the medical care has to be entrusted to him at home, *an appropriate set of written instructions should be given to him.* The clinician will find that the patient's compliance with the instructions will improve greatly by the use of this simple device, to his great benefit.

Further course

- If *ulcers or gangrenous spots* have already developed, a serious state exists. The part should be kept at rest. The ulcerated area is gently washed daily with lukewarm water and mild soap, and a dressing applied. The dressing should be kept in place by a bandage, adhesive plaster being avoided.

  Cultures of the area should be taken. Organisms will often be grown, but antibiotics should only be started if the ulcer is inflamed or there are systemic signs of infection. In most cases the ulcer can be managed by local cleansing and dressing.

- If *rest pain* occurs the patient should sleep with the foot side of the bed a little lowered in order to increase the arterial supply. If this fails to give relief from pain, analgesics and even narcotics should be used.
- If *ischemia* is present, indicated by intermittent claudication or ulceration, and the pulses are diminished, arteriography should be carried out to see if reconstructive surgery is feasible and if so, operation should be performed.

INFECTION IN A DIABETIC

If infection develops in a diabetic it must be treated energetically, because it can have serious consequences for the patient. If ischemia due to vascular disease is present, what might only be surface contamination in the normal patient can become invasive infection in the diabetic, because diabetes interferes with the ability of polymorphonuclear cells to kill bacteria.

When infection occurs the insulin requirement of the diabetic increases, and if not provided for, can rapidly lead to ketoacidosis. Therefore, firstly every effort should be made to prevent infection; and secondly, if infection does take place, effective medical and surgical treatment should be given to prevent ketosis.

If *elective surgery* is to be undertaken on a diabetic, every effort should be made to clear up any existing infection unless it is the reason for the operation. At the same time remote infections should be carefully searched for and eliminated before operation. If the infection cannot be eliminated, antibiotics should be started and continued for 3 to 4 days postoperatively.

Prophylactic antibiotics should be used only in contaminated and clean-contaminated cases. They must be started before operation, usually at the time of induction of anesthesia, and continued for only a few hours, or at the most a day or two. Lengthy courses of antibiotics do not confer any added benefit. Finally, antibiotics started after the operation are useless for prophylaxis.

Future developments in control of diabetes

Insulin pumps

Whatever the mode of administration of insulin, the glucose level in the blood fluctuates considerably. Damage to the blood vessels, nerves, and various other tissues occurs during the periods of hyperglycemia. In order

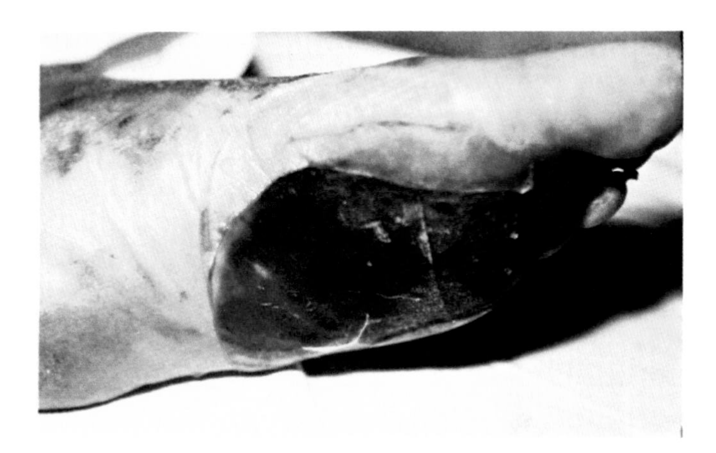

Fig.11.1 Diabetic gangrene. Note that the soft tissues of the sole of the foot have sloughed away, and the necrotic tissue is blackened.

to stabilize the glucose metabolism *implantable insulin pumps* are being developed. The most sophisticated of these pumps can constantly monitor the blood glucose and keep on releasing insulin according to need. Such pumps, when perfected, will be a major advance in the control of diabetes, and will help prevent many of the complications of imperfectly controlled diabetes.

Pancreatic transplantation

The only treatment of type 1 diabetes that establishes an insulin-independent euglycemic state consists of pancreatic transplantation. However, the price which has to be paid for achieving such a state is the need for immunosuppression. If the patient is uraemic from nephropathy, he is already on immunosuppression; in that case pancreatic transplantation should definitely be carried out.

PREPARING THE DIABETIC FOR SURGERY

Preoperative management

The signs and symptoms of diabetes and any associated pathology should be assessed. Laboratory tests should include a full electrolyte, urea and creatinine screen, blood count with white cell differential, chest x-ray and ECG. If the patient is receiving treatment for other conditions, e.g. alpha-blockers, calcium channel inhibitors, other antihypertensives, digitalis, etc., the situation should be optimized before surgery.

Plasma potassium levels may be decreased in uncontrolled diabetes, and may need to be supplemented.

Cardiac autonomic neuropathy

In about one-third of all diabetics the heart is the seat of an autonomic neuropathy, whose manifestations include:

- A lack of variation of the heart rate, with a higher than average resting heart rate.
- Postural hypotension.
- Intraoperative episodes of bradycardia and hypotension.

The presence of cardiac autonomic neuropathy is associated with a poor prognosis.

Perioperative management

The major hazard in diabetes is hypoglycemia. However, acute hyperglycemia during surgery may result in altered host defence mechanisms, extracellular dehydration and electrolyte imbalance, intracellular dehydration and impaired wound healing. The blood glucose level is best maintained in the range of 90–199mg/dl (5.5 to 11mmol/litre).

Fluid replacement should be given as normal saline solution; higher blood glucose levels (and hence higher insulin requirements) are seen in patients receiving either 5% dextrose or Ringer's lactate.

The operation

The diabetes must be controlled before the operation, which should be scheduled first thing in the morning. The patient should be on an empty stomach, and should omit insulin or oral antidiabetic:

- A patient who is not on insulin and is having minor surgery should simply be observed on the day of operation with three-hourly glucose level estimation.
- All other patients should get a glucose-potassium-insulin (GKI) infusion [500ml 10% dextrose, 15 units short-acting insulin and 10mmol KCL].

The blood glucose should be checked every two hours to keep the glucose level between 6 and 11mmol/kg. If the glucose level goes outside these limits, the dose of insulin should be increased or decreased by five units.

GKI should be continued till the patient starts on an oral diet.

Emergency surgery

Sometimes a patient is admitted in severe diabetic acidosis or coma secondary to an urgent surgical problem, e.g. a perforated appendix. The diabetes may get out of control before the patient realizes it; his cerebral function may be impaired and he may be admitted as an emergency.

Apart from urine analysis, the patient's blood sugar, serum acetone and electrolytes must be immediately determined. Normal saline with soluble insulin should be started through the intravenous line immediately. Half the dose is given intravenously and the other half subcutaneously. If the patient is in shock the entire dose of insulin should be given intravenously, because of the poor absorption of drugs in shock.

During the operation

- The blood glucose is measured every hour, and the state of fluid replenishment repeatedly assessed, with a central venous catheter and an indwelling urinary catheter.
- When the serum *electrolyte* levels are known the fluid may be changed to Ringer's lactate; the lactated buffer in the solution helps in correcting the acidosis.
- As soon as an adequate *urinary output* has been achieved, potassium which has been lost due to the osmotic diuresis should be added to the intravenous solution.
- Further, as soon as *acidosis* is corrected and dehydration reversed, the patient may undergo the emergency operation

Chapter

12 ULCERS AND SINUSES

ULCERS

An ulcer can be defined as a disintegration of the surface of the skin or a mucous membrane with necrosis of epithelial tissue. There is progressive destruction of the tissue cell by cell.

CLASSIFICATION AND CAUSATION OF ULCERS

Congenital

- Genetic.
- Sporadic.

Acquired

- Traumatic.
- Inflammatory:
    - Physical.
    - Chemical.
    - Infection.
        - Viral.
        - Bacterial.
        - Rickettsial.
        - Protozoal.
        - Fungal.
        - Heliminthic.
- Neoplastic:
    - Benign.
    - Malignant.
- Degenerative.
- Autoimmune.
- Proliferative.
- Metabolic.
- Hormonal.
- Mechanical.
- Ischemic.
- Self-induced.
- Psychosomatic.
- Iatrogenic.
- Peptic.

Life-history of an ulcer

This consists of three phases: extension, transition, and finally either repair or chronicity:

Extension

In the stage of extension the floor of the ulcer is covered with exudate and sloughs. The base is hard from active inflammation, the edge is sharply defined, the discharge is purulent or blood-stained, and the surrounding skin is red and inflamed.

Transition

At this stage the floor of the ulcer is clear, the sloughs separate, the base is less hard, and red granulation tissue develops, with a covering of a single layer of epithelial cells.

Chronicity

If conditions are not favourable for healing, the ulcer becomes chronic. The granulations are pale and the base, edge and surrounding areas are hard. The formation of weak granulation tissue may be due to a systemic disorder e.g. myxedema, malnutrition, long-term therapy with steroids, local ischemia or specific infections. Zinc-containing lotions e.g. red lotion and scarlet red, which stimulate granulation tissue formation, are useful in such situations.

CLINICAL EXAMINATION OF AN ULCER

During the clinical examination of an ulcer the following points must be noted:

Site. Most rodent ulcers occur on the upper part of the face. Carcinoma of the lip commonly arises on the lower lip.

Size and duration. A rodent ulcer grows extremely slowly, a carcinoma somewhat slowly, and an inflammatory ulcer rapidly.

Sape. A rodent ulcer is usually round, a syphilitic ulcer is irregular in shape.

Edge. A healing non-specific ulcer has a sloping edge, a tuberculous ulcer an undermined edge, syphilitic ulcer a punched-out edve, a rodent ulcer a rolled edge, and an epithelioma a raised and everted edge.

Floor. In tuberculosis the floor is covered by gelatinous granulations, so also in amebiasis.

Base. The base of the ulcer is hard in carcinoma, and fixed to the deep structures in a varicose ulcer. Syphilitic ulcers have a slough that looks like yellow grey wash-leather. Ischemic ulcers often contain poor granulation tissue, and tendons and other structures may lie bare in the base.

Discharge. In acute infection the discharge is purulent, in *Pseudomonas pyocyaneus* infection it is bluish green, and in tuberculosis it is often watery.

Pain. Non-specific ulcers in the stage of extension are painful. Tuberculous ulcers are painless except when they occur on the tongue.

Lymph nodes. In rodent ulcer the lymph nodes are not enlarged, except from secondary infection; in carcinoma they may be enlarged, hard, and fixed.

General examination. During the general examination the clinician must look for evidence of anemia, diabetes, tuberculosis, etc.

Pathology

Any discharge should be examined bacteriologically. If the diagnosis is not clear, a biopsy from the edge of the ulcer should be taken, including a part of the normal skin adjacent to the margin of the ulcer.

TREATMENT OF ULCERS

General treatment

In order to treat an ulcer successfully, it is essential to know its exact etiology. Clinical findings often provide essential clues to the underlying disease. For example, the distal part of a limb the seat of arteriosclerosis may be cold, while a limb affected by the neuropathy of diabetes shows loss of sensation. If doubt still remains as to its exact nature, a *biopsy* of the edge should be carried out. Once the cause is found, it is eliminated as far as possible. At the same time any anemia is corrected.

Local treatment

In the case of ulcers due to specific causes, the treatment varies according to the cause of the ulcer. However, in the case of non-specific ulcers the following applications have been found to be useful in dealing with different situations:

- If granulations are excessive and edematous, they can be made firm and pink by the application of *magnesium sulphate glycerine paste.* This paste is markedly hypertonic, and therefore withdraws fluid from the ulcer due to osmosis, making it less water-logged. It should not be applied over a fresh wound, as the effect of the salt on the raw nerve endings produces unbearable pain. When the endings get covered by a layer of granulation tissue this paste may be used; the patient still gets a twinge of pain but it soon passes away, as the paste gets diluted by the tissue fluid.
- If the excessive granulations occupy a small area, they can be discouraged by the caustic effect of a 10 to 15% solution of *silver nitrate,* or by direct application of a crystal of silver nitrate. If a crystal is used, care should be taken to touch only the raw area with it. If silver nitrate powder is used by mistake, and this spills out over the surrounding skin, a severe burn with unbearable pain is the result.
- If there is an excessive quantity of sloughs in the floor of the ulcer, gauze soaked in a solution of *Eusol* is a very useful dressing. Eusol is a clear watery solution of hypochlorite, with an odour like that of slaked lime. It clears up sloughs rapidly, and makes the ulcer look clean.
- If the ulcer is chronic and non-healing, *infra-red radiation* is helpful. The healing agent is the heat produced by the infra-red rays, which causes hyperemia. This brings in many times more blood to the part, which not only delivers more oxygen and nutrients but also carries away the waste products of metabolism more promptly. Unfortunately, since the advent of antibiotics the healing properties of heat applied to an inflamed part have been forgotten, and this method of treatment is underutilized. The healing effects of heat are complementary to those of antibiotics; both can therefore be used together with advantage.
- *Antibiotics.* In general, antibiotics are not required in granulating wounds, because healthy granulation tissue forms a very effective natural barrier against bacterial invasion, and is virtually impermeable to both topical and systemic antibiotics. Antibiotics are required only if the ulcer is infected with surrounding cellulitis, and in the case of ulcers of specific bacterial origin, e.g. syphilis or tuberculosis.

Decubitus ulcer (pressure sore)

These ulcers occur over the sacral area, the heels and the back. Such an ulcer is one of the most common complications in the chronic invalid who is bedridden, or the critically ill patient, most occurring in patients who are old and have impaired mobility and neurological disease, often along with incontinence of urine and feces due to sphincter disturbances. Localized constant pressure over a contact area causes ischemia, with eventual necrosis first of the subcutaneous fat and later of the skin. The gangrenous skin eventually separates, leaving necrotic subcutaneous tissue and fat, which overlies the developing granulation tissue. The ulcer may deepen to involve tendon and bone.

Frequency of pressure sores at different sites

Pressure spores at different sites can be listed as follows in descending order of frequency:

- Ischium.
- Greater trochanter.
- Sacrum.
- Heel.
- Lateral malleolus.
- Occiput.

Prevention

Prevention is much better than the long drawn-out healing process of the ulcer once it has formed:

- Normally, a person in bed keeps changing his side periodically. Patients who are unable to move themselves *must be turned in bed every two hours,* as uninterrupted pressure due to the body weight results in ischemia of the skin and the development of bedsores.
- Twice a day, meticulous skin cleansing should be carried out using methylated spirit or cetavlon solution, followed by gentle massage and application of talcum powder.
- *Ripple air beds* are available, in which alternate air cells are inflated and deflated by a motor every few minutes, and help to distribute pressure on the back. They are a great advance in the prevention and treatment of bedsores, and allow patients to be in bed for long periods without developing pressure ulcers.
- Anemia, uremia, diabetes and hypothyroidism delay the formation of granulation tissue and their correction helps in healing.

If an ulcer still develops, the above measures are continued. Slough and dead tissue are removed until capillary bleeding is just encountered.

Silicone foam cushion

A silicone foam cushion is created as follows: the solution for producing the foam is poured into the ulcer. It 'rises' to create the foam cushion which is the exact size and shape of the defect, and distributes the pressure of the bandage evenly. The cushion is removed, washed thoroughly and replaced in the ulcer, it is washed and replaced at every change of dressing. In most cases such treatment leads to healing of the ulcer, which gets accelerated as soon as the patient starts moving about.

In a bedridden patient the ulcer may be very resistant to treatment. In such a case rotation flaps of skin and fat may need to be brought over from the buttocks.

Vacuum-assisted closure

This is also known as negative pressure wound closure. The application of intermittent negative pressure of about minus 125mm of Hg appears to hasten debridement and formation of granulation tissue in chronic wounds and ulcers.

Stages of bedsores

If left untreated, a bedsore may pass through the following four stages:

- A small area becomes red but does not blanch on pressure. The skin is intact. This area usually lies over a bony prominence. It may be painful, and could be difficult to detect in dark-skinned persons.
- There is partial thickness loss of dermis with a pink wound bed. In other cases there may be a blister filled with serum.
- The bedsore advances to full-thickness skin loss exposing subcutaneous tissue but not bones or muscles. There may be some slough.
- Here, along with full-thicknes skin loss bone, tendon or muscle are exposed. Slough may be present, along with undermined edges and tunnelling.

Ischemic ulcer

The ischemic ulcer is usually initiated by minor trauma to a limb with impaired blood supply. The anterior tibial region just above the ankle is the most common site for these ulcers.

Clinical features

Intermittent claudication or rest pain, and previous trouble with healing of skin, should lead one to suspect the condition. These clinical findings are due to reduced blood supply. The skin is atrophic. The granulation tissue is pale. The limb feels cold and is hairless with deformed nails, often with a nail-fold infection. The pulses are weak or absent.

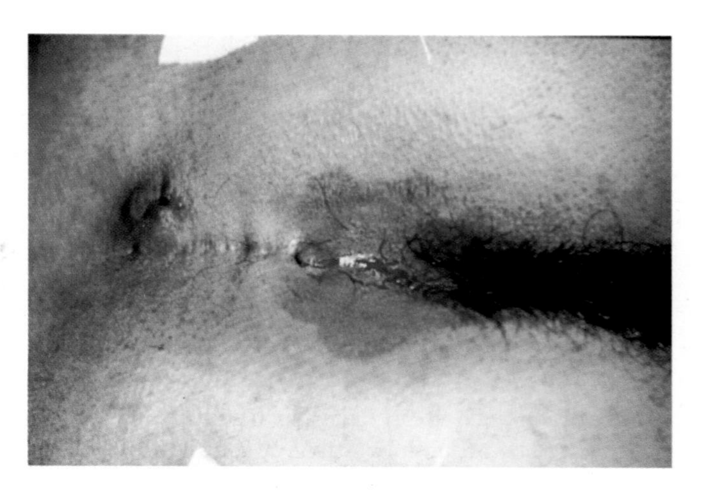

Fig.12.1 Pilonidal sinus, showing multiple sinuses with hair peeping out from some of them

Investigations

The *Doppler test* and *thermography* show reduced blood flow. The cardiovascular and respiratory systems should be examined.

Arteriography demonstrates the presence or absence of a surgically correctable arterial lesion.

Treatment

If angiography shows that *direct arterial surgery* is feasible, operation is carried out. Correction of a major vessel block may dramatically improve leg perfusion and lead to ulcer healing. Balloon angioplasty is not suitable due to the diffuse nature of the lesion.

SINUSES AND FISTULAE

Sinus

A sinus is a discharging blind-ended tract which opens onto an epithelial surface and often leads to an abscess cavity (Fig.12.1). The key to the correct treatment of a sinus is the detection of any associated deep abscess cavity or complex deep extensions of the sinus tract. Failure to do so will result in recurrence of the sinus in the same or an adjacent location.

The discharge from a sinus should always be submitted for bacteriological examination. Most of the pathogens isolated will be skin organisms or gut commensals. However, occasionally specific infections such as tuberculosis, actinomycosis or fungus (Fig.12.2 and 3) may be found. The sinus opening should be gently probed to assess the depth, direction and multiplicity of the tracts. If the opening is small, a fine tube may be introduced and a radiopaque dye injected for a 'sinogram' x-ray.

Fistula

A fistula is an abnormal communication between two epithelial or endothelial surfaces. Commonly, this communication is between two internal organs, or between an internal organ and the skin. The fistula usually derives its name from the organs which it joins together. Thus a fistula between the rectum and vagina is called a rectovaginal fistula, one between the bronchus and pleura is a bronchopleural fistula, and so on.

Causes of sinuses and fistulae

Sinuses and fistulae may be congenital or acquired:

Congenital

Examples of congenital sinuses and fistulae include preauricular sinus, tracheo-esophageal fistula, branchial fistula, etc. Most of these arise due to imperfect fusion of skin, or incomplete separation of hollow tubes from one another. Thus a preauricular sinus develops due to imperfect fusion between the auditory tubercles, and a tracheo-esophageal fistula due to incomplete separation of the trachea from the esophagus.

Acquired

These sinuses often result from inadequate drainage of an abscess, e.g. a perianal abscess may burst on the surface and lead to a sinus.

Causes of persistence of sinuses and fistulae

Congenital

Congenital fistulae are lined by epithelium, and will persist indefinitely unless surgically closed, with excision of the epithelial lining.

Acquired

Acquired sinuses and fistulae may persist due to one of many reasons:

- A *foreign* body may be present in the sinus. For example a piece of unabsorbable suture may be responsible. Again, a piece of dead bone, i.e. a sequestrum, may lead to the persistence of an osteomyelitic sinus.
- Inefficient drainage may prevent the healing of a sinus. Thus when a drain is introduced it should be placed in the most *dependent* part of a cavity, as otherwise some of the fluid remains undrained and stagnates in the cavity, resulting in persistence of the sinus.
- Irritating *discharges*, e.g. urine or stool, may prevent healing.
- Unrelieved *obstruction* of a hollow tube distal to a fistula can be the cause of non-healing of an intestinal fistula.

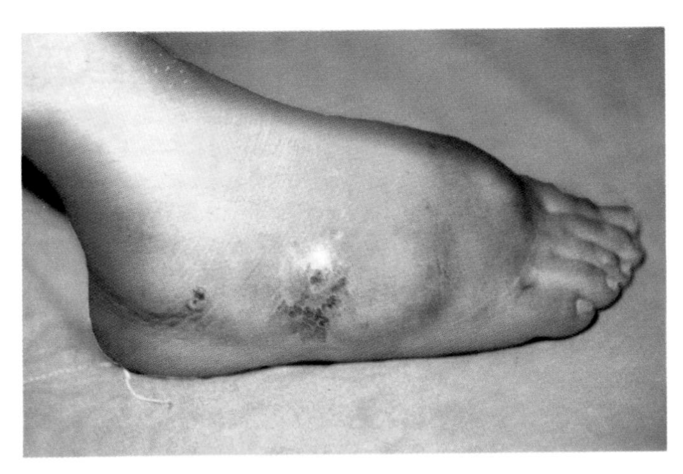

Fig.12.2 Madura foot. Grossly swollen foot with nodular fibrous masses and sinuses

- If dense *fibrous tissue* is present and prevents contraction of the cavity, the sinus or fistula will not heal.
- *Specific infections*, like tuberculosis or actinomycosis, may prevent healing.
- If the track is lined by *epithelium* the question of healing of a fistula does not arise unless and until the epithelium is excised at operation.
- If a fistula between two organs has developed due to extension of a *malignant ulcer* in one of the organs, it will not heal unless the ulcer is excised along with some healthy tissue around it. In fact, in such cases even more radical operations are usually required.

Treatment

In the treatment of a sinus or fistula, its cause must be removed. As far as the local operation is concerned: while treating any sinus, after proper evaluation the sinus is laid open or excised and a piece of tissue from the wall of the sinus sent for biopsy. In most cases this will be seen to be ordinary granulation tissue, but occasionally a metastatic deposit or a specific inflammatory condition like tuberculosis will be revealed, which would be missed if routine biopsy was not being practiced.

In the case of a fistula, if the track is lined by granulation tissue, laying it open with thorough curettage will often suffice. However, if the track is epithelialized, excision of the epithelial track is essential for healing.

ABSCESSES

An abscess is a local collection of pus which consists of a semiliquid debris of necrotic leucocytes and tissue cells. An acute abscess commonly starts as follows: a large inoculum of bacteria enters the tissues. Neutrophils are attracted to the area by chemotaxis; they surround the bacteria and liquefaction necrosis results. The lining of the abscess, which leads to the formation of more pus, consists of an inner layer of leucocytes surrounded by an outer zone of granulation tissue (*pyogenic membrane*). More neutrophils and macrophages are drawn into the cavity. At the same time the large protein molecules constituting the bodies of the bacteria and pus cells are broken down into smaller molecules which are more numerous and hence exert more osmotic pressure. Thus, both the size of the cavity and the pressure inside it continue to increase.

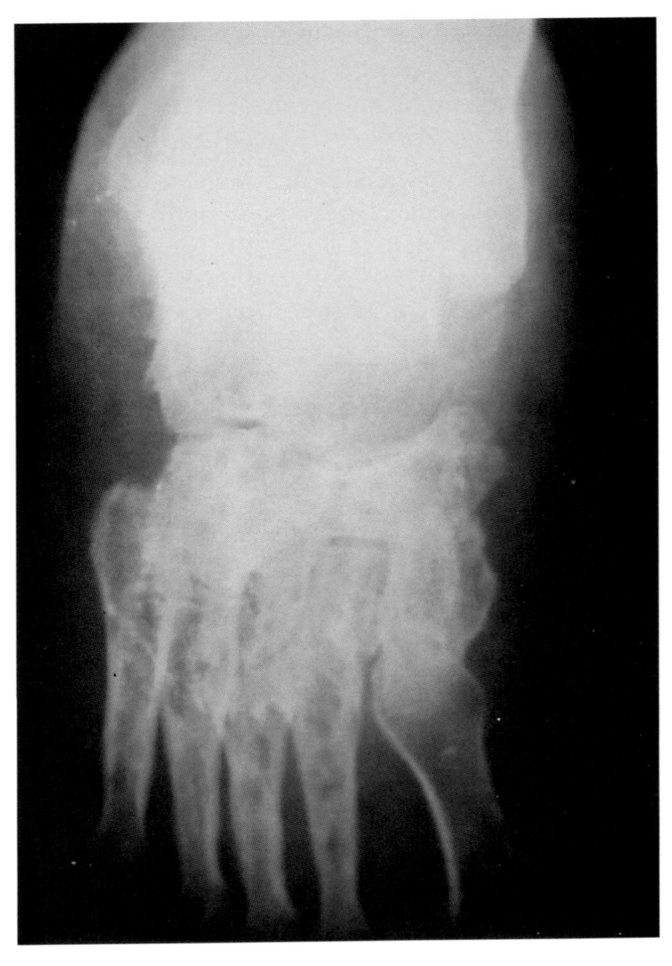

Fig.12.3 X-ray of Madura foot showing metatarsals riddled with cavities

Treatment

Antibiotics are not very effective in dealing with an abscess. The reasons for this are three:

- The granulation tissue prevents adequate levels of antibiotics penetrating the cavity.

- Many antibiotics are inactivated by different factors in the pus.
- The bacteria in the pus are in a resting phase. This reduces the uptake of the antibiotics by the bacteria.

All the above-factors render the antibiotic ineffective against the pus in the abscess. Now, antibiotics being relatively useless, drainage is the only proper method of dealing with most abscesses, and it is for this reason that such a great deal of stress is placed upon proper and adequate drainage.

Abscesses at different sites

Abscesses may form anywhere in the body, and the nature of the infecting organism varies with the site.

Abscesses in the *subcutaneous tissues* are most often caused by *Staphylococcus aureus*. With penetrating wounds as in stabs, gunshot wounds, car accidents and crush injuries, dirt and bacteria get inoculated into the tissues. In these cases the risk of infection with clostridial organisms is high, specially in the presence of dead or crushed tissue. These wounds therefore always require prompt surgical excision and toilet.

Intra-abdominal abscesses are usually caused by perforations in the gastrointestinal tract, as in cases of appendicitis, diverticulitis, peptic ulcer and malignant ulcer of the colon. In other cases a leaking surgical anastomosis may be responsible. Usually many organisms are present, commonly from the enteric group: coliforms, *Streptococcus fecalis*, clostridia and bacteroides.

Factors increasing the risk of infection

In cases of perforation of the colon and esophagus the risk of development of intra-abdominal abscesses is very high. The risk is less with perforation of the stomach and small bowel, as the normal resident count of bacteria in these organs is low. However, when the small intestine is obstructed or acid secretion is reduced in the stomach, bacterial overgrowth occurs. Other factors increasing the risk of sepsis include:

- Advancing age of the patient.
- Obesity.
- Malnutrition.
- Shock.
- Decreased immunocompetence.

Following surgical treatment of intra-abdominal abscesses in such cases the mortality rate is high, upto 20%.

Clinical features

There is usually a systemic reaction with toxicity and intermittent fever. Pain and tenderness are present. The pain may become severe and throbbing if the pus is under tension.

If an abscess is deep-seated and not under pressure, it may be silent even though large. However, the patient develops signs of toxicity and a hypercatabolic state, which may even progress to *multiple organ system failure*.

At the same time, the risk of rupture of an abscess into the bloodstream and *sepsis* is always present. Rupture of an intra-abdominal abscess results in widespread peritonitis.

Natural history

- An abscess may resolve after prompt and appropriate antibiotic therapy. The contents become liquefied by proteolytic digestion and the watery debris is gradually reabsorbed. The residual cavity occasionally calcifies.
- If the abscess is near an external or internal surface, it may drain spontaneously and resolve.
- The pressure effect of an expanding abscess may cause vascular thrombosis and cell death around it. The abscess may now track along fascial layers.

When an abscess gets drained, not only does this lead to evacuation of the pus and reduction of the bacterial load, but also it releases the pressure in the abscess and allows the penetration of antibiotics into the abscess cavity. The bacteria also start multiplying again and thus become more sensitive to antibiotics.

Treatment

The proper treatment of most abscesses consists of adequate drainage of the pus. After incision and drainage of the pus the abcess cavity should be thoroughly washed and curetted to break all the loculi and the cavity left open to heal by secondary intention; never should the abcess cavity be primarily closed.

Percutaneous drainage

In the past drainage always meant open drainage, but since the advent of ultrasound and computerized tomography, percutaneous drainage of the pus under ultrasound or CT control has become quite popular. The guidance provided by these imaging methods obviates the need for open operation. The catheter is left inside the cavity, and soon the drainage fluid from the abscess becomes more liquid. The rate of shrinkage of the abscess cavity can be monitored by x-rays taken after injection of a contrast medium. There may be more than one abscess, and if clinical improvement does not take place after adequate drainage of the abscess, the ultrasound examination should be repeated. An abscess may be secondary to a serious underlying disease; in that case appropriate treatment of the underlying condition should be carried out as soon as the abscess has been drained.

The onset of shock, rigors, a rising pulse rate and fever indicate sepsis. Blood cultures should be taken, fluids replaced and antibiotic therapy commenced. Evacuation of pus should not be delayed. A biopsy of the wall of the abscess should be sent in all cases if a malignancy is not to be missed. Pus should be sent for culture; a swab is less effective in obtaining an accurate culture unless sent in a transport medium.

Chapter

13 SURGICAL INFECTIONS

Infections are of great importance to the surgeon. If, after a major operation, the wound heals cleanly, the patient goes home in a few days. On the other hand if infection develops, the patient may be in the hospital for many weeks. If the infection remains localized to the area of the wound it will delay wound healing and at the same time lead to a broad ugly scar. If it spreads through the blood-stream it could even kill him by causing septicemia.

Historically, a surgical operation was a dreaded event, because almost all operation wounds became septic, and nearly half of all patients who had a major operation died as a result of invasive infection, so that compound fractures were treated by amputation!

It was only after Lister and others, from the 1860s onwards, introduced the concept first of antisepsis and later of strict aseptic precautions in surgery that infection rates fell to the present low levels. Sterilization of instruments, first by chemicals and later by steam, was introduced during the 1880s, followed shortly by hand washing and wearing of gowns, gloves, caps and masks. Before this time surgeons used to wash their hands after, not before, operations!

Antibiotics were first used in the treatment of infections in the 1940s, starting with penicillin and followed by streptomycin and others. Since then, an increasing number of antibiotics has become available, so that infections which in days gone by regularly resulted in mortality are treated successfully in the great majority of cases.

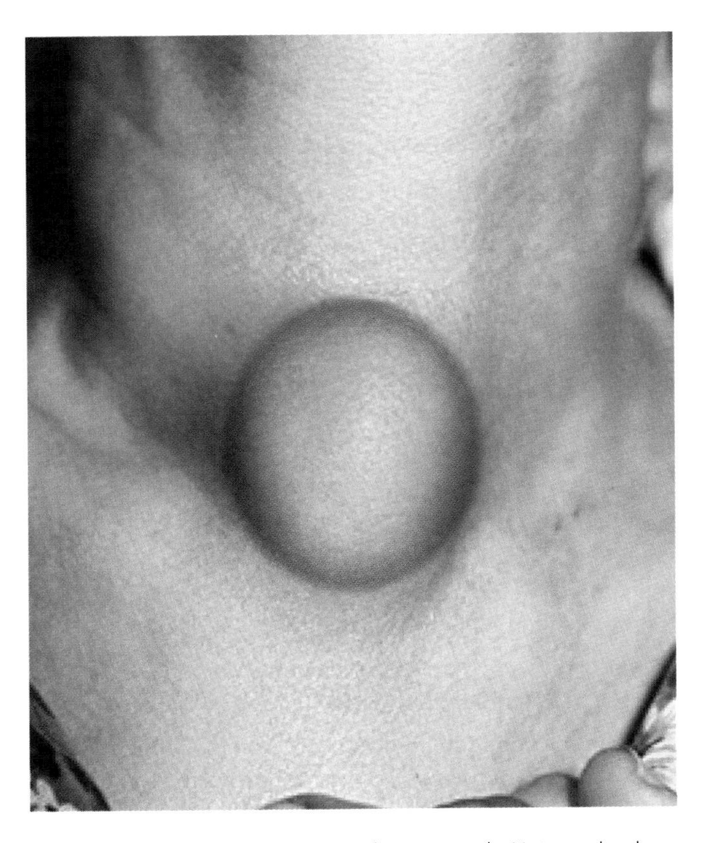

Fig.13.1 Acute subcutaneous abscess neck. Note red colour due to the hyperemia of inflammation.

Surgical infections

These include those infections that either require, or result from, operative treatment, and those that are hospital-acquired:

Infections ***requiring operative treatment*** include the following:

- Body cavity infections, e.g. peritonitis, pericarditis, empyema.
- Confined infections, e.g. abscesses, suppurative arthritis.
- Soft tissue infections resulting in necrosis.

Infections ***resulting from operative treatment*** include:

- Wound infections.
- Postoperative abscesses and peritonitis.
- Infections associated with prosthetic devices.

Hospital-acquired infections include:

- Pneumonias and infections resulting from catheters.
- Viral or fungal infections that can overwhelm a surgical patient who is immuno-compromised.

FACTORS IN THE DEVELOPMENT OF INFECTION

Soon after birth a variety of micro-organisms colonize both the external and internal surfaces of the body. They do no harm and in fact may be beneficial. For example the normal intestinal flora act as a barrier against infections with pathogens such as Salmonella and Shigella species.

Even in the case of pathogenic bacteria contamination becomes invasive infection only if either the micro-organism is excessively virulent or the resistance of the patient is reduced. The development of infection depends upon several factors, but predominantly microbial virulence and host defences.

Microbial virulence

Whether infection develops or not depends upon the balance between microbial virulence and host defences. Microbes that cannot cause infection in a normal host can result in serious infection in an individual with immunocompromised defences.

Enhanced pathogenicity

Some bacteria possess features that increase their pathogenicity:

- Certain bacteria have surface components which increase their pathogenicity by *inhibiting phagocytosis*, e.g. the capsule of Klebsiella.
- Other bacteria have surface components which are *toxic*, e.g. the enterobacteria.
- Still others, like clostridia and some strains of streptococci, produce *exotoxins*.

In clean wounds the common organisms found are skin bacteria like *Staphylococcus epidermidis*. In traumatic wounds the most common organisms are *Staphylococcus aureus* and *Streptococcus pyogenes*. When a body viscus is entered the resident flora become the expected pathogens.

Number of bacteria required to produce infection

Bacterial contamination with greater than 10^5 organisms commonly leads to infection, whereas contamination with less than this number usually does not. In traumatic wounds foreign bodies and devitalized tissues are often found; in their presence fewer organisms are required to produce infection than in normal tissues. This is the reason why foreign materials and dead tissues are disliked so much by surgeons, and every effort is made to get rid of them.

Bacterial toxins

Bacterial infection causes damage to the host cells and tissues at the site of invasion. At the same time bacterial toxins are transported by the blood and lymph to cause cytotoxic effects at distant sites.

Different micro-organisms vary in their ability to cause local and systemic damage:

- *Staphylococcus aureus* produces local damage but has little tendency to spread.
- *Streptococcus pyogenes* is both invasive and toxigenic.
- *Clostridium tetani* is almost solely toxigenic.

Types of toxins

Toxins are of two types:

Exotoxins

These are specific proteins produced by certain bacteria. When they are denatured they lose their toxicity but retain their antigenicity. Such modified exotoxins are called *toxoids*. Those produced from *Clostridium tetani* are used to induce active immunity in man.

Endotoxins

These are produced by gram-negative species. They are lipopolysaccharides of the bacterial cell wall, and are released only on dissolution of the bacterial cell. They do not form toxoids, so vaccines against them cannot readily be prepared.

Host defences

Local host defences

Epithelia

Epithelia surround the tissues of the body and protect them from invasion by microbes. The skin as well as the epithelia around body orifices, e.g. pharynx, esophagus and urinary tract, are multilayered for more effective protection. Mucous membranes are less resistant, but even here bacterial entry does not usually take place unless a small break occurs.

Breaches in epithelia

Many hospital-acquired infections result from therapeutic procedures which involve a breach in the skin or another epithelial surface. Prolonged use of indwelling urinary or vascular *catheters*, *tracheostomies* and *ventilators* are responsible for most iatrogenic infections.

Phagocytes

For effective function by phagocytes, firstly they have to be delivered at the site of infection, and secondly they have to ingest the infecting bacteria.

Delivery of phagocytes

Any condition which reduces the delivery of phagocytes to an area of bacterial contamination promotes the development of infection. Examples include the following:

- Reduced blood flow, e.g. in vascular occlusive states, in hypovolemic shock, or after the use of vasopressors.
- The presence of devitalized tissues, foreign bodies, hematomas and seromas.
- Decreased vascular reactivity, e.g. in old age, in uremia, and after the use of steroids.
- Decreased production of phagocytes, e.g. after irradiation or cytotoxic chemotherapy, and in granulocytopenia from drugs or other cause.

Ingestion by phagocytes

In certain disease states the ingestive phase of leucocyte function is defective. Examples include the following conditions:

- Uraemia.
- Ketosis.
- Hyperglycemia.
- Prematurity.
- Certain malignancies.
- Immunologic deficiency diseases.
- Malnutrition.
- In extensive burns and wounds, as well as in severe sepsis, a hypermetabolic state exists, which may lead rapidly to protein malnutrition. When this occurs, phagocytic function is impaired, leading to bacteremia and even severe sepsis.

Local environment

Each site also provides a local environment that is not conducive to the growth of microbes. These local factors include the flushing action of tears and urine, the action of the cilia in the respiratory tract, the low pH and mucus in the stomach, etc.

Disturbance in environment

- If *trauma* has resulted in devitalization of tissue, or if *foreign bodies* have become deposited in the wound, the likelihood of infection is greatly increased.
- *Fluid collections* inhibit phagocytosis and increase the likelihood of infection.
- *Peripheral vascular disease* as well as *shock* reduce the delivery of blood (and the systemic host defence factors it contains) to the infected part, and are accompanied by a greater incidence of infection.

Surgical technique

Last, but not least, surgical technique has a significant bearing on the incidence of postoperative infection. The chances of infection are decreased by:

- Gentle handling of tissues.
- Removal of devitalized tissue.
- Avoidance of excess use of cautery.
- Ensuring adequate blood supply to bowel ends before anastomosis, etc.

Systemic host defences

These consist of phagocytes; the immune system; and molecular cascades, such as the complement system, the coagulation system and the kinins. The phagocytes include polymorphonuclear leucocytes (PMNs) and macrophages.

Neutrophils

As a result of interaction with complement and other activators, neutrophils adhere to vessel endothelium, migrate across the endothelium, and move towards the microbe. They attach to and phagocytose the microbes. Finally lysosomes empty their enzymes into the phagosome and the microbe is digested.

Macrophages

Macrophages not only phagocytose microbes but also initiate the immune response and can elaborate cytokines, tumor necrosis factor, interferons, etc.

Impairment of host defences

Host defences are *impaired:*

- In the very young and the very old.
- In malnutrition.
- After major trauma and burns.
- After extensive operation.
- In advanced malignant disease, and after chemotherapy for the same.
- After immunosuppression to prevent rejection of organ transplants.
- In patients on steroids.

Superinfections

Superinfections with viruses and fungi usually occur when the resistance of the host is diminished. Apart from immunologically deficient patients, they occur mostly during a course of antibiotic therapy!

The cytokine cascade

Cytokines are factors released by activated cells that act as messengers in cellular communication, at times spilling over into the circulation to function as hormones in response to hemorrhage, sepsis, inflammation and other forms of injury. They are *proteins* that are stimulated by the host defence system, and have autocrine effects (in the cells), paracrine effects (adjacent to the cells), and endocrine effects (at a distance).

The two most important cytokines are interleukin-1 and tumor necrosis factor:

Interleukin-1 (IL-1)

Stimulants to the release of interleukin-1 include nearly all inflammatory, infectious and immunological processes. IL-1 acts on the central nervous system. It:

- Induces *fever* by stimulating release of prostaglandins in the anterior hypothalamus.
- Produces *anorexia* by direct action on the satiety center.
- Lessens *pain* perception by increasing beta-endorphan release.
- Promotes skeletal muscle *proteolysis*. The amino acids thus released are used by the liver for energy as well as for synthesis of new proteins.

Tumor necrosis factor (TNF)

This is a cytokine protein which acts synergistically with interleukin-1 to induce *hypotension*, *tissue injury* and *death* in animals subjected to experimental sepsis.

TNF probably mediates the early hypotension of sepsis, and IL-1 participates in the later phases of sepsis-induced shock.

DIAGNOSIS

Signs and symptoms vary according to the site and severity of infection. Diagnosis requires a composite of information, including history, physical examination, radiographic findings, and laboratory data. The commonest presenting features are fever, redness, swelling, pus discharge, increase in fluid from drains, wound dehiscence, diarrhea, cough, dysuria etc.

Sources of pathogens

The pathogen may be exogenous or endogenous:

Endogenous

Most of these microorganisms come from the patient's endogenous flora.

Exogenous

Occasionally, the pathogenic organisms are acquired from an exogenous source, such as:

- The air in the operating room.
- Surgical equipment.
- Implants or gloves.
- Medications administered during the operative procedure.

Laboratory

Specimen selection, collection, and processing

- The quantity of material must be *adequate*.
- Specimens are selected on the basis of signs and symptoms, and should be *representative* of the disease process.
- *Contamination* of the specimen must be avoided by using only sterile equipment and aseptic precautions.
- The specimen must be taken to the laboratory and examined *promptly*. Special transport media may be helpful.
- Meaningful specimens to diagnose bacterial infections must be secured before antimicrobial drugs are started.

Inflammatory markers

A recent rise in the inflammatory markers is a clue towards progress of the disease process. At the same time checking inflammatory markers at the start of treatment and again later indicates response to treatment and serves as a guide regarding duration of treatment. Common markers that are checked include:

- White cell count.
- C reactive protein (CRP).
- Erythrocyte sedimentation rate (ESR).
- Pro calcitonin levels.
- Galactomannan assays etc.

Leucocytosis

Leucocytosis accompanies an acute bacterial infection. In most surgical infections the count is only slightly or moderately raised. A very high leucocyte count (upto 35,000/mm^3) occurs in suppuration.

A *reliable* total and differential leucocyte count is of great help to a surgeon in the diagnosis of the not-so-obvious infection.

Leucopenia

However in the elderly, in the severely ill patient, and during therapy with antibiotics, some anticancer and immuno-suppressive drugs, white cell counts may be normal or even low. In overwhelming sepsis there may be leucopenia, due to suppression of the bone marrow and exhaustion of the supply of leucocytes.

In some cases the total number of leucocytes is normal. However, if there is a larger proportion of immature cells ('shift to the left'), this indicates an accelerated rate of production of white cells and points to the presence of an infection.

Pitfalls in diagnosis

It must be remembered that the only evidence of a chronic infection may be fatigue, low-grade fever and anemia. At the same time, massive pyogenic abscesses may occur without leukocytosis, fever or tenderness. So the clinician should be on his guard in patients presenting with vague symptoms.

Appearance of pus

The pus should be examined for colour, odour and consistency. Foul-smelling pus usually means infection with anaerobes. Thin pus often indicates spreading infection, while thick pus definitely means that the infection has been confined (the 'laudable pus' of the past).

Gram staining

Micro-organisms causing a surgical infection may often be seen under the microscope on a gram-stained smear. This is a simple, rapid and inexpensive method which *provides very valuable information* for the surgeon. It should be used more often. Pus from abscesses may be obtained by incision-drainage or, in the case of deep-seated abscesses, by needle aspiration. Antibiotics should be started only after the pus has been collected.

Acid-fast stain

The acid-fast stain is applied to sputum, other fluids, and tissue samples when AFB (acid-fast bacilli e.g., *Mycobacterium* spp.) are suspected. The identification of the pink/red AFB against the blue background of the counterstain requires expertise. This can also be used in scenarios where nocardia or actinomycosis is suspected.

Biopsy

In granulomatous lesions biopsy is useful in establishing the diagnosis, e.g. in tuberculosis, syphilis and the mycoses.

Cultures

Cultures can help in identifying the micro-organisms responsible for the infection. Special care should be taken while interpreting the reports, as at times normal flora is reported and treating that may end up in a failure. Similarly, colonization should also be ruled out by looking into further details on the smear report especially for specimens other than blood. However, even a specimen taken at the height of a chill and fever may be negative, because phagocytes rapidly remove bacteria, while chills and fever occur about an hour later.

The chances of detecting a bacterial pathogen are increased by:

- Increasing the volume of the blood sample collected.
- Obtaining multiple cultures (up to three per 24 hour periods).

Blood cultures if reported positive should be repeated frequently as in certain organisms the duration of antibiotic therapy depends on when the cultures became negative after the start of therapy.

Imaging

Focal abscesses necessitate immediate ultrasonography, CT or MRI as part of an evaluation for surgical intervention. The choice of imaging depends on the site of collection and availability. Antibiotics should be administered before imaging but only after blood for cultures has been drawn.

PRINCIPLES OF TREATMENT OF INFECTIONS

In the case of *acute spreading* infections, e.g., cellulitis and septicemia, antibiotics are the primary treatment, and should result in clinical improvement in 24 to 48 hours; when the blood culture report is received, a change to a more effective antibiotic may be indicated.

As far as *localized* infections are concerned, antibiotics may not penetrate inside abscess cavities, and therefore incision and drainage must be carried out. At the same time, *necrotic* tissues or foreign bodies prevent the proper functioning of host defenses, and have to be removed.

Perforations or anastomotic leaks of the gastrointestinal tract provide a continuing source of bacteria that overwhelm the defenses.

Surgical exploration

This is required to eradicate this constant source of infection by closing the perforation or, in the large bowel, by 'exteriorizing' it as in a colostomy.

Supportive measures to be taken for surgical infections include the following:

- Bed rest.
- Relief of pain.
- Immobilization of the infected region to provide rest.
- Elevation of a limb to promote venous and lymphatic drainage.

TYPES OF SURGICAL INFECTIONS

Soft tissue infections

Cellulitis

This is an acute inflammation of the skin, subcutaneous tissues and intercellular spaces. There is swelling, redness, warmth and pain without definite localization. The central area may undergo necrosis and suppuration. In severe forms, blebs and bullae form on the skin. The etiology is diverse and depends on the clinical setting, and history has an important role in determining the cause. For example the neutropenics, cases of bites, and the elderly diabetics, all have a predilection to one or more different pathogens.

Treatment

This consists of appropriate antibiotic therapy and rest. If there is no response in 48–72 hours, the patient may need imaging to rule out collections, and a broader antibiotic cover.

Lymphangitis

Lymphangitis is an inflammation of lymphatic pathways, and is usually visible as red streaks under the skin. Again the most common aetiological agent is the hemolytic streptococcus. Lymphangitis and the associated lymphadenitis are a normal defence reaction against bacterial invasion, and are often seen on the forearm of a patient with infection of the hand or fingers. Most cases will respond to antibiotic therapy and rest.

Erysipelas

This is characterized by an abrupt onset of fiery-red swelling of the face or extremities. The distinctive features of erysipelas are well-defined: indurated margins, particularly along the nasolabial folds, rapid progression, and intense pain. Flaccid bullae may develop during the second or third day of illness, but extension to deeper soft tissues is rare. Erysipelas is usually caused by hemolytic streptococci which gain entrance through a break in the skin.

Treatment

Treatment with penicillin is effective. Antibiotic therapy halts the spread of the infection, but the erythema disappears more slowly with desquamation.

Abscess

An abscess is a localized collection of pus surrounded by an area of inflamed tissue in which there is marked hyperemia and infiltration by leucocytes. Abscesses can be divided into two categories i.e. superficial and deep. Superficial abscesses mainly involve the skin and subcutaneous tissues, while deep abscesses include intraperitonial, visceral, perinepheric, psoas, brain and lung abscesses.

Boil or furuncle

This is an abscess in a sweat gland or hair-follicle. The course of a boil may be self-limited as it bursts and subsides, and may require no treatment. However, large boils and abscesses should be incised and drained and the patient treated with antibiotics.

'Dangerous area'

The area of the face bounded by the bridge of the nose and the angles of the mouth is called the 'dangerous area'. This is because the veins of this area communicate with the cavernous sinus, and a boil or other infection in their drainage area can produce septic cavernous sinus thrombosis, with serious consequences for the patient.

Carbuncle

A carbuncle is a multilocular suppurative extension of a boil into the subcutaneous tissues. The back of the lower part of the neck and the upper part of the chest are common sites. The carbuncle consists of a honeycomb of hundreds of tiny abscess cavities. When they rupture onto the skin, numerous sinuses develop. The most common organism concerned is *Staphylococcus aureus,* but streptococci and gram-negative bacilli may also be found. Incision of all the hundreds of cavities is impossible; therefore the only proper treatment of a carbuncle is to excise it completely. The wound contracts to a small scar, and a skin graft is usually not required. Carbuncles are almost always seen in patients suffering from diabetes mellitus; the diabetes should be brought under as effective control as possible before operation on the carbuncle.

Necrotizing soft tissue infections

Soft tissue infections that result in tissue necrosis are less common than other forms of infection but more serious because of extensive destruction of tissues and a higher mortality rate. Most are caused by mixed aerobic and anaerobic gram-negative and gram-positive bacteria. *Clostridium* species are common and cause the most severe infections, to which the term gas gangrene has been applied.

These infections must be recognized early and treated aggressively. If the overlying skin is normal, diagnosis may be difficult. Early mental confusion, toxicity and failure to respond to non-operative therapy may be the earliest clues to the presence of a necrotizing infection. Gas gangrene is described in detail later in this chapter.

Body cavity infections

These include peritonitis, intra-abdominal abscess, and empyema. They are described in the appropriate chapters.

Prosthetic-device associated infections

These are seen in cases with prosthetic cardiac valves, vascular grafts and artificial joints. They are accompanied by failure of the operation besides great morbidity, and even death of the patient. Although the prosthetic devices have occasionally been salvaged by adequate antibiotic use if infections occur early (approximately 1 month) after surgery, usually infected devices require removal. If removal is not possible in case of prosthetic joints, antibiotics in suppressive doses may have to be given for longer durations.

Hospital-acquired (nosocomial infections)

These are infections acquired during stay in a hospital and occur after 48 hours of admission. They lead to an increased hospital stay and a great deal of loss of time from work. Hospital-acquired infections are caused by viral, bacterial, and fungal pathogens; the most common types include:

- Bloodstream infection.
- Urinary tract infections (UTI).
- Pneumonia, e.g. ventilator-associated pneumonia.
- Vascular catheter-related infections.
- Surgical site infections.

Urinary tract infections

These account for 30% of hospital-acquired infections. Among UTIs acquired in the hospital, approximately 75% are associated with a urinary catheter.

The most important risk factor for developing a catheter-associated UTI is *prolonged use* of the urinary catheter. Therefore, catheters should only be used for appropriate indications and should be removed as soon as they are no longer needed. Catheters should be placed by properly trained persons using sterile equipment and an aseptic technique, and a closed drainage system should be maintained to prevent infection.

Lower respiratory tract infections

These constitute the third largest group of hospital-acquired infections. The common factors responsible include the following:

- Abolition of cough reflex by anesthesia permits aspiration of contaminated material.
- Pain from thoracic or upper abdominal operations interferes with coughing and deep breathing and allows retention of sputum in the tracheobronchial tree and atelectasis which predisposes to infection.
- Pulmonary edema or adult respiratory distress syndrome arising due to overinfusion, cardiac failure, trauma, sepsis, etc. predisposes to pulmonary infection.
- In intubated patients in critical care units, even low levels of aspiration may lead to pneumonia.

Ventilator-associated pneumonia

This is a lung infection that develops in a person who is on a ventilator, and accounts for one of the major contributors to morbidity in areas with poor infection control.

Vascular catheter-related infections

These are quite common, involving micro-organisms at the exit site of the catheter. Any evidence of phlebitis or cellulitis, or suspicion of septic complication due to an intravenous line, should be dealt with by immediate removal of the cannula in the case of a peripheral cannula.

In cases of central vascular catheters, the best course to follow is to confirm a central-line-associated bloodstream infection, and then manage accordingly.

WOUND INFECTIONS

Local factors

Local factors in wound infection have been discussed above as well as in the chapter on wounds.

Systemic factors in wound infections

Many systemic conditions have an influence on the healing of wounds:

Resistance

The resistance of the patient is deficient in a number of systemic conditions and diseases. These include:

- Old age.
- Prematurity.
- Advanced malignancy.
- Burn or traumatic injury.
- Diabetes mellitus.
- Uraemia.
- Inherited immunodeficiency diseases.
- Immunosuppressive therapies.

In these conditions extraordinary precautions should be taken to prevent the development of wound infections, including correction of the underlying defect whenever possible.

Malnutrition

Even when subclinical, malnutrition can greatly impair host defences. The surgeon must correct any malnutrition before surgery, or as soon thereafter as possible. Malnutrition is widely prevalent in underdeveloped countries. There are two main causes:

- Undernutrition due to poverty.
- The loss of valuable proteins in the diarrhea of repeated episodes of dysentery due to poor food hygiene and impure water supply.

Surgeons in these countries should be aware of this. The cause of malnutrition should be identified and corrected *before* elective surgery, as fas as possible.

Drugs

If steroids, anticancer agents or antimetabolites are used there is an increased incidence of septic complications.

The above list of factors predisposing to infection in wounds shows how important it is *to take a meticulous and detailed history about the general health* of any patient who is about to undergo a surgical operation.

PREVENTION OF WOUND INFECTION

Prevention of infection is far more practical than treating it once it has become established. Fortunately, strict adherence to the principles of wound care can prevent the vast majority of infectious complications in surgical practice.

In the hospital

Meticulous attention to every aspect of hygiene in every ward and operation theatre is important.

- *Toilets*, specially in operation theatres and surgical wards, should at all time be kept spotlessly clean.
- Severely infected cases should be *isolated* and barrier nursed.
- Surgical *audit* should be instituted to keep the infection rate under surveillance, so that adequate steps can be taken whenever necessary.
- If there is an *outbreak* of staphylococcal sepsis:
    - o Elective operations should be stopped.
    - o Nasal swabs should be obtained from patients and staff to detect carriers, who should be treated and not allowed to return to work until the organism has been eliminated.
    - o Patients with sepsis should be isolated and discharged as soon as possible.

Preparation of the patient

The longer a patient's preoperative stay in hospital, the higher is the incidence of infection even in his otherwise clean wound, due to micro-organisms accumulated by the patient during his hospital stay. Therefore, each patient should be operated upon as soon after admission as possible.

If a *remote* infection is present, the rate of wound infection is tripled; therefore elective operations should be delayed until the infection has been eliminated.

A *preoperative shower*, preferably with an antiseptic soap, such as chlorhexidine or povidone-iodine, reduces the resident skin bacteria.

In the operation theatre

Air

The theatre should be supplied with properly filtered *air*, using filters with a pore size of 2mm. If clean air is introduced into the operating room close to the ceiling, and allowed to exit near the floor, it helps in limiting airborne contamination to very low levels. The air should be brought in at positive pressure, so that the flow of air is from the theatre outwards and not vice versa. The number of air changes per hour should be kept at the prescribed rate for the theatre block. The *number* of persons in the operating theatre, their *movement*, as well as *conversation*, should be kept at a minimum.

Instruments

The instruments should be sterilized by autoclave, antiseptics or ethylene dioxide, and the adequacy of sterilization checked regularly.

Gowns

These should be properly designed, and *caps and masks* should be properly fitting. Recent studies have shown that when surgeons did not wear masks, wound infection rates did not increase. However, the above-named barriers should still be used, if only to prevent the patient's blood coming in contact with the operation room staff.

Hands

Hands should be washed for 5 minutes, using chlorhexidine or povidone-iodine. During operation a fair number of *gloves* get punctured; they should be immediately changed to avoid bacterial contamination of the wound.

Skin

The patient's skin around the operation area should be prepared with a soap, followed by painting with a bactericidal solution, e.g. 0.5 % chlorhexidine in 70% alcohol or 1 % povidone-iodine. The whole body apart from the operation area should be covered with cloth *towels* held in place by towel clips. An alternative is to apply a sterile, transparent, adhesive sheet to the operation area, with the incision made through the plastic sheet. This measure gained popularity; however, some recent work has shown the use of this method to have increased the incidence of infection due to the warmth and moisture under the impermeable sterile sheet!

During the operation

Dissection should be gentle, without bruising or forceful retraction of the tissues. *Hemostasis* should be adequate, as a hematoma acts as a foreign body. The surgeon should not spend an *unduly long* time over the operation, as the tissues are traumatized while the wound is open.

If *non-absorbable* sutures have to be left in the wound, as far as possible they should be monofilament materials.

Open drains should be avoided as far as possible; tube drains leading to bottles should be used instead. If open drains have to be used, they should be removed as soon as possible

GI and GU tracts

If the gastrointestinal, respiratory or urinary tract has to be transected:

- Before a hollow viscus is entered, the operative area should be carefully isolated by towels from the rest of the operative field.
- A different set of instruments should be used for that part of the operation until the hollow viscus is closed.
- All instruments, towels and sponges that may have come into contact with the contaminating bacteria should be discarded.
- The gowns and gloves of the surgical team should be changed before proceeding with closure of the wound.

WOUND CARE

Wounds should be taken care of meticulously, specially if there is an impairment of host defence:

- Gentle care of the tissues is important, as it minimizes local damage.
- Devitalized tissues and foreign bodies should be removed.
- If complete debridement is not possible the wound *should not be closed*.
- In contaminated wounds, monofilament suture materials, e.g. polypropylene, are preferable to multifilament sutures like silk. This is because bacteria can get lodged in the interstices of multifilament sutures, where they are safe from the action of macrophages and antibiotics. If infection takes place in the presence of a multifilament suture it will not subside until the offending suture is removed.
- The presence of hematomas, seromas or dead spaces favors bacterial localization and growth. If a large potential dead space results after an operation, it is best to provide a system of closed suction drainage.
- In heavily contaminated wounds the use of *delayed primary closure* will greatly reduce the chances of serious infection. The skin and subcutaneous tissues are left unsutured and packed loosely with gauze. The number of phagocytes at the wound edges increases to reach a peak in about five days. At the same time there is intense capillary budding. The exudate diminishes in quantity and becomes clear, and closure can usually be safely carried out at this time.

ANTIBIOTIC THERAPY

When used for the correct indications, antibiotics help reduce the incidence of post-operative infections. However, blind and indiscriminate use of antibiotics does more harm than good by developing resistant strains of bacteria in hospitals. As far as the likelihood of development of infections is concerned, wounds can be divided into three categories:

Clean surgical wounds

These are those:

- which are non-traumatic,
- where there is no break in aseptic technique,
- where the respiratory or alimentary tracts have not been entered.

In such wounds the incidence of infections is less than 1% when careful, gentle, meticulous aseptic technique is practised. Therefore there is no need to use prophylactic antibiotics in these cases. If infection occurs it is due to poor surgical technique or errors in aseptic routine.

Clean-contaminated cases

These are wounds in which:

- the gastrointestinal or respiratory tracts are entered without significant spillage,
- pharynx, vagina or non-infected genitourinary or

biliary tract are entered,

- there is a minor break in aseptic technique.

Contaminated cases

These are wounds:

- which are traumatic cases,
- where there has been a major break in aseptic technique,
- where gross spillage has occurred from the alimentary tract,
- where the genitourinary or biliary tracts have been entered in the presence of infected urine or bile.

The acceptable infection rates for clean, clean-contaminated and contaminated cases are less than 1%, 3%, and 5% respectively. If higher rates of infection are encountered, the matter should be investigated.

Prophylactic antibiotics

The idea behind prophylactic antibiotics is that if contamination with bacteria takes place during operation, the antibiotic should already be in position in the bloodstream and the tissues, so that it can destroy the small numbers of organisms before they get a chance to multiply to very large numbers. It should again be stressed that *prophylactic antibiotic therapy is no substitute for careful surgical technique* and aseptic surgical principles, and its indiscriminate or general use is not in the best interest of the patient.

Some points to note are the following:

- The antimicrobial agent should be started within 60 minutes before surgical incision; it is generally started at the time of the induction of anesthesia.
- Single-dose prophylaxis is usually sufficient.
- The duration of prophylaxis for all procedures should be less than 24 hours.
- For patients known to be colonized with methicillin-resistant *Staphylococcus aureus*, it is reasonable to add a single preoperative dose of vancomycin to the recommended agent.

Re-administration

If an agent with a short half-life is used (e.g., cefazolin, cefoxitin), it should be readministered if the duration of the procedure exceeds the recommended redosing interval (from the time of initiation of the preoperative dose).

MICRO-ORGANISMS IN THE BLOOD-STREAM

Bacteraemia

Bacteraemia is defined as the transient presence of bacteria in the blood with no toxemia or other clinical signs, as a result of local infection or penetrating injury. It usually lasts only a few moments, as the macrophage phagocyte system destroys these organisms under normal conditions. The normal person probably experiences bacteremia many times e.g. after tooth brushing, dental procedures, wounds etc. It is probable that infections in internal organs, e.g. osteomyelitis and subacute bacterial endocarditis, develop through this kind of bacteremia.

Systemic inflammatory response syndrome (SIRS)

This is the name given to a widespread inflammatory response to a wide variety of severe clinical insults related to sepsis.

SIRS criteria

SIRS is clinically recognized by the presence of two or more of the following criteria:

- Temperature: > 38°C or < 36°C
- Heart rate: > 90
- Respiratory rate: > 20 or PaCO2 <32
- WBC: > 12,000
  < 4000, or
  >10% immature forms

Criteria of sepsis and severe sepsis

For the diagnosis of sepsis and severe sepsis, additional criteria apply:

Sepsis: *SIRS criteria + evidence of infection, or:*

- White cells in normally sterile body fluid.
- Perforated viscus.
- Radiographic evidence of pneumonia.
- Syndrome associated with a high risk of infection.

Severe sepsis: *Sepsis criteria + evidence of organ dysfunction, including*:

- *CV*:
  - o Systolic BP < 90mmHg.
  - o MAP (mean arterial pressure) < 70mm Hg for at least 1 hour despite volume resuscitation.
  - o Use of vasopressors.
- *Renal*:
  - o Urine output < 0.5ml/kg body weight/hr for 1 hour despite volume resuscitation.

- *Pulmonary*:
  - o $PaO_2/FiO_2 < 250$ if other organ dysfunction is present.
  - o Or < 200 if the lung is the only dysfunctional organ.
- *Hematologic*:
  - o Platelet count < 80K
- *Metabolic*:
  - o pH < 7.3
  - o Plasma lactate > 1.5 x upper normal.

Pyemia

This is the serious situation when, in a case suffering from severe sepsis, organisms and neutrophil polymorphs embolize to many sites in the body producing abscesses. Therefore it is necessary not only to drain the abscesses but also to take steps to increase the patient's resistance to infection. Before the advent of antibiotics pyemia was uniformly fatal; the mortality rate is still high.

Toxemia

In toxemia toxins/bacterial products are circulating in the blood, and it is the physical condition resulting from these products; the bacteria themselves may not be present in the blood stream.

Scoring the severity of infection

The scoring systems that can be used to assess the severity and outcome of disease include:

Apache II system

Many scoring systems have been used to assess the severity of infections. The Apache II system has achieved the greatest measure of popularity. It judges the severity of the acute illness through an acute physiology score, while in the background it also assesses the general health of the patient utilizing chronic health evaluation points [**Acute Physiology** And **Chronic Health** Evaluation (APACHE II)].[1]

Simplified acute physiology score (SAPS II)

Sequential organ failure assessment (SOFA) scores).

CLASSIFICATION OF SURGICAL INFECTIONS

The location of a lesion often provides a clue to the identity of the causative organism. For example:

- Most wound infections are caused by *Staph. aureus* or a mixed flora.
- *Abdominal* infections with perforation of the gastrointestinal tract are always mixed, with aerobic and anaerobic gram-negative enteric bacteria, as well as gram-positive anaerobic bacteria.
- Infections in the *genitourinary* tract are mostly from gram-negative aerobes, specially *Escherichia coli.*
- A spreading cellulitis is usually due to *Streptococcus pyogenes.*

Staphylococcal infections

Most infections in surgical wounds are caused by *Staph. aureus*. They are localized, with thick creamy pus, which is odourless and yellow or cream-coloured. Hospital-acquired infections are usually caused by antibiotic-resistant bacteria of increased virulence. Their treatment is surgical drainage with rest and elevation of the part. If such an infection occurs in the incision after an operation, the wound should be opened widely to facilitate free drainage of pus. Antibiotics should be started before the operation for drainage.

Streptococcal infection

Of all streptococci, *Strep. pyogenes* is the one which is most commonly encountered in surgical practice. The lesions it produces are usually invasive, with a rapid course. There is cellulitis, lymphangitis, lymphadenitis and extension of the inflammation along fascial planes. The pus is thin and watery, abscess formation being rare. Thrombosis of small vessels may lead to gangrene of the tissues. Bacteraemia is common, with chills, high fever, thready pulse and signs of toxemia.

Streptococcal gangrene is a spreading subcutaneous infection in which thrombosis of nutrient vessels results in sloughing of skin and fasciae. Treatment is wide surgical drainage along with antibiotics.

---

1 **Acute physiology** score parameters include temperature, blood pressure, heart and respiratory rates; arterial oxygen and pH; serum sodium, potassium and creatinine; hematocrit and white cell count.

Every step-wise increase in the departure from the norm for each parameter adds a point to the score.

Neurology. Glasgow coma scale points are added.

Age. Every 10-year increase beyond 44 years adds 1 or 2 points.

Chronic health. Hepatic, cardiac, pulmonary, renal or immune dysfuntion each adds a point.

For patients with intra-abdominal infection a score of 21 indicates a mortality risk of 50 percent.

The microaerophilic streptococcus causes infections that develop slowly. Chronic burrowing ulcer and chronic cutaneous gangrene are good examples. Radical drainage is necessary for cure, antibiotics alone being useless.

It should be remembered that *where the correct treatment is drainage, any number of antibiotics will not produce a cure without drainage.*

Infections by gram-negative bacilli

A variety of gram-negative bacilli are indigenous to the gastrointestinal and genitourinary tracts. Most wound infections by these organisms result from operative contamination of spilled gastrointestinal contents, and are due to careless operative technique. In other wound infections, and in many systemic invasive infections, these organisms act as opportunistic invaders. This is specially the case when host defence is impaired, or when incompletely removed devitalized tissues are present, e.g. in extensive burns and wounds. These infections are usually mixed, with both aerobic and anaerobic organisms. However, they are often not recognized as such, because anaerobic cultures are not routinely carried out in many hospitals. *If foul-smelling pus is found and anaerobic cultures are not available, the presence of anaerobic organisms should be presumed* and drugs effective against them, e.g. metronidazole or clindamycin, added to the regimen.

CLOSTRIDIAL INFECTIONS

Infections due to anaerobic clostridia cause three diseases important in surgical practice: clostridial cellulitis, gas gangrene and tetanus.

Clostridial cellulitis

This is a serious septic process of areolar tissues caused usually by *Clostridium welchii.* The cellulitis spreads along fascial planes. On palpation crepitus is felt due to the gas produced by the anaerobes. There is sloughing of skin and fasciae due to thrombosis of blood vessels. Pain is present, along with a greyish white discharge.

Treatment

This should include surgical decompression with excision of dead skin and fasciae. At the same time, systemic antibiotics are administered in large doses, usually penicillin and one of the tetracyclines.

GAS GANGRENE

Unlike clostridial cellulitis, gas gangrene is a clostridial myonecrosis. The most common organism responsible is Clostridium perfringens, other less common organisms are C. septicum, C. histolyticum, and C. novyi. C. perfringens produces as many as 20 toxins responsible for its effects. In severe cases it may result in shock, hemolytic anemia, renal failure and jaundice, and may cause the death of the patient.

Other organisms can also cause gas gangrene, mostly aerobic gram negative bacteria like *Escherichia coli, Pseudomonas aeruginosa, Klebsiella pneuminiae and Proteus species*. The incubation period varies from 1 hour to 6 weeks, usually less than 24 hours. The infection primarily involves muscles, and is characterized by spreading gangrene and profound toxemia, which is rapidly fatal if untreated. The toxemia is due to the circulating exotoxins.

Clostridial spores are very widespread in nature, yet gas gangrene is extremely rare in civilian practice. This is because the condition develops only in the presence of reduced oxygen tension. Clostridial gas gangrene can be traumatic or spontaneous:

- **Traumatic gangrene** may result from severe contusion and laceration with necrotic tissue, devitalization of a wound by compression, or from an impaired blood supply.
  - Most cases arise from *contamination of large wounds* as in agricultural tractor injuries, severe comminuted compound fractures sustained in road traffic accidents, and battle casualties.
  - In the advanced countries gas gangrene is most commonly seen after *criminal abortion* and infections following *intestinal surgery*.
- **Spontaneous gas gangrene** is caused by C. septicum; the portal of entry is the gastrointestinal tract. Predisposing conditions are colon malignancies and neutropenic colitis.

Gas forms in muscles, which exhibit crepitation. The infected muscles are soft, swollen and dark red. The overlying skin goes through a series of changes, initially it is pale followed by bronze appearance and later purple or red discoloration occurs. The wound usually has no smell, or it may have a sweet smell. There is brown watery exudate with bubbles of gas, which contains many gram-positive rods when examined microscopically, thus giving an immediate definitive diagnosis.

The patient is listless, sweats profusely, and is pale due to marked anemia. Stupor and delirium develop near the end.

Imaging

CT scan and *MRI* are useful in determining whether infections are localized or spreading, and indicate accurately the extent of the tissue necrosis.

Treatment

Surgical treatment

This should be prompt, with extensive decompression of all involved muscle compartments by incision and fasciotomy. *Aggressive excision of all dead and infected tissue at the first operation is crucial to the survival of the patient.* If irreversible gangrenous changes have taken place in the extremity, amputation must be carried out. If amputation is the only way to save the patient's life from the severe toxemia, no hesitation should be shown in proceeding with the operation.

Medical treatment

The toxemia in gas gangrene is due to exotoxins, but antitoxin therapy is relatively ineffective. Antibiotics cannot prevent or cure gas gangrene, but are useful as an adjunctive measure to surgery. Antibiotic therapy consists of a combination of penicillin (3–4 million units IV four hourly) plus clindamycin (600–900mg IV eight hourly) or tetracycline. If the patient is allergic to penicillin, metronidazole or clindamycin may be used instead. Hyperbaric oxygen can also be a useful adjunct to surgical treatment.

Hyperbaric oxygen

If oxygen is inhaled at two or three times the normal atmospheric pressure, the oxygen tension in plasma, lymph and tissue fluids is increased about 20 times. This greatly increases the effectiveness of surgical and antibiotic therapy in anaerobic infection, e.g. in clostridial myonecrosis, and dramatic clinical improvement may be seen within 24 hours. Its role is controversial due to non-availability of randomized controlled trials. Large hyperbaric pressure chambers are available at only a few medical centres, but much less expensive single-patient chambers are now available and can be used. The regimen consists of repeated treatments of 90 minutes each at a pressure of 3 atmospheres two to three times a day.

TETANUS

This dangerous and sometimes fatal infection of wounds has been virtually eliminated from the advanced countries due to the universal practice of tetanus immunization in the neonatal period. However, in the remote and backward parts of the underdeveloped countries it is unfortunately still quite common.

The causative organism is *Clostridium tetani,* which is a Gram-positive spore-bearing bacillus. The spores require reduced oxygen tension for them to germinate and they are usually resistant to autoclaving at 121^0 C for 10–15 minutes. Thus, although the wound responsible for the development of tetanus is usually a minor one, it is nearly always *deep,* so that anaerobic conditions are produced in its depth. *Commonly the wound is located in the lower limb.*

Other causes of tetanus include the following:

- Cases of septic abortion.
- Septic umbilical stumps, where stump hygiene is less than perfect.
- Imperfectly sterilized non-disposable syringes.
- Unhygienic piercing of ear-lobes.
- Burns.
- Surgical operations on the gastrointestinal tract.
- Patients with dental infection.
- Patients with diabetes and infected extremity ulcers.

The tetanus bacillus produces two toxins: tetanolysin and tetanospasmin; the latter is a neurotoxin and is responsible for the clinical manifestations of tetanus. It reaches the central nervous system along the axons of motor nerve trunks, and blocks the inhibitory impulses at the motor synapses. Two types of contractions of striated muscles are produced by the toxin:

- Tonic (spasms) which are a feature of early disease.
- Clonic (convulsions) which indicate severe established disease.

Tetanus is a serious illness, its annual worldwide incidence is 0.5 to 1 million cases and its prevalence is highest in newborns and young persons. The overall mortality even in leading centers is as high as 10 to 15%. The mortality rate is higher if:

- The patient is either very young or very old.
- The incubation period is short.
- Convulsions start early.
- The illness is severe.
- There is delay in treatment.

Tetanus at different ages

Tetanus can occur at any age, including the neonatal period.

Neonatal tetanus

In the underdeveloped countries neonatal tetanus constitutes the majority of the total number of cases and causes a significant number of deaths in 2008 a total of 59,000 deaths were reported due to neonatal tetanus worldwide.

Clinical features

The clinical picture usually becomes manifest on about the eighth day of life. In fact as early as the 3rd day the infant fails to suckle. Shortly thereafter, spasm of the facial muscles develops (*risus sardonicus*). At the same time the masseter muscles go into spasm (*lock jaw*). Generalized clonic spasms finally commence.

Untrained birth attendants

Tetanus usually results because of the unfamiliarity of untrained traditional birth attendants (TBAs) with elementary principles of asepsis and hygiene. It has often been stressed at conferences that so long as TBAs are going to manage a significant number of births in these countries, they should at least be exposed to short courses where they could be taught the essentials of aseptic techniques. However, unfortunately not much progress has been made in this important field so far. Application of cow dung on the umbilical stump and use of non-sterile equipment during delivery contribute to neonatal tetanus.

Children and adults

The vast majority of patients who develop tetanus have not previously been immunized. The incubation period ranges from 5 to 10 days; the shorter the interval the more severe the disease. Muscle pains, headaches, irritability and restlessness are followed by risus sardonicus, lock jaw and dysphagia (the last being due to spasm of the muscles of deglutition).

Finally, generalized clonic convulsions come on, which are triggered by mild external stimuli (sound, movement of personnel, etc.). As the extensor muscles are more powerful than the flexors, the whole body, i.e. the back and the lower limbs, assumes a posture of hyperextension (*episthotonus*). The muscles do not relax between convulsive attacks; this distinguishes the convulsions of tetanus from those due to strychnine poisoning.

Degrees of severity

The Ablett classification of severity of tetanus is generally employed (Table 13.1).

Management

Prevention

Immunization

The best method of prevention of tetanus is by active immunization with tetanus toxoid. This is included in the routine immunization schedule in childhood along with diphtheria and pertussis vaccine (DTaP vaccine), O.5ml being the usual dose administered intramuscularly:

- Three doses are given at the age of 2, 4 and 6 months.
- First booster dose is recommended at age 18 months.
- A second booster is given at age 5 years.
- Booster doses should be given every 10 years.

At the time a wound is sustained:

- If the immunization status is not known, or fewer than three previous tetanus toxoid doses have been given, a vaccine containing tetanus toxoid should be administered.
- For dirty contaminated wounds, human tetanus immune globulins are administered in a dose of 250 units intramuscularly.
- If the patient has received three doses of tetanus toxoid, and the wound is minor and clean, give booster only if last dose was given 10 years ago.
- If the wound is dirty and contaminated, give a booster if the last dose was given five years back.

Care of wounds

Apart from active and passive immunization, prevention of tetanus requires that wounds should be looked after properly. In grossly contaminated wounds great care should be taken to remove all dirt, grit and foreign matter, after which the whole wound should be left open to be closed later by delayed primary suture.

Treatment

Specific measures

If a wound is present it should be excised, debrided and left open, being packed with hydrogen peroxide for creating aerobic conditions. Metronidazole (500mg IV 6 hourly) or penicillin G (2–4 million units IV 6 hourly) should be given for 7–10 days. Human tetanus immunoglobulin should be given to neutralize unbound toxin; it is given in a dose of 3,000 to 6,000 i.u. intramuscularly. In neonatal tetanus intrathecal tetanus immunoglobulin has proven of no benefit.

General measures

All patients should be managed in a dark and quiet room preferably in the intensive care unit (ICU):

- For *mild* tetanus sedation with diazepam is sufficient.
- In patients with *moderate* tetanus tracheostomy is usually required in addition to sedation.
- In *severe* disease the muscle spasms have to be abolished by curarization and the patient kept on intermittent positive-pressure ventilation.
- In *very severe* disease, sympathetic overactivity results in cardiac arrhythmias; these patients require

adrenergic blockade. The severe muscle spasms need to be abolished by the use of anesthesia and muscle relaxants; therefore the patient has to be placed on a ventilator for many days, until the effect of the toxins on the muscles is terminated.

OTHER INFECTIONS OF SURGICAL IMPORTANCE

Mixed bacterial infections

Many surgical infections are polymicrobial. The wound from a *human bite* contains oral spirochaetes as well as aerobic and anaerobic mouth bacteria, and produces a synergistic and locally destructive lesion. There is thick foul-smelling pus and necrosis of fasciae. Surgical decompression, antibiotics effective against both anaerobes and aerobes, and splinting are important in treatment.

Non-clostridial crepitant cellulitis

This usually occurs as a complication of wounds contaminated by gastrointestinal or genitourinary discharges. The common organisms are the residents of the GIT and GU tracts, namely anaerobic bacteroides, streptococci and the coliforms. There is necrosis of skin and fasciae due to thrombosis of vessels. Wide surgical decompression and intensive antibiotic therapy is required.

Bacterial synergistic gangrene

First described by Meleney, this condition is caused by synergism between an aerobic hemolytic *Staphylococcus aureus* and a microaerophilic non-hemolytic streptococcus. One or two weeks after operation a pale red cellulitis develops around the wound, with a blue or purple central area which becomes gangrenous and ulcerates. The ulcer enlarges as its purple and painful margin extends outwards.

Treatment requires radical excision of the lesion, systemic penicillin or erythromycin, and delayed skin grafting. Local bacitracin application is helpful. Prompt operation should be carried out to prevent increasing and sometimes fatal septicemia.

Peritonitis

Infections that follow perforations of the gastrointestinal or genitourinary tract or contamination by their contents are always polymicrobial, both aerobic and anaerobic bacteria being present. Unfortunately, anaerobes are usually not detected, because they are difficult to culture. A good combination of antibiotics for infection by bowel bacteria consists of gentamycin and clindamycin.

Table 13.1 Ablett classification of degrees of severity of tetanus

Grade 1 (Mild)	Mild trismus and general spasticity only, no dysphagia, spasm or respiratory distress
Grade 2 (Moderate)	Moderate trismus, rigidity, short spasm; mild dysphagia and respiratory distress
Grade 3 (Severe)	Severe trismus, generalized rigidity, severe dysphagia, prolonged spasm and apneic spells.
Grade 4 (Very severe)	Grade 3 plus autonomic instability

The mycoses

Actinomycosis israelii

This infection occurs rarely, producing a granuloma. The area becomes swollen and indurated, with multiple sinus tracts. The pus shows sulphur granules. The areas affected are cervicofacial, thoracic and abdominal. In the neck the lower jaw is commonly affected, in the thorax the apex of the lung. In the abdomen the infection enters through the cecum, and sinuses form in the right iliac fossa.

Treatment

This consists of incision and drainage of abscesses and prolonged therapy with penicillin or other antibiotic.

Moniliasis (Candidiasis)

Fungus infection occurs occasionally in the mouth and suggests that the patient's immune mechanisms are depressed. Nystatin four times a day or oral Fluconazole for 7–14 days thrice daily may help clear up the infection.

VIRAL INFECTIONS

ACQUIRED IMMUNODEFICIENCY SYNDROME (AIDS)

The acquired immunodeficiency syndrome consists of a spectrum of illnesses which are caused by infection with the human immunodeficiency virus (HIV) and which lead, over a number of years, to serious disease and death. At present *30.7* million adults are estimated to be infected worldwide *with 1.5 million deaths of adults in 2011 only* and many more are likely to be infected with the passage of time. The virus is transmitted mainly via semen, cervical secretions and blood. Transmission takes place via the following routes:

- *Sexual intercourse* (vaginal and anal). Heterosexual intercourse accounts for the vast majority of infections, followed by intravenous drug abuse.
- *Mother to child*. As more women become infected, more babies are likely to acquire HIV from them *in utero*, during childbirth or via breast milk.
- *Blood and blood products*. Transfusion of blood or clotting factors (e.g. in hemophilia) can be followed by HIV infection. Worldwide blood and its products are now screened and clotting factors are heat-treated, so that the risk of transfusion-related HIV infection is minimal. However, where such screening is not possible, the risk remains significant.
- *Contaminated needles*. Intravenous drug users sharing common syringes and needles are a major route of spread of HIV infection. Doctors and nurses have an approximately 0.3 % risk following a single needle prick with known HIV-infected blood.
- *Surgeons* run additional risks of infection due to the possibility of a needle-prick during the placement of sutures, or a spurt of blood from a divided artery directly into the conjunctival sac. Therefore, they need to take extra precautions, including the wearing of goggles.

There is no evidence that HIV is spread by social or household contact.

Immunology

The cellular receptor for HIV is the CD4 molecule, which defines the cells that are susceptible to infection. Many cells within the immune system bear this molecule, and include CD4+ lymphocytes (which are most affected). There is a progressive and severe depletion of CD4 'helper' lymphocytes, and it is this that leads to the clinical manifestations of HIV infection.

The spectrum of illness associated with HIV infection is broad. The Centres for Disease Control (CDC) classify patients into four stages. In (Table 13.2) the classification has been somewhat abbreviated for ease of understanding by undergraduates:

Clinical features

There are three main stages of HIV infection: acute infection, clinical latency and AIDS:

The acute stage starts with an influenza-like illness with fever, lymphadenitis, sore throat inflammation, and rash, besides, vomiting, diarrhea and peripheral neuropathy; this lasts for a couple of weeks, and is generally not recognized as HIV infection.

This is followed by a latent period which can last from 3 to 20 years, with mild symptoms off and on, and often with persistent generalized painless lymphadenopathy.

Finally, AIDS sets in, with opportunistic infections, specially pneumocystis pneumonia and esophageal candidiasis, resulting in cachexia.

Diagnosis

Enzyme linked immunoabsorbent assay (ELISA) is used for screening. If this becomes positive, further confirmation is carried out by Western blot test. If this is also positive then HIV PCR to check viral load and CD4 counts are checked.

Treatment

The aims of management are to maintain health, provide palliative support, and avoid transmission of HIV. Confidentiality must be strictly adhered to, and psychiatric support provided to the patient as well as his family. Drugs from the following five groups are used for the treatment of HIV infection:

- Nucleoside or nucleotide reverse transcriptase inhibitors.
- Non-nucleoside reverse transcriptase inhibitors.
- Protease inhibitors.
- Entry inhibitors.
- Integrase inhibitors.

Three or more drugs in combination from these groups are usually required for HIV treatment.

Prevention of AIDS

Educational programmes should provide factual information and strategies to avoid infection, including the use of condoms and access to clean needles and syringes among drug users.

ANTIMICROBIAL AGENTS

A number of different antibiotics and other antimicrobials are employed in the treatment of surgical infections.

Selection of antibiotics

Ideally, the identity and sensitivity of the organism should be known before an antibiotic is started. However it is quite proper, and in fact the usual practice, to send the pus for culture and immediately start an antibiotic which is likely to be effective. On receipt of the culture report, the drug may have to be changed.

Normally the culture and sensitivity report takes two or three days to arrive. However, in urgent situations information may be obtained much more quickly:

- *Immediate gram staining* of the purulent exudate will sometimes show the organism.
- *Direct sensitivity testing* may be carried out by plating the pus directly on a blood agar plate and simultaneously testing with sensitivity discs. Preliminary information can thus usually be obtained within 12 hours. *In critically ill patients this early receipt of information can make the difference between life and death* by guiding the clinician in the choice of the correct antibiotic. Unfortunately this is a greatly underutilized method, because many clinicians are not familiar with it.

Resistant strains

These emerge most often when contamination from external sources continues, as in open wounds, leg ulcers and burns.

Penicillins

Penicillins, as well as cephalosporins, have a beta-lactam ring fused to a thiazolidine ring. Penicillins block the cross-linking between alanine and glycine which is an important step in the final stages of formation of the cell wall. *Benzylpenicillin* can be given only parenterally, and is the drug of choice for serious infections including pneumonia, streptococcal and gonococcal infections, clostridial infections (tetanus, gas gangrene), actinomycosis, anthrax and spirochaetal infections e.g. syphilis.

Flucoxacillin is insensitive to bacterial penicillinase, and is therefore used in infections caused by penicillinase-producing staphylococci. *Ampicillin* is sensitive to penicillinase, but its activity includes Gram-negative organisms such as Salmonella, Shigella, *E. coli, H. influenza* and Proteus. It is useful in the treatment of urinary tract and upper respiratory infections. *Amoxycillin* has a similar activity to ampicillin, but is better absorbed if given by mouth. *Carbenicillin* and ticarcillin are active against Pseudomonas infection.

Generally, the penicillins are very safe drugs. However, hypersensitivity (skin rash, urticaria, anaphylaxis), encephalopathy and tubulo-interstitial nephritis can occur.

Cephalosporins

Like the penicillins, the cephalosporins inhibit bacterial cell-wall synthesis. Cephalexin, cephradine and cefixime can be taken by mouth. At the same time, highly potent parenteral preparations are available, in the form of cefuroxime, cefotaxime, ceftriaxone and ceftazidime. Cefipime (anti-pseudomonal cephalosporin) is a fourth generation, whereas ceftaroline, which is active

Table 13.2 Centres for Disease Control staging of AIDS (abbreviated).

	Aids-defining condition	Count of CD4+ T lymphocytes
Stage 1	No	≥500 cells/µL
Stage 2	No	200–499 cells/µL
Stage 3	Yes	<200 cells/µL
Stage unknown	No info	No info

against methyllin-resistant Staphylococcus-aureus (MRSA) is a fifth generation cephalosporin. Both are used parenterally. They are resistant to staphylococcal penicillinase and are active against both Gram-negative and Gram-positive organisms.

The cephalosporins are useful for the treatment of serious systemic infections. They are commonly used for serious postoperative sepsis and in immunocompromised patients.

Monobactams

The only member of this class in current use is *aztreonam*. Its spectrum of activity is limited to aerobic Gram-negative bacilli, it is inactive against gram positive and anaerobic bacteria. It is commonly used in combination with metronidazole, clindamycin (for anaerobes) and penicillin or erythromycin (for Gram-positive cocci).

Aminoglycosides

These antibiotics are derived from *Streptomyces* spp. They interrupt bacterial protein synthesis by inhibiting ribosomal function.

Streptomycin is not often used in the advanced countries. However, in the poorer communities it still has a place because of its low cost.

Neomycin is only used for the topical treatment of eye and skin infections and orally for preoperative 'sterilization' of the bowel.

Gentamycin and *tobramycin* are given parenterally. They are highly effective against many Gram-negative infections including *Pseudomonas*.

Other aminoglycosides include *amikacin, netilmicin, paromomycin* and *kanamycin*. Paromomycin is used to treat amebiasis whereas kanamycin is a second line anti-tuberculous drug.

Aminoglycosides are used in combination with other

drugs. Usually a single daily dose is recommended, with the exception of endocarditis caused by Enterococcus.

Aminoglycosides are *nephrotoxic and ototoxic*, specially in the elderly, therefore their blood levels should be checked.

Tetracyclines

These are bacteriostatic drugs. They inhibit bacterial protein synthesis by interrupting ribosomal function. They are effective against Gram-positive and Gram-negative bacteria. Tigecycline, a long acting third generation tetracycline, was approved in 2005. It is a derivative of minocycline, used for intra-abdominal infections and skin and soft tissue infections.

Macrolides

This group consists of erythromycin, azithromycin, clarithromycin and fidaxomicin. Macrolides inhibit protein synthesis by interrupting ribosomal function.

Erythromycin has a similar antibacterial spectrum to penicillin, and can be used both orally and parenterally. It is included in the treatment regimens of all pneumonias as many are due to Mycoplasma. Prolonged treatment with erythromycin can be followed by cholestatic jaundice.

Azithromycin and *clarithromycin* are active against gram negative organsisms as well as Listeria monocytogenes. At the same time they have enhanced tissue and intracellular penetration, and a longer half-life that allows once or twice daily dosage.

Carbapenems

These are broad-spectrum beta-lactams. This group includes *Imipenem, Meropenem, Ertapenem* and *Doripenem*. They cover most of the gram negatives including Pseudomonas and anaerobes except for Ertapenem which does not cover Pseudomonas. Organisms usually resistant to carbapenems are methicillin-resistant staphylococcus, Burkholderia cepacia and Enterococcus faecium.

Fusidic acid

The structure of fusidic acid resembles that of bile salts. It is used mainly for penicillinase-producing *Staph. aureus* infections such as osteomyelitis and endocarditis, and for other staphylococcal infections associated with septicemia. The drug is well absorbed orally, and is concentrated in bone. Resistance occurs rapidly; therefore it is used in combination with another antibiotic. It may occasionally be hepatotoxic, but is generally safe and can be given in pregnancy.

Sulphonamides

Sulphonamides block the synthesis of thymidine and purine. Trimethoprim also inhibits folic acid synthesis.

Sulphamethoxazole is used mainly in combination with *trimethoprim* (as co-trimoxazole) for *P. carinii* infection. Trimethoprim alone is now used for urinary infections and bronchitis

Sulphapyridine in combination with 5-aminosalicylic acid (i.e. sulphasalazine) is used in inflammatory bowel disease. Bacteria may become resistant to sulphonamides by altering bacterial cell permeability to these agents. Sulphonamides potentiate oral anticoagulants and hypoglycemic agents. They also cause thrombocytopenia, folate deficiency and hemolysis in individuals with glucose-6-phosphate dehydrogenase deficiency, and therefore should not be used in such persons. At the same time, co-trimoxazole should be avoided in the elderly.

Quinolones

Ciprofloxacin, norfloxacin and *ofloxacin* are useful oral broad-spectrum antibiotics related structurally to nalidixic acid. The latter achieves only low serum levels, and therefore its use is restricted to the urinary tract where it is concentrated.

Quinolones inhibit bacterial DNA synthesis by inhibiting DNA gyrase. They should be reserved for infections resistant to other drugs. The extended spectrum quinolones such as ciprofloxacin are active against Gram-negative and Gram-positive bacteria, and are useful in Gram-negative septicemia, skin and bone infections, gastrointestinal, urinary and respiratory infections, gonorrhoea and infection with *Chlamydia trachomatis*. *Levofloxacin, Moxifloxacin* and *Gamifloxacin* are newer quinolones. These are used for respiratory infections and complicated abdominal infections.

Toxic effects include gastrointestinal disturbances, photosensitive rashes, neuropathy, tendinopathy and prolongation of QT interval.

Nitroimidazoles

Metronidazole

This is the most important member of this group of drugs. Minor modifications in its structure have produced *tinidazole* and *nimorazole*. They act by breaking down the strands of DNA in the microbes.

Metronidazole is important in the treatment of anaerobic bacterial infection, particularly that due to *Bacteroides*. It is also widely used prophylactically in colonic surgery. Apart from this, it is the treatment of choice for amebiasis, giardiasis and *Trichomonas vaginalis*. It can be used both orally and intravenously. Nitroimidazoles result in a metallic taste, and produce peripheral neuropathy with prolonged use. They should be avoided in pregnancy.

Vancomycin

Vancomycin is a complex glycopeptide produced by *Streptomyces orientalis.* It exerts bactericidal activity against Gram-positive bacteria by inhibiting cell-wall synthesis. It is not a drug meant to be used routinely. It is given orally for pseudomembranous enterocolitis produced by *Clostridium difficile,* and intravenously for methicillin-resistant *Staph. aureus.* It is also employed in Gram-positive infections in patients allergic to penicillins.

Antifungal drugs

Amphotericin B is used intravenously in severe cases for most fungal infections. Common side effects include fever, renal failure, hypokalemia and hypomagnesemia.

Lipid preparation *Amphotericin B* is less nephrotoxic.

Nystatin is not absorbed through mucous membranes and is therefore useful in the treatment of candidiasis affecting the mouth, esophagus and vagina. It can be given orally or as pessaries.

Other antifungal groups include Triazoles and Echinocandins.

Triazoles include *Fluconazole, Itraconazole, Voriconazole* and *Posaconazole*. Posaconazole is approved for prophylaxis against Aspergillus and Candida infections in patients with prolonged neutropenia or stem cell transplantation.

Echinocandins include *Caspofungin* and *Micafungin*.

Griseofulvin is concentrated in keratin, and is therefore a useful remedy for chronic fungal infection of nails, as well as for ringworm.

ANTIVIRAL DRUGS

Acyclovir, valacyclovir and famcicyclovir

These compounds are used to treat herpes simplex and Varicella zoster infections. Only acyclovir is available intravenously.

Ganciclovir

This is a guanine analogue. It is used for cytomegalovirus retinitis and gastrointestinal disease in patients with HIV infection. The major complication is neutropenia.

Foscarnet

This is used for gancyclovir resistant herpes infection or as an alternative for CMV infection. Its side effects include electrolyte disturbance and renal failure.

Oseltamivir and zanamivir

These are neuraminidase inhibitors and they are used for the treatment of Influenza A and B infections.

Interferon

This is a naturally occurring substance produced by T lymphocytes during virus infection. It is produced in response to infection by many different viruses, and production stimulated by one virus may confer protection against a second viral invader. It is used in hepatitis B and C, as well as in certain malignancies.

Chapter

14 NEOPLASIA

Introduction

A neoplasm is a group of cells which have become unresponsive to control mechanisms, and which show excessive, useless proliferation.

Benign neoplasms are characterized by excessive cell growth but this remains localised. Their clinical features arise as a consequence of compression of surrounding normal tissue.

Malignant neoplasms (cancers), in contrast, not only show local growth and pressure symptoms, they also *invade* surrounding normal tissue and *spread (metastasize)* to other parts of the body. The cancer present at the site of origin is called the *primary tumor*. The primary tumor may spread to other organs giving rise to *secondary tumors (metastases)*.

This chapter will describe some of the mechanisms causing cancer and the biological behaviour of cancers. We will also describe methods of diagnosing cancer and discuss general principles of cancer management with emphasis on surgical management.

BIOLOGY OF CANCER

Normal growth and development of an organism depend on coordinated cell division and maturation. These processes are regulated by several genes which exert their effects through production of various proteins and hormones as well as expression of various growth receptors on the cell membrane. This complex interaction means that normally, cell growth occurs when required, and stops when it is no longer needed. The offspring of the cell division mature and perform their designated functions till a time when they undergo *'programmed cell death'* or *apoptosis*. Neoplasms develop when one or more of these control mechanisms relating to growth, maturation or cell death, fail. The most common underlying mechanism of neoplastic growth is development of mutations in the genes controlling these processes.

Defects in DNA replication and synthesis

The cell has very sophisticated and complex mechanisms to ensure correct replication and synthesis of DNA at cell division, minimising the chances of mutations. However, given that billions of cells in our body continuously undergo the processes of cell division and growth, replacing older cells which die out, it is not surprising that defects in DNA synthesis and replication may occur in a small proportion of these cells despite these mechanisms.

The cell has mechanisms to detect defective DNA synthesis. Detection of defective DNA triggers DNA repair mechanisms. However, if the defect cannot be repaired and is severe enough to threaten normal cellular function and growth, programmed cell death (apoptosis) is activated and the cell dies.

Accumulating mutations

Neoplasms develop when cells accumulate mutations in:

- The genes promoting proliferation and growth.
- The genes controlling DNA repair.
- The genes regulating growth suppression and apoptosis.

Proto-oncogenes are the genes that *promote cell proliferation* and growth. Cancers may develop when mutations in these genes result in enhanced activity (*activating mutations*).

Tumor suppressor genes are the genes that *inhibit cellular proliferation*. Cancers may develop when mutations result in loss of function of these genes (*inactivating mutations*).

CAUSES OF CANCER

Cancer-causing mutations can arise at random without an identifiable precipitant, but several factors have been identified which increase the risk of cancer development. These include:

- Inherited conditions resulting in familial cancers.
- Dietary factors.

- Reproductive and hormonal factors.
- Some chronic inflammatory conditions and infections.
- Exposure to chemicals and radiation.

Carcinogens

Any exogenous agent that promotes cell proliferation or causes DNA damage will potentially increase the risk of cancer. Such an agent is called a carcinogen. Several environmental carcinogens have been identified:

Physical carcinogenesis

Tumor induction by physical agents occurs by essentially two mechanisms:

- Induction of cell proliferation over a period of time, which increases the opportunity for events leading to transformation.
- Exposure to physical agents that induce changes in DNA replication.

A *foreign body* rarely induces a tumor itself. However, the irritation induced by the foreign body promotes cellular proliferation, thereby increasing the chances for errors in DNA replication that may lead to neoplastic transformation. A similar role is played by *chronic inflammatory conditions* such as inflammatory bowel disease.

Chemical carcinogenesis

Tobacco

One of the most well-known causes of cancer is *tobacco*. Tobacco use is associated with development of several cancers including cancer of the lung, oral cavity, oropharynx, larynx, esophagus and urinary bladder. Cigarette smoke contains several carcinogenic chemicals, mainly polycyclic aromatic hydrocarbons and aromatic amines, although other compounds including N-nitrosamines and heavy metals may also be involved.

Alcohol

As with cigarette smoking, a high intake of *alcohol* increases the risk of cancers of the upper respiratory and digestive tracts. The increased risk is particularly great for people who both smoke and drink heavily. Heavy and prolonged alcohol consumption is also associated with hepatocellular carcinoma via the development of cirrhosis and alcoholic hepatitis.

Industrial and occupational chemicals

Several such chemicals have been linked to increased risk of cancer. These include asbestos (lung cancer and mesothelioma), and aromatic amines found in the textile, rubber, and printing industries (bladder cancer).

Radiation

Radiation exposure causes DNA damage and predisposes to development of cancer in the exposed area.

At the time of discovery of X-rays by Roentgen and radioactivity by Marie Curie, the carcinogenic potential of radiation was not known. Excessive radiation exposure resulted in a high incidence of cancers in workers as well as patients exposed to radiation. Similarly, survivors of the atomic bombs from Nagasaki and Hiroshima showed a high incidence of several cancers.

Several clinical studies have shown increased risk of cancer in children exposed to even small doses of radiation used in diagnostic scans. Nowadays there are strict laws and precautions regarding industrial and clinical use of radiation to minimise these risks. Similarly, clinical use of even a small amount of radiation (e.g. x-rays, CT scan) needs to have a proper justification and indication so that the benefits outweigh the risk of carcinogenesis.

Infections

Several viral infections increase the risk of cancers. Infections with Hepatitis B and C viruses increase the risk of hepatocellular carcinoma. Other carcinogenic viruses include Human papilloma virus (cancer of cervix and oropharynx) and Epstein-Barr virus (Burkitt's lymphoma, nasopharyngeal cancer). Most of these viruses are thought to cause cancers by incorporating parts of their DNA (oncogenes) in the host cell's DNA, causing activation of proliferation-promoting genes.

Infection with Human Immunodeficiency virus (HIV) predisposes to several cancers including lymphomas, anal cancer and Kaposi's sarcoma. HIV is not directly oncogenic and it is thought to cause cancers by its immunosuppressive effects.

Bacterial infections like Helicobacter pylori (gastric cancer and gastric lymphoma), and parasitic infestations like schistosomiasis (bladder cancer) and liver flukes (cholangiocarcinoma) may also be carcinogenic.

Immunodeficiency

Immunodeficient individuals and immunosuppressed recipients of organ transplants are at a greater risk for neoplastic disease, mostly of the lymphoreticular system. In the normal host several types of lymphoid cells including T, B, and NK lymphocytes participate in the destruction of aberrant cells and prevention of neoplasia.

Inherited cancers

In all cancers, changes take place in the normal cellular genes:

- In the vast majority of cancers (especially in older people) these genetic changes occur in the somatic tissues of the individual and *do not enter the germ-line*, so even close relatives of the patient do not run an increased risk.

- In a few cancers close relatives may have an increased susceptibility to neoplastic change, but the cancer is not caused by a single gene defect; rather, multiple factors are responsible.
- Finally, in some very rare cancers the changes can be inherited as a single gene defect.

As an example, in Lynch syndrome increased risk of hereditary non-polyposis colorectal cancer, endometrial cancer, as well as other tumors, including ovarian, bowel and urothelial tumors, and gliomas, is a result of defective DNA repair due to a mutation in mismatch repair gene.

BRCA1 (breast cancer A1) and BRCA2 are tumor suppressor genes. Mutations in these genes lead to increased risk of breast and ovarian cancers.

Hormonal factors

Several endogenous hormones are powerful stimulants of growth and proliferation. Imbalances in hormonal production or exogenous administration may increase susceptibility to cancer. For example, established risk factors for breast cancer include:

- Early age at menarche.
- Low parity.
- Late age at first birth.
- Late age at menopause.

CARCINOGENESIS

In experimental tumors if the dose of the carcinogen is large the tumors are induced in a shorter period of time. In humans many tumors arise slowly, suggesting that they are the result of prolonged exposure to low doses of carcinogens. Tumorigenesis takes a long time to have its effect.

The progression of the cell to frank malignancy passes through different stages. These stages are characterized by increasing accumulation of mutations in the cells.

Hyperplasia

This is an increase in the number of cells. Following injury the local growth rate increases over the baseline in the normal process of wound healing. As wound closure is achieved, the rate of cell division returns to that of the adjacent tissue. Hyperplasia increases the chances of development of malignancy, but to a very slight extent.

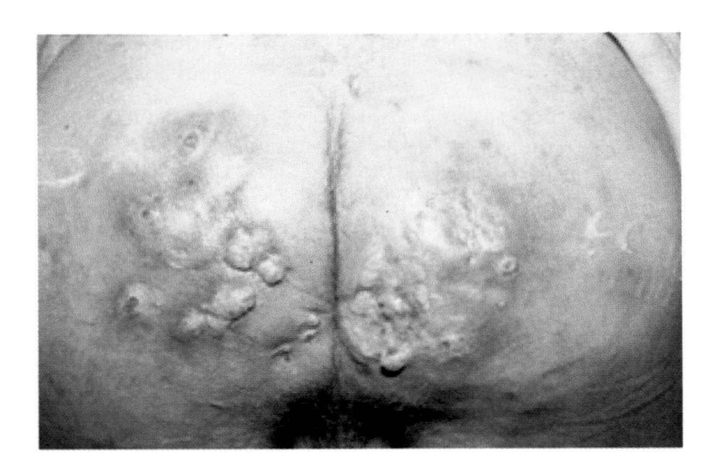

Fig.14.1 Very advanced cancer of rectum fungating on the surface of the buttocks. Note the nodules and the ulcerated skin.

Metaplasia

This is a reversible transformation of one mature cell type to another, the replacing cell type being present in an area where it is not normally found. For example, in gastro-esophageal reflux the normal distal esophageal squamous epithelium exhibits metaplasia to a 'gastric-type' columnar epithelium.

Dysplasia

In dysplasia the cell size, shape and organization is altered. The cells show polymorphism and hyperchromasia, often with complete loss of cellular and epithelial polarity. Mitoses are frequent. There is no penetration of abnormal cells through the epithelial basement membrane. High grade dysplasia (carcinoma in situ) has a high risk of progression to invasive cancer.

Invasive cancer

Final induction of invasive cancer takes place when cells accumulate mutations enabling them to continue uncontrolled proliferation despite withdrawal of the growth factor. Mutations also allow cancer cells to invade surrounding tissues leading to local infiltration and metastases.

Invasion and metastases

The hallmark of malignant neoplasms (cancers) is their ability to invade and destroy surrounding tissues (Fig.14.1) and to spread to other parts of the body (metastasize).

Spread of cancer

Cancer cells spread:

- Via lymphatic channels to locoregional lymph nodes.

- Via blood vessels (mostly following venous drainage) to other organs.
- Along body cavities (trans-coelomic spread in pleural or peritoneal cavities).

Tumor invasion and metastases is a stepwise process:

- The initial step is loss of cell-cell cohesion found in normal tissues.
- After an initial mass of malignant cells (primary tumor) has formed, its cells tend to break away from the main tumor mass and move into the surrounding tissues. This is facilitated by mechanical pressure, release of lytic enzymes and the increased motility of tumor cells.
- Cancer cells invade surrounding normal host tissue with penetration of small vascular channels or lymphatics, reaching their lumen. While circulating immune cells destroy some of these cells, some may survive.
- These surviving cancer cells reach local lymph nodes (via lymphatics) or capillary beds of distant organs (via blood vessels).
- In the lymph nodes and capillary beds, extravasation of cancer cells occurs, i.e. the cancer cells move out of the lumen of the arresting lymphatic or blood vessel.
- This is followed by growth of the disseminating tumor cells at the distant site resulting in established metastatic deposits.

Classification of tumors

Neoplasms can arise from any part of the body. Malignant neoplasms (cancers) are broadly divided into three main categories:

- **Carcinomas**. Cancers arising from the *epithelial* lining of various organs or from the epithelial layers of the skin are called carcinomas. For example adenocarcinoma of stomach, squamous cell carcinoma of skin. Carcinomas are the commonest cancers seen in human beings. Breast cancer (adenocarcinoma), lung cancer (adenocarcinoma or squamous cell carcinoma) and prostate cancer (adenocarcinoma) are the commonest cancers worldwide. Primary liver cancer (hepatocellular carcinoma) is usually associated with hepatitis B or C infection as well as chronic liver disease from other causes.
- **Sarcomas**. Cancers arising from the *fibrous and connective tissue* and from bones are called sarcomas. For example osteosarcoma of tibia, fibrosarcoma of the soft tissues of the arm.
- **Cancers of the blood and lymphoid tissues.** For example leukemia, lymphomas, myeloma.

PRINCIPLES OF MANAGEMENT

Surgical oncology is the discipline dealing with surgical management of cancers. Surgical oncologists are highly trained surgeons who work in close liaison with cancer specialists in other disciplines.

The modern management of cancer is best carried out in dedicated cancer centres or oncological departments within large hospitals by a *multidisciplinary team (MDT)* of specialists. In most cancer centres, there are dedicated MDTs for various tumor types, e.g. breast cancer, colorectal and upper GI cancer, lung cancer, sarcoma etc. The MDT usually consists of the surgeon and physician belonging to the relevant specialty, medical oncologist, radiation oncologist, pathologist and radiologist. The MDT meets regularly to review and to discuss the clinical data and investigations of patients and formulate a management plan. Specialist cancer nurses and ancillary specialists like physiotherapists, psychologists and social workers are part of these MDTs to provide holistic care to the cancer patient.

As in other branches of medicine and surgery, there is now increasing emphasis on ***evidence-based medicine*** in cancer management as well. Practising evidence-based medicine means using available evidence from research studies, critically appraising it and incorporating this into one's clinical practice. This approach places more importance on evidence gathered from well-conducted randomised controlled trials and systematic reviews of literature. Case control and cohort studies are sources of important but less robust evidence. Historical clinical practice and expert opinion are considered less reliable but remain useful guiding sources, particularly in areas where well-conducted studies are not available. Most cancers are now managed according to evidence-based guidelines prepared by various specialist organisations.

DIAGNOSIS

Diagnosis of cancer should be pursued in an orderly fashion. The diagnostic algorithm includes a very careful history, thorough physical examination, appropriate laboratory tests, x-rays, ultrasound examination, CT and radioisotope scans, and biopsy, as indicated by the clinical findings.

Clinical features

The symptoms and signs of neoplasia, both benign and malignant, are very variable and depend on the site of the primary tumor, presence of local invasion and distant metastases, as well as systemic symptoms arising from a number of chemicals and hormones produced by the tumors.

Local signs and symptoms

Benign neoplasms primarily cause symptoms by pressure on adjacent tissues. Tumors of the testis (Fig.14.2) skin and soft tissue may present as a lump. Deep seated tumors may cause compression of vital blood vessels or nervous tissue.

Cancers, in addition to pressure symptoms, may cause ulceration and invasion of blood vessels and nerves leading to bleeding and/or neurological deficit.

Brain tumors may present with signs of raised intracranial pressure or focal neurological deficit, e.g. hemiplegia. Lung cancer may present with hemoptysis or superior vena caval obstruction. Colon cancer may present as iron deficiency anemia due to chronic blood loss or sometimes as an emergency with large bowel obstruction.

Expansion of the tumor may result in destruction of host tissues. Examples are seen when tumor cells replace bone and result in a pathological fracture. Similarly, malignant cells may replace the greater part of the liver parenchyma and result in hepatic insufficiency.

Not infrequently, the symptoms from the primary tumor may be absent or minimal but the secondary tumors (metastases) may cause the presenting symptom. For example pathological bone fracture from metastatic prostate cancer, brain metastases from lung cancer, tender hepatomegaly from liver metastases from colon cancer, may be the presenting features.

Systemic signs and symptoms

Several cancers produce systemic symptoms like weight loss, anorexia, cachexia or fever. These symptoms are mediated by a number of cytokines produced by cancer cells.

Some tumors, particularly benign neoplasms, may exhibit hyperactivity of the normal physiological function of their parent tissue. For example pituitary adenoma may produce excessive growth hormone, causing gigantism or acromegaly. An adrenal cortex adenoma may produce excessive aldosterone resulting in signs and symptoms of hyperaldosteronism.

Para-neoplastic syndromes

Some cancers are associated with specific paraneoplastic syndromes. These result from production of various biologically active peptides/hormones by the cancer cells. Examples are ectopic ACTH production, secretion of parathormone related peptide, or syndrome of inappropriate anti-diuretic hormone. Some paraneoplastic syndromes are mediated by autoimmune antibodies e.g. myasthenia gravis with thymoma.

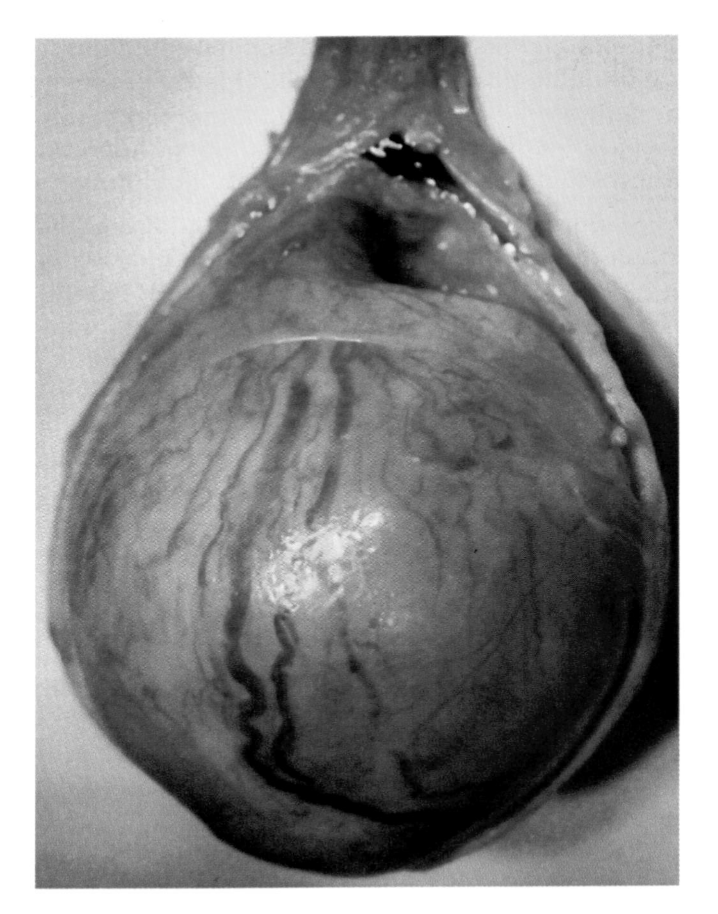

Fig.14.2 Seminoma testis

INVESTIGATIONS

Pathology

The aim of investigations in a patient with suspected cancer is to confirm the diagnosis and define the extent of disease (stage of the cancer). With very few exceptions, the diagnosis of cancer requires demonstration of malignant cells from the tumor on microscopic examination of a biopsy specimen. Biopsies may be obtained in a number of ways and the most appropriate approach to biopsy is determined by the location of the tumor and suspected diagnosis.

Fine needle aspiration cytology (FNAC)

This is usually the easiest way to obtain a biopsy. A fine (usually 22G) needle mounted on a 10cc syringe is introduced in the tumor either under direct vision or with ultrasonic or CT guidance and suction is applied.

Three to four passes are usually required. The cellular aspirate thus obtained is spread on a glass slide. A cell block may be prepared by adding the specimen to a solution (usually 50% ethanol). Aspiration of suspected malignant pleural or ascitic fluid may also be done.

Microscopic examination of this cellular aspirate by a trained cytopathologist can give information about cell shape, size, nuclear/cytoplasmic ratio etc. FNAC is now increasingly used as the initial test to confirm the diagnosis in a case of suspected cancer.

Exfoliative cytology

Exfoliative cytology specimens may be obtained from the surfaces of some neoplasms arising in epithelial-lined body cavities and orifices, such as the vagina, cervix, bronchus etc. Pap smear from the cervix is a classic example of exfoliative cytology used for screening and diagnosis of cancer.

Core/Tru-cut biopsy

This uses a similar technique as FNAC but a bigger guage hollow needle or a special tru-cut needle is used so that the specimen obtained is a tiny core/piece of the tissue. The advantage of this technique over FNAC is that the specimen gives more detail about malignant cells and tissue architecture. After an initial FNAC has shown malignant cells, core/tru-cut biopsy is now the technique of choice in many cancers for final diagnosis and characterization of tumor type.

Endoscopic biopsy

These are obtained for accessible tumors of the hollow viscera. For example lung cancer involving trachea or main stem bronchi, esophageal and gastric tumors, colorectal tumors and endometrial tumors are amenable to endoscopic biopsies. A biopsy forceps is used to obtain a punch biopsy consisting of a small piece of tumor tissue.

Surgical biopsy

This can be either *incisional* when a small piece of the tumor is removed surgically, or *excisional* when the whole tumor is excised and submitted for histological examination. It is now used very rarely and has largely been superseded by core/tru-cut biopsy. An important exception is lymph node excision biopsy in suspected lymphoma, when needle biopsies are usually inadequate for characterization of lymph node architecture and lymphoma type. Also, for ulcerating skin lesions, a *cutaneous punch biopsy*, using a small surgical blade is usually employed to obtain the tissue specimen.

Minimally invasive techniques

Major surgical procedures like laparotomy or thoracotomy are now very rarely used to obtain a diagnostic biopsy. If a surgical biopsy is required, minimally invasive surgical techniques are usually employed, e.g. laparoscopy, thoracoscopy or video assisted thoracoscopic surgery. More commonly, these procedures are used to define the extent of disease (i.e. cancer staging).

Selecting the approach

The approach to biopsying a tumor should be selected carefully. While FNAC is usually a low risk procedure, with core/tru-cut and surgical biopsies, the risk of needle track seeding or seeding of the surgical biopsy scar by cancer cells is significant for some cancer types like mesothelioma, ovarian cancer and sarcomas.

The biopsy approach should be selected so that the biopsy track/scar can easily be excised later at the time of definitive surgical resection. An incorrectly placed scar may compromise definitive resection. For example in limb sarcomas, an incorrectly placed biopsy scar may make resection of the tumor with limb salvage impossible and an amputation may become necessary.

Frozen section

Frozen section examination of a biopsy specimen is a technique to identify cancer cells quickly in a biopsy specimen, but it is less accurate than formal histological examination of a paraffin-embedded specimen. It is, however, useful when the diagnosis is required *during the surgical procedure*, so that the decision about the type of resection can be guided by it.

Paraffin section

If the diagnosis is not required during a surgical procedure, a paraffin section is always preferable, for which the most common technique remains hematoxylin/eosin staining and light microscopy examination. Further specific stains may be applied to identify specific cell types.

Histopathological examination

Histopathological examination of the biopsy specimen comments on:

- Cell type.
- Cell and nuclear size.
- Pleomorphism (variability in shape).
- Presence of mitotic figures.
- Tumor grade (degree of differentiation).
- Specific cytoplasmic inclusions.
- The pathologist also looks for presence of invasion

of surrounding tissue, lympho-vascular or peri-neural invasion by cancer cells.

If the specimen is a surgical resection, the pathology report must also include description of:

- Tumor size.
- Intactness or otherwise of the tumor mass.
- Presence/completeness of any surrounding capsule.
- Very importantly, the extent of resection margins, to indicate completeness of excision.

Immunohistochemical staining (IHC)

This is a technique where specific antibodies are used to stain cancer cells. The antibodies will react with and stain the cancer cell only if it expresses its specific antigen. This is particularly helpful in identifying the type and tissue of origin in poorly differentiated cancers.

Cytogenetic analysis

With increasing sophistication in diagnosis, techniques like cytogenetic analysis to detect specific chromosomal abnormalities (e.g. translocations) and to identify specific mutations are now used in several cancers. These techniques may help in:

- Identifying a particular cancer type (diagnosis).
- Predicting the biological behaviour of the cancer (prognosis).
- Choosing a specific type of drug for a cancer (response prediction).

For example:

A breast cancer biopsy may be stained for expression of estrogen receptors (ER), progesterone receptors (PR) or expression of a growth factor c-Erb B2 (Her-2 neu staining):

- o Cancers which are positive for ER or PR are treated with hormone receptor blocking drugs (tamoxifen, letrozole) after surgery to reduce the risk of cancer recurrence.
- o Cancers showing positive results for Her-2 neu staining are treated with a specific antibody against the growth receptor to reduce the risk of recurrence after surgery.
- o Cancers which are negative for all three receptors show a more aggressive behaviour and poorer outcomes with treatment.

Mutation analysis

A very important use of mutation analysis is in hereditary cancers where identification of a known heritable genetic mutation may trigger screening for other cancers in the same patient or in his/her family.

Tumor markers

These are chemical substances secreted by tumor cells or other cells in response to cancer, which can be measured by laboratory testing. Several of these markers are peptides that are usually expressed by primitive cells in the embryonal/fetal stage but not by adult mature cells:

- *Diagnosis.* These markers may be used for diagnosis of a cancer. For example elevated serum levels of alpha feto protein (AFP), beta-human chorionic gonadotrophin (beta-hCG) or lactate dehydrogenase (LDH) in a young male with a testicular mass are diagnostic of germ cell tumor. Other tumor markers that may help in diagnosis include:
  - o Carcino-embryonic antigen (CEA) for gastrointestinal cancers.
  - o AFP for hepatocellular carcinoma.
  - o CA-125 for ovarian cancer.
- *Prognosis.* Tumor markers are also useful in *predicting prognosis and for assessing response to treatment.* For example very high levels of AFP, beta-hCG or LDH in germ cell tumors, and elevated CEA in colorectal cancer are bad prognostic signs. Decline in the blood levels of these tumor markers with chemotherapy or after resection of tumor indicates response to treatment.
- These are also useful for monitoring during the follow up after initial treatment to detect a *recurrence* at an early stage when the patient may be asymptomatic. It is important to be aware of the limitations in the use of tumor markers. Not all cases of a cancer type will exhibit elevated tumor markers (*sensitivity* less than 100%) and occasionally an elevated tumor marker may be due to a non-cancer cause (*specificity* less than 100%).

Imaging

Radiological examination

This is an extremely important part of diagnostic work-up for cancers. Various imaging modalities are used to:

- Identify the primary tumor.
- Plan the best route for biopsy.
- Define the local extent of the tumor.
- Assess for resectability of the tumor.
- Assess the extent of disease spread to other parts of the body.

A range of modalities ranging from plain X-rays and 2-D conventional ultrasonography, through to computerized tomograpgy (CT scan) and magnetic resonance imaging (MRI) are used depending on the cancer type and site.

Nuclear medicine imaging techniques like bone scan, octreoscan etc. are useful in defining distant metastatic disease.

Positron emission tomography (PET scan)

This uses several radioisotopes but radiolabelled fluoro-deoxy-glucose (^{18}FDG) is the commonest agent employed. This isotope is preferentially taken up by cancer cells because it is metabolically more active than surrounding tissue and therefore primary tumor and metastases appear as areas of hyperactivity on PET scan. Combined PET-CT scan is now an integral part of staging and follow up for several cancers.

Interventional imaging techniques

These include:

- Endoscopic retrograde cholangio-pancreaticography (ERCP).
- Endoscopic ultrasound (EUS).
- CT angiography.

These are particularly useful in defining the local extent of the tumor, its relation to surrounding structures and details of vascular supply. For the surgeon, this information is vital in planning the correct surgical procedure for the cancer.

CANCER STAGING

The spread of a tumor including its locoregional extent and distant metastases is called stage of the tumor.

Clinical stage

This is determined by clinical parameters of physical examination, laboratory testing including tumor markers, and radiological investigations.

Pathological stage

Surgical excision and histopathological examination provide further information about accurate tumor size, involvement of adjacent organs and regional lymph node involvement. This information forms the basis of the pathological stage.

Importance of staging

Staging is important for several reasons:

- It helps *predict prognosis and expected survival.* Patients with more advanced stage have poorer survival. This is important for counselling the patient and the family about disease.
- Information about cancer stage helps in *choosing the most appropriate treatment* strategy. For example, in managing a patient with lung cancer, it is important to know the local extent of the tumor to decide if it is resectable. However, in addition, it is also important to know if any locoregional lymph nodes are involved or if there are any distant metastases. A patient with a small resectable primary lung tumor but with bone or liver metastases will not benefit from resection of the primary tumor as the metastatic disease is very likely to progress over the following few months and the expected survival would not be affected by removing the primary tumor. The morbidity of the surgical procedure may therefore be avoided in such a patient and treatment aimed at systemic control of disease and improving quality of life will be more appropriate.
- Stage of a cancer is also helpful in *predicting the risk of recurrence* after surgical resection of the primary tumor and locoregional lymph nodes. Patients with higher stage may be at a higher risk of recurrence due to the presence of subclinical microscopic metastases. These patients are usually treated with *adjuvant chemotherapy or radiation* to achieve long-term control.

Staging systems

Historically, several staging systems have been in place for different cancers. These systems reflected the nature and biology of the disease, the diagnostic tests available and the availability of the various treatment options. Over the last three decades or so, there has been an effort to devise a uniform staging system for cancers across the world. The benefit is that it will be easier to compare the results of various diagnostic and therapeutic strategies for similar stages of cancer across the various cancer centres and be able to make recommendations about standards of care.

While specific staging systems for some cancers remain in use, most of the solid cancers are now staged according to the *Tumor Node Metastases (TNM) staging system* proposed by the International Union for the Control of Cancer (UICC). UICC reviews and publishes detailed and updated staging for each cancer type periodically. Some general principles of TNM staging are as follows (Table 14.1):

TNM system

"**T**" denotes the size and extent of the primary tumor. Small tumors are designated T1. Increasing size of tumors is denoted by T2 and T3. T4 usually describes a tumor invading adjacent organs.

"**N**" denotes the status of locoregional lymph nodes. N0 means no lymph node involvement. N1, N2 and N3 denote increasing burden of locoregional lymph node involvement by cancer.

Table 14.1 TNM system of staging of cancer (as for carcinoma colon)

Primary tumor (T)	
Tis	Carcinoma in situ
T1	Invades submucosa
T2	Invades muscularis propria
T3	Invades serosa
T4	Invades other organs
Regional lymph nodes (N)	
NO	No regional node metastases
N1	Metastases in 1 – 3 regional nodes
N2	Metastases in 4 or > nodes
Distant metastases (M)	
MO	No distant metastases
M1	Distant metastases

"**M**" is for metastases to other organs. M0 means no distant metastases. M1 denotes the presence of metastases in other organs.

The actual staging

The various TNM combinations are then grouped into stages I, II, III and IV (Table 14.2). Generally M1 status means that the cancer will be in stage IV category. The TNM stage can either be a *clinical stage* (cTNM), based on clinical and radiological findings, or a *pathological stage* (pTNM), if based on surgical exploration and results of histopathological examination of resected tumor and locoregional lymph nodes.

TREATMENT OF CANCER

Effective management of cancer, through all the stages of diagnosis, treatment and follow up requires close cooperation between several disciplines. As mentioned above, this is best done under the auspices of a multidisciplinary team of specialists.

The methods available for the treatment of cancer include surgery, radiotherapy, chemotherapy and immunotherapy. So long as the tumor is localized to the primary site and the regional lymph nodes, surgery and radiotherapy are the most successful means of dealing with it. Once the disease has metastasized beyond the local region these methods cannot be considered curative, although they may be used for palliation.

On the other hand, chemotherapy and immunotherapy represent systemic forms of treatment effective against tumor cells which have already metastasized. These methods have a greater chance of curing patients with a minimum number of tumor cells than those with clinically evident disease. Thus, though surgery and radiotherapy cannot be curative unless the disease is confined locally or regionally, they can be used to decrease the patient's tumor burden so that chemotherapy or immunotherapy may become more effective. Treatment combining surgery, radiotherapy, chemotherapy and possibly immunotherapy significantly improves cure rates above those achieved with any single method of treatment. This *multimodality treatment* approach underlines the importance of the multidisciplinary team (MDT) of specialists in the management of cancer.

Intent of treatment

Once the diagnosis of malignant disease has been made, before any treatment is started, *intent of treatment (curative/ palliative)* and expected outcome should be discussed clearly within the MDT and with the patient and his/ her family. The benefits and risks of the proposed treatment strategy need to be considered very carefully and discussed openly with the patient and the family. This is particularly important because most cancer treatments, radical surgery, radiotherapy, chemotherapy, have significant morbidity associated with them. If there is a chance of long-term cure, one may have to accept morbidity or even a risk of mortality. Under-treatment as

Table 14.2 TNM staging of cancer (Definitive/post op)

Stage	Tumor	Nodes	Metastases
I	T1	NO or N1	MO
II	TO	N1b	MO
	T1	N1b	
	T2	NO	
		N1a	
		N1b	
III	T3	Any N	MO
	T4	Any N	
	Any T	N2 or N3	
IV	Any T	Any N	M1

well as futile over-treatment is to be avoided. Whatever strategy is adopted, the importance of a considered, deliberate approach by the surgeon, discussion with colleagues, and obtaining a truly informed consent to ensure patient participation in decision making, cannot be overemphasized.

SURGERY

Surgical treatment represents the most effective method of cancer eradication and long term control. However, only about one third of cancer patients are cured by surgery alone, because surgical treatment is effective only when the disease is localized to the primary site and regional nodes.

Most malignancies, after starting from a single cell, have a relatively long latent period. Unfortunately, during this period they often shed cells into the blood vessels as they grow. Surgery is a means of local control of the disease, and obviously can have no effect on the cells which have been swept away into the blood stream and have produced metastases at distant sites. However, the decrease in tumor burden following local resection can alter the host-tumor balance to favour the patient with minimal metastases, so that it can become easier to deal with these micrometastases by adjuvant treatment.

In the case of skin cancers the resulting skin defect is usually immediately covered by skin grafting; a full-thickness graft (Fig.14.3) gives a better cosmetic result.

Indications

Indication of surgery in a particular patient needs to be defined clearly. This in turn will determine the type of surgical procedure that will be undertaken. Apart from obtaining a diagnostic surgical biopsy in suspected cancer, a surgical procedure may be indicated in any of the following situations:

- ***Attempting long-term cure.*** In the case of benign neoplasms or localised, non-metastatic cancer, the usual aim is complete resection of the neoplamm with long-term cure as the expected outcome.
- ***Achieving local control of disease.*** In some situations of locally advanced or even metastatic disease, a curative resection may not be possible but surgery may reduce the disease burden, improve local symptoms and allow adjuvant treatment with radiation or chemotherapy to be more effective. The benefits and risks/morbidity of surgery need to be very carefully considered in such situations. A detailed discussion with the patient should ensure that the aims and risks of surgery are well understood.
- ***Debulking disease.*** In some situations, for example stage III ovarian cancer with disseminated peritoneal deposits and omental involvement, complete removal of all the disease is not possible. However, there is good evidence to show that debulking surgery in this situation, with maximal removal of as much disease as possible improves survival, presumably by increasing the effectiveness of chemotherapy on residual disease.
- ***Metastatectomy.*** In most cases the presence of distant metastases signifies systemic spread of cancer that is usually beyond the scope of surgical cure. However, in selected situations with *oligometastatic disease*, when the metastases may be confined to just one organ and are very few in number, surgical excision of metastases in combination with chemotherapy or radiation may result in long-term control of cancer. For example resection of liver-only metastases followed by chemotherapy in colorectal cancer, or resection of a solitary brain metastasis followed by cranial radiation in breast cancer.
- ***Palliative bypass surgery.*** This may be undertaken in cases of intestinal obstruction when the primary tumor cannot be resected. Examples of such surgical procedures include gastrojejunostomy for stomach cancer, or defunctioning ileostomy for colon cancer.

Pre-operative preparation

In advanced cancer the patient's condition may be relatively poor. Many cancers have a greater degree of toxic effect on the host than would be expected from their size. In cancers of the esophagus and intestinal tract there may be malnutrition due to interference with normal alimentary function. Anemia, vitamin deficiencies, defects in the coagulation mechanisms and hypoproteinemia must be corrected before an operation can be safely performed. The treatment of any co-morbid conditions like diabetes mellitus, hypertension or ischemic heart disease needs to be optimized and a careful assessment of surgical risk undertaken.

The operation

The operative procedure for a case of cancer must be very carefully planned, because *the best, and often the only, opportunity for cure is at the time of the first operation.* If the tumor is incompletely excised at that time, tissue planes, lymphatics and blood vessels are violated and tumor cells seeded throughout the wound. Therefore, enucleation of tumor masses is never the correct treatment for a cancer.

En bloc excision of tumor, including *wide resection margins* of surrounding normal tissue is the preferred technique. Several precautions need to be taken to *prevent dissemination of cancer cells during operation*. During the operation, cancer cells should not be transferred by inoculation into the surrounding tissues:

- If preliminary biopsy is done and the tissue sent for frozen section, the entire operative field should be prepared again after the biopsy incision is closed. The instruments and gloves, and even the saline used during the biopsy, are not used again, because they may have been contaminated.
- During the operation cancer cells can also be disseminated via the blood stream. To prevent this, manipulation of the tumor during the operation is avoided. At the same time, the vascular pedicle of the tumor is ligated early during the operation to prevent venous spread.

Surgical management of locoregional lymph nodes

Several cancers, particularly carcinomas, first spread to local lymph nodes along the normal lymphatic drainage of the region. Surgical management of locoregional lymph nodes is an extremely important component of oncological surgery. It is necessary for accurate nodal staging (N stage of TNM system). It also has a therapeutic benefit in several situations, so that removal of nodal metastases reduces the risk of local recurrence and distant metastases. Traditionally this consisted of methodical surgical exploration of the locoregional lymph nodes and:

- Either removing a few lymph nodes for histological examination *(lymph node sampling)*.
- Or complete dissection and removal of all the lymph nodes *(lymph node clearance)*.

Examples include axillary sampling or axillary clearance for breast cancer, and total mesorectal excision for rectal cancer to ensure removal of peri-rectal lymph nodes.

Sentinel node biopsy

Lymph node dissection can, however, sometimes lead to significant morbidity in the form of nerve injury and lymphedema. Recently, there has been a trend to reduce this morbidity by performing a sentinel lymph node biopsy in a number of cancer types. The sentinel lymph node is supposed to be the first in the series of lymph nodes draining a particular region. The concept is that if the sentinel lymph node is not involved by cancer, the chances of spread to other lymph nodes are very low and the patient can be spared the morbidity of more extensive lymph node dissection. However if the sentinel lymph node is positive for cancer, a formal regional lymph node dissection is usually required. The sentinel lymph node can be identified pre-operatively by injecting a radiolabelled or fluorescent dye in the tumor and tracking the lymphatic flow. This technique is now the standard of care for breast cancer and cutaneous melanoma.

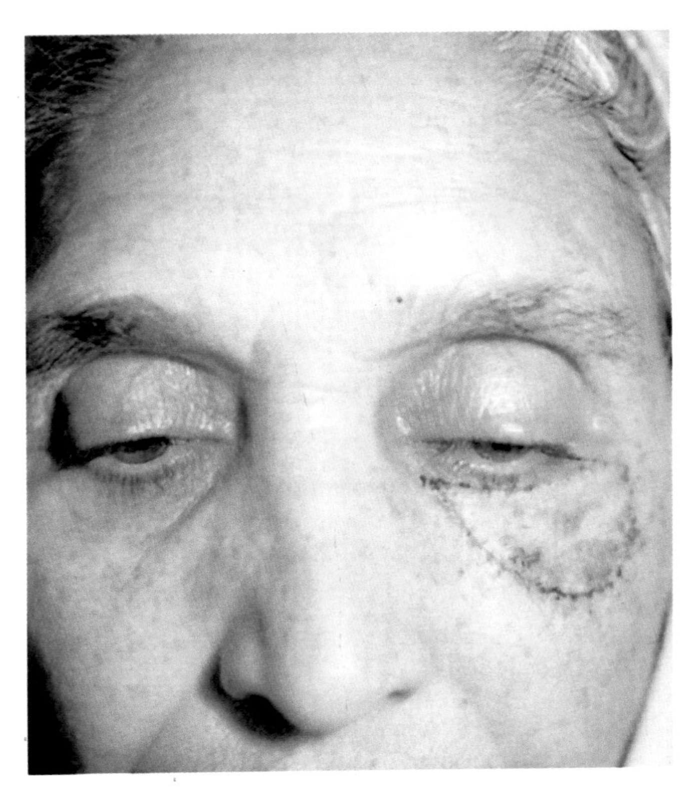

Fig.14.3 Basal cell carcinoma excised and full-thickess retroauricular skin graft applied. Immediately after removal of stitches.

RADIOTHERAPY

Radiotherapy is the use of ionising radiation to treat cancers and occasionally some non-malignant conditions:

- Radiotherapy administration from an external source (e.g. linear accelerator or Cobalt) in the form of a focused beam that is directed to a specific part of the patient's anatomy is called *external beam radiotherapy* or *teletherapy*.
- Radiation can also be delivered by *brachytherapy* whereby a radioactive source is inserted inside a body cavity or radioactive needles inserted directly in the tumor. The most well-known example is brachytherapy for cancer of the cervix where radioactive sources are placed in the uterine cavity and vagina.

- *Radioisotopes may also be injected intravenously* to achieve a cytotoxic effect. One example is use of radioactive iodine to treat differentiated thyroid cancer which is preferentially taken up and concentrated in the thyroid tissue and so achieves a high dose of radiation delivered at the site of the tumor while sparing the rest of the body.

Mechanism of action

Radiation exposure produces a large number of fast electrons due to ionization. These electrons can cause:

- *Direct damage* to DNA, or.
- *Indirect damage* by interacting with other atoms or molecules in the cell to produce free radicals that are able to diffuse far enough to reach and damage DNA. This is called indirect action of radiation.

A free radical is an atom or molecule carrying an unpaired orbital electron in the outer shell.

Clinical uses and indications

Radiosensitivity

Radiotherapy may be used alone or as part of a multimodality treatment strategy along with chemotherapy and surgery. Cancers show a wide range of radiosensitivity, with some tumors responding very well to even small doses of radiation (e.g. lymphomas) while others showing little or no response to even high doses (e.g. osteosarcoma).

Concurrent chemoradiation

Quite often radiation is combined with concurrent chemotherapy administered as a *radiosensitiser*. The two modalities act synergistically to produce DNA damage and cytotoxicity. Concurrent chemoradiation is now an integral part of treatment of several cancers like cancer of the cervix, esophagus and rectum.

External beam

External beam radiation is typically given in daily fractions over several days to weeks. The total dose given depends upon:

- Intent of treatment (curative versus palliative).
- Radiosensitivity of the tumor.
- Radiation tolerance of surrounding normal organs.

In most clinical situations the total dose to the tumor has to be curtailed at a level beyond which there is an unacceptably high risk of damage to normal tissue.

Different forms of radiotherapy

Adjuvant

Radiation may be given to the tumor bed and locoregional lymph nodes after surgical resection of the primary tumor as an 'adjuvant' treatment to eradicate residual micrometastatic disease and reduce the risk of recurrence.

Neo-adjuvant

It may be used pre-operatively as 'neo-adjuvant' treatment to reduce tumor bulk and improve the chances of complete resection.

Radical

A 'radical' course of radiation usually implies that a high dose of radiation is being used as the sole modality to cure a cancer.

Radiosurgery

Radiosurgery is a technique where a very high dose of radiation is given in a very focused way to a small area. The result is ablation and necrosis of tissue within that area. It is used in the treatment of brain metastases or other small solid tumors when surgical resection is not feasible. The whole those is given in a single sitting measured in seconds.

Palliative

Radiotherapy is also very useful in palliation, to improve cancer symptoms related to pain, bleeding, pressure or luminal obstruction.

Complications of radiotherapy

Radiotherapy causes acute toxicity in the exposed area in the form of skin desquamation, mucositis or enteritis. Long-term toxicities to tissues and organs within the radiation field include fibrosis, loss of bone density and risk of secondary cancers.

Although radiation therapy is not usually associated with any immediate mortality, *the morbidity, complications and long-term effects of radiotherapy may be considerable.* The acute changes are caused by edema and inflammation, the chronic changes by scarring, fibrosis and ischemia. Megavoltage radiation has mostly eliminated the skin changes seen in the past with lower voltage radiation.

Radiation sickness

Many patients undergoing radiotherapy develop malaise, nausea, vomiting, weakness and weight loss. These symptoms are directly related to dose, volume and rate of delivery. Antiemetic drugs help prevent and treat this *radiation sickness.*

Table 14.3 Common chemotherapeutic agents

Class	Type	Action	Example
Alkylating agents	Non-cell cycle-specific	Contribute unstable alkyl group to cross-link nucleic acids	Cyclophosphamide, Cisplatin
Antibiotics	,,	Interfere with synthesis of nucleic acids	Doxorubicin, Actinomycin D
Plant alkaloids	Phase-specific	Bind microtubules and cause arrest in metaphase	Vincristine, Vinblastine, Etiposide
Antimetabolites	,,	Interfere with DNA and RNA synthesis	Methotrexate, 6-Mercaptopurine

Late carcinogenic effects

These may be seen from time to time. In the early days after the discovery of x-rays, before the malignant potential of radiation became known, radiologists used to take no precautions to protect themselves from x-rays. It was only when they started developing skin cancers on their hands, and leukemias, that rigid protocols for the protection of the personnel of x-ray departments were instituted, and are now in routine use. Similarly, some decades ago radiotherapy was freely prescribed for benign conditions in the neck in childhood, specially in the USA. It was only when these children grew up, and a large number of them started developing thyroid cancers, that the practice was discontinued. With proper precautions, such problems are seen much less often nowadays.

SYSTEMIC TREATMENT OF CANCER

Systemic therapy may be divided into four broad categories, though some drugs have actions related to more than one category: chemotherapy, hormonal agents, targeted biological therapy and immunotherapy.

CHEMOTHERAPY

There are several classes of cytotoxic drugs and the vast majority of these exert their biological effects by:

- Disrupting critical enzymatic pathways of DNA synthesis and replication, or.
- Causing direct DNA damage, thereby disrupting cell division and inducing apoptosis.
- However, a number of important drugs act on other targets like microtubules and cytoskeleton to disrupt mitotic cell division.

Table 14.3 summarises some of the commonly used chemotherapeutic agents and their mechanism of action.

Clinical uses of chemotherapy

Chemotherapy may be used independently, or before or after surgery or radiotherapy. Some cancers are particularly chemosensitive and are cured by chemotherapy alone:

- Leukemias.
- Lymphomas.
- Trophoblastic tumors.
- Germ cell tumors.

Adjuvant chemotherapy

This describes the use of systemic or regional chemotherapy after local-regional tumor ablation by surgery or radiotherapy

All adjuvant chemotherapy is the treatment of presumed micrometastases. This kind of treatment is given only to patients considered to be at moderate-to-high risk of local or distant recurrence. The risk of relapse and therefore the potential benefit of adjuvant treatment is estimated usually by the pathological stage of the tumor including tumor size, extent of locoregional lymph node involvement (TNM stage) and the histological grade of the tumor.

Induction or neo-adjuvant chemotherapy

This is used before definitive resection or radical radiation to reduce the bulk of primary tumor and eradicate subclinical micrometastatic disease and thus make local treatment more effective at a later stage.

The method has obvious attractions:

- Locally advanced tumors may be down-staged before operation.
- Tumor responsiveness can be determined while gross tumor is still present, and can guide postoperative chemotherapy; if the response is poor, other methods can be used.

- Possible micrometastases are treated immediately, instead of after several weeks' delay due to surgery or radiotherapy.

However, there are also important drawbacks:

- If chemotherapy produces its effect on the tissues, it may cause confusion in the pathological staging of resected tissues, complicating future treatment decisions and prognosis.
- If there is no response, local-regional treatment of the tumor may be delayed.
- If the tumor progresses despite chemotherapy, a safe resection may become impossible.

In clinical practice the decision to use neoadjuvant treatment is based on:

- The relative chemo-sensitivity or radio-sensitivity of the tumor.
- The risk of incomplete upfront resection.
- The risk of presence of subclinical micrometastases.
- The available evidence from clinical trials about the effectiveness of this approach.

Neoadjuvant treatment is now employed successfully in several cancers. For example at present pre-operative and post-operative chemotherapy is considered standard treatment for muscle invasive gastric cancer as a clinical trial has shown that this improves survival compared to upfront surgery.

Palliative chemotherapy

Unfortunately, quite often patients present with metastatic disease which is not curable. In such situations the role of local treatments, like surgery and radiotherapy, is usually limited to providing relief of local symptoms. Palliative chemotherapy is now used in several cancers in this situation to improve systemic cancer-related symptoms, improve quality of life and prolong survival.

Complications and toxicities of chemotherapy

Most, but not all, chemotherapeutic drugs are emetogenic and cause significant *nausea and vomiting* and therefore require routine use of pre-emptive anti-emetics.

Other common toxicities are due to damage to rapidly dividing normal cells which are more sensitive to chemotherapy drugs. These include:

- Alopecia.
- Mucositis.
- Enteritis and myelosuppression.

Still other toxicities include:

- Risk of infertility due to gonadal damage.
- Nephrotoxicity.
- Cardiomyopathy.
- Neuropathy.
- Induction of secondary cancers.

HORMONAL AGENTS

Breast cancer and prostate cancer are typical examples of cancers driven by hormones.

Breast

A significant proportion of breast cancers express estrogen and progesterone receptors (ER, PR). In hormone receptor positive breast cancer, various strategies to reduce the level of circulating estrogens or to block the receptors directly are useful to reduce the risk of relapse after surgery or to control metastatic disease. Ovarian ablation, estrogen receptor antagonists (e.g. tamoxifen), and aromatase inhibitors (e.g. letrozole) are in clinical use in breast cancer.

Prostate

The growth of prostate cancer is driven by testosterone:

- Castration, either surgical or hormonal (the latter with gonadotrophin-releasing-hormone agonists like goserelin) is the most effective systemic treatment for prostate cancer.
- Direct testosterone receptor antagonists like bicalutamide are also used as adjuncts with castration for *total androgen blockade*.

Targeted biological therapy

With our increasing understanding of the various genes and molecular pathways that drive cell growth and proliferation, as well as neoplastic angiogenesis and metastases, there has been an interest in developing drugs that target these specific pathways.

Imitanib

The first major breakthrough was the development of imatinib for chronic myeloid leukemia (CML). The basic genetic abnormality in CML is the reciprocal translocation between chromosome 9 and 22, manifesting as the Philadelphia chromosome. The biological consequence of this translocation is that an epidermal growth factor receptor (EGFR), found on the cell membrane of CML cells, remains continuously active and stimulates cell growth and proliferation despite the absence of any growth factor. Imatinib is a specific inhibitor of this receptor and by blocking it produces excellent response and long-term control in CML.

Since the development of imatinib, several other agents have been developed that target various cellular pathways. There is a huge list of potential cellular targets and their respective antagonists which includes various EGFR inhibitors, vascular endothelial growth factor inhibitors and anti-angiogenic agents.

One of the major attractions of these agents is that they do not have the usual toxicities of emesis, alopecia and myelosuppression associated with chemotherapy. Addition of more drugs to this list will represent great advancement in the treatment of cancers.

IMMUNOTHERAPY

One of the central tenets of cancer biology is the ability of cancer cells to avoid detection and destruction by the immunological systems. Strategies to boost host immunity have long been employed to treat cancer, with variable success. For example, interferon alpha and interleukin-2 in combination with chemotherapy have been used in melanoma and renal cell cancer with infrequent but occasionally dramatic responses.

More recently, development of synthetic antibodies against various receptors on cancer cells has shown great promise. Anti-CD20 antibody (rituximab) for lymphoma and anti-EGFR antibody (trastuzumab) for breast cancer are the most well-known examples. Synthetic antibodies against various other receptors and cell types are now in clinical use for treatment of several cancers.

PALLIATIVE CARE

Cancer pain

Advanced, infiltrating cancer produces a great deal of pain and distress. A patient suffering thus needs all the support and sympathy the doctor can give him, apart from the analgesics and other drugs that are administered to him. In the terminal stages of cancer one should not be miserly in respect of the use of analgesics and narcotics.

To treat cancer pain effectively, it is important to determine the cause of pain. Cancer pain may be due to:

- Bone metastases.
- Pressure or infiltration of nerves.
- Visceral distension.
- Inflammation and ulceration associated with the tumor mass.
- Often the pain results from a combination of these components.

Table 14.4 WHO's pain relief ladder

FREEDOM FROM CANCER PAIN
3 Strong opioid (morphine) for moderate to severe pain +/-non-opioid drug
PAIN PERSISTING or INCREASING
2 Mild opioid (codeine) for mild to moderate pain +/-non-opioid drug +/-adjuvant
PAIN PERSISTING or INCREASING
1 Non-opioid drug +/-adjuvant

Analgesia

Analgesic use based on the WHO pain relief ladder (Table 14.4) and the application of the following principles provides adequate pain control in most patients:

- **Analgesics.**
  - o Prompt administration of *non-opioids* (aspirin and paracetamol) is the first step.
  - o If pain control is suboptimal, *mild opioids* (codeine) are used.
  - o If still required, *strong opioids* such as morphine are given, until the patient is free of pain.
- **'Adjuvant' drugs.**

'Adjuvant' drugs like non-steroidal anti-inflammatory drugs (NSAIDs), anxiolytics, nerve stabilising agents (amitriptyline, gabapentin) should be added at any step as required by the type of cancer pain and the clinical condition of the patient.

- To maintain freedom from pain, drugs should be given at regular intervals (e.g. 3–6 hourly), rather than 'on demand'.
- Adequate *'breakthrough' analgesia* for top-up use in addition to the regular medications should be prescribed.
- Additional measures, for example:
  - o *Palliative radiation* for painful bone metastases or enlarging tumors causing pressure symptoms or nerve compression/infiltration.
  - o *Nerve blocks*, for example celiac plexus block with alcohol injection.

Rehabilitation

The clinician should be concerned not only with eradication of the disease but also with reconstruction of any loss of symmetry or contour of the body and full return of function.

Counselling

Most patients take an active part in decision-making about their illness; others need more guidance and support. Sympathetic listening and discussion reassures the patient. Sufficient time should be available to the clinician to discuss all aspects of the patient's illness and to advise him about the best course to be followed. This should be the practice not only in cases of cancer but in all major illnesses.

Should the patient suffering from cancer be told the truth? Clearly it is the ethical and legal obligation of the treating doctor to obtain an 'informed' consent before embarking on a course of treatment. This involves explaining to the patient the diagnosis of cancer, the various treatment options, the likelihood of these being successful and potential toxicities and complications. All this needs to be done in a sensitive and gentle manner, taking into account the patient's emotional state and level of understanding. One must be prepared to deal with the patient's feelings of anger, blame, grief and guilt. Questions should be encouraged and answered in clear terms avoiding medical jargon. The help of the patient's family, with the patient's consent, should be sought but one has to be careful not to reveal confidential medical information unless appropriate consent has been sought from the patient. It may take more than one session to ensure that the patient has an appropriate level of understanding.

Prognosis

Predicting the future course of a cancer is a difficult matter. However, a number of factors are important in determining prognosis. These include:

- Site of origin.
- Stage of the disease.
- Histology.
- Host immune factors.
- Age of the patient.
- Centre where the treatment is carried out.

Cancer screening

Identification of dietary and hormonal risk factors for cancer and exogenous carcinogens has given us the opportunity to avoid high risk diets, modify our life style and avoid exposure to carcinogens to reduce risk of cancer. Examples include:

- Maintaining a high fibre diet.
- Taking regular exercise.
- Observing laws and regulations controlling radiation exposure.
- Avoiding smoking.
- Avoiding alcohol.

The clinical model of stepwise progression from normal cells to hyperplasia, metaplasia, dysplasia and finally, invasive cancer provides the opportunity to identify these pre-cancerous lesions, thereby preventing progression to invasive cancer. Cancer screening means using a clinical test in an asymptomatic population to detect a pre-cancerous lesion or early stage cancer before the development of symptoms. The assumption is that the treatment of these pre-cancerous lesions or early cancer is likely to be more effective and the chances of long-term cure will be higher.

For screening to be effective:

- The cancer in question must have a long period of tumorigenesis.
- A clinical test which reliably detects pre-cancerous/early stage cancer should be available.
- An effective treatment should exist to manage detected lesions.

Screening is usually directed at a population with a sufficiently high risk of cancer incidence to justify the administration of the screening test. Examples include:

- Annual mammography (breast cancer).
- Regular cervical smear examination (cancer of cervix).
- Regular colonoscopic/sigmoidoscopic examination (colorectal cancer).

Enhanced screening

Identification of an inherited form of cancer in one family member may mean that relatives are at a very high risk of developing cancer at a later stage. Such individuals will merit either enhanced screening (for example annual colonoscopy in siblings of a patient with Lynch syndrome) or even prophylactic treatment (for example prophylactic mastectomy/oophorectomy in individuals with BRCA mutations).

SOFT TISSUE SARCOMAS

Introduction

Soft tissue sarcomas are discussed here as the chapters in Part II of the book are organ-specific, while these tumors are not confined to any one organ.

These tumors are relatively rare and histologically diverse, arising from cartilage, muscles, ligaments and connective tissue. They share a common embryologic origin, arising primarily from tissues derived from the mesodermal germ layers.

Classification

Soft tissue sarcomas are classified as follows, primarily by the dominant tissue type seen on histological examination:

Histological grade

Histological grading of sarcomas is of utmost importance as the clinical behaviour of low-grade (grade 1) sarcomas (slow growth, low risk of metastases) can be very different from high grade (grade 3) sarcomas (rapid growth, early onset of metastases). The histological grade of sarcomas is decided on the basis of three parameters:

- Cellular pleomorphism.
- Mitotic count.
- Presence/absence of necrosis.

Clinical features

With such diverse sites of origin, soft tissue sarcomas can present with a variety of symptoms and signs. When they arise in the retroperitoneum or deep in the thigh they may be quite large before they are noticed. The larger and more rapidly growing the mass the more likely it is to be a sarcoma. This diagnosis should be considered for any mass that lies under the deep fascia. The misleading feature of soft tissue sarcomas is their 'benign' presentation that induces a false sense of security.

The risk of distant metastases increases with increasing size and more advanced grade of the tumor. Unlike carcinomas, which tend to show spread and metastases first to lymph nodes and then to distant organs, soft tissue sarcomas usually metastasize via the hematogenous route. The most common sites of metastases are bones and lungs. Regional lymph node metastases are uncommon, though they may be seen in some sarcomas, e.g. epithelioid sarcomas and rhabdomyosarcomas.

Diagnosis

To confirm the diagnosis in a suspicious soft tissue mass, a biopsy is required.

Biopsy

For sarcomas, fine needle aspiration cytology (FNAC) is usually not adequate as it does not provide details of tissue architecture, and a core/tru-cut needle biopsy provides the answer in most cases. If the diagnosis remains in doubt, a surgical biopsy (incisional or excisional) may be carried out.

Approach to biopsy

The approach to biopsying a tumor should be selected carefully. While FNAC is usually a low-risk procedure, with core/tru-cut and surgical biopsies, the risk of needle track seeding or seeding of the surgical biopsy scar by cancer cells is significant. Particularly for soft tissue lumps of the limbs, it is absolutely essential that an assessment by an orthopedic surgeon is carried out *before* a biopsy approach is selected so that the biopsy track/scar can easily be excised later at the time of definitive surgical resection. An incorrectly placed scar may compromise definitive resection. For example in limb sarcomas, an incorrectly placed biopsy scar may make resection of the tumor with limb salvage impossible and an amputation may become necessary.

MRI

The imaging modality of choice for soft tissue sarcomas is magnetic resonance imaging (MRI).

This is used to define:

- The local extent of the tumor.
- Its relation with the fascial compartments, neurovascular bundle and bone.

This would decide resectability and the type of operation (e.g. limb salvage vs amputation).

MRI before biopsy

Quite often, for skin lumps, if the clinical suspicion of malignancy is high, local imaging with MRI may be obtained *before biopsy*, so that a clear surgical plan is in place.

Staging

Systemic staging requires CT chest and bone scan as lung and bone are the commonest sites of metastases.

Treatment

Soft tissue sarcomas are uncommon and comprise a diverse group of tumors with widely varying clinical behaviours. Successful management requires individualized treatment by surgeons and oncologists with experience in managing sarcomas.

For non-metastatic disease, radical resection is the treatment of choice. This consists of tumor excision with either en bloc removal of the involved tissue compartment or with a generous margin of apparently normal tissue. For low-grade tumors this may be as little as 1cm of clear margin; for high-grade tumors 4cm. Such margins cannot be provided in all tumors; in such cases amputation is required.

Radiotherapy

Post-operative radiotherapy after a wide local excision reduces the risk of local recurrence for high-grade tumors larger than 5cm. Post-operative radiotherapy is also recommended if repeated surgical excisions are required for tumor recurrence. *Pre-operative* radiotherapy or pre-operative chemoradiotherapy may be used to downstage the disease, if there is a reasonable chance that reduction in the size of tumor will allow clear resection margins or may allow limb salvage surgery rather than amputation.

Chemotherapy

For some *high-grade* soft tissue sarcomas (e.g. rhabdomyosarcoma and extra-skeletal Ewing's sarcoma), systemic chemotherapy is an integral part of the treatment regimen because the risk of systemic metastases is very high.

The outlook for *metastatic* soft tissue sarcoma is generally poor. Systemic chemotherapy, local radiation and palliative amputation (e.g. for bleeding control) are primarily aimed at improving the quality of life.

Chapter

15 TRANSPLANTATION

Transplantation of entire organs is one of the most impressive advances in the field of surgery. However, before this stage could be reached, scientific progress spread over many fields and many decades was required.

During the first few decades of this century sufficiently fine suture materials were produced, and techniques of anastomosis of arteries and veins were perfected. However, some very important problems remained to be solved before whole organs like the kidney or the heart could be transplanted:

Cooling

Firstly, it was necessary that after removal from the cadaver and before being transplanted, the organ should not suffer such damage as would affect its function or its viability in the recipient's body. For this purpose methods were devised by which the organ could be perfused with a physiological solution e.g. plasma at low temperatures. The cooling greatly reduced its metabolic needs, while the plasma contained most of the nutrients, including fatty acids, required for its metabolic activity. If the plasma was passed through a membrane oxygenator, oxygen could also be supplied.

Immunosuppression

Secondly, it was necessary to ensure that once the organ was transplanted it was not rejected by the recipient's body through an antigen-antibody reaction. For this purpose such methods had to be devised which could suppress the immune response to the transplant (*immunosuppression*).

Extracorporeal circulaton

Thirdly (in the case of the heart) it was essential that during the period between removal of the patient's diseased heart and its replacement by the new heart the circulation be carried out artificially. Therefore heart transplantation could only be attempted when *heart-lung machines* had not only been developed but their use had become commonplace.

Organ preservation

It is important that graft damage be minimized from the time the organ is removed from the donor to the time it is implanted into the recipient, i.e.:

- While the graft is still within the donor in preparation for graft procurement.
- During removal, storage and transport of the graft.
- During the transplantation operation.

Continuous cold perfusion

Many different measures help in organ preservation:

Cooling from 37° C to 0° C, by reducing the metabolic rate, extends the storage time of most organs from 1 to 2 hours to about 12 hours.

The large-molecule and impermeant sucrose provides osmotic force to oppose cellular edema.

Phosphate provides a buffer to counter intracellular acidosis. Continuous cold perfusion combines all these benefits:

- Hypothermia.
- Continuous buffering.
- Continuous provision of oxygen and nutrients.
- Continuous washout of accumulating toxic metabolites.

If during storage the organ could be treated to deplete it of antigen-presenting cells, this could dramatically improve results and would be a major advance in the future.

Types of grafts

Grafts may be classified in different ways:

By source

- *Autograft* is an organ or tissues taken and transplanted into the same individual.
- *Isograft* is a transfer of tissues between genetically identical individuals i.e. identical twins.

- *Homograft (allograft)* is an organ or tissues transplanted from one individual to another from the same species.
- *Xenograft* is an organ or tissue transplant that occurs between the members of two different species.

By site of placement

- *Orthotopic graft* is a graft placed in its normal anatomical position.
- *Heterotopic graft* is a graft placed in a site different from that where the organ is normally located.

By function

Structural grafts act as a non-living scaffold. e.g. DACRON vascular prosthesis, cardiac valve grafts.

Graft rejection

Unless immunosuppressive measures are taken, allografts are rejected by a process called the *allograft reaction*. In an acute allograft reaction, vascularisation of the graft is normal initially but in 11 to 14 days marked mononuclear cell infiltration and reduction in circulation occurs with eventual necrosis. This is called *primary (first set) reaction*. In most grafts, rejection is mediated by T-cells, but antibodies sometimes contribute to the rejection, as in the case of bone-marrow transplants.

In experimental animals, the rejection of the graft is mediated by cells and not by serum. Also, T-cell deficient animals do not reject allografts but B-cell deficient animals reject them.

If a second allograft from the same donor is applied to a sensitized recipient, it is rejected in 5–6 days. This is *accelerated(second-set) reaction* caused primarily by presensitized cytotoxic T-cells.

Major histocompatibility complex proteins (MHC proteins)

The acceptance or rejection of a graft is mainly determined by class I and II major histocompatibility complex proteins (MHC proteins) on donor cells, because these activate the helper and cytotoxic T-cells which cause killing of the donor tissues. Foreign MHC proteins activate more T-cells than the foreign proteins that are not MHC proteins.

Chronic graft rejection

An allograft that survives an acute rejection can nevertheless become non-functional as a result of chronic rejection which occurs months to years after the transplantation. The main pathological process is the atherosclerosis of the graft endothelium. The immunological reason is not well known; however, the minor histocompatibilty factors and the side-effects of long-term immunosuppression can be responsible.

Hyperacute graft rejection

This typically occurs within minutes and is due to the reaction of preformed anti-ABO antibodies in the recipient with ABO antigens on the surface of the endothelium of the graft. Hyperacute reaction is often called 'white graft' reaction because the graft turns white as the result of vasospasm and occlusion of blood supply to the graft. In view of this the *ABO blood group of the donor and the recipient must be matched carefully*.

Prevention of rejection

The most important problem in organ transplantation is not the surgical problem of removing the organ and joining the arteries, veins, and excretory ducts of the donor organ to the vessels of the recipient. The most difficult matter is to ensure that the foreign proteins introduced into the recipient's body in the form of the donor organ are not rejected. Before methods could be devised by which rejection of transplants could be prevented or suppressed, it was necessary to understand the process of rejection.

Major histocompatibility complex

The ideal transplant is one where there is no antigenic difference between the donor and the recipient, as in the case of identical twins. If the tissues of the transplanted organ are 'foreign' to the recipient they will elicit an antigen-antibody response and the organ will be rejected. The strongest transplantation antigen is expressed in a single chromosomal region called the major histocompatibility complex (MHC), which in human beings is located on chromosome 6. Transplantation antigens were first investigated on leucocytes and were therefore named human leucocyte antigens (HLA).

The less antigenic the graft, the less the host will react against it:

- When the donor and recipient are identical twins, there is no antigenic difference and the tissues are accepted.
- When they are siblings or if a parent is the donor, there is a greater likelihood of antigen-sharing between donor and recipient.
- When an unrelated donor is used, the chances of rejection are the greatest.

Demonstrating antigenic similarities

Several methods have been developed for *demonstrating* similarities of antigens between donor and recipient, so that donor and recipient pairs which are relatively histocompatible may be selected. This lessens the need for large doses of immunosuppressive drugs and increases the likelihood of a successful outcome. The common methods include:

- Leucocyte typing.
- Mixed leucocyte culture.

The role of the small lymphocyte

Mature lymphocytes lie in a state of immunological readiness. The small lymphocyte can recognize whether or not a molecule is foreign and can react to it. It does so by producing antibodies that can react with the antigen, and can recruit other mediators of the immune response. In addition, lymphocytes carry immunologic memory.

The most striking feature of the immune response is its specificity. For each unique stimulus a distinctive population of antibodies or immune cells is elicited.

Graft destruction

The recognition of antigens by sensitized cells or antibodies marks the beginning of the active disposal of the foreign graft. However, the reaction of an antibody with a graft will not by itself destroy the graft. The recognition merely triggers the activation of several cascading enzyme systems, which include the complement pathway. The process of allograft rejection thus has two phases:

- *Recognition phase*. In the first phase the foreign material is recognized as such. This process is immunologically specific, and is called the recognition phase.
- *Amplification* phase. The second phase consists of the actual process of rejection, which is greatly enhanced or amplified in the presence of complement. This process is immunologically non-specific, and is called the amplification phase.

When an unsensitized patient is allografted:

- The first change is perivascular infiltration of round cells, followed by macrophages.
- Antibody and complement are deposited in the area of the capillaries, and the lymphocytes produce immunoglobulins. Thus both recognition molecules (antibodies) and sensitized cells (lymphocytes, etc.) are present.
- On recognizing the foreign tissue, sensitized cells release mediators of inflammation and cell damage. Complement is fixed, producing chemotactic factors and finally cellular damage.
- Capillary permeability is increased by anaphylotoxins and kinins. Damaged cells release additional compounds that attract polymorphonuclear leucocytes. These release vasoactive amines (histamine and serotonin) and other factors increasing vascular permeability.
- The small vessels become plugged with fibrin and platelets. The intima and media of vessels is thickened, and the lumen narrowed as a result. These changes reduce perfusion and prevent function.

Highly specialized cells

The myocardial cell of the transplanted heart, the tubular cell of the kidney, and the acinar and islet cells of the pancreas are highly specialized structures which require an abundant supply of oxygen. If destroyed, they cannot be replaced by further cell division. Therefore, compromise of oxygen supply by endothelial and medial hypertrophy, intravascular platelet aggregation, and interstitial edema result in their atrophy and death, with replacement by fibrous tissue.

Immunosuppression

If an allograft is to be successful one must make sure that the rejection response described above will be suppressed. In theory many different methods can be employed towards this end. However, in practice the common methods depend upon destroying the immunocompetent cells and inhibiting their differentiation and proliferation.

At the same time, to be most effective immunosuppression must be commenced *before* the time of transplantation, because once the immune response is under way it is more difficult to suppress it.

Immunosuppressive agents

Immunosuppressive therapy plays a very important role in organ transplantation by preventing rejection of grafts. The important agents in use include antiproliferative agents, cyclosporin and corticosteroids.

Antiproliferative agents

Most of the commonly used immunosuppressive agents have been borrowed from cancer chemotherapy for their antiproliferative activity. They prevent the differentiation and division of the immunocompetent lymphocyte after it encounters the antigen, and thus inhibit the full expression of the immune response

Antiproliferative agents fall into two broad categories:

- *Antimetabolites* structurally resemble needed metabolites.
- *Alkylating agents* and *toxic antibiotics*, combine with certain cellular components, such as DNA, and thereby interfere with cell function.

Antimetabolites

These are structurally similar to the normal cell metabolites, e.g. purine, pyrimidine and folic acid. They get incorporated during synthesis to produce faulty molecules:

- The purine analogue *azathioprine* has been the most widely used immunosuppressive drug in organ transplantation. Its toxicity is due to bone marrow suppression leading to leucopenia.
- The folic acid antagonist *methotrexate* prevents the conversion of folic acid to tetrahydrofolic acid, a step which is necessary for the synthesis of DNA, RNA and certain coenzymes. It has been used in bone marrow transplantation but not much in kidney transplants.

Alkylating agents

The usefulness of alkylating agents like *nitrogen mustard* and *cyclophosphamide* is limited by their toxicity. Even so, cyclophosphamide has been used in kidney transplants when liver toxicity prohibited the use of azathioprine.

Antibiotics

The immunosuppressive antibiotics include *actinomycin D* and *mitomycin C*. However, none of these is clinically useful as an immunosuppressive agent for transplantation.

X-rays

Total body irradiation has not been used much in transplantation because the toxicity is too high. It is utilized only to reduce the immune reactivity of patients before bone marrow transplantation. The toxicity of total body irradiation is predictable. The rapidly multiplying cells of the skin and gastrointestinal tract are affected most and nausea, vomiting, diarrhea and skin changes occur.

Late problems also occur due to damage to the cellular genetic apparatus:

- Growth retardation.
- Sterility.
- Cataracts.
- A higher incidence of cancer.

Cyclosporin

Cyclosporin represents an entirely different class of immunosuppressive agents. It selectively inhibits the activity of T lymphocytes, leading to inhibition of IL-2 production.

It is not antiproliferative, and therefore it does not suppress the bone marrow. *This lack of myelosuppression is a major advance over other immunosuppressants.* It is therefore one of the most frequently used immunosuppressive agents, and its use made liver and heart transplantation feasible.

In combination with modest doses of prednisolone and/or azathioprine, it provides effective control of graft rejection with fewer side effects. Stopping the drug permits rejection to proceed again, so that it does not lead to permanent tolerance.

Specially in liver transplants FK 506, a macrolide antibiotic, has given results as good or better than cyclosporin.

Corticosteroids

These are the immunosuppressants which have been most often used in clinical practice. Glucocorticoids have many anti-inflammatory actions, which make them potent immunosuppressants:

- Steroids cross the cell membrane and bind to specific receptors in the cytoplasm of most cells, including lymphocytes.
- The steroid-receptor complex then enters the nucleus and interacts with DNA. In lymphocytes the synthesis of DNA, RNA and proteins is inhibited, with degeneration and lysis of lymphocytes, specially of T cells. Within a few hours of administration of steroids a profound fall in the blood lymphocyte count occurs.
- Furthermore, the ability of macrophages to respond to lymphocyte-derived signals is blocked by steroids.

Steroids alone cannot prevent allograft rejection, but along with other compounds, they help in preventing and reversing rejection reactions.

Side effects of steroid therapy include a cushingoid appearance, hypertension, weight gain, peptic ulcers and gastrointestinal bleeding, personality changes, cataract formation, diabetes, pancreatitis and osteoporosis.

Transplantation will be greatly facilitated when more specific immunosuppressants are developed and the present steroid dosages can be reduced.

Monoclonal antibodies

The development of monoclonal antibodies *recognizing different cell markers on lymphocytes* has made immunosuppression increasingly specific and precise. Already OKT3, a monoclonal antibody against T cells, is being used to treat steroid-resistant rejection.

Multimodal therapy

The introduction of *multimodal therapy* using a combination of drugs which act synergistically allows maximum immunosuppression with a minimum of side effects, because lower doses of each drug are required.

Complications of immunosuppression

Immunosuppression is not obtained without paying a significant price in terms of side effects. The most frequent complications encountered with the use of non-specific immunosuppressive agents are infection and malignancy:

Infection

Transplant recipients who receive immunosuppression encounter a greatly increased incidence of infection, which remains the most common cause of mortality. Most deaths used to be due to invasive infections. These have been controlled by antibiotics. Nowadays most infections are caused by opportunistic pathogens, including fungi, protozoa and viruses, the latter being specially common among kidney transplant patients.

Fungi

Candida albicans and *Aspergillus* species are the most common fungi encountered in transplant patients. The latter produces upper lobe pulmonary cavities. The protozoan *Pneumocystis carinii* is also a frequent cause of pulmonary infection, producing an alveolar infiltrate with severe dyspnoea and cyanosis. However, it is seen less often since the use of prophylactic trimethoprim and sulfamethoxazole in transplant recipients.

Viruses

Among the viruses, cytomegalovirus (CMV) and Epstein-Barr virus (EBV) commonly infect transplant patients. CMV is the most important virus infection seen in immunosuppressed transplant patients. The virus itself produces severe immunosuppression, rendering the patient susceptible to bacterial and fungal opportunists. The prophylactic use of acyclovir has caused a significant reduction in the incidence of viral infections.

Prevention of infection

The following measures help reduce the incidence of severe infections:

- Sources of infection should be sought by routine preoperative cultures and eliminated.
- Organs should be obtained from well-matched cadavers as far as possible.
- If the white cell or platelet count drops, the dose of azathioprine should be reduced.

Isolation of the patient is probably ineffective and imposes much psychological stress; it is therefore not recommended.

Malignancy

Cancer is seen more often in transplant recipients than in the general population, but not so often as to contraindicate transplantation. Most cancers are either epithelial or lymphoid. The former, consisting of carcinomas of the cervix and lip and basal cell carcinomas, constitute about one half of these; B-cell lymphomas form the other half. Many lymphomas are not true cancers, as they are not monoclonal. They represent proliferation of B cells in response to EBV infection, and respond to treatment with acyclovir.

The reasons for the high incidence of malignancies in immunosuppressed transplant patients probably include the following:

- Normally, surveillance by lymphocytes may be responsible for elimination of tumor cells as they arise; when lymphocyte function is suppressed, tumors arise.
- Azathioprine may cause mutations in the cells of the patient.
- Herpes virus, to which the immunosuppressed patient is susceptible, could induce these malignancies.

Other complications are mostly considered to be due to the use of steroids: Cushing's syndrome, cataracts, gastrointestinal bleeding, hypertension, pancreatitis, and avascular necrosis of the femoral heads.

Graft vs host reaction

This reaction occurs because grafted immunocompetent T-cells proliferate in the irradiated, immunocompromised host and reject cells with 'foreign' proteins resulting in severe organ dysfunction. The donor's cytotoxic T-cells play a major role in destroying the recepient's cells. Among the main symptoms are a maculopapular rash, jaundice, hepatosplenomegaly and diarrhea. Many graft-versus-host reactions end in overwhelming infections and death.

The graft-versus-host (GVH) reaction can be reduced by treating the donor tissues with anti-thymocyte globulin or monoclonal antibodies before grafting; this eliminates the mature T-cells from the graft. Cyclosporine is also used to reduce GVH reaction.

TRANSPLANTATION OF INDIVIDUAL ORGANS

KIDNEY

Indications

All patients with end-stage renal failure are potential candidates for renal transplantation, there being no absolute contraindications. The patient should have a normal urinary outflow tract, and should not have:

- Active infection.
- Severe malnutrition.
- Disseminated malignancy.
- Incapacitating systemic disease.

As far as the actual cause of the irreversible renal failure is concerned:

- Type I diabetes is the most common cause, accounting for 10 to 20 percent of all patients coming to transplantation.
- *Chronic glomerulonephritis* and *chronic pyelonephritis* similarly provide many candidates for transplantation. Often patients do not present a classic history of either disease, and the kidney lesions are so far advanced by the time biopsy is performed that the pathogenesis is not definite. Rather than make a definitive diagnosis suggesting a cause it is best to regard such patients as having end-stage renal disease of unknown cause. Recently however, with the more widespread use of renal transplantation, patients arrive at earlier stages of their illnesses.
- A patient with a malignant tumor arising in a solitary kidney can be treated with nephrectomy followed by dialysis and later transplantation.
- Among children, patients with *congenital obstructive disease* of the urinary tract with an advanced degree of renal damage are suitable candidates for renal transplantation.
- *Renal vascular disease.*
- *Sytemic lupus erythematosus.*
- *Analgesic nephropathy.*

Recipient operation

Through an oblique incision in either iliac fossa, the muscles are divided in the line of the incision.

The peritoneum is reflected upwards and medially to expose the iliac vessels. The renal vein of the donor kidney is anastomosed end-to-side to the external iliac vein, and the renal artery end-to-end to the internal iliac artery. The ureter is implanted in the bladder through an anterior cystostomy with a submucosal tunnel (Fig.15.1). The wound is usually closed without drainage, and an indwelling catheter left in the bladder for a few days.

A kidney from a living related donor always starts functioning immediately, that from a cadaver donor only about 70% of the time. During the first 24 hours the urine output varies from 5 to 25 liters, and requires careful replacement employing a central venous pressure line for 2 or 3 days.

Results. Most grafts carried out in the Western world are cadaveric, most of those in the underdeveloped countries are from living related donors. Around 80% of grafts are functioning at 1 year, and about 65% at 5 years. Patient survival rates are around 90% at 1 year and 80% at 5 years.

Complications

- *Vascular.* Renal artery thrombosis (1%), renal vein thrombosis (upto 5%). Renal artery stenosis presents late and affects about 10% of patients, and presents as increasing hypertension and decreasing renal function. Angioplasty or vascular reconstruction should be carried out to cure it.
- *Urological.* These affect about 5% of patients and usually result from improper ureteric implantation into the bladder resulting in ureteric stricture, dilatation of proximal ureter and hydronephrosis. This can be prevented by leaving a ureteric stent in situ for a few days.
- *Lymphocele.* Peritransplant lymphoceles are usually asympomatic, but larger ones may impinge on and obstruct the ureter resulting in hydronephrosis.
- *Infections.* Cytomegalovirus infection from the graft tissue.
- *Rejection.* Acute, hyper-acute and chronic.

Indications for renal replacement therapy

The need for renal replacement therapy must be evaluated in each individual patient. Commonly, the following are considered threshold values:

- Potassium > 6mmol/l
- Blood urea > 40mmol/l
- pH < 7.2

However, the overall clinical status needs to be considered. The aim of therapy is to remove uraemic toxins and maintain fluid, electrolyte and acid-base balance. In the patient with uncomplicated renal failure a plasma urea level below 30mmol/l is generally considered acceptable. In the critically ill patient lower target values close to 20mmol/l are preferred.

Transplant or dialysis?

Renal transplantation is nowadays the treatment of choice for most patients with renal failure, hemodialysis and peritoneal dialysis serving as temporary substitutes. Even if renal transplantation is planned, usually the patient is kept on hemodialysis while the investigations and preparation for transplantation are proceeding.

In the poorer communities kidney transplants sometimes cannot be used because of the cost of the immunosuppressive agents, which are required thereafter for the rest of the patient's life.

When it is successful, transplantation provides a greater degree of rehabilitation to the uraemic patient than dialysis. The risk is also slightly greater because of the immunosuppression required indefinitely. Transplantation is superior to dialysis with respect both to quality of life and medical costs. In children growth is more active; similarly diabetics have fewer problems. Most patients who have had a transplant–even one that has failed–prefer life with a renal transplant to life on dialysis.

HEART

A few decades ago no one could have imagined that it will ever become possible to take out a living person's heart, replace it with another, and make it work. Because if Shylock had known it, he would not have insisted upon the heart as his chosen pound of flesh. Today, thousands of heart transplants are being done every year around the world, with 5 year survival rates of around 70%. At the same time, a high degree of rehabilitation is achieved in as many as 90% of the surviving patients in some centres.

Before a heart could be successfully transplanted, researchers had encountered and tackled the following technical problems:

- They had developed a technique of resuscitation and preservation of the cadaver heart.
- They had developed a surgical technique for the actual transplantation, consisting of anastomoses of the pulmonary artery, aorta and the atria.
- They had demonstrated that the denervated heart would function adequately after operation.
- They had devised methods of early detection and prevention of homograft rejection.

It was only after all the above hurdles had been overcome that the first heart transplants were attempted. The successes achieved were most impressive.

Indications

A heart transplant is indicated only if the patient is suffering from terminal heart disease for which all alternative methods of treatment have been exhausted:

- Most patients have severe *coronary artery* disease with multiple infarctions and extensive loss of left ventricular myocardium.
- Another group includes patients with *cardiomyopathy* who do not respond satisfactorily to medical therapy.

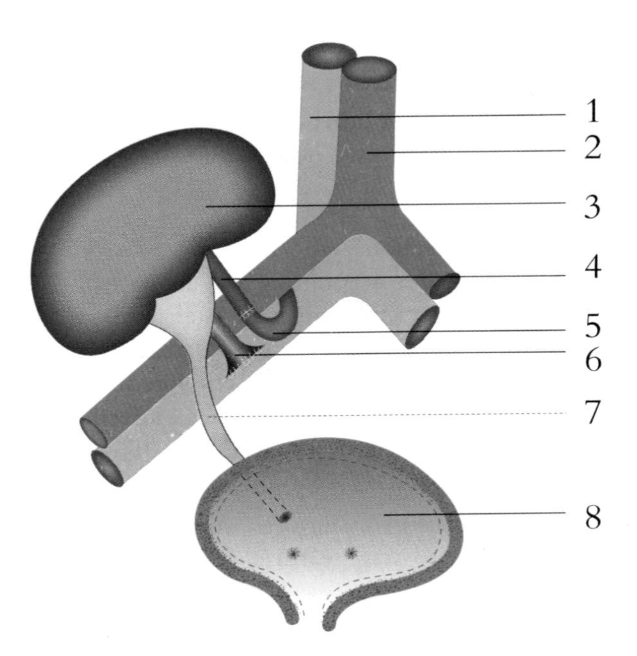

Fig.15.1 Kidney transplant, recipient operation: 1. Inferior vena cava 2. aorta 3. donor kidney 4. renal artery 5. internal iliac artery 6. renal vein 7. ureter 8. urinary bladder.

- Valvular and congenital heart disease provide the remaining few patients.

Recipients are usually less than 60 years of age, although patients are now accepted for the operation upto the age of 70 years. The patient should not have irreversible systemic illness or active infection, and should be emotionally stable, so as to be able to comply with a rigid postoperative protocol of immunosuppressive drugs. The pulmonary vascular resistance should not be unduly elevated; if it is, a *heart-lung transplant* might be more suitable.

After a median sternotomy the aorta and venae cavae are encircled and controlled. The patient is heparinized and cannulae placed into the superior and inferior venae cavae. The aorta is cannulated and cardiopulmonary bypass commenced. Systemic cooling to 29^0 C is initiated. An aortic cross clamp and snares are applied and the heart excised, dividing the aorta, pulmonary artery and the middle of the atria.

The donor heart is placed in position and anastomoses carried out with running sutures successively of the left and then right atrium, aorta and finally pulmonary artery. The last-named is anastomosed with the heart beating, and is vented for about 20 minutes to allow reperfusion of the new heart, before weaning the patient from the cardiopulmonary bypass. The patient is resuscitated, with pressor support as necessary.

Heterotropic cardiac transplant

In this method the donor heart is placed adjacent to and augments the recepient's own heart.

Complications

Rejection and infection are the most common complications, together accounting for about half the deaths in cardiac transplant recipients. After one year the incidence of both these complications decreases greatly. Rejection is managed by intravenous methylprednisolone and if necessary monoclonal antibodies; infection is controlled by the aggressive use of antibiotics. If rejection still persists, retransplantation should be considered.

Results. Cardiac transplantation is very effective in the treatment of end-stage cardiac failure, over 70% surviving at five years.

LIVER

Liver transplant has become a standard procedure in patients suffering from congenital and acquired disorders of the liver:

- The grafted liver may be placed in the normal anatomical position after total hepatectomy of the recipient *(orthotopic transplantation)*.
- Alternatively, the donor organ is placed in an ectopic site *(heterotopic transplantation)*, usually with retention of the host's liver *(auxiliary transplantation)*.

Most clinicians prefer orthotopic transplantation.

Indications

The indications for liver transplantation are the following:

In infants

In infants *biliary atresia* which is incorrectable surgically is the most common indication. If the initial Kasai portoenterostomy fails, the baby should be immediately considered for transplantation, as multiple attempts at revising biliary drainage compromise the likelihood of success of the transplant.

In later childhood

- Inborn errors of metabolism.
- Postnecrotic cirrhosis.
- Unresectable hepatic neoplasms.

In children, the non-availability of suitable-sized donors has led to the development of *reduced-size liver transplants*, one lobe of the liver being used.

In adults

- The leading indication has been *postnecrotic cirrhosis*. Patients with high levels of hepatitis B antigen are at a higher risk of developing recurrence, and are often excluded from consideration for transplantation.
- On the other hand hepatic replacement for other conditions leading to end-stage cirrhosis, such as primary biliary cirrhosis, sclerosing cholangitis, and autoimmune hepatitis, is highly successful. The recent trend is to carry out the operation early, instead of allowing the patient to deteriorate to the point of repeated gastrointestinal bleeding, malnutrition, sepsis and coma.
- Patients with small-sized *primary carcinomas of the liver* with pre-existing cirrhosis, which precludes partial hepatic resection, should be offered hepatectomy and liver transplantation; 50% survive disease-free in the long term.
- *Acute liver failure* represents a difficult indication for liver transplantation. If stage III-IV encephalopathy has set in, the mortality rate will be forbiddingly high. To be successful, therefore, hepatic replacement should be carried out before stage IV coma is established.

Contraindications

Contraindications to liver transplantation include the following:

- Widespread malignancy.
- Concurrent disease seriously impairing survival.
- Irreversible infection.
- A high risk of recurrent disease in the organ to be transplanted.

Complications

- Hemorrhage.
- Hepatic artery thrombosis.
- Biliary stenosis.

At centres with considerable experience of liver transplantation, five year *survival* rates of over 60% are obtained. Most deaths occur in the first three months after operation, due to early graft dysfunction or infection. Most of the surviving patients are adequately rehabilitated, 80% resuming their previous occupations. Some of the earlier patients have survived for over 20 years, and death in patients who survived over 5 years has occurred only rarely. This suggests that the prognosis of those expected to survive 5 years is excellent.

PANCREAS

In spite of the availability of insulin and oral hypoglycemic agents, diabetics are 17 times more liable to kidney disease, 5 times to gangrene of the extremities, and twice as likely to develop heart disease, for the simple reason that the control of the blood sugar level is both inaccurate and intermittent. If control could be continuous as well as accurate, it would be a very great advance. Transplantation of whole pancreas or islets provides precisely that.

The major problem in pancreatic transplantation is difficulty in establishing drainage of the pancreatic duct. In the most popular technique the whole pancreas and the second part of the duodenum are taken from a cadaver. The superior mesenteric artery of the donor is anastomosed to the external iliac artery of the patient, while the portal vein is joined to the recipient's inferior vena cava. The duodenum is anastomosed to the urinary bladder, so that the pancreatic juice is drained via the urinary tract (Fig.15.2). An important advantage of the technique lies in the ease with which urinary amylase levels can monitor the survival and function of the graft.

The immediate effect of successful pancreatic transplantation is dramatic. Within 24 hours the allograft provides a self-regulating source of insulin: the patient does not require any intra-or postoperative insulin. As far as long-term prospects are concerned, as many as 60% are still functioning at three years.

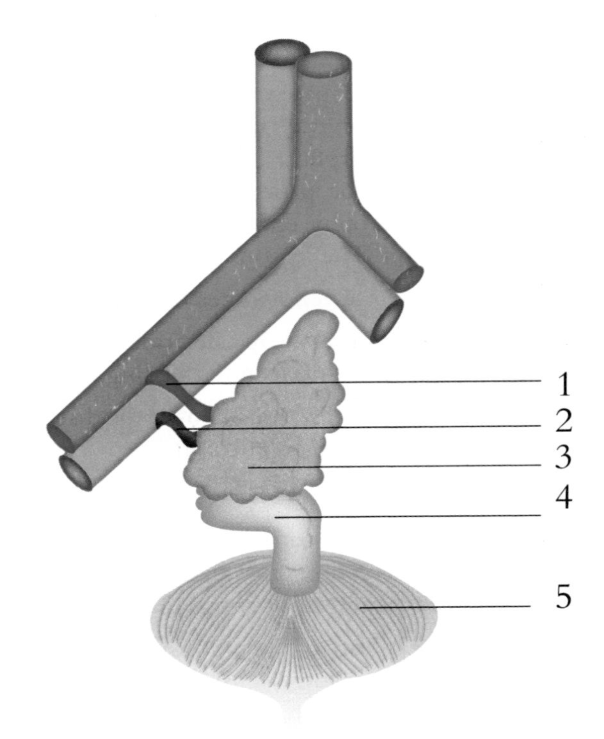

Fig.15.2 Pancreas transplant, recipient operation. 1. Superior mesenteric artery anastomosed to right external iliac artery 2. pancreatic vein anastomosed to right external iliac vein 3. pancreas 4. duodenum 5. urinary bladder.

Pancreas and kidney transplants

Thousands of clinical pancreatic transplants have been performed, and an International Human Transplant Registry is maintained, in order to pool together the experience gained world-wide. Most recipients have end-stage diabetic renal disease; therefore the kidney is also transplanted at the same operation. Combined pancreas and renal transplant should be carried out before renal function deteriorates to the stage of dependence on dialysis, because the restoration of normal glucose metabolism at this earlier stage of the disease will more effectively prevent microangiopathy. With the passage of time, pancreatic transplants are being carried out before advanced renal disease occurs.

Transplantation of islets

The results of transplantation of the vascularized pancreas now compare reasonably with those of other organ transplants. However:

- To transplant an entire organ to cure a non-lethal condition when all that is required is a small fraction of the organ, i.e. the islets, does not sound proper.
- Transplantation late in the disease does not reverse the complications of diabetes. And yet, a young diabetic cannot be expected to agree to transplantation with the necessary life-long immunosuppression.

It is therefore gratifying to note that it is not necessary to transplant the entire pancreas in order to cure diabetes; transplantation of pancreatic islets suffices. In this method the pancreas is mechanically disrupted and digested by enzymes, and the islets are separated. Isolated islets infused into the portal vein produce long-lasting control of diabetes in rats.

Autotransplantation of islets

This technique has been applied successfully to the autotransplantation of islets in patients who require total pancreatectomy for chronic painful pancreatitis, their own islets being used for the purpose. When it comes to transplantation from a human donor, rejection poses a problem. However, the evidence from animal experiments that islet tissue graft can prevent, halt, and even improve the vascular and neurological lesions of diabetes provides an incentive for research despite the difficulties.

SMALL GUT

Improvements in total parenteral nutrition have significantly improved survival of patients with short-bowel or severe malabsorption syndromes. However, prospects remain poor for patients whose remaining bowel does not hypertrophy enough to allow at least partial enteral nutrition. The reasons are mainly two:

- Recurrent infections at venous sites take their toll.
- Liver function progressively deteriorates from prolonged high-calorie intravenous feeding.

The only viable alternative is replacement of the diseased or absent bowel by a functioning allograft.

Indications

- Adult candidates include patients who have survived massive bowel resection for extensive Crohn's disease, vascular compromise or trauma.
- In children the short-gut syndrome commonly results from resection for extensive atresia, midgut volvulus or necrotizing enterocolitis.

Problems

Three main problems make small bowel transplantation difficult:

- The allograft inevitably becomes colonized by microbes.
- Huge numbers of immunocompetent donor lymphocytes are necessarily transplanted.
- The incidence of thrombotic complications is high.

A few transplants have succeeded in the short term. The procedure as yet is only to be considered in highly selected patients in whom all other options have been exhausted.

Cellular transplantation

Cellular transplantation is a newly emerging specialty. Historically, bone marrow was the first successful cellular allograft. Grafting of pancreatic islets is now accepted as a clinical approach to the treatment of diabetes. Grafting of liver, muscle and nerve *cells* is the next likely field of research, with exciting possibilities in the treatment of hitherto incurable illnesses.

Chapter

16 IMAGING AND ENDOSCOPY

Upto the middle ages the only way a clinician could diagnose a patient's illness was by the use of his five senses, specially sight (inspection), touch (palpation and percussion), and hearing (auscultation). Compared to the medical worker of today he was at a very serious disadvantage. Great advances in the science of physics have changed all that during the last two centuries. These advances could not even be imagined in those days. In order to understand the rationale and concept of each advance it is best to see how each method evolved to its present state of refinement. To a greater degree than in the case of internal medicine, the surgeon depends upon imaging and endoscopic techniques rather than biochemical investigations. These techniques are considered in the following pages.

IMAGING TECHNIQUES

X-RAYS

Before the advent of x-rays the only way the human body could be examined was by inspecting or palpating it from outside, or by examining the blood or various excreta. The discovery of x-rays was one of the most important milestones in the history of medicine. It is difficult to imagine the thrill felt by Roentgen when he was able to take an x-ray picture of his own hand. What was concealed uptil now became revealed. Pathological processes in bones and joints could be elucidated without exposing them at operation. The lungs were now like an open book, and most pulmonary diseases could be diagnosed by a simple chest x-ray. Changes in the outline of the heart could indicate cardiac pathology. Urinary tract stones and opaque gallstones could be seen. The distribution of air bubbles in obstructed intestines could point to the site of obstruction. Soft tissue shadows of the kidney, etc. could provide valuable information. And so on and so forth.

Conventional and digital x-rays

X-ray pictures can be taken either by conventional or digital methods. In the latter, digital equipment is used instead of photographic film. Advantages of the latter include the following:

- Instant production.
- Less radiation.
- Images can be transferred, enhanced, lightened, darkened, etc.

Digital methods have replaced the conventional in the advanced countries, and are gradually taking over in the developing world.

Contrast media in radiography

Soon after the discovery of x-rays researchers thought of outlining the various body cavities by radio-opaque media:

- The first system to be explored was the *gastrointestinal tract,* and barium sulphate became accepted as the standard medium to outline it. Again it is not easy to imagine the excitement of those early workers when they found they could see the whole outline of the esophagus (by a barium swallow), the stomach and intestines (by a barium meal follow-through), or the colon and rectum (by a barium enema). In any of these hollow tubes, a stricture, an ulcer, a tumor etc. could now be easily shown up.
- Soon after this an opaque medium (a precursor of the modern day lipiodol) was prepared, suitable for introduction into the *bronchial tree.* Cases of bronchiectasis, tumors of bronchi, etc. could be investigated by this method.
- Similarly, radiopaque dyes suitable for introduction into the *spinal theca* through a lumbar puncture (in myelography) were invented. The cause of compression of the spinal cord could now be detected with a fair degree of accuracy.
- Next, such radiopaque dyes were prepared which could be safely injected *intravenously,* and which had the property of being excreted by the kidney into the urine (for intravenous urography) or by the liver

into the bile (for intravenous cholangiography). The whole of the urinary tract could now be outlined, showing up any stricture with dilatation above it, any diverticulum, the filling defect produced by any tumor or radiolucent stone, and any congenital anomaly of the urinary tract. Intravenous urography also indicated the function of each kidney.

- Dyes suitable for injection into *arteries* (in arteriography) were next produced. Because a dye injected into an artery is quickly washed away, rapid-changing x-ray cassettes had to be produced before arteriography could be usefully employed.

Arteriography is used in two types of conditions:

- o In diseases of arteries, e.g. aneurysm, coarctation, atherosclerosis etc., to outline the artery itself.
- o Where a tumor is thought to be present which may be displacing the arteries to one side, or have a characteristic pattern of circulation in its mass. This application of arteriography is employed in many different parts of the body.

- *Mammography* is a more recently developed technique. It is really just plain x-rays of both breasts, using rays of a strength suitable for soft tissues. Benign tumors show up as smooth rounded shadows, cancers with shadows of variegated density and irregular borders, and with stippled calcification. Chronic mastitis casts a dense shadow and may mimic carcinoma.

Fluoroscopy

In this elaboration of x-ray technique, a fluorescent screen shows moving ('real-time') images of the organs being studied. Examples of its use include:

- Fluoroscopy of the chest, which shows moving images of the beating heart and the expanding and contracting lungs.
- Barium studies of the GI tract: as the barium passes through the esophagus, stomach and small and large intestine, it shows the caliber of, and any filling defects in, the gut; also, it highlights the movements of the gut, so that motility of the gut can be assessed.

Because many more pictures are taken during flouroscopy than with the conventional x-rays, the hazard of radiation with this technique is significantlyincreased.

SECTIONAL IMAGES

Although x-rays provide good images, the x-ray tube is positioned on one side of the body while the film is on the other. In the x-ray picture the images of various structures overlap, and cannot be distinguished from, each other; also, the less opaque structures are not visualized at all.

Cross-sectional images

If an image could be created where the structures in the body could be seen as if a section had been cut across the body, it would be a very major advance. The section of each structure would lie side by side with the other organs; there would be no overlap, and each viscus would be seen clearly.

In an attempt to obtain cross-sectional images, three different forms of energy have been used, namely:

- Ultrasound waves (in ultrasonography).
- X-rays (in computerized tomography i.e. CT scan).
- Magnetic waves (in magnetic resonance imaging, i.e. MRI).

Ultrasonography

In this technique sound waves of a frequency higher than that which is suitable for hearing *(ultrasound* waves) are beamed at the selected part of the body. If they encounter an interface between two tissues of different density, some of the waves are reflected back in the form of *echoes,* which produce images on the screen. By measuring the time lag between different wave fronts and their direction, it is possible to construct an image. The higher the frequency of the sound wave, the greater is its resolution but the lesser its depth of imaging. The usual frequency used for medical ultrasonography ranges between 3–20 MHz, while abdominal imaging is best carried out in the range of 3–7MHz.

If the waves come across a clear fluid, they pass right through it so that no echoes, and therefore no images, are produced and the area appears quite black on the screen. While passing through turbid fluids, and even more so when they encounter solids, some of the waves are reflected back and the area appears as a dark or light shade of grey, depending upon the number of echoes produced. If the waves come across a dense solid, such as a stone, they are all reflected back, so that a dark area appears on the screen on the far side of, i.e. behind, the stone. This area is called an *acoustic shadow,* and its presence confirms the presence of the stone (Fig.16.1).

Air acts as a barrier to the passage of ultrasound waves. This has significance in at least two respects.

- To avoid the layer of air between the probe and the patient's skin, a jelly-like material has to be smeared on the skin before the probe is moved over it.
- The gas contained in the intestines usually prevents good visualization of the pancreas and the lower end of the common bile duct, both of which lie behind the intestines.

Endoluminal ultrasound

Sometimes we need to have a higher resolution and at the same time need to study the deeper structures. In such a case the transducer is mounted on the probe and introduced per-rectum or per-vaginum. The rectal probe is used to examine the prostate (transrectal ultrasound–TRUS). This modality is known as endoluminal ultrasound.

Doppler ultrasound

The principles of physics dictate that if sound waves are reflected from a moving object, there is a change in the frequency of the waves. This principle is used in doppler ultrasound, where the moving objects are blood cells. By measuring the changes of frequency it is possible to estimate the speed and direction of the flow of blood.

Doppler imaging is usually used in the assessment of arterial and venous diseases where any obstructive lesion alters the direction and the speed of flow.

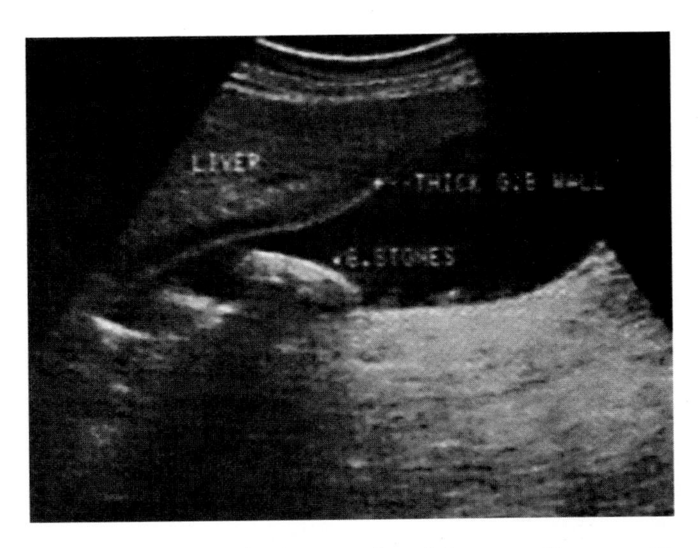

Fig.16.1 Ultrasound picture of gallstones with acoustic shadows behind them. The thickness of the gallbladder wall can also be assessed.

Applications

The most common applications of ultrasound are to be seen in the gastrointestinal (GI) tract and the urinary tract.

- In the *GI tract,* conditions of the liver, gallbladder, spleen and pancreas lend themselves to elucidation by this technique. The intestines are not ideally suited to investigation by this method. However, dilated intestines and thickened walls of gut loops can be shown up, and can be interpreted in the light of the clinical findings.
- In the *urinary tract,* ultrasound examination has nearly replaced intravenous urography, except in respect of the following:
    - o Ultrasonography cannot tell us anything about kidney function.
    - o If a plastic repair on the renal pelvis i.e. a pyeloplasty is contemplated, intravenous pyelography gives a very clear picture of the anatomy of the pelvis and helps in planning the surgery.
- Apart from the gastrointestinal and urinary tracts, cystic lesions in the thyroid and breast can be examined by the ultrasound probe.
- Similarly, in the newborn the open anterior fontanelle provides a window through which dilated ventricles can be visualized.

Shear wave elastography

Most normal tissues have a certain elasticity. In chronic fibrosis from whatever cause, and in the case of malignant tumors with their induration, this elasticity is diminished or lost. Shear wave elastography measures this elasticity. In this recently introduced method an ultrasound pressure wave produces waves in the tissue. The velocity of the waves is proportional to the elasticity of the tissue, and enables its hardness to be assessed. Cancers, diseased livers, etc., are more stiff than normal tissues. Incidentally, this method has had a mixed reception and is not an established procedure.

Caution

Ultrasound examination findings should be interpreted intelligently. This requires knowledge of basic anatomy, and of the changes produced by different diseases in the ultrasound pictures of the various organs. Some time ago the author came across an ultrasound report on a swelling of a testis. It stated that, as the swelling contained fluid, it was either a hydrocele or a meningocele! The finding of fluid in the swelling was correct; the interpretation was wide off the mark. Thus the main disadvantage of ultrasonography is that it is totally user-dependant; if the person carrying out the examination misses or misinterprets a finding, the whole report is faulty.

Computerized tomography (CT scan)

In computerized tomography an x-ray tube rotates around the body in the transverse plane. During this process x-rays are beamed across the body from different angles and pictures taken. A computer synthesizes these different images to produce a single picture which makes it appear as if the body had been sectioned transversely and one was looking at the section from below (Fig.16.2). A series of

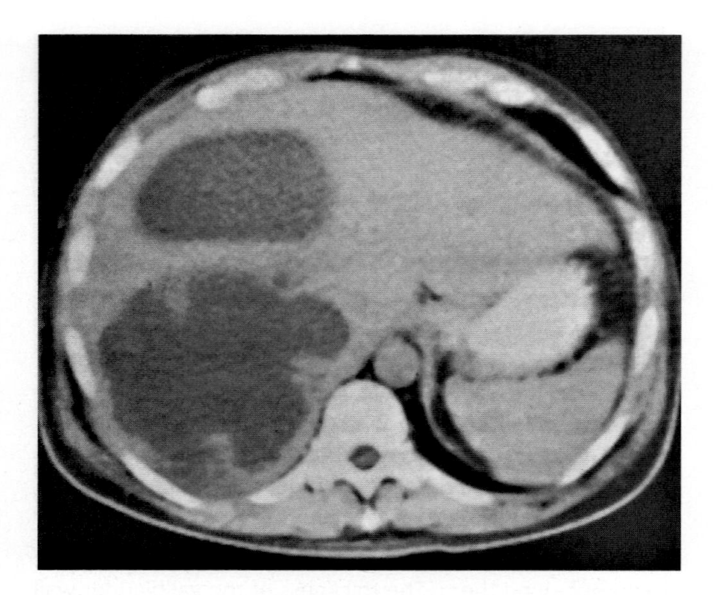

Fig.16.2 CT scan through liver showing a large multilocular liver abscess. Note the transverse section of the vertebra, and the oblique sections of the ribs. In front of the vertebra lies the aorta, and behind it the mass of the erector spinae muscle. The spleen is seen at the back on the left side.

sections are taken at different thicknesses, such as 8mm, 10mm, and so on, according to the requirement.

Applications

A CT scan can be used for most of the conditions for which ultrasonography is used. It allows transverse sections to be taken at regular distances, allowing a standardized record of the lesion to be kept. At the same time, 3-dimensional reconstruction of an image can be done from the CT image, which can provide valuable information to plan the surgery.

Spiral CT

This is a more advanced method, where the tube moves spirally around the body:

- Thus the machine rotates uninterruptedly, saving much time.
- The images can be used by the computer to build a coronal image, which can be useful in examination of the abdomen etc. (Spiral CT scan with coronal reconstruction). (Fig.16.3).
- The fastest scanners can produce an image in less than a second and thus show the heart and coronary vessels as if in a still picture.

Finally, whereas ultrasound waves cannot penetrate through the skull, the CT scan is one of the most useful methods of investigation of the cranial contents.

However, it must be mentioned that CT scan is a good deal more expensive method of investigation than ultrasonography. In other words the latter can be called the poor man's CT scan, and has great relevance in the poorest communities. However, this is not to underestimate its very considerable utility.

Magnetic resonance imaging (MRI)

In magnetic resonance imaging the selected part of the body is placed in the field of a very powerful magnet. When the magnet is switched on, the protons in the body tissues get aligned according to the magnetic field. The magnet is now switched off. The protons return to their original positions and a signal is emitted, which results in the creation of the image.

MRI produces a picture with a sharper resolution than CT, *specially in the case of the soft tissues*. However, it is more expensive than a CT scan.

The problems with MRI are the following:

- The image is easily distorted by the slightest movement as those of breathing and heart pumping, for which cardiac and repiratory gating has to be used.
- Patients with any kind of metal in their body cannot be assessed by this method.

CT scan and MRI have completely revolutionized the process of imaging throughout the body. For example, before their advent carotid angiography, air encephalography, and myelography were the only imaging methods available for gaining information about the brain and spinal cord. All three were invasive and potentially dangerous investigations. CT and MRI have replaced those techniques.

NUCLEAR MEDICINE

In this discipline a radioactive isotope is tagged to a substancs that is taken up by the cells of the organ inder investigation. This is introduced into the blood and is taken up by the concerned organ. The radiations emitted by it are recorded graphically.

Radio-nuclides are put to the following uses:

- *Diagnostic*. This includes the use of radio-isotopes which can be imaged by a gamma-camera after distribution in the body. This includes the relatively recent *PET Scanning*.
- *Therapeutic*. As an example, use of radioactive Iodine-131 to treat hyperthyroidism, or certain types of metastatic thyroid carcinomas.

PET scan

PET SCAN or positron emission tomography is a type of nuclear medicine study in which a positron-emitting substance like 18F is tagged and used to assess the metabolic rate of different tissues. The most commonly used tracer is 18F-2 flouro-2-deoxy-D-glucose.

PET-CT scan

Though very sensitive in picking up metastatic disease, PET scan has a very poor spatial resolution. So, to overcome this problem, PET scan is often combined with CT-scan (PET-CT scan) to pick up the fine metastases in the CT scan.

SPECT

Single photon emission computed tomography (SPECT) is a tomographic technique employed in nuclear medicine using gamma rays, which provides three-dimensional images that are projected as cross-sectional slices.

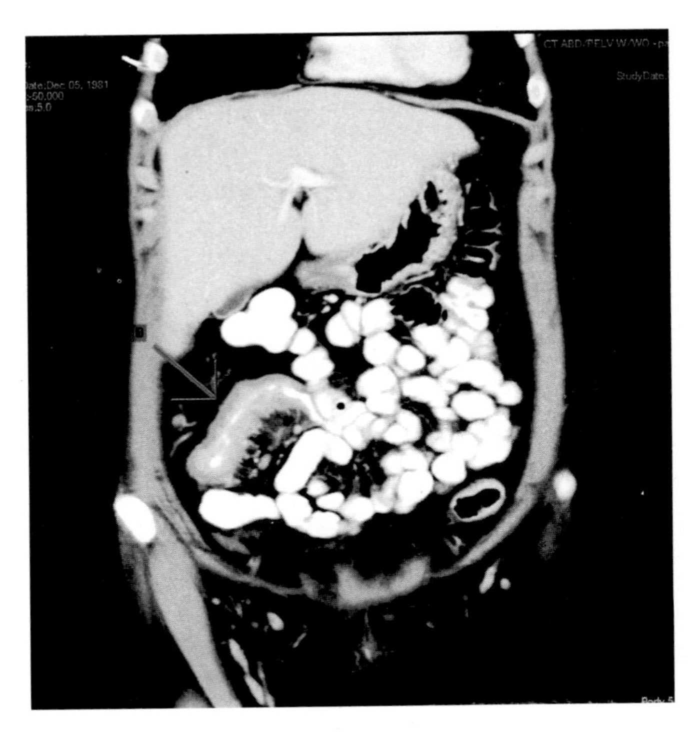

Fig.16.3 CT scan with barium and coronal reconstruction, showing segment of terminal ileum with wall thickened and lumen narrowed by Crohn's disease (upper arrow)

ENDOSCOPY

The electric bulb

Before the advent of electricity no reliable and accurate source of light was available for looking inside the various body cavities. The development of the electric bulb placed such a source at our disposal at the flick of a switch. Further, as smaller and smaller bulbs were crafted, these could be mounted on the tips of slim endoscopes, so that narrower and narrower body tubes could be illuminated and investigated. This led to the design first of *sigmoidoscopes,* and later of *esophagoscopes* and *bronchoscopes,* of which the last-named have the narrowest lumen and require the smallest bulbs. However, these tiny bulbs frequently broke down, and this was a great nuisance.

Fibreoptics

The realization that fine, transparent synthetic fibres could transmit light though their substance led to great advances in endoscopic techniques. As these fibres were flexible, the endoscopes no longer needed to be rigid; they could go around bends and could be passed more comfortably and for much longer distances. In fact the modern colonoscope can be passed all round the colon to the cecum and terminal ileum. Secondly, as the light source could be kept outside, much larger and more powerful bulbs could be used. This not only led to greater intensity of illumination, but also made sure that the bulbs did not break down as frequently as in the past.

As the endoscopes became finer, it became easy to swallow them for gastroduodenoscopy or bronchoscopy. Through the lumina of these endoscopes fine forceps could be passed for biopsy of lesions and for short procedures under diathermy. Catheters could also be passed up the bile duct and pancreatic duct for injection of radiopaque dyes for cholangiography and pancreatography respectively.

With these brilliantly lit endoscopes, the interior of the hollow viscus under investigation can be inspected by direct vision, leaving no doubt about the presence or absence of a suspected lesion. As their tips can be bent backwards through 180^0, every nook and corner of the viscus under investigation can be visualized. Similarly, the procedure of cystoscopy has benefited greatly from the introduction of fibreoptic cystoscopes.

Modern endoscopes play an ever-increasing role in the diagnosis of surgical conditions. The common endoscopes used by surgeons include bronchoscopes, esophagoscopes, gastro-duodenoscopes, colonoscopes, sigmoidoscopes, proctoscopes, cystourethroscopes, and last but not least laparoscopes. The different types of endoscopic procedures are described in the relevant chapters.

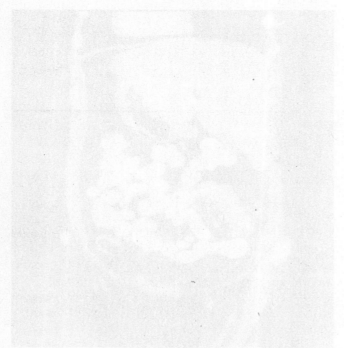

Chapter

17 SURGICAL MATERIALS

With each passing decade, advances in optics, metallurgy, plastics, etc., are continuing to make hospital equipment more and more efficient. Some illustrative examples follow:

Metals

In the old days needle-holders could not hold the more delicate curved needles, as their crude jaws would crush them. Nowadays these jaws are covered with a layer of tungsten carbide which is softer, and therefore more gentle than stainless steel; thus, the finer needles can be held more firmly yet delicately, so that finer sutures can be used.

Plastics

A few decades ago only red rubber tubes were available. The rubber had a rough surface, and also caused a marked inflammatory reaction around it. Also, as the material was not very strong, the wall of the catheter had to be thick, so that the lumen was narrow and clogged easily. At the same time very fine tubes could not be made out of this rather brittle material.

Modern plastic materials have changed all that:

- These materials are strong, so that very fine tubes can be made from them.
- The wall can be thin, so that the bore can be made wider for a better flow of fluids.
- The surface can be very smooth, so that the lumen does not clog easily.
- The tube can be transparent, so that the flow of fluids through it can be monitored visually.
- Finally, when placed in the tissues the tubes induce very little reaction.

Because of such properties of these tubes it has become possible to carry out much more refined procedures than in the past.

SUTURES

Sutures are required to accurately appose the wound edges and to hold them together until the reunited tissue has acquired a sufficient degree of strength to support itself. However, as they are foreign bodies they irritate the tissues and increase the chances of development of infection. In this connection, the following characteristics of sutures are of special significance:

Thickness

About a century ago only crude suture materials were available. Three sizes of sutures were made, and were called sizes 1, 2 and 3. Later, when surgeons wanted to carry out more delicate suturing they started asking for finer materials. The thinner silk which was made was given the number zero. When even more fine sutures were produced they called them 2/0, 3/0 and so on until today some of the finest sutures are 10/0 or so. However, this numbering by zeroes was illogical and cumbersome, therefore the metric system of numbering was introduced. Table 17.1 shows the equivalent numbers of

Table 17.1 Equivalence between old and new systems of numbering of suture sizes

Old system	Metric system	
	Silk Polypropylene Polyglactin	Catgut
6/0	0.7	
5/0	1	
4/0	1.5	2
3/0	2	3
2/0	3	3.5
0	3.5	4
1	4	5

the two systems. Students would be well advised to learn the metric system, as in the next many decades of their expected working life this system will be employed more commonly.

The thicker the suture, the more foreign body is introduced into the tissues. Therefore, sutures should be selected at the finer end of the range. Modern synthetic sutures are generally stronger than the natural ones, so finer sizes can be used without sacrificing strength.

Number of filaments

Monofilament sutures cause less reaction than multifilament threads, because their smoother surface presents less of an area to the tissues. They are also attractive because infection does not persist if it occurs; with multifilament sutures bacteria lodge in the recesses of the suture and are outside the reach of phagocytes and antibiotics, so that infection persists until the offending suture is removed, thus requiring another operation. However, monofilament sutures have two important disadvantages:

- They are difficult to knot, and the knot can slip unless extra ties are thrown.
- The larger-sized sutures are more stiff than multifilament sutures in equivalent sizes. This property is a drawback in two situations:
    - When used to close the muscular abdominal wall, the end of the stiff suture can sometimes erode through the skin and result in a sinus.
    - Removal of skin sutures can be painful due to the stiffness of the suture.

Absorbability

In the beginning surgery was limited in its scope to superficial operations. The commonly available threads namely linen and silk were employed. It was only when surgeons started proceeding deeper into the body that the need arose for sutures which would get absorbed spontaneously, rather than result in longstanding granulomas around them. Only then was catgut, consisting of collagen from the submucosa of sheep, employed. Having served its purpose of bringing tissues or walls of hollow tubes together for union, it got absorbed.

It should be remembered that absorbable sutures generally cause more reaction than non-absorbable ones in equivalent sizes, because nature's vultures, the macrophages, collect in large numbers to devour them. Over a period of time a large number of both non-absorbable and absorbable sutures have been synthesized, the more commonly used sutures being listed in Tables 2 and 3.

Different sutures

Non-absorbable sutures

Silk

Before the introduction of synthetic sutures, silk was the most commonly used non-absorbable suture. It had adequate tensile strength. Further, being flexible and having a matt surface, it was easy to knot and its knot did not slip. Finally, silk is a soft suture, and stitch removal was painless.

The main problem with silk as with other multifilament sutures arose from the fact that if infection developed, it was very difficult to eradicate it because of the bacteria lurking in the interstices of the suture. Because of this important drawback, multifilament sutures have mostly been supplanted by monofilament sutures.

Polypropylene

This is an extremely useful suture.

Advantages

- It has great tensile strength, so that smaller sizes can be used. At the same time where extra strength is required as in the repair of tendons, it is a suitable suture.
- Because it is monofilament, it has no interstices into which bacteria could lodge and hide away from the body's defences.
- It also causes very little reaction in the tissues.
- For all these reasons the incidence of infection after its use in clean cases is very low.

Because of these qualities it is a popular suture today.

Disadvantages

The smooth surface of polypropylene, however, creates problems:

- The knot slips, and therefore not only does the thread have to be pulled rather tight, many loops of the knot have to be thrown. When pulled tight, it can result in more pain, edema and venous congestion, and a greater likelihood of infection.
- Further, polypropylene is stiff, specially in the larger sizes. When used to repair the muscular abdominal wall its ends can burrow through the overlying skin, specially in a lean person, and result in bothersome sinuses.

Multifilament nylon

This type of suture has most of the advantages and disadvantages of silk, and is similarly used less often than monofilament sutures.

Table 17.2 Absorbable suture materials

Suture	Absorbed in (weeks)	Strength	Knotting
Plain Catgut	2		+-Loose
Chromic Catgut	3	+	Reasonable
Polyglactin	6	+++	Good
PDS	8	++++	Good

Table 17.3 Non-absorbable suture materials

Type of suture	Number of filaments	Strength	Knotting
Silk	Multiple	++	Good
Multifilament nylon	Multiple	+++	Good
Polypropylene	Single	+++	Slips*

*The surface of monofilament sutures is smooth, therefore the knot often slips, so this often requires extra throws of the knot.

Absorbable sutures

Catgut

Catgut is used in the deep structures when it is desired that the suture should get absorbed within a few weeks.

Plain catgut

This lasts only two to three weeks. It is best for use in the subcutaneous tissues, where fat has a poor blood supply and a suture is required which is easy to absorb.

Chromic catgut

On the other hand chromic catgut chromic lasts approximately twice that long. It is used to suture intestines, urinary bladder, bile duct etc. In the last-named two structures its early absorbability is attractive, as it ensures that there is no foreign body around which stones could form afresh. It is not a very strong suture, and is not suitable for bringing together tissues requiring strength, such as aponeuroses. Catgut is attractive in communities where the higher cost of polyglactin is significant.

Polyglactin

This is a synthetic suture. It is a great deal stronger than catgut, hence much finer sizes can be employed. It lasts in the tissues for many more weeks, and for this whole period lends its strength to the tissues it has joined. It is suitable not only for the gastrointestinal tract but also for joining together the muscular layers of the abdominal wall.

PDS

This is another synthetic suture which is even stronger than polyglactin, but more expensive.

NEWER SUTURING MODALITIES

Many new advances have been made in the field of tissue approximation, anastomosis and wound care. Some of them are listed below:

Steristrips

These are used to approximate the skin when there is no tension between the edges of the wound and the wound is clean and tidy, with sharply incised margins. The benefits are better cosmetic results, and psychologically the patient feels better in the absence of visible sutures.

'Opsite'

This is a transparent adhesive film which providea a dual action: first of holding the edges of the wound, the second to provide an aseptic environment and the facility of inspecting the wound without the need of removing the dressing. However, recent work has shown cases where infection took place under the film due to the warm and humid environment produced by it.

Glues

Fibrin glues are sometimes used; when applied to a wound, they polymerise to form a firm adhesive bond. They are rapid-acting and no local anesthesia is needed for their application. Infection rates are said to be low with their use.

Skin clips

These are often used to minimize the time of suturing, and they produce good eversion of the wound edges to avoid overlapping. The infection rate is lower as compared to conventional sutures because the metallic limb of the clip does not traverse the whole thickness of the tissue. They are expensive and require a specific instrument for their removal but they save a surgeon's time.

Stapling devices

A number of different types of staplers are used for anastomosis of the bowel. They are used for end-to-end anastomosis, intra-luminal anastomosis and side-to-side ansatomosis. They apply two rows of staples and divide the bowel in between. These devices are of prime importance in anastomosis at difficult sites i.e. in the pelvis and in esphagectomies.

Ligasure

This is a tissue fusion technology used to seal a vessel to prevent it to bleed and to achieve hemostasis. It fuses the vessel wall to create a seal. The newer variant of this technology are so designed that they could sense when the vessel has been sealed and then discontinue its energy dissipation. A vessel of upto 7mm can be sealed within a matter of 2–4 seconds.

Harmonic scalpel

This instrument uses an ultrasound transducer to produce vibrations at the rate of 20000–50000 Hz. These vibrations cause the denaturation of proteins and cut, coagulate and seal the tissue without producing heat. As no smoke is produced during its use so the visibility of the tissues remain good during the procedure, although it takes longer for the harmonic scalpel to cut and coagulate. It is claimed that harmonic dissection improves the post-operrative pain, swelling, operative time and complication rate.

Chapter

18 MISCELLANEOUS

In this chapter it is proposed to discuss the importance of clinical methods in surgical practice, a few basics of operative surgery, the use of lasers in surgery, and clinical audit.

CLINICAL METHODS

This is not a book on clinical methods, for which the reader is referred to various excellent volumes on the subject. However, the author would impress upon the surgical trainee the over-riding *importance* of clinical methods in diagnosis. Unless a clinician is thoroughly conversant with the correct methods of examining a patient, he cannot elicit the different physical signs on which the diagnosis of the patient's illness is based. The *history* and the *physical signs* each have their importance.

History

It is axiomatic that about 80% of diagnoses are made on the basis of the history alone. The reason is this: physical examination tells us only about the state of affairs at the present moment. On the other hand the *history gives us information about all the events that have taken place since the onset of the illness,* which may be as far back as many years ago.

If the patient has been having epigastric pain off and on, it has significance. If the pain has recently increased greatly in severity it has added importance. If he has, in addition, had hematemesis repeatedly, it has further significance. Now, it is self-evident that physical examination, however thorough, cannot tell us about these things; *it is only history which can.* Every medical teacher stresses upon the students the value of listening to the sick person patiently, methodically and skilfully, because each sentence uttered by the patient narrating his story is likely to unfold an event in the development of the illness.

Physical signs

A few centuries ago the only way in which a clinician could find out about a patient's physical condition was by the use of his five senses. Modern investigative methods have placed many very effective tools at his service. However, the value of the use of physical signs for diagnosis is still undiminished. At the same time, these signs are available to the clinician even where sophisticated investigations are not; for example, away from the hospital setting.

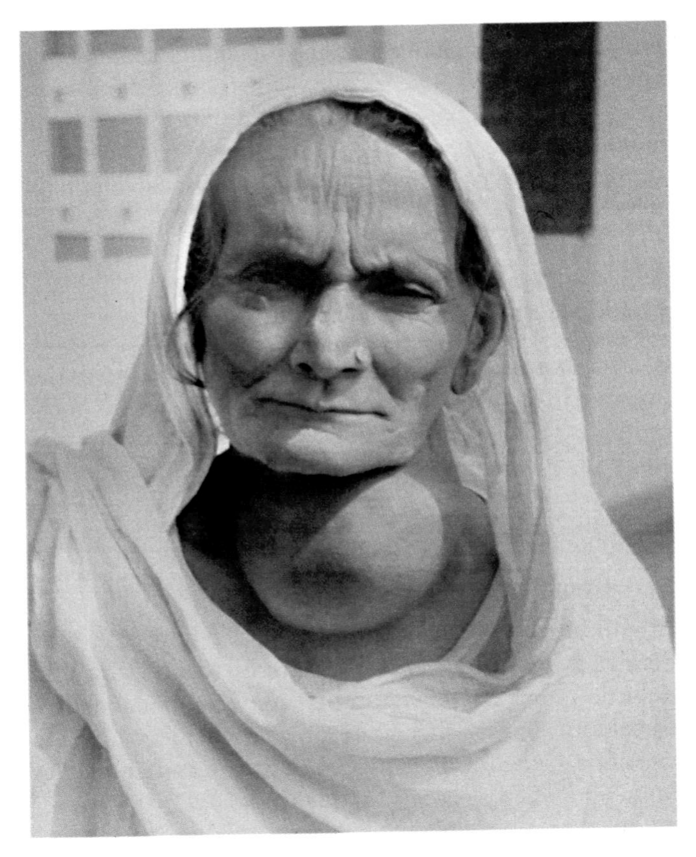

Fig.18.1 Large swelling due to multinodular goitre in middle-aged woman

Swelling as a physical sign

The importance of a swelling as a physical sign in surgery cannot be over-emphasized, for the simple reason that *the majority of surgical conditions result in the development of a swelling.* (Fig.18.1) If a kidney is diseased a swelling appears; if the thyroid is abnormal it is swollen; if the testis is diseased a swelling is the result. Therefore, it behoves the surgical trainee to thoroughly familiarize himself with the methods of physical examination of a swelling in any organ or part of the body. If he knows how to examine a swelling it means he has mastered at least half of all clinical surgery.

The student should thoroughly familiarize himself with all the important points to be remembered while taking the *history* of a case with a swelling. Next he should commit to memory all the points of importance in both *inspection* and *palpation* of a swelling, and should constantly practice the methods of eliciting the relevant signs. Only thus will he be able to form a correct opinion about the nature of the swelling and the underlying illness. *Complete familiarity with the methods of examination of a swelling will pay him rich dividends throughout his clinical career.*

SOME BASICS OF OPERATIVE SURGERY

Being allowed the privilege of helping restore the function of a person's most precious possession, his body, every surgical operation should be carried out gently and with attention to detail. Only general guidelines are given below, while special situations may require special steps.

Sterilization

Attention to the fine points of sterilization pays rich dividends by ensuring the healing of wounds by first intention, and by preventing the development of life-threatening sepsis. Sterilization can be achieved by the use of heat, chemicals, gamma-irradiation and ultraviolet light.

Heat

Boiling kills bacteria but not spores, therefore for effective sterilization temperatures have to be raised above the boiling point of water. This can be achieved either by hot air oven or the autoclave:

- A *hot air oven* can raise the temperature to 120°C and beyond. It is used for the sterilization of *blunt instruments* and *glassware*. However, fabrics get burnt in such an oven, therefore a different method of sterilization is required for linen.
- In the *autoclave* steam is generated at similar high temperatures. This is suitable for *linen*, as the steam penetrates through all its layers. However, the linen should be packed loosely to allow this to happen. At the same time, certain sensitive chemicals on paper strips are placed in the deep part of the linen. These change colour, and show the effectiveness of sterilization.

Chemicals

The sharp edges of *cutting instruments* are damaged by all kinds of heat. Therefore *chemical* methods have to be employed, and these instruments are kept dipped in appropriate solutions for varying periods of time. The time-honoured liquid is pure phenol (carbolic acid). Recently other solutions, like glutaraldehyde and phthalaldehyde have come into use, which are milder in spite of having a rapid action on the microorganisms.

Gamma rays

Instruments can also be sterilized by *gamma-irradiation.*

Ultraviolet rays

Finally, the interior of the *operation theatre* can be exposed to *ultraviolet light* from a lamp overnight.

Position on the table

It is often not realized that a proper position on the table is of the utmost importance. One of the important reasons for the apparent difficulty of an operation is the unsuitability of the patient's position on the table for the particular procedure.

Lighting

Good theatre lights contain numerous bulbs for shadowless viewing. Further, they can be rotated through large arcs to provide light from almost every conceivable angle. Before the operation starts one should have the light fixed at the best angle. Working under imperfect illumination can have dangerous consequences.

Assistants

Most average-sized operations can be carried out with one assistant and one scrub nurse, apart from a runner. In the usual type of case it is more convenient for the assistant to stand across the table, so that both the nurse and himself can assist the surgeon more efficiently. (Fig.18.2)

If an operation is proving to be unexpectedly difficult, the surgeon should check to see if the position of the patient on the table, position of the lights and of the assistants, even the method of draping, are all as they should be.

Shaving and scrubbing

Hair should be shaved off from the area of the operation. However, care should be taken that cuts are not produced in the skin, which could become infected.

At the operation table the area to be operated upon should

be scrubbed with a detergent to remove any grease etc. The time-honoured detergent is ordinary soap, which is perfectly adequate for the purpose. However, antiseptic detergents are available, like cetavlon, and should be employed. This should be followed by painting with methylated spirit, povidone iodine or other antiseptic.

Draping

Autoclaved linen sheets are used to drape the patient, leaving only the area of the operation exposed. An adhesive transparent plastic sheet may be fixed to this area to completely exclude bacteria from the wound; however, recent work has shown *higher* infection rates following its use, due to the warm and humid environment under the impervious plastic.

Incisions

These are made keeping in view the requirements of exposure. As far as possible they should follow the lines of skin tension, as healing then takes place with the least conspicuous scars. The length of the incision should be quite sufficient for adequate exposure to enable the operation to proceed smoothly.

Diathermy

During surgical operations diathermy is used both for closing down small bleeding vessels and for hemostatically cutting tissues.

A diathermy machine passes electric current through the body:

- One electrode, which is applied at an area away from the site of the operation and commonly at the lateral surface of the thigh, has a large flat surface.
- The second electrode is the active electrode. This is used in the wound, and is pinpoint. The large quantity of current converging on this point acts on the tissue: if a low frequency current is passed through the tissue, it coagulates it; if a high frequency current is passed, it cuts it:
    - *Coagulating current.* The tip of the electrode is made to touch an artery forceps which is holding a small vessel, and the tissue gets coagulated, producing hemostasis. Only a minimum amount of tissue should be taken into the grip of the hemostat, so as to minimize the amount of tissue coagulated.
    - *Cutting current.* A higher frequency of diathermy can also be employed. This cuts the tissue, acting in place of the 'cold' knife. Even the cutting current produces a hemostatic effect, so that there is minimal loss of blood.

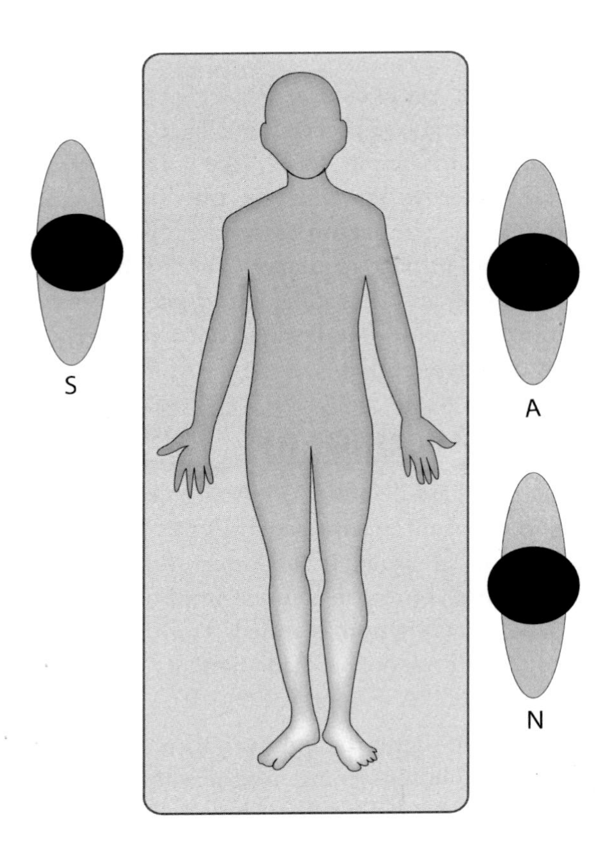

Fig.18.2 An example of the positions of members of the surgical team around the operation table. S: surgeon, A: assistant, N: nurse

Whether using it for coagulation or for cutting, one should hold the active electrode like a pen, not like a sword.

Closure of wounds

This should be carried out meticulously. The edges of the skin should not be allowed to overlap each other, otherwise a granulating broad ugly scar results.

Drainage

If a large cavity is left behind after the operation, drainage of the wound should be employed. These drains are mostly made of transparent synthetic material:

- *Tube* drains are most commonly used, leading to a collection bag.
- *Corrugated* drains function smoothly and rarely get blocked; however, they can allow introduction of infection from outside, specially if left in for long.
- *Suction* drains evacuate fluid before it can collect, allowing the walls of the wound to come together. They thus greatly expedite healing.

Speed

Some surgeons can operate at a faster speed than others. In driving a car, if one proceeds at a pace slightly slower than one's comfortable speed, the journey proceeds most satisfactorily; the same is true during surgical operations. The temptation to rush the pace should be avoided. The utmost gentleness should be exhibited while handling and dissecting the tissues; it pays rich dividends in trouble-free healing and a relatively pain-free postoperative period.

LASERS IN SURGERY

If a photon (a particle of light) hits an atom, it can either get absorbed, or it can stimulate the emission of another photon from the atom. If the latter event takes place, this stimulated emission causes amplification of the light. The phenomenon is called 'Light Amplification by Stimulated Emission of Radiation' and the light thus emitted is called LASER light.

Unlike ordinary light, the light produced from lasers is coherent, the photons being in step with each other in both time and space. Therefore there is little divergence of the beam which can be focused onto a very small spot, producing enormous irradiance and localized power.

On striking a tissue if the light is reflected, transmitted through or scattered in a tissue, it produces no biological effect. It is only if the light is absorbed in the tissue that a biological effect is produced. The effect of absorption in a tissue depends on its constituents such as hemoglobin, myoglobin and water; lasers of different wavelength are preferentially absorbed by different tissues. For example carbon dioxide laser is particularly absorbed by water, argon laser by hemoglobin and other pigments.

Biological effect

The biological effect is dependent on the temperature attained in the tissue:

- Upto 45°C, selective hyperthermic destruction of malignant tissues takes place.
- Above this all cells are rapidly killed.
- Further heating causes contraction and coagulation of proteins.

Hemostasis

As the tissue shrinks, small vessels can be sealed, arresting hemorrhage; thrombosis of the vessel then follows. The Nd YAG laser is able to seal vessels upto 1mm in diameter.

Tissue ablation

If more energy is used tissue necrosis occurs, with vaporization and tissue ablation.

Applications

Gallstones

Nd YAG laser is used for lithotripsy (breaking down stones) in the endoscopic fragmentation of *biliary calculi.* Laser beams are transmitted down flexible optical fibres, the ends of which are placed just touching the stone. The laser pulses produce a localized shock wave that pulverizes the stones.

Liver and pancreatic cancers

Interstitial laser hyperthermia is utilized for unresectable *liver and pancreatic cancers.* Multiple fibres are inserted into the tumor under ultrasound control. The progression of the damage to the tumor can be monitored by ultrasound or MRI, and the area of destruction can be matched to the size of the lesion.

Upper GI hemorrhage

In cases of upper GI hemorrhage, surgery can be avoided if the laser is used as an endoscopic hemostatic device to produce thermal contraction of the bleeding vessel. The bleeding vessel is identified, any clot washed off, and the lesion ringed with several pulses of laser energy. The tissue turns white when it is coagulated and the feeding vessel has been occluded. The method is associated with a 1 percent mortality compared with a 12 percent mortality in control patients.

Esophageal cancer

Laser therapy is now widely used for the *palliation of* malignant dysphagia caused by esophagogastric cancer. Treatment is entirely local and is used at high power to coagulate and vaporize the tumor. In the *esophagus* laser treatment is most useful for the treatment of totally obstructing tumors and for tumors which are unsuitable for endoscopic placement of prosthetic tubes. It is not suitable if a tracheo-esophageal fistula is present; in that case intubation is to be preferred.

Colorectal cancer

A few colorectal cancers have advanced metastatic spread or severe concomitant disease that render them unfit for surgery. In such cases laser therapy aims to remove all of a cauliflower tumor, improving bleeding, discharge and obstructive symptoms.

Ureteric stones

The laser fibre is passed through the operating port of a ureteroscope. The small fibre size, accuracy and safety allow successful *ureteric stone fragmentation* with minimal invasiveness. The low energy pulse, the selective absorption of the particular wavelength by the stone, and its minimal absorption by the tissue, makes this a safe and effective method of stone fragmentation. This is thus a better method than Extracorporial Shock Wave lithotripsy (ESWL).

Prostate

Laser prostatectomy is the method which probably holds the most promise for the future. The laser probe directly touches and vaporizes the prostatic tissue, the result being the immediate removal of obstructing tissue in a manner similar to transurethral prostatectomy. Improvement in the urinary stream is usually prompt. It is expected that reduced bleeding may lead to reduced requirement for transfusion and the possibility of avoiding cathĕterization. If this can materialize, selected patients could be treated in this way in a day surgery unit.

CLINICAL AUDIT

Clinical audit is a process that has been defined as a quality improvement process that seeks to improve patient care through systematic review of care against explicit criteria. Perhaps the first ever medical audit was carried out by Florence Nightingale in 1853 during the Crimean War. She found very insanitary conditions and high death rates among injured troops. She enforced strict adherence to hygiene and kept records; mortality rates fell precipitously and proved the value of her methods. Then in 1912 Codman scrutinised patients' histories after surgical operations to detect mistakes made by surgeons.

During the 1990s the idea of auditing clinical work arose out of morbidity-mortality conferences. Today clinical audit has become a routine followed in all properly accredited hospitals, and this is leading to better patient care.

Steps of clinical audit

The process of clinical audit moves through the following steps:

- Identify the problem.
- Define standards.
- Collect data.
- Compare performance with standards.
- Implement change.

Part II

PRACTICE

Section

1

GASTROINTESTINAL TRACT AND ABDOMINAL WALL

Chapter

19 ESOPHAGUS

Investigations

Endoscopy

A flexible gastroduodenoscope provides much of the information required in esophageal disorders. It also allows the clinician to carry out a biopsy or take an aspiration cytology specimen, remove a foreign body, dilate a stricture, and band-ligate esophageal varices. The stomach and duodenum are examined during the same session.

Endosonography

Trans-esophageal endo-ultrasound-guided FNAC (fine-needle aspiration cytology) can be used to take a biopsy of the mediastinal lymph nodes.

Esophageal manometry

In motility disorders, a multilumen catheter records esophageal pressures at different levels.

24-hours pH monitoring

In patients with suspected gastroesophageal reflux, a pH probe produces a 24-hour recording of pH.

ESOPHAGEAL ATRESIA

Atresia is defined as the congenital absence or closure of a normal body orifice or tubular organ. Esophageal atresia is a serious illness of the newborn, and occurs in 1 in 4,000 births.

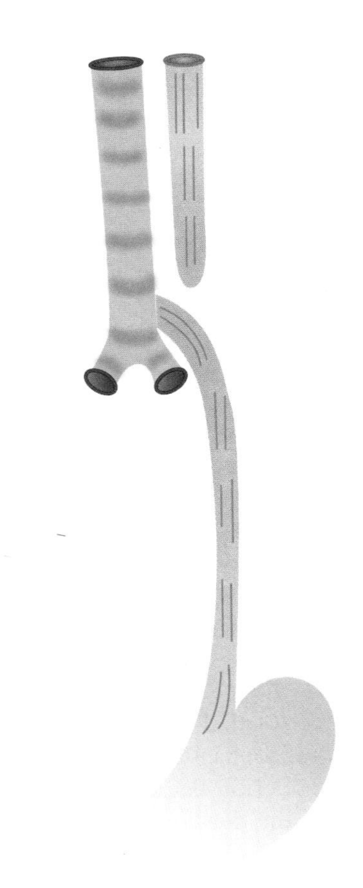

Fig.19.1 Esophageal atresia of the common type. The upper end is blind, the lower is communicating with the trachea.

In the common type of this abnormality, which accounts for about 85% of the cases, the upper pouch ends blindly, while the lower communicates with the trachea (Fig.19.1). Because of the upper blind pouch, the infant cannot swallow his saliva. When the baby breathes and the air goes in and out through the pharynx, it mixes with the saliva to create froth, and therefore the baby is seen to blow bubbles. He also gets repeated attacks of coughing, choking and cyanosis. Because the lower pouch communicates with the trachea, some of the air breathed in goes into the stomach and can cause abdominal distension. At the same time, reflux of gastric juice can occur into the lungs, resulting in bronchitis and pneumonia.

If a baby presents in this manner, esophageal atresia should be suspected. The diagnosis can be confirmed by passing a stiff size 10 catheter through the mouth, when its passage will be arrested at 10cm from the gums. 0.5ml of meglumine diatrizoate can be injected down the catheter and an x-ray taken, which will outline the blind pouch. However, the contrast medium must be immediately and completely aspirated from the pouch, otherwise it can spill over into the lungs and cause pneumonia.

Prognosis

The following conditions make the prognosis worse:

- if the baby's birth weight is low,
- if pneumonia has already set in, or
- if there is, at the same time, a congenital heart lesion, an anorectal anomaly or a duodenal atresia.

Treatment

This is by urgent operation. If the baby has been born in hospital and the diagnosis made within a few hours, operation should be carried out immediately. If pneumonia has already set in, 12 to 24 hours may be required to control the lung infection with intensive antibiotic therapy.

Replogle tube

During this waiting period the secretions from the upper pouch must be dealt with very carefully. A double-lumen (Replogle type) tube is ideal for this purpose. It is passed into the pouch and connected to a low-pressure suction pump. The advantage of the second lumen lies in the fact that when suction is applied air can go down this lumen. Otherwise, with the usual single-lumen catheter the blind pouch collapses onto the catheter and no suction can take place. If a double-lumen tube is not available an ordinary catheter should be passed and aspiration ordered every 5 minutes by a dedicated nurse.

Operation

Operation is performed through a right thoracotomy (Fig.19.2). If the esophagus is approached extrapleurally the results are superior, because if any leakage occurs it does not lead to the development of an empyema. The fistula is divided and the tracheal end closed. End-to-end anastomosis using fine PDS sutures is carried out between the upper and lower pouches.

Most surgeons carry out a *gastrostomy* as a safety valve, as otherwise the air belched up through the esophagus can disrupt the delicate anastomosis. After the operation oral feeds are withheld for 8 to 10 days. In a few cases a narrowing develops at the site of the anastomosis, which requires dilatation.

Awareness

Awareness about this anomaly is important in order to diagnose and treat it in time. *All medical students and midwives should be taught to pass a size 10 catheter if the condition is suspected.*

Before concluding, two other uncommon forms of this anomaly may be mentioned:

- Esophageal atresia without fistula. Both ends are blind in this form. The abdomen is airless.
- Tracheo-esophageal fistula without atresia, i.e., an H-type fistula. Choking and coughing after feeds are almost always present, and respiratory infections are common.

Detailed description of the repair of these types is outside the scope of this book.

Foreign bodies in the esophagus

Coins, pins and dentures are the most common foreign bodies in the esophagus. If the swallowed object is radiopaque, an x-ray confirms the position. If not, a barium swallow may outline it. It is removed by passing an esophagoscope. Occasionally, a denture may require cervical esophagotomy for removal.

Esophagoscopy

Two types of esophagoscopes are available:

The *classical* instrument is straight and rigid and has a large lumen. It is more useful for removing foreign bodies.

The *modern* version employs fibreoptics and is flexible. It is used much more commonly because of the ease with which it is swallowed.

The patient is sedated with a small dose of diazepam given intravenously immediately before the procedure. He is asked to lie down on his left side. The throat is sprayed with a local anesthetic solution, and he is asked to swallow the scope, the instrument being advanced under vision. The only difficult point is the upper esophageal sphincter; once it is passed the instrument moves quite easily onwards, and the whole of the lumen of the esophagus can be visualized. Suction is employed as necessary to clear the saliva. The presence of a polyp, a diverticulum, a growth, a stricture, esophagitis, etc. can be noted. Biopsy of a suspicious mass can be taken, and esophageal varices injected if present.

DYSPHAGIA

Dysphagia is the sensation of swallowed material sticking on its journey from the mouth to the stomach. Painful swallowing is unusual, but it occurs if esophagitis or spasm is present.

Causes

The causes of dysphagia are many. They may lie in the lumen, in the wall, or outside the wall of the esophagus:

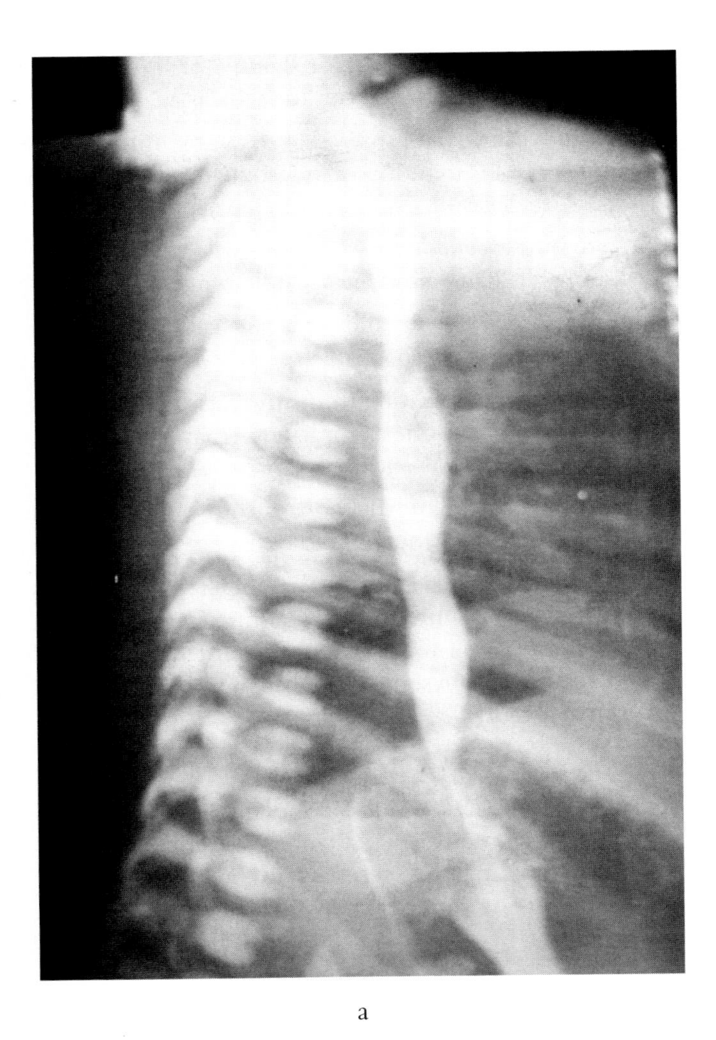

a

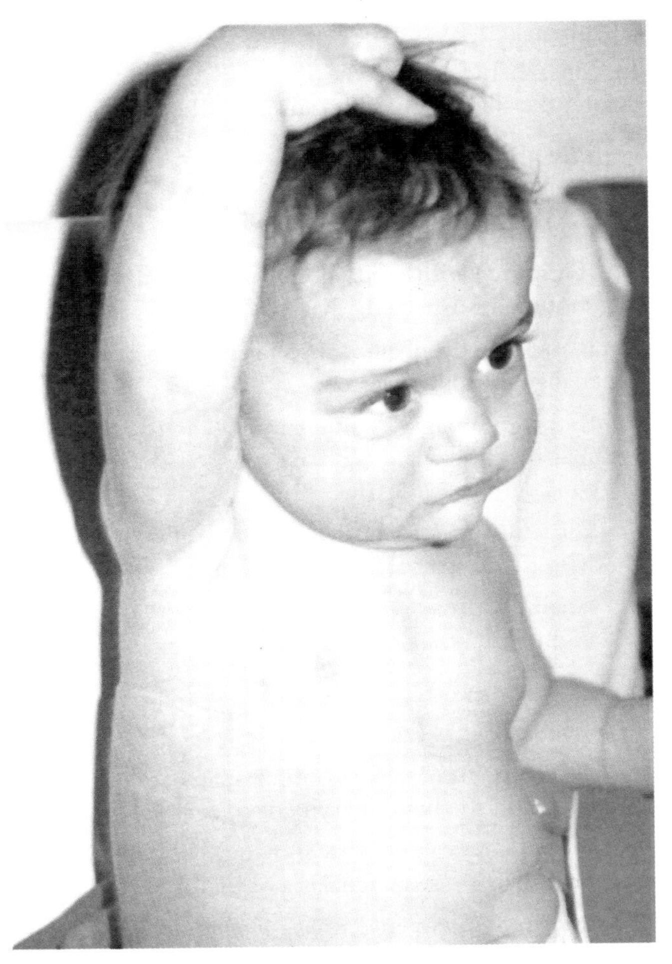

b

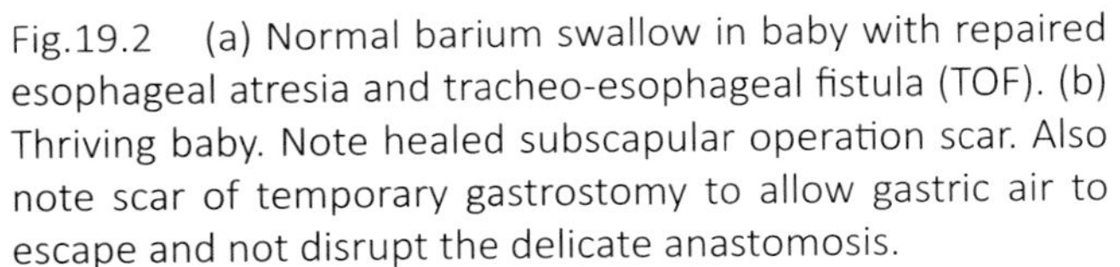

Fig.19.2 (a) Normal barium swallow in baby with repaired esophageal atresia and tracheo-esophageal fistula (TOF). (b) Thriving baby. Note healed subscapular operation scar. Also note scar of temporary gastrostomy to allow gastric air to escape and not disrupt the delicate anastomosis.

- In the lumen, swallowing may be made difficult by:
  - o Foreign bodies.
  - o Polyps.
- In the wall:
  - o Esophagitis may render swallowing not only difficult but also painful.
  - o Tumors produce dysphagia by mechanical blockage.
  - o Achalasia leads to dysphagia by the failure of the cardia to relax.
  - o Neurological disorders make swallowing difficult by the failure of the esophagus to propel its contents forwards.
- Outside the wall:
  - o A goitre, an aortic aneurysm, or a rolling hiatus hernia may produce dysphagia by compressing the esophagus.
  - o A bronchial carcinoma may produce dysphagia by infiltrating it.

Dysphagia at different ages

- In infants, dysphagia is caused by esophageal atresia.
- In children, foreign bodies, diphtheria and retropharyngeal abscess are common.
- In middle age, most cases are due to strictures and achalasia.
- In old age, especially in males, dysphagia is commonly seen due to malignancy.
- Esophageal webs in Plummer Vinson syndrome are seen mainly in females.

Duration

In general, the longer the duration of dysphagia, the greater the chances that it is caused by a benign condition.

Liquids and solids

- If dysphagia commenced for both solids and liquids together, a motor disorder is likely.
- If it started with solids alone, mechanical obstruction should be suspected.
- If an initial dysphagia for solids progresses to liquids, malignancy is suggested.
- If the dysphagia is intermittent, achalasia, diffuse spasm or impacted food above a stricture should be considered.
- Difficulty in *starting* the act of swallowing usually arises from neurological disorders.
- Finally, diffuse esophageal spasm may simulate angina pectoris.

Investigations

A *barium swallow* is carried out first.

Cinefluoroscopy allows visualization of any abnormality of swallowing at the hypopharynx or upper esophagus.

A *plain chest x-ray* can help, by showing a large mediastinal gas shadow in a case of achalasia or hiatus hernia.

If a stricture is discovered, *esophagoscopy* and *biopsy* should be carried out.

Motility disorders should be evaluated by esophageal *manometry*.

Treatment

Once the cause is determined, it must be treated. Carcinoma is best treated by resection, and benign stricture by dilatation with or without an anti-reflux procedure. Achalasia is best dealt with by myotomy, although some cases respond to pneumatic dilatation.

PERFORATION OF THE ESOPHAGUS

Causation

Perforation of the esophagus may be seen in the following situations:

- Perforation most commonly occurs from inexpert use of an esophagoscope or gastroscope in 1 in 1,000 endoscopies.
- Esophageal *dilatation* with bougies results in a number of perforations. The risk is increased:
  - o when early dilatation is carried out after a caustic burn, because it is performed through friable tissues; and
  - o when forceful hydrostatic or pneumatic dilatation is carried out for achalasia.
- *Celestin plastic tubes* passed transorally through an unresectable carcinoma of the esophagus as a palliative measure occasionally end up in a perforation.
- Forceful *endotracheal intubation* can perforate the esophagus just below the cricopharyngeus muscle.
- *Hiatal hernia* repair and *vagotomy* can occasionally result in perforation.
- After forceful vomiting from any cause, spontaneous perforation of the esophagus may take place (*Boerhaave's syndrome*).
- Foreign bodies, mostly bones, coins, and artificial dentures, can perforate the esophagus.

If the injury takes place just above the cricopharyngeus or just above a stricture, it may go unnoticed. However, severe chest pain, fever, dysphagia, mediastinal and subcutaneous emphysema and ultimately dyspnoea and sepsis may occur.

Imaging

X-ray may show widening of the mediastinum along with surgical emphysema. Pleural effusion or hydro-pneumothorax may be seen, usually on the left side. If gastrografin is swallowed it may leak out and be seen on x-ray.

A *CT scan* after contrast swallow may visualize a tiny perforation which has been missed by conventional x-ray studies.

Treatment

If perforation has occurred, urgent operation is required to repair it, through a cervical incision or a thoracotomy. It should be carried out under full antibiotic cover for aerobes and anaerobes. After the repair, a pleural pedicled flap may be wrapped round the esophagus, suturing it firmly over the area of leakage. A gastrotomy may be performed at the same time for drainage, as well as a jejunostomy for feeding.

Morbidity and *mortality* result from extensive mediastinal or pleural infection as well as if the surgery is delayed beyond 24 hours.

Mallory-Weiss syndrome

If repeated vomiting or retching takes place due to any cause, a mucosal tear may occur at the gastroesophageal junction resulting in upper gastrointestinal (GI) bleeding. This condition is called the Mallory-Weiss syndrome, and is responsible for about 10% of severe upper GI bleeds.

Endoscopy

The diagnosis is confirmed by upper GI endoscopy, which should be delayed in shocked patients until resuscitation is achieved by volume-replacement blood transfusion. If bleeding is continuing, the tear may be electrocoagulated at the same time. The treatment is conservative, with proton pump inhibitors.

Surgery

This is required only if the hemorrhage continues or recurs after the above measures, the bleeding mucosal tear being suture-ligated through a generous gastrostomy. In poor-risk patients such as cirrhotic individuals, percutaneous embolization of the left gastric artery may be carried out.

Corrosive esophagitis

Ingestion of strong acids, alkalies, etc. produces extensive chemical burns with severe esophagitis. Sloughing of the mucosa, inflammation of the submucosa, thrombosis of esophageal vessels, perforation and mediastinitis may develop. In severe cases, the patient looks toxic, with high fever, prostration and shock. Swelling of the lips, tongue and pharynx may produce respiratory distress and severe dysphagia.

Complications include perforation, mediastinitis and tracheesophageal fistulas. Circular burns result in strictures.

Treatment

Patients are hospitalized and resuscitated with I/V fluids and I/V antibiotics. Urgent endoscopy is carried out to assess the degree of burn and a nasogastric tube is placed as a stent. Nutrition is maintained by the parenteral route. Further treatment depends on the degree of esophageal injury and whether a stricture develops. The use of corticosteroids to reduce fibrous tissue formation and stricture is controversial.

The esophagus may be replaced by stomach at a later stage.

Benign strictures

The most common cause of a benign stricture is corrosive esophagitis. Other causes include congenital esophageal atresia, indwelling nasogastric tubes, radiation therapy, and postoperative (anastomotic) stricture. Corrosive strictures are usually multiple, the narrowest being at the level of the crossing of the left bronchus. The presenting symptom is increasing dysphagia. Diagnosis is established by barium swallow x-ray and esophagoscopy.

Investigations

Barium swallow

This can help assess the length and diameter of the stricture as well as provide clues to other causes of dysphagia. If the stricture is longer than 20mm and located in the upper or middle esophagus, if it looks like an 'apple core' and reflux is absent, it raises the suspicion of neoplasia.

Endoscopic biopsy and cytological brushings

These are essential to rule out malignancy.

Esophageal pH studies

With 24-hour ambulatory pH monitoring, these studies help detect gastroesophageal reflux disease as a cause of esophageal stricture.

Treatment

Medical

In cases due to reflux, *anti-reflux measures* include:

- Elevation of the head of the bed.
- Avoiding eating before bedtime.
- Antacids.
- Omeprazole is a *proton pump inhibitor* that inhibits acid production in the stomach. It is very effective against gastroesophageal reflux disease, most cases of esophagitis healing at a daily dose of 20 to 40mg.
- *Metoclopramide* and *cisapride* increase the lower esophageal sphincter pressure and improve gastric emptying, correcting two factors responsible for gastroesophageal reflux disease. These two agents may be used with a proton pump inhibitor for maximal effect.

Dilatation

Bougie-dilatation plays an important part in stricture management. The aim is to break up the fibrous stricture and improve dysphagia and alimentation. Dilatation is also used to allow endoscopic inspection and biopsy. Objective results of dilatation are transient, lasting less than 12 weeks.

Surgical

This is reserved for patients who fail to improve from conservative management or suffer complications from dilatations. The operation carried out is *resection of the esophagus* and replacement by stomach or a segment of jejunum. This is required in cases of non-dilatable, long or multiple strictures. The jejunum has a better blood supply than the colon, and is a more firm tube. At the same time the jejunum avoids the need for vagotomy and gastric drainage which is required if gastric pull-up is used for reconstruction.

HIATUS HERNIA AND REFLUX DISEASE

Physiology

The esophagus passes through the esophageal hiatus of the diaphragm into the abdomen and travels downwards and to the left for a distance of 3 to 4cm before it enters the stomach at the cardia. Normally, reflux of gastric contents back into the esophagus is prevented by the following factors:

- The lower esophageal sphincter, which measures 3–4cm in length, has a resting tone (pressure 15–24mm Hg) and relaxes on swallowing. Transient lower sphincter relaxation occurs periodically during the day due to gastric distension, and any reflux occurring then is considered physiological reflux.
- The muscle fibres of the right crus exert a pinch-cock type of action.
- When the gastric fundus distends, the valvular action of the angle between the abdominal esophagus and the fundus of the stomach has the effect of closing the esophagus.
- The folds of mucosa at the cardia help further in closing it tightly.

Pathophysiology of reflux

Some reflux is normal, and therefore pathological reflux is defined as more reflux than 95% confidence limits for the population, (or simply stated, more reflux than occurs in 95% of the normal population). In actual figures, reflux is pathological if the lumen of the distal esophagus is at a pH below 4 for more than 4% of the day, or if there are more than 10 reflux episodes (i.e. pH below 4) per 24 hours. Prolonged exposure of the esophagus to acid is caused by:

- Frequent episodes of reflux.
- Large volume reflux.
- Defective esophageal clearance.
- A combination of all three.

Anatomical changes at the hiatus such as a *sliding hernia* or *resection of the distal esophagus* make reflux more likely. *Obesity* often accompanies sliding hernias and contributes to the development of reflux by raising the intra-abdominal pressure. *Age* is important, reflux being common at the extremes of life. In infancy the gastroesophageal mechanism is not fully developed. In old age not only does this mechanism become degenerate, peristalsis is also less efficient; further, a sliding hiatus hernia is often present.

Reflux is both painful and damaging to the esophagus. Gastric contents are corrosive and burn the esophageal squamous epithelium. Gastric and duodenal juices together are more destructive than either alone, indicating that the damage is not purely pH dependent. Deep chronic ulcers or peptic strictures may be produced. The esophagitis is graded macroscopically from 0 (normal) to grade 4, although there is poor correlation between severity of inflammation and symptoms.

Types of hiatus hernia

There are two types of hiatus hernia, the sliding and the rolling (paraesophageal) (Fig.19.3).

SLIDING HIATUS HERNIA

More than 90% of hiatus hernias are of this type. The upper stomach slides up into the thorax through the hiatus, so that the cardia lies in the chest (Fig.19.3a).

Of the above-mentioned factors, preventing reflux, the first three are operative only so long as the cardia lies in the abdomen. When it slides up into the chest, they are put out of action and reflux occurs. Reflux is increased by lying down, and by anything which raises the intra-abdominal pressure e.g. stooping, straining, overeating, late pregnancy and advanced obesity.

Clinical features

Most patients are above the age of fifty, this being a disease of middle and old age. Half the cases have no symptoms. When symptoms do occur, they can be classified into three types:

- *Typical symptoms.*

  Retrosternal and epigastric burning pain i.e. 'heartburn' often occurs after meals or while lying down. It is relieved by drinking water or by antacids.

- *Atypical symptoms.*
  - Nocturnal reflux with frequent aspiration may present in the elderly as recurrent respiratory tract infection.
  - In rare cases, reflux may be responsible for attacks of asthma in younger patients.
  - Laryngitis from the refluxed acid may lead to hoarseness.
  - The acid acting on the teeth may cause loss of enamel.
  - Chest pain and night sweats may be seen from time to time.

Complications

Peptic strictures present in older patients with gradually progressive dysphagia, but little weight loss.

In contrast, *carcinoma* of the esophagus presents with marked weight loss despite the brief history.

Diagnosis

History

The history is important in diagnosis. Symptoms resembling those of sliding hiatus hernia can be produced by gallstones, peptic ulcer, achalasia and coronary artery disease.

Endoscopy

Confirmation of the diagnosis is obtained by endoscopy. This demonstrates the esophagitis or the columnar transformation of the distal esophageal mucosa. A hiatus hernia is often visible, with the squamocolumnar junction between stomach and esophagus lying at a variable distance above the crura of the diaphragm.

pH

If history strongly suggests reflux but esophagitis is absent, *24-hour ambulatory esophageal pH measurement* may demonstrate pathological reflux.

Acid infusion test

If the symptoms are atypical, an acid infusion test may help. The test is positive if the patient complains of pain when 0.1 M hydrochloric acid is infused into the esophagus and the pain disappears when the infusate is changed to saline.

Esophageal manometry

Rarely, esophageal manometry helps in the diagnosis of diffuse esophageal spasm due to reflux as a cause of non-cardiac chest pain in the presence of a normal ECG and exercise test.

Barium swallow

This shows up a hiatus hernia.

Cineradiography

This helps in the diagnosis of dysphagia caused by neurological or pharyngeal muscular disorders, some of which may be secondary to pathological reflux.

Complications

The main *complication* of sliding hiatus hernia is esophagitis, which can lead to ulceration and stricture formation.

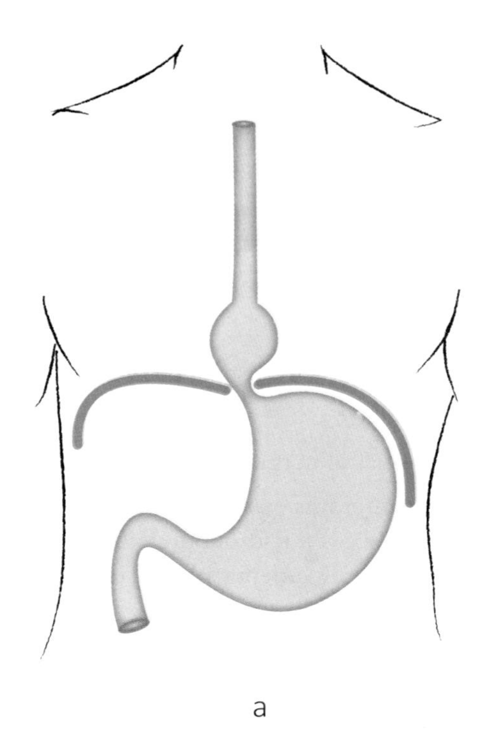

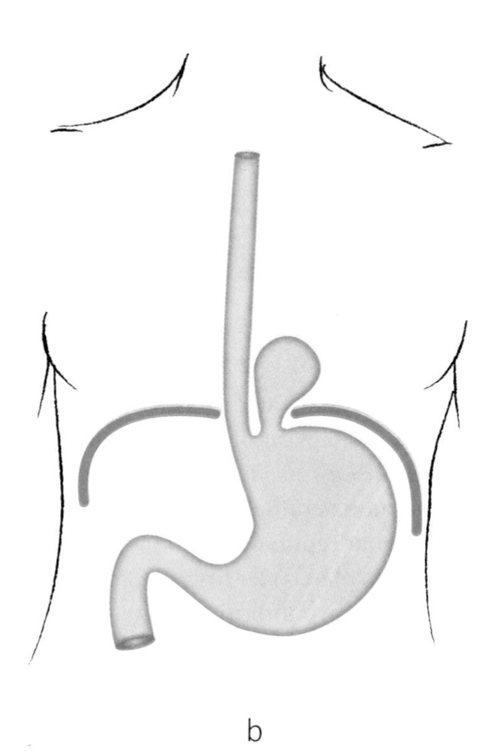

Fig.19.3 Hiatus hernia. (a) sliding; the gastro-esophageal junction (GEJ) is above the diaphragm. (b) paraesophageal (rolling); the GEJ is below the diaphragm. The gastric fundus has rolled up into the chest by the side of the esophagus.

Treatment

Medical

Half the cases have no symptoms and require no treatment. Of the other half, the great majority can be managed conservatively.

In *moderate* cases, the following general corrective measures alone are usually sufficient:

- Weight reduction.
- Avoidance of heavy meals just before retiring to bed.
- Stopping smoking.
- Avoiding anticholinergic drugs and excess alcohol.

More *severe* symptoms and esophagitis require, in addition to the above, acid suppression with a *proton pump inhibitor* such as omeprazole, as it provides more complete acid suppression.

If symptoms still persist, a *prokinetic drug* such as metoclopramide may be used to enhance gastric emptying and esophageal clearing.

For *maintenance therapy*, 40mg of omeprazole daily prevents recurrence over a period of five years in 80% of cases.

Surgical

Surgery is indicated in the few patients in whom:

- Severe symptoms are present which cannot be controlled medically.
- Complications arise, e.g. esophagitis, hemorrhage, or stenosis.
- Associated lesions are present, e.g. gallstones, peptic ulcer etc., which require operation in any case.
- 10% of the patients with gastro-esophageal reflux disease show metaplasia of the esophageal epithelium, also called *Barrett's esophagus*; this is the replacement of the squamous epithelium of the distal esophagus with columnar epithelium. This metaplasia may progress to dysplasia over time. High-grade dysplasia is a pre-malignant condition and may eventually lead to adenocarcinoma.

Operative treatment

The aim of surgical management is to prevent excessive reflux while allowing physiological reflux. Most operations are performed through the abdomen. The guiding principle of repair is to ensure a length of at least 4cm of intra-abdominal esophagus, and to prevent this segment from returning to the chest

Nissen's fundoplication

The most popular operation is that by Nissen where the abdominal esophagus is mobilized and the fundus of the stomach wrapped around it. It ensures an intra-abdominal segment of esophagus and also re-constitutes the esophagogastric angle. The Floppy Nissen fundoplication is a 270 to 360° fundal wrap. Modifications of the operation vary the wrap to as little as 180° around the distal esophagus. The more the wrap, the better is reflux prevented; however, the greater also are the risks of gas bloat and dysphagia.

90% of patients have a good result after operation; the remainder have persistent reflux. Currently, this procedure is performed laparoscopically.

PARA-ESOPHAGEAL ('ROLLING') HERNIA

Here the fundus or the whole stomach herniates into the thorax to the left of an undisplaced gastroesophageal junction (Fig.19.3b). Para-esophageal hernias are of two types:

- In the first type the gastroesophageal junction is undisplaced and the fundus herniates through the hiatus. These patients do not have reflux and therefore no symptoms unless the herniation produces mechanical obstruction.
- In the other more common type, the gastroesophageal junction is also displaced upwards along with the herniation (as in the sliding type), and hence there are more symptoms.

If left untreated, the intrathoracic stomach may undergo volvulus or acute dilatation, which are dangerous complications; therefore such a hernia should be repaired early.

Clinical features

Symptoms rarely appear until the hernia attains a large size, and are mostly due to pressure on adjacent organs by a recurrent gastric volvulus. There may be a good deal of belching.

- The patient may complain of difficulty in swallowing.
- Palpitations may occur due to cardiac arrhythmias.
- Hiccough may result from irritation of the phrenic nerve which passes near the hernia before reaching the muscle of the diaphragm.

Diagnosis

Barium swallow will show the anatomy and the type of the hernia. *Esophagoscopy* is required for further evaluation and to rule out neoplasia.

Complications

Hemorrhage, incarceration, obstruction and strangulation

Treatment

Medical treatment is of no avail.

Surgical correction

This is required in most cases since the complications are frequent and associated with high mortality and morbidity. In the latter type with a gastric volvulus, rapid fluid replacement, gastric decompression, oxygen therapy and intravenous antibiotics are important preoperative measures.

Operation

Elective

An elective operation in an old patient is best performed through an upper midline incision. The stomach is reduced into the abdomen, the hernia sac excised, and the crura approximated by non-absorbable sutures to close the hiatus around the esophagus. An anterior gastropexy, fixing the lesser curve of the stomach to the anterior abdominal wall with three or four non-absorbable sutures, prevents recurrence. In the advanced centres laparoscopic surgery has replaced open procedures. In patients with reflux, partial fundoplication may be added.

Acute

In acute cases it is dangerous to attempt to draw the stomach down from the thorax through an abdominal incision because of the risk of gastric rupture. For these cases, a left thoracotomy through the bed of the 7th rib is the best approach, and provides good access to decompress and mobilize the stomach. The left chest is opened, the hernia reduced, the sac excised and the hernial orifice repaired by overlapping sutures of a non-absorbable material. However, this operation is much more traumatic for elderly and frail patients and carries a greater risk of complications.

Gastro-esophageal reflux in children

Besides middle age, gastroesophageal reflux occurs in newborns. There is effortless vomiting of small amounts, usually blood-tinged, soon after birth. The cause of this reflux is the absence of both an intra-abdominal segment of esophagus and an acute angle between the esophagus and the gastric fundus.

Management

The baby should be nursed in an upright position in a legless chair made of Plaster of Paris or other material. In most infants, all symptoms disappear when they start to walk; some others require the Nissen fundoplication procedure. In this operation, the gastric fundus is wrapped around the lower esophagus to prevent reflux.

Plummer-Vinson syndrome

This condition occurs nearly only in middle-aged women. The patients complain of dysphagia which can be shown on endoscopy and radiography to be due to a fibrous web partially obstructing the esophageal lumen a few millimeters below the cricopharyngeus muscle. Severe retching spells may occur. On examination, the tongue is smooth and pale, the corners of the mouth are cracked, the finger-nails are spoonshaped and brittle. The spleen is enlarged and the bone marrow is devoid of stainable iron stores. There is hypochromic anemia and usually achlorhydria. The lesion is precancerous.

Treatment. The condition has been shown to be due to iron deficiency, and responds to oral iron and bougie dilatation of the web. Ferrous sulphate with vitamins is prescribed. Hyperalimentation through a nasogastric tube accelerates the regeneration of the desquamated epithelium of the esophageal mucosa.

ACHALASIA

This is a primary esophageal motility disorder which is characterized by impaired peristalsis, and in which the lower esophageal sphincter fails to relax in response to swallowing. Due to this functional obstruction, the esophagus dilates and hypertrophies, without organic stenosis. The dilatation terminates abruptly at the cardia. There is marked stasis and retention esophagitis due to the presence of the foul-smelling stagnant fluid. The incidence is 1:100,000. Achalasia is a risk factor for cancer.

Etiology

There is atrophy of ganglion cells in Auerbach's plexus. The cause of the loss of ganglion cells is not known, but may be due to a neurotropic virus.

Clinical features

Achalasia occurs in middle age. There is progressive *dysphagia* of many years' duration. Although the patient says she vomits, in fact there is regurgitation of undigested food several hours after the meal.

The retention esophagitis results in *retrosternal discomfort*.

The retained food stagnates and putrefies, so that there is *foul-smelling belching*. Due to malnutrition the patient remains in *poor health*.

Some of the fluid overspills into the bronchi, producing *aspiration pneumonia*.

A *'rheumatoid' arthritis* due to toxic absorption may occur.

In *infants,* respiratory problems due to overspill may be the first symptom to prompt evaluation and diagnosis.

Investigations

Plain X-ray

Characteristic features on x-ray include:

- Widening of the mediastinum.
- A posterior mediastinal air-fluid level.
- Chronic aspiration may produce abnormalities of the lung fields.

Barium swallow

This demonstrates:

- Dilatation and tortuosity of the esophagus.
- A smooth pencil-shaped narrowing of the lower end of the esophagus (bird's beak deformity).
- Lack of a gas bubble in the stomach.

An esophageal diameter of less than 4cm qualifies as mild disease, 4 to 6cm as moderate, and greater than 6cm as severe disease ('mega-esophagus').

Esophageal manometry

The most reliable and accurate method of diagnosis consists of *esophageal manometry*. In this method, pressure-sensitive catheters (transducers) are used to measure the intra-esophageal pressures and to detect and record the occurrence of peristaltic activity. If it is found that organized peristaltic activity is absent throughout the intrathoracic esophagus, and that the lower esophageal sphincter does not relax, the diagnosis of achalasia is confirmed.

Endoscopy

On endoscopy, the esophagus appears as a cave filled with dirty water.

Differential diagnosis

Achalasia may be confused with:

- Benign stricture.
- Carcinoma at the cardia.

In both these cases, the huge dilatation of the esophagus seen in achalasia does not occur. Also, in carcinoma the lower end of the barium column is irregular (rat-tail appearance).

Treatment

Different types of treatment my be helpful:

Medical treatment

- Calcium channel blockers are used to decrease LES pressure; this is used in elderly patients.
- *Botulinum toxin (Botox).* The intrasphinteric injection of botulinum toxin to block the release of acetylecholine and relax the lower esophageal sphincter is effective in 50% of patients though the response is short-lived. Hence it is used only in the elderly, high risk patients.

Surgery

Myotomy

Division of the circular muscle of the distal 4–5cm of the esophagus, with or without fundoplication, is the procedure of choice in the majority of young and middle-aged patients. The success rate is about 90% and long-lasting.

The aim of treatment is to relieve the functional obstruction at the cardia. This can be accomplished by disruption of the constricting fibres of the LES, either from within by an inflatable bag, or from without by Heller's myotomy. Neither method can restore coordinated peristalsis of the esophageal body. However, disruption of the sphincter relieves the dysphagia and regurgitation:

- **Pneumatic balloon dilatation.**

Forceful balloon dilatation involves rapid pneumatic expansion of an inflatable bag placed at the esophagogastric junction. Usually three or four dilatations are required. This is effective in 70–75% of cases and, in patients who are not fit for major surgery, is a useful alternative.

- **Heller's operation.**

In Heller's operation, the muscle coat of the lower end of the esophagus is divided longitudinally, care being taken to divide all the muscle fibres, and to reach proximally to include all the dilated esophagus. Distally, the incision should extend upto 1cm onto the stomach wall. Results are good to excellent in 90% of patients. Laparoscopic technique is preferred and hence more popular these days

Benign tumors

Benign tumors of the esophagus are rare. They produce dysphagia, and are discovered on barium swallow as indentations of the esophageal lumen. Esophagoscopy with biopsy confirms the diagnosis.

A *leiomyoma or lipoma* may be removed transthoracically. A *papilloma*, as it is pedunculated, may be excised by diathermy through an esophagoscope. A *cavernous hemangioma* may cause hematemesis; injection of a sclerosing agent may help

CARCINOMA OF THE ESOPHAGUS

Incidence

Carcinoma of the esophagus is more common in males, occurring most often between 50 and 70 years of age. The incidence varies considerably around the world, from 5 per 100,000 in the United States to 100 per 100,000 in some parts of China. Squamous cell carcinoma is the most common type. However, in the distal esophagus, adenocarcinoma is seen more often.

Risk factors

The important risk factors include the following:

- Heavy alcohol use.
- Smoking, the risk being even greater when combined with excessive alcohol intake.
- Malnutrition, specially:
    - o Plummer-Vinson syndrome, from iron and vitamin B deficiencies.
    - o Coeliac disease, due to multiple deficiencies from malabsorption.
    - o Molybdenum, zinc and magnesium deficiencies.
- Chronic irritation:
    - o Chronic corrosive strictures.
    - o Achalasia.
    - o Esophageal diverticula.
- Barrett's esophagus: Gastroesophageal reflex disease (GERD) is the most common predisposing factor for adenocarcinoma.

Pathology

The vast majority of tumors are squamous cell carcinomas, from the squamous epithelium of the esophagus. However, tumors arising at the cardia are usually adenocarcinomas, mostly of gastric origin. Three gross patterns of growth are commonly seen:

- *Ulcerating* type has a well-defined ulcer with a raised margin.
- *Fungating* type has a large intraluminal protrusion with an irregular surface.
- *Infiltrating* type shows extensive circumferential intramural growth without ulceration.

Table 19.1 TNM staging of esophageal cancer

TO	No tumor
Tis	Carcinoma-in-situ
T1	Invades submucosa
T2	Invades muscularis propria
T3	Invades periesophageal tissues
T4	Invades adjacent structures
NO	No node metastases
N1	Regional node metastases
MO	No distant metastases
M1	Distant metastases

The tumor spreads:

- by direct invasion into the surrounding structures;
- through the blood stream;
- by lymphatic dissemination.

Lesions of the lower esophagus metastasize primarily to the coeliac *lymph* nodes. As far as *blood-borne* metastases are concerned, they develop mostly in the lungs, bones, liver and brain.

Mass screening

In a high-risk population in China, extensive mass screening was carried out by *abrasive cytology* using a swallowed balloon which is inflated and pulled back through the esophagus, thus collecting a sample of epithelial cells. Dysplastic cells were almost always found in association with carcinoma.

When patients were followed for 12 years:

- No patient with normal cytology progressed to carcinoma.
- 1% of patients with mild dysplasia developed cancer.
- As many as 15% with severe dysplasia developed cancer.

Importance of early diagnosis

Surgical treatment of early, cytologically diagnosed, asymptomatic cancers provided over 90% survival at five years, emphasizing the importance of early diagnosis.

TNM staging is given in (Table 19.1).

Clinical features

Progressive dysphagia is the most prominent symptom, causing marked weight loss. At first, solid foods cause difficulty, later even liquids are difficult to swallow. This is a late symptom and usually indicates that two-thirds of the lumen is involved. There is weakness and anemia.

Signs of spread

- Steady deep chest pain usually indicates mediastinal invasion.
- Cough and hoarseness are common in upper esophageal tumors from invasion of the airway or recurrent laryngeal nerve.
- Aspiration pneumonia may be present due to:
  - Obstructive overspill.
  - Malignant esophageal-airway fistula.

Complications

- Occult anemia is frequent, though massive bleeding is rare.
- There may be invasion of:
  - superior vena cava or aorta, producing fatal hemorrhage;
  - pericardium, producing cardiac arrhythmias;
  - trachea, producing:
    - tracheal obstruction,
    - a fistula with the trachea, producing aspiration pneumonitis and lung abscess.

Investigations

Radiology

Barium meal x-ray

- This may show an irregular mass whose upper border is roughly horizontal like a 'shelf'.
- Annular lesions show a narrow lumen with an irregular mucosal outline.
- Angulation of the long axis of the esophagus suggests mediastinal invasion and predicts unresectability.

Chest x-ray may show:

- An esophageal air-fluid level.
- Lung infiltrates suggesting aspiration.
- Mediastinal widening from tumor or lymphadenopathy.
- Pulmonary nodules suggesting lung metastases.

CT scan

- This shows the esophageal wall, mediastinal structures and metastatic sites clearly.
- Gross distortion of a mediastinal structure indicates invasion.
- The presence of a fat plane between the tumor and the structure indicates the absence of invasion.
- CT chest and abdomen is used for staging and assessment of resectibility.

Endoscopy

Esophagoscopy

Esophagoscopy with biopsy confirms the diagnosis and helps measure the length of the lesion and the distance from the incisors for staging and treatment planning. *Endoscopic ultrasound (EUS)* is very sensitive in assessment of 'TNM' staging, because the probe lies right on the lesion and gets a close-up view. It improves the ability to determine wall penetration and abnormal lymph nodes, thus greatly improving preoperative staging.

Bronchoscopy

This is necessary in upper and middle third carcinomas to detect involvement of the trachea or bronchi.

Laparoscopy

This is carried out if indicated by ultrasound or CT scan, and allows biopsy of the liver, perigastric lymph nodes and peritoneum.

Treatment

There are only two methods of treatment proved to benefit patients with carcinoma of the esophagus: surgical resection and irradiation. Most patients present with advanced disease (Stage III) with full-thickness invasion of the esophageal wall and lymph node metastases; this precludes cure, so that the aim is palliation.

Irradiation

Squamous cell carcinoma of the esophagus is a radiosensitive and theoretically radiocurable tumor. Unfortunately, although the primary lesions may be controlled, failures result from the presence of tumor outside the irradiated fields, and few permanent cures are obtained. Radiotherapy for *adenocarcinoma* of the gastroesophageal junction is much less effective.

Radical radiotherapy (5,000 to 6,000 rads) is followed by only 5 to 10% five year survivals. At the same time, the complications of such radiotherapy are many: radiation pneumonitis, local recurrence, stricture, trachoesophageal fistula, perforation, spinal cord injury and pericardial effusion.

Chemoradiation. Neoadjuvant chemotherapy plus radiation is given to selected patients with locally advanced disease to down-stage the disease and achieve better local control.

Surgery

Surgical treatment quite effectively controls local disease and restores normal swallowing.

Five year survival rates are as follows:

Stage	I	85%
Stage	II	34%
Stage	III	15%
Overall		22%

This shows the importance of early diagnosis.

Today, the most popular operation is resection of the esophagus and its replacement by the mobilized stomach. Because of its thick and tough wall, its richer blood supply, and the absence of bacteria in its lumen, the stomach is better than colon for use as replacement for the esophagus. Colon is used only when stomach is not available for some reason.

The stomach is taken up either through the right chest, or through the posterior mediastinum i.e. the normal route of the esophagus. It can be taken all the way to the neck, and can therefore be used in cases of carcinomas arising anywhere along the thoracic esophagus.

Approaches

The different *approaches* are as follows:

Left thoracoabdominal approach

This is made through the left 7th interspace, the diaphragm being divided circumferentially to avoid injury to the phrenic nerve; this is best for lower third lesions and tumors of the cardia.

Laparotomy and right thoracotomy

This is best suited for middle or lower third lesions. Through an upper midline laparotomy, the stomach is first mobilized on the right gastric and gastroepiploic arteries. The hiatus is enlarged and the lower esphagus mobilized. The patient is now turned on his left side. Through a right thoracotomy the esophagus can be mobilized right upto the apex of the right chest, resected, and anastomosed obliquely to the fundus of the stomach that is drawn up into the chest.

Right thoracotomy

This is suitable for tumors of the mid-esophagus. The right chest is opened and the esophagus mobilized. The hiatus is enlarged and the stomach drawn up through it, successive branches of the left gastric and gastroepiploic arteries being divided to enable this. The esophagus is resected, the upper end being cut obliquely and anastomosed to the stomach a little below the fundus.

Trans-hiatal esophagectomy

The chest is not opened. Dissection is carried out downwards from the neck and upwards from the abdomen. The middle third of the esophagus has to be dissected by the fingers.

The advantage of the method consists of the avoidance of a thoracotomy. The disadvantage lies in the necessity of blind dissection of the middle third of the esophagus, and the possibility of injury to thoracic duct, trachea, azygos vein and recurrent laryngeal nerve.

Cancers of the cervical esophagus and hypopharynx

In these cases, radiotherapy is superior to surgery and has the added advantage of preserving the voice if the local tumor is controlled. However, if the tumor recurs, the surgeon has to carry out en bloc removal of the larynx, pharynx and esophagus in an irradiated field, which is a difficult undertaking.

Chemotherapy

Chemotherapy alone has very little effect in palliating patients with either squamous cell carcinoma or adenocarcinoma of the esophagus. Because of the belief that this disease is often systemic at the time of diagnosis, combined modality treatment using chemotherapy, irradiation and resection has gained popularity. At the same time, preoperative adjuvant chemotherapy has shown promising results, partial and complete response rates upto 66% being reported.

Palliation of inoperable esophageal cancer

In patients with far advanced malignancies, distant metastases, or recurrence after radiotherapy, the aim is palliation, so that the patient can swallow. This was achieved in the past by placing a plastic tube in the lumen of the esophagus and passing it down through the growth. However, these tubes used to slip or be obstructed by food and pose problems. The following methods have therefore displaced them:

Expandable metallic stents

These can be placed endoscopically across the tumor under fluoroscopic control. Stents are best suited for patients with tracheo-esophageal fistulas

Laser ablation

Endoscopic Nd:YAG laser relieves dysphagia in the majority of the patients by vaporization of the tumor. Multiple sessions are required.

The average survival after such palliation is less than six months.

Causes of death

If the growth is not removed, death is caused by:

- Progressive cachexia and dehydration.
- Pneumonia from perforation into the bronchial tree.
- Mediastinitis.
- Erosion into the aorta.

Chapter

20 STOMACH AND DUODENUM

INFANTILE HYPERTROPHIC PYLORIC STENOSIS

This condition results from hypertrophy of the muscle of the pylorus and distal antrum of the stomach. The cause is not known. However, there is a strong familial element, with a 5% incidence in children whose mothers suffered from the condition. Males predominate 4:1. The condition is seen in the newborn, and is more common in first-born infants.

Clinical features

The baby is usually full-term, and *feeds well for one or two weeks.* At that time occasional regurgitation of some feeds starts. In a few days the vomiting becomes more frequent, forceful, and projectile. However, in the weak premature infant there may be effortless regurgitation of stomach contents. The vomitus contains no bile. Shortly after the vomiting the infant wants to feed again. Because of the obstruction at the pylorus, constipation with hard feces develops. Due to diminished absorption from the intestines, weight is lost. Gastric peristaltic waves can usually be seen moving across the epigastrium from left to right. In some cases the thickened pylorus can be palpated as a lump when the baby is relaxed by sedation or by feeding clear fluids.

X-rays

If the pyloric tumor cannot be palpated, an x-ray picture is taken after giving a small amount of meglumine diatrizoate. The pyloric canal may be outlined by a 'string sign' or a pyloric 'beak' may be seen where the pyloric entrance from the antrum occurs. X-rays taken two or three hours later show most of the dye still lying in the stomach.

Differential diagnosis

Repeated vomiting in the newborn may also be due to feeding problems, intracranial lesions, an incompetent cardiac sphincter, pyloro-spasm, duodenal atresia, malrotation of the bowel or adrenal insufficiency. It is

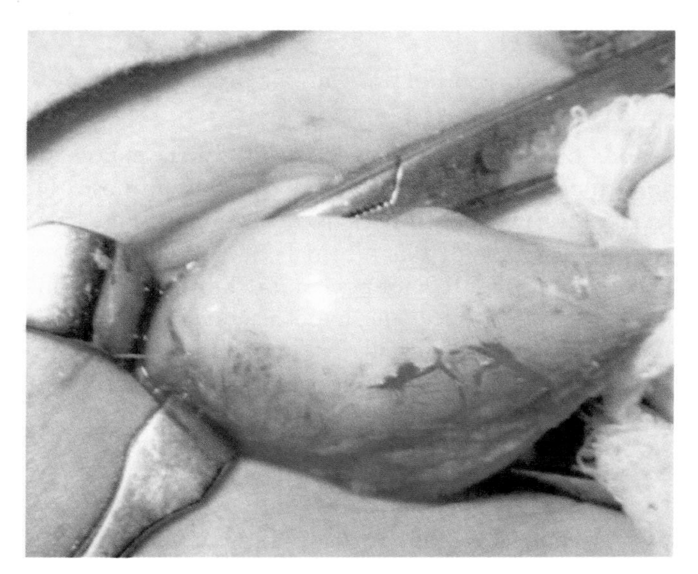

a

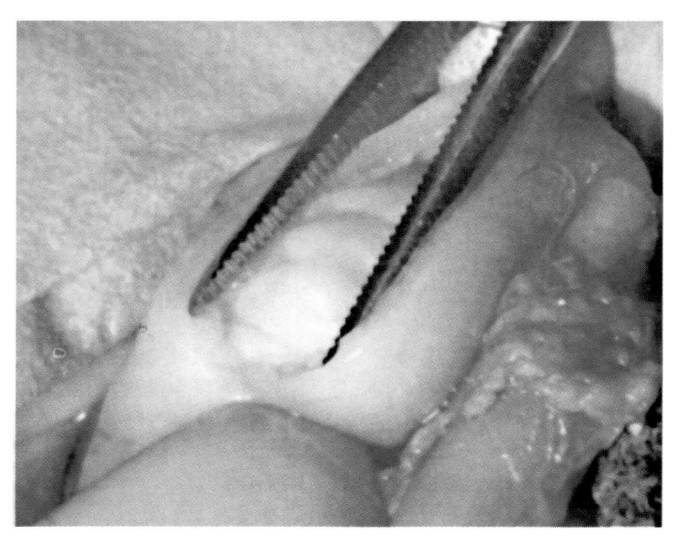

b

Fig.20.1 a. Hypertrophied pylorus delivered through the abdominal incision. b. Pyloromyotomy; note the mucosa bulging through the hypertrophied muscles.

extremely important to remember that *the vomiting of infantile pyloric stenosis does not start at birth but one or two weeks later.* This fact helps distinguish this condition from duodenal atresia.

Complications

Repeated vomiting leads to loss of water and nutrients producing dehydration and starvation with weight loss. Chloride and potassium are lost in the vomitus, resulting in hypochloraemic hypokalemic alkalosis. Aspiration of vomitus can produce pneumonia.

Treatment

Medical treatment is of no avail; the proper treatment is surgery.

Before operation, the deficiency of water, potassium and chloride must be corrected; for this purpose the level of serum electrolytes is determined. The baby is resuscitated with 0.5 Normal saline solution (0.45 percent NaCl) with 2g of potassium chloride per 500ml bag initially to correct the hypokalaemia and alkalosis. When the bicarbonate falls below 30mmol/1 the baby is taken to the theatre. A nasogastric tube is placed in position before operation to empty and wash out the stomach.

Rammstedt's operation

Operation is carried out through a right upper transverse incision. The pyloric tumor, which is an olive-shaped mass upto 2cm in diameter, is delivered and a longitudinal incision made over it, from the pyloroduodenal junction at least 2cm on to the antrum, dividing all the muscle fibres and exposing the mucous membrane, which bulges into the incision (Fig.20.1). Some air is squeezed from the stomach into the duodenum to demonstrate adequate division of the muscle. The cut in the muscle is left unsutured. The abdominal wall is repaired. This procedure, which is essentially a pyloromyotomy, is called Rammstedt's operation.

Small feeds of 5ml hourly are started next morning and rapidly increased over a period of one or two days. If diagnosed and treated promptly, the mortality rate in this condition approaches zero. However the greater the delay the worse the prognosis.

Duodenal atresia and stenosis

In duodenal atresia there is congenital occlusion of the second part of the duodenum, usually just distal to the ampulla of Vater; in stenosis there is a narrowing (but not complete occlusion) often due to an annular pancreas. The baby starts vomiting right from birth, and the vomitus contains bile. This is in contradistinction to the situation in infantile pyloric stenosis, where vomiting starts one or two weeks after birth, and the vomitus contains no bile (Fig.20.2).

The *plain x-ray* shows just two gas shadows: a large one in the stomach, and a small one in the duodenum (the double-bubble sign).

Operation should be carried out urgently, through an upper right transverse incision. The most suitable procedure is a duodenojejunostomy, i.e. joining up the distended duodenal loop to a collapsed loop of the proximal jejunum.

Volvulus of the stomach

This is a serious though rare condition. The stomach usually rotates around the axis made by its two fixed points--cardia and pylorus. The greater curve with the colon moves up to lie under the diaphragm. A paraesophageal hiatus hernia often occurs with it. Rotation around the transverse axis is rare.

There is severe abdominal pain, vomiting, retching, epigastric distension and inability to pass a nasogastric tube. Immediate laparotomy is required to untwist the volvulus and prevent death from acute gastric necrosis and shock.

PEPTIC ULCER

Peptic ulcers result from the corrosive action of acid gastric juice on a vulnerable epithelium:

They are commonly seen in the duodenum and stomach and occasionally in the esophagus. They may also be encountered uncommonly in the jejunum after a gastrojejunostomy, or rarely in the ileum in a Meckel's diverticulum adjacent to ectopic gastric mucosa.

Thus it will be seen that peptic ulcers normally arise at sites adjacent to acid-secreting epithelium. The common locations are the lesser curvature of the stomach and the first part of the duodenum. Realization of the central role of acid has led to therapy by proton pump inhibitors, and to operations that reduce acid secretion.

Peptic ulcer is a very common condition nearly all over the world. Men are affected 3 times as often as women. Duodenal ulcer is 10 times more common than gastric ulcer. Duodenal and gastric ulcer are fundamentally different diseases whose major common feature is acid-pepsin-dependent ulceration.

Pathophysiology of peptic ulcers

Ulcers of the stomach and duodenum are caused chiefly by the effects of hydrochloric acid produced by the parietal cells of the stomach, and by lack of protection of the mucosa against this acid by what is known as the mucosal barrier.

Duodenal ulcer

In *duodenal ulcer, increased acid production* is by far the most important factor. However it cannot be the only factor, because the severity of duodenal ulcers does not vary directly with the amount of gastric acid secreted.

Role of helicobacter pylori

A major advancement in the elucidation of pathogenesis of peptic ulcer has been the realization of the role of Helicobacter pylori in both duodenal and gastric ulcers. This is a microaerophylic gram-negative bacillus that colonizes the gastroduodenal mucosa, and by damaging the mucosal barrier prepares the ground for the ulcerogenic effect of acid pepsin. H. pylori is found in the duodenal mucosa in about 90% of the patients with duodenal ulcer. At the same time only 10–15% of the infected persons develop ulcers.

H. pylori is also implicated as an important factor in the development of gastritis, gastric ulcer, MALT lymphoma[1] and even gastric carcinoma. H. pylori is now considered by WHO as a class I carcinogen.

Other factors

Duodenal ulcer is somewhat more common in persons with blood group O. At the same time stress and anxiety, irregular and highly spiced meals, inadequate mastication, alcohol, caffeine and excessive smoking are all considered to have some role in causation.

Gastric ulcer

Mucosal barrier

The gastric mucosa is protected from the damaging effect of the hydrochloric acid which it secretes by an adherent layer of mucus. Further, under the mucus lies a layer of bicarbonate which neutralizes any acid diffusing back through the mucus layer. The mucus layer also protects the mucosa from other noxious agents such as bile, alcohol and aspirin and other irritating drugs and constitutes the mucosal barrier.

This mucosal barrier is damaged by Helicobacter pylori and by different drugs: non-steroidal anti-inflammatory drugs (NSAIDs), steroids, alcohol, tobacco etc.

Gastric ulcers at different locations

The causes of *gastric ulcers* vary with the location of the ulcers. In this respect two categories of ulcers are seen:

1 MALT lymphoma: a type of lymphoma involving the mucosa-associated lymphoid tissue (MALT), most commonly in the stomach.

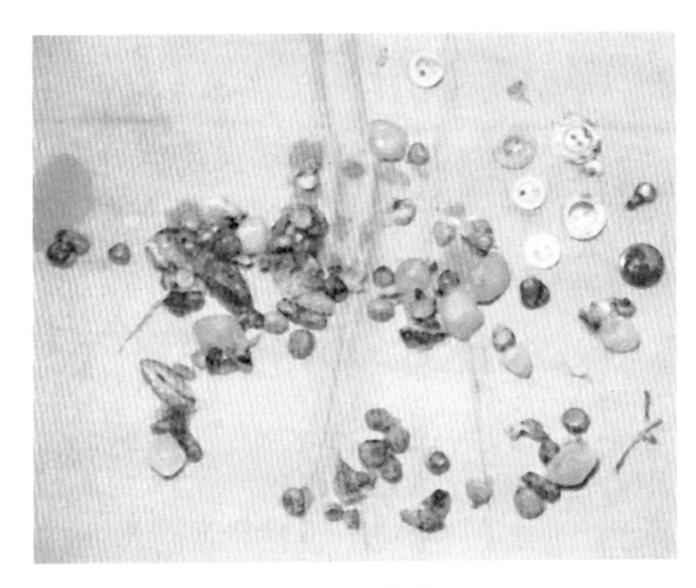

Fig.20.2 A large number of objects—seeds, buttons, trinkets—recovered at operation from the dilated upper loop of duodenum in a case of duodenal stenosis, showing the type of items a toddler puts in his mouth from time to time.

- To the first category belong *Type 1* ulcers, i.e. ulcers which are located *in the body of the stomach*. These are seen in cases of chronic gastritis due to H. Pylori infection. In these cases gastric acid secretion levels as determined by secretory tests are normal or low. Hence it is the loss of mucosal barrier with back diffusion of HCl into the mucosa that seems to be involved, rather than a high level of acidity.
- In the second category we find two types of ulcers:
  - o *Type 2* gastric ulcers are those *combined with a duodenal ulcer*.
  - o *Type 3* describes ulcers *in the prepyloric area*.

In both these types the effects of increased acid production are more important.

Ulcers that develop *after gastroenterostomy*, and those which recur *after various operations* for duodenal and gastric ulcers, are due to persistent secretion of hydrochloric acid. Finally, *extragastric* lesions can lead to increased levels of serum gastrin and consequent excess acid production. Thus, in the Zollinger-Ellison syndrome, a non-beta cell tumor secreting large quantities of gastrin occurs in the pancreas, and produces multiple extremely intractable duodenal ulcers.

Diagnosis

Duodenal ulcer

Duodenal ulcer is most common in the young and the middle-aged (20–45 years), and occurs more often in

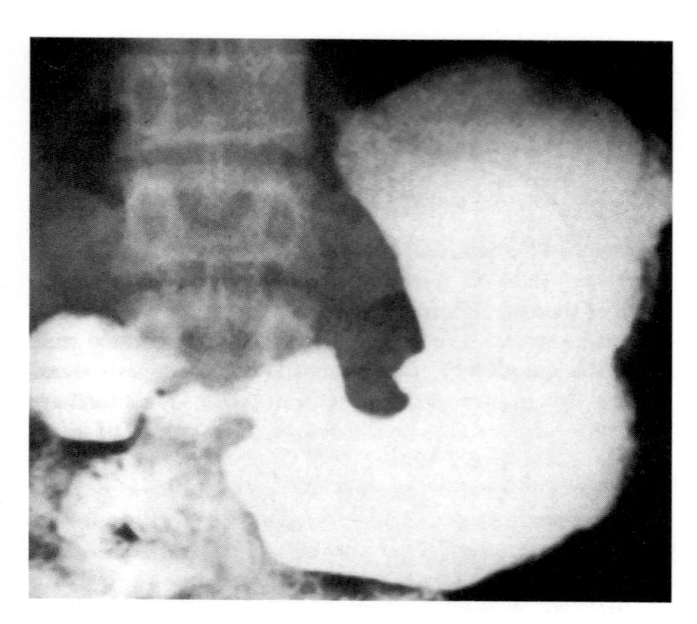

Fig.20.3 Barium meal x-ray showing benign gastric ulcer located at the typical site on the lesser curvature.

men than women. 95% occur in the duodenal bulb i.e. the first 2cm of the duodenum.

Clinical features

Aching, burning or gnawing pain occurs in the epigastrium. Pain occurs either early in the morning or one hour or more after breakfast. The pain is relieved by lunch, but recurs in the afternoon. It is most likely to occur at night, several hours after food. Food, milk or antacids give temporary relief. When the ulcer penetrates posteriorly into the head of the pancreas, the pain bores through to the back and may become more persistent. On examination there may be tenderness in the epigastrium to the right of the midline.

The symptoms typically come and go, each relapse lasting for several weeks. This *periodicity* of pain is an important feature of duodenal ulcer.

Investigations for a suspected peptic ulcer

Gastroduodenoscopy

Fibreoptic gastroduodenoscopy has completely replaced barium meal x-ray (Figs. 3 and 4) for the diagnosis of peptic ulcer, as the whole interior of the stomach and proximal duodenum can be clearly visualized. Endoscopy can also accurately localize the site of bleeding in hematemesis and assess the response to therapy. As the end of the gastroscope can be turned backward on itself through 180°, the area of the fundus can also be visualized.

Laboratory findings

If the Zollinger-Ellison syndrome is suspected the serum gastrin level is determined (for details see under the Z-E syndrome).

Differential diagnosis

The most common diseases simulating duodenal ulcer are the following:

- *Chronic cholecystitis.* This is usually seen in females. In this condition pain is usually felt more to the right side i.e. in the right hypochondrium. Also, if pain radiates backwards it does not bore through to the back but spreads around the chest to the inferior angle of the scapula and often to the right shoulder. Ultrasound examination shows up the stones in most cases.
- *Pancreatitis.* In severe acute forms of this illness shock is present to a degree out of proportion to the severity of pain, and serum amylase is raised to a very high level.
- *Reflux esophagitis.* In this condition the pain commonly radiates upwards retrosternally.

Complications

Besides the distress caused by pain, the common complications of duodenal ulcer are hemorrhage, perforation and duodenal obstruction. They are discussed later jointly with gastric ulcer.

Gastric ulcer

Gastric ulcer is most common between the ages of 40 and 60 years. 95% of the ulcers occur on the lesser curvature. A few gastric ulcers occur near the pylorus at the same time as a duodenal ulcer; their treatment should follow the guidelines for duodenal ulcers. Most gastric ulcers, however occur by themselves, without a duodenal ulcer.

Clinical features

The main symptom of gastric ulcer is epigastric pain relieved by food or antacids, as in duodenal ulcer. Epigastric tenderness usually occurs. Contrary to the situation in duodenal ulcer, the pain tends to occur early after eating, within about 30 minutes. Sometimes vomiting, anorexia and aggravation of pain by food is more frequent than with duodenal ulcer. However, the two diseases cannot be distinguished on the basis of the history, and endoscopy is required.

Gastroscopy

On gastroscopy the rolled-up margins of a malignant ulcer can be distinguished from the flat edges of a benign ulcer. *Endoscopic biopsy is the mainstay of diagnosis of peptic ulcers.* Biopsies are taken from the edges of the ulcer in each quadrant (four-quadrant biospy).

Differential diagnosis

Dyspepsia due to hiatus hernia, atrophic gastritis, chronic cholecystitis, irritable colon syndrome and functional problems can mimic gastric ulcer. The clinical features of each of these conditions differ somewhat from those of gastric ulcer. Endoscopy helps distinguish the first two conditions, and gallstones are shown up on ultrasound examination.

Complications

The common complications of gastric ulcer are the same as those of duodenal ulcer, namely hemorrhage, perforation and stenosis. They are discussed in detail later jointly with duodenal ulcer.

MANAGEMENT OF PEPTIC ULCER

This is now possible with the elimination of H. pylori with chemotherapy and prevention of reinfection by public health measures. Ulcerogenic drugs and other substances, e.g. caffeine, alcohol, nicotine and highly spiced foods, should be avoided in susceptible individuals. In this connection it should be remembered that nearly all non-steroidal anti-inflammatory drugs (NSAIDs) are ulcerogenic, and should be avoided.

Medical treatment

Medical treatment is similar for gastric and duodenal ulcer and includes the use of specific medications and elimination of known gastric irritants. At the same time attempts are made to relieve social problems and irregular habits of eating, working and sleeping.

Gastric irritants

These include tobacco, alcohol, caffeine, aspirin, ibuprofen, indomethacin and salicylates, as well as most other non-steroidal anti-inflammatory drugs (NSAIDs).

Diet

In the past *diet* was considered as closely related to ulcer disease; this is not true. Normal food taken at regular intervals is best. Food buffers gastric acid, so during acute episodes the patient should take frequent meals, or snacks between the three main meals. A drink of milk and a few biscuits are valuable at bedtime and also for rapid control of pain that appears in the middle of the night, if no medicine is available.

Medicines

Traditional antacids e.g. aluminium hydroxide and magnesium carbonate have today a very limited role, mainly confined to patients seeking relief off the counter at pharmacies.

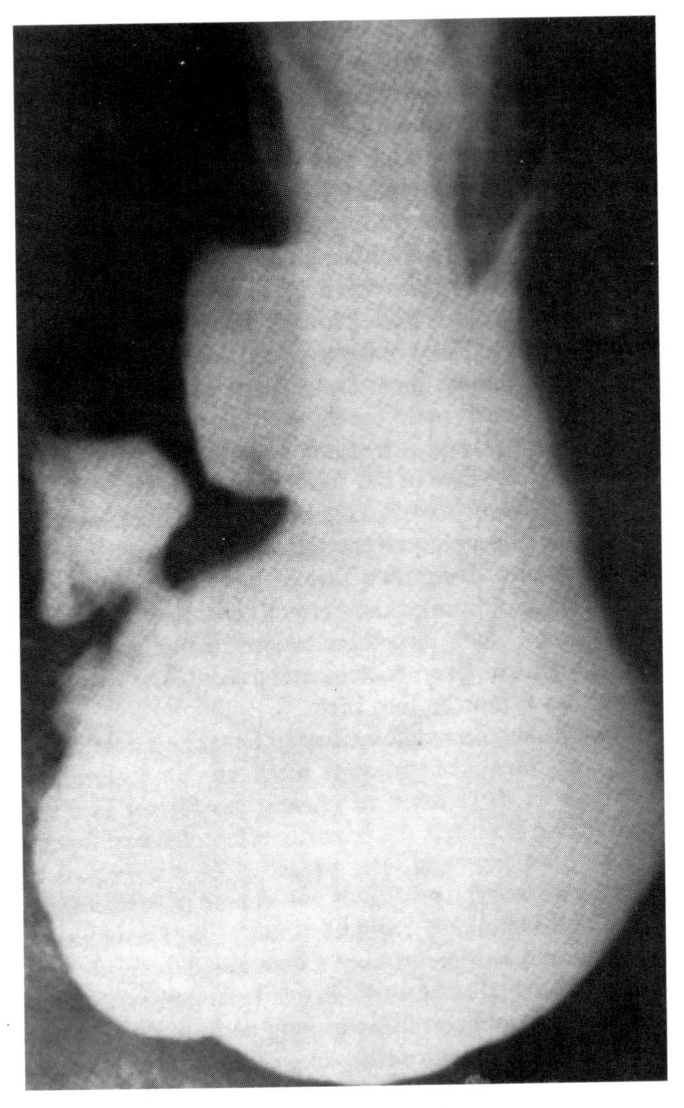

Fig.20.4 Malignant gastric ulcer on the lesser curvature, diameter greater than 2cm.

H2 receptor antagonists

These drugs were a great advancement in the treatment of both duodenal and gastric ulcers, as most ulcers healed with a few weeks of treatment by them. However, a few cases proved refractory.

Proton pump inhibitors

Finally, the treatment of peptic ulcers has been revolutionized by proton pump inhibitors (PPIs), because PPIs can make the patient achlorhydric, restricting the role of surgery to the complications of the ulcers. Omeprazole and other PPIs inhibit the intracellular *proton pump* and can eliminate gastric acid production altogether.

Mucosal coating agents

These are also useful medicines for peptic ulcers, the most effective *coating agent* being sucralfate (lg four times daily).

Prostaglandins

These increase the blood supply to the gastric mucosa and decrease the damaging effect of NSAIDS. The only prostaglandin approved by the FDA[1] is misoprostol.

On medical treatment 80% of ulcers heal within one month, although gastric ulcers take longer to heal. A certain number recur within 6 months.

Eradication therapy

If a case of peptic ulcer tests positive for presence of H. pylori, a course of a proton pump inhibitor plus two antibiotics (commonly amoxicillin and clarithromycin), for two weeks, completely eradicates the microorganism and cures the illness; hence it is referred to as eradication therapy. Further, reinfection is uncommon. This treatment is a great deal safer than surgery, and shorter than long courses of PPIs.

Non-healing gastric ulcer

A *gastric ulcer* which is unhealed after a full course (6–8 weeks) of medical treatment could either be simply an intractable ulcer, or it could be a malignant one. Multiple endoscopic biopsies should now be carried out. Ulcers located in the body of the stomach and beyond the lesser curvature should also undergo biopsy:

- If the biopsy shows *malignancy*, operation is the only method of treatment which offers hope of cure, and should be carried out, unless contraindicated by evidence of widespread disease or very poor general condition of the patient.
- If the biopsy shows that the ulcer is *benign* the decision has to be made between continuing medical treatment or resort to surgery. Gastric ulcers are generally difficult to cure medically, recur frequently and cause more severe symptoms than duodenal ulcers. Therefore, surgery should be offered earlier than in the case of duodenal ulcers. However, in the elderly high-risk patient medical treatment should be continued.

Surgical treatment

An overall decrease in the incidence of peptic ulcer and the advent of effective medical treatment has reduced the need for surgery very greatly. If medical treatment has been properly carried out, an ulcer that fails to heal may be judged intractable, and surgical treatment will be required. Each surgeon will have his own ideas about how many episodes of recurrence make operation mandatory. The patient and the surgeon should discuss this matter to arrive at a decision. Hemorrhage, perforation or obstruction are also manifestations of intractability.

Excision of the ulcer itself is not sufficient for either duodenal or gastric ulcer; recurrence always takes place following such a procedure. *Therefore all the different operations available for peptic ulcer aim at reducing the level of acidity in the stomach.*

The procedures available are of two types : methods of reducing acidity, and drainage or diversion procedures.

Methods of reducing acidity

The objective of reducing gastric acidity may be achieved by:

- Abolishing the nervous phase of gastric secretion.
- Draining the acid gastric contents into the duodenum or jejunum.
- Providing for reflux of alkaline duodenal or jejunal contents into the stomach to neutralize the acid.
- Removing the gastrin-secreting area i.e. the antrum.
- Removing the whole or a part of the acid-secreting area i.e. the parietal-cell-bearing regions of the stomach.

Operations available

The operations available are vagotomy, drainage procedures and gastric resections:

Vagotomy

This abolishes the nervous phase of gastric acid secretion. There are two types of vagotomy:

- *Truncal vagotomy.* (Fig.20.5a) 1 to 2cm of each vagal trunk is excised, just below the esophageal hiatus. This procedure denervates the entire stomach and the gastrointestinal tract to the midcolon. Combined with other operations, it is highly effective in reducing the number of recurrent ulcers. However, it carries some deleterious side-effects and disadvantages:
    - o It reduces the ability of the stomach to empty.
    - o It is followed by other late motility disturbances like diarrhea and reflux alkaline gastritis.
    - o Further, as it is followed by gastric stasis it cannot be used alone; it has to be combined with a drainage procedure.
- *Highly selective vagotomy.* The branches of both anterior and posterior vagi running from the main

1 FDA: Food and Drug Administration of the USA.

trunks to the lower 7cm of esophagus and the upper stomach down to 6–7cm proximal to the pylorus are divided, those supplying the antrum (nerve of Latarjet) being spared. The main trunks are also left intact. Thus the antrum remains innervated so that gastric emptying takes place normally, and this type of vagotomy does not have to be supplemented by a drainage procedure.

Drainage procedures

These are required with truncal vagotomy, which denervates the stomach and delays gastric emptying:

- *Gastrojejunostomy.* (Fig.20.5b) A side-to-side anastomosis is made between the posterior wall of the stomach and the most proximal loop of the jejunum.
- *Pyloroplasty*. A longitudinal incision divides the pyloric sphincter and renders it incompetent; the wall of the stomach and duodenum is then repaired in the transverse axis. Pyloroplasty is preferred to gastrojejunostomy as the former is more physiological.

Incidentally, all drainage procedures–whether gastroenterostomy, pyloroplasty or gastrectomy— also provide for reflux of alkaline intestinal contents into the stomach to neutralize acid. Therefore they should properly be called 'drainage and alkalinization' procedures.

Resections of the stomach

- *Antrectomy*. (Fig.20.5c) The gastric antrum is removed. The stomach is anastomosed to the duodenum (Billroth I operation).
- *Partial gastrectomy*. (Fig.20.5d) The distal 2/3rd to 3/4th of the stomach is excised. The stomach is joined to a loop of proximal jejunum, the duodenal stump having been closed (Polya operation).

The ways in which these operations achieve the objective of reducing acidity are given in (Table 20.1). Sub-total gastrectomy is used only for the extremely severe hyperacidity produced by the Zollinger-Ellison syndrome if a gastrinoma cannot be localized.

To sum up, the operations used commonly are the following:

- Highly selective vagotomy.
- Truncal vagotomy and gastrojejunostomy (or pyloroplasty).
- Partial gastrectomy (distal 3/4 stomach).
- Vagotomy and antrectomy.

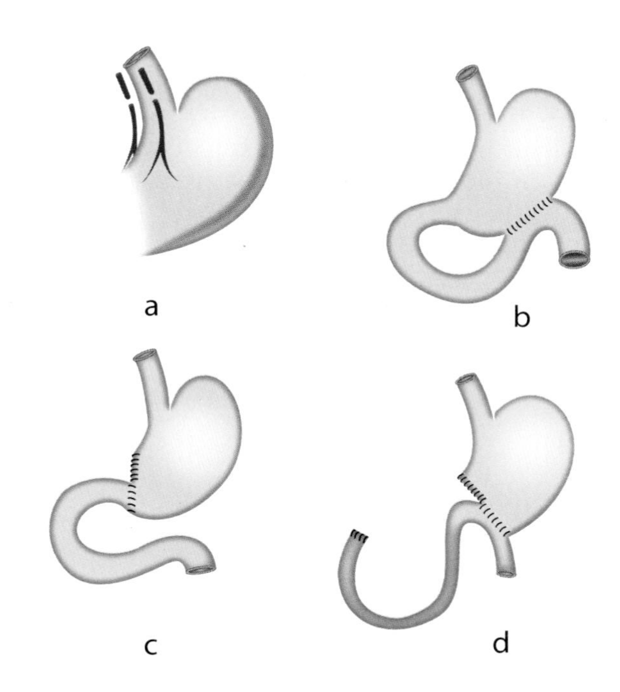

Fig.20.5 Different operations for petic ulcer a: vagotomy, b: gastrojejunostomy, c: antrectomy (Billroth I), d: partial gastrectomy (Billroth II). In the Polya operation the full circumference of the open stomach is anastomosed to the jejunum.

Choice of operation

Duodenal ulcer

In highly selective vagotomy only the parietal cell mass of the stomach is denervated. The mortality rate, the incidence of side effects and the recurrence rate are all low. However, the number of these operations performed fell precipitously after the advent of eradication therapy by the use of antisecretory agents.

Out of the resection operations for duodenal ulcer, vagotomy and antrectomy has mostly displaced partial gastrectomy.

Gastric ulcer

Billroth I gastrectomy is the operation of choice for gastric ulcer. Excision of the ulcer is an important component of the surgery, and if the ulcer is high on the lesser curve the distal gastrectomy is combined with local excision of the ulcer.

For patients with gastric ulcer *without* duodenal ulcer, a 50% gastrectomy with Billroth I reconstruction is advised. The recurrence rate is low (2%) and the long-term results excellent.

In patients with a prepyloric ulcer *along with* a duodenal

ulcer, the duodenal lesion should be regarded as the primary one, and the case should be dealt with as described under duodenal ulcer, i.e. by vagotomy plus drainage or vagotomy plus antrectomy. The recurrence rate after the former operation is a good deal higher than after the latter; therefore, it is used only in poor-risk patients.

All these procedures can now be carried out laparoscopically except in emergency situations.

Recording the results

Visick's criteria allow us to record the postoperative result objectively.

They are as follows:

Visick I:	Totally asymptomatic.
Visick II.	Minor symptoms.
Visick III.	Symptoms interfering with daily life.
Visick IV.	Totally incapacitated.

Prognosis after treatment

Duodenal ulcer patients who do less well with *medical* treatment are those with a high acid secretion. Bleeding occurs in 15% and perforation and obstruction each in about 5%. The onset of back pain is a bad prognostic sign. The results of *surgery* are good in 90% patients. The mortality rate following elective surgery is 1–2%. In ulcers that fail to heal, malignancy cannot be excluded. For these reasons, and because gastrectomy cures *gastric ulcer* so efficiently, *surgery* is advised in many of these patients.

Complications after gastric operations

Apart from the usual pulmonary, cardiac and thrombotic complications which can follow any major upper abdominal operation, a variety of specific complications can occur after operations on the stomach and duodenum.

Post-vagotomy diarrhea

This is seen more often with truncal vagotomy, in 10–15% of patients. Most patients will have increase in the frequency of stools but a minority will have profuse diarrhea. The exact cause is not known.

Recurrent ulcer

A recurrent ulcer usually occurs at the primary site or just distal to the anastomosis (anastomotic ulcer) and arises due to insufficient reduction in gastric acidity. As duodenal ulcer is far more common than gastric ulcer, the recurrence is seen more often in duodenal ulcer. The recurrence rate varies widely from 5–25% depending upon the type of procedure and aetiological factors involved. There is severe persistent boring pain. If the stoma is adequate and acid hypersecretion is present, vagotomy will cure the ulcer.

If an anastomotic ulcer remains untreated it may erode into the transverse colon and produce a *gastrojejunocolic fistula*. There is severe diarrhea after every meal, with foul eructations. The fistula should be resected and the colon and jejunum repaired. At the same time, vagotomy or a high partial gastrectomy should be carried out.

A gastric ulcer in the body (Type 1) does not produce much acid. If it is dealt with by gastric resection even without vagotomy, the operation is followed by a low rate of recurrence.

On the other hand a gastric ulcer with a duodenal ulcer (type 2), or a pyloric or prepyloric ulcer (type 3), has a high acid output. If it is treated by highly selective vagotomy, the recurrence rate is high; these ulcers should therefore be treated by antrectomy plus bilateral truncal vagotomy.

The lowest recurrence rate is seen after gastric resection and bilateral truncal vagotomy, the highest after proximal gastric vagotomy. However, today recurrent ulcers after proximal gastric vagotomy can be successfully treated by anti-secretory drugs.

Postgastrectomy syndromes

After partial gastrectomy or gastro-jejunostomy the food passes rapidly into the small intestine:

- This may sometimes give rise to the *early dumping syndrome* (sweating, palpitations, abdominal cramps and diarrhea) within half an hour after a meal; this is seen particularly after liquids with a high osmolality, such as milk shakes.
- The *late dumping syndrome* is also related to the intake of carbohydrates. About 2 hours after the meal, the hyperglycemia induces an oversupply of insulin which then leads to a reactive hypoglycemia with symptoms of sweating and extreme weakness. Moderation of carbohydrate intake usually controls the symptoms.

Reduced acidity in the proximal intestines impairs calcium absorption, leading to *osteoporotic* changes in bones. Other less specific symptoms have been included in this category, e.g. early satiety, regurgitation and reflux gastritis.

Steatorrhoea and anemia

In the Billroth I type of gastrectomy the stomach is anastomosed directly to the jejunum, and the duodenum is bypassed. Here two additional problems arise:

- The poor mixing of food with bile and pancreatic juice may cause *steatorrhoea*.

Table 20.1 Ways in which different operations on the stomach reduce acidity.

	Abolishes nervous phase (a)	Drains acid contents (b)	Allows alkaline reflux (c)	Removes gastrin secreting area (d)	Removes parietal cell area (e)
Vagotomy	+				
Gastrojejunostomy		+	+		
Vagotomy plus gastrojejunostomy	+	+	+		
Antrectomy		+	+	+	
Vagotomy plus antrectomy	+	+	+	+	
Total gastrectomy	+	+	+	+	+

- At the same time, bypassing the duodenum hinders iron absorption and results in *anemia*.

Weight loss

The combined effect of all the above factors is diminished absorption, with weight loss.

COMPLICATIONS OF PEPTIC ULCER

The three most important complications of peptic ulcer include hemorrhage, perforation and stenosis.

Upper gastrointestinal hemorrhage

Upper gastrointestinal (GI) hemorrhage may be mild or severe, but *should always be taken seriously* and investigated thoroughly. Bleeding is the most common serious complication of peptic ulcer, portal hypertension and gastric erosions, and these conditions account for most episodes of upper GI bleeding.

Hematemesis

Vomiting of bright red or dark blood indicates that the source of bleeding is proximal to the duodenojejunal junction. Vomitus looking like ground coffee (*'coffee-ground vomiting'*) indicates that blood has been in the stomach long enough for gastric acid to convert hemoglobin to methemoglobin.

Melena

Melena can be produced by blood entering the bowel at any point from mouth to cecum, but most patients with melena are bleeding from the upper gastrointestinal tract. The red cells in the blood disintegrate, and the released hemoglobin is broken down into haem and globin. Intestinal and bacterial enzymes now oxidize haem to hematin, which gives melena stools their black colour. Bright red blood from the rectum is not called melena but hematochezia.

Hematochezia

This means the passage of bright red blood from the rectum; the blood comes from the anus, rectum or colon. But if very brisk bleeding is occurring in the upper intestine, bright red blood may be passed in the stool due to rapid transit.

Management of upper GI hemorrhage

If in a healthy looking patient melena has continued for a week or more, it suggests slow bleeding. Such a case should be admitted to hospital and investigated.

On the other hand, hematemesis or sudden melena should be regarded as a much more serious emergency, and urgent resuscitative measures should be taken as follows:

- The circulatory status should be assessed. The pulse rate and blood pressure are recorded, and one should look for the presence of pallor, cold extremities and air hunger, which indicate loss of a large volume of blood.

- The amount of blood lost and the rate of bleeding should be estimated, and the deficit made good by rapid blood transfusion. Crystalloid resuscitation should precede transfusion.

Emergency endoscopy

This should be carried out to detect the site of bleeding. If possible, the hemorrhage should be arrested:

- By sclerosing injection into esophageal varices, or
- By diathermy or laser coagulation of a bleeding artery in the base of an ulcer.

Patients are admitted to an ICU or a high dependency unit and managed by a team consisting of gastroenterologist, surgeon and intensivist.

The following findings indicate that surgical treatment will probably be required:

- The presence of hypotension on admission.
- Continued bleeding.
- Recurrent bleeding during hospital stay, after initial control by non-invasive measures.
- Age above 60 years, because these patients tolerate continued blood loss less well.
- Endoscopic features such as visible clot, visible vessel in ulcer base, or lack of facilities for hemostasis.

Bleeding ulcers in the duodenum are usually located on the posterior wall. As the ulcer becomes deeper the gastro-duodenal artery may get eroded, leading to very severe hemorrhage.

Treatment of bleeding peptic ulcer

Most patients with bleeding peptic ulcer can be managed medically or by endoscopic means, whereas about 25% require emergency surgery.

Upper GI endoscopy

Early upper gastrointestinal endoscopy is the most valuable diagnostic procedure. However, profuse bleeding may make it useless; the diagnosis of the source of bleeding sometimes has to be made by laparotomy. If available, peroperative endoscopy will identify the source of bleeding. If necessary, a wide gastrotomy incision that extends across the pylorus gives the best exposure to help find the source.

Patients over the age of 60 do not tolerate massive bleeding well; they respond much better to early operation. Under that age mortality is not increased by the delay imposed by attempts to control the bleeding by endoscopic techniques such as electrocoagulation, Argon laser coagulation, Bicap or heater probe.

Embolization

In high risk patients not suitable for surgery, *arterial embolization* of the bleeding pancreaticodudenal artery by the interventional radiologist can be life saving.

Operation

Early *operation* is indicated in patients bleeding from the gastroduodenal artery or a gastric ulcer. If the patient's general condition is good, a bleeding gastric ulcer is best treated by a partial gastrectomy, and a duodenal or prepyloric ulcer by a vagotomy and antrectomy. In an emergency situation, suture-ligation of the bleeding vessel with or without vagotomy will suffice.

Perforated peptic ulcer

A perforated peptic ulcer is a very serious emergency. Most perforated ulcers are on the anterior surface of the duodenal bulb, much less often on the anterior surface of the stomach. In most cases there is a long history of peptic ulcer. In a few cases a 'silent' ulcer perforates, especially if the patient has been on steroids.

Clinical features

At the moment of the perforation either gastric acid, or (in the case of a duodenal ulcer) bile and pancreatic enzymes, suddenly pour into the peritoneal cavity. Due to the intense chemical peritonitis the patient cries out in agony. Peritoneal fluid is now secreted in liberal amounts. This dilutes the irritants and gives temporary relief. However in a few hours the stage of bacterial peritonitis sets in. The patient is in severe pain. The temperature may be subnormal. The abdomen is held still. The whole abdomen is tender and rigid like a board. The escaping gas may change the normal liver dullness to a tympanitic note. Peristaltic sounds are absent due to paralytic ileus.

It should be noted that in occasional cases the presentation may not be as dramatic, and diagnosis may be missed because the clinical manifestations are not sufficiently severe, especially in the elderly.

X-rays

Plain x-rays in the erect posture show free air under the diaphragm in the great majority of patients. If no air is seen, gastrografin is given by mouth and x-rays may show escape of contrast material from the lumen.

Differential diagnosis

The differential diagnosis of a perforated peptic ulcer includes:

- Acute cholecystitis.
- Acute pancreatitis.
- Strangulating intestinal obstruction.
- Acute appendicitis.
- Mesenteric thrombosis.

In pancreatitis there is more shock than would be expected from the degree of pain. In cholecystitis pain often radiates to the inferior angle of the scapula and the right shoulder.

Treatment

The treatment of a perforated peptic ulcer is immediate operation. A right paramedian incision is commonly employed. All pus and food debris are removed and the peritoneal cavity irrigated with saline. The perforation is closed by interrupted sutures of Vicryl or PDS, taking care to avoid the sutures cutting through the edematous and friable edges of the ulcer. A patch of greater omentum is sewn over the suture line to provide further protection from leakage. Drains are placed in both paracolic gutters.

If the patient is young and in good condition and the operator is experienced, the definitive operation for the ulcer may be carried out instead of simple closure of the perforation. Of patients treated by simple suture, one-third remain free of symptoms. Of the other two-thirds, about half require a definitive operation.

Most perforated gastric ulcers are located in the prepyloric area. They behave as perforated duodenal ulcers and require similar treatment. However, perforation of an ulcer elsewhere in the stomach introduces the possibility of malignancy, and immediate definitive resection of the stomach is recommended. If the patient's condition is poor, only excision of the ulcer is carried out; biopsy of the margin of the ulcer should be taken to rule out malignancy.

Pyloric stenosis

Gastric outlet obstruction is due to stenosis of the bulbar part of the duodenum and pyloric canal. Most patients have a long history of dyspepsia. The ulcer pain gets worse, and there is anorexia and vomiting. *The vomitus contains food taken many hours or a day before.* There is *no bile in the vomitus*. Weight loss and dehydration are obvious.

A *succussion splash* may be elicited from retained gastric contents in the dilated stomach. Occasionally, peristalsis in the distended stomach may be visible, *passing from left to right in the epigastrium*.

Tetany may occur due to advanced alkalosis. *Anemia* is common.

Metabolic disturbances

Prolonged vomiting causes dehydration and alkalosis. Vomiting depletes the patient of sodium, potassium and chloride. The loss of hydrochloric acid in the gastric juice causes the extracellular bicarbonate level to rise. The kidney excretes this excess bicarbonate, which takes large amounts of sodium with it as sodium bicarbonate. The loss of sodium activates aldosterone. In order to maintain the extracellular fluid volume, sodium is conserved and potassium and hydrogen are excreted instead. The glomerular filtration rate falls and produces prerenal azotaemia. A marked deficit of Na^+, $Cl^-$and H_2O is the result.

Replacement of fluids

While replacing the fluid and electrolyte losses the usual practice is that water and NaCl are replaced first till a satisfactory urine flow starts; KCl replacement is only then started. If potassium is given before a good flow of urine is obtained, dangerous hyperkalaemia may result.

Treatment

In the vast majority of cases of pyloric stenosis operation is required to relieve the obstruction and reduce acidity. Operation is carried out only after the electrolyte disturbances have been corrected and the stomach cleared of the food residue by gastric lavage. Apart from chronic duodenal obstruction the other most important cause of gastric outlet obstruction is gastric cancer, and endoscopy and biopsy is required to settle the issue.

The common operations carried out are: either vagotomy and gastroenterostomy, or partial gastrectomy. Elderly patients in poor condition who are considered to have burned-out ulcers can be treated by gastroenterostomy under local anesthesia.

Zollinger-Ellison syndrome

The Zollinger-Ellison syndrome consists of peptic ulcer disease caused by a gastrin-producing tumor (gastrinoma). These are mostly non-beta islet cell carcinomas or adenomas in the head of the pancreas, or more commonly in the 2nd part of the duodenum. Rarely the condition is associated with multiple endocrine neoplasms (MEN syndrome Type I).

Clinical features

Symptoms result from the extremely severe hyperacidity. Abdominal pain occurs due to the peptic ulcer. Diarrhea is common, and is due to hypersecretion of acid. The duodenum is flooded with acid. This destroys pancreatic lipase and produces steatorrhoea and also damages the small bowel mucosa. Anastomotic ulcers appear even after surgical operations that would heal ordinary ulcers.

Laboratory findings

If the Zollinger-Ellison syndrome is suspected the serum gastrin level is determined.

Levels above 200 pg/ml are abnormal. These levels are raised in two different conditions:

- Serum gastrin is markedly increased in the Zollinger-Ellison syndrome; in this condition a gastrin-secreting islet cell tumor (gastrinoma) produces a greatly increased quantity of gastric acid and results in peptic ulceration. The *serum gastrin* level may be *many times the normal* upper limit of 200 pg/ml.
- Serum gastrin levels are also raised in atrophic gastritis and pernicious anemia. It happens like this: achlorhydria occurs, and the absence of acid in the stomach results in a loss of the normal inhibition for gastrin release, thus raising the gastrin level. However, these levels are not raised as high as in the Zollinger-Ellison syndrome.

On *gastroduodenoscopy* an ulcer may be seen in the duodenal bulb. Occasionally the ulcer may be in the distal duodenum or upper jejunum; an ulcer in that location is diagnostic of gastrinoma, as the 'normal' duodenal ulcers occur only in the first part of the duodenum.

Treatment

In the past total gastrectomy was the only effective treatment for the Zollinger-Ellison syndrome, and was the standard treatment. After total gastrectomy most patients lose weight and suffer from nutritional deficiencies. Life-long iron e.g. ferrous sulphate 1 tablet b.d. and parenteral vitamin B12 are required.

However, these days most gastrinomas can be localized by CT scan, endo-ultrasound, and selective angiography. Exploratory laparotomy with duodenal illumination and duodenotomy finds many more gastrinomas. Therefore, the treatment of choice today consists of excision of the tumor.

Gastric surgery for morbid obesity

If the weight is more than twice the ideal body weight (200 to 225% to be exact) for the patient, he is defined as *morbidly obese*. If his weight is more than 225% of ideal body weight, he is classified as *superobese*. In such cases the complications related to obesity are severe; at the same time, long-term weight reduction cannot be achieved by conservative methods and surgery is required. In the past, short-circuiting of the small intestine used to be employed for this purpose. However, this was found to lead to extremely severe nutritional and metabolic deficiencies, and has been given up.

The most successful method of dealing with morbid obesity and superobesity consists of restricting the surface area of the stomach available for contact with food (*gastric restrictive surgery*). Not only does this kind of surgery cure morbid obesity, it also helps in connection with the different obesity-related complications. For example, Type II diabetes and hypertension related to morbid obesity may be cured in as many as two-thirds of the patients. The two most commonly performed procedures are:

- Gastric banding.
- Gastric bypass.

Both can be carried out laparoscopically.

CARCINOMA OF THE STOMACH

Carcinoma of the stomach is an important cause of death from cancer. The highest incidence is between 45 and 65 years of age. The disease has wide geographical variation, from 10 cases per 100,000 persons per year in the USA to 70 cases per 100,000 per year in Japan. Premalignant conditions are gastric polyps and pernicious anemia. More than half the tumors arise in the pyloric region. Microscopically the tumors are nearly always adenocarcinomas. A few squamous cell tumors are seen at the cardia, but they actually arise from the esophagus.

Two distinct types of gastric cancers are identified:

- *Early gastric cancers*. These are confined to the mucosa and submucosa, are diagnosed only on endoscopy, and have an excellent prognosis. This type is more often seen in Japan, where it is extremely common.
- *Late gastric cancers*. These tumors have invaded the muscle wall and serosa. This type is far more common in the West as well as the South Asian subcontinent. They have a low resectability rate and much worse prognosis.

Macroscopically there are five types:

- A cauliflower-like growth.
- An ulcer with irregular indurated edges.
- Colloid carcinoma.
- Scirrhous carcinoma.
- Carcinoma secondary to gastric ulcer.

Aetiological factors

Familial and racial factors play a part in the causation of gastric carcinoma. 4 percent of the patients give a family history of the disease, which is slightly more common in patients with *blood group A*. Other risk factors are *smoking, alcohol, gastric surgery and H. pylori*. In Japan gastric cancer occurs in almost epidemic proportions, being responsible for nearly half the deaths from all malignancies.

Atrophic gastritis, along with its resultant achlorhydria, is associated with an increased incidence of the condition.

Finally, *nitrates* as food preservatives have been incriminated. It may be mentioned that in the advanced countries, recently there has been a remarkable decrease in the number of cases of carcinoma of the body and antrum. While the reason for this dramatic decrease is speculative, it could be due to better refrigeration and more rapid transport of commercial meat prior to ingestion.

Spread

Extension of carcinoma of the stomach occurs by spread in the wall, direct spread to adjacent organs, and lymphatic metastases. Transperitoneal implantation may occur; these cells gravitate to the pelvis and produce tumors there. Vascular spread is to the liver and later to lungs and bones.

Clinical features

The first symptom is gastric distension with inability to take a normal meal. Anorexia and weight loss develop. Epigastric pain is persistent. The patient is anemic and weak, and gets tired easily. He may present with obstruction at the cardia (dysphagia), or at the pylorus (fullness, belching and vomiting).

A lump in the epigastrium may be palpated incidentally without any symptoms. Carcinoma in the body of the stomach is usually silent, but may give rise to features in other organs e.g. obstructive jaundice (from secondary deposits in the liver), ascites (from carcinomatosis of peritoneum), etc.

Investigations

A thorough investigation should be undertaken in every case of persistent indigestion, specially in middle and old age. Anemia is present in 40%, achlorhydria in 20% and occult blood in stools in 80% of cases of gastric carcinoma. The E.S.R. is raised in 70% cases.

Gastroscopy

Gastroscopy has replaced conventional radiology.

All patients with a newly discovered gastric ulcer should undergo fibreoptic gastroscopy. Carcinoma is recognized by its:

- Nodularity.
- Multi-coloured base.
- Immobility.

Multiple biopsies must always be taken. Usually, biopsy is taken from each quadrant of the mass or ulcer *(four-quadrant biopsy).* Fibre-optic gastroscopy has revolutionized the diagnosis of carcinoma as well as of other mucosal lesions of the stomach, and has replaced barium meal x-rays.

Exfoliative cytology

Exfoliative cytology has become much less important since the introduction of excellent fibreoptic gastroscopes through which biopsies can be taken.

Treatment

Surgical resection is the only curative treatment for carcinoma of the stomach. Emaciated patients should be nutritionally resuscitated by a 2–3 weeks course of high-calorie parenteral nutrition (3,000 to 3500 kcals/day) before surgery. In the advanced countries 90% of patients are operable. At operation the lesions are resectable in 60% of cases. Of these more than one half are potentially curable, i.e. there are no signs of spread beyond the limits of resection.

Pyloric tumors require distal 2/3rd gastrectomy with removal of omentum and nearby lymph nodes, all *en bloc.* Restoration of continuity may be achieved by the Billroth I procedure; in this procedure the remnant of stomach is joined to the duodenum.

Tumors of the *proximal half* of the stomach require total gastrectomy. After removal of the stomach a loop of jejunum is taken up to the hiatus and joined to the esophagus.

Tumors of the *cardia* require resection of the distal esophagus and proximal stomach, with esophagogastrostomy.

For *palliation* of a pyloric tumor a limited resection utilizing a Billroth II resection is better than a diverting gastrojejunostomy.

For advanced disease chemotherapy with a combination of methyl-CCNU and fluorouracil (5-FU) gives objective improvement in nearly half the cases.

Prognosis

Early gastric cancers have survival rates approaching 80%, whereas in the case of the more common advanced gastric cancers, the overall survival is 10–20%.

In the absence of lymph node involvement the 5-year survival rate is as high as 50%; with lymph node involvement 12%. Death may follow dissemination to other organs or be the result of progressive obstruction and malnutrition (malignant cachexia).

Acute gastritis (Erosive gastritis)

This condition has been recognized with greater frequency since the use of fibre-optic gastroscopy in acute upper gastrointestinal bleeding. Ingestion of large amounts of alcohol, salicylates or non-steroid anti-inflammatory drugs (NSAIDs) etc. are important causative factors.

There may be acute epigastric pain, or no symptoms. Tiny mucosal ulcers develop and occasionally cause massive hemorrhage. Diagnosis is made by gastroscopy and biopsy.

Gastric lavage with cold solutions and proton pump inhibitors (PPI's) usually halt blood loss. Surgery is rarely required. If hemorrhage continues undiminished, operation may have to be performed. Subtotal or rarely total gastrectomy might be necessary to save the patient's life.

Duodenal diverticula

These are fairly commonly seen in autopsies and barium meal series. But only 1% of those detected by x-ray require surgery. Dyspepsia may occur and require antacids and anticholinergics. Complications are hemorrhage, perforation and biliary obstruction.

Duodenal fistula

A duodenal fistula may occur:

- Due to traumatic rupture of the duodenum.
- As a complication of Polya gastrectomy: this used to be the most common cause. However, with the very great decrease in the number of gastrectomies carried out since the advent of proton pump inhibitors, it is taking second place.
- Due to injury to the duodenum during nephrectomy or colectomy.

Both bile and pancreatic juice are discharged in large quantities through the fistula and produce excoriation of the skin. Dehydration, electrolyte depletion and hypoproteinemia can quickly arise if the fistula is a large one.

Treatment

This consists of

- Protection of the skin with a barrier cream.
- Drainage of the fistula, which may be aided by the patient lying on his right side.
- Total parenteral nutrition until the fistula heals.

In common with other intestinal fistulae one must ensure that there is no distal obstruction if the fistula is to heal on conservative treatment.

Chapter

21 LIVER

INJURIES TO THE LIVER

Liver injuries may penetrating or blunt.

Penetrating injuries

The common *penetrating* injuries are stabs and bullet wounds. Stabs usually cause less damage; high velocity bullet wounds shatter the parenchyma over a wider area.

Blunt injuries

More commonly, liver injuries are *blunt.* They are most often sustained during traffic accidents. They may produce bursting wounds with much damage. Problems are caused by hemorrhage, bile leakage, and devitalization i.e. infarction of liver tissue. Overlying ribs may be fractured.

Bleeding may be profuse and free into the peritoneal cavity producing collapse, or it may occur within the liver as a large hematoma. This may become infected to form an abscess, or may burst into the bile duct to give rise to hemobilia.

Bile leakage can cause chemical biliary peritonitis with abscess formation. *Infarction* of the liver can also result in an abscess.

Clinical features

If the liver is badly shattered, there may be hypovolemic shock with hypotension, decreased urinary output, and low central venous pressure. Abdominal distension may be present.

Hemoperitoneum may produce shifting dullness. If liver rupture is suspected on clinical grounds, diagnostic peritoneal lavage may be carried out to look for blood-staining of the aspirate.

Diagnosis

This is based on a history of trauma to the right lower chest or upper abdomen and signs of hypovolemia. Principal investigations are abdominal ultrasound and CT with I/V contrast.

CT scan

In the past nearly all liver injuries were treated by laparotomy. CT scans have revolutionized the treatment; they have shown that in many of these injuries blood loss is less than 500ml. For these stable and relatively minor injuries observation alone is satisfactory. If, in an injury to the right hypochondrium, a CT scan shows that the hepatic flexure of the colon and the right kidney are not damaged, the case can be treated conservatively; if more extensive injuries are shown, immediate laparotomy would be the appropriate course to follow.

Treatment

The principal objective of treatment is to arrest bleeding and debride devitalized liver if required. As mentioned above, any patients with minor or stable intermediate injuries are managed conservatively if bowel injuries can be ruled out. Most lacerations have stopped bleeding by the time operation is performed. These should not be sutured, because stagnation of blood and serum in the closed space thus created could lead to abscess formation. Active bleeding may be managed by ligation or suture of bleeding points. If the hepatic flexure of the colon is also injured the bowel should be exteriorized, i.e. a colostomy performed.

Cases with extensive damage to the liver parenchyma are difficult to manage. Debridement involves piece-meal removal of dead tissue rather than lobar resection. However, a particularly severe crushing injury may require lobectomy. At the end of the operation suction catheters should be placed and brought out through separate incisions.

A few other points to remember are the following:

- The body temperature must be maintained, if necessary by having the room temperature above 26° C. The core temperature will then remain within a physiological range, allowing normal enzymatic processes to work, particularly those responsible for coagulation of blood.

- If bleeding persists and the site of origin cannot be found, it should be remembered that a tear in the inferior vena cava could be responsible.
- An effort should be made to get the liver on to the abdominal wall for better exposure, by dividing the falciform and triangular ligaments.
- If more than 5 units of blood have to be given, 10 packs of platelets and 5 units of packed cells should be given for every additional 5 units of blood transfused.

If all else fails or the patient's condition deteriorates the bleeding area should be packed and the abdomen closed. A day or two later, when any coagulopathy, hypothermia or acidosis has been dealt with, the abdomen can be re-opened and the packs removed.

Prognosis

The mortality rate after liver injury is about 10–15%. Only 1% of stabs are lethal, but as many as 20% of blunt injuries result in a fatality. This is because stabs result in a puncture-like wound in the liver, whereas blunt injuries produce more widespread disruption of the hepatic tissue. If three major organs are damaged, the death rate is as high as 70%. Most deaths are due to bleeding.

LIVER ABSCESS

Hepatic abscesses may be bacterial, parasitic or fungal. In the advanced countries the common abscesses are pyogenic; in the poorer communities amebic, due to poor hygiene.

Pyogenic liver abscess

Incidence

The incidence of pyogenic liver abscesses has not changed much over the last 50 years. However, fifty years ago most patients were under the age of 40 and the most common cause was appendicitis. Today the average age lies between 50 and 60, and the most common cause is biliary tract disease, with an increasing incidence of malignant disease in these cases.

Examples

Pyogenic abscesses may be solitary or multiple, are distributed throughout both lobes of the liver, and usually follow suppuration elsewhere. Examples of some conditions resulting in pyogenic liver abscesses follow:

- *Cholangitis,* whenever bile flow is obstructed. Typically:
  - *Total obstruction* raises the pressure in the biliary tree, producing an acutely septic course and miliary microabscesses throughout the liver—'acute suppurative cholangitis'.
  - *Incomplete obstruction* usually results in a subacute course and a single abscess.
- *Suppurative thrombophlebitis* in the *portal* venous system secondary to appendicitis, diverticulitis, infected hemorrhoids, etc.
- *Direct extension* from infections involving the gallbladder, subphrenic space or pleural cavity, and sites of bowel perforation.
- *Trauma* to the liver, hemorrhage or bile extravasation into liver tissue, or areas of hepatic necrosis, produce devitalized tissue which can become infected.
- *Hepatic arterial infection.* In leukemias and chronic granulomas, systemic bacteremias may seed the liver. Again, in liver transplantation in children the hepatic artery anastomosis may become thrombosed with local or systemic micro-organisms.

Clinical features

Irregular fever with spikes occurs. The liver is usually enlarged and tender.

Laboratory

Leucocytosis is commonly present. Serum alkaline phosphatase and bilirubin levels may be raised in multiple abscesses.

Imaging

On *x-ray* the right dome of the diaphragm may be raised, with basilar atelectasis or pleural effusion.

CT scan (Fig.21.2, chapter 16) and *ultrasound* are extremely useful and accurately indicate the presence, size, number and location of the abscesses. Special needles passing through the centre of the ultrasonic probe are available for aspiration of abscesses under ultrasound control. The radio-isotope scan gives less clear-cut demarcation.

Treatment

Open drainage

The classical treatment of pyogenic liver abscesses consisted of *open* drainage of the abscess, correction of the underlying pathology if possible, and a 4-to 6-week course of antibiotics, usually a beta-lactam, an aminoglycoside and metronidazole.

Percutaneous drainage

However, in the recent past most patients have been treated by antibiotics and percutaneous drainage with benefit:

- The extensive abdominal wall wound in open drainage, with its attendant pain and likelihood of involvement in the suppurative process, is avoided.
- Contamination of the peritoneal cavity is avoided. Thus, further surgery is dispensed with in an individual who is usually immunocompromised due to extensive sepsis.

Percutaneous drainage is carried out under ultrasound or CT guidance, with the insertion of a pigtail catheter using the *Seldinger technique*: the abscess is punctured with a sharp hollow needle. A guidewire is passed through the needle and the needle withdrawn. A pigtail catheter is passed over the guidewire into the abscess and the guidewire withdrawn.

Samples of pus are taken for microbiological examination, the cavity is gently irrigated with saline, and the catheter left in place to provide continuing drainage.

It should be remembered that in about 15% of patients percutaneous drainage fails. This may be due to:

- Incorrect placement of the catheter.
- Excessive viscosity of the pus plugging the catheter.
- Thick abscess walls that do not collapse with drainage.

Open drainage is then necessary.

The overall mortality rate is high, and is due to delay in diagnosis and the presence of multiple abscesses. If jaundice is present, and if the serum albumin level is falling, the prognosis is bad. Even if the abscess is solitary and is treated promptly there is still a significant mortality rate, upto 10%.

Amebic liver abscess

Amebic dysentery is endemic in most underdeveloped countries. In a few cases of amebic dysentery the ameba passes into the radicles of the portal vein and lodges in the liver to produce an amebic liver abscess. The amebae produce liquefaction necrosis. A proteolytic enzyme produced by the ameba causes coalescence of the invaded areas and abscess formation.

80% of the abscesses are located in the right lobe, probably because venous return from the right side of the colon, where the ameba commonly lodges, is predominantly delivered to the right lobe.

The pus is not yellow but brown or chocolate-coloured. It consists of broken-down liver cells, leucocytes and red blood cells. In many cases the pus contains staphylococci, streptococci and *Esch. coli* in addition to the amebae. If the freshly aspirated pus is examined under the microscope for the presence of motile amebae, usually none are seen; they are mostly to be found in the walls of the abscess.

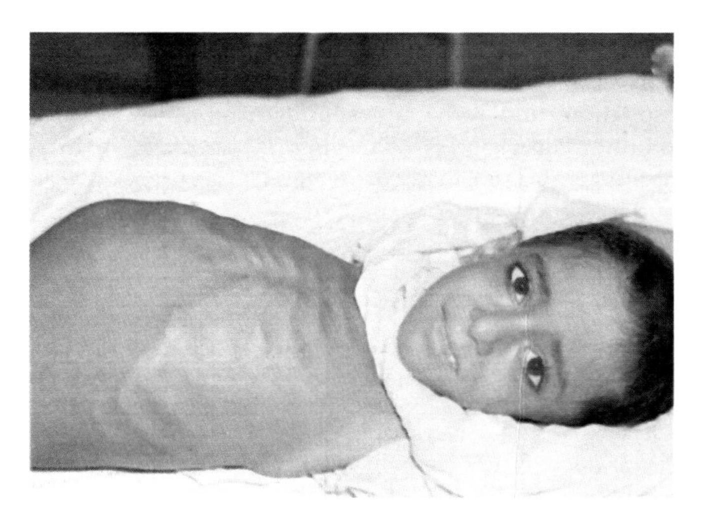

Fig.21.1 Huge amebic liver abscess causing bulging of the chest wall. The child is emaciated from the toxemia.

The *further course* may be along any one of the following lines:

- The abscess may resolve under treatment with metronidazole.
- It may become encapsulated.
- It may continue to enlarge.
- It may rupture into the right lung, the peritoneal cavity or the pleural cavity.
- Secondary bacterial infection may occur, specially if the abscess is treated by open drainage.

Clinical findings

There may or may not be a history of recent dysentery. Young males are the most common sufferers.

In early cases the patient complains of discomfort and fullness in the liver region. The liver enlarges and becomes tender. Fever develops, at first intermittent, later unremittent. Sweating is severe specially at night. The patient loses appetite and weight. The enlarged liver may cause bulging of the chest wall (Fig.21.1). Chest movement is restricted on the affected side and deep breathing is painful. The liver dullness is increased upwards. Jaundice is uncommon but may occur.

Diagnosis

The diagnosis of hepatic amebiasis may be difficult, as the history of dysentery is present only occasionally.

Chest x-rays

These often show changes: raised diaphragm on the right side with reduced movement on screening, basal collapse and pleural effusion.

Utrasound

This examination is invaluable both in diagnosis and aspiration, and serial ultrasound scanning is used to monitor the progress of healing. It can diagnose liver abscess with a sensitivity of 98% and an accuracy of 99%, and is as good as a CT scan.

Laboratory

A *polymorph leucocytosis* is nearly always present.

The *stool* may show amebae or cysts, and sigmoidoscopy may sometimes show the ulcers.

Liver function tests are not often helpful.

Serological tests are accurate. The *indirect hemagglutination test* is positive in 95% of patients with an amebic liver abscess, and in areas of low prevalence a positive result strongly suggests the presence of acute infection. However, antibody levels remain elevated for many years after infection; therefore, the test is not of much use in endemic areas, as nearly half the general population may be seropositive. On the other hand levels of antibodies detected by indirect immune-fluorescence and counterimmuno-electrophoresis become undetectable within a few months of acute infection; these tests are therefore more useful in endemic areas.

Treatment

The treatment of choice is metronidazole 500 or 750mg orally or intravenously three times daily for 10 days, although there are still a few failures. In those cases dihydroemetine is given in a dose of 1mg/kg/day intramuscularly four times daily for five days. This should be accompanied by chloroquine phosphate 600mg base/day orally four times daily for four days, followed by 300mg/day for a total of 14–21 days. Small abscesses respond to this regimen.

Aspiration

Abscesses larger than 5–8cm usually require aspiration under ultrasound control. Repeat aspiration is better than catheter drainage on account of the risk of secondary infection and bleeding. If an abscess does not resolve on medical treatment alone it will require percutaneous drainage or repeated aspiration, under ultrasound or CT guidance. A smaller volume of pus is obtained at each successive aspiration until the cavity completely dries up.

In *deep-seated abscesses* a long needle must be used at a level below the pleural reflection to avoid infection of the pleural cavity. The needle is passed under ultrasound control. Ultrasound probes are available which feature a track for the needle down the middle of the probe, for extremely accurate placing of the needle. After aspiration a full course of specific antiamebic drug therapy should be used. A leaking or ruptured abscess can be managed laparoscopically.

For cysts

The above-mentioned medical regime may be followed by treatment with an agent that can eradicate cysts which persist in the intestine after treatment with metronidazole. Such luminal amaebicidal agents include:

- Diloxanide furoate 500mg orally three times a day for 10 days.
- Iodoquinol 600mg daily three times a day for 20 days.
- Paromomycin 25 to 30mg/kg/day orally three times a day for 7 days.

It should be stressed that as far as possible an amebic liver abscess should be treated by drug therapy plus aspiration, or at most percutaneous drainage. Open drainage should be reserved for those cases where aspiration has failed. It is interesting to mention that even aspiration needle tracks sometimes get infected by amebiasis cutis.

HYDATID DISEASE OF THE LIVER

Hydatid disease is common in sheep-rearing areas e.g. Australia, South America, Greece, Turkey, Iran and Iraq. In Pakistan it is seen more often in areas of Southern Punjab and Baluchistan. The most common form is caused by *Echinococcus granulosus* which occurs in the form of a cyst in the liver or lung.

E. multilocularis is uncommon. It occurs in an invasive form in the liver. The lesion does not have a well-demarcated cystic structure, may spread via the blood vessels, and in fact behaves almost like a malignancy, with a bad prognosis.

Life-cycle

The hydatid has two forms, the adult and the larval. The adult is a short flat worm in the primary host, usually a *dog*. It lives in the small bowel of the host, and has 3 to 5 segments. The last is the gravid segment, containing a few hundred ova which are shed in the feces. The ova resist drying and remain viable for weeks.

A grazing animal like *sheep* swallows the ova. The outer coating of the ovum is digested, allowing an embryo to hatch in the small intestine of the sheep, penetrate the bowel wall and enter the portal circulation. Most embryos are trapped in the liver and grow into cysts; some pass into the lungs and onwards to other parts of the body. The life-cycle is completed when a dog eats the contaminated liver of the sheep.

Human beings usually contract the disease during childhood or adolescence, when ova are swallowed after contact with an infected dog. The embryo reaches the portal circulation and develops into a cyst. Man is an occasional intermediate host, and represents a dead end for the parasite, since dogs seldom have access to human viscera. It should be remembered that human beings are not infective to other humans.

Pathology

A typical hydatid cyst has three layers:

- It is lined inside by a single layer of cells, the germinal epithelium *(endocyst)*. This secretes internally the hydatid fluid, which is a crystal-clear watery fluid. Brood capsules develop from the germinal epithelium and are attached to it by stalks. Within these capsules the heads of future worms *(scoleces)* develop. Spillage of the fluid into the peritoneum or pleural cavity can allow further hydatids to develop.
- On its outer aspect the germinal epithelium secretes the laminated membrane *(ectocyst)* which looks like a water-filled balloon.
- The outermost adventitia *(pseudocyst)* consists of fibrous tissue produced by the reaction of the liver to the parasite. It is not really a part of the cyst proper.

Clinical features

The patient commonly presents with a *painless, symptomless* mass in the right upper abdomen, which has been present for many years, as this cyst grows very slowly.

If it *ruptures* into the bile duct, biliary colic and jaundice can occur. Rarely, *secondary infection* occurs in the cyst with fever as the presenting symptom.

Hydatids can cause *allergic* phenomena like urticaria, pruritus, asthma and anaphylaxis. Hepatomegaly (usually tender) may be the only sign.

Complications

- *Secondary infection* may occur into the cyst, as in any other collection of relatively stagnant fluid in the body.
- *Rupture* may result from trauma, operative intervention or infection. Rupture may also occur into the gallbladder, biliary tree, pleural cavity or hepatic veins.
- Severe *allergic* manifestations may occur as a result of rupture, and constitute a grave complication of abdominal hydatid disease.

Laboratory

Although the cyst is isolated from the liver by an adventitial layer, there is an absorption of parasitic products which acts as an antigenic stimulus:

- This is manifested by *eosinophilia* in as many as one fourths of the patients.
- The *hemagglutination* test is a great deal more reliable.
- The detection of circulating scolex antigen by counter-current immunoelectrophoresis *(CIE)* or the enzyme-linked immunosorbent assay *(ELISA)* give the most reliable results.

Imaging

The cyst is readily and clearly demonstrated both by *ultrasound* and *CT scan. X-ray chest* is required to rule out lung hydatid disease.

Treatment

Medical

It should be remembered that medical treatment is only partially effective and multiple courses are required.

Indications

- Multiple cysts or a centrally placed cyst which cannot be removed intact.
- Recurrence after surgery.
- Patient not fit for surgery.
- Pre-or post-operatively in patients with large and multiple cysts in which the risk of spillage and peritoneal contamination is high.

Although the only effective treatment is surgical, albendazole (10mg/kg/day in two divided doses for 4 weeks) is specifically available for hydatid. After liver function tests and blood counts have been checked, the cycle is repeated after an interval of two weeks. Penetration of the cyst by the drug is uncertain and although many cysts decrease in size, not all scoleces are killed. In Australia, where the disease is common, the drug is used:

- Only for disease which is recurrent or surgically inaccessible.
- If there are serious associated medical conditions.

Surgical

If the cyst ruptures and the hydatid fluid spills into the peritoneal cavity, it can produce anaphylactic shock and implantation of cysts throughout the abdomen. Therefore surgical treatment involves removing the intact cyst *without contaminating the patient's tissues*.

The cyst is exposed at laparotomy. A long transverse or oblique abdominal incision gives wide exposure. Black drapes soaked in hypertonic saline isolate the cyst from the peritoneal cavity. The cyst fluid is aspirated and replaced by a scolicidal agent like hypertonic sodium chloride.

Formalin or phenol, which were used previously, should not be injected into the cyst, because:

- They can severely damage the bile ducts if a communication exists.
- There is little evidence of the effectiveness of these fluids. They would have to reach an adequate concentration within the cyst, and it is impossible to predict the degree of dilution caused by residual cyst contents.

The cyst can usually be shelled out intact by developing a plane of cleavage between the ectocyst and pseudocyst. Otherwise the contents have to be removed piecemeal. After evacuation the cavity should be examined for the presence of daughter cysts or any bile leaks which should be closed.

The best way of dealing with the cavity left behind in the liver is *omentoplasty*. The greater omentum is mobilized from the transverse colon preserving its blood supply, and is laid into the cavity.

Complicated cysts

- Cysts *superinfected* with bacteria are best considered as abscesses and treated by drainage and antibiotic therapy.
- For *E. multilocularis,* hepatic resection is the best treatment, as there is no central cavity to be emptied, nor is there a clear margin for pericystectomy.
- Cysts with *extensive calcification* are usually sterile and are probably best left alone.
- If jaundice develops due to *intrabiliary rupture*, the common bile duct needs to be opened with clearance of cysts followed by T-tube drainage.

Recurrence

The risk of recurrence is 10–15% which may be due to reinfestation or true recurrence.

Hydatid cysts in other organs

Hydatid of the *lung* occurs in about one third of the cases with liver cysts.

In the *brain* hydatid cysts usually present as space-occupying lesions.

Hydatid disease of the *heart* may be discovered at autopsy. During life the cysts may rupture into the chambers of the heart with pulmonary metastases or systemic embolization causing infarction.

In the *kidney* the cysts may rupture into the renal pelvis producing renal colic and dysuria with the passage of hydatid material into the urine.

Finally, echinococcus may rarely involve any other site like orbit, ovaries, broad ligament and uterus, and even the limbs (Fig.21.2).

Cirrhosis of the liver

Cirrhosis is defined as diffuse fibrosis with nodule formation in the liver. The common causes of this condition are different in children and adults:

In children

- *Congenital atresia of the bile ducts.* Most patients used to survive only a few months. However, Kasai's operation has increased longevity. If it is carried out within 8 weeks and the bilirubin level falls to normal, the great majority live till the age of 10 years.
- *Nutritional.* This occurs in protein-deficient infants. Examples are found in Africa among the undernourished infants of very poor parents, and in India among the babies of high-caste Hindu vegetarians, whose religion does not allow them to eat meat.
- *Infective* i.e. viral hepatitis. A history of severe jaundice in early infancy is obtained.

In adults

- Overindulgence in alcoholic beverages.
- Virus hepatitis, particularly of the B and C classification.
- Chronic (surgical) biliary obstruction (secondary biliary cirrhosis).
- Schistosomiasis (in Egypt, etc.).

The outlook in cirrhosis depends upon the severity of the associated hepatocellular disease.

PORTAL HYPERTENSION

Normally the portal pressure is upto 12mm Hg. A portal vein pressure of >15mm Hg or 20cm of water constitutes portal hypertension. If the flow of blood through the portal system is obstructed it may lead to an increase in portal venous pressure.

Classification

The obstruction may be classified as follows:

Prehepatic (20%)

Most patients are children. The common causes are the following:

- Congenital absence of portal vein.
- Thrombosis of the portal vein:
    - o Due to extension of the normal obliterative process of the umbilical vein at birth.
    - o Secondary to a hypercoagulable state or thrombosis of the splenic vein.

Intrahepatic (80%).

- The most common cause is *cirrhosis.*
- In a few countries like Egypt, *schistosomiasis* is a very important cause.
- *Idiopathic* fibrosis may rarely be the cause.

Posthepatic

The common conditions responsible include:

- Constrictive pericarditis.
- Veno-occlusive disease.
- Thrombosis of hepatic veins or vena cava.
- Congenital caval valve (Budd Chiari syndrome).

Due to the raised pressure in the tributaries of the portal vein, blood flows across anastomotic channels at the lower esophagus and anal canal to areas of lower pressure. When the portal vein is absent or thrombosed collaterals proximal and distal to the vein enlarge. When the obstruction is intrahepatic, anastomotic channels between portal and systemic veins become engorged.

The only anastomoses which are dangerous to life are those in the submucosa of the lower esophagus (*esophageal varices*); the hemorrhoidal veins do not get engorged in portal hypertension. Even if hemorrhoids are present in these cases they are idiopathic, and not caused by the raised portal venous pressure.

Splenomegaly and ascites develop as late features of portal hypertension.

Clinical features

Portal hypertension is responsible for some of the most severe cases of hematemesis. If the patient is known to have cirrhosis, hemorrhage should be assumed to be coming from esophageal varices until proved otherwise. In most cases the spleen is palpably enlarged.

Prehepatic

The patient is usually a *child or a young adult*. He may be brought for a sudden hemorrhage or for weakness due to anemia. The liver is impalpable but the spleen is obviously enlarged. Anemia is due partly to hypersplenism. Liver function tests remain normal as the disease advances. *Splenoportography* displays the site of the block.

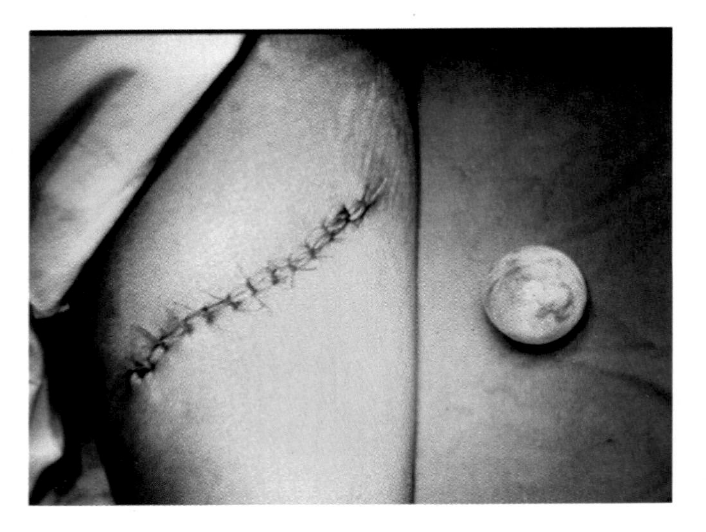

Fig.21.2 Hydatid cyst removed from thigh of young woman, showing that such a cyst can be found anywhere

Intrahepatic

The patient is normally an *adult* and suffers from hepatic cirrhosis. Enlargement of the veins of the abdominal wall radiating from the umbilicus may be present (*Caput medusae*). As long as hypertrophy of liver tissue is sufficient to compensate for cellular destruction by cirrhosis, the liver function tests remain normal. The varices can be seen through an esophagoscope.

Modified child's classification (C.T.P. score)

This classification is useful for evaluation of the severity of the liver disease and prediction of the risk of death. This is based on:

- Serum albumin and bilirubin levels.
- Ascites.
- Encephalopathy.
- Prothrombin time.

Investigations

Laboratory

Operative procedures in patients with compromised liver function carry significantly increased risk. Therefore, evaluation of the patient's hepatocellular reserve is important when selecting treatment for bleeding varices. Recommended laboratory investigations include the following:

- Full blood count for anemia, leucopenia and thrombocytopenia.
- Liver function tests to indicate primary cause of liver disease.
- Serum albumin and prothrombin time to determine efficacy of synthetic function.

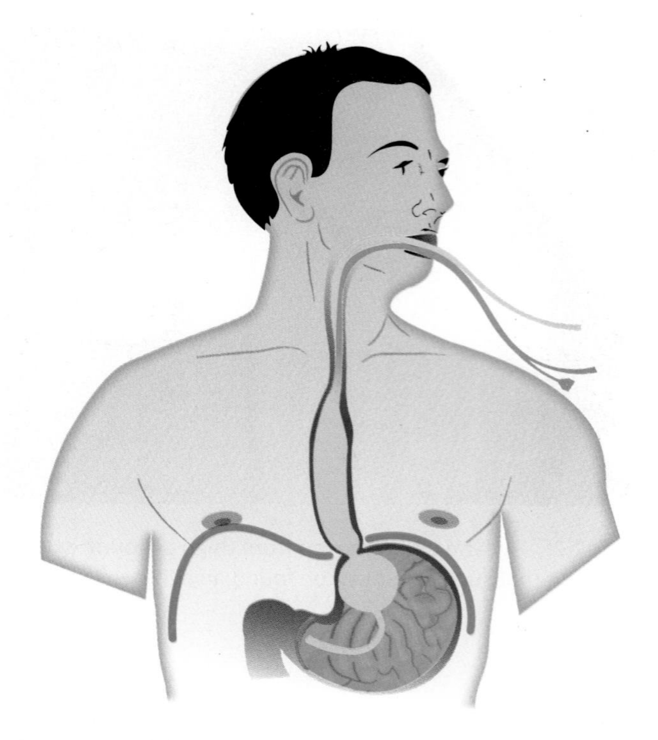

Fig.21.3 Balloon tamponade by a Sengstaken tube. The pressure in the esophageal balloon should be 40mm Hg. The stomach balloon should contain at least 300ml of air.

- Autoantibodies: in primary biliary cirrhosis and chronic active hepatitis.
- Serological markers of hepatitis B and C.
- Blood grouping.

Endoscopy

- This not only *confirms* the presence of varices but also determines whether or not they are bleeding, and therefore removes any doubt about the source of the hemorrhage.
- It is of vital importance in *excluding* other causes of bleeding, such as peptic ulcer, gastritis, duodenitis, or an esophageal tear.
- At the same time the varices can be band ligated to cause them to fibrose, band ligation having replaced sclerotherapy.

Imaging

Numerous imaging methods help the clinician in cases of portal hypertension. When operative intervention is planned, information about the anatomical details of the portal circulation is needed. In the past this was provided by angiography, but non-invasive methods like *ultrasound, CT and MRI* are being increasingly employed.

Angiography

Coeliac and *superior mesenteric angiography* Using a trans-femoral Seldinger catheter the coeliac trunk and superior mesenteric artery are selectively cannulated. Contrast medium is injected. X-rays are taken while the medium is in the arteries and also when it enters the veins.

The arterial phase can show up hemangiomas as well as tumor circulation in the case of liver malignancies. The venous phase allows evaluation of the splenic vein and can demonstrate esophageal varices.

Ultrasound

Because it is non-invasive and provides detailed and accurate information, ultrasound scanning is now the first-line investigation in portal hypertension. It clearly shows up thrombosis of the portal vein and its tributaries, as well as the resulting large collateral veins. Portasystemic shunts can be measured and graft occlusion demonstrated.

CT scanning

This can also demonstrate the above lesions, but ultrasound and MRI can do so more easily and accurately, therefore CT is rarely the procedure of choice.

MRI

This allows excellent parenchymal visualization, imaging in any plane and better blood vessel imaging than CT. It is limited by long imaging times. However, it gives better definition of soft tissues than computed tomography, and is displacing it in this as in many other fields.

Treatment

The following methods of treatment are available for dealing with esophageal varices resulting from portal hypertension:

- ***Oral propranolol*** in a dose sufficient to reduce the resting pulse rate by 25% reduces portal pressure, both by a decrease in cardiac output and by causing constriction of the splanchnic arteries. It reduces the frequency of re-bleeds and some studies show it to be as effective as sclerotherapy.
- ***Vasoconstrictor therapy***. The main use of this is for emergency control of bleeding while waiting for endoscopic band ligation. Vasoconstrictors restrict portal inflow by splanchnic arterial constriction:
  - o Vasopressin is given by intravenous drip, 25 units/hour, preferably by a central venous catheter to avoid local spill and necrosis. It is contraindicated in patients with angina, as generalized vasoconstriction results.

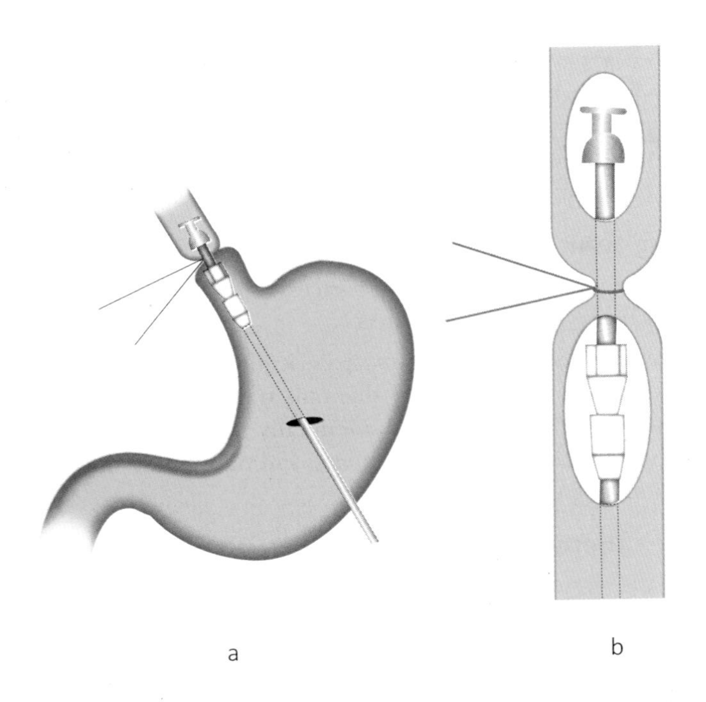

Fig.21.4 Esophageal transaction and reanastomosis with circular stapler. (a) Through a gastrotomy the stapler has been introduced and passed up into the esophagus. Between its jaws a thread is being tied around the esophagus. (b) The thread is tied; the stapler will now be fired, its jaws will come together, and will transect and reanastomose the esophagus.

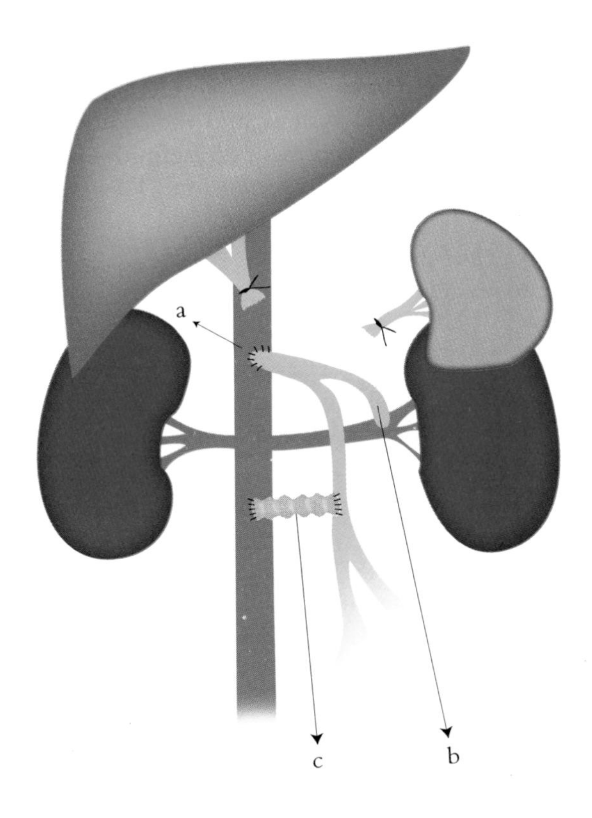

Fig.21.5 Different kinds of porta-systemic shunts: (a) Portocaval, (b) Splenorenal, (c) Mesocaval

- o Octreotide, a somatostatin analogue, 50mm Hg bolus followed by 50 μgm/hour for 48 hours, produces splanchnic vasoconstriction without systemic effects, and therefore should now be used as first-line treatment.
- Band-ligation. Each varix is ligated with a band.

  Although both sclerotherapy and band–ligation are effective, ligation is better, and is the preferred option.
- ***Balloon tamponade.*** If the bleeding is so brisk that endoscopic evaluation is impossible, tamponade is carried out by a Sengstaken tube (Fig.21.3). This tube has a rounded inflatable balloon near its tip and a long cylindrical balloon just proximal to it. The tube is passed into the stomach and the distal balloon inflated with 300ml of air. The tube is now gently withdrawn until the balloon impinges on the cardia. The long proximal balloon is now lying in the distal esophagus. It is inflated to a pressure of 40mm Hg, causing pressure on the varices and arresting hemorrhage. When the esophageal balloon is deflated after some hours bleeding has often stopped. A couple of days after this, band ligation can be carried out through esophagoscopy.
- ***Esophageal transection and re-anastomosis.*** Through a gastrotomy a circular stapler is passed up the lumen of the esophagus. A thread is tied around the esophagus opposite the groove in the stapler. When the stapler is fired, the instrument divides the esophagus and re-anastomoses it with a circular row of staples, so that the vessels across the anastomosis are disconnected (Fig.21.4). With this, the high-pressure portal system of veins is disconnected from the low-pressure systemic veins. It is used as an emergency surgical procedure in bleeding varices.
- ***Transjugular intrahepatic portacaval stent shunt* (TIPSS).** This method has revolutionized the emergency treatment of variceal hemorrhage, and has become the main treatment of hemorrhage from the varices that have not responded to drug treatment and endoscopic therapy. This is a most ingenious method to reduce the portal venous pressure, and is used with local anesthesia and fluoroscopic and ultrasonic control. A guide wire is passed from the jugular vein downwards into the liver and an expandable metal shunt is forced through the liver substance to form a channel between the portal and systemic venous systems. It is used in cases where

the bleeding cannot be stopped by any other method.

- ***Portosystemic shunts.*** These shunts drain the high pressure portal system into the low-pressure systemic veins. They represent the definitive surgical procedures for portal hypertension. They can be carried out at three sites (Fig.21.5):
  - o *Portocaval* shunt. The portal vein is anastomosed end-to-side or side-to-side to the inferior vena cava.
  - o *Splenorenal* shunt. The spleen is removed. The proximal end of the splenic vein is anastomosed end-to-side to the left renal vein.
  - o *Mesocaval* shunt. The superior mesenteric vein is anastomosed to the inferior vena cava, the distance between the two being bridged by a vascular graft made of PTFE (polytetrafluoroethylene). Physiologically and hemodynamically this is similar to the side-to-side portacaval shunt.

Indications for surgery in portal hypertension

- **Variceal bleeding.**
  - o *In emergency* when non-operative measures fail, the following procedures may be life-saving:
    - ▪ Esophageal transection.
    - ▪ Esophago-gastric devascularization.
  - o *Re-bleeding* may be prevented by shunts:
    - ▪ Portocaval.
    - ▪ Mesocaval.
    - ▪ Splenorenal.
- **Ascites**: In severe ascites, peritoneo-venous shunts may be employed.
- **End-stage liver disease**: Liver transplantation.

Emergency treatment

If the patient comes into the emergency department with massive hemorrhage from varices, initial resuscitation is carried out by *urgent transfusion*, colloids being used while waiting for blood to be arranged. Vasoconstrictor therapy using vasopressin appears to be valuable. The addition of nitroglycerine is advantageous, as it reverses the adverse systemic cardiovascular effects of vasopressin.

Emergency endoscopy should be available round the clock. This is required for confirming the diagnosis of bleeding varices, and a sclerosing agent should be injected into the varices at the time of the emergency endoscopy. If this successfully controls hemorrhage a Sengstaken tube will not be required, and the patient will be spared the inconvenience and the dangers of balloon tamponade by this tube.

If emergency sclerotherapy fails to control the hemorrhage a *Sengstaken tube* should be inserted to arrest the bleeding. It is only rarely that *esophageal transection* will be required for emergency control of variceal hemorrhage; usually sclerosing injection treatment suffices for this purpose.

Long-term control of varices

For the long-term control of varices, oral *propranolol* on a daily basis has been suggested.

*Repeated sclerothera*py into varices is the most popular method today. However if this fails transection, or one of the shunts, can be used. Generally speaking, shunts are used in the better-risk patients, and transection in the poorer-risk cases.

The different shunts

Of the various shunts the *portacaval shun*t is the most effective. However, it diverts the venous drainage of the intestine away from the liver and prevents prompt metabolism of the products of digestion, such as ammonia and the various amines; it therefore results in a high incidence of encephalopathy, with confusion, drowsiness, jaundice, and hypoglycemia.

The *more peripheral shunts*, i.e. splenorenal and mesocaval, are less often followed by encephalopathy. However, they are also somewhat less effective in reducing portal pressure and the frequency of variceal bleeds. In children with portal vein thrombosis only the peripheral shunts can be utilized.

Finally, in patients with *end-stage liver disease* and marked hepatic dysfunction, after the bleeding has been controlled with sclerotherapy or TIPS, liver transplantation is often appropriate.

TUMORS OF THE LIVER

Benign tumors

The most common benign hepatic tumor is *cavernous hemangioma.* Women are affected six times more commonly than men. These tumors are solitary subcapsular growths. Spontaneous rupture may cause severe hemorrhage. A large hemangioma may occasionally behave like an arteriovenous fistula and produce cardiac hypertrophy and congestive heart failure. Symptomatic hemangiomas can be excised, but this is rarely necessary.

Primary malignant tumors

Hepatocellular carcinoma (HCC)

Pathology

Primary carcinoma of the liver [hepatocellular carcinoma (HCC)] is one of the most common cancers in the world. It arises mostly as:

- A complication of cirrhosis resulting from chronic hepatitis B and C.
- Secondary to hemochromatosis, primary biliary cirrhosis, alcohol etc.

The *histological varieties* are hepatocellular carcinoma (HCC) and cholangiocarcinoma.

Macroscopically, a carcinoma of the liver can take one of three forms:

- A single large mass.
- Multiple nodules, commonly in cases with cirrhosis.
- Diffuse infiltration of tumor throughout the liver.

In 70% of patients distant spread has already occurred when the condition is first diagnosed. The tumor may be highly vascular. This sometimes leads to massive intraperitoneal hemorrhage from rupture of the tumor.

Clinical features

The diagnosis is not easy especially in the early stage. Abdominal pain, anorexia and distension are the most common symptoms. Pain may be felt in the epigastrium and right hypochondrium, and may be referred to the tip of the right shoulder. Weight loss and jaundice are common.

The liver is enlarged in 80% of cases, and a mass is palpable in most of the rest. An arterial bruit may be heard over the liver, and is a good clue to the diagnosis. Ascites or gastrointestinal bleeding from varices may occur. Fever may be present, and in tropical countries a diagnosis of amebic liver abscess may be made. A primary site should be looked for, because secondary carcinoma of the liver is very much more common than the primary variety.

Investigations

- *Alpha-fetoprotein* may be elevated. This glycoprotein is normally present only in the plasma of the fetus. It is produced by the cells of carcinoma of the liver because they have de-differentiated and reverted to their fetal type of metabolism. An AFP of over 200 ngm/ml is strongly suggestive of HCC.
- *Ultrasound* is a very useful investigation. It distinguishes between solid and fluid-containing areas, and also between solids of different densities.
- *CT scan* and *MRI* give an even better image than ultrasound.
- *Fine needle aspiration cytology (FNAC)* establishes the histological diagnosis, but care must be taken not to cause a secondary hemorrhage, which can assume dangerous proportions in occasional cases.
- In high-risk patients (with cirrhosis), screening and surveillance with serial ultrasound and alpha-fetoprotein (AFP) is helpful in early diagnosis.

Complications

The complications that can arise in cases of hepatic carcinomas consist of sudden intraperitoneal hemorrhage and portal hypertension from portal vein obstruction. Liver failure is a common cause of death.

Treatment

Only surgical resection offers a possibility of cure. Hepatic resection if possible is the treatment of choice but is possible in only 25–30% of the patients. In cirrhotic patients only segmental resection (1–2 segments) is advisable. If the tumor extends to the opposite lobe or if cirrhosis is present, which increases the risk of liver failure, resection is not feasible, but transplantation can be considered. Many 5-year survivals have been reported after hepatic lobectomy. Otherwise the average life expectancy after diagnosis is only 6 months.

A small primary carcinoma of the liver occurring in the presence of cirrhosis, which precludes even partial resection of the liver, is an indication for total hepatectomy and transplantation. If the effects of chronic hepatic failure and portal hypertension are absent, the patient is a good surgical candidate. Cancer recurs in about half the patients within 1 year of liver replacement; long-term disease-free survival is seen in the other half.

Palliation

In patients who are not candidates for resection:

- *Intra-lesional ablation* using ethanol may be employed.
- In other cases *transarterial chemoembolization* (TACE) is utilized. In this method a combination of a chemotherapeutic agent and lipiodol is injected into the tumor, followed by artificial emboli to produce ischemia and tumor necrosis.

Metastatic tumors

In the liver, metastatic tumors are 20 times more common than primary tumors. Cancers of the breast, lung, pancreas, stomach, large intestine, kidney, ovary and uterus account for most of the cases. Weight loss, fatigue and anorexia are the common complaints, with right upper abdominal pain, ascites and jaundice. The liver is usually enlarged and may be nodular.

If ultrasound scanning is used to direct the needle, biopsy can establish the diagnosis. CT with I/V contrast will confirm the diagnosis and is helpful in selecting patients for surgery.

Hepatic resection if possible is the only effective treatment modality. Metastatic tumors from colorectal cancer and some neuroendocrine tumors are major indications for surgery. If confined to one lobe, lobectomy may be considered, and 40% 5 year survival rates have been reported if the primary tumor was in the colon. Systemic chemotherapy does not improve survival. Hepatic artery perfusion by cytotoxic agents has benefited some patients temporarily.

Chapter

22 GALLBLADDER

CONGENITAL ANOMALIES

Embryology

The hepatic diverticulum arises fom the ventral wall of the foregut and elongates to form the bile duct. This divides into many branches which join up with the canaliculi attached to the liver cells. At the same time the bile duct gives off a lateral bud which forms the gallbladder.

Anomalies

The gallbladder may be *absent.* It may have a *mesentery.* In rare cases there may be a *double* gallbladder. Most of the anomalies pertain to cystic duct and cystic artery. *The cystic duct may be absent.* In such cases injury to the common duct can occur during cholecystectomy.

BILIARY ATRESIA

In this condition the bile ducts are obliterated and the newborn suffers from obstructive jaundice. Biliary atresia is classified into three types (Fig.22.1):

- Type I — Atresia restricted to the common bile duct.
- Type II — Atresia of the common hepatic duct.
- Type III — Atresia of the right and left hepatic ducts.

The common causes of jaundice in the newborn are three: physiological jaundice, neonatal hepatitis and congenital biliary atresia. If the jaundice is physiological it should clear up in two or three weeks. If it persists after that period, a thorough evaluation should be carried out.

Management of suspected biliary atresia

Ultrasound scan is the basic and non-invasive investigation. Biliary atresia should be suspected if the gall bladder is shrunken or not seen.

Hepatobiliary isotope scan can differentiate biliary atresia from other conditions. Diisopropyliminodiacetic acid scan (DISIDA) is generally used for this purpose:

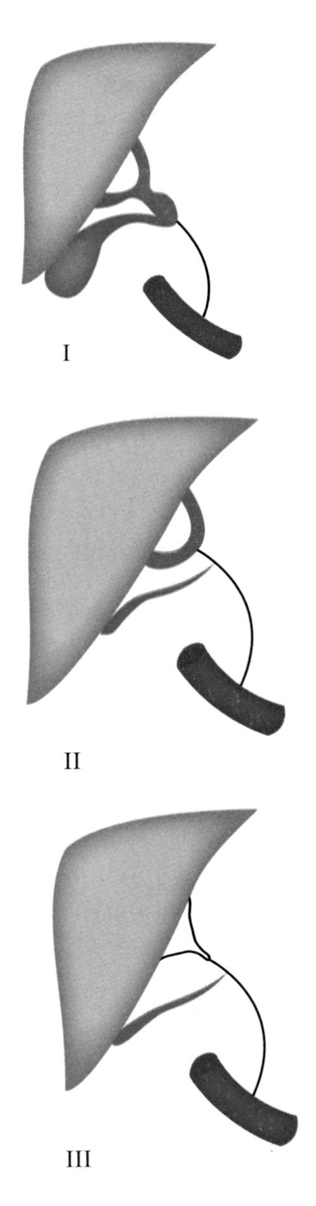

Fig.22.1 Different types of biliary atresia (see text opposite).
I. Restricted to common bile duct
II. Atresia of common hepatic duct
III. Atresia of right and left hepatic duct

- If the isotope is detected in the intestine, it confirms ductal patency and excludes biliary atresia.
- Non-visualization of the isotope in the intestine after 24 hours indicates biliary atresia.

Percutaneous liver biopsy is an essential part of the investigations.

Operation

If radionuclide scan indicates biliary atresia the abdomen is explored, usually by a right paramedian incision:

- In *type 1 lesions* a patent proximal bile duct is found. A *Roux-en-Y hepaticojejunostomy* is followed by bile flow in three-fourths of the cases.
- *Type 2 and 3 lesions* cannot be dealt with by hepoaticojejunostomy and have to be treated by the Kasai operation.

  Kasai operation. Before this procedure these types were considered inoperable. However, Kasai from Japan showed that the porta hepatis can be transected to demonstrate bile passages of a diameter of about 200 microns. All bile duct tissue upto the porta hepatis is radically excised. A loop of jejunum is now anastomosed to the porta (*portoenterostomy*). As bile starts to flow the bile passages gradually dilate. In three fourths of the cases the bilirubin level falls to normal; the great majority of these infants survive for 10 years or more.

  Portoenterostomy is successful only if carried out within the first six weeks. After this, so much cirrhosis has taken place that the previously existing bile passages inside the liver have become obliterated. Thus awareness of this condition is important, because only then can diagnosis be made early enough to be of any use. Both undergraduates and pediatric residents should be taught that *if a case of neonatal jaundice has not been sorted out by the age of six weeks the abdomen should be explored.*
- *Liver transplantation* should be considered in infants in whom the portoenterostomy is unsuccessful. As many as 75% of the patients are alive 2 to 5 years after the transplant.

JAUNDICE

Jaundice is caused by an increase in the level of bilirubin in the serum so that the tissues, including the conjunctivae, become stained yellow. This can arise in the following different ways:

- Increased bile pigment load on the liver cells (hemolytic jaundice) (Prehepatic).
- Disturbed diffusion of bilirubin from the sinusoids into the liver cells (caused by some drugs).
- Defective conjugation of bilirubin (e.g. Gilbert's syndrome).
- Defective transport of bilirubin to the cell membrane for excretion into the bile canaliculi (intrahepatic cholestasis).
- Obstruction of the large bile ducts, e.g. from a gallstone or cancer of the head of the pancreas (extrahepatic cholestasis).

Only the last type of jaundice can be relieved surgically, and it is therefore called 'surgical jaundice'.

Symptoms

A carefully taken history helps in indicating the cause in certain cases. Drug addiction may suggest viral hepatitis from shared hypodermic syringes. In some patients with cirrhosis chronic alcoholism is responsible. Obstructing gallstones or tumors are more common in older people.

Patients with gallstone jaundice may have attacks of biliary colic, fever and chills and a history of similar attacks. On the other hand, the pain in malignant obstruction is a late feature and deep-seated and dull. In extrahepatic obstruction the stools are light in colour and the urine dark; pruritus also occurs and causes discomfort. Its exact cause is not known.

Signs

The liver is enlarged in both hepatic and posthepatic jaundice. Secondary stigmas of cirrhosis are spider angiomas, ascites, caput medusae and splenomegaly

Courvoisier's law

If the gallbladder is enlarged and non-tender this suggests malignant obstruction of the common duct. Conversely, if in a case of obstructive jaundice the gallbladder is not palpable this suggests that the cause of the obstruction is a stone in the common bile duct, the gallbladder having contracted in size due to chronic cholecystitis (Courvoisier's law). However, this law does not hold good in every case, so that absence of a palpable gallbladder does not rule out malignancy.

Laboratory tests

Serum bilirubin level

In *hemolytic* disease the increased bilirubin is mainly in the unconjugated indirect fraction. Because it is insoluble in water it does not pass into the urine (*acholuric* jaundice). The total serum bilirubin rarely exceeds 5mg/dl, because the rate of excretion in the stool increases as the bilirubin level rises, and a plateau is reached. Higher values suggest that parenchymal disease is also present.

In *hepatic* jaundice both unconjugated and conjugated bilirubin are increased. An increase in the conjugated fraction always means disease within the hepatobiliary system. Since conjugated bilirubin is water soluble it is excreted in the urine.

With complete *extrahepatic obstruction* the total bilirubin may rise upto 30mg/dl. At this point loss in the urine equals the additional daily production. If the values are still higher it suggests that either hemolysis is occurring so that a very large quantity of bile pigment is being produced, or the renal function is impaired so that these pigments are not being excreted. Obstruction of a single hepatic duct does not usually produce jaundice.

In malignant extrahepatic obstruction the serum bilirubin level usually exceeds 10mg/dl and may go upto 30mg/dl. On the other hand in gallstone obstruction the values are rarely above 15mg/dl.

Serum levels of other substances

As far as the level of fecal *urobilinogen* is concerned, hemolysis increases it; on the other hand complete biliary obstruction decreases both fecal and urinary urobilinogen.

In extrahepatic obstruction the serum *transaminase* levels (AST, ALT) are raised only slightly. High levels may occur, but only for a few days. Transminase levels above 1,000 units suggest viral hepatitis.

Hepatic *alkaline phosphatase* is produced by the epithelial cells of the cholangioles. The raised level is due to overproduction and not under-excretion. So it may occur even with focal hepatic lesions, e.g. solitary metastasis or abscess, and in the absence of jaundice. Alkaline phosphatase is also produced by bone. Therefore bone disease may complicate the interpretation of abnormal alkaline phosphatase levels. In such a case serum calcium and phosphorus levels should be determined.

In cirrhosis the serum *albumin* level falls and the level of *globulin* rises, so that the albumin/globulin ratio is abnormal.

Liver biopsy

If hepatic *parenchymal* disease is suspected a liver biopsy should be carried out.

Imaging

In patients with persistent jaundice, an *ultrasound* and a *CT scan* with I/V contrast is required in malignant obstruction for diagnosis as well as staging of the disease.

Cholangiogram

If on the other hand a *ductal* obstruction is more likely, a percutaneous transhepatic cholangiogram or endoscopic retrograde cholangiopancreatogram may be performed.

Percutaneous transhepatic cholangiogram (PTC)

A 22-gauge flexible Chiba needle is advanced through the skin and well into the liver under local anesthesia. Contrast medium is gently injected as the needle is slowly withdrawn. The procedure is watched on an image intensifier; when contrast enters a bile duct withdrawal is stopped. More contrast medium is then injected to fill the biliary tree. If the ducts are dilated the test is successful each time; if not, about two-thirds of the time.

Major *complications* include bile leakage into the peritoneum, cholangitis and hemorrhage. Therefore, it is best to plan to relieve any obstruction immediately or soon after the examination.

With the advent of magnetic resonance cholangiography (MRCP) which is far less invasive, diagnostic PTC is now less commonly performed.

Endoscopic retrograde cholangiopancreatogram (ERCP).

The sedated patient lies on his right side under fluoroscopic control. The duodenoscope is introduced into the stomach, passed along the greater curvature, and its tip lifted and passed into the duodenum. The ampulla is found on the medial wall of the duodenum. The pancreatic and bile ducts are cannulated in turn. Contrast medium is injected and x-rays taken. Diagnostic ERCP is carried out in patients where the obstruction is distally located in which case the obstruction can be relieved with the help of a stent. Another indication for ERCP is biopsy of a periampullary lesion.

Management

The foremost objective in the diagnosis of jaundice is to distinguish surgical (obstructive) from non-surgical jaundice. In most cases the history, physical examination, laboratory data and minimally invasive imaging tests allow a diagnosis to be made without invasive tests like liver biopsy or direct cholangiogram. Once obstruction is definitely demonstrated, either open operation or an appropriate minimally invasive procedure is employed for its relief.

GALLSTONES

Gallstone disease is one of the most common major surgical illnesses affecting the abdomen. It occurs mostly among women. Gallstones usually consist of cholesterol or calcium bilirubinate, or much more commonly alternate layers of these. Protein is another constituent:

Cholesterol stones

A cholesterol stone is usually single (cholesterol solitaire). It is oval or rounded, 1–2cm in diameter, pale yellow and translucent. On section it shows radiating

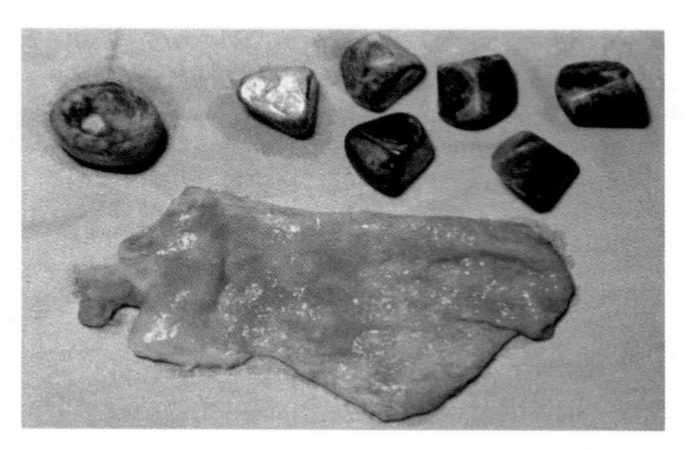

Fig.22.2 Gallbladder with one large, rounded cholesterol stone and numerous faceted mixed stones of the next generation.

crystals. About 6% of gallstones are of this type. They form in aseptic but static bile. If an oval cholesterol stone blocks the neck of the gallbladder and causes infection, the resulting numerous gallstones are faceted due to mutual pressure (Fig.22.2).

Sometimes cholesterol stones are numerous; in that case they look like mulberries. If a mulberry stone blocks the neck of the gallbladder, the resulting stones are similarly faceted (Fig.22.3)

Pigment stones

These are those stones that have less than 30% cholesterol. They are black or brown.

Black stones account for 25% of all stones. They contain a bile pigment mixed with calcium phosphate. They occur in cases of hemolysis, usually sickle cell anemia or hereditary spherocytosis.

Brown stones contain calcium bilirubinate and stearate, and cholesterol. They usually form in the bile duct due to stasis and infection, and in the presence of foreign bodies like parasites or stents.

Mixed stones

These constitute the majority of gallstones (75–80%). They are multiple and faceted due to mutual pressure. Dozens or hundreds may pack the gallbladder to capacity (Fig.22.4). On section each one is laminated; alternating layers of cholesterol and calcium bilirubinate/calcium carbonate are seen around a central nucleus of debris or bacteria.

Factors in the causation of gallstones

Metabolism

Normally phospholipids and bile salts keep cholesterol in solution in the bile. When the quantity of cholesterol in the bile increases, or exceeds the binding capacity, it precipitates out and forms calculi. In different hemolytic anemias excessive hemolysis may lead to the formation of pure pigment stones.

Bile stasis

Without stasis stones would not grow to the sizes commonly found. They would be voided while still in particulate or gravel form. Stasis is usual during pregnancy. In the formation of gallstones in multiparae, stasis probably plays an important part.

Infection

Organisms have often been found in gallstones and have long been blamed as a cause. However, gallstones can develop in the absence of infection; this shows that infection cannot be an essential factor in their development.

Clinical features

Age and sex distribution

A fat, fertile, flatulent female, forty years of age is the classic patient. However, gallstones form in both sexes. They may form at a much earlier age, and they are also common in old age. They are said to occur in 15–20% women in the child-bearing period. In old age upto 20% persons of both sexes may have gallstones.

Gallstones may remain *silent* for long periods, and are often found only at autopsy after death from some other cause. They may cause *flatulent dyspepsia*, which usually improves after cholecystectomy. Approximately one third of the individuals with silent stones develop symptoms over time.

Biliary colic

The most characteristic symptom is *biliary colic* due to gallstone obstruction of the cystic duct. Severe pain starts abruptly in the right hypochondrium, lasts for a few minutes to several hours and subsides gradually. It may also be felt in the epigastrium. It very often radiates around the costal margin to the inferior angle of the right scapula. In many cases it radiates to the tip of the right shoulder. In a severe attack the patient usually curls up in bed in agony.

During an attack of biliary colic it is difficult to examine the patient properly. Later, palpation may reveal an enlarged gallbladder. If pressure is exerted over the right hypochondrium while the patient takes a deep breath, there is a catch in the breath just before the end of inspiration (*Murphy's sign*).

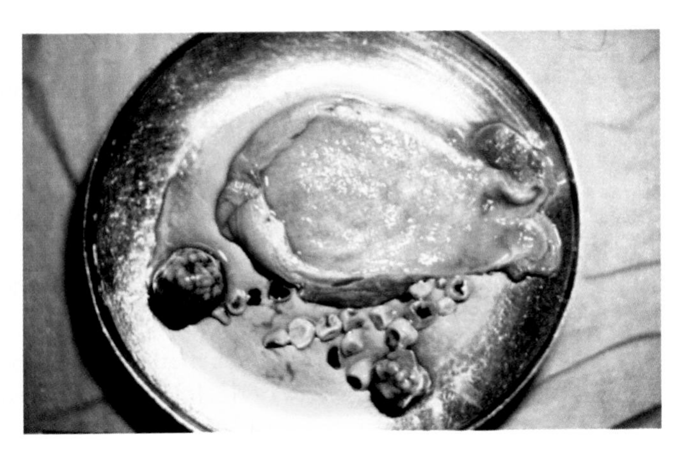

Fig.22.3 One of the two original mulberry stones blocked the neck of the gallbladder and resulted in the formation of faceted stones.

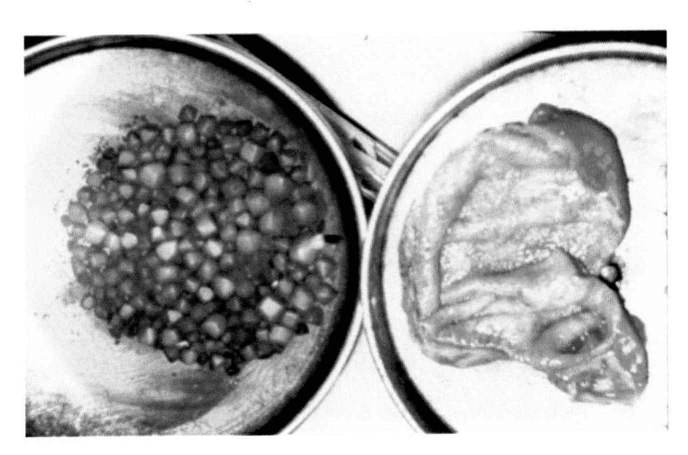

Fig.22.4 Hundreds of small faceted stones of different sizes due to repeated attacks of infection

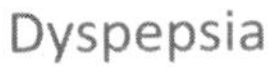

Dyspepsia

Fatty food intolerance, dyspepsia, indigestion, heartburn, flatulence, nausea and *eructations* also occur in gallstone disease. However, they are also frequent in the general population. Therefore their presence in any given patient is not necessarily due to the gallstones. Occasionally the patient may be jaundiced, as in acute cholangitis and Mirizzi's syndrome[1].

Acute cholecystitis

This results when obstruction of the cystic duct produces severe inflammation of the gall bladder with persistent pain, fever and marked tenderness in the right upper quadrant.

Investigations

Plain x-ray

This shows radiopaque gallstones in only 10% of cases, because most gallstones are radiolucent. About 50% of pigment stones are radiopaque.

Ultrasound examination

This method has revolutionized investigation of gallbladder disease. It has replaced oral cholecystography. Ultrasound is highly sensitive and specific in detecting gallstones, dilatation of intra and extra hepatic biliary ducts and in acute cholecystitis (edema/thickening of gallbladder wall with pericholecystic fluid). The cavity of the gallbladder appears black on the screen, while stones and debris look white. The ultrasound waves cannot penetrate the stone, therefore a linear shadow is seen on the side of the stone away from the ultrasound beam (*acoustic shadow*) (Fig.22.5 and 6). The thickness of the gallbladder wall can be measured to assess the degree of any inflammation, the maximum normal being 3mm. Carcinoma of the gallbladder shows up as an irregular thickening of the wall. The test takes only a few minutes, is non-invasive and without the hazard of radiation or iodine sensitivity. It is therefore the first investigation to be undertaken in a patient suspected of suffering from gallstone disease as well as in obstructive jaundice.

Treatment

Medical treatment

Dissolution by the use of the bile salt chenodeoxycholic acid is a very lengthy treatment (1–2 years) and still the recurrence rate is very high (>50%), hence it is not indicated.

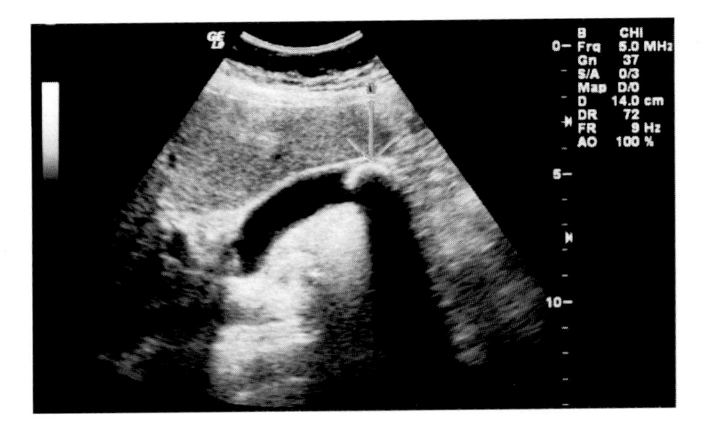

Fig.22.5 Ultrasound of the gallbladder showing gallstone with dark acoustic shadow below it

1 Mirizzi's syndrome is a rare condition in which a gallstone becomes impacted in the cystic duct, compressing the common bile duct (CBD) or common hepatic duct and resulting in obstruction and jaundice.

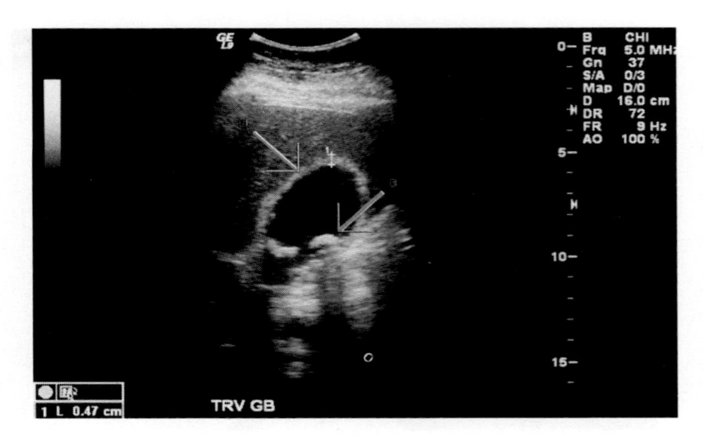

Fig.22.6 Ultrasound of gallbladder showing stone and its acoustic shadow

Surgical treatment

Cholecystectomy should be performed in most patients with symptoms. This operation removes not only the stones but also the gallbladder; if the gallbladder was left behind, the stones would form in it again.

Cholecystectomy

There are two methods of performance of chelocystectomy: laparoscopic and open.

Laparoscopic cholecystectomy

This is the commonly performed operation today. It was first carried out in France in 1987. From then on, an ever-increasing number of surgeons around the world learned this method and are utilizing it. It is currently the gold standard of treatment for gallbladder disease.

In this technique, cholecystectomy is carried out without making a full abdominal incision. Three, or sometimes four, small incisions, only 5 to 10mm in length, are made, one each in the epigastrium and umbilical scar, and two in the right hypochondrium. The umbilical scar is punctured by a Veress needle (designed to prevent injury to the gut), and the abdomen insufflated with CO_2. A laparoscope is now introduced through the umbilical port. The hypochondrial ports are used to introduce forceps to hold up the fundus and the Hartmann's pouch respectively.

Through the epigastric port a dissecting forceps exposes in turn the cystic duct and the cystic artery, which are divided between clips. Small blood vessels are sealed by diathermy. The gallbladder is finally dissected off its bed, and removed through the umbilical wound, after sucking out the bile from it.

The *advantages* of the procedure include:

- The avoidance of an abdominal wound with its attendant pain and possibility of infection.
- A short hospital stay.
- Early recovery. The patient can usually go home on the first or second postoperative day.

The *disadvantages* include:

- Insufflation with carbon dioxide with a possibility of embolism.
- The inability to dissect formally in the region of the porta hepatis due to a two-dimensional view.
- Lack of touch, and the fact that the method cannot be used in cases where the area of the hilum is obscured by dense adhesions and fibrosis.

Laparoscopic cholecystectomy should only be employed by those who have received proper training in the method. Finally, every surgeon should familiarize himself with the technique of open cholcystectomy (described below), as this may be needed if the going becomes difficult during laparoscopic cholecystectomy.

Single incision laparoscopic surgery

Research is going on to reduce the trauma of multiple ports by employing a single umbilical port for inserting all the instruments for the operation. The technique requires specially manufactured multichannel ports, is difficult to learn, and needs further corroboration before being employed for general use, but promises considerable advancement if it proves practicable.

Open cholecystectomy

A *right subcostal* or *transverse* incision can be used. A gallbladder holding forceps is applied to the fundus of the gallbladder, which is drawn up. A Lahey's forceps is applied over Hartmann's pouch and draws it up. The peritoneum is divided over Calot's triangle close to the gallbladder and the fat dissected to display the cystic artery and cystic duct. The duct is followed down to its T-junction with the common bile duct. This is important, in order to avoid ligating the common bile duct by mistake. The cystic artery and the duct are now divided between ligatures. The gallbladder is dissected away from its bed in the liver, and the resulting raw area needs hemostasis.

The common bile duct is explored:

- If stones have been shown in the duct on ultrasound examination or ERCP.
- If stones can be palpated in the duct.
- If during operation a per-operative cholangiogram is carried out through a catheter in the cystic duct, and it shows up any stone in the common bile duct clearly.

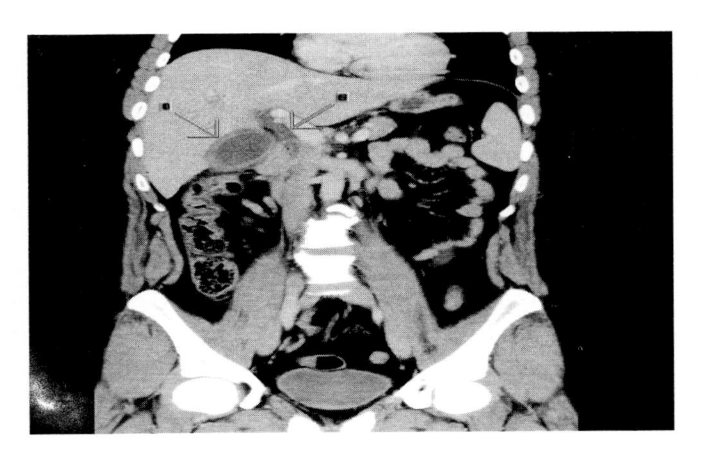

Fig.22.7 CT scan showing acute cholecystitis.

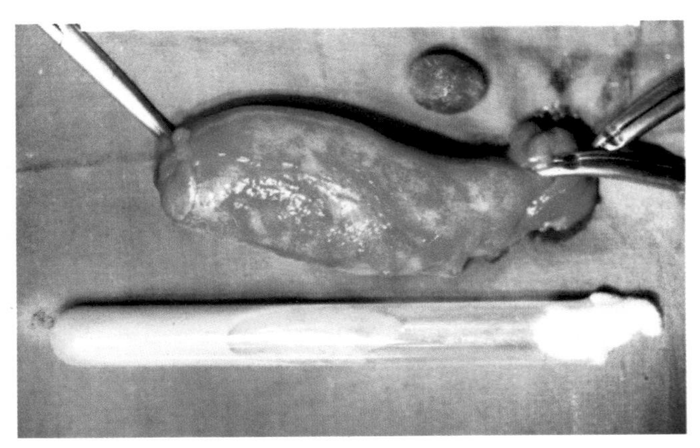

Fig.22.8 Empyema of the gallbladder removed by cholecystectomy. Note the inflamed wall of the gallbladder, the stone which was impacted in its neck, and the pus in the test tube for culture.

Per-operative cholangiogram. This procedure is performed selectively, but is almost obligatory in USA. Other indications of per-operative cholangiography include:

- A history of jaundice.
- Dilated common bile duct.
- Elevated alkaline phosphatase.
- Unclear anatomy of Calot's triangle.

Routine use of this investigation is desirable. Although it adds a few minutes to the operating time, it reduces the incidence of overlooked common bile duct stones considerably.

Asymptomatic gallstones

What advice should be given to the patient who undergoes medical examination for some other condition and where gallstones are found incidentally? The fact that only about 1/3rd of the patients with gallstones develop symptoms suggests that the decision to operate can be selective. The presence of any of the following indicates a more serious course and should serve as a reason for cholecystectomy:

- Non-functioning gallbladder, as it is more likely to be the seat of infection due to stasis.
- A calcified gallbladder ('porcelain gallbladder') because it may be associated with carcinoma.
- Diabetic and immune-compromised patients, because of the high morbidity and mortality in acute cholecystitis.

In general the tendency is to operate on most patients, on the plea that if left alone over time, they are prone to different complications; but to treat the elderly patients conservatively. If coexistent cardiopulmonary or other problems greatly increase the surgical risk, operation should be avoided.

Complications of gallstones

If stones remain in the gallbladder for any length of time, the following complications can arise: acute cholecystitis sometimes leading to perforation, chronic cholecystitis, stones in the bile ducts leading to jaundice, and occasionally carcinoma. Besides, stone in the bile duct may cause cholangitis, strictures and acute pancreatitis, which is a potentially fatal condition.

Acute cholecystitis

If a stone gets impacted in Hartmann's pouch the gallbladder becomes intensely inflamed and distended (Fig.22.7), with its mucous membrane swollen and wall edematous. Occasionally, gangrene occurs in patches. The further course of the illness may be along one of the following lines:

- The stone may get *disimpacted* as the gallbladder distends further. The mucopurulent contents of the gallbladder escape via the cystic duct and the inflammation subsides.
- Less frequently, the impaction persists and an *empyema* of the gallbladder results (Fig.22.8).
- Rarely the distended inflamed gallbladder *perforates*, with the formation of a local abscess. Unlike the situation in appendicitis, perforation into the general peritoneal cavity is fortunately rare (only 0.5% of cases), probably because the intestines and omentum get adherent to the inflamed gallbladder before it perforates, and localize the infection so that an abscess results.
- *Gallstone ileus.* Occasionally a large stone may erode through adherent walls of the gallbladder and duodenum and enter the small bowel. This stone

may cause small bowel obstruction if impacted proximal to the ileocecal valve ('gallstone ileus').

Clinical findings

The onset of acute cholecystitis is sudden. Agonizing pain occurs in the right hypochondrium. Severe nausea and vomiting occur. Fever is usual, and in fulminating cases rigors also occur. There is marked tenderness, and may be some rigidity, in the right hypochondrium. The inflamed, tender gallbladder may be palpable. Differential diagnosis is from:

- Leaking duodenal ulcer.
- High retrocecal appendicitis.
- Acute pancreatitis.
- Coronary thrombosis.
- Liver abscess.

Treatment

Conservative treatment

In 90% of cases symptoms of acute cholecystitis subside with conservative treatment. The patient is kept on nothing by mouth. Fluids and electrolytes are given intravenously. Analgesics e.g. pethidine with atropine are administered, along with broad-spectrum antibiotics. When the temperature, pulse and physical signs show that the inflammation is subsiding, glucose drinks are started, and oral feeding commenced, going on to a fat-free soft diet within a few days. About two months later when the inflammation has subsided and the adhesions resolved, cholecystectomy is carried out.

Surgery

If one of the following conditions is present *immediate operation* is advised:

- If there is uncertainty about the diagnosis e.g. when perforated duodenal ulcer or acute appendicitis cannot be ruled out.
- In typhoid cholecystitis, because perforation is common in this condition.
- In empyema of the gallbladder and suspected perforation.
- If pain and tenderness spread across the abdomen, or the pulse rate rises, conservative treatment is abandoned and cholecystectomy performed.

However, in the very ill and the elderly *cholecystostomy* may be preferred, in order to shorten the operative procedure.

Prognosis

The overall mortality rate in acute cholecystitis is 3–5%. Nearly all the deaths are in patients over the age of 60 or those with diabetes mellitus. In the older age groups secondary cardiovascular or pulmonary complications contribute to an increased mortality rate.

Gallstones in the bile ducts

(Choledocholithiasis)

Most stones in the ducts have arisen in the gallbladder; a very few (usually sludge or concretions) have formed in the bile ducts. 10–15% of patients with gallstones have their stones in the bile ducts, the figure being higher in old age.

Clinical findings

There is no great difference between the biliary colic due to gallbladder stones and that due to stones in the common bile duct. However, in the latter condition obstructive jaundice may supervene. The urine becomes dark with bile, and the stools become pale. The skin starts itching. There may be tenderness in the epigastrium. Usually the gallbladder cannot be felt because it is shrunken due to repeated attacks of inflammation. After an attack the patient may remain well for many months or may get another attack soon. Occasionally stones in the common bile duct cause acute cholangitis. In acute cholangitis due to obstruction from stones, the patient is toxic, jaundiced with high fever and chills, and leukocytosis.

Charcot's triad of symptoms is characteristic of common bile duct stones: intermittent jaundice, intermittent pain and intermittent fever. These recurring symptoms are produced as follows: the stone becomes impacted, it floats free when the duct dilates, but later impacts again.

Differential diagnosis of a stone in the common bile duct is from viral hepatitis and carcinoma of the pancreas or ampulla of Vater.

Complications

If obstruction of the bile duct is unrelieved, the following complications may ensue:

Worsening liver function

When the bile duct remains obstructed the pigments in the bile are absorbed by the mucosa of the bile ducts, which secretes some mucus. The resultant clear mucoid fluid is called *white bile*, and its presence is a bad sign as it indicates long-standing biliary obstruction. However, brisk recovery may occur after relief of the obstruction. Unrelieved obstruction lasting over four weeks causes liver damage, and the operative mortality rises greatly.

Acute suppurative cholangitis

This is a dangerous complication causing pyogenic liver abscess, liver failure, septicemia and death, and requires timely surgical drainage of the biliary tree along with antibiotic therapy.

Acute biliary pancreatitis

This results from obstruction of the ampulla of Vater due to a stone; this is an agonising complication with a high mortality.

Treatment

The treatment of calculous obstruction of the biliary tract is removal of the stones and drainage of the obstructed duct by therapeutic ERCP, or surgery if necessary. In jaundice the prothrombin level in the blood is low, due to failure of absorption of vitamin K_1, therefore this vitamin is given intramuscularly or intravenously before operation. Antibiotics are administered. Adequate hydration is required to promote diuresis and prevent the renal failure which can occur in obstructive jaundice. If the jaundice is subsiding, a few days may be allowed before operation. In the absence of endoscopic facilities and if jaundice is increasing and specially when there is fever, operation should be performed within a day. In cases with an advanced degree of jaundice the postoperative course is usually stormy.

Operation

At operation it is advantageous to mobilize the duodenum by incising the posterior parietal peritoneum lateral to it, so that it can be lifted forwards (Kocher's maneuvre). The common bile duct is opened in its supraduodenal part. Next, stone-removing forceps (of the Desjardin's type) are passed in both directions. They are advanced with their jaws open to catch any stones, and then withdrawn with the stone or stones. The bile ducts are finally flushed out, using normal saline as irrigating fluid. A choledochoscope is passed in to ensure that all stones have been removed.

The common bile duct is closed around a T-tube, the short limb of which lies in the bile duct, while the long limb is led via a tubing to a bag suspended from the side of the bed. The T-tube provides a safety valve. By the time the tube is removed after 10 to 12 days, adhesions have formed around the tube and therefore the bile does not leak into the peritoneal cavity.

With the availability of endoscopic removal of stones from the common bile duct choledocholithotomy is performed less often.

Endoscopy (Therapeutic)

This is a less invasive and safer alternative to surgery. Following clearance of the duct endoscopically, the gallbladder if present can be removed laparoscopically. Alternatively, at some specialized centres laparoscopic duct exploration can be performed along with cholecystectomy.

Injury and stricture of the common bile duct

The most common cause of stricture of the common bile duct is *damage to the duct during cholecystectomy* (open or laparoscopic).

Ductal injuries during laparoscopic cholecystectomy

The number of bile duct injuries following surgery (iatrogenic) rose sharply during the early laparoscopic surgery era (1990s). This high rate declined during the last decade on account of extensive experience and specialized training, but still the rate of bile duct injury during laparoscopic surgery is higher than in open surgery. It may be noted that currently in the USA as well as UK laparoscopic injuries are a major source of mal-practice claims.

There are two ways in which this accident commonly takes place:

- If the T-junction between the cystic duct and bile duct is not displayed, the ligature may be applied to the common bile duct by mistake.
- If sudden hemorrhage occurs and an artery forceps is blindly plunged in to arrest it, the common hepatic duct may be damaged.

Management varies with the timing of diagnosis:

- If the damage is *recognized at operation* :(10–15%)
    - o There may be a short incision in the duct; this should be closed with fine absorbable sutures, over a T-tube if necessary.
    - o The bile duct may be divided across but there is no loss of length. This should be repaired with fine delayed absorbable Polydioxenone (PDS II) sutures with a T-tube left through a separate stab incision, to minimize the chances of a stricture at the site of the division.
    - o A portion of the duct may have been excised. Here the best course is hepaticojejunostomy to a Roux loop of jejunum.
- If the damage is *unrecognized at operation* (80–85%)
    - o Persistent bile leakage may occur from the wound.
    - o If bile cannot escape through the wound, it may leak into the peritoneal cavity and produce bile peritonitis.
    - o Deepening obstructive jaundice may follow due to complete blockage or stricture of the duct.

Treatment is by re-operation:

- If the common bile duct or the common hepatic duct is divided, it is joined to a Roux loop of jejunum, which is prepared as follows: the jejunum is divided a suitable distance distal to the duodeno-jejunal flexure. The end of the proximal loop is anastomosed to the side of the distal, while the distal loop is brought up to the hilum of the liver and joined to the divided bile duct (Roux-en-Y).
- If the duct injury is very high, there is no duct available to which the jejunum may be anastomosed. In such cases the best results are obtained when the left hepatic duct, which is dilated due to the obstruction, is exposed by dissection in the groove behind the quadrate lobe ('lowering of the hilar plate') and joined to a Roux loop of jejunum. Because mucosa-to-mucosa union is brought about, there is no chance of fibrosis occurring and causing jaundice due to stenosis at the anastomosis.

In these cases it is no use trying to bring up the divided distal end of the common bile duct for anastomosis. The loop of jejunum is much more easily mobilized, has a much wider lumen and better blood supply. As such, it provides the best available replacement for the common bile duct.

Carcinoma of the gallbladder

This tumor occurs mostly in cases with gallstones. Therefore it is most common in women. The longer the history of stones the greater the chances of development of carcinoma. Most primary tumors of the gallbladder are adenocarcinomas: scirrhous, papillary or mucoid. Spread occurs early; directly to the liver and hilar structures, and by metastases to the liver and lungs. Nearly all cases have spread before symptoms appear. This tumor is not as uncommon in the East as in some western countries. These are primarily adenocarcinomas, which spread both directly as well as by lymphatics and veins. Prognosis is poor as the disease is not diagnosed early.

Clinical findings

There is pain in the right hypochondrium similar to the previous episodes of biliary colic, but more persistent. Obstructive jaundice may arise from involvement of the common bile duct. A hard mass is usually palpable in the gallbladder area. Ultrasound examination or CT scan may show gross and irregular thickening of a part of the gallbladder wall or infiltration of the liver.

Treatment

Radical cholecystectomy

If a *localized* carcinoma is found at laparotomy the most common and effective treatment is removal of the gallbladder with en bloc removal of an adjacent 2–3cm of normal liver and dissection of the lymph nodes in the hepatoduodenal ligament.

If, however, tumor is *limited to mucosa only* (as rarely happens) cholecystectomy is enough.

If gall bladder cancer is diagnosed *after* cholecystectomy for stone disease (incidental cancer), in most cases reoperation should be carried out to remove part of the liver and lymph nodes. As such cases have early disease, they have good chances of long-term survival and even cure.

If in any patient it is found that surgery is not possible, some surgeons advise endoscopic stenting of the biliary tree to reduce jaundice and a stent in the stomach to relieve vomiting.

In most *cases with liver metastases or distant spread*, surgery cannot offer much. Nor is radiotherapy or chemotherapy effective. Most patients die within a year of diagnosis.

Malignant tumor of the common bile duct

(Cholangiocarcinoma)

These tumors are less common than carcinoma of the gallbladder. They are not more common in patients with gallstones. Most are adenocarcinomas. Obstructive jaundice due to these tumors is *painless and progressive* due to increasing narrowing in the duct; in gallstone disease it is intermittent, with pain and fever. Hepatomegaly is common.

Depending upon the site of the obstruction of the common bile duct tumor the gallbladder may or may not be palpable. If cholangiocarcinoma is located at the hilum or common hepatic duct, the gall bladder is not palpable. If the biliary obstruction remains unrelieved cirrhosis, splenomegaly, ascites and bleeding varices may be seen.

Treatment

Tumors of the distal common duct should be treated by *pancreaticoduodenectomy* i.e. removal of the head of the pancreas and duodenum. At operation, it has to be decided first of all whether the tumor is resectable or not. If the growth is adherent to the portal vein, the operation has to be abandoned because this vein cannot be sacrificed.

Palliation. Palliation is required in the majority of the cases, as well as in patients not fit for surgery.

Endoprosthesis. Stents (temporary plastic or permanent self-expanding) can be placed across the tumor endoscopically by the gastroenterologist or transhepatically by the interventional radiologist.

Chapter

23 PANCREAS AND PERITONEUM

Pancreas

Annular pancreas

The pancreas develops from a dorsal and a ventral segment. Normally the ventral segment also rotates and comes to lie dorsally. If it fails to do so a collar of pancreas surrounds the second part of the duodenum and may constrict it.

Clinical features depend on the extent of the obstruction. There may be complete or partial duodenal obstruction in the newborn, or obstruction arising later in life. Because of the duodenal obstruction the infant cannot absorb the amniotic fluid swallowed by him and maternal polyhydramnios results. Therefore if polyhydramnios is present, one of the conditions which should be kept in mind is obstruction of the gastrointestinal tract at some level. If, as is usual, the constriction is distal to the entrance of the common bile duct, there is bile in the vomitus. X-rays show a dilated stomach and proximal duodenum (*double-bubble* sign).

Treatment. Fluid and electrolyte depletion is corrected, and the obstruction is bypassed by a *duodeno-jejunostomy*. The pancreas should not be divided or dissected, as a pancreatic fistula often develops.

ACUTE PANCREATITIS

Acute pancreatitis is caused by non-bacterial inflammation caused by activation, release and auto-digestion of the pancreas and peripancreatic tissue by its own enzymes. Acute pancreatitis is a serious illness with a mortality rate which may be as high as 20%.

Etiology

In acute pancreatitis, the trypsinogen and phospholipase in the pancreas get activated and cause auto-digestion of the organ.

Most of the cases of acute pancreatitis are caused by:

- Alcohol.
- Gallstones.

Other causes include:

- Metabolic i.e. hypercalcemia, hyperlipidemia.
- Iatrogenic:
  - o Surgery, ERCP.
  - o Drugs (steroids, contraceptives, estrogens, diuretics).
  - o Familial, malignancy and infections.

Pathogenesis

Previously, trypsin and other proteases were thought to initiate the process of autodigestion. Now it is phospholipase A, lipase and elastase which are considered responsible, whereas trypsin is required to activate phospholipase A. In biliary pancreatitis phospholipase A and bile salts produce lysolecithin which causes severe pancreatitis. Elastase when activated can digest vessel walls and lead to hemorrhage.

Alcoholic pancreatitis results from a combination of factors such as ductal obstruction, secretory stimulation and finally its direct toxic effect on the parenchymal cells.

Acute pancreatitis may present in two different ways:

- Acute edematous pancreatitis.
- Acute necrotizing pancreatitis (previously called hemorrhagic pancreatitis).

Pathology

In edematous pancreatitis there is mainly edema and inflammatory cell infiltration. In necrotizing pancreatitis there is bleeding into the pancreas and peripancreatic tissues, and extensive pancreatic necrosis. When pancreatic lipase is liberated it splits fats into glycerol and fatty acids. The fatty acids combine with calcium to form soaps. These calcium soaps get deposited on the peritoneum and omentum, so that these surfaces are studded with small white tubercles, which are called areas of *fat necrosis*.

In severe cases the pulmonary alveolar capillary membrane is rendered excessively permeable. This damage is supposed to occur either from fatty acids generated from serum triglycerides by lipase, or because of destruction of pulmonary surfactant. Finally, activated pancreatic proteolytic enzymes are capable of initiating intravascular coagulation.

Clinical features

The attack usually begins after a large meal. There is severe epigastric pain which radiates to the back. The pain is persistent. Vomiting and retching usually occur. *In severe cases the patient collapses from shock.*

There is profound dehydration, hypotension and tachycardia. Tenderness is most marked over the epigastrium, but may be generalized. Rigidity develops slowly. Bowel sounds are decreased or absent, and the abdomen slowly distends because of the paralytic ileus. If a mass is felt it may be the swollen pancreas (phlegmon) or a *pseudocyst.* In severe pancreatitis the blood may dissect retroperitoneally into the flank *(Grey Turner's sign)* or into the periumbilical area *(Cullen's sign).*

Laboratory findings

There is commonly a moderate *leucocytosis. Liver function* studies are usually normal, but serum bilirubin is slightly elevated (below 2mg/dl).

A serum *amylase* level above 500 I.U. is strongly suggestive of acute pancreatitis and a rise over 1,000 I.U. is diagnostic. A raised serum lipase is suggestive of alcoholic pancreatitis. In biliary pancreatitis liver enzymes (AST and ALT) and bilirubin are usually abnormal. However, acute pancreatitis can occur without a rise in serum amylase. At the same time, the level of this enzyme can be raised in other acute abdominal conditions. Therefore, the value of this test is limited. The serum *calcium* level may fall due to a combination of calcium with fatty acids (liberated from retroperitoneal fat by lipase).

Laboratory investigations are important for evaluation of the severity and outcome as in various prognostic scoring systems.

Imaging

Radiology

There may be an air-fluid level due to a dilated loop in the region of the duodenojejunal junction (*sentinel loop*). X-ray changes in the lungs are non-specific: raised diaphragm, atelectasis and pulmonary infiltrates, especially on the left side.

Ultrasound

Ultrasound examination may show a swollen pancreas and gallstones, but gives abnormal findings in only about 60% of patients with acute pancreatitis. In the rest, the pancreas cannot be adequately seen because of gas in the overlying intestines.

CT scan

This is very useful for the definitive diagnosis of acute pancreatitis as well as the presence and extent of pancreatic necrosis. It may also show stones in the gallbladder and an early pancreatic tumor. A CT scan visualizes retroperitoneal structures including the pancreas better than ultrasound, regardless of the presence of intestinal gas.

Differential diagnosis

Acute pancreatitis should be remembered as a possible cause in every case of severe upper abdominal pain, and a serum amylase estimation carried out. The following conditions may have similar features:

- Coronary thrombosis.
- High intestinal obstruction.
- Perforated peptic ulcer.
- Gallstone colic.

Prognostic markers

The risk of complications or death may be assessed by Ranson's criteria (Table 23.1). Other severity scoring systems i.e. Glasgow and APACHE II are more commonly used these days along with CT scan for estimating the extent of pancreatic necrosis.

Complications

Local

The important local complications of acute pancreatitis include:

- Infected pancreatic necrosis.
- Abscess formation.
- Pseudocyst of the pancreas.

Systemic

These include:

- Respiratory dysfunction.
- ARDS.
- Renal failure.
- DIC and multiple organ system failure leading to death.

Hypoxia develops quite often, and in severe cases

respiratory insufficiency may occur. The following steps may improve the prognosis:

- Early endotracheal intubation.
- Assisted ventilation.
- Attention to fluid and acid-base balance.
- Peritoneal lavage to wash out the exudate.

Treatment

Most attacks of acute pancreatitis are self-limiting and subside spontaneously. For a mild attack, a conservative approach with nothing by mouth, intravenous fluids, and frequent non-invasive observations, is adopted. If vomiting persists nasogastric aspiration will be required.

The principles of treatment of more severe attacks are as follows:

- Pain relief: pethidine or its synthetic analogues.
- Volume replacement with crystalloids and colloids.
- Regular arterial blood gas analysis for detection of respiratory failure and its management.
- If cardiocirculatory compromise develops, a Swan-Ganz catheter for pulmonary artery wedge pressure and cardiac output estimation.
- Management of local complications i.e.:
    - o Pseudocyst.
    - o Infected pancreatic necrosis.
    - o Abscess.
- Detection of etiological factors i.e. gallstones and alcohol, and their management.
- Nutritional support via parenteral or nasojejunal feeding tubes.

Medical treatment

The goals of medical treatment are: reduction of pancreatic secretory stimuli and correction of fluid and electrolyte derangements. Proton pump inhibitors are given as prophylaxis against hemorrhagic gastritis to which these patients are prone.

Total *parenteral nutrition* should be started and continued till the patient starts looking well. In severe pancreatitis secondary infection is likely, therefore *antibiotics* are used to prevent it; in mild cases they are not required.

The role of surgery is reactive and responsive to particular complications as they evolve in a minority of patients. In fulminant pancreatitis, during the first few days *peritoneal lavage* can remove the dark brown toxic ascitic fluid which contains kinins and other vasoactive amines, and this frequently leads to rapid improvement.

Table 23.1 Ranson's criteria of severe acute pancreatitis

On admission

Age greater than 55 years.

White cell count >16 000/mm^3.

Fasting blood glucose > 11.2mmol/l (200mg %).

Serum LDH >350 iu/l.

SGOT > 250 S.F. Units %.

Within 48 hours of admission

A hematocrit decrease > 10 %.

BUN increase >1.8mmol/l (5mg/dl).

Serum calcium < 2mmol/l (8mg/dl).

Arterial pO^2 < 7.98 kPa (60mm Hg).

Base deficit > 4 meq/l.

Estimated fluid sequestration > 6 litres.

Mortality rates are as follows:

< 3 signs:	1 %
3–4 signs:	18 %
5–6 signs:	50 %
> 6 signs:	90 %

Indications of surgery in acute pancreatitis

These are as follows:

- Treatment of a pseudocyst: a mature non-resolving or persistently symptomatic cyst will have to be drained usually internally via cystogastrostomy or cystojejunostomy.
- Treatment of gallstones or common bile duct stones.
- Drainage/debridement of infected pancreatic necrosis and abscess.
- Management of hemorrhage and peritonitis due to bowel perforation.

PANCREATIC PSEUDOCYST

This is a common complication of acute pancreatitis, occurring in about 10–20% of patients towards the end of the first week. It develops like this: in acute pancreatitis part of the exudate collects in the lesser sac. In some cases the opening into the sac gets closed by edema. The closed lesser sac then distends with more exudate and produces a smoothly rounded swelling which is dull on percussion. This is called a pseudocyst because it is devoid of any epithelial lining.

An ultrasound scan can show that the swelling contains fluid. Such a collection usually gets absorbed spontaneously within a few weeks. Although ultrasound is diagnostic, CT scan confirms the diagnosis and indicates cyst wall thickness as well as its proximity to a viscus suitable for drainage.

Management

Mature cysts (wall thickness >3mm) which do not resolve within 8–12 weeks and remain symptomatic are drained internally via cystogastrostomy or cystojejenostomy. In the former operation the stomach is opened and its posterior wall incised over the cyst. The fluid is sucked out, and sutures placed all around the edges of the opening to join the gastric mucosa to the wall of the cyst. The anterior wall of the stomach is then closed. After such free drainage the pseudocyst seldom causes any trouble. Only infected cysts are drained externally without waiting for resolution.

CHRONIC PANCREATITIS

Chronic pancreatitis is characterized by structural damage to pancreatic parenchyma leading to calcification and dysfunction. The parenchyma of the pancreas is destroyed and replaced by fibrous tissue, with formation of calculi in the ducts, which show areas of stenosis and dilatation.

Etiology

The most common *cause* of chronic pancreatitis is chronic *alcoholism*. However, a few cases are due to *metabolic* disorders e.g. hypercalcemia and hyperlipidemia. Gallstone disease can cause repeated attacks of acute pancreatitis, but rarely does it cause chronic pancreatitis.

Two types of chronic pancreatitis are commonly recognized; a common 'calcific' form and a less common 'obstructive' form. The former type is associated with alcohol abuse.

Clinical features

Chronic pancreatitis may produce no symptoms. Alternatively, there may be abdominal pain, malabsorption with steatorrhoea, or diabetes mellitus. The pain is felt deep in the upper abdomen radiating through to the back. It may last for days or weeks and may come on after intervals lasting many months. Splenic vein thrombosis may occur due to the proximity of the vein to the chronically inflamed pancreas, and may produce features of hypersplenism.

Investigations

Laboratory findings

Serum and urinary amylase may be elevated. Due to damage to the islets, insulin-dependent diabetes mellitus occurs frequently. Due to fibrosis around the lower end of the bile duct the serum alkaline phosphatase and bilirubin levels may rise. Pancreatic pseudocyst and abscess may cause leucocytosis and elevated amylase levels.

Ultrasonography

This should be carried out first. Pancreatic size is assessed; in the early stages inflammation causes enlargement with an irregular outline, while in the advanced stages atrophy may ensue. Calculi produce bright echoes.

CT scan

This is more sensitive than ultrasound in the diagnosis of chronic pancreatitis, and may distinguish between pancreatitis and pancreatic cancer.

Endoscopic retrograde pancreatography

This helps establish the diagnosis by outlining the pancreatic ducts which are irregular, with stenoses and dilatations ('multiple lakes'). *However, it can itself aggravate pancreatitis.* Occasionally a pancreatic stent can be placed across a stricture to relieve mechanical obstruction.

Treatment

Medical treatment

Diabetes and malabsorption are treated. An enteric-coated pancreatic enzyme tablet is given with each meal to improve digestion by making good the deficiency of pancreatic ferments. Anemia is corrected.

The patient should be strongly advised against the continued use of *alcohol*, and if he heeds the physician's advice, he will find considerable relief from pain. When there are also problems arising from alcoholism, social deprivation and personality disorders, management can be very difficult.

Surgical treatment

Surgery is required if pain still persists after alcohol has been abandoned. The aim of surgery is to facilitate drainage of the dilated pancreatic duct, or to resect diseased pancreas. Chronic pancreatitis with a dilated duct (6mm or above) and strictures can be treated by side-to-side pancreatico-jejunostomy; the duct is opened along the whole body of the pancreas and anastomosed to a loop of jejunum.

If the disease is even more widespread, a *subtotal pancreatectomy* is occasionally performed, leaving a remnant of the head of the gland attached to the duodenum. Suspicion of malignancy is also an indication for pancreatic resection.

CARCINOMA OF THE PANCREAS

This is a moderately common tumor which usually occurs in middle-aged people, specially in their fifties and sixties. The better-established risk factors include:

- Cigarette smoking.
- Intake of fats.
- Diabetes mellitus.
- Chronic pancreatitis.
- Prior gastrectomy and cholecystectomy.

The neoplasm may arise in the head, the body, or the tail of the gland. Two thirds of the tumors are located in the head, the rest in the body and tail. Most are adenocarcinomas, and at the time of diagnosis 85% have extended beyond the limits of the organ, most commonly to liver and peritoneum. The tumor spreads early to adjacent structures, regional lymph nodes and the liver. Distant spread occurs late.

Carcinoma of the head of the pancreas

As this carcinoma arises close to the termination of the common bile duct, it may present with *painless, progressive jaundice*. Sometimes pain in the back occurs due to infiltration of the tumor into the surrounding structures. There is also usually some loss of weight. The liver is enlarged, being distended with bile.

When the tumor obstructs the common bile duct, the gallbladder being normal distends greatly. On the other hand in obstructive jaundice due to gallstones the gallbladder being the seat of chronic cholecystitis cannot distend. Thus in jaundice due to carcinoma of the head of the pancreas the gallbladder is palpable, whereas in calculous jaundice it is not *(Courvoisier's law)*; however, there are exceptions to this rule.

Clinical features

Early features are painless progressive jaundice and anorexia. Abdominal pain radiating to the back is a late feature; so is vomiting due to duodenal obstruction and weight loss. Clay-coloured stools and itching are characteristic of obstructive jaundice. Hepatomegaly and palpable gallbladder are seen in about half of the cases (Courvoisier's sign).

Laboratory findings

Alkaline phosphatase and bilirubin levels are raised due to common bile duct obstruction. The bilirubin levels average 18mg/dl, being higher than those seen in benign obstruction. Serum transaminase levels as well as prothrombin times are also raised.

Imaging

Ultrasound

This is the initial investigation in patients with obstructive jaundice.

Endo-ultrasound (EUS)

In this test a gastroscope is passed, with an ultrasound probe being passed through the scope to lie over the bile duct opening in the duodenum. Being in direct proximity to the ampulla of vater and the head of the pancreas, it provides an excellent image of these structures; thus it is very helpful in detecting early tumors.

Endoscopic retrograde cholangio-pancreatography (ERCP)

This is helpful in the diagnosis as well as biopsy of periampullary tumors. In patients with biliary obstruction ERCP and stent placement is required for the temporary relief of obstruction.

CT scan with I/V contrast is very useful in the diagnosis and staging of pancreatic tumors; it is invaluable in the evaluation of the patient as regards resectability of the tumor.

Laparoscopy

This can demonstrate even 2–mm nodules on the surface of the liver, peritoneum or omentum, which cannot be shown up by any other method.

Periampullary tumor

Tumors which are located within 1cm of the ampulla of Vater are called periampullary tumors irrespective of their origin (pancreatic duct, bile duct, or common channel). This tumor obstructs the common bile duct early. The history and clinical presentation are similar to those of carcinoma of the head of the pancreas. However, it differs from the latter in the following respects:

- It occurs at a somewhat earlier age.
- It spreads locally and metastasizes more slowly.
- Jaundice occurs early, so the tumor is *often diagnosed while still curable*. Weight loss and pain are less prominent.
- The stool often contains occult blood due to ulceration of the tumor.

- In occasional cases the only symptom is persistent nausea. Ultrasound shows some dilation of common bile duct. Endo ultrasound may show a 1cm tumor, with positive brush-washing. Such a tumor has an excellent prognosis.

Treatment

Whipple's operation

The only treatment offering any prospect of cure for either carcinoma of the head of the pancreas or periampullary carcinoma is excision of the head of the pancreas. As the duodenum is so intimately related to, and has a common blood supply with, the head of the pancreas, it has to be removed with it. The operation is called pancreatico-duodenectomy (Whipple's operation).

The standard procedure for a carcinoma of the head of the pancreas or the ampulla is a pylorus-preserving pancreatoduodenectomy. After the excision the stomach is joined to a Roux loop of the jejunum, to which the pancreatic and bile ducts are also anastomosed. The operation carries a high morbidity and mortality rate. The 5-year survival rate after surgery is quite low. In the case of carcinoma of the head of the pancreas it is only about 10–20%; with periampullary tumors it varies from 30–40%.

Palliation

As 3/4th of the pancreatic head tumors are unresectable, palliation to relieve the jaundice may be required in the majority of cases. The different modalities available for palliation are:

- Biliary-enteric bypass can be carried out in the form of choledochojejunostomy or cholecystojejunostomy.
- Self-expanding metallic stents are placed endoscopically across the tumors in those cases that are either not fit for surgery or refuse surgery.
- For the relief of pain from pancreatic tumor, transcutaneous blockage of the coeliac axis can be carried out under fluoroscopic control.

Carcinoma of the body and tail

As these carcinomas lie at a distance from the common bile duct, jaundice is uncommonly seen in these cases. The presenting features are pain, weight loss, and finally the appearance of a mass. Unfortunately, by the time a mass becomes palpable it is too late. If the patient has only vague pain and weight loss he may be labelled a psychoneurotic. If back pain dominates the clinical picture, orthopedic or neurological illness may be suspected.

If a pancreatic mass is detected on ultrasound examination, *percutaneous fine needle aspiration biopsy* may be carried out under ultrasound or CT scan control, for evaluation by cytological examination. For employing this method the help of a competent cytologist is required. The only curative treatment is surgery which is possible in only 5–10% of cases due to late diagnosis.

Pancreatic islet cell tumors: Insulinoma

The islets of Langerhans contain five types of cells:

- α-cells produce glucagon.
- β-cells produce insulin.
- γ-cells produce somatostatin.
- F cells produce pancreatic polypeptide.
- Enterochromaffin cells produce serotonin.

The majority of these tumors are functioning, and among the non-functioning tumors a significant percentage is malignant.

Insulinoma

The most common tumor arising from the islet cell of the pancreas is an insulinoma. It arises from the beta cells and produces insulin.

Clinical features

- The tumor gives rise to signs of hypoglycemia. Symptoms arise due to the brain being deprived of glucose: bizarre behaviour, lapses of memory, and unconsciousness. The patient may be diagnosed as suffering from a psychiatric illness.
- Profuse sympathetic discharge may cause palpitations, sweating, and tremulousness.

Whipple's triad

This consists of three criteria (called Whipple's criteria) that suggest a patient's symptoms result from hypoglycemia which may indicate insulinoma:

- Hypoglycemic symptoms known to be produced by fasting.
- Blood glucose level below 50mg/dl during symptomatic episodes.
- Relief of symptoms by intravenous glucose.

Since most insulinomas are less than 2cm in diameter, CT scan and ultrasound fail to detect about half of them. Arteriography demonstrates upto half of the tumors due to their being hypervascular.

Other endocrine tumors are vipoma and somatostatinoma.

Investigations

With the help of helical CT and MRI, localization can be achieved in about 90% of cases. Intraoperative ultrasound is invaluable.

Treatment

Surgery should be performed promptly, because with hypoglycemic attacks permanent cerebral damage occurs, and also the patient becomes very obese. If a tumor is found it is enucleated. If not, the body and tail of the pancreas are excised and multiple sections made to detect the tumor.

Peritoneal Cavity

ACUTE PERITONITIS

Nearly all varieties of peritonitis are due to bacterial infection of the peritoneum. This is so true that when the term peritonitis is used without qualification, bacterial peritonitis is normally meant. Traditionally there are two types: the less common primary peritonitis and the more common and severe secondary peritonitis.

Bacteriology

Acute peritonitis is commonly caused by bacteria which normally reside in the alimentary tract. However, a few cases occur due to non-enteric bacteria.

Bacteria from the alimentary canal

This variety is many times more common than the other. Bacteria may enter the peritoneal cavity:

- From an inflamed organ, e.g. in acute appendicitis or cholecystitis.
- By perforation of a viscus, e.g. in a case of duodenal or gastric ulcer.
- By perforation in typhoid fever.

Usually the infection is a mixed one. The most common invaders are *Escherichia coli,* aerobic and anaerobic streptococci, and the bacteroides. Less often *Clostridium welchii* is found, besides staphylococci and *Klebsiella pneumoniae.* Many strains of E. coli, bacteroides and *Cl. welchii* produce toxins which cause severe illness or even death when they are absorbed from a large area like the peritoneum.

Bacteroides are gram-negative non-sporing bacilli resident in the lower intestine. They are strictly anaerobic and grow slowly on culture media unless there is sufficient CO_2 tension in the anaerobic apparatus. With increasing use of anaerobic cultures, their frequency and importance in the causation of peritonitis has been recognized. They are resistant to penicillin and other commonly used antibiotics but sensitive to metronidazole and clindamycin.

Bacteria not from the alimentary canal (Primary peritonitis)

Pelvic infection through the fallopian tubes is responsible for a significant number of cases. Examples of such bacteria include pneumococcus, beta-hemolytic streptococcus and gonococcus, and mycobacterium tuberculosis. If the infecting organism is the pneumococcus, the pus is slimy due to the mucopolysaccharide of the bacterial capsule. Such infection occurs:

- Mostly in patients with *impaired immunity*, specially those with ascites or with renal failure that is being treated with peritoneal dialysis.
- Also in poorly nourished young girls who squat naked on the floor; the infection is presumed to reach the peritoneal cavity by ascending via the genital tract.

Primary peritonitis can be treated with antibiotics and other medical measures.

Presentation

Acute peritonitis may present as:

- *Localized* peritonitis e.g perforated appendix, diverticulitis and pelvic peritonitis.
- *Generalized* (diffuse) peritonitis.

Spread of the infection

Infection tends to spread widely if:

- An inflamed appendix or other hollow viscus perforates before localization has taken place.
- A purgative induces violent peristalsis.
- The organisms are very virulent.
- The omentum is small, e.g. in children.
- The host defenses are compromised.

Abscess formation

If peritoneal defences cannot completely eliminate the bacteria but succeed in localizing the infective process, an abscess results. Mechanical barriers also help prevent the spread of the exudate. For example, the transverse colon and mesocolon divide the abdomen into supracolic and infracolic compartments, and discourage spread of infection from the one to the other.

Clinical features

Severe *pain* of a cutting or burning type occurs, and is made worse by moving or breathing. The patient therefore lies still. The pain is at first localized to the site of the lesion, but soon spreads out from this point. Vomiting may occur.

Marked *tenderness* and board-like *rigidity* are present if the peritonitis affects the anterior abdominal wall, otherwise both these signs are present to a lesser degree. The abdomen is *silent* due to paralysis of the intestines from the toxins of the bacteria. The *pulse* rises gradually.

Multiple organ dysfunction syndrome

Without treatment acute generalized peritonitis may *rapidly progress* to marked ileus with increasing abdominal distension, hypotension and septicemia, with ultimately respiratory, renal, hepatic and cardiac failure. This condition is called multiple organ dysfunction syndrome. In such a case death may occur even after the primary focus of infection has been controlled.

On the other hand the condition *may resolve*. The pulse rate falls and the pain and tenderness diminish. The condition may localize, producing one or more abscesses, or may completely clear up. The peritoneum heals very rapidly after injury, so that mesothelial regeneration is complete within a week to ten days.

Localized peritonitis

In localized peritonitis the initial symptoms and signs are those of the causative lesion:

- If inflammation is under the *diaphragm*, pain is felt at the tip of the shouler.
- In *pelvic peritonitis* from a pelvic appendix or salpingitis the abdominal signs are often slight, but a rectal or localized peritonitis usually resolves. In 20% cases an abscess forms.

Investigations

Diagnostic *aspiration* of the peritoneal cavity may be helpful but is usually unnecessary.

Plain x-*ray* of the upper abdomen in the erect posture may show gas under the diaphragm in a case of perforated peptic ulcer.

Very high *serum amylase* levels support the diagnosis of pancreatitis, but can also occur in other acute abdominal conditions.

CT scan abdomen may be required in some patients to establish the diagnosis. CT is also useful for the drainage of localized intra-abdominal collections.

- If the cause can be established with certainty as *primary* peritonitis the treatment is conservative.
- If not, as in the vast majority of cases, operation is necessary:
  - o In *early* peritonitis treatment consists of removing the source of infection by operation. Thus the most common operations in the control of early peritonitis are appendicectomy, cholecystectomy, closure of perforated peptic ulcer and resection of gangrenous intestine. Combined with antibiotic therapy, early operation is associated with a very low mortality rate in this situation.
  - o *Advanced* and established peritonitis also requires surgery for its control.
  - o Sometimes, however, patients are seen in whom the peritonitis is *localizing,* and a period of careful observation and conservative treatment may be advised.

Treatment

The essential principles in the treatment of peritonitis are the following:

- *Fluid resuscitation*. These patients have a great deficit of fluids. The peritoneal exudate contains nearly the same electrolytes as plasma, so replacement should be by lactated Ringer's solution. Inflamed peritoneum leaks proteins, and thus plasma proteins may need to be replaced with colloids (albumin).
- *Nasogastric tube aspiration*. This is carried out until the paralytic ileus resulting from the peritonitis has recovered. In seriously ill patients the aspirate is chocolate-coloured. This colour originates as follows: in the dilated stomach and intestine, due to hypoxia and toxemia, minute erosions form in the mucosa. Small quantities of blood are lost into the lumen from these. The hemoglobin is broken down by the gastric and intestinal enzymes. Hematin is produced, which has a dark brown colour.

  When the patient's condition improves and the hypoxia and toxemia are corrected, the above process is halted. No more blood leaks into the gut, so that the colour of the nasogastric aspirate changes back from chocolate to the *normal light green or yellow. This is an extremely important sign of recovery.* Enough emphasis is not placed on this fact in the literature.
- *Antibiotics.* These prevent the multiplication of bacteria and the release of endotoxins. As the infection is usually polymicrobial, initially parenteral third generation cephalosporins or ciprofloxacin, and metronidazole, may be given. In more serious

infections with impending septic shock, imepenem or meropenem are preferred.

- *Surgical correction* of the cause should be carried out as soon as the patient is fit for operation. At surgery, after the cause has been dealt with, the pus in the peritoneal cavity is all sucked out. The cavity is then irrigated with normal saline and sucked dry.

With modern treatment diffuse peritonitis carries a mortality rate of 10%. The lethal factors include:

- Bacterial toxemia.
- Paralytic ileus.
- Electrolyte imbalance.
- Bronchopneumonia.

The very advanced case

Rarely, specially in the aged and debilitated, the patient's condition has deteriorated to the point where anesthesia and surgery would be lethal:

- An interventional radiologist may be able to drain all intraperitoneal collections under CT guidance with appropriately placed catheters.
- If such help is not available, a corrugated drain should be placed into the peritoneal cavity at the flank on either side through a small incision under local anesthesia. A large quantity of pus is thus drained away. This reduces the toxemia sufficiently to save the patient's life, and render him fit in a day or two for laparotomy under general anesthesia for the full surgical treatment of the condition.

Complications of peritonitis

Besides the complications of any bacterial infection, there may be:

- *Intestinal obstruction* due to adhesions. *Fluid levels* are seen to be larger as one proceeds distally, till the site of obstruction is reached. Thus in upper jejunal obstruction there are only a few levels in the left upper abdomen; in the lower ileum the levels are distributed all over the abdomen, being larger at the lower levels.
- *Paralytic ileus*. Air-fluid levels of equal size are distributed throughout the small and large intestine, because the whole of the intestine is paralysed. The abdomen is silent.

  If organic obstruction is clearly shown to be absent, the following regimen should be employed:

  - The *serum electrolytes* are estimated. If the potassium level is low, the deficiency is made good. Any other electrolyte imbalance is also corrected.
  - Now three injections of *neostigmine* 0.5mg are given intramuscularly at intervals of two hours. In a significant number of cases wind is passed and the distension subsides.
- *Residual abscesses*. Intra-peritoneal collections of pus are an important cause of post-operative paralytic ileus and toxemia; in suspected cases ultrasound or CT-guided drainage may be required. The common sites are subphrenic, pelvic and midabdominal (paracolic and central).

Peritonitis after abortion

The abortionist has usually pushed an instrument through the uterine vault and streptococcal peritonitis occurs:

- If the infection is *confined* to the pelvis the treatment is conservative with antibiotics, nasogastric aspiration and intravenous fluids. If a pelvic abscess forms it is drained through the vagina.
- If peritonitis is *generalized* a laparotomy is required. Commonly a loop of small or large intestine has been perforated, and requires repair or resection. As the treatment of the generalized peritonitis is sometimes neglected in this situation because of social factors, multiple organ dysfunction syndrome can supervene.

Meconium peritonitis

This is the term applied to any antenatal intestinal perforation:

- When the perforation occurs *early* in intrauterine life the meconium causes an inflammatory reaction and calcification within the peritoneal cavity. The baby vomits bile and shows all the signs of intestinal obstruction. X-ray shows air-fluid levels and calcification. At operation there are widespread adhesions and a localized mass of intestines encased in a dense inflammatory reaction. The bowel has to be dissected out of the adhesions and the perforated loop exteriorized.
- When the perforation occurs *late* in intrauterine life there is no calcification. The infant is born with a hugely distended abdomen which interferes with respiration. Ultrasound shows an abdomen full of fluid, with little gas. Prompt *paracentesis* is performed to decompress the abdomen and relieve the respiratory distress. The perforated loop of intestine is *resected*. The prognosis is bad, but recovery follows prompt operation in some cases.

INTRA-ABDOMINAL ABSCESSES

Subphrenic abscess

There are four important intraperitoneal subphrenic spaces, two on either side. On the right side there are the right subphrenic and the right subhepatic spaces. On the left side lie the left subphrenic space and the lesser sac. Besides these there is an extraperitoneal space, the bare area of the liver.

The right subphrenic space lies between the liver and diaphragm, bounded posteriorly by the coronary and right triangular ligaments. Abscesses here are commonly due to a perforated duodenal ulcer, a perforated gallbladder, and appendicitis.

The right subhepatic space (Morrison's pouch) lies between the liver and the right kidney, with the duodenum medially and the hepatic flexure below. It is the most common site of a subphrenic abscess, which usually arises from appendicitis, cholecystitis, perforated duodenal ulcer, or after upper abdominal surgery.

The left subphrenic space. This space lies between the diaphragm and liver, bounded posteriorly by the triangular ligament. Common causes of an abscess here include complications after operations on the stomach, tail of pancreas, spleen or splenic flexure of colon.

The lesser sac. This cavity lies below the liver, with the lesser omentum and stomach lying in front. The causes of abscesses here include pancreatitis and perforated posterior gastric ulcer or cancer.

Clinical features

The symptoms and signs of a subphrenic abscess are often obscure. The old saying 'pus somewhere, pus nowhere, pus under the diaphragm' is often appropriate.

Symptoms

Commonly the history is as follows: after an infective focus in the abdomen has been dealt with, the patient's condition improves temporarily, but after a few days symptoms of toxemia reappear. The condition steadily deteriorates. Sweating, wasting and anorexia are present. There may be epigastric fullness and pain, or pain in the shoulder from irritation of the phrenic nerve referred to the cervical plexus.

Signs

If the abscess is anterior, the abdominal examination will reveal tenderness, rigidity or even a palpable swelling. Examination of the chest may reveal collapse of a lower lobe or a pleural effusion.

Course

If left unrecognized and untreated, a subphrenic abscess may rupture into a bronchus, or the peritoneum or pleura, with serious consequences. The mortality rate in neglected cases is very high.

Investigations

A marked leucocytosis is usually present. A plain x-ray may show an air-fluid level below the diaphragm with a pleural effusion above it. Ultrasound and CT scans are diagnostic.

Treatment

The treatment of subphrenic abscess is drainage under antibiotic cover. Ultrasound-guided or CT guided *percutaneous aspiration catheter drainage* has largely replaced open drainage in the management of subphrenic abscesses. With this method the large wounds and postoperative pulmonary complications associated with open trans-abdominal drainage have diminished greatly.

Pelvic abscess

The common causes of a pelvic abscess include pelvic appendicitis, salpingitis and generalized peritonitis from any cause. *Neisseria gonorrhoeae* and *C. trachomatis* are the primary pathogens responsible for salpingitis in sexually active women. This abscess is easily recognized if suspected. There is fever, lower abdominal discomfort, and diarrhea with passage of mucus. The abscess may subside or progress to a tense mass bulging into the vagina or the anterior rectal wall. Rectal examination discloses tenderness and a fullness in the pouch of Douglas.

Ultrasound

Pelvic ultrasound is valuable in corroborating the diagnosis and distinguishing an abscess from a phlegmon.

Treatment

A pelvic abscess may be drained through the rectum or the fornix (vagina). In general such drainage provides a very gratifying result with rapid recovery. In patients with a ruptured tubo-ovarian abscess, laparotomy with unilateral salpingo-oophorectomy is required.

Midabdominal abscess

These abscesses may occur anywhere within the abdomen from just below the transverse colon to the pelvis. The right and left paracolic gutters are the most common sites but an abscess may form wherever a collection of blood or foreign material has occurred. Midabdominal abscesses are particularly difficult to identify. Repeated gentle palpation for a developing mass may give the first clue.

Ultrasound and CT scan help greatly in localizing the fluid collection, and should be utilized in every case of suspected abdominal abscess. A progressively enlarging mass is an indication for drainage.

A word of warning about ultrasound: the person carrying out the examination must be properly trained and skilled. Otherwise his report may be worse than useless; it may be misleading

Tuberculous peritonitis

Tuberculous peritonitis is commonly a chronic condition. It presents with abdominal pain, fever and night sweats, loss of weight, ascites or an abdominal mass. The infection originates from tuberculosis of ileocecal region, mesenteric lymph nodes, fallopian tubes or through the blood stream from pulmonary tuberculosis. It may take the form of a generalized or encysted ascites, or may present as a plastic peritonitis.

In cases with generalized *ascites* the peritoneal cavity becomes filled with pale, straw-coloured fluid. The fluid is rich in lymphocytes, and *Mycobacterium tuberculosis* can be cultured in it. The onset is gradual. There is loss of energy, pallor and loss of weight. The patient seeks advice because of enlargement of the abdomen. A transverse solid mass can often be palpated in the upper abdomen; this is thickened and rolled up greater omentum. Treatment is by a full course of antituberculosis chemotherapy.

In the *encysted* form the fluid is walled off in a part of the abdomen. A diagnosis of mesenteric or ovarian cyst may be made.

In the *plastic* form there are widespread adhesions which cause coils of intestine, specially ileum, to become matted together and distended. These distended coils act as 'blind loops' and give rise to steatorrhoea, wasting and attacks of abdominal pain. The first indication of disease may be subacute or acute intestinal obstruction. At operation adhesions are divided and stenosed segments of gut resected. Antituberculosis drugs are used for the full prescribed period. Remarkable improvement takes place after setting the whole small gut free of the adhesions.

Tuberculosis of mesenteric lymph nodes

Tubercle bacilli are ingested and reach the mesenteric lymph nodes by way of Peyer's patches. In the developed countries following universal pasteurization of milk the bacilli are usually human, in the underdeveloped countries usually bovine. Sometimes only one lymph node may be infected, usually there are several. Occasionally massive involvement occurs. Abdominal tuberculosis is a common cause of a 'chronic abdomen' in the less affluent countries. Tubercular mesenteric lymph nodes may present clinically in one of many forms:

- A *calcified lymph node* may be seen on x-ray. The shadow is round or oval and mottled. The infection may still be active, because other uncalcified nodes may also be present. Central abdominal pain may occur. If there is tenderness in the right iliac fossa, appendicitis may be impossible to exclude, and operation may occasionally be performed.
- A coil of intestine may become adherent to a caseating lymph node and be angulated to cause *intestinal obstruction.*
- Tuberculous pus from caseating mesenteric nodes may collect between the leaves of the mesentery and be mistaken for a *mesenteric cyst.*
- Evening pyrexia, pallor, anorexia and weight loss may occur; these non-specific symptoms are seen in abdominal tuberculosis in any form.

Treatment

If the certain diagnosis of tubercular infection has been made, treatment is essentially medical.

Chapter 24 SPLEEN

Anatomy

The spleen is a purple green bean-shaped organ of the reticulo-endothelial system that lies under the left hemidiaphragm. It is covered on all its surfaces by peritoneum. However, its hilum is connected to the kidney by a fold of peritoneum, the lienorenal ligament, which contains the splenic artery and vein. Similarly it is connected to the stomach by the gastrosplenic ligament, which contains the short gastric vessels. During splenectomy each of these ligaments has to be divided and the vessels contained therein ligated.

Accessory spleen

An accessory spleen is present in 10% of the normal population, usually within the ligamentous attachments of the spleen, i.e gastrosplenic, lienorenal and gastrocolic ligaments. It is important because inability to remove it during splenectomy for various hematological disorders may lead to relapse of the original disease.

Physiology

The spleen is comprised of white pulp and a peripheral red pulp. The white pulp consists of lymphatic tissue with T-cells and B-cells; the red pulp consists of vascular structures and is responsible for the filtration of the red cells.

The endothelial *macrophages* in the spleen remove from the circulation worn-out and damaged red cells, as well as particulate foreign matter, microbes, antigens and cellular debris.

The spleen contains the largest collection of both *T and B lymphocytes* in the body. Antigen is taken up by follicular cells and presented to immunocompetent cells leading to antibody production by the plasma cells.

The normal spleen contains about 8% of the *red cell mass*, which is discharged into the circulation during emergencies such as anoxia.

The spleen is a center of *hematopoiesis*, although a minor one.

TRAUMA TO THE SPLEEN

Rupture of the spleen most often occurs in industrial or traffic accidents of the crushing or run-over type. Other organs may be injured at the same time. The spleen may also be injured during operations on the stomach, esophagus, vagus nerves etc.

Clinical features

Symptoms

The symptoms vary from minimal or no symptoms to hypovolemic shock. There may be severe left upper abdominal pain. Referred pain may be felt in the left shoulder due to irritation of the diaphragm *(Kehr's sign)*.

Signs

The signs indicate low-grade peritoneal irritation, i.e. tenderness and slight rigidity. Abdominal distension occurs due to intestinal paresis. The area of splenic dullness may be increased. With marked bleeding there is tachycardia, hypotension and shock. Tenderness may be present over the left ninth and tenth ribs.

In a few cases a subcapsular hematoma forms. The red cells gradually disintegrate and the hematoma liquefies. Increased osmolarity of contents causes expansion of the blood-filled cavity and finally rupture. This is probably how *delayed rupture* takes place days or weeks after the injury.

X-ray

On x-ray there may be obliteration of the splenic outline and of the psoas shadow, and indentation of the left side of the stomach air-bubble. Fracture of one or more ribs on the left side may be seen.

Ultrasound and CT scan

If the diagnosis of splenic trauma is suspected in a patient whose cardiovascular system is stable, an ultrasound or CT scan can be carried out to obtain information about the presence and severity of the splenic injury.

Treatment

In the past immediate laparotomy was regarded as the only reliable course of action whenever splenic injury was strongly suspected. The ruptured spleen was removed, blood evacuated, injury to other viscera excluded and the abdomen closed.

However, in due course it was found that after splenectomy the patient, specially if a small child, is very vulnerable to overwhelming infections, particularly with pneumococci. Therefore the recent trend is to treat minor injuries non-operatively and moderate injuries with suture (*splenorrhaphy*) or partial splenectomy, reserving splenectomy for extensive lacerations of the spleen. If this course is followed, different measures can be employed at operation to achieve hemostasis:

- For trivial trauma pressure can be combined with topical agents to arrest bleeding:
  - *Fibrin glue*, a highly concentrated form of fibrinogen and clotting factors, can be sprayed onto the injury or over a fractured surface. It can also be used along with sutures to seal the splenic surface after a partial resection.
  - *Microfibrillar collagen* forms a firm, adherent coagulum which traps and activates platelets. It can be packed into cracks and fissures.
- If the short gastric vessels are intact, the splenic artery can be ligated in continuity for hemostasis without infarction of the spleen.
- Sutures tend to cut through, but can be applied over collagen or teflon pledgets, or over omentum.
- The spleen may also be wrapped in omentum.

It should be emphasized that such a patient must be nursed in a critical care unit for a few days and a close watch kept for recurrent bleeding.

Rupture of a malarial spleen

If in a tropical country the spleen is greatly enlarged as a result of malaria, even minor trauma can result in its rupture. Bleeding may be extremely profuse. The operation of splenectomy in this condition is much more difficult than in a ruptured normal spleen. To avoid going through the hematoma the splenic vessels may first be ligated as they run along the upper border of the body of the pancreas.

CONDITIONS REQUIRING SPLENECTOMY

Indications for splenectomy

Always indicated:

- Splenic Abscess.
- Hydatid cyst.
- Hereditary spherocytosis.

Sometimes indicated:

- Chronic immune thrombocytopenic purpura.
- Splenic vein thrombosis causing gastric varices.
- Splenorenal shunt in portal hypertension.
- Primary hypersplenism.
- β-thalassaemia.
- Trauma to the spleen.
- Autoimmune hemolytic anemia.

In certain blood diseases, as described below, the spleen may have to be removed as part of the treatment of the illness.

HEMATOLOGICAL DISORDERS

Splenectomy may be required in idiopathic thrombocytopenic purpura, certain hemolytic anemias, and in hypersplenism from different causes.

Idiopathic thrombocytopenic purpura (ITP)

This is a syndrome characterized by a low platelet count. The platelets of affected patients become sensitized by antiplatelet IgG autoantibodies and are then removed from the circulation. The term ITP should be applied to a hemorrhagic disorder only if the subnormal platelet count is found in the presence of bone marrow containing normal or increased numbers of megakaryocytes, and in the absence of any systemic disease or history of ingestion of drugs capable of inducing thrombocytopenia.

There is a greatly reduced number of platelets, so that purpuric hemorrhages take place. The increased platelet destruction takes place in the macrophage phagocyte system, specially the spleen. As a response to this shortage of platelets, and in an effort to make good the deficiency, the number of megakaryocytes is increased.

Clinical features

Most patients are young women.

Acute form

The onset may be acute, with ecchymoses, petechiae, and bleeding from gums, vagina, urinary tract or gastrointestinal tract. In the intestine the swollen, hemorrhagic mucosa may lead to the development of intussusception or intestinal obstruction. In some patients symptoms regularly get worse during menses. The spleen is rarely palpable and if it is enlarged, the diagnosis should be reconsidered.

Chronic form

The chronic form may occur at any age. There is a gradual onset. The patient bruises easily, and may have menorrhagia.

The *platelet count* is always below 100 x 10^9/l, and at times approaches zero. Many patients need no treatment if the platelet count remains over 50 x 10^9/l. If the count falls below 20 x 10^9/l the risk of bleeding increases.

Because of the thrombocytopenia, the bleeding time may be prolonged, but the clotting time remains normal. The bleeding results in an iron deficiency anemia. The marrow shows large numbers of abnormal megakaryocytes. Before a definitive diagnosis of ITP can be made, different causes of nonimmunologic thrombocytopenic purpura, such as leukemia and aplastic anemia, must be ruled out.

Mild cases

If the patient has only *mild* symptoms, he should avoid rough sports, elective surgery and non-essential drugs.

Moderate or severe cases

In these cases corticosteroids are used, when 80% of patients go into remission on 60mg prednisolone/day. Steroids make the capillaries less permeable. However, if the disease does not respond to corticosteroids, or relapses after a remission, splenectomy is required. Although the platelet count is low, platelet transfusion is not commenced until the splenic vessels have been ligated, when 6 to 8 units of platelets may be transfused.

Prognosis

In children with acute ITP, as many as 80% have a complete and permanent spontaneous remission; this occurs in only 25% of adults. Overall, splenectomy is successful in 85% of patients, but more often in idiopathic cases than in those secondary to another disorder.

Hemolytic anemias

Hemolytic anemias in which splenectomy may be helpful include hereditary spherocytosis, β-thalassaemia, and autoimmune hemolytic anemia.

Hereditary spherocytosis

This is the most common congenital hemolytic anemia. It is transmitted as an autosomal dominant trait. In this condition the red cell membrane is more permeable to sodium ions than normal. As the sodium leaks into the cell it swells and becomes more rounded and therefore more fragile. Thus a large number of red cells are destroyed. Significant red cell destruction takes place only in the presence of the spleen. The hemolysis results in the production and excretion of excessive amounts of bilirubin, so that bile pigment stones often form in the bile ducts. During infancy the condition may resemble hemolytic disease of the newborn due to ABO incompatibility.

Clinical features

As a result of excessive hemolysis the patient is jaundiced. Due to the anemia he is pale and gets tired easily. The spleen is enlarged. Exacerbations of hemolysis may occur from time to time. During a crisis there is sudden fever, abdominal pain, nausea, vomiting and extreme pallor with increased jaundice. The red cell count may fall to 1.5 million/cu mm.

In adult cases there is often a history of attacks of gallstone colic. The gallbladder may contain pigment stones. *Whenever gallstones are seen in a child the patient should be investigated for presence of hereditary spherocytosis.*

Laboratory findings

The diagnosis is made on examination of a peripheral blood film where spherocytes and reticulocytes are seen. The red cells are more *fragile* than normal. Hemolysis occurs in 0.6% saline or even stronger solutions, whereas normally it occurs only in much more dilute solutions. The reticulocyte count is high. The patient's own red cells are *labelled with 51Cr* and reinjected; scanning over the spleen shows increased radioactivity due to sequestration of red cells.

Treatment

The spleen does not allow the defective red cells to survive long enough to be of much use, therefore it must be removed. After splenectomy, although the red cells are still abnormally shaped, they have a normal life span, so that the anemia is rectified.

In children the optimum age for operation is about seven years. Before this age splenectomy is followed by a greatly increased vulnerability to infections; after this age gallstones start to form. At operation if gallstones are present, the gallbladder is also removed. Following splenectomy the anemia and jaundice disappear. It should be remembered that *special care must be taken to treat infections in the splenectomized child promptly.*

Thalassaemia

The thalassaemias are anemias originally found in people living on the shores of the Mediterranean (Greek *thalassa*

= sea) but now affect people throughout the world. This is an autosomal dominant disorder. One of the globin chains of the hemoglobin molecule is defective. Fetal hemoglobin (HbF) persists, and can be detected by serum electrophoresis; its presence is diagnostic. This produces abnormal red cells.

Minor and major thalassaemia

- Heterozygotes have only mild anemia *(thalassaemia minor)*.
- On the other hand homozygotes have severe chronic hemolytic anemia with jaundice, gross splenic enlargement and retarded growth *(thalassaemia major)*. The peripheral blood film reveals target cells, nucleated red cells and a hypochromic microcytic anemia. The hemolysis produces an excess of bile pigments, so that 25% of patients have gallstones.

Treatment

Minor thalassaemia requires no treatment. The hemoglobin level remains at the lower limit of normal throughout life, but poses no major problems.

In *major* thalassaemia, due to excessively rapid hemolysis, blood transfusion may be required every few weeks. In order to prevent immunization to leucocyte antigens as a result of frequent transfusions, leucocyte-depleted red cell concentrates may be employed.

Splenectomy

When hemolysis becomes so severe that transfusion has to be given every 7 to 10 days, recourse must be had to splenectomy. The operation reduces hemolysis and transfusion requirements, and removes an enlarged, uncomfortable spleen (Fig.24.1).

Autoimmune hemolytic anemia

If a patient develops antibodies against his own red cells, the condition is called *autoimmune hemolytic anemia.* Both warm and cold antibodies have been described. Only patients with warm antibodies (IgG) require splenectomy. Those with cold (non-gamma) antibodies do not benefit from this operation.

Autoimmune hemolytic anemia can occur due to high doses of penicillin, quinidine or methyldopa, besides other chemical and physical agents and bacteria. Antibodies are produced which are hemagglutinins. The immunologically altered red cells are trapped in the macrophage phagocyte system including the spleen, and are destroyed.

Clinical features

The condition is most common after the age of 50. There is an acute onset of anemia, mild jaundice and sometimes fever. The spleen is usually enlarged, and pigment gallstones are often present. Coombs test is positive.

Treatment

This includes removal of the offending drug or other agent, administration of corticosteroids, and blood transfusions. Associated diseases responsible for the condition are sought and treated. Corticosteroids produce a remission in 75% of patients, but only 25% of remissions are permanent.

Splenectomy is indicated in the following situations:

- If there is no response to six weeks of high-dose corticosteroid therapy.
- If the condition improves with treatment, but a relapse occurs.
- For patients in whom corticosteroid therapy is contraindicated.

Hypersplenism

One of the important functions of the spleen is to destroy worn-out blood cells especially RBCs and platelets. If the spleen enlarges greatly for whatever reason, this function is greatly exaggerated and there is excessive destruction of the different blood cells leading to anemia and thrombocytopenia. Such a state is called hypersplenism, which is nearly always *secondary* to some other condition.

- It may result from *excessive destruction* of red cells from one of the following causes:
  - The red cells may be defective in structure, as in hereditary spherocytosis.
  - Autoimmunity may result in excessive destruction of red cells in auto-immune hemolytic anemia.
- In many diseases the spleen may be greatly enlarged for *different reasons:*
  - In portal hypertension, due to venous congestion.
  - In various neoplastic conditions involving the spleen, e.g. Hodgkin's disease, lymphomas and leukemia, due to deposition of the malignant tissue.

The common indications for *splenectomy* for hypersplenism include lymphoma and chronic lymphatic leukemia. After splenectomy for these conditions about 80% of cases achieve hematological correction; this allows chemotherapy to be commenced and partial or complete remission to be obtained. α-Interferon is used for patients with little or no splenomegaly or in those in whom splenectomy is contraindicated.

Other indications for splenectomy

The spleen may be removed for hydatid cyst of the spleen; for schistosomiasis, splenic abscess and as part of a cancer operation because of local extension of tumors of the stomach, colon or pancreas.

Schistosomiasis

This is common among Egyptian peasants in the Nile delta and elsewhere in Africa, as well as in Venezuela, who stand in the water where the embryos of *Schistosoma mansoni* or *S. hematobium* cause infestation of the human being by penetrating the skin of the feet. Periportal fibrosis in the liver occurs first. The spleen then enlarges due to the portal hypertension and the products of disintegrated worms and ova which are filtered by the spleen.

In advanced cases the liver is shrunken with ascites, and the spleen may be so large as to extend to the pelvic brim. The urine and feces should be examined for ova. Early cases of schistosomiasis respond to treatment by antimony salts. In advanced cases, after careful preoperative preparation with blood transfusions and antibiotics, splenectomy is undertaken and confers a great deal of benefit.

Splenectomy

Preoperative preparation

In view of the risk of post-splenectomy sepsis, all patients should receive vaccines against the pneumococcus, meningococcus and *Hemophilus influenzae type b.* In patients with idiopathic thrombocytopenic purpura, platelets should be available for use after splenectomy if thrombocytopenic bleeding occurs. The blood and blood products should be warmed before use, specially in chronic lymphocytic leukemia and lymphoma, because the patient may have developed cold hemagglutinin disease and may have an increased risk of hemolysis.

Technique

Either a left subcostal or upper midline incision can be used to expose the spleen. A midline incision is preferred in two situations:

- In a ruptured spleen because it allows a better examination of other viscera which may have been injured at the same time.
- In a case where the spleen is huge, because the incision can be extended greatly if required.

The spleen is mobilized by dividing its posterior ligamentous attachments, which contain blood vessels requiring ligation. The short gastric vessels are next divided and ligated. Finally, the hilum of the spleen is dissected, and the splenic artery and vein ligated and divided individually, to avoid the possibility of the development of an arteriovenous fistula.

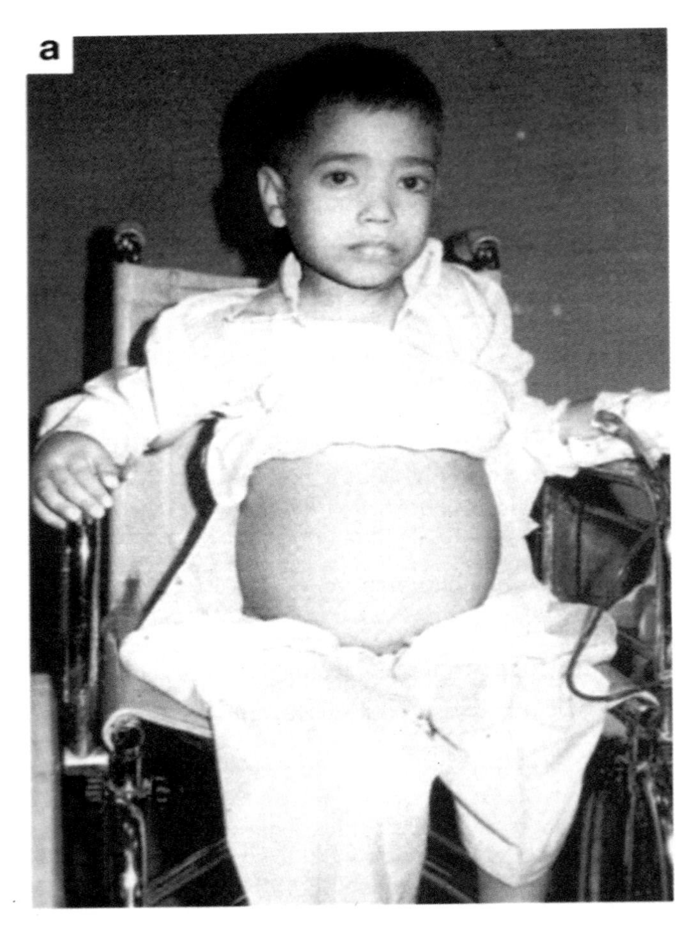

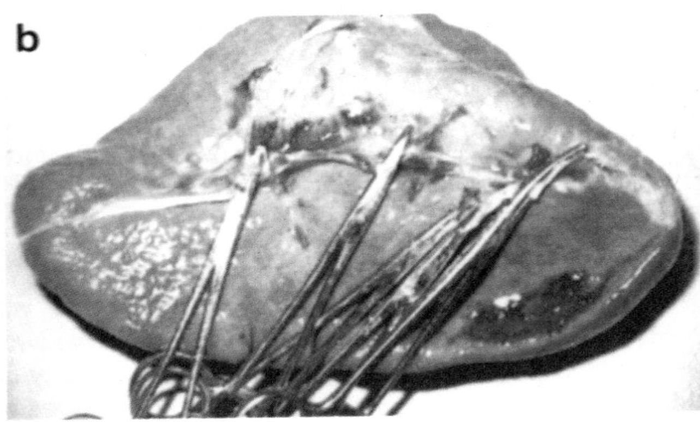

Fig.24.1 (a) Young boy with major thalassaemia. The abdomen is distended due to the splenomegaly. (b) The spleen removed

In a case with a huge spleen, it is desirable to reduce its blood supply before mobilizing it. This can be achieved by exposing the splenic artery through the gastroplenic ligament and ligating it as it runs along the upper border of the pancreas. When splenectomy is carried out for a hematological disorder, a careful search should be made for accessory spleens, which should be removed. The left upper quadrant is not drained routinely. If there has been injury to the tail of the pancreas or if hemostasis is incomplete, closed suction drainage should be employed.

Laparoscopic splenectomy. Splenectomy can nowadays be performed by laparoscopic techniques. This may take a little longer, but carries all the advantages of minimally invasive surgery.

Complications

Most patients tolerate the operation well.

The most common postoperative complication of splenectomy is *collapse* of the lower lobe of the left lung. Other more serious complications include:

- Postoperative hemorrhage.
- Subphrenic abscess.
- Injury to the pancreas causing fistula or pancreatitis.
- Portal and mesenteric vein thrombosis.
- Wound infection.

Chemoprophylaxis

On account of increased risk of infection following splenectomy, prophylactic antibiotics are given for a variable period of time, there being no consensus on the duration of chemoprophylaxis. Children are given oral penicillins or long-acting injectable penicillins up to age 8 to 10 years, and in adults most authorities recommend antibiotics for two years post-operatively.

After splenectomy every febrile episode should be investigated thoroughly and treated actively.

Chapter

25 SMALL INTESTINE

In the intestines food is digested and absorbed. In the small intestines the various enzymes break down the constituents of food into smaller molecules which are then absorbed. In the large intestine some further absorption of nutrient materials takes place, and water is absorbed so that the residue is firm and relatively dry for easier disposal. In such conditions of the intestines where digestion or absorption is at fault, malnutrition results.

INVESTIGATION OF SMALL BOWEL DISEASE

The function of the small intestines being digestion and absorption, this is the aspect which is the subject of most tests carried out in small gut disease.

Radiology

Supine and erect films

These are useful mainly in acute intestinal obstruction and perforation. In plain x-ray in the erect posture, obstruction shows air-fluid levels in distended bowel loops. Perforation shows the ground glass appearance of fluid.

Barium meal follow-through

This is more useful for the chronic disorders.

Small bowel enema

To increase the diagnostic yield, specially for small bowel tumors, Crohn's disease and in patients with occult gastrointestinal hemorrhage, the barium may be instilled directly via a tube into the upper jejunum (small bowel enema). In malabsorption the contrast medium appears flocculated and segmented, the mucosal folds thickened, and the intestinal loops dilated. However these changes are non-specific and must be confirmed by other more specific tests.

Selective splanchnic angiography

This is the best method of detecting angiodysplastic lesions (vascular malformations) which present with occult gastrointestinal bleeding. A Seldinger catheter is passed up from the femoral artery. Its tip is placed opposite the origin of the coeliac or superior mesenteric artery and the dye injected.

CT scan of the small gut

The distance between the shadows of barium in adjacent loops is due to the two thicknesses of bowel wall between them. Thus, CT helps in detecting thickening of the bowel wall by disease.

Ultrasound

In intestinal obstruction ultrasound scan can distinguish between fluid-filled dilated bowel loops and other cystic structures as well as free fluid.

Isotope scintigraphy

Intestinal bleeding

In patients with intestinal bleeding due to a suspected *Meckel's diverticulum*, polyp or tumor, isotope methods are helpful. *Technetium pertechnetate* is injected intravenously; the ectopic gastric mucosa in Meckel's diverticulum excretes it into the lumen, where it appears as a hot spot in the scan.

Active bleeding

In active bleeding in an emergency situation, *99msulphur-colloid* (Tc Sc) is preferred. After intravenous injection, Tc Sc is cleared from the circulation by the macrophage system within 15 minutes, so that radioactivity at the bleeding site increases, allowing its detection as a hot spot.

Small bowel transit time

This can be estimated by administering isotope-labelled meals. The end-point is reached when radioactivity is detected over the cecum.

Fecal fat

Quantitative estimation of fecal fat is the most sensitive and reliable test of disorders of digestion and absorption, the normal upper limit of fecal fat output on a standard diet, containing 80 to 100 g of fat, being 6.0 g/day.

Jejunal biopsy

This is the definitive test for most cases of malabsorption. It is essential for the diagnosis of celiac disease, tropical sprue, amyloidosis and giardiasis. Endoscopic biopsies from the distal duodenum have been shown to be as useful as jejunal biopsies. The steerable Medi-tech biopsy capsule is much quicker than the Crosby capsule and two or three biopsies can be taken.

Colonoscopy and terminal ileum

In the past colonoscopes could be passed only upto the cecum, and could thus visualize only the large bowel. However, the latest colonoscopes are more flexible than the older models. Therefore, during the last 15 years colonoscopes have been routinely passed into the terminal ileum, going up to 30–35cm, with a 95% success rate. This is a most valuable advancement, as most disorders of the small gut, e.g. tuberculosis, Crohn's disease, etc., involve its terminal portion, and can be directly visualized and biopsied.

SMALL BOWEL OBSTRUCTION

This is one of the most common conditions seen in surgical practice. Many diseases of the intestines, both congenital and acquired, end up by obstructing the passage of intestinal contents and present to the clinician as cases of intestinal obstruction. This results in an emergency situation which requires prompt treatment. For appropriate management one has to decide whether obstruction is present and if so, what is the likely cause. In many cases the exact cause is found only at operation.

Intestinal obstruction may be classified into two types, mechanical and paralytic, also called dynamic and adynamic.

Mechanical obstruction

There is a mechanical block to the passage of intestinal contents. The block may be:

- In the lumen, e.g. inspissated feces or gallstones, worms etc.
- In the wall, e.g. inflammatory or malignant strictures, polyps etc.
- Outside the wall, as in hernias or adhesions and bands.

Clinically, there are three types of mechanical obstruction:

- *Acute obstruction*, with severe pain, vomiting, distension and absolute constipation (i.e. no feces and no flatus), and coming on suddenly.
- *Chronic obstruction*, with abdominal colic at first, and absolute constipation and distension after a few weeks; this is intermittent or episodic in presentation.
- *Acute-on-chronic obstruction*, in which acute (complete) obstruction supervenes on a longstanding chronic i.e. incomplete obstruction.

Paralytic obstruction

In this condition peristalsis ceases. This is called *paralytic ileus* (ileus means colic), e.g. in mesenteric vascular occlusion, peritonitis, etc.

Pathology

If obstruction is unrelieved for several days the increasing distension causes the peristalsis to diminish and finally cease, the intestine now being flabby and toneless, because when a smooth muscle fibre is stretched beyond a certain limit, it loses the power to contract.

The intestine *below* the obstruction shows normal peristalsis and absorption. When the residue of its contents has been passed onwards, it becomes contracted, pale and immobile.

Distension occurs proximal to the obstruction due to both gas and fluid:

- *Gas* is derived from swallowed air, diffusion from the blood, and products of digestion. The carbon dioxide and oxygen get absorbed into the blood-stream, leaving behind nitrogen and foul-smelling hydrogen sulphide.
- Every day many liters of *fluid* are secreted into the upper part of the gastrointestinal tract as follows: saliva (1,500ml), gastric juice (2,500ml), bile (500ml), pancreatic juice (1,000ml), and succus entericus (3,000ml). However, the same is also absorbed mainly in the small intestine.

Reduction in extracellular fluid volume occurs due to:

- Vomiting.
- Defective absorption.
- Loss of the above-mentioned secretions into the lumen of the bowel. This fluid, although within the body, is outside both the compartments (spaces) of body fluid i.e. the intracellular and extracellular spaces. It is therefore said to be *sequestrated* into a *third space*.

Fluid depletion is severe and occurs early in proximal small intestinal obstruction, later in ileal obstruction, and even more slowly in colonic obstruction. This is because the lower the obstruction the greater the absorptive area available above it.

Strangulation

Strangulation of the bowel occurs when its blood supply is interfered with due to its being trapped in a hernia or involved in a volvulus or intussusception. It is a dangerous condition and demands early treatment. First the veins are compressed and the gut becomes blue or purple. Later the arterial supply is affected. The peritoneal coat loses its shine, the mucosa is ulcerated, and gangrene is imminent.

Loss of blood volume into the congested segment is proportional to the length of the segment. If a long loop of intestine is strangulated, the patient may go into oligaemic shock, and his life may be in danger.

When the wall of the gut is devitalized, first bacterial toxins and later bacteria pass into the peritoneal cavity and are absorbed into the circulation. Therefore strangulation in an external hernia is far less dangerous than intraperitoneal strangulation, because in the former case the toxic transudate is confined to the relatively small hernia sac. Unless the strangulation is relieved promptly it progresses to gangrene and perforation of the bowel leading to peritonitis.

Toxic absorption

It should be remembered that in most cases of strangulation the obstruction is of the *closed-loop* type. After relief of strangulation, toxic substances in the strangulated loop may pass on to normal intestine and become absorbed. This may cause a deterioration in the patient's condition or even death.

Clinical features

The clinical features of intestinal obstruction consist of pain, vomiting, distension and absolute constipation.

Acute obstruction

Abdominal pain

This is the first symptom, and it starts suddenly. It recurs at intervals of a few minutes. These colicky attacks spread all over the abdomen, but are localized mainly at the umbilicus. Such attacks of pain are absent only in paralytic ileus. The pain from ischemic bowel is continuous, severe and gripping with tenderness and rigidity appearing over the abdomen.

Vomiting

In high jejunal obstruction vomiting starts after several hours of pain, except that the first attack of pain may be accompanied by a vomit. As the obstruction progresses the character of the vomiting changes. First it contains partly digested food, then mucoid gastric juice, then yellow fluid from regurgitation of bile, and finally dark brown fluid. The dark colour is produced as follows: blood oozes out of the congested gut mucosa; its hemoglobin is acted upon by the alkaline intestinal juice to produce chocolate-coloured hematin.

The lower down the gut the site of obstruction, the later does vomiting commence.

Distension

This takes several hours to develop. Visible peristalsis may be seen in thin individuals. Peristaltic sounds may be loud enough to be audible *(borborygmi)*. The hernial sites must be examined to exclude strangulated hernia.

Constipation

After the contents of the bowel below the obstruction have been evacuated, there is *absolute constipation* i.e. neither feces nor flatus is passed. This absolute constipation distinguishes obstruction from simple constipation.

Dehydration

Loss of absorptive power by the intestine and repeated vomiting leads to dehydration. The skin and the tongue are dry, the eyes are sunken, the urine is scanty and concentrated.

Chronic obstruction

The common cause of chronic intestinal obstruction in the large intestine is a carcinoma, in the small intestine in underdeveloped countries a tubercular stricture. Constipation appears, increases gradually over weeks or months, and finally may become absolute. Abdominal distension then occurs. In small gut obstruction intestinal loops are seen lying one above the other __ the *ladder pattern*. In large gut obstruction, on palpation a tumor can occasionally be felt in the line of the colon. Pain occurs in the form of bouts of colic.

Acute-on-chronic obstruction

This condition starts as chronic obstruction, but the narrowing of the lumen increases so much that it ends up as acute obstruction.

Strangulation

This must be distinguished from non-strangulating obstruction, because strangulation requires immediate operation to avoid gangrene. The picture is usually that of an obstruction together with a degree of shock. Pain is more severe and constant. Tenderness and rigidity may be present. If strangulation occurs in an external hernia, the lump is tense, tender and irreducible, with no cough impulse.

X-rays

A plain x-ray of the abdomen is taken with the patient erect and supine. Distended jejunum shows valvulae connivantes. In contrast, the haustral folds of the colon are spaced further apart and the indentations are not placed opposite each other; at the same time these lines do not extend right across the shadow of the bowel loop.

Fluid levels appear at a late stage (Fig.25.1). The lower the site of obstruction in the small bowel and the longer its duration, the larger the number of fluid levels. Obstruction low in the colon does not commonly produce fluid levels in the small gut.

Treatment

This resolves itself into three steps:

- Gastroduodenal suction.
- Replacement of fluids and electrolytes.
- Relief of the obstruction, usually by operation.

Suction

The first step is to empty the stomach and keep it empty by an indwelling *nasogastric tube*. By relieving distension and reducing the size of the distended coils of intestine, aspiration facilitates the operation and closure of the wound. Also, toxic intestinal contents, which would have been absorbed after the relief of obstruction, are evacuated beforehand. The outer end of the nasogastric tube should not be closed but left open, so that air continues to escape constantly, as the air pressure in obstructed intestine is higher than the atmospheric pressure. The end of the tube should be connected to the tubing of a collecting bag, which should be suspended from the side of the bed.

Fluid replacement

The fluid and salt lost must be replaced. If signs of dehydration are present, three to four liters of normal saline with KCl are commonly required. A fluid balance chart must be maintained.

Relief of obstruction

When the stomach has been deflated and as soon as any fluid deficit has been made good, operation for the relief of the obstruction is usually carried out. There are two exceptions to this standard practice:

- In case of strangulation (even if suspected) the operation should be done *on an emergency basis* after a short period of resuscitation.
- In adhesive bowel obstruction which is usually the commonest cause in young adults and in postoperative situations, *non-operative conservative treatment may be continued for 48 hrs*, if strangulation or closed loop obstruction can be ruled out. Continuous close monitoring of the patients is very important in this situation.

INTESTINAL OBSTRUCTION IN THE NEWBORN

The common causes of this condition are congenital anomalies. These include atresias at various levels, arrested rotation, volvulus of the midgut and meconium ileus.

Atresia and stenosis of the duodenum

In atresia the duodenum is completely blocked; in stenosis its lumen is greatly narrowed. Vomiting starts immediately after birth. If the atresia lies below the duodenal ampulla the vomitus is bile-stained, otherwise it is colourless. Visible peristalsis may be seen in the epigastrium passing from left to right. A plain film shows a large bubble in the stomach and a smaller one in the duodenum (*double-bubble sign*). To relieve the obstruction the dilated proximal duodenum is anastomosed to the most proximal loop of the jejunum (*duodenojejunostomy*).

Jejunal and ileal atresia

In this condition either the ileum is blocked by a septum, or a whole segment of the gut is missing. Vomiting starts within a day or two after birth. If not diagnosed early, the increasing distension impairs the blood supply of the gut, causing gangrene and perforation. Central distension comes on within 24 hours of birth.

Plain *x-ray* shows many more fluid levels in ileal than in jejunal atresia.

The grossly distended ileal segment does not function, due to its smooth muscle having been overstretched and put out of action. *Therefore it must be resected* before anastomosis is performed. Before this point was appreciated, newborns usually suffered continuing obstruction even after anastomosis, and often died of it.

Malrotation

In this condition, after the midgut returns to the abdomen, it fails to undergo rotation:

- The cecum remains in the left hypochondrium instead of rotating to the right iliac fossa. A peritoneal band runs from it to the right across the duodenum and obstructs the latter.
- At the same time the cecum and the whole of the small intestine, which has a narrow attachment, may revolve around its pedicle resulting in a volvulus of the midgut.

Midgut volvulus is a dangerous condition. If it remains untreated it results in gangrene of the *whole small gut*, a condition which is incompatible with life. At the same time it leads to serious hypovolaemia due to loss of fluid into the very long segment of gut. *Therefore recurrent obstruction in the newborn should be carefully investigated.*

Meconium ileus

This is the neonatal presentation of mucoviscidosis of the pancreas. Due to the absence of pancreatic enzymes from the gut, the terminal ileum is filled with meconium mixed with viscid mucus to produce a hardened mixture which may be felt as a rubbery mass. The infant is born with intestinal obstruction.

Operation

At laparotomy the affected coil of gut is irrigated with 1% hydrogen peroxide or 1 to 4% N-acetylcysteine through a short incision to loosen the glue-like mass. If this method fails, the coil is resected.

Meconium peritonitis

This is the term applied to any antenatal intestinal perforation.

Early perforation

When the perforation occurs early in intrauterine life the meconium causes an inflammatory reaction and calcification within the peritoneal cavity. The baby vomits bile and shows all the signs of an intestinal obstruction. X-ray shows air-fluid levels and calcification.

Operation

At operation there are widespread adhesions and a localized mass of intestines encased in a dense inflammatory reaction. The bowel has to be dissected out of the adhesions and the perforated loop exteriorized. At a later stage continuity of the bowel is restored.

Late perforation

When the bowel perforates late in intrauterine life there is no calcification. The infant is born with an abdomen that is hugely distended with fluid which interferes with respiration. X-ray shows an opaque abdomen with little gas.

Treatment

Prompt paracentesis is performed to decompress the abdomen and relieve the respiratory distress. The perforated loop of intestine is resected. The prognosis is bad, but recovery has followed prompt operation in some cases.

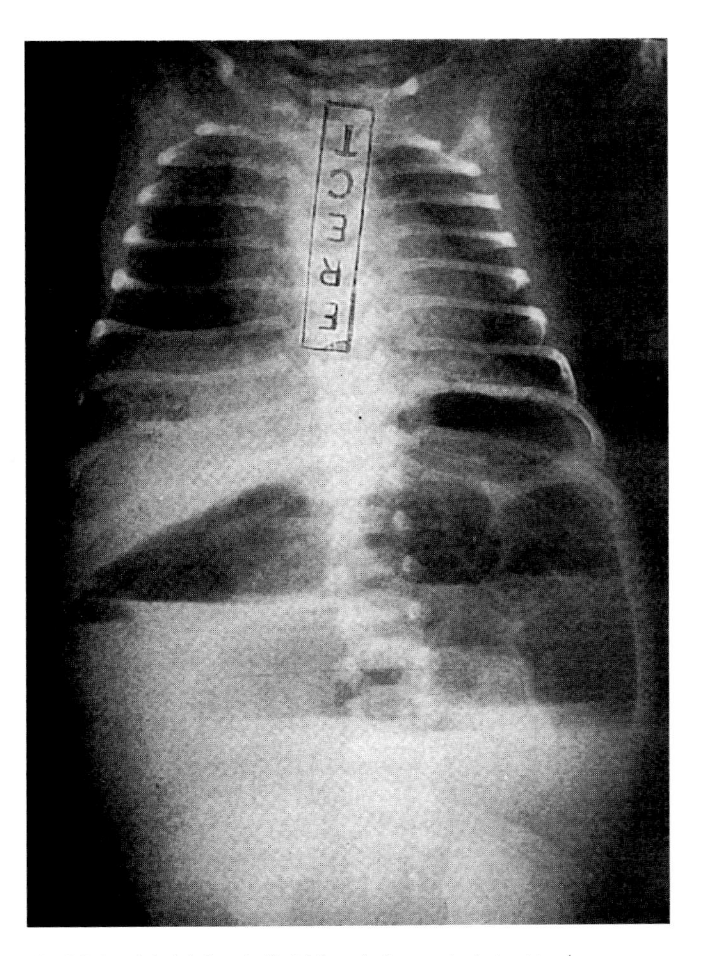

Fig.25.1 Multiple air-fluid levels in acute intestinal obstruction due to ileal atresia in a newborn

ACUTE INTUSSUSCEPTION

In this condition a segment of the gut becomes invaginated into the one immediately distal to it. There may be an obvious cause which initiates the intussusception, e.g. a polyp, a submucous lipoma, an inverted Meckel's diverticulum, etc. The outer tube is called the intussuscipiens, the inner and middle layers together form the intussusceptum. The blood supply of the inner layers may be impaired due to pressure, resulting in gangrene. The ileocolic type accounts for about 77% of cases, other types being ileo-ileal, ileo-ileo-colic; colo-colic etc.

Intussusception of infants

In the intussusception of infants there is no obvious cause. It is thought that a change in the diet predisposes to inflammation of the intestine and causes swelling of Peyer's patches. Such a swollen patch becomes the focus of commencement of the intussusception.

Clinical features

Usually the patient is a male child aged six to nine months. The reason for this particular age incidence is probably to be found in the fact that the lymphoid tissue in the submucosa of the small gut is most plentiful at this time.

The onset is sudden with attacks of severe abdominal pain each lasting a few minutes, the baby lying pale and listless between the attacks. He may vomit at the onset, but only after twenty-four hours is vomiting a conspicuous feature. In the early stages a normal stool may be passed; later, blood and mucus are evacuated.

On examination the abdomen is not distended. A lump may be felt if the child is quiet or asleep, and if the swelling is not lying under the costal margin. The right iliac fossa feels empty. In a rare case where the intussusception has travelled far enough, its apex may be felt by rectal examination, otherwise blood and mucus are found on the examining finger.

After twelve to twenty four hours the abdomen starts to distend. If untreated, death may occur due to the obstruction or due to peritonitis secondary to the gangrene. Very rarely a natural cure occurs after sloughing of the intussusceptum.

Imaging

X-rays

Plain films of the abdomen reveal increased gas shadows.

Barium enema may show up an ileocolic intussusception. The column of barium ends abruptly in a convex filling defect occupying the whole lumen of the gut.

Ultrasound scan

This is a non-invasive and reliable investigation. The characteristic appearance, when the intussuscepted loop is seen end-on, consists of two rings of low echogenicity separated by a hyperechoic ring (target or doughnut sign).

Differential diagnosis

Acute intussusception must be distinguished from the following conditions:

- In acute *enterocolitis* diarrhea is a leading symptom, and fecal matter or bile is always present in the stool.
- In *prolapse* of the rectum the mucosa can be felt to be continuous with the perianal skin.
- In *purpura* with intestinal symptoms intussusception often coexists.

Treatment

Non-operative management

This involves reduction using either hydrostatic or air enema under continuous fluoroscopic control. The pressure of the air or barium emulsion reduces the intussusception, and the reduction can be observed on the screen. This method is applied in those babies who do not show signs of peritonitis or pneumoperitoneum:

- Hydrostatic reduction is carried out using barium enema.
- Pneumatic reduction involves insufflation of air under controlled pressure. Successful non-operative reduction obviates open surgery.

It should be emphasized that these non-operative methods should be employed only *where the baby arrives at hospital within a few hours and without any complications, and expert x-ray screening is available.* Further, in the case of failure of non-operative management, immediate operation must be carried out.

Operative management

This is indicated in patients with signs of peritonitis or shock, and in patients where non-operative reduction has either failed or its use has been decided against.

After rehydrating the baby with saline, laparotomy is carried out and the sausage-shaped mass delivered on the surface (Figs.25.2 and 3). The lowest part of the mass is squeezed to reduce the intussusception. The last portion is the most difficult to reduce, and should be gently compressed in a warm saline pack to rèduce the edema. If reduction proves impossible the affected loop is resected, with end-to-end anastomosis. Postoperatively, gastric aspiration and intravenous fluids are continued for a day or two, after which sips of water and later mother's milk are started. Recurrent intussusception is very rare but does occur.

Recurrent intussuseption is rare because it is only at the age of a few months that the submucosa of the terminal ileum is so overloaded with lymphocytes that it is liable to be dragged onwards by peristaltic waves, taking the intestine with it.

Blind (stagnant) loop syndrome

If a blind loop of small intestine is formed, or is made at operation, stasis is the result. This can happen when a loop of gut is bypassed at operation. Stasis produces an abnormal bacterial flora which leads to defects of absorption:

- If the blind loop is in the *jejunum* the defect is of fat absorption leading to pale, bulky, greasy stools (steatorrhoea).

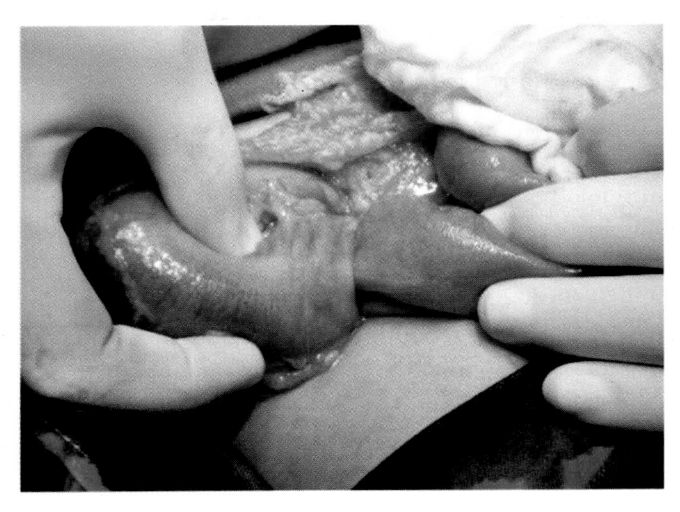

Fig.25.2 The common ileocolic intussusception being reduced

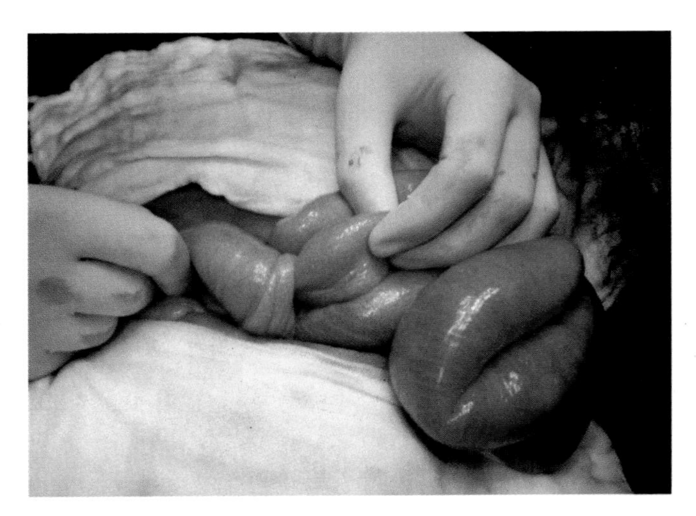

Fig.25.3 Ileoileal intussusception being reduced

- If it is in the *ileum*, vitamin B12 deficiency results, with macrocytic anemia. Sometimes bacterial overgrowth develops in the absence of a local cause. This may occur in patients with malnutrition or immune deficiency.

Clinical features

These are non-specific and include weakness, nausea, vomiting and weight loss. Diarrhea is frequent. Other features include stomatitis, anemia, hypoproteinemia, edema, tetany, rickets and osteomalacia, and retardation of growth in children.

Treatment

Cure is obtained only by surgical removal of the blind loop. However, in certain cases where the underlying disease is either systemic like scleroderma, or very extensive like jejunal diverticulosis, temporary improvement follows the use of antibiotics to destroy the abnormal bacteria. Tetracycline and metronidazole are the common agents used, for about two weeks at a time. Soon after the antibiotic is stopped, bacteria again colonize the gut. However, symptomatic relief lasts for many months. This is fortunate because intermittent therapy can be employed, obviating the need of continuous long-term treatment with its side-effects.

Short gut syndrome

This is the most serious form of intestinal decompensation, and is seen:

- In some patients subjected to jejuno-ileal *bypass* for morbid obesity.
- After massive *resection* of the small bowel, e.g. in intestinal atresia, Crohn's disease, mesenteric infarction, radiation enteritis, midgut volvulus and small bowel tumors.

In some western countries Crohn's disease is the most common cause, requiring repeated resections over a number of years, and culminating in the short-gut syndrome; therefore resections for this condition should be as conservative as possible.

An assessment of how much length of gut *remains behind* is more important than knowing how much has been removed. As a general rule 50 percent of the small intestine can be resected without causing severe or persistent malabsorption.

As more intestine is removed the effects of malabsorption become more severe, but life can be continued more or less normally if more than 1 to 1.5 meter remains. Below this figure, metabolic and nutritional consequences develop, the condition being called short bowel syndrome, and the patient requires *life-long home parenteral nutrition*. It is important to retain the following:

- The last few centimetres of the terminal ileum, because vitamin B12 and bile salts are absorbed in this part of the gut.
- The ileocecal valve, because it both slows down the transit time and limits colonization of the residual intestine by an overgrowth of colonic bacteria.

The short-gut syndrome may be followed by:

- Malabsorption of fats and proteins as well as lactose intolerance.
- Formation of gallstones and urinary stones.
- Rise in the levels of hepatic enzymes.
- Impairment of renal excretion.

With time, structural and functional changes occur in the residual bowel as an adaptation to the reduced absorptive area. The remaining intestine gets dilated and lengthened, and the villi enlarge in size.

Treatment

Medical

Enteral or parenteral nutrition is provided according to the situation as indicated above. Loperamide and diphenoxylate + atropine are used to decrease the motility. Anti-secretory drugs like proton pump inhibitors and octreotide are also helpful.

Surgical

Reversed intestinal segment

A segment of small intestine about 10cm in length is isolated, its direction *reversed*, and continuity restored. Because of its reverse peristalsis, it delays transit and allows more time for absorption from the gut proximal to it.

Intestinal lengthening

Bianchi's intestinal lengthening operation is ingenious, and has been used on a number of infants. It relies on the fact that each side of the small gut is supplied independently by alternating terminal branches of the mesenteric arteries. The leaves of the mesentery, each with its contained vessels, are separated and the intestine divided longitudinally by a stapling device. The two tubes are joined end-to-end to double the length of the intestine which also dilates in due course, increasing its absorptive surface.

The future

Small bowel *transplantation* has been carried out successfully from an HLA compatible sibling. Multiple rejection episodes requiring aggressive immunosuppression and life-threatening infections were encountered, but long-term survival and health independent of parenteral nutrition was achieved. However, the results are inferior to kidney and liver transplantation. In any case, this is a major breakthrough and points towards the likely developments in the future.

Meckel's diverticulum

This is the most common intestinal diverticulum, being present in 2% individuals. It is a remnant of the vitello-intestinal duct, and is situated on the antimesenteric border of the ileum about 60cm from the ileo-cecal valve (Fig.25.4). In a few cases the diverticulum contains abnormally located (i.e. ectopic) epithelium, which may be gastric or colonic, or occasionally pancreatic tissue. It is usually asymptomatic and found incidentally on abdominal exploration.

Complications

A Meckel's diverticulum usually remains symptomless throughout life. If encountered during an operation it should be removed, because the following complications can arise in it, the risk of complications being about 5–10% throughout life:

- *Bleeding* per rectum due to peptic ulceration in abnormally placed gastric mucosa. This can pose a difficult problem in differential diagnosis.
- *Intussusception*, which can occur at any age, and result in intestinal obstruction.
- *Meckel's diverticulitis* due to lodgement of coarse food residue etc. Symptoms are very similar to those of appendicitis. If perforation occurs, the very severe peritonitis may simulate perforated peptic ulcer.
- *Intestinal obstruction*. If a band connects the diverticulum to the umbilicus, a coil of intestine may get twisted around it.

Surgical complications of typhoid

Because of poor food hygiene typhoid fever is still common in certain parts of the world. Therefore, from time to time surgeons receive patients where a typhoid ulcer has perforated or bled. At the same time, acute typhoid cholecystitis and a chronic carrier state is occasionally seen.

Perforated typhoid ulcer

A typhoid ulcer develops over a Peyer's patch in the terminal ileum. In cases of typhoid the wall of the bowel is extremely friable due to the effect of the bacterial toxins. It is not surprising therefore that it sometimes breaks down at the site of an ulcer. Such a perforation usually occurs during the second week of the fever, and the patient presents with severe abdominal pain and tenderness, along with some rigidity.

The *diagnosis* is relatively easy, and can be made fairly confidently if the usual course of the disease is remembered and the history taken carefully. This is the only type of peritonitis where a few days of high fever *precedes* abdominal pain and tenderness. In all the other forms of peritonitis, whether due to a perforated peptic ulcer, a perforated appendix, etc., fever comes on *after* the onset of pain. *The occurrence of many days' high fever before pain is diagnostic of typhoid.* Although the Widal test or typhidot is usually positive in these cases, it is not required for diagnosis.

The patients are usually critically ill with septicemia from the generalized peritonitis, dehydration and electrolyte imbalance, specially potassium deficiency. They should be resuscitated in an intensive care unit. Blood transfusion may be required to correct severe anemia.

Treatment

The treatment of any perforation of the small intestine is closure of the opening by surgical operation, and this is carried out by laparotomy. However, in typhoid as mentioned above, the wall of the bowel is as friable as wet blotting paper. Therefore the incidence of breakdown of the repair with formation of an ileal fistula is fairly high. Various measures have been employed to prevent this serious complication:

- Unabsorbable sutures are used.
- An omental patch may be sewn over the repair.
- The worst affected segment of ileum may be resected.
- A temporary catheter ileostomy may be carried out proximal to the repair, to decompress the ileum.
- The perforated segment may be brought out as a loop ileostomy.

The results of closure of typhoid perforations are so poor that some advise a non-operative management for this condition. However, this is too extreme a view. Specially in gravely ill patients, a compromise between operative repair of the perforation and conservative treatment can be arrived at:

Under local anesthesia a corrugated drain is placed into the peritoneal cavity on each side in the paracolic gutter. Large quantities of pus are evacuated and the fever and toxemia subside. As the patient's general condition improves greatly, the perforation often gets walled off and closes itself; if it does not, surgical repair is carried out.

Fortunately such hopeless cases seen until the 70's and 80's are less common nowadays. This may be due to improvement in primary health care and freely available chemotherapy against typhoid.

Bleeding typhoid ulcer

Very occasionally a typhoid ulcer may bleed massively. Blood transfusions along with antibiotics effective against typhoid are indicated. The situation where resection of the terminal ileum has to be carried out for uncontrollable hemorrhage is very rare indeed. This condition should be considered in a patient with a lower GI bleed.

Typhoid cholecystitis

Acute typhoid cholecystitis occurs from time to time and perforation can occur. Ultrasound examination is helpful in these cases. If in a case with fever and tenderness in the right hypochondrium the wall of the gallbladder is thick indicating acute cholecystitis but no stones are seen, this is substantial evidence in favour of typhoid cholecystitis, as this is the only common cause of acalculous cholecystitis.

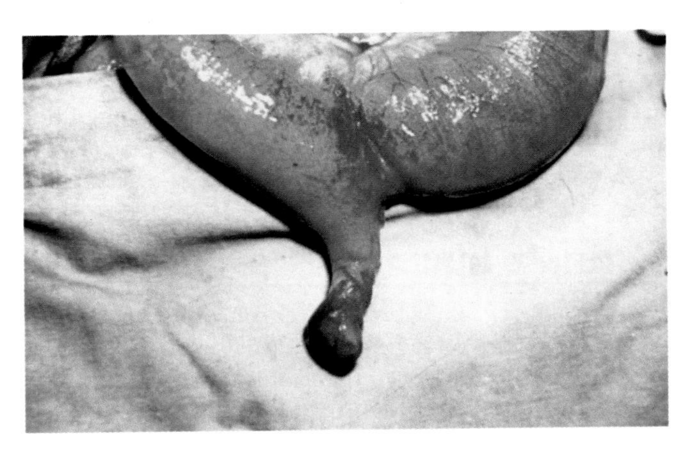

Fig.25.4 Meckel's diverticulum arising from anti-mesenteric border of small intestine. Treated by excision

Chronic typhoid cholecystitis can result in a *carrier state*, with bacteria being discharged with the feces from the gallbladder reservoir. If such a carrier state is proved by examination of the stools, cholecystectomy is indicated. If gallstones or chronic cholecystitis are present, cholecystectomy is the treatment of choice.

INFLAMMATORY BOWEL DISEASE-

The term inflammatory bowel disease includes two major entities, namely ulcerative colitis and Crohn's disease. Although these two diseases differ from each other in many ways, they also have common features. Both conditions are common in the West, specially among Jews, and uncommon in the Eastern and developing countries. The lymphoid tissue of the gut is active in both conditions: in Crohn's disease as a granuloma, in ulcerative colitis in the form of an Arthus reaction[1]. Both conditions show autoantibody production and raised serum levels of gammaglobulins. Finally, the extraintestinal manifestations of inflammatory bowel disease are present in other immunologically mediated diseases.

Recent work suggests that these conditions arise due to a *hyperactivation of the immune response*, including lymphocyte proliferation, cytokine release, excessive

[1] Arthus reaction is a local, immune-complex-mediated, hypersensitivity reaction in vessel walls, serous linings and glomeruli.

neutrophil products, specially leukotrines and reactive oxygen metabolites, and ultimately tissue injury. The actual tissue damage is probably in the nature of a non-specific injury to an 'innocent bystander'. Crohn's disease is described next, while ulcerative colitis is discussed in chapter 27.

CROHN'S DISEASE

Crohn's disease consists of a chronic granulomatous inflammation involving the gut. It may affect any part of the alimentary canal from the mouth to the anus, but is seen most often in the ileum and colon. An interaction between genetic, environmental and immunological factors plays a part in the pathogenesis, with activation of the mucosal immune system. Some constituents of the intestinal contents may be responsible because:

- Defunctioning of the colon by an ileostomy helps the condition to subside.
- Elemental diets are as effective as steroids in providing relief.

There is much evidence to show that immunological mechanisms play a role in pathogenesis. Intestinal macrophages and T lymphocytes are activated within the inflamed intestine and release cytokines and inflammatory mediators, which alter epithelial permeability, damage endothelium, activate fibroblasts and initiate fibrosis.

The disease is characteristically discontinuous, affecting a number of segments with normal mucosa in between. The mucosa undergoes inflammation and fibrosis, accompanied by ulceration. The inflammation is predominantly submucosal although it often goes right through the bowel wall. It usually commences at the ileocecal junction and extends proximally for an average distance of 30cm. Above this there may be another separate area of diseased intestine–a *skip* lesion. The intestine is swollen and bright pink with a fibrinous exudate. The mesentery is thickened and its lymph nodes are fleshy. The distal ileum is the most frequent site followed by the colon, and the anal and perianal regions.

Clinical features

Acute

In the acute condition, which is seen in only 5% of cases, the appearances are similar to those of acute appendicitis, except that diarrhea nearly always commences before the attack of pain.

Chronic

The chronic condition is divided into three stages:

- In the *1st* stage there is prolonged diarrhea and colic, with fever and a tender mass. Stools show mucus and occult blood.
- The *2nd* stage presents as acute or chronic intestinal obstruction.
- In the *3rd* stage adhesions develop and sometimes slow perforation occurs, which may result in fistulae into surrounding viscera e.g. pelvic colon or bladder, or to the exterior through the scar of a previous operation e.g. appendicectomy.

Complications

These include:

- Perforation, acute dilatation and hemorrhage.
- Uveitis and arthritis, but less often than in colonic disease.
- Gallstones and renal stones occur more commonly than in the general population.
- Amyloidosis occurs rarely.

Perianal disease i.e. ulcers, chronic fissures, perianal abscess and fistulae, occur in association with both ileal and colonic disease.

Diagnosis

Barium meal x-ray

This shows straightening of the valvulae connivantes. If ulcers are present, multiple specks of barium are left behind after the gut segment has emptied of barium. In advanced cases the terminal ileum is stenosed–the *string sign* of Kantor.

If available, a *small bowel enema* (instillation of contrast material through a tube passed into the duodenum) allows a much better definition of the mucosal pattern, as well as of strictures, than a conventional barium meal follow-through. If this confirms the diagnosis of Crohn's disease, a full examination of the colon should be made by colonoscopy and biopsies.

CT scan sometimes shows the lumen narrowed and the gut thickened at many places (Fig.25.5 a and b). Further, both CT and *MRI* are useful in the assessment of fistulae and pelvic abscesses.

Laboratory

Hemoglobin, platelet count, albumin, ESR and serum levels of the acute-phase proteins, help assess the severity of the disease.

Treatment

Since Crohn's disease cannot be cured, the clinician's role is to:

- Control the inflammation.
- Correct the nutritional deficiencies.
- Ameliorate the symptoms.

Surgery is often required, and most patients undergo at least one operation during their lifetime.

Medical treatment

In general, medical treatment should be dictated by symptoms.

Early stages

If the activity of the disease is shown only by laboratory data, large doses of corticosteroids or immunosuppression are not indicated. In the early stages medical treatment is given a trial with *bed rest*, a diet rich in *proteins and vitamins*, and iron. Oral *iron* is poorly tolerated by these patients and the total dose may have to be given intravenously, with preparations to deal with the rare case of anaphylaxis.

Magnesium and *zinc* deficiencies can also occur, and serum concentrations should be measured in patients with extensive chronic disease. Oral *elemental diets* and supplementary *parenteral nutrition* will provide rest to the bowel.

Mild disease

Patients with mild disease are given 5-ASA (aminosalicylate) which is now available along with other *aminosalicylates* as Asacol, Mesalamine etc.; they are used for maintaining remission. Alternatively, oral prednisolone is given in a dose of 20mg daily for six weeks.

Severe disease

Patients with severe disease require *intravenous hydrocortisone*, 100mg every six hours, intravenous fluids, and blood.

Chronic active disease

If such a patient goes into relapse on reducing the dose, it means he has *chronic active disease*, and immunosuppression by *azathioprine* 2mg/kg/day should be employed over a long period, with regular blood counts to monitor possible marrow suppression.

Surgical treatment

Approximately 50–70% patients with Crohn's disease require surgery during their lifetime for the following reasons:

- Obstruction, being the most common indication.
- Perforation, abscess, fistula (internal/external).
- Perianal disease.
- Failure of growth in children.

Remember that surgery does not cure Crohn's disease; it only relieves obstruction or removes a diseased segment. As the disease keeps recurring over a period of time, resections of intestines should be very conservative. At the same time, bypass operations should be avoided as they result in malabsorption by creating blind loops.

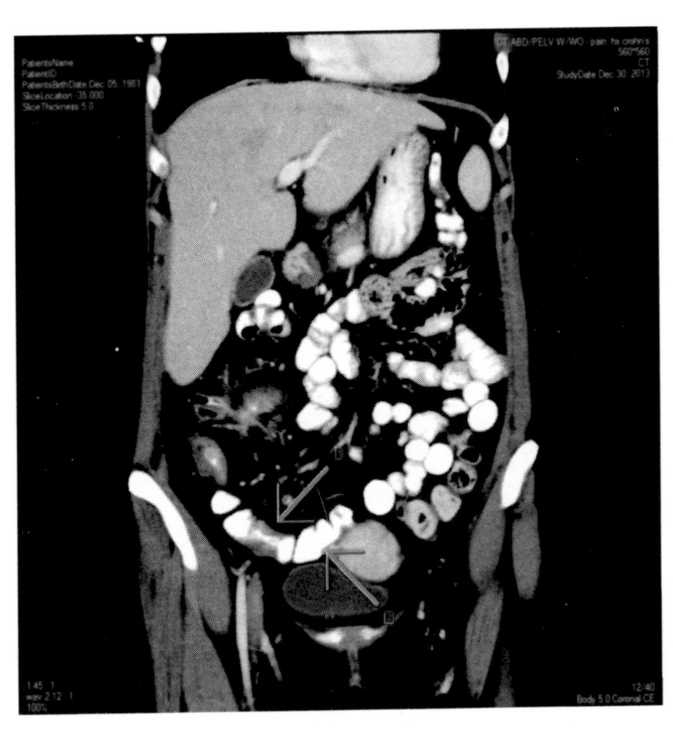

Fig.25.5 CT scan with barium and coronal reconstruction, showing segment of terminal ileum with wall thickened and lumen narrowed by Crohn's disease.

ABDOMINAL TUBERCULOSIS

This term includes tuberculous infection of the gastrointestinal tract, mesentery, peritoneum, liver and spleen. Genitourinary tuberculosis is a separate entity and is not discussed here.

The *primary* type of intestinal disease is caused by ingestion of milk contaminated by *Mycobacterium bovis*.

The *secondary* type occurs due to swallowing of sputum infected with *Mycobacterium tuberculosis* from an active primary focus in the lung.

In the advanced countries abdominal tuberculosis is nowadays rarely seen because of:

- Improvement in living conditions and nutrition.
- Tuberculin testing of cows.
- Pasteurization of milk.
- Effective treatment of pulmonary tuberculosis.

However, elsewhere in the world intestinal tuberculosis is still common. At the same time, HIV patients have a high risk of developing TB.

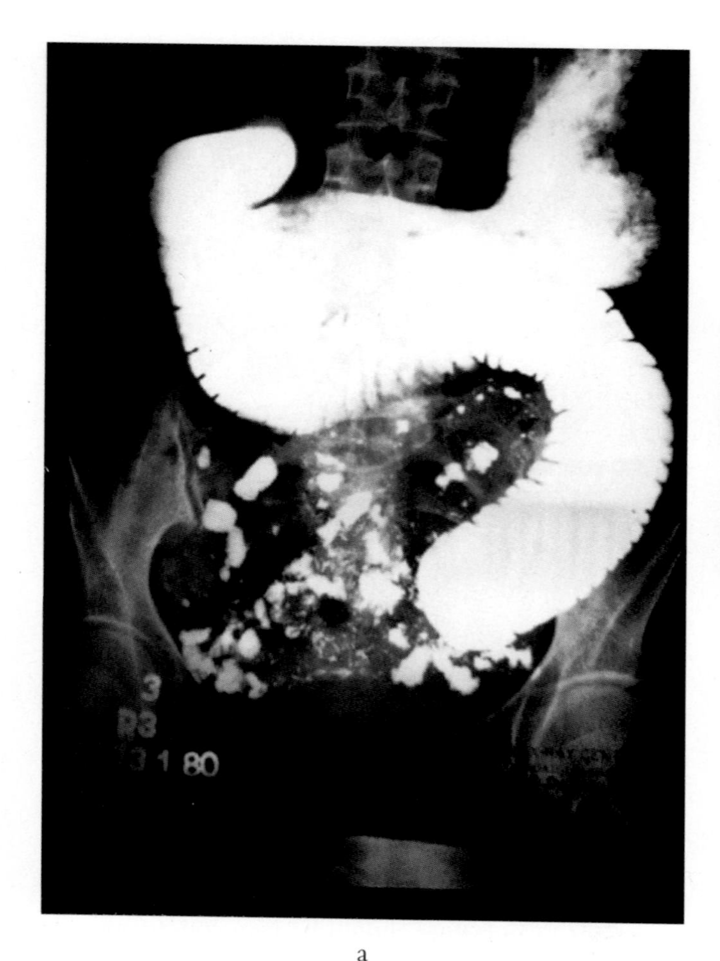

a

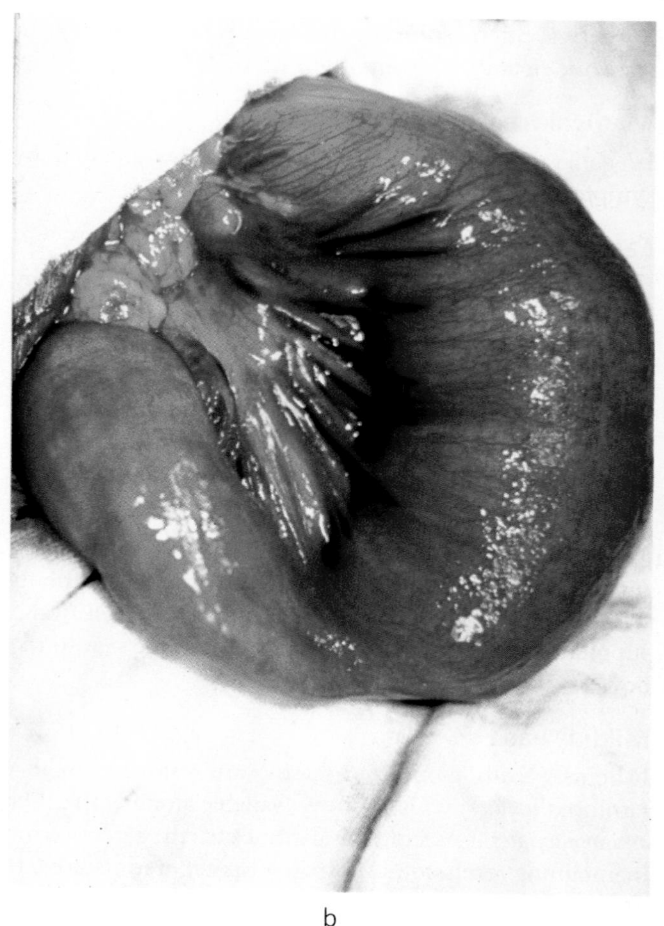

b

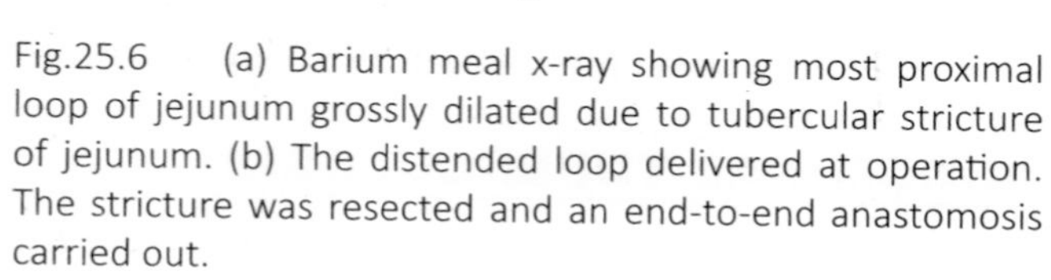

Fig.25.6 (a) Barium meal x-ray showing most proximal loop of jejunum grossly dilated due to tubercular stricture of jejunum. (b) The distended loop delivered at operation. The stricture was resected and an end-to-end anastomosis carried out.

Tuberculous peritonitis

Chronic

In most cases chronic tuberculous peritonitis results from reactivation of a primary peritoneal focus, and is therefore hematogenous in origin. It causes malaise, weight loss, fever and ascites. Active intestinal infection is usually not present, but infections of other serous cavities, e.g. the pleura and pericardial cavity are commonly seen. The dry plastic type of disease which gives a doughy abdomen is rare.

Acute

Acute tuberculous peritonitis is sometimes seen as part of miliary disease, or following rupture of a tuberculous mesenteric lymph node.

Intestinal tuberculosis

This condition occurs in two main forms, the ulcerative and the hyperplastic.

Ulcerative

Ulcerative intestinal tuberculosis is secondary to pulmonary tuberculosis due to swallowing tubercle bacilli. Ulcers form in the terminal ileum, the long axis of the ulcers lying transversely along the lymphatics. Diarrhea with pus and blood occurs. Often the patient has had treatment for pulmonary tuberculosis.

Barium meal may fail to visualize the terminal ileum and cecum due to hypermotility.

Treatment. A prolonged course of chemotherapy heals the ulcers. However, if a stricture forms, operation may be required for intestinal obstruction (Fig.25.6 a and b).

Hyperplastic

This occurs most often in the ileocecal region. There is much thickening of the wall of the cecum and consequent narrowing of the lumen. Besides fibrous tissue there is a great deal of fatty tissue. This accumulation of fibrofatty tissue around the gut is a characteristic but non-specific feature of chronic disease of the large bowel.

Lymph nodes enlarge, and may caseate. Abscess and fistula formation is rare. Although this condition is usually called ileocecal tuberculosis, the lesion is in fact confined to the cecum and should therefore be called tuberculosis of the cecum.

Clinical features

Attacks of abdominal pain with stoppage of wind occur. Stasis and infection of the ileal contents may cause steatorrhoea, anemia and loss of weight.

A firm mass is palpable in the right iliac fossa. This has to be differentiated from an appendix mass, a carcinoma of the cecum, Crohn's disease and an actinomycotic granuloma. A mass in the epigastrium may be due to thickened and rolled up omentum.

Barium meal x-ray

This shows a long narrow filling defect, consisting of cecum and ascending colon. The latter is shortened due to fibrosis and the cecum lies at a higher level.

Treatment

Chemotherapy

If obstructive symptoms have not developed and the diagnosis is certain, chemotherapy may completely cure the condition. The course lasts for 9–12 months. Therapy is started with four drugs: rifampicin, pyrazinamide, isoniazid and ethambutol. The patient is monitored periodically for hepatotoxicity. If liver enzymes get raised, one or both out of rifampicin and pyrazinamide are stopped; in that case the remaining drugs have to be taken for a longer time. Pyridoxine 10mg/day must be given with isoniazid to prevent peripheral neuropathy.

Surgery

The indications for surgery are the following:

- Intestinal obstruction.
- Perforation.
- Abdominal mass.
- Occasionally to confirm the diagnosis.

If obstruction is present *resection* of the involved segment of gut is the treatment of choice.

Mesenteric cysts

These cysts are developmental in origin and are common during the first two decades of life:

- The cyst may produce a painless, fluctuant abdominal *swelling* (Fig.25.7) which moves freely in a plane at right angles to the attachment of the mesentery.

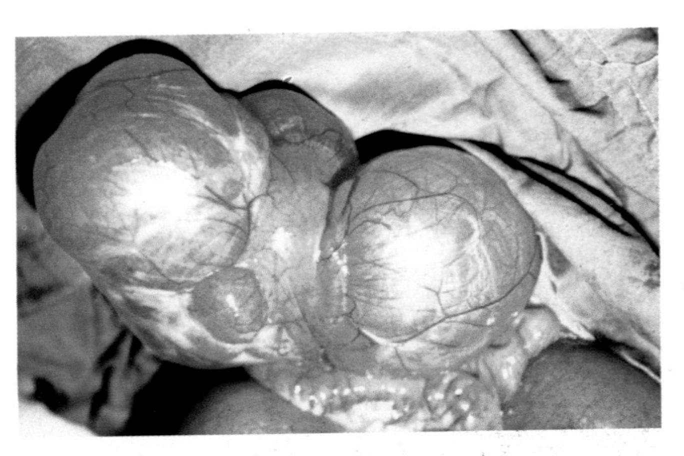

Fig.25.7 Multilocular mesenteric cyst, with loop of small gut carrying it, treated by resection of the segment of gut.

- There may be attacks of abdominal *pain* due to impaction of a food bolus in a segment of bowel narrowed by the cyst.
- The cyst may *rupture,* or *infection* or *hemorrhage* may occur into it.

A mesenteric cyst in the mesocolon contains serous fluid, unless it is blood-stained due to hemorrhage. A cyst in the small bowel mesentery contains chylous fluid, possibly due to congenital lymphatic obstruction--a chylolymphatic cyst (Fig.25.8). These cysts resemble enteric duplications in their location within the mesentery. However, they do not have any mucosa or muscular wall.

Treatment

This is by surgical resection. The cysts are mostly benign and enucleation or excision is curative. This can now be carried out laparoscopically. Because of the intimate proximity of the cysts to the bowel, a segmental resection of the involved loop of intestine is usually required.

TUMORS OF THE SMALL INTESTINE

Benign tumors

Adenoma and lipoma are rare. They may produce intussusception. The first-named may also produce melena. Gastrointestinal stromal tumors (GST) have replaced such tumors as leiomyoma and leiomyosarcoma.

Peutz-Jegher's syndrome

This consists of:

- Familial intestinal polyposis of the jejunum, causing melena or intussusception.
- Melanosis of the oral mucosa and lips.

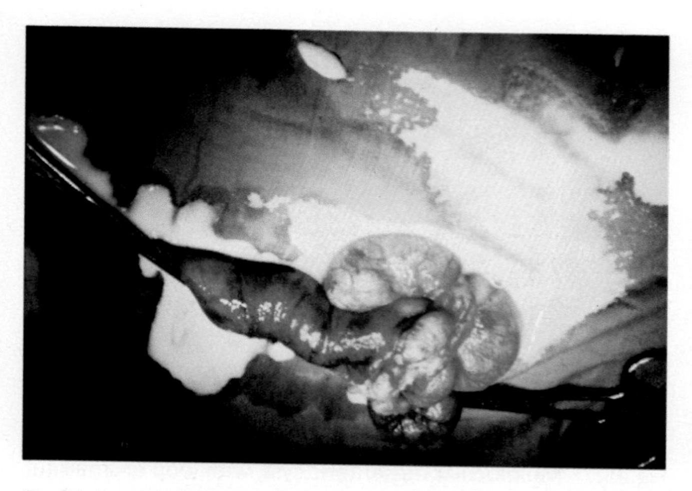

Fig.25.8 Chylolymphatic cyst. It forms due to blockage of lymphatics in the mesentery. Rupture of the cyst has led to milky fluid being spilt. Removed by resection of a segment of the small intestine.

Malignant tumors

Carcinoid tumors

These are [1]APUDOMAS which arise from the enterochromaffin cells in the gut, and may be associated with MEN I and II syndromes. These occur in the gastrointestinal tract and also in the bronchus, testis and ovary. The appendix and the ileum are the most common sites. Carcinoids are seen in about 0.5% of appendicectomy specimens.

Carcinoids produce vasoactive substances: serotonine, amines (histamine, dopamine, and prostaglandins. Approximately 10% patients with small bowel carcinoids produce the carcinoid syndrome.

Biologically active substances

- Those substances listed above and produced by *intestinal carcinoids* are inactivated in the liver.
- Those produced by *liver metastasis and primary carcinoids of the ovary and lungs* are released into the systemic circulation and cause the carcinoid syndrome.

Carcinoid syndrome

This is comprised of the following:

- Diarrhea.
- Bronchospasm.
- Flushing.
- Valvular disease of the heart.

Symptoms

These including the following:

- Reddish blue cyanosis and flushing attacks of the face.
- Loud peristaltic sounds with bouts of diarrhea.
- Asthmatic attacks and ultimately pulmonary and tricuspid stenosis.

The tumor, specially if it has arisen from the ileum, may metastasize to the liver.

Treatment

As carcinoids are malignant tumors which metastasize, a radical operation, e.g. right hemicolectomy should be performed. Appendicular carcinoids are usually benign, but a tumor larger than 2cm or associated with enlarged lymph nodes should be treated as a malignant tumor (by right hemicolectomy). All resectable tumors in the bowel, mesentry and peritoneum should be resected. Localized liver metastases should also be resected.

If metastases have occurred to the liver:

- Considerable palliation can be obtained by *reduction of the tumor burden* by:
  - o *Surgical extirpation*.
  - o *Hepatic arterial embolization*. In this procedure, a Seldinger catheter is passed up until its tip lies in the origin of the hepatic artery. The arteries supplying the metastases are blocked by injecting bits of gelatin sponge.
- Lesser degrees of palliation can be obtained by *chemotherapy* using cyclophosphamide, adriamycin and 5-fluorouracil singly or in combination.
- Better results are obtained by *prolonged infusion directly through the hepatic artery*. For prolonged access to the hepatic arterial tree a stainless-steel chamber with a silicone diaphragm can be implanted into the subcutaneous tissues; this allows intermittent and prolonged infusions, the chamber being refilled by repeated percutaneous puncture of the diaphragm.
- **Octreotides** (somatostatin analogues) inhibit the activity of many gastrointestinal and other hormones. They can be used to relieve symptoms of carcinoid syndrome as well as to suppress tumor growth.

1 An apudoma is an endocrine tumor that arises from APUD cells that are derived from neural crest cells.

Chapter

26 APPENDIX

Anatomy

The vermiform appendix is inconstant in position, its common positions being retrocecal (74%) and pelvic (21%). The other positions are paracecal, preileal and postileal. *McBurney's point* lies at the junction of the lateral with the middle third of a line joining the anterior superior iliac spine and the umbilicus; the grid-iron incision in appendicectomy is commonly centred around it. The appendix is usually looked for by following one of the taeniae coli downwards on the cecum until the appendix is reached at the junction of the three taenia.

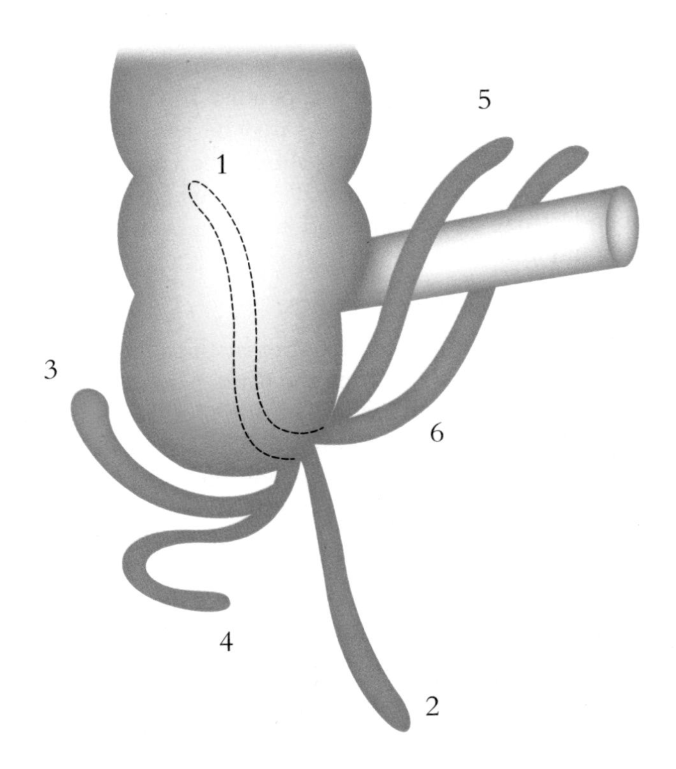

Fig.26.1 Different positions of the appendix. 1. retrocecal 2. pelvic 3. paracolic 4. subcecal 5. preileal 6. postileal

ACUTE APPENDICITIS

Etiology

Appendicitis is more common in the developed countries. It is thought that this is due to the change from a traditional diet rich in the bulky cellulose of whole bran cereals to one rich in meat and fats, so that constipation is common, with its resulting stagnation of large bowel contents. Quite often the actual precipitating cause is a faecolith, which consists of inspissated fecal material. The infection in the appendix is usually a mixed one, the most common organisms being Esch. coli (85%), enterococci, and streptococci. Anaerobic organisms, especially Bacteroides often play an important role in the infection.

Pathology

Appendicitis may be non-obstructive or obstructive.

In the *non-obstructive* type the inflammation varies from quite mild to really severe forms. In the *mild* form the appendix looks virtually normal from outside, but on being slit open the mucosa is unmistakably inflamed; it is purple in colour, with blood, blood clot, and sometimes pus in the lumen.

In the *obstructive* type of appendicitis the products of inflammation become pent up. Therefore inflammation proceeds more rapidly to gangrene and perforation, adhesions have no time to develop, and generalized peritonitis often results.

Clinical features

Rare before the age of two, acute appendicitis is common during childhood, adolescence and adult life, being less common in advanced age. More than half the patients give a history of previous, though usually milder, attacks.

Usually the first symptom is *pain*:

- The pain may be umbilical, epigastric or generalized. This pain is *mediated through the visceral nerves*. It is colicky in obstructive cases, but constant in the non-obstructive type.
- The inflamed appendix irritates the overlying parietal peritoneum, so after a few hours the pain shifts to the

right iliac fossa. This latter pain is *mediated through the somatic nerves*, and is therefore accurately localized and constant. In a few cases the pain is located in the right iliac fossa from the start.

In *obstructive appendicitis* the symptoms are more severe, and their onset more sudden. There may be generalized abdominal colic with vomiting.

Pylorospasm occurs and may cause anorexia, nausea, vomiting, a furred tongue and a foul breath. The *temperature* and *pulse* usually remain unaltered during the first few hours after the onset of the attack. Later, they are both raised slightly, or in severe cases moderately.

Tenderness occurs at McBurney's point or elsewhere according to the site of the appendix. In the case of a pelvic appendix the tenderness may be confined to the pelvis, so rectal examination should be carried out in every case of lower abdominal pain. A high retrocecal appendix may cause pain and tenderness in the right flank and loin.

Rebound tendernesss

If after deep palpation in the right iliac fossa the pressure is suddenly released by lifting the hand, pain may be felt. This is called rebound tenderness and is elicited in cases where the parietal peritoneum is irritated by an inflamed appendix. With a retrocecal or pelvic appendix it may be difficult to elicit the signs of peritoneal irritation.

The appendix at different sites

- If the inflamed appendix is lying over the psoas there may be spasm of this muscle, so that extension of the right hip causes pain (*Psoas test*).
- If a pelvic appendix is lying over the obturator internus muscle, pain may be produced when the right hip is flexed and internally rotated (*Obturator test*).
- If a pelvic appendix is lying over the *bladder* there may be *dysuria*.
- An appendix lying over and irritating the *rectum* may result in *diarrhea* with mucus and tenesmus.
- Diarrhea is also seen in cases where the appendix is lying behind the *terminal ileum* and irritating it (post-ileal appendix).

Diagnosis of appendicitis

Appendicitis is most reliably diagnosed by a carefully taken history and by physical examination to elicit tenderness.

Leucocytosis is common, but occurs only once the condition is well established, and the illness should generally be diagnosed before that happens.

Plain x-rays are so non-specific as to be of no value.

In doubtful cases *ultrasound* can help exclude ureteric stone, ovarian cyst and ectopic pregnancy, and can sometimes indicate a swollen appendix.

Contrast CT scan can show a thickened wall, dilated lumen (Fig.26.2), and sometimes periappendicular fluid.

However, most cases of appendicitis are straightforward, yet precious time is often wasted while awaiting the results of unnecessary tests.

Differential diagnosis

The conditions from which acute appendicitis commonly requires to be distinguished include the following:

- *Acute cholecystitis*. If the appendix is highly placed it may be confused with acute cholecystitis. However, in the latter condition the pain commonly radiates to the inferior angle of the scapula, and to the right shoulder.
- *Perforated peptic ulcer.* In this condition pain starts in the epigastrium and quickly spreads to the right iliac fossa, because the irritating stomach contents spill over into the right paracolic gutter. However, here the pain is diffuse, with board-like rigidity.
- *Right ureteric colic*. In this condition pain often radiates down to the groin. Microscopy of the urine reveals red blood cells. Ultrasound examination or plain x-ray may show a stone in the line of the ureter.
- *Enterocolitis*. In dysentery there may occasionally be pain in the right iliac fossa. However, diarrhea is the most important feature of dysenteries, whereas it is normally absent in cases of appendicitis.
- *Non-specific mesenteric lymphadenitis*. This condition is supposed to be responsible for pain in children in those cases where operation is carried out but a normal appendix is found, and mesenteric lymph nodes are seen to be enlarged. It is difficult to be certain whether such an entity actually exists.
- *Intestinal obstruction*. Here the pain usually remains around the umbilicus. Bowel sounds are loud and plain x-ray in the erect posture shows many fluid levels.
- *'Diabetic abdomen'*. In diabetic ketosis severe abdominal pain and vomiting sometimes come on before coma sets in, and cause confusion. The urine should therefore be tested in every acute abdominal emergency.
- *Right-sided pneumonia or pleurisy*. The lower part of the chest wall is supplied by the 7th to the 12th thoracic nerves. These nerves then proceed onwards to supply the abdominal wall. Therefore in basal pneumonia or pleurisy pain is sometimes felt in the

abdomen. However, in pleurisy the respiratory rate is increased, inspiration causes severe pain, a pleural rub may be heard, and a chest x-ray may show up the effusion or consolidation.

Appendicitis in the young female

The diagnosis in young females aged 18–40 is difficult due to gynaecological causes of lower abdominal pain as discussed below:

- Torsion/hemorrhage in an ovarian cyst.
- *Ectopic gestation*. A ruptured ectopic gestation is associated with signs of severe internal hemorrhage, and is unlikely to be mistaken for appendicitis. However, unruptured right tubal pregnancy may cause pain in the right iliac fossa. Thus if the patient is a female in the childbearing period, the menstrual history must always be enquired into. In cases of ectopic gestation usually only one period has been missed.
- *Ruptured ovarian follicle*. When an ovarian follicle in the right ovary ruptures, it may produce pain in the right iliac fossa. This always comes on in the middle of the menstrual period. Occasionally, when operation is carried out the appendix is seen to be normal and a ruptured follicle is found, having caused diagnostic confusion.
- *Salpingitis*. In this condition the pain is usually bilateral; in cases of doubt an ultrasound examination can show up the distended fallopian tubes.

Ultrasound

In a doubtful case ultrasound examination helps by showing a distended edematous appendix. A faecolith if present may also be highlighted along with its acoustic shadow, although the mere presence of a faecolith does not prove the case is one of acute appendicitis.

Appendicitis in pregnancy

Acute appendicitis is as common in pregnant as in non-pregnant women, whereas the risk of perforation of the appendix is somewhat higher, especially during the 2nd half of pregnancy.

The treatment of appendicitis at any stage of pregnancy is appendicectomy. However, the following points may be mentioned in this connection:

- During the *first six months* of pregnancy symptoms of appendicitis do not differ from those in the non-pregnant woman.
- During the *third trimester* the enlarged uterus displaces the appendix, so that it lies at a higher position, and this fact should be kept in mind. At the same time the abdominal wall is lifted from the appendix by the gravid uterus, and the signs of peritoneal irritation may therefore be minimal. Also, leucocytosis is a normal response to pregnancy and cannot be relied upon to help confirm the diagnosis of appendicitis.
- If appendicectomy is carried out before the appendix perforates, upto 30% of cases could proceed to premature labour. If it has already perforated, this figure rises as high as 50%. Therefore, if acute appendicitis develops during pregnancy it should be diagnosed and treated promptly.

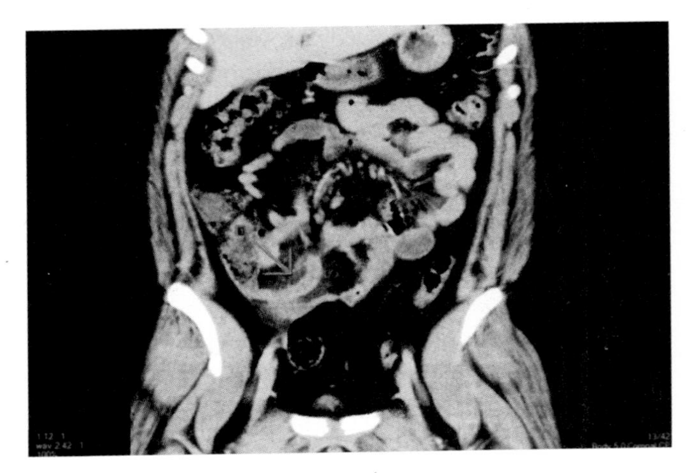

Fig.26.2 Acute appendicitis. The acutely inflamed and swollen appendix is indicated by the arrow.

Appendicitis in the elderly and obese

In elderly patients the diagnosis of appendicitis may be missed. There are two reasons for this: firstly, as the condition is uncommon at this age, it may not be suspected. Secondly, as the abdominal wall is lax, rigidity may not be present even though the appendix is gangrenous.

In obese patients the signs of an inflamed appendix may be masked. If serious doubt exists operation should be carried out.

A word of caution

When a clinician receives a patient suffering from an acute abdominal condition about whom a diagnosis of acute appendicitis, ureteric colic, or other acute condition has been made by someone else, he should consider the patient as suffering from an 'acute abdomen' until his own interrogation and investigation reveals the exact diagnosis. He should not rely on a diagnosis made elsewhere, because having undertaken the patient's treatment he is responsible for the accuracy of the diagnosis and the correctness of the management. In fact this rule should be followed throughout one's clinical practice, otherwise one will be treating patients on the basis of diagnoses made by other people, which may or may not be correct.

Untreated appendicitis

Appendix mass

If a severely inflamed appendix remains untreated for a few days the edematous omentum and intestines adhere to the appendix and result in the formation of an inflammatory mass, the appendix mass. The presence of the mass indicates that the infection has become walled off and that generalized peritonitis is unlikely to supervene. If left alone an appendix mass can follow one of two courses:

- It can become smaller and subside slowly as the inflammation resolves.
- It can enlarge and become an appendix abscess.

Appendix abscess

If an appendix perforates but the infection remains confined to the right iliac fossa, an appendix abscess may result. If the pus is under tension there may be a swinging temperature. If the pus is 'pointing' through the abdominal wall, there may be overlying edema, with induration and greatly increased tenderness. A marked polymorphonuclear leucocytosis is the rule.

Treatment of acute appendicitis

The treatment of acute appendicitis is appendicectomy. If the case is seen before a mass has formed, there is universal agreement that the appendix should be removed immediately.

Conventional appendicectomy

Appendicectomy is commonly performed through a right grid-iron incision. A transverse skin-crease incision at the McBurney's point also gives adequate access and may be even better. Laparoscopic appendectomy is another option with its potential advantages especially if there is any doubt in the diagnosis as in young females.

In the grid-iron incision each of the three muscles of the anterolateral abdominal wall are split along the line of their fibres. The incision is best placed parallel to the skin creases in this region, when it results in a more inconspicuous scar.

After the peritoneum has been opened the cecum is withdrawn and the appendix hooked out by the finger and held in a Babcock forceps. If any difficulty is encountered, the taenia coli on the cecum are traced downwards, and will lead the operator to the base of the appendix.

The mesoappendix is clamped in an artery forceps, divided and ligated. The base of the appendix is crushed in a hemostat, which is removed and reapplied a little distal to the crushed portion. A vicryl (absorbable) suture is tied round the crushed portion near the cecum. A silk purse-string suture is placed in the cecum around the appendix base. The appendix is amputated with a knife, and the lumen of the appendix stump cleaned out with a small swab on a holder. The stump is not normally invaginated.

The peritoneum and abdominal wall muscles are repaired in layers with absorbable sutures, usually employing chromic catgut for the peritoneum and polyglactin for the muscles. The skin is sutured using fine polypropylene or staples. In an occasional case, if there is much pus in the peritoneal cavity, a drain may be placed through a separate stab incision. This ensures that the main wound heals undisturbed.

Laparoscopic appendicectomy

The operation table is placed in a moderate Trendelenberg position to facilitate delivery of bowel from the pelvis. Operating ports are placed at points considered suitable. The operation then proceeds through the same steps as in the conventional procedure and the appendix is removed through one of the ports. A single stitch closes the linea alba and the skin of each port.

After laparoscopic appendicectomy patients have less pain and a much speedier return to normal living than those who have had conventional appendicectomy. The operation is specially suitable for use in obese patients, in whom the conventional operation imposes a large wound, with delayed convalescence and higher rates of infection.

After removal, *if an appendix appears normal,* it should be slit open. If the mucosa is pale, this was a normal appendix; if the lumen contains purple blood clot and inflamed mucosa, this is an inflamed appendix. Incidentally, such an occasion should occur only occasionally.

Antibiotics

The bacterial flora in the appendix are the same as in the colon. The use of antibiotics effective against both aerobic and anaerobic organisms therefore reduces the incidence of postoperative wound infection. In early acute appendicitis without pus and gangrene, a short course consisting of the first dose just before operation followed by one dose 6–8 hours post-operatively should suffice. In perforated appendicitis 7 to 10 days of antibiotic therapy is advisable. Effective regimens include third generation cephalosporin i.e. cefoxitin or ampicillin-sublactam with metronidazole.

If the diagnosis is in doubt, it is best to admit the patient overnight for observation. During this period it should be possible to determine whether exploration for appendicitis should be carried out or the patient discharged. If the diagnosis is still doubtful, laparoscopy may be indicated to help determine the cause of the illness.

Treatment of an appendix mass

If an appendix mass has already formed before the patient presents, the treatment is traditionally conservative. This is because an attempt at appendicectomy at this time would require separation of the adhesions; this could result in perforation of the intestine and lead to the formation of an intestinal fistula. Besides, it may be impossible to find the appendix in the inflammatory mass.

Oschner sherren regimen

In such a situation the patient is best placed on an Oschner Sherren regimen. Antibiotics are started parenterally; for example, a third generation cephalosporin for the Gram-negative bacteria, and metronidazole for the anaerobes. Fluids are given intravenously, though clear fluids may be allowed by mouth as tolerated. The pulse, temperature, degree of tenderness and rigidity, and size of the mass are monitored every few hours. Normally the symptoms and signs abate in a day or two, and the inflammation subsides over a few weeks. '*Interval appendicectomy*' is then carried out after about four weeks.

However, if the abdominal pain spreads widely, vomiting becomes copious and chocolate-coloured, the pulse rate continues to rise, and the size of the mass increases, operation has to be carried out. The causes of failure of conservative treatment of an appendix mass include abscess formation and small bowel obstruction from adhesions.

Treatment of an appendix abscess

If in a case of appendix mass the temperature continues to swing, the pulse rate remains high and the swelling becomes larger and more tender, it means that an abscess has formed, and incision-drainage must be carried out. During this operation no effort should be made to remove the appendix unless it is lying free in the abscess cavity.

If a USG/CT scan shows the abscess to be lying immediately deep to the abdominal wall, ultrasound-guided tube drainage can be carried out. After successful closed or open drainage of an appendix abscess, appendicectomy must be carried out after 3 or 4 months, as otherwise the patient will remain prone to further attacks of appendicitis.

TUMORS OF THE APPENDIX

Carcinoid tumor of the appendix

This tumor arises in the Kulchitsky cells of the crypts of Lieberkuhn. These cells have a special affinity for silver stains, therefore they are called argentaffin (L. argentums = silver), and the tumor is called an argentaffinoma. It can arise anywhere in the gastrointestinal tract; however, the most common site is the appendix, followed by the small intestine. The tumor is found once in about 200 appendices submitted for histology. Most patients are female. Most carcinoid tumors of the appendix are found incidentally at the time of appendicectomy, usually at the tip of the organ. The muscular coat of the appendix is often involved, but more distant metastases are quite rare.

Carcinoids are mostly benign and are treated by appendicectomy unless:

- There are enlarged lymph nodes.
- The size of the tumor is more than 2cm.
- The tumor is located at the base of the appendix, in which case right hemicolectomy should be carried out.

Adenocarcinoma

This is a rare tumor of the appendix. It presents as acute appendicitis or intestinal obstruction, and is best treated by right hemicolectomy.

Chapter

27 COLON AND RECTUM

Absorption of foods takes place mainly in the small gut; the colon is primarily a conduit for the residue. However, sodium and potassium are absorbed in the colon and potassium, bicarbonate and mucus are secreted. Certain carbohydrates and proteins are also digested and an environment provided for the production of vitamin K by bacteria. Water is absorbed along the whole length of the colon. The fibrous residue is thus rendered firm and dry for easier disposal, and is stored in the descending and sigmoid colon before being expelled at the time of defecation.

MEGACOLON

Megacolon is defined as an abnormally dilated colon. It may be primary or secondary.

PRIMARY MEGACOLON

(Hirschsprung's disease)

In this condition there is delay in passing meconium after birth, resulting in severe constipation.

Pathology

The constipation is due to complete absence of parasympathetic ganglion cells in the wall of the rectum and sigmoid colon, which arises as follows: the ganglion cells of the bowel migrate from the neural crest along the vagus nerves within the bowel wall to reach the anus by birth. If this migration fails to reach the anus, the result will be a segment of bowel without ganglion cells. This segment extends upwards from the anus for a varying distance. The segment of bowel without proper innervation by the autonomous nervous system cannot conduct a peristaltic wave and acts as a physiological obstruction to the onward passage of bowel contents. The more proximal colon becomes greatly dilated and hypertrophied. The mucosa of the dilated intestine is chronically inflamed due to the stagnant contents, and often ulcerated. The aganglionic bowel contracts down to a small size. This is the *narrow segment* seen on barium enema.

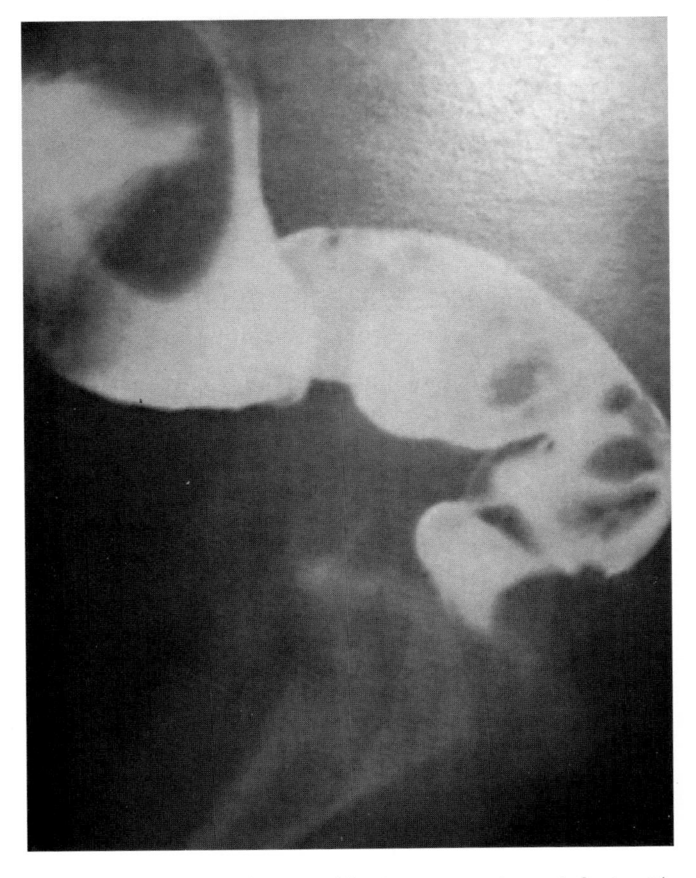

Fig.27.1 Left lateral view of barim enema in an infant with Hirschsprung's disease, showing dilated sigmoid colon and contracted segment of rectum.

Clinical features

The condition is much more common in males, with a familial tendency. Symptoms always appear within a few days of birth. The baby fails to pass meconium during the first two or three days of life. He suffers from severe constipation, and passes meconium only after the passage

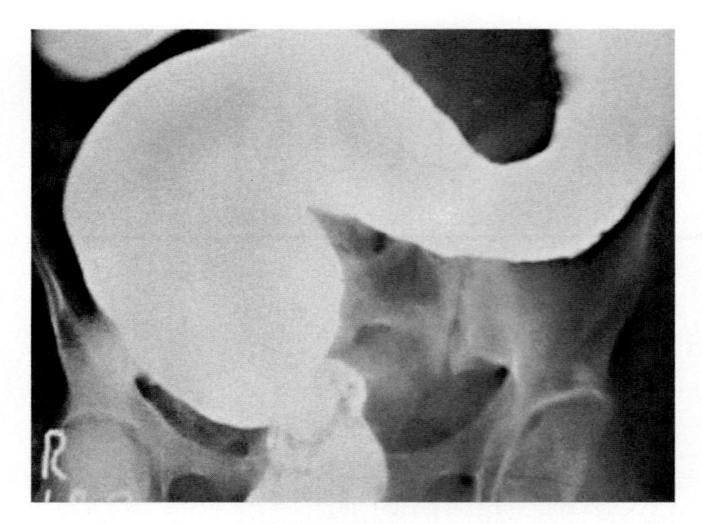

Fig.27.2 Hirschsprung's disease in adolescent showing narrow rectum and dilated sigmoid colon. The patient suffered from severe constipation since birth.

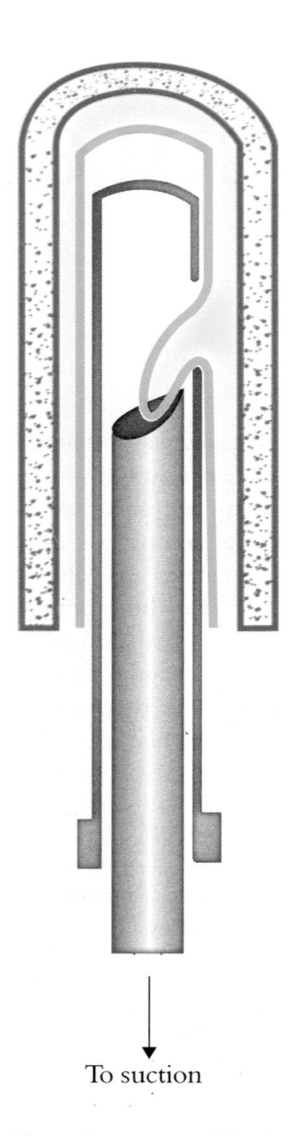

Fig.27.3 Suction biopsy instrument. The instrument has been passed in the rectum. Suction is being applied, and it has sucked mucosa into the instrument through a side window. Now the knife will be advanced; it will cut a piece of mucosa and suck it into the bottle.

of a finger into the rectum. The infant strains to bring out toothpaste-like stools in small amounts.

Abdominal distension appears within the first few days of life, with loud borborygmi and visible peristalsis. The rectum is empty and grips the examining finger. Complete intestinal obstruction may occur. The baby fails to thrive, with malnutrition and stunted growth. Severe constipation in the newborn is a very serious condition, and could be due to Hirschsprung's disease. If this fact is overlooked the consequences can be grave.

Investigations

Gastrografin enema

X-ray of the abdomen and pelvis is taken after giving an enema of barium or Gastrografin solution. A lateral view of the pelvis is also taken, as it shows the rectum better. The enema shows the dilated colon and the contracted aganglionic segment of the rectum (Figs.27.1and 2).

Rectal suction biopsy

If Hirschsprung's disease is suspected on the basis of the contrast enema, a rectal suction biopsy should be performed. This can be carried out without anesthesia as an outpatient

Procedure

The cylindrical suction biopsy instrument (Fig.27.3) is passed into the rectum. When suction is applied a small piece of mucosa of the rectum is sucked into the lumen through a side opening. The built-in blade is now advanced forwards. This cuts off the mucosa, which is sucked into the bottle attached to the biopsy instrument.

As serious bleeding can occasionally occur, the infant should be kept in hospital for a few hours after the procedure. Only mucosa and submucosa can be obtained by this method. The tissue is examined microscopically after paraffin section and staining. If ganglion cells are present this means that the bowel wall is normal and Hirschsprung's disease is not present. If on the other hand, ganglion cells are absent and there is hypertrophy of the nerve fibres, the case could be one of Hirschsprung's disease. Recently, *punch biopsy forceps* are being used to obtain rectal biopsies under local anesthesia.

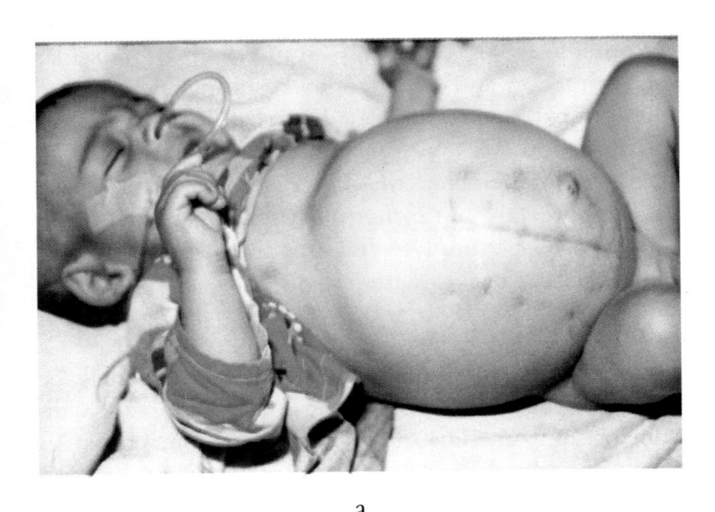

a

Fig.27.4 (a) Unsuccessful laparotomy for Hirschsprung's disease

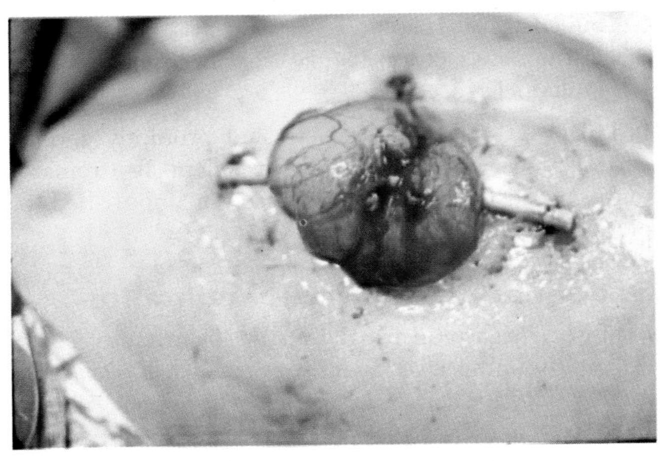

b

Fig.27.4 (b) Right transverse colostomy to decompress the colon. In due course barium enema x-ray, rectal biopsy and a Duhamel operation was performed.

However, a firm diagnosis cannot be made on the basis of suction biopsy alone. For this purpose:

- *Full-thickness rectal biopsy* has to be carried out under general anesthesia, in order to prove that ganglion cells are absent from the muscle layers also. The tissue is examined histochemically for the presence of increased acetylcholine esterase activity.
- *Anorerctal manometry.* In normal persons if the rectum is distended the internal sphincter is reflexly inhibited. In Hirschsprung's disease this inhibition does not occur, and this can be demonstrated by anorectal manometry.

Treatment

Although the severe constipation of Hirschsprung's disease can be temporarily tided over by repeated enemas, the only curative treatment is excision of the non-functioning aganglionic segment which acts as a peristaltic block. In the newborn, a loop colostomy is carried out just above the cone area to relieve the obstruction.

When laparotomy is carried out for resecting the aganglionic area, the only way in which the upward extent of the aganglionic segment can be determined with certainty is by frozen-section examination of biopsies taken at different levels, which should be carried out. When the upper limit of resection has been decided upon, the further operative procedure can take one of three forms:

- **Swenson operation**. In this procedure the entire aganglionic segment of large bowel is removed, and the normal ganglionic colon anastomosed to the anal canal.
- **Duhamel procedure**. Here the lower part of the rectum is preserved. The ganglionic colon is brought down behind the rectum and out through the internal sphincter. To the adjoining walls of the colon and rectum is applied a specially designed stapler, which crushes, staples and divides them to produce a single cavity. The posterior part of this tube consists of ganglionic colon, providing propulsive activity; the anterior part is rectum which, although it is aganglionic, provides the rectal sensation of fullness.
- In both the above operations the nervi erigentes are in danger of damage leading to impotence; this is prevented by staying close to the colonic wall during the pelvic dissection.
- **Soave operation.** During the 1980's this procedure had become the most popular procedure. In this operation the muscular tube of the rectum is left in place, while its mucosal layer is excised. The normal colon is passed down through the rectal muscular sleeve, and sutured to mucosa at the anorectal junction. Any possibility of damage to the nervi erigentes is thus eliminated by dissecting inside rather than outside the rectum.

The Soave operation is best carried out in early infancy, when it can be performed without a covering colostomy. The other two operations normally require a preliminary colostomy. The Soave operation has now gone out of favour because the rectal muscle sleeve often contracts around the pulled-through colon to produce a severe stricture of the new rectum. Its place has been taken by the Duhamel procedure.

If Hirschsprung's disease is treated promptly and by correct surgery, the prognosis is excellent. If it remains undiagnosed the infant gets severely malnourished, or dies of enterocolitis.

Secondary (acquired) megacolon

Acquired megacolon usually results from faulty bowel care and training. *Symptoms can be traced from infancy, but never from birth; in this way it differs from Hirschsprung's disease.* In contrast to the situation in Hirschsprung's disease, the rectum and sigmoid are also dilated, and barium enema shows no contracted rectal segment. Similarly, rectal biopsy shows normal ganglion cells, i.e. the rectum is developmentally normal.

Etiology

If the bowel wall is normal, what then is the cause of acquired megacolon? Inadequate toilet training in infancy and emotional deprivation are probably responsible. Both these factors are often present in orphans, and in children from broken homes. As the infant is not made to pass stools at the normal times, he does not develop a regular bowel habit. The stools accumulate in his bowels and lead to their chronic dilatation.

Social aspects

An important cause of an emotional disorder is seen when another child is born into the family, the family moves to a new town or a different house, or the child is shifted to a new school. When the history is being taken this aspect should be carefully enquired into.

Treatment

Treatment consists of emptying the greatly dilated colon of its contents by repeated enemas or, if that is not feasible, by manual evacuation under anesthesia. This should be followed by careful toilet training, along with as much emotional support and encouragment as possible.

DIVERTICULAR DISEASE OF THE COLON

This condition is relatively uncommon in the East, possibly because the diet contains natural fibre which has been removed from the food consumed in the more advanced countries. It is commonly seen in middle and old age. The diverticula protrude outwards through the circular muscle coat at the point where blood vessels penetrate the colonic wall. In the vast majority of cases the sigmoid colon is involved. 5% of the patients have associated gallstones and hiatus hernia.

Diverticulosis is probably caused by muscular incoordination and hypertrophy resulting in increased intraluminal pressure. Diverticulitis involves inflammation of one or more diverticula due to stagnation of their contents. These episodes may occur at varying intervals, but symptoms usually get worse with the passage of time. Diverticulitis is not precancerous, but cancer can coexist with it.

Clinical features

Diverticulosis may be symptomless, or there may be distension and heaviness in the lower abdomen, with pain off and on. Diverticulitis causes more persistent pain. Fever, malaise and leucocytosis may be present. There may be diarrhea or constipation. The left iliac fossa is tender, and the sigmoid colon may be thickened with overlying fibro-fatty tissue. Diverticular disease occurs predominantly in the elderly who often have associated diseases that complicate diagnosis and influence treatment.

Diverticulitis has to be distinguished from carcinoma. As compared to carcinoma, in diverticulitis the history is longer and pain and bleeding more common.

Complications

The complications to which sigmoid diverticula are prone include the following:

- Recurrent inflammation.
- Perforation with generalized or localized peritonitis and septic shock.
- Intestinal obstruction from progressive fibrosis.
- Hemorrhage.
- Fistula formation with bladder, vagina, small bowel or skin.
- Intractable disturbance of bowel function (distension, cramps, diarrhea, or constipation) and persistent pain, occasionally requiring surgical treatment even in the absence of the more defined complications listed above.

Investigations

Diverticulosis

Often, diverticulosis of the sigmoid colon is present without causing any symptoms. Therefore, symptoms should be ascribed to diverticulosis only if other causes have been excluded by colonoscopy and barium enema.

Barium enema confirms the presence of diverticula, provides evidence for or against the diagnosis of diverticulitis, and helps exclude the presence of carcinoma. As against cancer, in diverticular disease:

- The length of the affected segment is greater.
- The mucosa is intact.
- Spasm is often present.
- The ends of the narrowed segment are tapering rather than blunt.

Diverticulitis

In diverticulitis barium enema or colonoscopy should be carried out only when the inflammation has subsided, in order to avoid perforation.

Treatment

Diverticulosis

This should be managed with a high residue diet. When the large gut is well filled with abundant residue it functions better, and the mild symptoms of diverticulosis disappear:

- If necessary, supplementary bulk may be added by about 20 g of wheat bran daily.
- The stool may be softened and moisturized by powdered psyllium seed (ispaghula) husk (5–10 g daily). This should be dissolved in a glass of water; if it is taken dry, the powder may choke the patient.
- Drugs that inhibit peristalsis (such as propantheline bromide 7.5mg thrice daily) may give symptomatic relief.

Diverticulitis

This requires bed rest, fomentation, antispasmodic drugs and a week-long course of broad spectrum antibiotics, usually a cephalosporin and metronidazole. Only a few patients require resection of the sigmoid colon.

Surgery

If obstruction is present, the feces are first diverted by a transverse colostomy. This gives rest to the sigmoid and allows the inflammation to subside. After a few weeks resection is carried out, and after another few weeks the colostomy is closed. This is the safest course to follow in this condition with chronically infected large bowel.

INTESTINAL AMEBIASIS

Amebiasis is defined as infestation with Entameba histolytica with or without overt clinical symptoms.

Pathology

The disease is contracted by consuming food or drinks contaminated with the cysts of the parasite. In countries where the condition is endemic there are innumerable carriers of the disease, because the vast majority of infestations are asymptomatic.

The active form of the ameba lives in the mucous membrane of the large intestine, where it ingests red blood cells. If it becomes pathogenic it invades the submucosa and produces ulcers with undermined edges and a necrotic floor. These ulcers are usually confined to the rectum and sigmoid colon. Some of the amebae migrate to the surface, become transformed into cysts and pass out with the feces. The most common symptom is dysentery, with or without blood and mucus.

Diagnosis

The stool should be examined for amebae. At the same time the suspected area of rectal mucosa may be scraped and the tissue examined immediately for the presence of amebae.

Treatment

Metronidazole is the drug of choice for amebiasis.

Asymptomatic intestinal amebiasis

This can be treated by diloxanide furoate 500mg orally thrice daily for 10 days, or di-iodohydroxyquinoline 600mg thrice daily for 21 days.

Acute amebic dysentery

This is treated by metronidazole 400mg orally thrice daily for 5 days.

An alternative regimen consists of emetine hydrochloride 1mg/kg intramuscularly in two divided doses daily for 4 to 10 days. This drug should not be used in cases of cardiac disease, and the patient should be confined to bed.

Complications

From time to time a case of intestinal amebiasis may present with one of the following complications:

- *Typhlitis* (i.e. inflammation of the cecum). This may be mistaken for appendicitis.
- *Perforation of the colon with peritonitis*. The wall of the colon becomes a white slough and multiple perforations result. The commonly affected sites are the cecum and the ascending and sigmoid colon. The condition has a very high mortality rate. Three types of perforation occur:
  - o Extraperitoneal perforation.
  - o Perforation of a granuloma or ulcer without acute dysentery.
  - o Perforation in a case of fulminant disease.

  Anti-amebic therapy is commenced. If the patient's condition deteriorates and rupture appears imminent, an ileocolostomy may be carried out to divert the fecal stream. However, if perforation is associated with gangrene, resection is the best course of treatment.

- *'Amoeboma'*, i.e. a mass of amebic granulation tissue. This may need to be distinguished from an appendix mass, a neoplasm, ileocecal tuberculosis and an actinomycotic granuloma.
- *Fulminant amebic colitis*. This type of colitis is seen in malnourished individuals and in patients with coincident debilitating disorders, also in patients on steroids and other immunosuppressive therapy. Indications for surgery include:
  - o Deterioration in spite of medical therapy (with severe diarrhea, toxicity and abdominal tenderness) with x-ray evidence of toxic colonic dilatation.
  - o Onset of an acute episode of perforation or bleeding.

  The best operative treatment is primary resection with exteriorization of the bowel ends. In the past the mortality rate was nearly 100%; this has been reduced to about 50% with improved medical treatment, early and aggressive surgery, and exteriorization.
- *Massive hemorrhage* from erosion of a large vessel in the bowel wall; this complication is quite rare.
- *Amebiasis of the skin*. If an amebic abscess is treated by open drainage the ameba may colonize the drainage tract, and can be quite difficult to eradicate even with intensive anti-amebic therapy. In fact, even if the abscess is treated with closed drainage by aspiration, the needle track may not heal because of amebiasis cutis.
- *Amebic liver abscess* is described in chapter 21.

ULCERATIVE COLITIS

Ulcerative colitis is a condition in which the mucosa and submucosa of the colon are the seat of chronic inflammation, with the formation of large numbers of ulcers over wide areas of the mucosa.

Etiology

The cause of this condition is not known. It may be related to the autoimmune diseases but this is not certain. There is some evidence that the patient may be prone to allergic reactions in the gastrointestinal tract. At the same time, in the mucous membrane there is a deficiency of type IV mucin and hydrolase, both of which have a protective function. Therefore the mucosa becomes more permeable and susceptible to injury by intraluminal irritants. When ulcers develop, secondary infection plays a large part in the disease process.

Pathology

Ulcers

In early cases hemorrhagic inflammation is seen, with petechial hemorrhages and bleeding. In more advanced disease, small ulcers form all over the mucosa of the colon and later join up to form larger ones. When they extend into the submucosa they cause reflex muscle spasm, and the false appearance of a stricture.

Pseudoplyps

When fibrosis occurs during the process of healing, the epithelium gets piled up between the ulcers, producing the so-called pseudopolyps, and also permanently shortening the affected part of the colon. When remission takes place, the normal structure of the mucosa may be restored, but some atrophy of the mucosa is often seen.

Dysplasia

In the long term, certain areas in the mucosa become dysplastic; this is an important change, as it predisposes to the development of carcinoma of the colon.

Clinical features

Ulcerative colitis is a disease of adult life, women being affected more often than men. The first symptom is watery diarrhea occurring day and night. Mucus with pus or blood is very common. The symptoms come and go.

Mild disease

The disease is defined as mild if fewer than four motions are passed daily, and there are no systemic symptoms or signs. This is the most common form of the disease, and the inflammation is usually confined to the rectum and sigmoid. The long-term prognosis is good, the patients rarely requiring admission to hospital, and the life expectancy is not affected by the disease.

Moderate disease

If between four and six stools are passed daily, the disease is defined as moderate. The stools invariably contain blood. Abdominal pain, low grade fever, and iron-deficiency anemia are in evidence, with loss of appetite and weight. The disease responds well to corticosteroids, but the long-term prognosis is not good, and rapid deterioration with the development of local complications e.g. toxic megacolon, massive bleeding and colonic perforation may occur at any time.

Severe disease

Severe ulcerative colitis is responsible for most of the deaths from the disease. The diarrhea is accompanied by tenesmus and rectal bleeding, with severe dehydration, electrolyte depletion, acidosis and anemia.

Fulminant disease

A fulminant type of disease also occurs. In this type there is fairly high temperature, continuous diarrhea with blood, mucus and pus, and a toxic appearance. Toxic paralysis of the colon may produce abdominal distension (toxic megacolon). This condition must be distinguished from dysentery and typhoid by examination of the stool and by blood culture or Widal test.

Chronic disease

The chronic type of disease is much more common. The initial attack is moderately severe, but exacerbations occur at variable intervals. The patient is wasted and anemic. The greater the area of colon affected the more frequent the motions, and the greater the degree of ill-health due to protein loss and the toxemia of bacterial infection. When the whole colon is involved the patient may be bedridden, due to the combined effects of malnutrition, electrolyte depletion and toxemia.

Prognosis

A bad prognosis is indicated in the following situations:

- If the initial attack is severe.
- If the disease involves the entire colon.
- If the age is above sixty.

Investigations

X-rays

The earliest x-ray sign is loss of haustrations in the distal colon. Later changes include a narrow contracted colon, ulcers with undermined edges, and pseudopolyposis. In long-standing cases the acute angles of the hepatic and splenic flexures are lost, resulting in a rounded course for the colon due to its shorter length.

Colonoscopy

On colonoscopy, at first the mucosa is hyperaemic and bleeds on touch, and there is a good deal of exudate. Later, tiny ulcers form and may join up. In amebic dysentery, on the other hand, there are large deep ulcers with fairly healthy mucosa in between. Biopsies are taken.

Rectal biopsy

Rectal biopsy establishes the diagnosis and shows the effects of treatment.

Complications

Systemic

These are common to both ulcerative colitis and Crohn's disease. They include:

- Liver changes e.g. cirrhosis.
- Skin lesions e.g. pyoderma gangrenosum.
- Arthritis.
- Anemia.

Local

Carcinoma

If the patient has suffered from ulcerative colitis for 10 years the risk of carcinoma developing is 1 %; if for 10 to 20 years, then as high as 5 %. Therefore, if the disease has been present for over ten years, regular colonoscopy should be carried out.

Cancer in cases of ulcerative colitis occurs at a younger age than in non-colitic patients. The tumors tend to be less well-differentiated and are more often multiple.

Dysplasia is regarded as predictive of neoplastic change. If moderate to severe dysplasia is present, prophylactic proctocolectomy is advised because of the risk of malignant change.

However, regenerative changes in the epithelium should not be mistaken for dysplasia. For this purpose, several *'mucosal markers'* have been developed to detect dysplasia, for example:

- Enzyme activity (G6-PDH).
- Antigen expression by the epithelial cells, like *carcinoembryonic antigen*.

Other local complications include:

- Massive hemorrhage.
- Toxic megacolon.
- Perforation.
- Perianal suppuration.
- Fibrous stricture.
- Hemorrhoids.

Toxic megacolon

In this condition the inflammation spreads to all coats of the colonic wall, with gross distension and resultant thinning of the bowel wall. The patient's general condition deteriorates, with absent bowel sounds due to paralytic ileus, severe toxicity, fever, tachycardia, and fluid and electrolyte depletion leading to hypovolaemia. The risk of perforation is very high; therefore, most cases are treated by emergency colectomy after resuscitation.

Toxic megacolon is sometimes also seen in Crohn's disease and in the pseudomembranous colitis which occasionally follows antibiotic therapy.

Treatment of ulcerative colitis

Mild and moderate cases of ulcerative colitis often respond to medical treatment; severe cases usually require surgery.

Medical treatment

The type of medical measures required depend on the severity of the disease:

Mild disease

These patients require sulphasalazine in a daily dose of 3–4 g, along with steroid enemas containing 20mg of prednisolone-21-phosphate. Some add low-dose oral prednisolone (20mg/day).

For *maintaining a remission* low-dose steroid therapy is ineffective, and sulphasalazine is the most effective agent in a dose of 2 g daily; in fact this is the most important indication for the use of this drug. Its *side effects* include headache, vomiting, diarrhea, skin rashes, male infertility, and hemolytic and aplastic anemia.

Moderate disease

Here, suphasalazine and steroid enemas should be accompanied by 40mg daily of oral prednisolone. If a remission is not achieved within two weeks, the patient should be hospitalized and treated as a case of severe disease.

Severe disease

Intensive medical therapy and monitoring should be provided. The fluid and electrolyte losses, the acidosis, and the hypovolaemia are corrected. Blood transfusions and human albumin solutions are often required to restore the hemoglobin level and protein content.

Intravenous prednisolone-21-phosphate is given in a dose of 64mg/day. Hydrocortisone drip enemas (100 g in 100ml of water) are administered twice daily. Some add tetracycline and metronidazole to the regimen. Codeine phosphate, belladona etc. are not recommended. Not only are they ineffective, they may also contribute to the development of toxic megacolon by aggravating any paralytic ileus.

Daily clinical and radiological assessment enables the clinician to monitor the progress of the case. Sudden deterioration of the general condition, increasing abdominal girth and absent bowel sounds indicate failure of medical therapy and the need for an emergency colectomy. If improvement is not obvious within a few days, surgery is indicated. The factors suggesting a poor prognosis include :

- Fever higher than 38^0 C.
- Pulse rate greater than 100/min.
- Motions more frequent than 12 per day.
- Serum albumin level lower than 3 g/dL.

About 70% of patients respond favourably. However, in the long term as many as 50% require proctocolectomy.

Surgical treatment

Emergency treatment

Subtotal colectomy and ileostomy

In an emergency situation, as in toxic megacolon, colonic perforation or massive hemorrhage, the treatment of choice is a subtotal colectomy and ileostomy. The rectum is left behind, the rectal stump being brought out as a mucous fistula. This course avoids a pelvic dissection and allows the possibility of joining the ileum to the rectum later on, when the patient has recovered from the systemic illness and is well-nourished.

Elective surgery

This is carried out in the following situations:

- If medical treatment has failed.
- If extraintestinal disease is present.
- If growth is retarded, in the young.
- If dysplasia, villous ademomas or carcinoma have developed.

Operations

The operations available as elective procedures are the following:

- ***Subtotal colectomy and ileostomy*** (as decribed above).
- ***Proctocolectomy and permanent ileostomy.*** In this operation the whole colon and rectum are removed in one stage, eliminating any risk of colorectal carcinoma or symptoms of colitis, but it leaves the patient with a permanent stoma. It is indicated for patients who cannot opt for restorative surgery because of anal sphincter problems.
- ***Restorative proctocolectomy.*** The whole of the colon and rectum are removed. To replace the rectum a pouch is formed from the terminal ileum by folding it on itself and anastomosing the limbs together as a 'J pouch' (Fig.27.5). This new rectum is joined to the anal canal, restoring the natural route for the passage of feces. Its advantages include the following:

- o The patient is spared the need for a permanemt ileostomy stoma.
- o The pouch takes the place of the colon as a reservoir, so that the number of movements of the bowel is reduced, making life more comfortable.

- ***Total colectomy with ileorectal anastomosis.*** In a few patients where the rectum is not diseased, the whole colon is removed but the rectum is preserved, with ileorectal anastomosis. After operation the patient passes stools through the normally placed anus. However, because of the absence of the colon the frequency of the stools is greater than normal. The operation has lost a good deal of its popularity since the advent of restorative proctocolectomy.

Care of ileostomy

There are thousands of patients all over the world who are living with permanent ileostomies. If the ileal stoma is made properly and looked after with due care, a fairly reasonable life can be led by the patient. The patient can also benefit by joining one of the *ileostomy associations* in his area. These groups, which are quite active in some countries, provide much-needed support in the form of comradeship, besides very useful literature.

Ischemic colitis

Ischemic colitis is an inflammatory condition of the mucous membrane of the colon produced by interruption of its blood supply insufficient to cause full thickness tissue death. It commonly affects those in the seventh and eighth decades of life.

Etiology

Its causes include:

- Occlusion of a major artery.
- Minor vessel disease.
- Venous obstruction.
- 'Low flow' states.
- Intestinal obstruction.

Pathology

Ischemia reduces the integrity of the mucosa and allows invasion by pathogenic organisms such as clostridia, which are normal constituents of the colonic flora. Inflammation and ulceration result, which may resolve completely, or may cause permanent injury with healing by fibrosis, and stricture formation.

Clinical features

The patient complains of acute *pain* starting in the left iliac fossa, with loose stools containing dark blood as well as clots. There may be low-grade *fever*. The affected colon is *tender* and may be palpable. Submucosal *edema* and *hemorrhage* produce swellings that bulge into the bowel lumen and are seen on barium enema as 'thumb printing'. Mucosal *ulcers* develop.

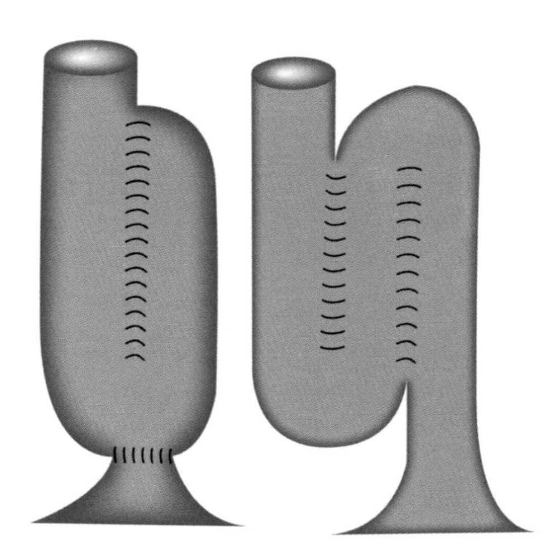

Fig.27.5 J-and S-pouches to increase the capacity of the new rectum after restorative proctocolectomy.

If a *stricture* results, it may be difficult to distinguish it from carcinoma. In ischemic colitis strictures are often long, uniform and smooth. If doubt exists colonoscopic biopsy should be carried out.

Treatment

Conservative management with bed rest, analgesics and intravenous fluids is the mainstay of treatment for those presenting with acute symptoms. In the rare case of stricture a resection and end-to-end anastomosis should be carried out.

Rectal prolapse

Prolapse of the rectum is a relatively rare condition in which some or all of the layers of the rectum protrude through the anus. The prolapse may be mucosal or full-thickness.

Mucosal prolapse

In mucosal prolapse only the mucous membrane prolapses out, for a distance of not more than 3.5cm. When it is palpated between finger and thumb it becomes obvious that it consists of no more than a double layer of mucosa. A mucosal prolapse can be easily distinguished from prolapsed internal piles due to the following differences:

- Prolapse forms a continuous ring all round, whereas piles constitute three or more separate masses.

- Prolapsed mucous membrane is red, whereas piles are purple in colour.

Full-thickness prolapse

In full-thickness prolapse the full thickness of the rectal wall comes down. It is more than 3.5cm in length, and may be as long as 10–15cm.

Rectal prolapse occurs at the extremes of life:

- In *children* below the age of five: it often follows a bout of diarrhea, and may disappear spontaneously. Simple bowel training is adequate treatment (Fig.27.6).
- In the *elderly,* specially females, full-thickness prolapse may be due to muscular degeneration. There is weakness of the pelvic fascia, the muscles of the pelvic floor, and the anal sphincter (Fig.27.7).

The prolapsed mucous membrane may be edematous or ulcerated. It secretes mucus, which soils the clothes and causes perianal dermatitis. On examination the sphincter is lax. The majority of cases are incontinent of feces. They regard themselves as social outcasts, and are ashamed to mention this symptom unless asked.

Treatment

Mucosal prolapse

This requires submucosal injections of a sclerosing solution e.g. 5% phenol in almond oil, in each of the four quadrants, to cause the submucosa to undergo fibrosis and adhere to the underlying muscle layer. Injections are quite adequate treatment for this type of prolapse.

Full-thickness prolapse

For full-thickness prolapse various operations have been devised:

- ***For poor-risk patients***. The simplest procedure, which is used only in the elderly and poor-risk patients, is the *Thiersch operation*. A circumferential suture of nylon is placed subcutaneously around the anal canal. The anal orifice is left large enough for the feces to pass, but not wide enough for prolapse to occur. This operation is effective provided the patient empties the rectum adequately; however, impaction often develops.

For good-risk patients many operations have been devised but none is perfect:

- *Polyvinyl alcohol sponge.* In the most popular operation the rectum is wrapped in a polyvinyl alcohol sponge, which is fixed to the front of the sacrum.
- *Rectosigmoidectomy*. Alternatively, the redundant sigmoid and upper rectum may be excised in a rectosigmoidectomy. The success rate of these repairs is upto 80%.
- *Submucosal injections.* In children, even full-thickness prolapse can be managed by submucosal injections of phenol in almond oil. However, unlike the injections given for the treatment for piles in adults, these are given under general anesthesia. Injections are given into each quadrant, a longer needle being used so that the oil can be deposited in the submucosa upto higher levels.

Fecal impaction

Hard dried stools impacted in the rectum and unable to pass through the anal canal are commonly seen in elderly and debilitated patients. This may be seen after orthopedic, pelvic or abdominal operations. A painful anal fissure may also inhibit defecation to the extent that overloading occurs.

Clinical features

The symptoms are those of chronic intestinal obstruction. Liquid stool passes around the fecal mass and leaks out in an uncontrolled manner (spurious diarrhea). Fecal masses may be palpable in the abdomen and can be distinguished from other abdominal lumps by the fact that they can be indented. On rectal examination the single large rock-like mass of stool can be felt.

Treatment

Enemas are usually insufficient. A *stool softener*, like dioctyl in mineral oil solution, can be left in the rectum overnight and may disimpact the feces. If it does not, the anal sphincter must be stretched under general anesthesia and the mass *removed manually*. Enemas are then given for a few days to allow any remaining hard stools to be expelled.

Diet

After the evacuation, advice is given about diet. Foods containing roughage, e.g. salads, vegetables and fruits should be taken in abundant quantities. Their bulk provides the most effective stimulus to peristalsis, so that the gut empties efficiently. Psyllium seed (ispaghulla) husk, 10gm in a glass of water at bedtime for a few days, softens the stools for easier evacuation; it should not be taken indefinitely. At the same time, 1 to 2 glasses of water taken before proceeding to the toilet help in defeacation because of the gastro-colic reflex.

Radiation proctitis

Exposure to radium, Cobalt-60 or x-rays during treatment of carcinoma of the cervix, uterus or bladder may cause inflammation in the adjacent rectum. This may subside,

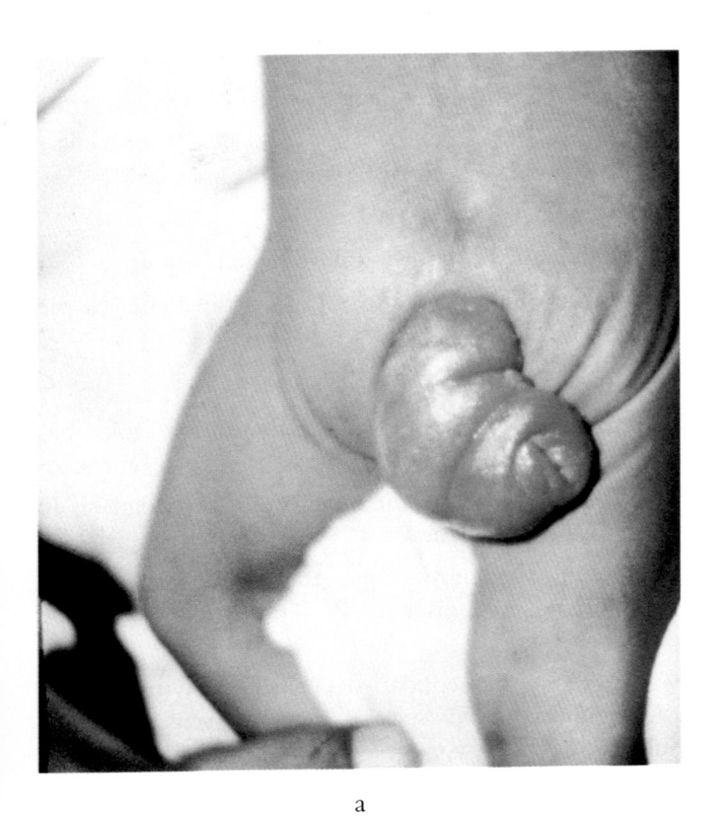

a

Fig.27.6 Full-thickness prolapse of rectum in a young boy

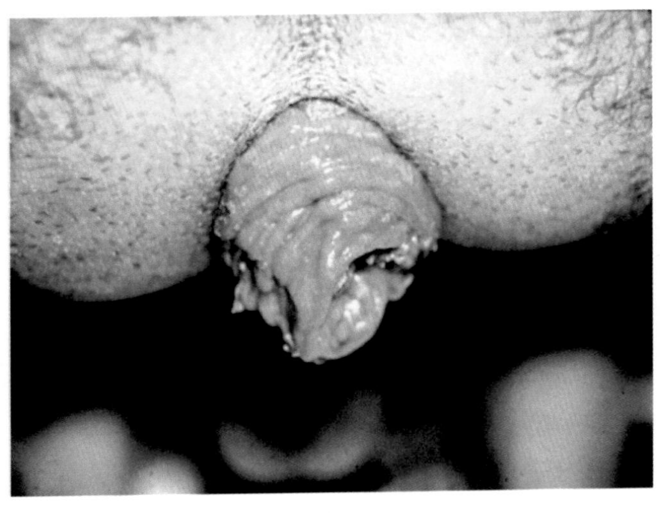

b

Fig.27.7 Full-thickness rectal prolapse in an adult

or may persist in a chronic form for many years and lead to stenosis. Treatment is rarely required. Occasionally a stricture requires dilatation, or a rectovaginal fistula needs repair.

VOLVULUS

Volvulus means axial rotation of a portion of the alimentary tract. It occurs commonly in the pelvic colon, and occasionally in the small intestine and cecum. As both ends of the twisted loop are closed it behaves as a closed loop obstruction.

VOLVULUS OF THE SIGMOID COLON

This condition is common in Eastern Europe, Peru, Uganda, etc., and in Pakistan among the Pathans[1]. Elsewhere in the world the condition is uncommon, except in inmates of mental institutions, in whom the enlargement of the sigmoid colon occurs due to neglect of regular evacuation of the bowel.

Pathology

The sigmoid colon is long with a narrow attachment of the pelvic mesocolon. If it twists around this narrow pedicle, it becomes a closed loop. It distends mostly with air and some feces, and balloons out to fill the whole abdomen.

Clinical features

The patients are adult, often middle-aged, and mostly males. There may be a previous history of attacks of left-sided colicky pain. When volvulus occurs there is sudden severe abdominal pain, with rapid onset of marked distension. There is absolute constipation. The obstruction being in the distal large bowel, vomiting occurs late.

Xray

Plain xray abdomen shows the greatly distended loop of sigmoid: filling the whole abdomen.

Treatment

If the diagnosis is certain and the case is of only a few hours' duration, a sigmoidoscope should be passed into the rectum, and an attempt made to pass a flatus tube into the distended sigmoid loop through the sigmoidoscope. If this is successful a great deal of wind is passed and the obstruction is relieved. If the flatus tube fails to pass into the sigmoid, immediate laparotomy should be carried out and the obstructed loop untwisted to allow the wind to pass.

However, this is not the end of the matter. Due to the greatly increased length of the sigmoid, the patient remains liable to repeated attacks of volvulus. Therefore,

1 Volvulus of the sigmoid colon among Pathans, I. Ahsan et al, Brit. Med J; 1 (5531) 1967.

a few weeks after untwisting the volvulus, the gut should be prepared and the sigmoid colon resected, eliminating the possibility of further attacks.

If *gangrene* has already set in before the patient presents, immediate resection of the gangrenous sigmoid colon must be carried out. In such a case the ends are not anastomosed together; they are brought out i.e. exteriorized, because if they were joined together, this would result in a high incidence of leakage at the anastomosis and spell disaster for the patient. The resulting colostomy is closed a few weeks later. In cases of gangrene the operative mortality rate is very high, due mainly to the toxemia of anaerobic infection.

Tumors of the colon

Benign. Adenomatous polyps are dark red pedunculated neoplasms. They are common.

Malignant. Carcinoma.

CARCINOMA OF THE COLON

Pathology

Microscopically, the tumor is a columnar-celled carcinoma. Macroscopically, it assumes one of the following forms:

- Annular.
- Tubular.
- Ulcerative.
- Cauliflower.

The annular variety causes early obstructive symptoms and is treated promptly, so the prognosis is good. The cauliflower type often commences as a benign adenoma. The most common sites are the pelvic colon and the rectosigmoid junction.

Spread

The neoplasm grows slowly, and if it is removed thoroughly at an early stage, a cure can be hopefully expected.

Local spread

The growth spreads at a slow rate, and usually causes intestinal obstruction before it has penetrated adjacent structures. Penetration may produce an internal fistula, or a local abscess and an external fistula.

Lymphatic spread

This occurs first to the epicolic lymph nodes lying on the colonic wall, and then successively to the paracolic, intermediate and 'main' lymph nodes.

Blood spread

This occurs late, and to the liver.

Grading

Dukes has classified colorectal cancers into the following histological grades:

- Low grade i.e. well-differentiated tumors.
- Average grade tumors.
- High grade i.e. poorly-differentiated tumors.

The more differentiated the tumor, the better is the prognosis.

Staging

As regards the extent of spread of the tumor, Dukes has also provided a system of staging of colorectal cancers:

A: Growths limited to the rectal wall: the prognosis in these cases is excellent.

B: Growths extending into the extra-rectal tissues, but with no metastases to the lymph nodes: here the prognosis is good.

C: Growths with secondary deposits in the lymph nodes: the prognosis in this stage is bad. This stage is further sub-divided into two:

C1: Only local para-rectal nodes are involved.

C2: Nodes accompanying the supplying blood vessels are implicated.

In recent years a stage D has been added which was not described by Dukes; it signifies the presence of metastases, usually hepatic.

Dukes vs TNM staging

The TNM staging is more precise, and allows useful division into subsets without being unduly complex. For this reason it is the most suitable system for clinical trials. Yet, because of its great simplicity Dukes' classification is attractive for clinical practice. As future generations of surgeons will use the TNM system from the beginning, they will find it easy to work with. Therefore this system is likely to displace all other methods of staging in times to come.

Clinical features

Except for occasional cases the patient is over fifty years of age. Over a quarter of the patients present with intestinal obstruction or peritonitis.

In carcinoma of the *left colon* the symptoms are often those of increasing intestinal obstruction due to the narrower lumen and more solid fecal contents.

Pain is usually of the nature of a colic. Increasing constipation may be present with distension. The carcinoma itself, or impacted feces, may be palpable.

Carcinoma of the *cecum* may present as an undiagnosed anemia, a mass, or an intussusception.

Carcinoma of the *transverse colon* may be mistaken for a neoplasm of the stomach due to its position.

In the *sigmoid colon* a papilliferous growth may produce a feeling of the need for evacuation, tenesmus, mucus and blood.

Investigations

Radiography

Barium enema x-ray

This may show a constant irregular filling defect (Fig.27.7).

Air contrast enema

If the barium is partly evacuated and air injected into the colon *(air contrast enema)* the walls of the colon become delineated, and even a small lesion may be shown up.

CT

Virtual CT colonoscopy can pick up small polyp/s, but if a biopsy is needed, endoscopy will still be required.

Endoscopy

Early growths in the lower pelvic colon may be missed by radiography, but are shown up on sigmoidosocopy.

Colonoscopes can go all the way to the cecum and are the most definitive ivestigation for carcinoma of the large bowel.

Exfoliative cytology

Exfoliative cytology of the colon is a laborious procedure, but successful diagnoses used to be made in growths situated in all parts of the colon. Since the advent of colonoscopy exfoliative cytology has lost its applicability.

Treatment

The treatment of carcinoma of the colon is by operation, to remove the segment of colon carrying the lesion as well as the whole of the primary lymphatic field draining the area of the lesion.

Preoperative preparation

For 48 hours before the operation the patient is allowed only clear fluids by mouth, and enemas are given twice daily to cleanse the bowel. However, some recent opinion suggests that mechanical preparation of the bowel increases the chances of infection.

Operation

At operation the first job is to ascertain the extent of spread of the tumor by examining the liver, the lymph node groups and the peritoneum to detect any secondaries, and the tumor to determine whether it is fixed or free.

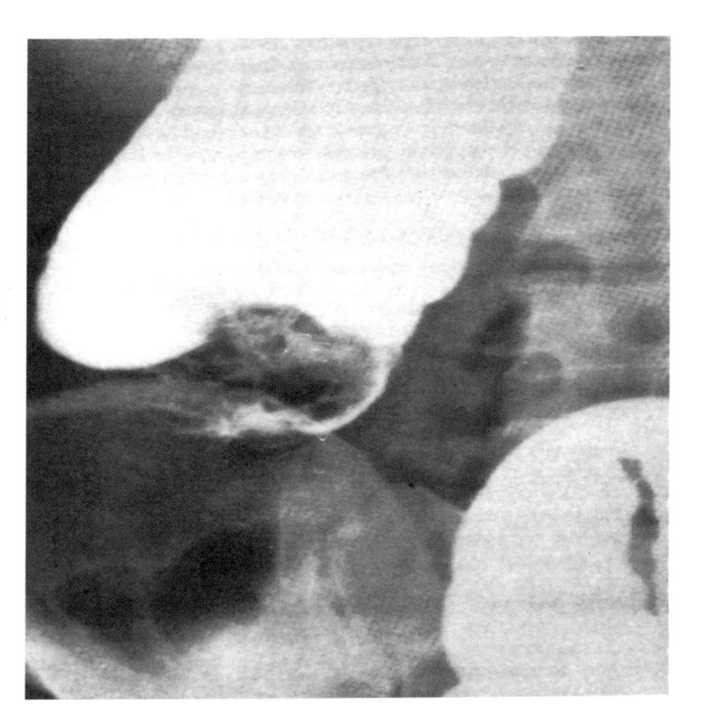

Fig.27.8 Barium enema x-ray showing irregular filling defect in cecum due to a cauliflower carcinoma.

While removing the colonic cancer the lymph nodes which drain the tumor must be removed, because they may be involved by metastases. As these lymph nodes lie along the regional veins and arteries those vessels, and therefore obviously the whole segment of colon supplied by them, has to be removed. Thus it comes about that during any particular resection a segment of the colon supplied by one or more of the following arteries is removed: the ileo-colic and right colic, the middle colic, the left colic and the sigmoid arteries. If the tumor lies at the junction of segments supplied by two different arteries, both segments are removed.

Inoperable growth

If a growth is *inoperable* surgery may still be carried out to relieve or prevent obstruction. In the ascending colon an ileo-transverse colostomy is carried out. In the upper left colon a transverse colostomy, and in the pelvic colon a high left iliac colostomy is performed. This provides for unhindered passage of feces through the maximum available length of the colon in each case, for the remaining period of the patient's life.

Laser therapy

If the patient has advanced metastatic spread or severe concomitant disease that render him unfit for surgery, *laser therapy* can be employed. It aims at removing all of a cauliflower tumor, improving bleeding, discharge and obstructive symptoms. Treatment is entirely local and is used to coagulate and vaporize the tumor.

Metastases in the liver

Colorectal cancer metastatic to the liver is highly resistant to systemic chemotherapy. However, portal venous perfusion of 1g of 5-fluorouracil immediately after the operation, has been shown to reduce the risk of development of hepatic metastases.

TUMORS OF THE RECTUM

Rectal tumors may be benign or malignant.

Benign tumors

Juvenile rectal polyp

If an infant between two and four years of age passes bright red blood per rectum, without pain and in the absence of dysentery, it is very likely a case of rectal polyp. It commonly arises from the posterior wall of the rectum as a pedunculated bright red rounded mass. The diagnosis is easily confirmed by digital rectal examination, which is best carried out after giving the infant a sedative like tricloryl syrup. A juvenile rectal polyp does not exhibit any tendency to become malignant, but should be removed per rectum under general anesthesia. Incidentally, sometimes it falls off itself, but one should not wait for that to happen.

Pseudo-polyps

These are just tags of mucosa which have hypertrophied due to chronic inflammation, commonly in ulcerative colitis.

Villous adenomas

These adenomas are often very large, and contain villi on the surface. They tend to become malignant, when the tumor becomes hard. These polyps secrete a good deal of mucus, which has a high potassium content. If the tumor is large, potassium depletion may result.

Familial polyposis coli

In this condition multiple polyps develop in the colon during adolescence and cause rectal bleeding. The polyps in the rectum and sigmoid can be seen by the sigmoidoscope. However, to assess the full extent of the disease and the total number of polyps, either colonoscopy or an air-contrast barium enema are required. In time some of these polyps become malignant. The malignant potential of any one polyp is very small. However, when it is remembered that in these cases there may be hundreds of polyps, it becomes obvious that the chances of any one of them becoming malignant are very great. In fact if left untreated, the patient is sure to develop a carcinoma in one of the polyps.

Treatment

In view of the above, the only proper treatment for familial polyposis coli is removal of the whole colon and rectum (total proctocolectomy). However, if the polyps in the rectum are regularly excised by diathermy the rectum can be preserved, sparing the patient the inconvenience of life with a colostomy. If malignancy develops in one of the rectal polyps in spite of repeated diathermy, the rectum would also require to be removed.

CARCINOMA OF THE RECTUM

Rectal carcinoma is one of the most common malignancies in both men and women. It used to occur only in middle and old age; however, during recent decades younger and younger patients are being seen, some even in their twenties.

Pathology

The tumor commonly starts as a nodule. The less malignant of these nodules project into the lumen, the more malignant tend to infiltrate the wall and ulcerate. The ulcer feels hard and has everted edges like malignant ulcers elsewhere. When a segment of large bowel is removed for carcinoma, often there are in addition one or more adenomas or papillomas. This suggests that these latter are pre-malignant lesions.

Histological sub-types

Dukes has classified colorectal carcinomas into the following grades:

- Well-differentiated adenocarcinomas.
- Averagely-differentiated adenocarcinomas.
- Anaplastic, undifferentiated adeno-carcinomas.

The more differentiated the tumor, the better is the prognosis.

Spread

Carcinoma of the rectum spreads locally, via the lymphatics, via the blood-stream, and by peritoneal dissemination.

Local spread

This occurs circumferentially rather than longitudinally. It takes a tumor about six months to spread around a quarter of the circumference, and about two years to go all round. Spreading outwards, the tumor infiltrates through the muscle of the rectal wall, then fat, then perirectal fascia. If the tumor is located anteriorly, in the male the prostate, seminal vesicles or bladder become involved, in the female the vagina or uterus. In either sex a lateral tumor may infiltrate into a ureter; similarly, extension backwards may involve the sacrum and the sacral plexus. Spread in a downward direction is uncommon.

Lymphatic spread

From the upper and middle thirds of the rectum lymphatic spread occurs almost entirely upwards along the inferior mesenteric vein and artery. From the lower third spread can also occur laterally along the middle rectal vein. Downward spread to the groin lymph nodes is very uncommon.

Venous spread

As a rule spread via the veins occurs late. However, anaplastic and rapidly growing tumors in younger patients often spread in this way. The most common sites for blood-borne metastases are the liver (because blood from the rectum is drained via the portal system), the lungs, the adrenals, and the brain.

Peritoneal dissemination

This can occur when a high-lying rectal carcinoma penetrates the peritoneal coat. The malignant cells set free into the peritoneal cavity can lodge on the surface of any organ, so that there may be small nodules everywhere if the case comes late.

Staging of rectal carcinoma

As regards the extent of spread of the tumor, Dukes has classified rectal carcinomas into three stages:

A. Growths limited to the rectal wall: the prognosis in these cases is excellent.

B. Growths extending into the extra-rectal tissues, but with no metastases to the lymph nodes: here the prognosis is good.

C. Growths with secondary deposits in the lymph nodes: the prognosis in this stage is bad. This stage is further sub-divided into two:

C1: Only local para-rectal nodes are involved.

C2: Nodes accompanying the supplying blood vessels are implicated.

Clinical features

Rectal bleeding

This is the earliest and most common symptom. Unfortunately, it often closely resembles the bleeding due to piles. Thus it is bright red in colour, and the blood is usually smeared on the surface of the mass of stools. Therefore it is often not taken seriously, and the rectum is not properly examined.

Sense of incomplete defecation

After the patient has passed stools he still feels the desire to pass more feces. This is because after defecation the tumor is still present in the bowel, which cannot distinguish between the mass produced by feces and that resulting from a tumor. The patient may try to empty the rectum several times a day, usually with the passage of some blood-stained mucus (spurious diarrhea).

Increasing constipation

This may set in if the carcinoma is annular, i.e. one which has gone all round the rectum and is causing increasing constriction.

Pain

Colicky pain may be seen due to some degree of intestinal obstruction. Severe constant pain occurs when the tumor infiltrates the surrounding structures. For example, pain in the back or sciatica occurs when the growth invades the sacral plexus.

Examination

Abdominal examination

This is positive only in advanced cases. For example, distension may be present due to intestinal obstruction, ascites due to peritoneal deposits, and nodularity of the liver due to secondaries.

Rectal examination

Digital rectal examination is an essential investigation in every case of rectal bleeding or unexplained alteration of bowel habit. Most carcinomas of the rectum can be felt by the finger. In an early case a hard nodule may be felt; more commonly the tumor has already ulcerated, the ulcer having a raised and hard edge. If an ulcer is felt, the finger on withdrawal is usually found to be blood-stained. In females a vaginal examination should also be performed, to find out if the tumor is adherent to the vagina.

Investigations

Sigmoidoscopy

This should be carried out in the knee-elbow position, so that the rectum hangs forwards and straightens out and the endoscope can be passed up further. If a tumor is seen, a biopsy forceps should be used for taking a biopsy, including a portion of the edge of the tumor.

Colonoscopy

This should be performed to rule out adenomas or synchronous carcinomas at higher levels in the large bowel.

Treatment

The only proper treatment for a carcinoma of the rectum is removal of the rectum along with its primary lymphatic field.

Anterior resection of the rectum

This is the most commonly performed operation for cancer of the rectum today. It is employed for tumors in the upper two thirds of the rectum, where there is a sufficient length of normal rectum below the tumor.

The sigmoid colon and rectum are removed from above, leaving a short segment of rectum below. The inferior mesenteric artery is ligated at its origin from the aorta; in this way the pelvic mesololon and its contained lymph nodes are taken away along with the artery. Finally, the descending colon is mobilized and anastomosed to the fringe of rectum. Thus the sphincters are saved and the patient spared the very considerable inconvenience of life with a permanent colostomy.

This operation can be performed laparoscopically with similar oncological results. However, it is technically difficult, and should be carried out only by properly trained and experienced surgeons.

Abdominoperineal resection

This procedure is most often used to treat cancers located in the lower third of the rectum or in the anal canal. The sigmoid colon, rectum and anal canal are all removed. Besides, the pelvic mesocolon containing the inferior mesenteric artery upto its origin, and the levators ani, are also removed *en bloc* with the gut. A permanent end colostomy is fashioned in the left iliac fossa. As the operation requires dissection both in the abdomen and the perineum, it is called abdominoperineal resection.

More extensive operations

When the rectal carcinoma has spread to neighbouring organs, the radical operation can usually be extended to remove these structures. Thus, in the male a total cystectomy can be added to the operation where indicated, in the female a hysterectomy. If necessary, all the pelvic organs may be removed, together with the pelvic lymph nodes (pelvic evisceration). However, this operation is justified only when the surgeon is confident that the disease can be removed in toto.

More limited operations

In a very old and debilitated patient, in whom there is a concern about anal sphincter function or possible breakdown of an anastomosis, a Hartmann's excision can be employed. Through an abdominal incision the rectum is excised down to within 2.5cm of the anus and an end colostomy performed. The peritoneal floor is closed and the perineal wound drained through the anal canal. In the elderly, where the tumor is usually slow-growing, and spread is late, this is a most useful operation.

Laser therapy

If the patient has advanced metastatic spread or severe concomitant disease that renders him unfit for surgery, laser therapy can be used to coagulate and vaporize a cauliflower tumor improving bleeding, discharge and obstructive symptoms.

Stenting

In high rectal tumors an endoluminal stent can be used:

- As a palliative.
- To relieve obstruction and allow elective surgery.

Palliative colostomy

This is indicated where there is gross infiltration by the tumor. Sometimes, after chemoradiotherapy, it becomes possible to resect the tumor, with occasional cure.

Prognosis

In specialist institutions the resectability rate may be as high as 90% and the operative mortality less than 5%. The overall 5 year survival rate for rectal carcinoma is about 50% in the advanced countries. In the underdeveloped countries due to late presentation the overall figures are more dismal.

When 10-year survivals after surgery for early and advanced cancers are examined, the figures in Dukes' four stages are as follows:

Dukes'

A	85%.
B	65%.
C	40%.
D	0–5%.

These figures show the overwhelming importance of early diagnosis.

Fecal fistula

A fecal fistula usually results from leakage of an intestinal anastomosis, or after operation on a case in which the gut wall is necrosed due to one cause or the other. Examples of the latter are found after surgery for the following conditions:

- Gangrenous appendicitis.
- Appendix abscess.
- Strangulated hernia with gangrene of the gut.

- Actinomycosis.
- Amebiasis.
- Regional enteritis.
- Abscess connected with diverticulitis or colonic carcinoma.

The track of the fistula may be lined by granulation or fibrous tissue, but in long-standing cases becomes epithelialized.

The higher the fistula the greater the extent of both fluid loss and skin digestion, because the duodenum and jejunum contain large volumes of potent digestive enzymes. In fistulas of the ileum or cecum the discharge is fluid; in the distal colon it is semi-solid or solid fecal matter.

In cases of doubt *methylene blue* given by mouth gives the discharge a blue colour.

To determine the site of the leak and the length of the fistula a *barium meal* or *barium enema* may help, or lipiodol may be injected into the outer opening.

Treatment

Fecal fistulae tend to heal spontaneously if there is no distal obstruction. The abdominal wall should be protected by the use of disposable ileostomy bags. Duodenal and jejunal fistulae cause dehydration and hypoproteinemia, and intravenous parenteral feeding is required. In order for surgical closure of an intestinal fistula to be successful, three conditions have to be met:

- The patient should be in positive nitrogen balance.
- There sould be no infection.
- There should be no distal obstruction.

A fecal fistula with an epithelial track will not heal until the track is removed. At operation an incision is made around the track which is dissected up through the abdominal wall and peritoneum, and the segment of gut bearing the fistula is resected.

Chapter

28 ANAL CANAL

ANORECTAL ANOMALIES

In the embryo the terminal part of the hindgut (before its division into rectum, bladder and genital primordia) is called the cloaca. The anal canal and rectum develop from the cloaca and proctodaeum in stages:

- First the cloaca gets divided by a transverse septum into an anterior urinary and a posterior alimentary part.
- Next the anus migrates backwards along the perineum.
- Finally, the lateral genital folds or anal tubercles fuse at their posterior ends.

Arrested or distorted development at any of these stages can lead to an anorectal anomaly.

The anomalies fall into two groups, the high and the low. In the high type the rectum ends above the puborectalis muscle; in the low type it has traversed this muscle and come down.

High anomalies

The common high anomalies include the following:

- The undivided ***cloaca*** may persist as such. The bladder enters this cavity from in front, the rectum from behind, and the uterus from above (Fig.28.1).

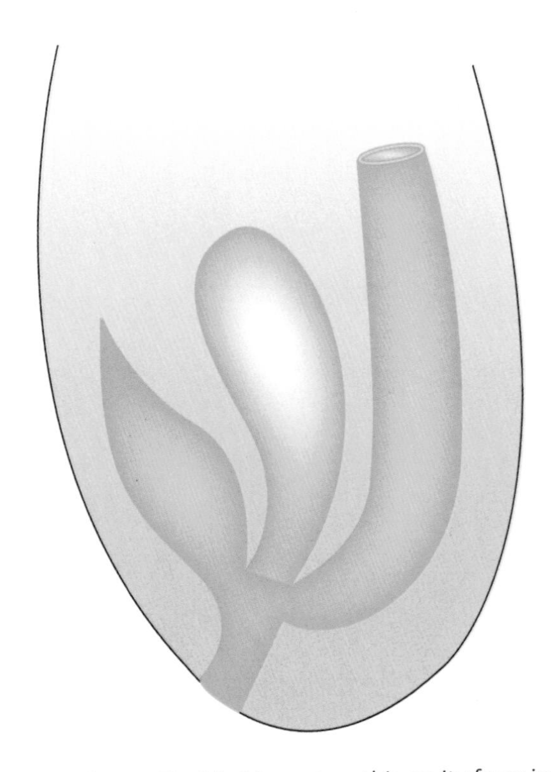

Fig.28.1 Cloaca. The bladder enters this cavity from in front, rectum from behind, uterus from above. The single opening in the perineum discharges greenish urine.

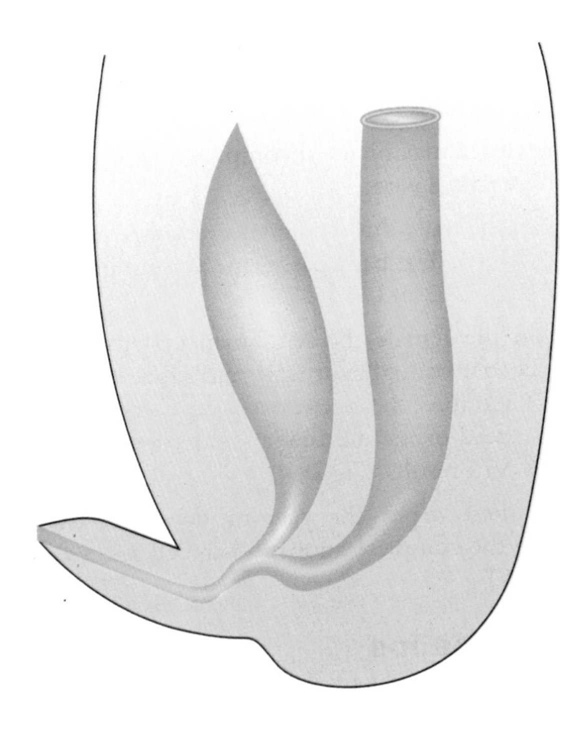

Fig.28.2 Recto-urethral fistula

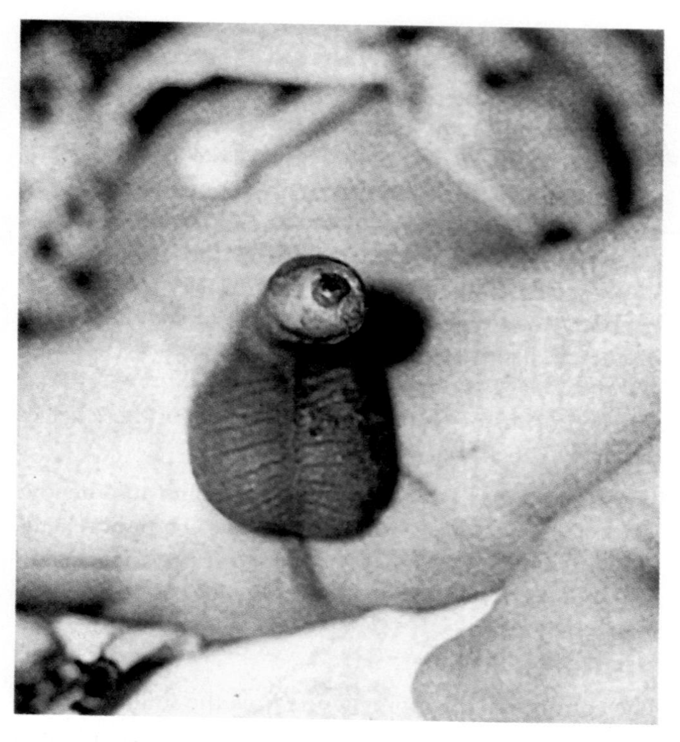

Fig.28.3 Recto-urethral fistula. Note meconium at external urinary meatus.

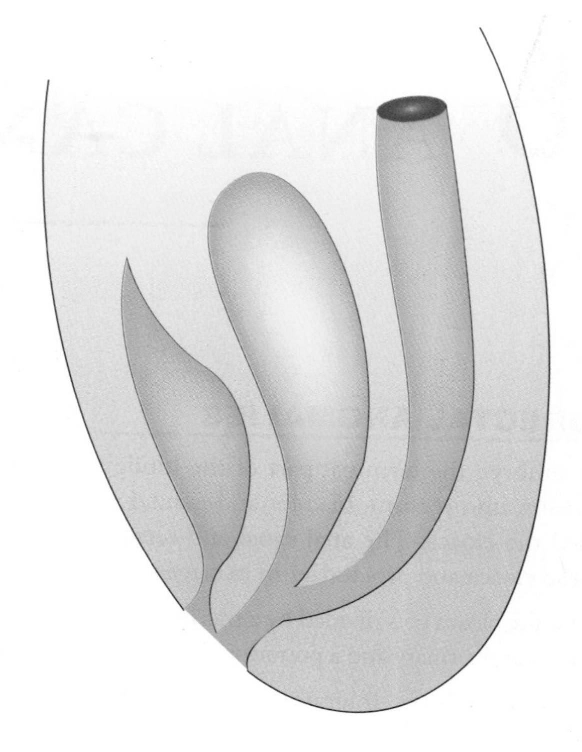

Fig.28.4 Rectovaginal fistula

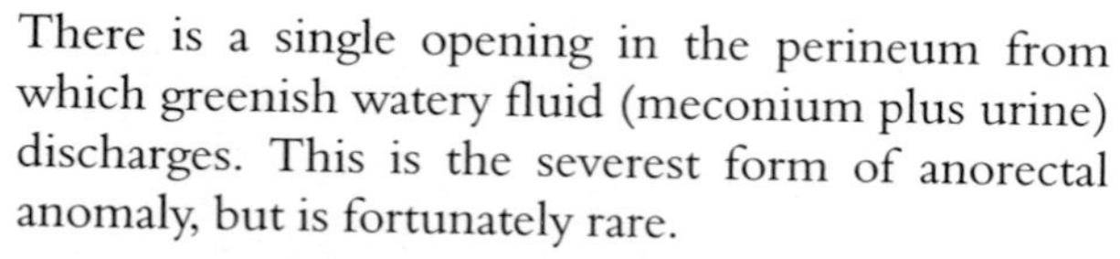

There is a single opening in the perineum from which greenish watery fluid (meconium plus urine) discharges. This is the severest form of anorectal anomaly, but is fortunately rare.

- The cloaca may divide incompletely into its urinary and intestinal parts.
    - In the male this results in a ***recto-urethral fistula*** (RUF). The baby passes meconium in his urine (Figs.28.2 and 3).
    - In the female the Mullerian system comes to lie between the urinary and alimentary tracts. Therefore the rectum opens into the vagina instead of the urethra, and a ***rectovaginal fistula*** (RVF) results (Fig.28.4).

In both these types the rectum does not develop. Therefore the complete anomaly is rectal agenesis with RUF or RVF.

Low anomalies

Low anomalies may take one of many forms:

- If the anus fails to migrate backwards the anal orifice is located far forwards. The result is as follows:
    - In the male the anus opens far forwards in the perineum—an ***anterior perineal anus*** (Fig.28.5)

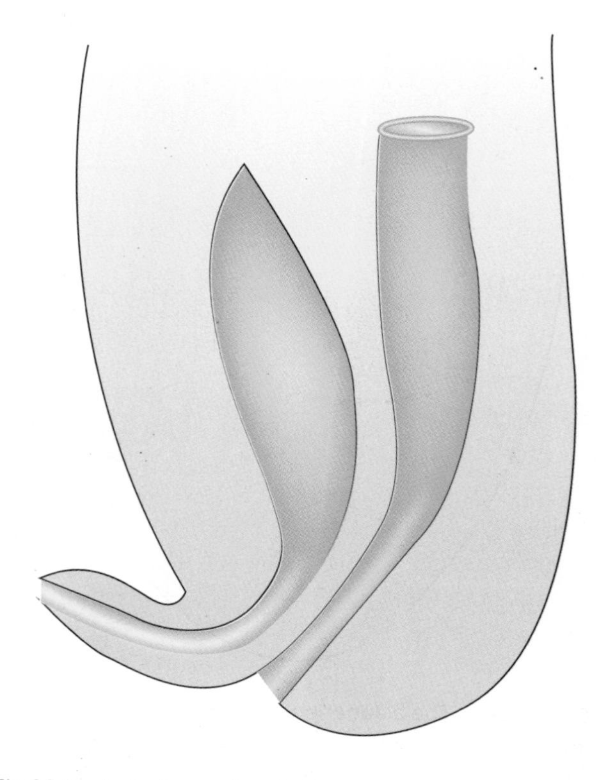

Fig.28.5 Anterior perineal anus in male.

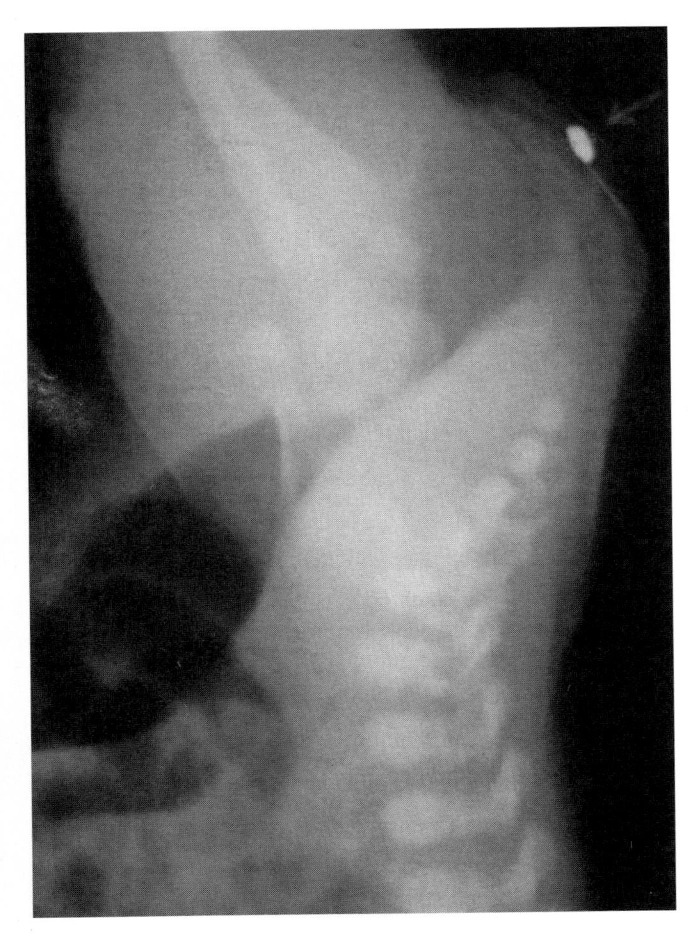

a

Fig.28.6 (a) Invertogram. Gas shadow extends to the metal object in the perineum, therefore this is a low anomaly.

- In the female the anus opens into the vulva or vestibule—a ***vulvar or vestibular anus***.
- If overfusion of the lateral genital folds or anal tubercles occurs, the anus becomes covered from behind by skin—a ***covered anus***. There are various forms of this anomaly:
  - A ***microscopic anus***.
  - A ***membrane*** occludes the normal anal site.
  - The fusion extends still further forwards:
    - In the male it carries a ***track*** in the skin along the perineal raphe. In this track a streak of meconium may be seen extending onto the scrotum or even the penis.
    - In the female the track may end in the vulva as a ***vulval ectopic anus***.

In all these cases of overfusion the anus beneath is practically normal.

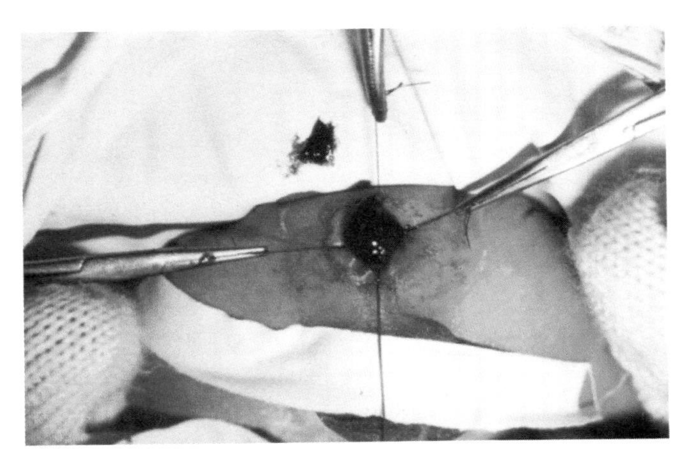

b

Fig.28.6 (b) Perineal operation on patient shown in Fig.28.6 (a). A membrane was occluding the anal canal. This was excised and meconium is coming through.

Clinical features

The most important method for establishing the type of anomaly is by physical examination of the perineum. In low anomalies in males, an ectopic opening of the rectum can be detected in the perineal raphe. In females this opening lies in the lower vagina, vestibule or fourchette. In many cases of anorectal anomalies other congenital abnormalities are also present, and should be looked for.

X-rays

It takes 12 to 18 hours after birth for swallowed air to reach the rectum. The baby is now held upside down to enable the gas to ascend to the rectum, and a lateral x-ray of the pelvis is taken (*invertogram*). The distance between the gas bubble in the rectum and the anal dimple (marked by a little barium paste) helps distinguish between high and low anomalies. For more exact differentiation, a straight line is drawn on the x-ray film joining the pubis with the coccyx. If the air bubble extends distal to this pubococcygeal line it is a low anomaly (Fig.28.6 a), if not, it is a high anomaly (Fig.28.7 a).

Treatment

Low anomalies are repaired by a simple perineal operation at birth:

- The microscopic anus needs dilatation.
- A membrane is excised.
- For the other varieties the orifice is cut backwards with a scissors blade in the opening.

Daily dilatations are carried out for about three months after the operation.

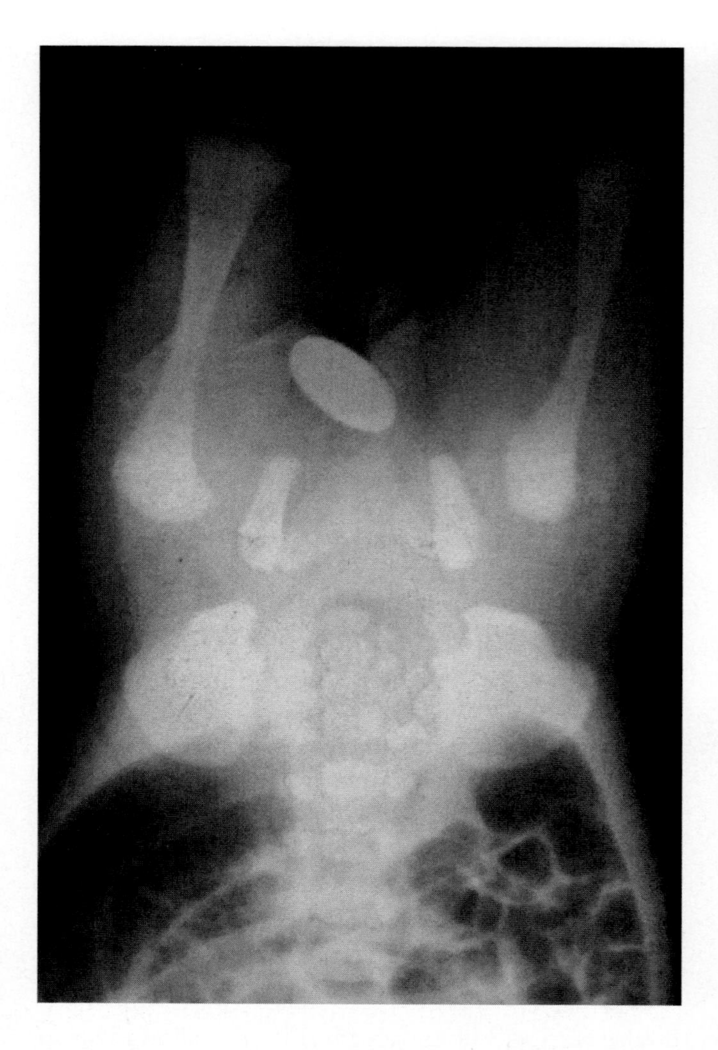

a

Fig.28.7 (a) Invertogram. No gas in pelvis, therefore high anomaly

In the ***high anomalies*** a colostomy is performed in the newborn. At the age of about one year the abdomino-perineal pull-through procedure is performed. In this operation the bowel is mobilized, brought down anterior to the puborectalis muscle and sutured to the perineum. A few weeks after the pull-through operation the colostomy is closed.

In high anomalies the puborectalis muscle is poorly developed. Therefore after operation continence is not always perfect. Many different operations have been tried; none has given complete satisfaction.

Posterior sagittal anorectoplasty (PSARP)

This latest operation consists of mobilization of the rectum through a posterior sagittal approach. Better results have been obtained than with other methods.

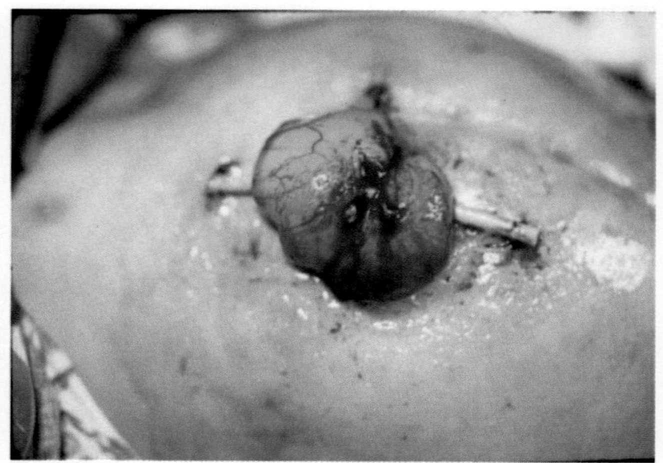

b

Fig.28.7 (b) Patient in Fig.27.8 (a) treated, as a newborn, by right transverse colostomy. A pull-through or posterior sagittal anorectoplasty will be done later.

HEMORRHOIDS (PILES)

The development of piles

In normal individuals a plexus of sponge-like veins lies under the mucosa in the anal canal above the mucocutaneous junction. They form vascular *hemorrhoidal cushions.* These cushions provide a spongy 'washer' on which the sphincter can act, assisting its closure and playing an important role in continence in respect to flatus and feces; collectively they are called the hemorrhoidal plexus. If with the passage of time the cushions swell up, they are called hemorrhoids or piles.

Important factors in the development of piles include:

- Chronic constipation. This is often due to the low-fibre diet which is popular in modern societies.
- Pregnancy.
- Hemorrhoids are frequently seen in members of the same family; here a congenital deficiency in the supporting tissues of the hemorrhoidal cushions is probably at work.

The term ***'external hemorrhoids'*** causes some confusion. It is used to signify pile masses that lie below the mucocutaneous junction underneath the anal epithelium and the perianal skin. It is better to regard the piles as disrupted vascular cushions, and observe whether the anodermal part is also involved.

The *reason* why the main pile masses always arise at 3, 7 and 11 O'clock is probably as follows: the superior rectal artery divides into a left and a right branch. The left branch runs down along the left side of the rectum (at 3

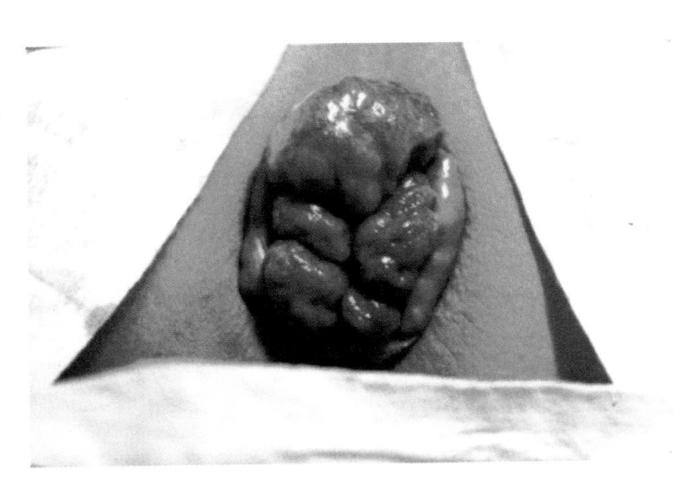

Fig.28.8 Third degree piles at 3, 7 and 11 O'clock. As usual, the largest pile is at 11 o'clock. Note secondary piles between main piles. Note rim of raised skin, the 'external piles'

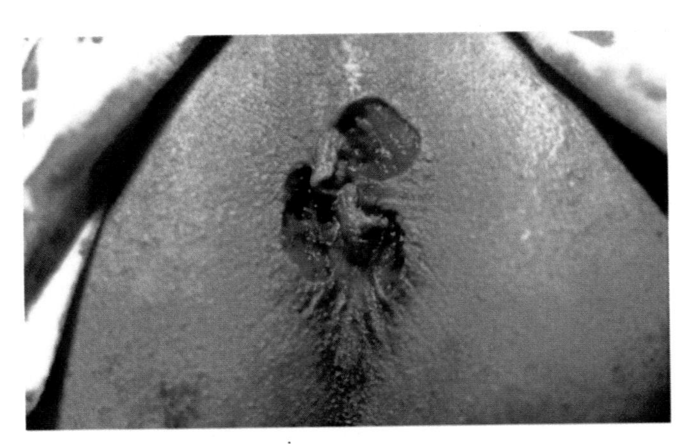

Fig.28.9 Three raw areas left after hemorrhoidectomy on patient shown in Fig.28.8.

O'clock with the patient in the lithotomy position). The right itself divides into two branches which descend at 7 and 11 O'clock respectively. Because the corresponding veins accompany the arteries, internal hemorrhoids occur at 3, 7 and 11 O'clock, corresponding to the branches of the artery. In between these three primary hemorrhoids there may be smaller secondary hemorrhoids.

Clinical features

Symptoms

Bleeding

This is the first and most important symptom. At first it is slight. It is bright red and occurs during defecation. Drops of blood may fall into the pan.

One type of bleeding is very typical of piles: when the stool mass passes over a pile it compresses it, so that blood spurts out through a tiny puncture in the mucosa as if it was being ejected from a syringe, and gets sprinkled around the inside of the commode. This kind of bleeding is rarely seen except in cases of hemorrhoids, and makes the diagnosis of piles virtually certain.

Degrees of hemorrhoids

First degree

Hemorrhoids that bleed but do not prolapse out of the rectum are called first-degree hemorrhoids.

Second degree

Prolapse usually starts later. At first prolapse occurs only at stools and reduces itself; these are second-degree hemorrhoids.

Third degree

At a more advanced stage the pile masses protrude with straining and have to be reduced manually; these are called third-degree hemorrhoids (Fig.28.8 and 9).

Fourth-degree

These are hemorrhoids that are permanently prolapsed.

Mucoid discharge occurs only when the piles are prolapsed and the mucosa exposed to the exterior. The discharge is followed by pruritus due to irritation of the skin.

It should be remembered that *pain* is always absent in hemorrhoids unless complications e.g. strangulation or thrombosis occur. The presence of pain in the history should make one think about strangulated piles (Fig.28.10), fissure, abscess, or fistula. Physical examination easily settles the matter.

Anemia may be present if the bleeding is persistent and profuse.

Signs

On *inspection* of the anal region external hemorrhoids may be seen as skin tags; internal hemorrhoids are not visible. On rectal examination internal hemorrhoids cannot be felt unless they are thrombosed.

Proctoscopy

The patient lies down in the left lateral position. He is asked to draw his knees up and advised to breathe gently though his open mouth and relax. A gloved and lubricated finger is always passed first. A proctoscope is next passed to its fullest extent and the obturator removed. The instrument is slowly withdrawn. At the level of the anorectal ring hemorrhoids, if present, bulge into the lumen of the proctoscope. Diazepam 5mg oral an hour before the examination allows the procedure to

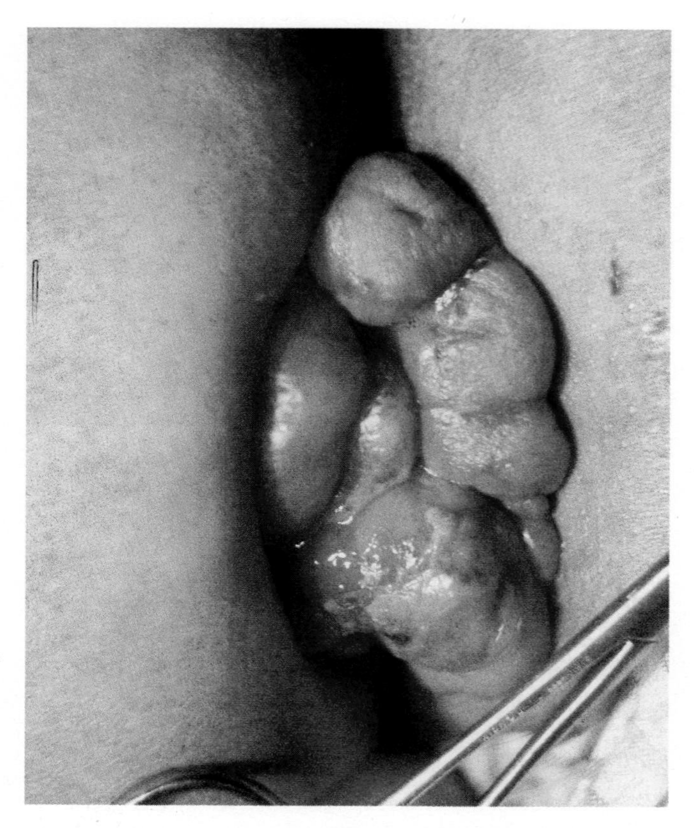

Fig.28.10. Strangulated piles. Note gross edema and leakage of rectal mucus.

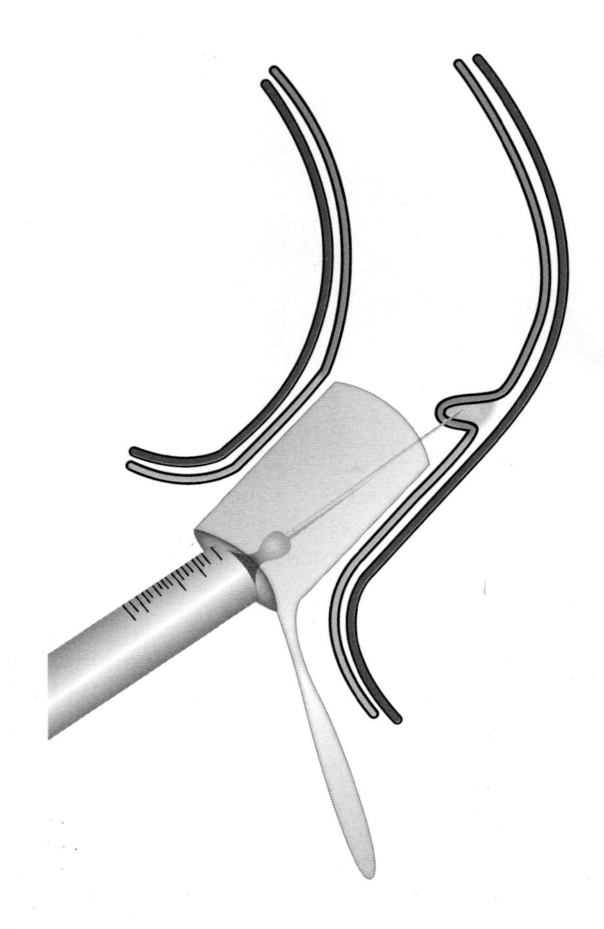

Fig.28.11. Injection of a hemorrhoid

be carried out smoothly.

Complications of hemorrhoids

Profuse bleeding with anemia is less common.

Strangulation. One or more hemorrhoids prolapse and are gripped by the sphincter. Venous return is impeded and congestion follows with pain, and thrombosis may result, the hemorrhoids becoming purple with considerable edema. Ulceration and gangrene with sloughing may follow. After thrombosis the pile gets fibrosed. Due to repeated traction at defecation, a *fibrous polyp* may form.

Treatment

In very early cases a high-fibre diet (vegetables, salads, fruits) helps. It softens the stools, so that there is no need to strain. If active treatment is required, it takes the form of injection, band-ligation or hemorrhoidectomy.

Injection treatment (Sclerotherapy)

This treatment is ideal for first-degree hemorrhoids. Early second-degree hemorrhoids are also usually cured, but a few of them relapse later. 5% phenol in almond oil is used. 2–3ml is injected into the submucosa at the upper pole of each pile. Injection is performed with a special syringe and a long needle through a proctoscope (Fig.28.11). All three primary hemorroids should be injected at the same time.

For second-degree or prolapsed hemorroids usually a second and a third set of injections have to be given, with intervals of a month between injections.

The injection causes inflammation, followed by fibrosis and shrinkage of the piles. Due to the fibrosis surrounding the submucosal veins, the bleeding stops. At the same time the overlying mucosa gets adherent to the internal sphincter. *Complications* are rare but include local sloughing of the mucosa, infection, and sensitivity reaction to the injected material. Pain after sclerotherapy occurs if injection is given at the level of the dentate line.

Rubber band ligation

This is an effective simple outpatient procedure for 2nd and early 3rd degree hemorrhoids. It has gained in popularity and has partly replaced injections. A constricting rubber band is placed around the upper part of the hemorrhoid.

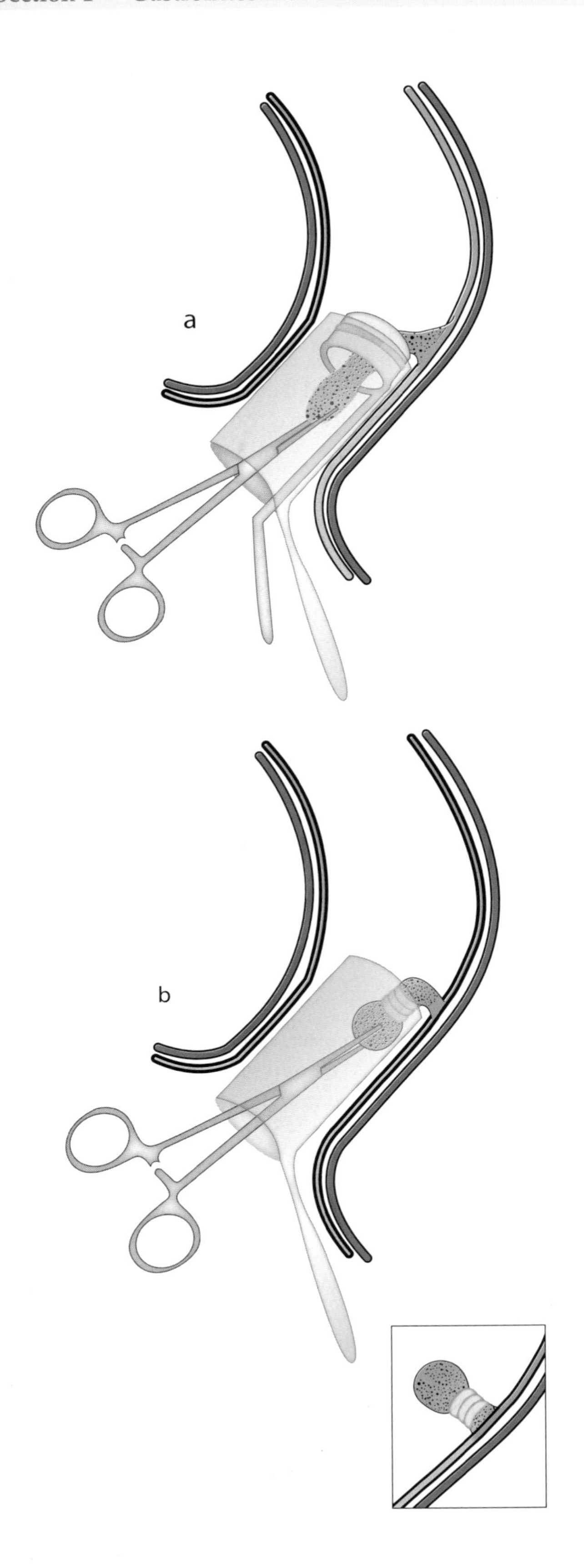

Fig.28.12 Rubber band ligation. ***Inset*** shows the ligated hemorrhoid

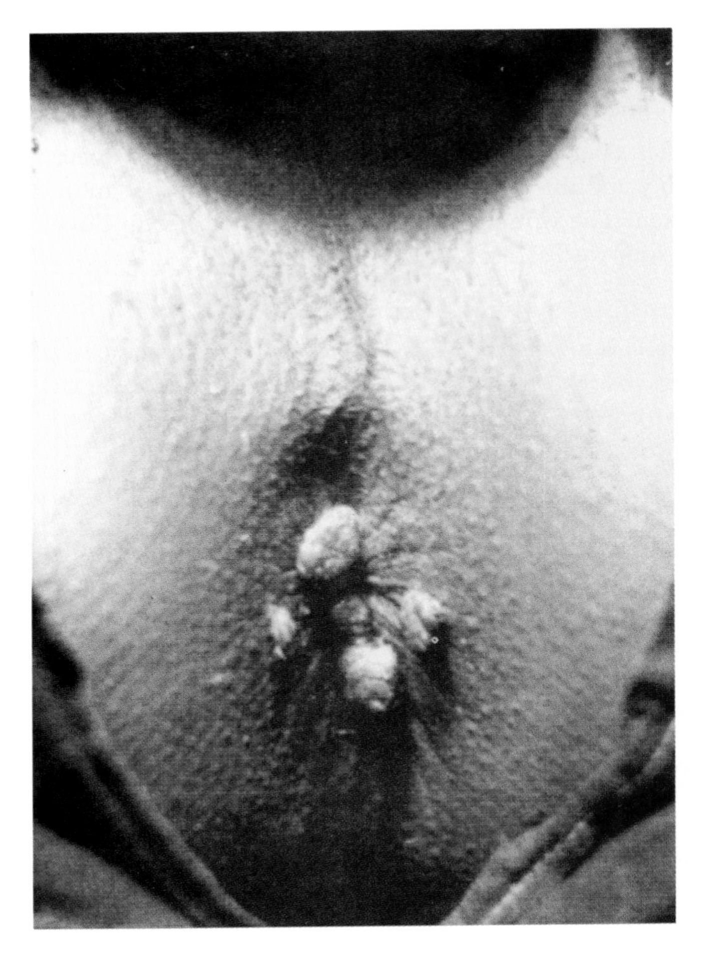

Fig.28.13 Anal warts

The tissue distal to the rubber band undergoes necrosis and sloughs off in a week's time. The result is more permanent than that of injection therapy, because there is precisely controlled loss of redundant mucosa. The patient should be warned that some bleeding occurs when the sloughs separate in 7 to 10 days (Fig.28.12).

Ultrasonic arterial ligation

In a recently introduced method, using endo-ultrasound, the artery suppling the pile is identified and ligated.

Finally, the techniques of cryotherapy and infrared photocoagulation have gone out of favour.

Hemorrhoidectomy

This is usually reserved for patients with third or fourth degree piles. Thrombosed hemorrhoids should be treated by hemorrhoidectomy after a few weeks of conservative treatment, after the edema has subsided.

At operation each hemorrhoid is dissected from the underlying tissues. Its pedicle is securely ligated and the hemorrhoid excised. *Adequate columns of mucosa and anoderm must be left behind between adjacent piles,* otherwise stenosis results. The margins of the skin wounds are trimmed so as not to leave overhanging edges (Fig.28.9).

After operation sitz baths should be employed twice daily and the cotton pad changed thrice daily or more often. The wounds granulate and epithelialize in three to four weeks.

Postoperative complications

Retention of urine occurs rarely. Reactionary and *secondary hemorrhage* can occur, but with careful technique are quite uncommon. *Stricture* results only if an excessive amount of mucosa is removed, which should be avoided.

Treatment of thrombosed piles

Bed rest and analgesia with frequent sitz baths cause the pile mass to shrink in size in a few days. Hemorrhoidectomy is then carried out two to three weeks later. However, in the rare event of necrosis supervening, debridement hemorrhoidectomy (cutting away the dead tissue) speeds recovery.

Thrombosed external hemorrhoid

This is also called a perianal hematoma. It is a small clot occurring in the perianal subcutaneous tissues. It arises due to rupture of a small vein while straining at stool. It is a tense, tender, hemispherical swelling about 1cm in size. Untreated it usually resolves and undergoes fibrosis, and may or may not produce a skin tag. Occasionally it suppurates, or extrudes the clot. It has been called a 'five-day, painful, self-curing lesion'. If seen within 24 hours of onset the hematoma is best evacuated under local anesthesia. However, even if left alone it usually resolves.

Conditions which simulate external hemorrhoids

The differential diagnosis of external hemorrhoids includes the following:

- ***Anal warts***. These are raised above the level of the skin and have a dry tufted surface (Fig.28.13). They are best removed by diathermy.
- ***Condylomas*** have a smooth surface and are moist.

Anal fissure

An anal fissure is a longitudinal tear of the skin-lined part of the anal canal. It commonly occurs in the posterior midline. The angle between the rectum and the anal canal causes the mass of stool to damage the anal epithelium at this site. A few anal fissures occur at the anterior midline.

Pathology

An *acute anal fissure* is a longitudinal tear through the skin of the anal margin. There is severe spasm of the internal sphincter, but as yet little inflammatory reaction.

A *chronic anal fissure* has indurated margins and a base consisting of scar tissue. In some cases the lowermost fibres of the internal sphincter may be seen running transversely across its floor. At the lower end of the fissure small bits of feces burrow under the skin. An edematous tag of skin forms, which is called a *sentinel pile*, because it stands as a sentinel below the fissure. Infection spreading from the fissure may cause abscess or fistula formation.

Clinical features

Anal fissures are commonly seen in adults. They are very painful because they lie below the mucocutaneous junction. Occasionally in an infant a fissure may cause severe constipation due to avoidance of defecation because of the pain, and result in acquired megacolon.

Examination is carried out in the left lateral position. The buttocks have to be separated gently to display the fissure. In chronic cases a sentinel pile may be seen. Digital rectal examination cannot be carried out in acute cases due to the pain. In chronic cases examination may be carried out, when the indurated edges of the ulcer can be felt.

Differential diagnosis

Very early carcinoma of the anus may simulate a chronic fissure. Excision-biopsy should be carried out. In *procto-colitis* multiple fissures are seen.

Treatment

Conservative treatment. An *acute* anal fissure with a short history (4–6 weeks) is treated conservatively with a smooth muscle relaxant e.g. 0.2% glyceryl trinitrate or 2% diltiazem applied locally 2–3 times a day. An alternate treatment is injection of Botulinum toxin (Botox) into the internal sphincter.

Surgery. In a *chronic* anal fissure, or where conservative treatment has failed, the lowermost fibres of the internal sphincter from the dentate line distally are divided under general or regional anesthesia *(Lateral internal sphincterotomy)*. This abolishes the spasm of these fibres and allows the fissure to heal promptly. Sphincterotomy was in the past carried out in the posterior midline. However, lateral sphincterotomy allows the operation to be carried out through a clean field.

ANORECTAL INFECTION

Anorectal infection has two phases: an acute phase i.e. anorectal abscess formation, and a chronic phase i.e. fistula-in-ano.

ANORECTAL ABSCESSES

An anorectal abscess results from the invasion of a pararectal or perianal space by pathogenic micro-organisms. A mixed infection usually occurs, mostly with Escherichia coli, Proteus vulgaris, streptococci, staphylococci and bacteroides. Anaerobes are often present. The abscess contains a good deal of foul-smelling pus. Anorectal abscesses are much more common in men.

Sources of infection. Infection usually extends from an anal crypt into the anal gland, and thence into one of the pararectal spaces. A perianal abscess may result from a thrombosed external hemorrhoid, or an infection of a hair follicle or sweat gland.

Classification

Anorectal abscesses are classified according to the anatomical space they occupy:

- ***Perianal or subcutaneous abscess.*** This lies immediately beneath the perianal skin (Fig.28.14. i). *This is the most common anorectal abscess.* Constitutional symptoms are less severe than in an ischiorectal abscess because the pus can expand the walls of the space easily. It forms a tender rounded cystic mass about 1.5cm in size at the anal margin.
- An ***ischiorectal abscess*** lies in the ischiorectal space (Fig.28.14 ii). The fat in this space has a poor blood supply, therefore the whole space becomes involved soon. The ischiorectal fossa communicates with that of the opposite side via a passage just behind the anal canal. Therefore, if untreated, infection spreads to the fossa on the opposite side. A tender, firm swelling may or may not be seen, but constitutional symptoms are severe with fever upto 39^0 C.
- A ***submucous abscess*** (Fig.28.14. iii) lies in the submucosa above the dentate line. It usually results from injection for hemorrhoids, and nearly always resolves itself; if not, it requires incision.
- A ***pelvirectal abscess*** lies above the levator ani and below the peritoneum (Fig.28.14. iv). It is really a pelvic abscess and usually secondary to appendicitis, salpingitis or parametritis.
- ***Intermuscular abscess.*** As mentioned above, in anorectal abscesses the infection starts from an anal gland, which lies in the intermuscular space. If infection remains confined to this site, an intermuscular abscess is the result (Fig.28.14. v). It can cause severe throbbing pain like that of a fissure. On examination no fissure is present, and the diagnosis may be overlooked because of the deep location of the pus.

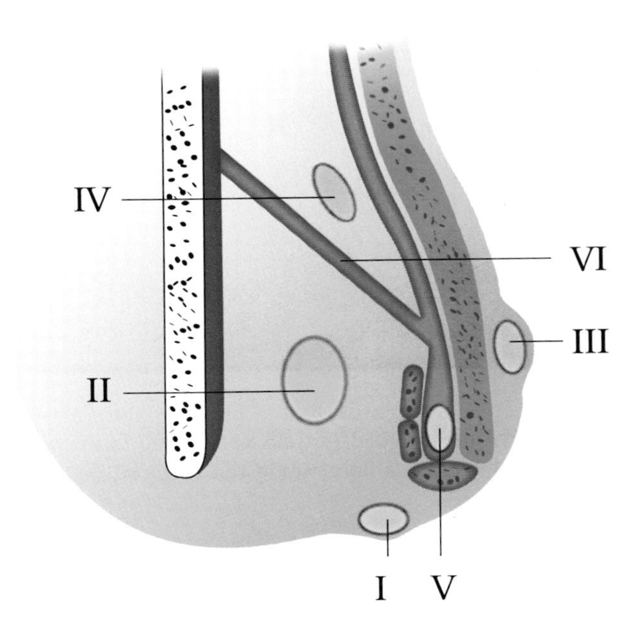

Fig.28.14 Anorectal abscesses. i. perianal, ii. ischiorectal, iii. submucous, iv. pelvirectal, v. intermuscular.

Treatment

The management of anorectal abscesses is relatively straightforward; they should all be drained as soon as diagnosed. In the case of perianal and ischiorectal abscesses a cruciate incision is made and the resulting flaps of skin over the whole abscess are excised. If a fistula track to the anal canal is found leading from the inner wall of the abscess it is opened, provided too much of the sphincter does not lie below it; in other words fistulotomy is performed at the same time. If no fistula track is found and opened up, the patient should be warned that after the wound fills up there may be a persistent discharge due to the unopened track, which may require a second operation; this will ensure that he is not disappointed and demoralized if this should happen.

FISTULA-IN-ANO

A fistula-in-ano is a track lined by granulation tissue which opens internally into the anal canal or rectum, and externally onto the skin around the anus. It usually results from an anorectal abscess which either burst spontaneously or was opened without laying open the entire track, as mentioned above.

Origin of anal fistulae

Infection enters through an anal crypt. An abscess forms in an anal gland which lies between the external and internal

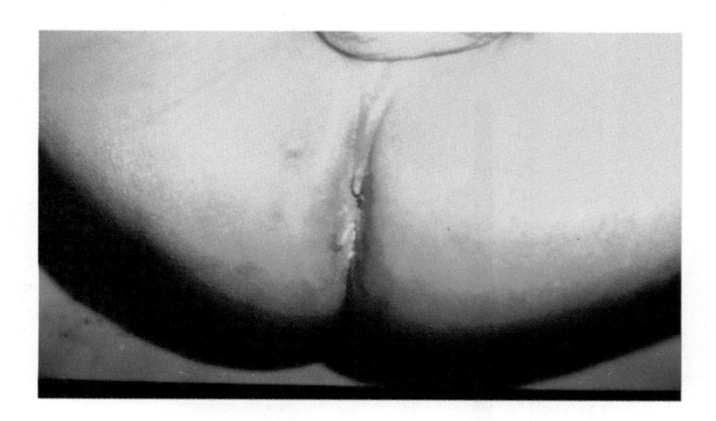

Fig.28.15 Fistula-in ano. The track can be felt by moving the finger firmly across a line joining the fistulous opening with the anus.

sphincter muscles (intersphincteric abscess). From this abscess pus can spread in various directions, producing the different types of fistulae (cryptograndular). Other causes include tuberculosis, Crohn's disease etc.

Clinical features

The main symptom of an anal fistula is a persistent discharge of a mixture of pus and serum which irritates the perianal skin and causes discomfort. If the opening gets closed, pain and sometimes fever occur till the collection of exudate bursts and discharges itself.

Palpation

The subcutaneous fibrous track can often be palpated under the skin, specially in low fistulae. For this purpose the finger should be moved firmly *across a line joining the fistula opening to the anal orifice* (Fig.28.15). The track is easier to feel in its outermost part where it lies close to the skin; in the inner portion it usually lies more deeply. The author has found this method of palpation very useful; however it is not stressed sufficiently in textbooks.

Goodsall's rule helps in predicting the site of the internal opening in cases of anal fistulae. It states that fistulae with the external opening in front of a transverse line drawn through the anus proceed in a straight line towards the anus. Those with the external opening behind this line have curved tracks and open into the anal canal in the posterior midline.

On ***digital examination*** the internal opening of the fistula may sometimes be palpated as a nodule. On ***proctoscopy*** the same opening may be seen. If a probe is passed one must be very gentle, otherwise a simple transsphincteric fistula may be converted into an extrasphincteric fistula, with serious consequences for the patient.

Classification

The most widely used classification of fistulae is that by Allan Parks:

- ***Subcutaneous.*** This uncommon type of fistula runs just beneath the perianal skin.
- ***Intersphincteric***. This is the most common type of fistula, the track runs through the lower part of the internal sphincter (Fig.28.16 i).

Treatment

The above two types can be treated simply by laying open the track (Fig.28.17). In the intersphincteric fistula the lower fibres of the internal sphincter are divided, but this does not lead to incontinence.

- ***Transsphincteric.*** The track runs across both sphincters (Fig.28.16 ii).
- Intersphincteric and transsphincteric are the most common types comprising more than 80% of fisluae-in-ano.
- ***Suprasphincteric***. Here the track passes upwards in the intersphincteric space over the puborectalis and down through the ischiorectal fossa to the the skin (Fig.28.16 iii).

Treatment

In both the preceding types, laying open the fistula would lead to incontinence as it would divide the sphincters. Therefore, a method has to be found to avoid such an eventuality:

- o Multiple silk or polypropylene threads may be passed through the fistula and left in place; to prevent them from getting dislodged, their ends are tied together. A thread utilized in this manner is called a *seton*. The mechanism of its action is often not properly understood; it allows constant drainage of the discharge of the fistula, and in this way often leads to healing.
- o A *mucosal advancement* technique may be employed. The external part of the track is first cored out. Inside the anal canal a flap of mucosa and submucosa is now raised and advanced over the orifice of the fistula, thus closing down its internal opening.

Alternative techniques

Delayed healing of the fistulous wound, a high recurrence rate with surgery, and the risk of incontinence, have led to adoption of less invasive procedures. The fistula track is curetted and then biological glues and plugs are used to keep the track open.

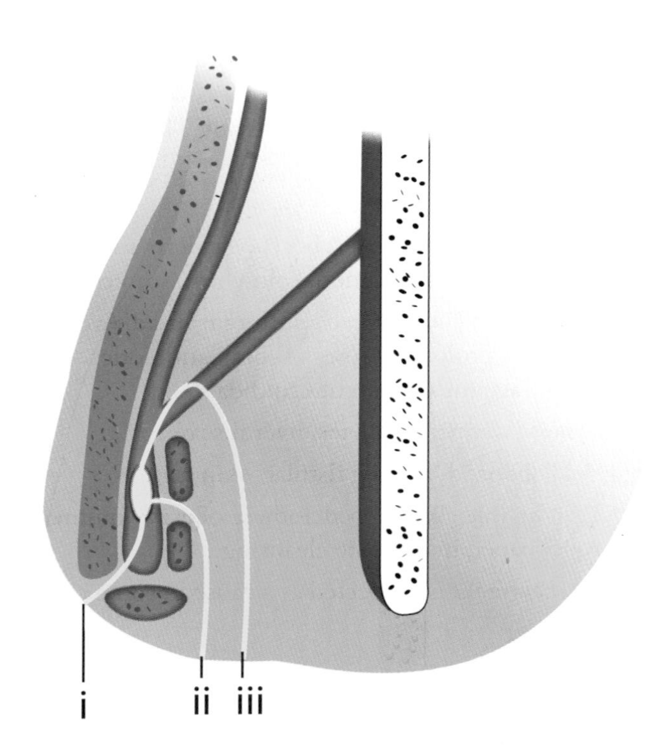

Fig.28.16 Fistulae-in-ano. i. inter sphincteric ii. transsphincteric iii. suprasphincteric

Post-operative care

Fistulotomy leaves behind a wound looking like a groove, which is packed and heals from the floor and the edges (Fig.28.17). The wound takes three to four weeks to fill up with granulations and epithelialize, depending upon its size.

One of the important reasons for recurrence of anal fistulae after operation is the lack of meticulous postoperative care. Usually the margins of the innermost part of the wound come together before the groove itself has filled up with granulations, so that the fistula is formed again. Therefore it is important that the surgeon should carry out the postoperative dressings himself; if this is not possible he should inspect the wound at least once a week.

Recurrence rate

The recurrence rate following fistulotomy is high. Failure of treatment may be due to one of the following reasons:

- The internal portion of the fistula is not removed.
- Collateral tracts are missed.
- The underlying cause i.e Crohn's disease, tuberculosis, actinomycosis, is missed.
- Postoperative care is inadequate.

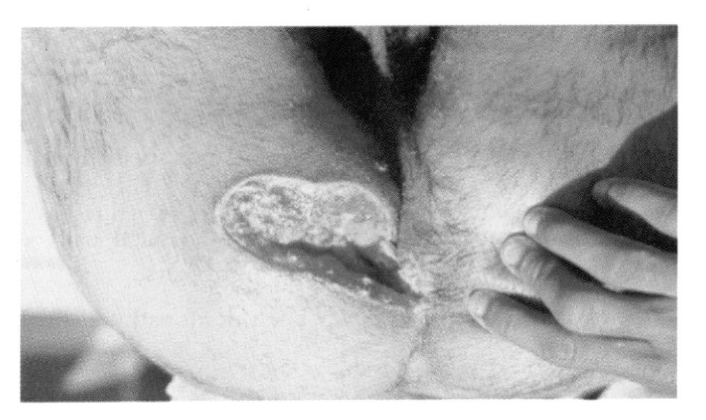

Fig.28.17 Fistula-in-ano. After excision of the track the wound has been left open to granulate. It will be treated by sitz baths and a cotton pad changed twice daily or more often.

Perineal wounds

Wounds in the perineum are different from wounds elsewhere. Whether they result from trauma or surgery, they heal slowly and with difficulty. The reasons are not far to seek. As the buttocks come together, the secretions of the skin are retained. At the same time the stools, which soil the perianal skin daily, contain millions of anaerobes, as well as both Gram negative and Gram positive bacteria.

A few clinicians close perineal wounds with suture in an effort to obtain prompt healing. Most others consider this too risky in the unhygienic environment of the anus, and leave the wounds open to granulate (Fig.28.17). After operation sitz baths are employed twice daily. The wound is dressed with a cotton pad, which should be changed by the patient himself twice a day or more often, as it gets soggy and foul-smelling. Elastic underpants can be worn over the pad to keep it in place. If the granulations are edematous, a 15% solution of silver nitrate may be applied to the wound as an astringent. The wounds normally granulate and epithelialize in three to four weeks.

Pilonidal sinus

A pilonidal sinus presents either as a sinus or an acute abscess over the coccyx and lower sacrum. There is granulation tissue, fibrous tissue, and often a tuft of hair. The sinus extends into the subcutaneous tissues. Branching side channels are frequent. Stratified squamous epithelium is found in patches along the walls of the sinus.

Etiology

Some believe this to be a congenital condition. However, the general opinion is that most cases are acquired due to trapping of hair which fall down along the midline groove at the back. Some arguments in favour of the acquired theory are the following:

- The disease mostly affects men, and specially hairy men.
- The common sites apart from the natal cleft are between the fingers, specially in barbers.
- Hair follicles have never been demonstrated in the wall of the sinus.
- Recurrence is common even after adequate excision of the track.

Clinical findings

Symptoms usually start in the third decade. Hirsute males with deep natal clefts are more often affected. There is a persistent or recurring sinus in the midline at about the level of the first piece of the coccyx. Typically, a tuft of hair projects from its mouth (Fig.12.1). The discharge is often foul-smelling due to stagnant contents and may contain hair. Secondary openings may be present on the sides where recurrent abscesses have burst through the skin.

Treatment

Both the acute abscess and the chronic sinus can be dealt by excision of the whole track along with half a centimeter of skin on either side of the sinus tract. This allows full drainage and formation of healthy granulation tissue, resulting in healing from the depths of the cavity.

Postoperative care

The wound edges are kept apart by an acriflavine gauze roll which is left in place for a day or two. During this time the patient takes baths. When the dressing is removed, a clean granulating wound is found. This allows healing from the bottom by contraction of the wound. The skin edges must be kept apart by daily packing with a gauze roll by a nurse, or by the patient at home if he is provided with a silastic foam dressing prepared to size. These methods prevent the edges coming together until the wound has filled up with granulation tissue.

The wide excisions of the past are no longer practiced; they used to leave behind large raw areas which took a long time to heal. Alternatively, the resulting wound can be closed primarily with or without lateral release, or marsupialized to reduce healing time. Whichever way the wound is managed, *its healing must be personally supervised by the surgeon*, otherwise a fair number of recurrences will occur.

Pruritis ani

Pruritus is defined as itching of the skin, specially without visible eruption. When this is confined to the perianal area it is known as pruritus ani. The skin may be thickened, red and moist.

The ***causes*** are numerous:

- *Skin diseases*. Psoriasis, seborrhoeic dermatitis, atopic eczema, fungus infections, pinworm, scabies.
- *Drugs*. Local anesthetic ointments used over long periods; prolonged use of oral antibiotics which encourage the growth of Candida.
- *Systemic diseases*. Diabetes, liver disease.
- *Anal diseases*. Draining fistulae, skin tags.
- *Poor hygiene*. Warm bedclothes, obesity, trauma by toilet paper, inadequate cleansing.
- *Psychoneurosis* is suspected as a cause in some cases.

Treatment

Any underlying cause is treated. Soap should not be used in the perineum; soap is alkaline, whereas the perineal area is slightly acid. The area should be cleaned after each bowel movement by washing with plain water. Consultation with a dermatologist may be required.

Non-malignant strictures of the anal canal

Anal canal strictures may be congenital or acquired.

Congenital

- A *microscopic anus*.
- *Postoperative*. After operation for an anorectal deformity the anal canal may be narrow and require repeated dilatation.

Acquired

- A chronic *anal fissure* produces some fibrosis in the sphincter.
- If during an operation for *piles* adequate vertical columns of mucosa are not left between the hemorrhoidectomy wounds, stenosis may result.
- *Irradiation* for carcinoma of the cervix or bladder can produce fibrosis in the anal canal.

Clinical features

There is increasing difficulty in defecation with toothpaste-like stools, and the patient requires increasing doses of laxatives. Rectal examination reveals the stricture, when biopsy should be undertaken.

Management

Prevention

Strictures following operations for hemorrhoids and low ano-rectal anomalies can be prevented by meticulous technique and by regular dilatations carried out a few weeks after the operation if required.

Treatment

In the case of many benign strictures of the anal canal repeated dilatations at regular intervals prove adequate. If dilatations fail, the stricture may be incised and the resultant wound covered by a split-skin graft, which is sutured in place. If a stricture has caused intestinal obstruction, colostomy has to be undertaken, specially in strictures complicated by anal fistulas.

MALIGNANT TUMORS OF THE ANAL CANAL

The anal canal extends from the anorectal ring to the dentate line; the area from then onwards to 5cm beyond the anal verge is properly called the anal margin. Tumors of the anal canal include squamous cell carcinoma and malignant melanoma.

Squamous cell carcinoma

This occurs at the anal verge (anoderm) or the perianal region, and behaves like a skin cancer. It is more common in men and responds equally well to surgery and radiotherapy. This is the most common tumor of the anal canal. However, it is much less common than adenocarcinoma of the colo-rectum. The tumor starts as a hard nodule which may be ulcerated. Rectal pain and bleeding are the most common symptoms.

Many cases are misdiagnosed as benign lesions, e.g. hemorrhoids or anal fissure, and treatment delayed. Early diagnosis is made by careful examination of the anal canal and is confirmed by biopsy. Endo-ultrasound, CT scan or MRI can be used to assess muscle invasion. Anal carcinoma spreads to the superior rectal, pelvic and inguinal lymph nodes.

Treatment

There has been a fundamental change in the treatment of anal canal tumors. Currently the treatment of choice is chemotherapy (5FU + Cisplatin) + Radiation, whereas surgery is reserved for failures and recurrences. The 5-year survival rate approaches 80% or above depending upon the stage of the tumor. The prognosis is even better with squamous cell carcinoma.

This combined modality treatment, i.e. chemotherapy and radiation, has the major advantage of allowing anal sphincter preservation.

Malignant melanoma

Malignant melanoma of the anal canal has a very poor prognosis. Fortunately it is rare. It presents as a dark mass protruding from the anus, and may be mistaken for thrombosed hemorrhoids.

Chapter

29 HERNIA AND ABDOMINAL WALL

Hernia

A hernia is the protrusion of a viscus or part of a viscus through an abnormal opening or a weak area in the wall. It is a very common condition; approximately 2–5% of the population suffer from hernias. The most common hernias are inguinal, umbilical and femoral.

Etiology

Indirect inguinal hernia

This occurs in a congenital preformed sac which develops as the peritoneum accompanies the testis during its descent through the inguinal canal into the scrotum.

Other hernias

Predisposing factors in the formation of other acquired hernias include the following:

- Increased intra-abdominal pressure, e.g. in chronic cough or urethral obstruction.
- Stretching of the abdominal muscles, e.g. in pregnancy and obesity.
- Degenerative changes in muscles and fascia (collagen failure) in middle and old age.

Complications of hernias

If left untreated, hernias are subject to the complications of irreducibility, obstruction and strangulation.

Irreducibility (Incarceration)

This usually occurs due to adhesions between the sac and its contents, or from overcrowding within the sac. It predisposes to obstruction and strangulation.

Obstruction

The intestine in the hernia is obstructed, but the blood supply to the bowel is not interfered with. There is vomiting, abdominal distension and absolute constipation, i.e. no passage of flatus or feces. The symptoms are less severe than in strangulation. However, the safe course is to assume that strangulation is imminent, and to operate at once.

Strangulation

In this condition the intestine is obstructed, and at the same time its blood supply is constricted. First the veins are obstructed, so that the intestine becomes congested and purple. Later, the arteries are also blocked. The serosa now becomes dull and covered by a fibrinous exudate. The intestine feels flabby and friable. The lowered vitality of the intestine allows bacteria to pass through its wall. Gangrene appears at the constriction rings (the points where the intestine is being constricted at the tight neck of the sac) and spreads, resulting in perforation.

Clinical features

There is sudden, severe pain over the hernia, spreading to the whole abdomen, with forceful, repeated vomiting. The hernia is tense, tender and shows no cough impulse. The patient is seriously ill and operation should be carried out urgently. If the constriction remains unrelieved, ultimately pain disappears due to the onset of paralytic ileus and endotoxic shock.

Treatment

The treatment of a strangulated hernia is by immediate operation, to avoid ischemic necrosis of the gut and peritonitis. For incarcerated hernias without signs of obstruction or vascular compromise, non-operative treatment used to be given a chance, with the foot of the bed raised. However, as nothing is to be gained by delay, operation should immediately be carried out.

Operation

At operation for a strangulated hernia the sac is first exposed and opened. Usually some blood-stained or dirty coloured fluid escapes, which has oozed out from the congested intestines; this is mopped up. The constricting neck of the sac is now divided, and the intestines drawn gently downwards. 100% oxygen is administered and the gut examined.

Viable gut is pink and undergoes peristalsis, and its arteries throb briskly. Gut which has lost its blood supply looks purple or black, does not exhibit peristalsis, and the mesenteric arteries do not pulsate; in fact thrombi may be palpated in them.

If the gut is found to be viable it is returned to the abdomen. If it is decided that the intestine is non-viable, the dead portion is resected and an end-to-end anastomosis carried out. Finally, the sac is ligated and hernia repair carried out. After operation, fluids are administered intravenously. Oral fluids are started once bowel sounds return.

INGUINAL HERNIA

There are two types of inguinal hernia, the indirect and the direct.

Indirect hernias come out through the internal inguinal ring, and direct hernias through the Hasselbach's triangle.

Hasselbach's triangle

Direct hernias come out through the lower part of Hasselbach's triangle, which is bounded by the inguinal ligament, inferior epigastric artery, and the lateral margin of the rectus muscle.

INDIRECT INGUINAL HERNIA

This is by far the most common of all the hernias. The sac into which this hernia descends is probably always congenital i.e. present at birth, due to non-obliteration of the processus vaginalis. However, intestine cannot descend into the sac because its neck is very narrow. During childhood or early adult life a bout of straining stretches the neck. Intestine or omentum comes down and a hernia is the result.

An indirect (oblique) inguinal hernia comes out through the internal inguinal ring, (Fig.29.1) which lies 1.5cm above the midpoint between the anterior superior iliac spine and the pubic symphysis (not the pubic tubercle). Its coverings include skin, subcutaneous tissue, external spermatic fascia (from the external oblique aponeurosis), cremaster muscle and fascia, and transversalis fascia.

Clinical features

An indirect inguinal hernia can appear at any age, and males are twenty times more commonly affected than females (But see fig.29.2). In the early stages, when the sac is limited to the inguinal canal, diagnosis can present some difficulty. At first the swelling appears intermittently, but as time goes by the hernia comes down as soon as the patient assumes the erect posture. In large hernias there is a sense of weight, and dragging on the mesentery may produce epigastric or umbilical pain.

Differential diagnosis

- *Direct vs indirect hernia*. The patient lies down supine. The hernia is reduced. A finger compresses the internal ring. The patient is asked to cough. In the case of the direct hernia the swelling reappears; with the indirect hernia it does not (*Internal ring occlusion test*).

  Incidentally, the differentiation between direct and indirect hernias is mainly of historical interest, because both types of hernias are treated in the same way in adults (by hernioplasty).
- *Vaginal hydrocele.* Here the swelling is dull, fluctuant and transilluminant, and unlike hernia, one can get above the upper pole of the swelling.
- *Encysted hydrocele of the cord*. If the testis is drawn gently downwards, this swelling also moves downwards.
- *Spermatocele.* This swelling lies just above the upper pole of the testis.
- *Femoral hernia.* This hernia reduces downwards (instead of upwards and laterally, as in the case of inguinal hernia), and its neck is found to lie below and lateral to the pubic tubercle (instead of above and medial to it as in inguinal hernia).

DIRECT INGUINAL HERNIA

Direct inguinal hernias are much less common than the indirect type, accounting for only 10% of all cases. About half of these hernias are bilateral. They are acquired, and commonly make their appearance in middle age.

Predisposing factors are those causing an increase in intra-abdominal pressure, e.g. chronic cough, straining and heavy work.

In a direct hernia there is no congenitally preformed sac; rather the whole posterior wall of the inguinal canal bulges forwards diffusely. These hernias do not commonly descend to the scrotum, whereas indirect hernias often do. The reason for this difference is to be found in the anatomy of the two lesions. The sac of an indirect hernia is narrow and elongated, and slides down covered by the cremaster muscle and fascia. Therefore it finds it easy to slip out of the external ring. The direct hernia sac on the other hand, being a broad structure,

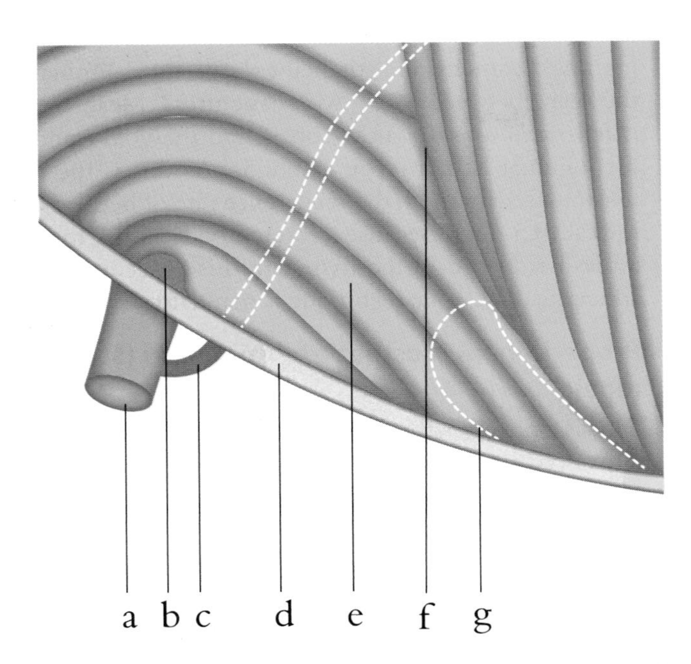

Fig.29.1 The posterior wall of the inguinal canal (a) femoral artery (b) internal inguinal ring (c) inferior epigastric artery, (d) inguinal ligament (e) conjoint tendon (f) margin of rectus abdominis (g) external inguinal ring

finds it more difficult to pass through the external ring; in any case it finds its passage blocked by the bulk of the spermatic cord filling the external ring.

At the same time, because the sac of a direct hernia has a very wide neck, it rarely strangulates.

TREATMENT OF INGUINAL HERNIA

Operation is the treatment of choice for an inguinal hernia. A truss should not be used, except in cases where operation is contraindicated because of severe cardiac, pulmonary or other systemic illness, or because of advanced senility.

The essential *steps* of any operation on an inguinal hernia are two: dealing with the sac, and repair of the posterior wall of the inguinal canal if required.

1. Dealing with the sac

- ***Indirect hernia.*** The sac of an indirect inguinal hernia is long and narrow, making the hernia prone to incarceration and intestinal obstruction. It therefore needs to be excised by herniotomy, which is thus *an essential part of every operation on an indirect hernia*.
- ***Direct hernia.*** On the other hand a direct hernia sac is a diffuse bulge, which can be simply pressed backwards before repairing the posterior wall of the inguinal canal. In this case, therefore, one can proceed directly with repair of the posterior wall.

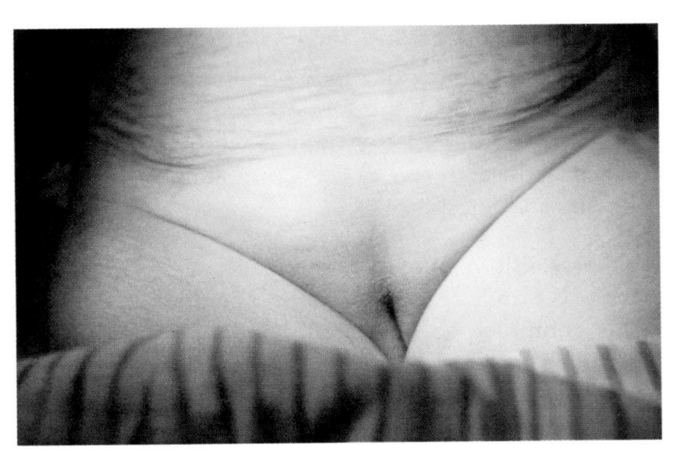

Fig.29.2 Unusual inguinal hernia in a female (the bulge on the right side)

Herniotomy

This operation consists of high ligation and excision of the hernia sac. This is an essential part of every operation on an *indirect* inguinal hernia.

The main *steps* of this operation are as follows:

- An incision is made parallel to and above the medial half of the inguinal ligament. For a better cosmetic effect the inner part of the incision is often curved slightly upwards.
- The inguinal canal is opened by incising the external oblique along its fibres.
- The envelope of cremaster muscle and fascia is opened.
- The hernia sac is separated from the pampiniform plexus and the vas. It is dissected upto its neck, opened to ensure that it is empty, ligated at its neck, and excised.
- The cremaster muscle and external oblique aponeurosis are now repaired and the skin sutured.

In children and adolescents this is all that is required.

In adults and old people it is usually necessary to strengthen the posterior wall of the inguinal canal, as described below under herniorrhaphy or hernioplasty.

2. Repair of the posterior inguinal wall

Repair of the posterior wall of the inguinal canal can be done in two ways:

A. By approximation, i.e. tissue repair.
B. By filling the gap, i.e. mesh repair.

A. Approximation (herniorraphy)

In this procedure the body's own tissues are joined together, the conjoint tendon being sutured to the posterior border of the inguinal ligament. Thus it is called a tissue repair. The common methods include Bassini and Shouldice:

1. Bassini

Since Bassini's description of his operation in the 1880s, this continued to be the most popular procedure for repair of inguinal hernias. In this method the elliptical gap in the posterior wall of the inguinal canal is obliterated, strengthening the abdominal wall over this area (Fig.29.3). A continuous suture using polypropylene is suitable. To prevent tension in the repair, a relieving incision in the inferolateral part of the anterior rectus sheath (*'Tanner slide'*) may be required.

2. Shouldice

Shouldice described his repair in 1945. He incised the fascia transversalis from the deep inguinal ring to the pubic tubercle and then overlapped one flap over the other, as in double-breasting. The external oblique aponeurosis was finally sutured to the inguinal ligament in similar manner, i.e. double-breasted.

However, the fascia transversalis is not the type of tissue that is easy to dissect and suture. This was a technically difficult repair, and the claimed recurrence rate (<1%) could not be duplicated outside the Shouldice clinic. Therefore this repair has been replaced with mesh repair either open or by laparoscopic methods.

Recurrence rate

The recurrence rate in these methods of approximation remains upto 5%, due to tension produced when approximating structures by drawing them together. For this reason surgeons have sought methods where the *gap is filled* either by the body's own materials or synthetic ones.

B. Filling the gap (hernioplasty)

Two types of material are used for filling the oval gap between the conjoint tendon and the inguinal ligament:

- *Darning.*

By darning[1], i.e. weaving into the gap:

  - o A synthetic suture, or
  - o A strip of the patient's own fascia lata.

- *Mesh.*

In this method a mesh of synthetic material is placed in the oval gap between the conjoint tendon and the inguinal ligament, and stitched to both, thus eliminating the gap between the two structures. Mesh repair *(Litchenstein repair)* is now considered the gold standard for inguinal hernia repair in adults. As this is the only tension-free method, the recurrence rate of hernia is the lowest (0.5–1%). Because a foreign body in the form of a mesh is placed in the tissues in this procedure, strict adherence to aseptic technique is mandatory.

Properitoneal prosthetic hernioplasty (Stopa's repair)

This is a novel method of performance of a hernioplasty. Through a Pfannensteil's incision the peritoneum is exposed and the whole pelvic peritoneal sac reflected upwards. A bowl-shaped prosthesis of prolene is placed in position in the pelvis, its edges extending up to the umbilicus. The peritoneal sac with its contents is allowed to fill it and the abdominal wall closed. The mesh becomes incorporated in the abdominal wall. As it lies permanently in position it prevents the occurrence or recurrence of inguinal as well as femoral hernias on both sides. It may be noted that before it can be placed in position an inguinal hernial sac, if present, should be ligated and divided. The vas and spermatic cord should be separated from the sac and pushed back, where they lie against the posterior abdominal wall.

Laparoscopic hernia repair

Using laparoscopic methods, after ligating the hernia sac a prosthetic mesh is placed in the properitoneal space behind the inguinal canal. This is now an established technique for the repair of all ventral hernias i.e. inguinal, para-umblical and incisional hernias.

Total extraperitoneal repair (TEP)

This is the most popular laparoscopic inguinal hernia repair today. The surgeon creates a space just deep to the abdominal muscles stretching from across the midline and into the retropubic space to 5cm beyond the internal inguinal ring. Having created the space, he places the 10x15cm mesh in place and repairs the abdominal wall.

Recurrence rates are low. Chronic pain, probably due to the mesh irritating nerves, may cause some trouble. In this connection the nerves passing along the inguinal canal must be meticulously protected.

Suture materials

Nowadays polypropylene suture is the most popular. Being monofilament, it is not associated with the problem of persistent infection; being non-absorbable, it gives permanent strength to the repair.

1 Darn: to mend (a hole in knitted material) by interweaving yarn with a needle

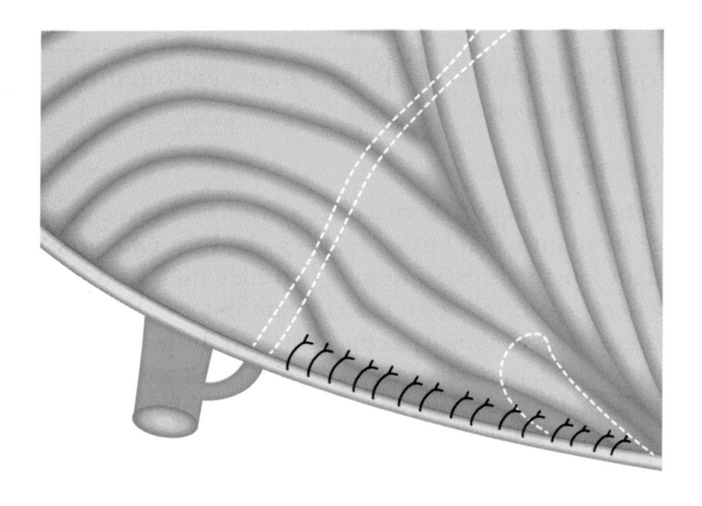

Fig.29.3 Bassini repair i.e. interrupted sutures between conjoint tendon and inguinal ligament

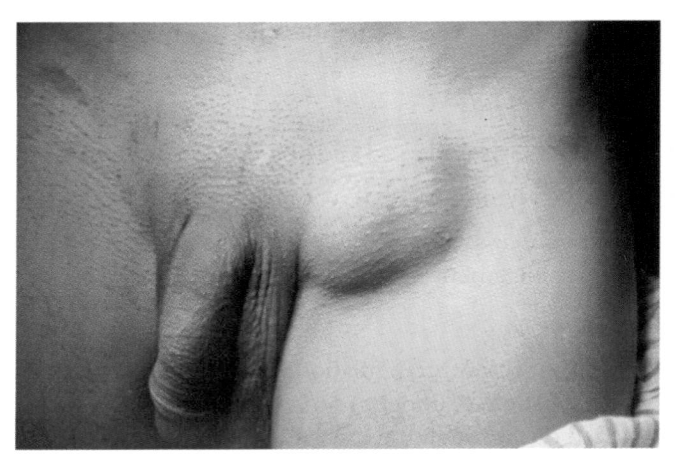

Fig.29.4 Femoral hernia

Day care surgery for hernias

Classically, hernias have been repaired under general anesthesia. However, due to the rising cost of hospital admission, an increasing number of hernias are being repaired under local anesthesia and discharged the same evening from a 'day care area' instead of being admitted to a hospital ward.

Recurrence of inguinal hernias

The causes of recurrence

The common causes of recurrence of inguinal hernias are the following:

- Faulty selection of cases e.g. patients with chronic bronchitis.
- Faulty technique, e.g.:
  - Failure to ligate the sac at the neck.
  - Imperfect hemostasis leading to hematoma.
  - Missing an indirect sac in a direct hernia repair.
  - Infection etc.
- Persistent cough, heavy lifting before three months after hernia repair, urethral obstruction.
- Tissue repair under tension.

The treatment of recurrence

In the *preperitoneal approach* an oblique incision is made over the lower part of the rectus sheath. The sheath is incised and the rectus retracted medially, thus entering the preperitoneal space. A piece of prosthetic mesh is *inlayed*, securing the mesh to cover the inner aspect of the defect. It is better than an onlay mesh placed in the inguinal canal, because abdominal pressure plasters an inlay mesh against the abdominal musculature, while it tends to push out an onlay mesh.

The main hazard of insertion of a mesh is infection. Scrupulous asepsis and prophylactic administration of antibiotics are essential.

Sliding hernia

A sliding hernia is said to be present when a viscus with a partial peritoneal covering, e.g. cecum or urinary bladder, slides down into the inguinal canal, so that it forms the posterior wall of the sac. Sliding hernias are seen commonly in large complete hernias in middle-aged men, and should be treated by operation. The viscus does not lie *within* the sac; the sac is applied to *part* of its surface. The viscus is likely to be damaged if the sac is dissected off its surface, and this type of hernia is best managed by a plicating suture, to eliminate the raw area, after which the viscus is returned to the abdominal cavity. The internal ring and posterior inguinal wall are next repaired as usual.

FEMORAL HERNIA

Femoral hernia is much more common in women but the inguinal hernias are still far more common (fig.29.4). The hernia descends into the femoral canal through the femoral ring, which is bounded anteriorly by the inguinal ligament, laterally by the femoral vein, posteriorly by the pubic bone and medially by the pectineal part of the inguinal ligament. As the femoral ring is very small, of all hernias this is the most liable to become strangulated. A small femoral hernia may be unnoticed by the patient for many years until it strangulates.

The *differential diagnosis* of femoral hernia includes the following conditions:

- Inguinal hernia.
- Saphena varix (enlarged end of long saphenous vein).
- Enlarged lymph node.
- Psoas abscess presenting in the groin under the inguinal ligament.

Treatment

The constant risk of strangulation is sufficient reason for urging the patient to undergo surgery. The operation may be carried out through the low and the high approach.

Low operation

The sac is exposed below the inguinal ligament (the low operation). The sac is exposed and opened, the contents reduced, the neck ligated, the sac excised, and the inguinal ligament stitched to the pectineal line by unabsorbable sutures.

High operation

Alternatively, the incision is extended higher up to open the inguinal canal, so that the neck can be ligated at a higher level through the posterior wall of the inguinal canal (the high operation). If the hernia is strangulated, the only structure which can be divided to release the constriction at the femoral ring is the pectineal part of the inguinal ligament. This division should always be carried out from above, because occasionally an 'abnormal' obturator artery i.e. one arising from the external iliac artery, runs on its upper surface and can be injured if the ligament is divided from below, resulting in dangerous hemorrhage. In other words upon a strangulated femoral hernia should always be operated from above.

VENTRAL HERNIA

The term ventral hernia denotes hernias of the anterior abdominal wall; however, inguinal and femoral hernias are not included, probably because they lie low down in the groin. The list of ventral hernias includes:

Spontaneous

- Umbilical-paraumbilical.
- Epigastric.
- Lumbar.
- Spigelian.

Traumatic

- Incisional.
- Parastomal.

UMBILICAL HERNIA

Hernias at the umbilicus take three forms, each occurring at a different age:

Exomphalos

This type of umbilical hernia is seen in *newborns*. It occurs once in about 6,000 births. It arises like this: when the midgut lengthens, the intestine extrudes itself into the extra-embryonic coelom. Later, as the abdominal cavity enlarges, the gut returns to the abdomen. If this process is arrested the portion of the abdominal wall around the umbilicus fails to come together. The resultant gap is covered by a semitransparent membrane which consists, from outside in, of amniotic membrane, Wharton's jelly and peritoneum.

Sometimes this sac ruptures during delivery and intestines are extruded.

Treatment

Exomphalos minor

If the sac is small, with a diameter less than 5cm, the condition is called exomphalos minor. Its treatment is simple; the cord is twisted to reduce the contents through the narrow umbilical opening, and strapping applied to keep them reduced for about two weeks.

Exomphalos major

In case the sac is large, the diameter being greater than 5cm, operation must be carried out within a few hours of birth, otherwise the sac will burst and lead to severe peritonitis.

Surgery

- If the abdominal cavity is too small to accomodate the whole midgut, respiratory embarrassment may result from complete repair of the hernia. In such cases *only the skin is sutured*, and repair of the resulting incisional hernia postponed for a few months or years, when the abdomen is large enough.
- Sometimes even the skin cannot be sutured without raising the intra-abdominal pressure to such heights as to greatly embarrass both respiration and venous return. In such a case *a patch of synthetic mesh is sutured over the gap* to produce a pouch. (Fig.29.5). Every few days a new line of sutures is applied to shrink the pouch. In this way the intestine is gradually returned to the abdomen until it has all been accomodated. The synthetic pouch is now excised and the abdominal wall repaired. Following such a staged procedure it may be weeks before normal intestinal activity returns, and prolonged intravenous feeding may be necessary.

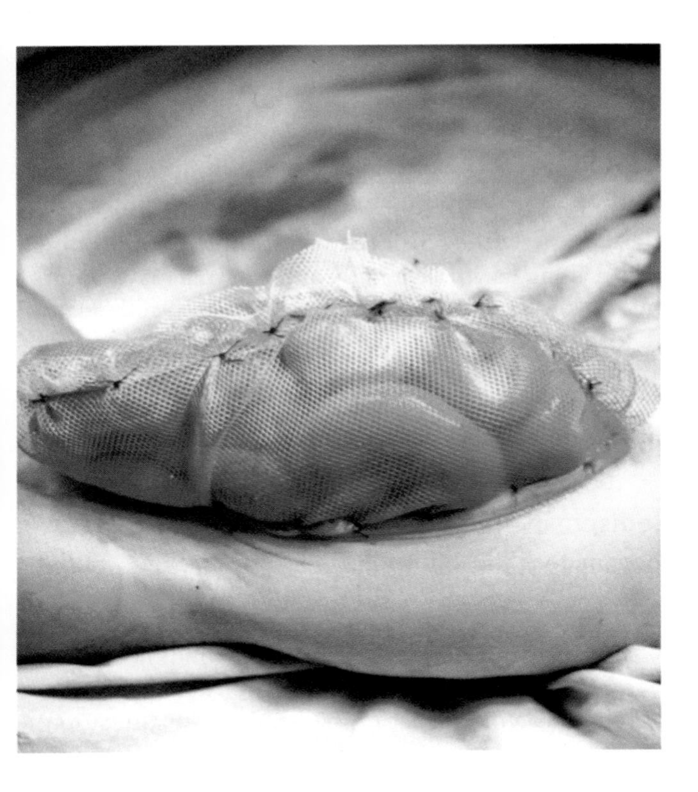

Fig.29.5 Major exomphalos. The abdominal wall is insufficient to cover the intestines. A synthetic mesh has been sewn over the defect. Every few days some of this pouch will be squeezed off and some more gut accommodated in the abdomen. Ultimately the remaining mesh will be cut off and the abdomen closed.

Infantile umbilical hernia

This is a hernia through a weak umbilical scar. These cases with a protruding umbilicus can be seen in small naked children in a poor locality in any tropical country. Small hernias are hemispherical; those that increase in size become conical. Obstruction or strangulation is rare.

Left alone, a very high percentage of cases disappear spontaneously during the first year or two of life. This is suggested by the fact that though these strictly umbilical hernias are very common in infants they are hardly ever seen in adults, although very few adults bear scars showing repair of such a hernia in childhood. It is likely that the thickening of the rectus muscles with growth obliterates the opening.

In the event, operation is only rarely required. If the tip of the little finger cannot enter the hernial orifice it will certainly close down itself, and operation is not required. If the hernial opening admits the little finger operation may be considered.

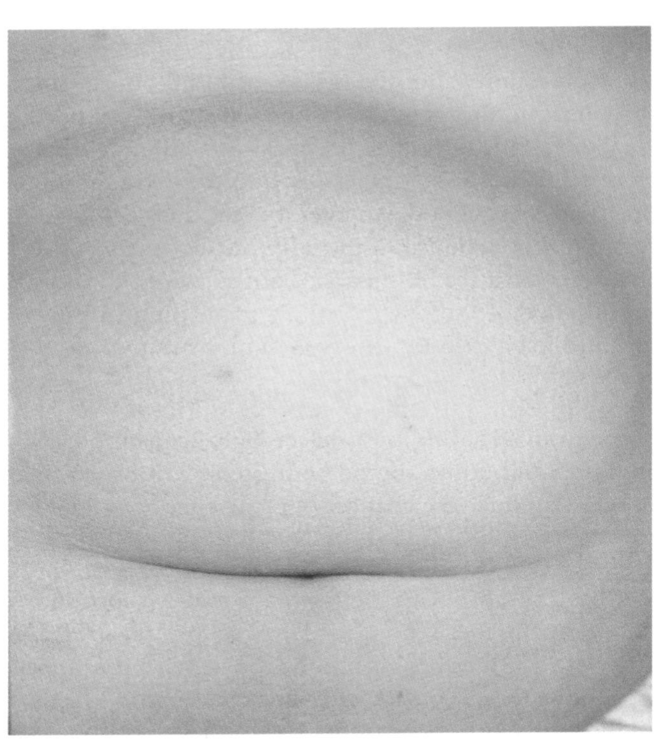

Fig.29.6 Large paraumbilical hernia. As always, the lower border of the hernia is at the umbilicus.

Paraumbilical hernia

This is the umbilical hernia of the *middle-aged* person. It protrudes through the linea alba just above the umbilicus. As it enlarges it tends to sag downwards, but its lower margin is always exactly at the umbilicus (Fig.29.6). The contents usually consist of greater omentum, often accompanied by small intestine or transverse colon. In old-standing cases the sac becomes loculated due to adhesions. The patient is usually an obese, multiparous woman between thirty-five and fifty years of age. These hernias often become irreducible due to omental adhesions within the sac. They may attain a very large size; in the past the hernia sometimes enlarged so much as to hang down to the knees. In such cases there may be dragging pain and nausea due to pull on the stomach or transverse colon. At the same time, constant friction between the lower abdominal wall and the skin of the under surface of the hernia can lead to a severe, persistent and often foul smelling dermatitis.

Treatment

The treatment of a paraumbilical hernia is by operation, to avoid increasing size and possible complications, e.g. irreducibility and strangulation.

Mayo's operation

In this procedure, after the hernia sac has been excised, the defect in the anterior rectus sheath is extended laterally on both sides. The lower flap of abdominal wall is inserted beneath the upper flap and sutured to it; the upper flap is brought down over it to produce a double-breasting. The removal of the large sac leaves a sizeable subcutaneous space. A suction drain is placed to avoid the collection of a seroma or hematoma. Redundant skin may need to be excised before the skin is sutured.

Mesh repair

Except for small hernias with defects upto 2cm, umbilical/paraumbilical hernias should be treated by mesh repair, in order to reduce the chances of recurrence.

Laparoscopic repair

This has the advantage of less pain and a short stay. However, the mesh used in laparoscopic repair is a composite mesh rather than polypropylene, and cannot be placed in direct contact with the bowel as gut is likely to adhere to it and get distorted and obstructed.

Very large hernia

Occasionally the hernia is so immense in size that nearly all the abdominal contents lie in it. In such a case reduction of these contents into the abdominal cavity which has adaptively contracted in size is not possible, and the patient might have to be told to live with his hernia. Alternatively, repeated insufflations of gas into the peritoneal cavity may be tried. If the cavity can be sufficiently enlarged by this method, operative reduction and repair may be attempted.

EPIGASTRIC HERNIA

An epigastric hernia comes out through a small defect in the linea alba usually midway between the umbilicus and the xiphoid process. It commences as a protrusion of extraperitoneal fat through the linea alba; if it enlarges it drags a pouch of peritoneum after it.

The patients are usually between thirty and forty years of age. The hernia may be symptomless, or there may be attacks of local pain, worse on physical exertion. If in an obese patient the small hernia has been unnoticed, a peptic ulcer may be suggested. Conversely, a patient suffering from peptic ulcer may attribute all his symptoms to an epigastric hernia.

This hernia can be distinguished from a para-umbilical hernia. Not only is it usually much smaller, but also unlike para-umbilical hernia there is always a gap between its lower border and the umbilicus (Fig.29.7)

The *treatment* of an epigastric hernia is by excision of the sac and repair of the abdominal wall.

INCISIONAL HERNIA

If after a laparotomy the wound in the abdominal wall fails to heal properly, the repair may be disrupted at one point or even along its whole length, and a hernia may appear. This is known as an incisional hernia. Occasionally it becomes obvious in the early postoperative period. However, more often it makes its appearance a few months after operation. Almost 80% of incisional hernias appear within 1–2 years of the operation. Lower midline incisions are notorious for incisional hernias.

Predisposing factors

These include the following:

Preoperative factors

- Hypoproteinemia, so that the building blocks of repair, i.e. the proteins, are deficient. The hypo-proteinaemia can be due to malnutrition, malabsorption, malignancies, etc.
- Administration of steroids and cytotoxic drugs (immunosupressed state).
- Jaundice and uremia.

Operative factors

- Absorbable sutures.
- Careless suturing technique, tension on suture line.
- Infection, leading to sloughing of wound margins.
- Layered closure of the abdominal wall: this is more often followed by wound disruption and incisional hernia than mass closure.

Postoperative factors

- Increased intra-abdominal pressure: due to obesity, chronic cough, pregnancy, postoperative distension due to paralytic ileus, etc.
- A hernia through a lower abdominal scar tends to assume a large size, and more and more of its contents become irreducible (Fig.29.8).

Treatment

The proper treatment of incisional hernia is by operative repair, unless the patient's poor general condition is a contraindication to surgery. Non-absorbable sutures are used, and according to the situation different methods of repair of the abdominal wall are employed:

- ***Mass closure*** using No. 1 nylon. Since the common employment of mass closure rather than layered closure of the abdominal wall, the incidence of

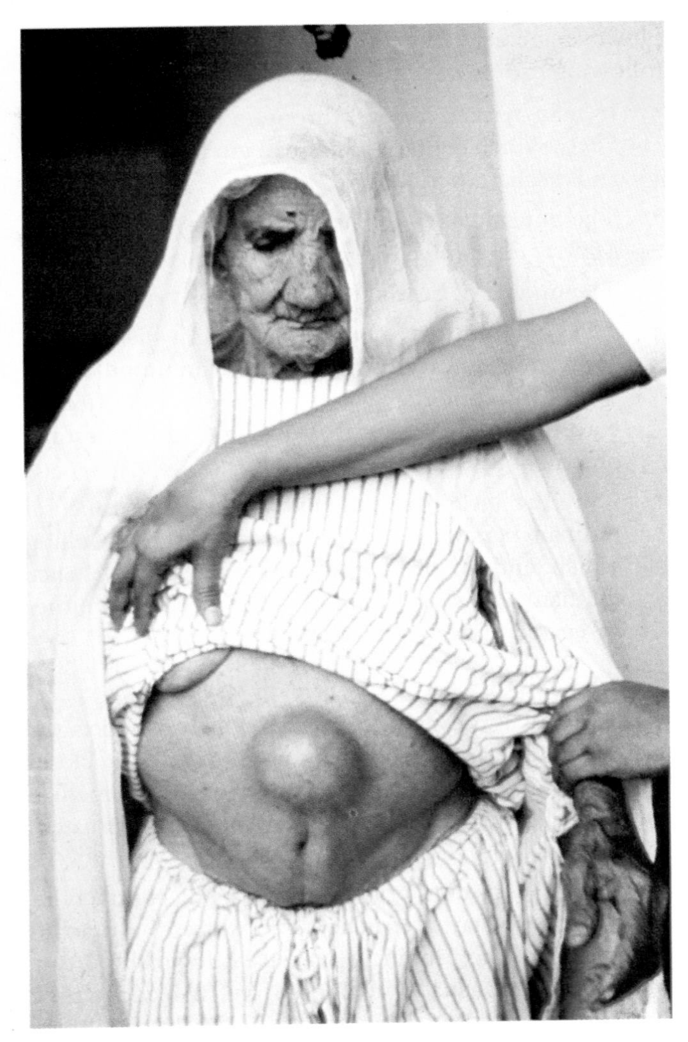

Fig.29.7 Epigastric hernia; unlike a paraumbilical hernia its lower edge is away from the umbilicus.

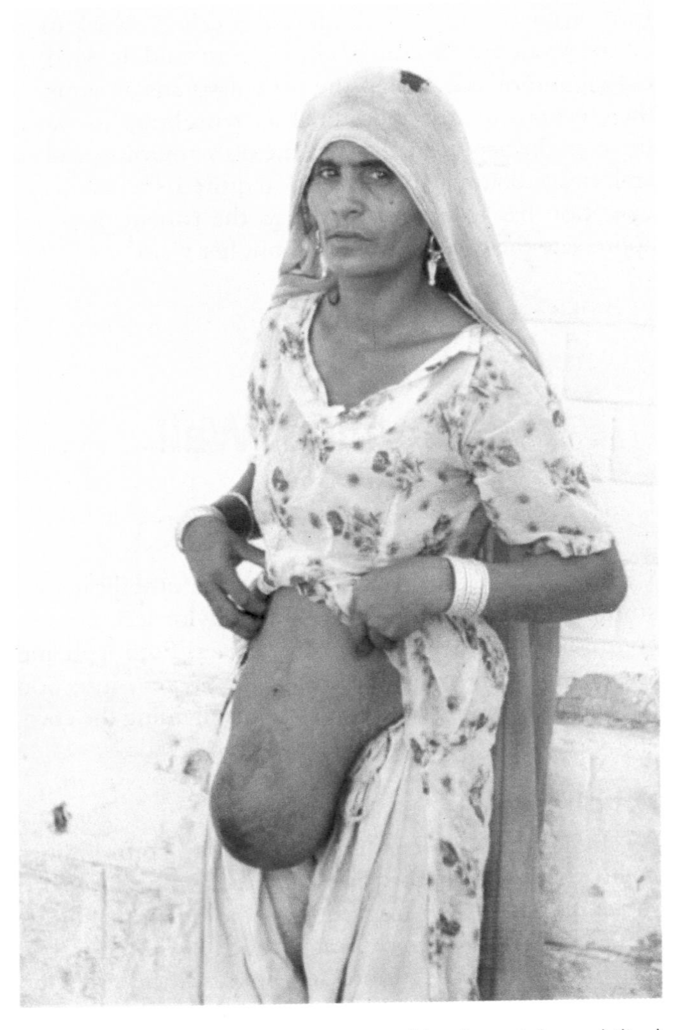

Fig.29.8 Large incisional hernia resulting from infraumbilical midine incision.

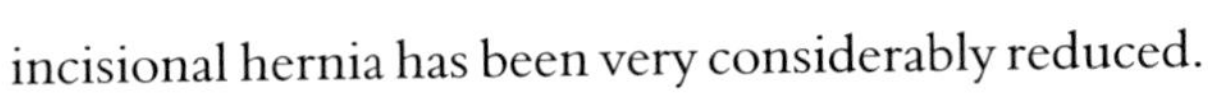

incisional hernia has been very considerably reduced.

- ***Overlapping*** of the rectus sheath, as in the 'double-breasting' of the Mayo repair.
- Implantation of a non-absorbable ***mesh*** of prolene or polytetrafluoroethylene (PTFE), or a composite mesh.

Recurrence rate

The recurrence rate after operation for incisional hernia is extremely high, of the order of 25 to 40%, and second repairs are equally unsuccessful. The operation should therefore not be undertaken lightly, and the patient should be informed about the real possibility of recurrence. The way in which the author explains this to his patients is as follows: he tells them that no man-made suture or material can equal the strength of the muscular grid consisting of three layers of abdominal muscles designed by nature, and with the fibres of each layer running in a different direction for added security.

Operation

The sac is isolated, ligated at the neck and excised. The gap in the linea alba is closed by a few non-absorbable sutures.

Parastomal hernia

This is a type of incisional hernia that occurs at the site of a stoma or immediately adjacent to the stoma.

Divarication of the recti abdominis

Due to stretching of the abdominal wall during repeated pregnancies, the recti abdominis sometimes get separated from each other. This condition is called divarication of the recti, and is commonly seen in middle-aged or elderly multiparae. When the patient strains or assumes the erect posture the abdominal contents bulge forwards through the gap. Usually there are no symptoms, and an abdominal belt may be all that is required. Occasionally, operation has to be carried out as the patient does not appreciate the excessive bulge about her waist.

Abdominal Wall

Within three or four days after birth the umbilical cord stump is found to be carrying staphylococci, or less commonly streptococci, in many babies. Esch. coli and Cl. tetani also occur occasionally. To prevent infection strict asepsis should be enforced while dividing the cord, and 1% chlorhexidine used locally for a few days.

Omphalitis

An infected umbilicus is common in communities where the umbilical cord is not divided aseptically. Warm moist dressings help resolution of the inflammation. If exuberant granulations form, a touch of silver nitrate discourages them. In more serious cases the infection may spread to the following parts:

- The abdominal wall, forming an abscess.
- The umbilical vein. This may result in one or more of the following complications:
    - Septicemia.
    - Portal vein thrombosis, with portal hypertension in later childhood.

Umbilical fistulae

As the umbilicus is a central weak point in the abdominal wall *a slow leak* from any viscus may surface here, e.g.:

- A septic discharge from a perforated carcinoma of the transverse colon.
- Stones from an inflamed gallbladder.

Secondly, the vitellointestinal duct or urachus may *remain patent*, with discharge of mucus or urine respectively.

Vitello-intestinal duct

In fetal life the vitello-intestinal duct connects the midgut with the yolk sac. Later it completely disappears. However, occasionally it may persist and take one of the following forms:

- It may remain patent throughout as an *umbilical fistula,* which connects the small gut to the umbilicus and discharges mucus.
- The intestinal end of the duct may persist as a *Meckel's diverticulum*.
- The middle of the duct may persist as a *cyst*.
- The whole duct may persist as a *fibrous cord* connecting the terminal ileum to the umbilicus. A coil of intestine may get twisted around the fibrous cord, and the patient may present with intestinal obstruction.
- Only the umbilical end may persist. The mucosal remnant persists as a pedunculated moist red swelling which tends to bleed. It looks like a raspberry, hence the name 'raspberry tumor' (Fig.29.9). It can either be ligated or excised by diathermy.

Patent urachus

The urachus is a canal in the fetus which connects the urinary bladder with the allantois. Normally it closes down and is replaced by a fibrous cord—the median umbilical ligament. Occasionally it persists in its patent form.

A patent urachus does not leak, because the contractions of the bladder start from the apex, where the urachus is attached to the umbilicus, and pass down the organ. It reveals itself usually in middle age, if bladder neck obstruction from some cause arises. In such a case there may be leakage of urine from the umbilicus.

Treatment

The bladder neck obstruction is dealt with. If leakage still persists, the urachus is excised and the bladder closed.

Burst abdomen (Dehiscence)

Sometimes a laparotomy wound breaks down and viscera are eventrated. This happens in about 1–2% of cases, the peak incidence being about one week after operation. Predisposing factors fall into three categories:

- *Poor suturing techniques*, with carelessly applied sutures. Dehiscence used to be common before the introduction of the method of mass closure of the abdominal wall.
- Conditions resulting in *excessive intraabdominal pressure* or abdominal distension, e.g. chronic cough and paralytic ileus.
- Conditions in which the process of *healing is impaired,* e.g. hypoproteinemia, anemia, malignancy, sepsis and infection.

- Sepsis, as in peritonitis.
- Long midline incisions are more prone to dehiscence.

In most cases dehiscence of the deeper layers (*partial dehiscence*) occurs some days before the wound actually bursts open. There may be a discharge of blood-stained serum. This is a clear indication that the wound is about to disrupt. The patient often says that 'he felt something give way'. If skin sutures have been removed, omentum or coils of intestine may be forced through the wound and will be found lying on the skin (*complete dehiscence*). Pain and shock are often absent.

Treatment

For midline laparotomy closure, No 1 prolene or PDS II are used for en mass closure. Sutures should pass through the anterior and posterior rectus sheaths rather than the linea alba. It should be remembered that closure of the abdomen under tension may lead to dehiscence, incisional hernia, or even an abdominal compartment syndrome.

Abdominal compartment syndrome

This syndrome occurs when tissue fluid pressure within the abdomen rises unduly due to the excessive accumulation of edema fluid, retroperitoneal blood, or free fluid in the abdomen. If the pressure rises over 20 mm Hg organs begin to fail, and the syndrome progresses to the end-stage highly fatal process termed abdominal compartment syndrome.

When abdominal compartment syndrome is anticipated, the abdomen should be closed with the help of a non-adhesive mesh or a *Bogota Bag*. This is a sterilized, 3 liter urinary bag that is slit open and sewn to the fascia of the anterior abdominal wall. It is used to tide over the period while the pathologic elevation of intra-abdominal pressure subsides over a week or so and the swelling subsides, after which it is removed and the abdominal wall closed.

Prophylaxis of burst abdomen

Sutures should be placed very carefully. In debilitated patients the intake of vitamin C and protein should be kept high. Since the last few decades the whole muscular abdominal wall is usually being sutured in a single layer, by the method of mass closure. This has very greatly reduced the incidence of burst abdomen, compared to the days when layered closure was employed.

Treatment

An emergency operation is required to replace the bowel and resuture the wound. While awaiting operation the wound should be covered with a moist sterile towel

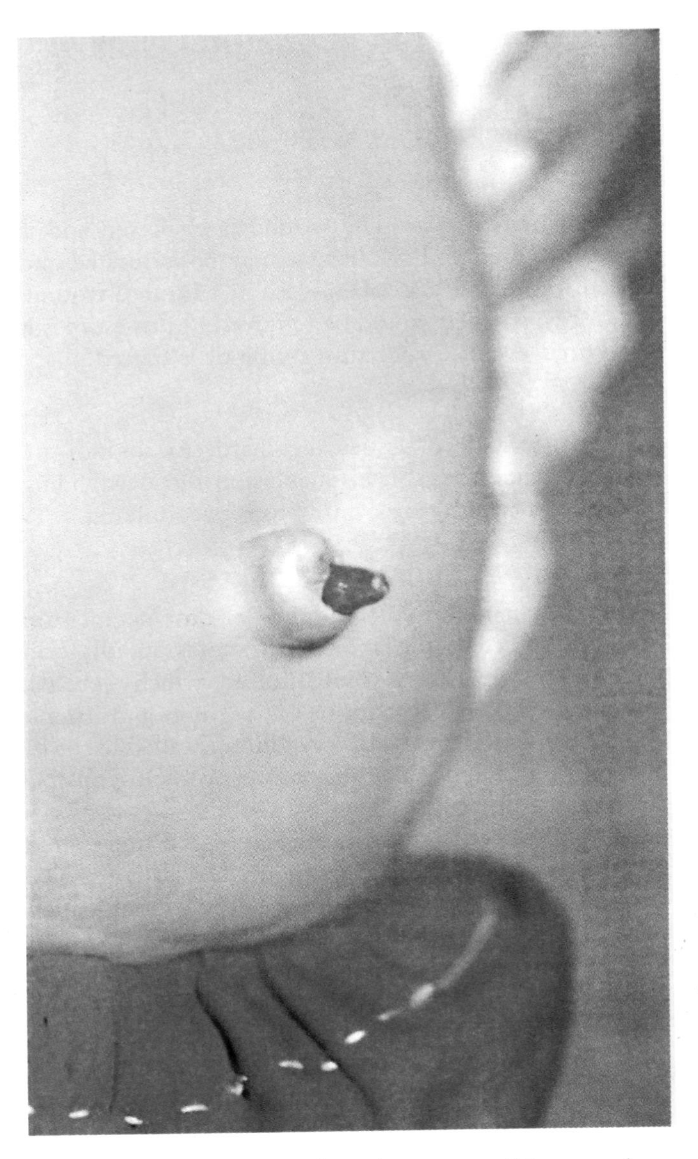

Fig.29.9 Enteroteratoma ('Raspberry tumor') in young boy

and the patient reassured. Nasogastric aspiration and intravenous fluids are started. At operation coils of intestine are gently washed with saline and replaced in the abdomen. All layers of the abdominal wall are approximated by through-and-through sutures of No.1 monofilament nylon. The abdominal wall may be supported by strips of adhesive plaster across the wound. Antibiotic therapy is started. Healing usually takes place satisfactorily.

One reason for prompt healing in these cases is the fact that the lag period of inactivity in the wound is already past and capillaries, fibroblasts etc. are available in abundance in the area.

Infections of the abdominal wall

Cellulitis

This may be superficial or deep:

Superficial cellulitis

The patient has fever. The wound is inspected and is found to be red and swollen. It may be indurated and tender. If infection has taken place in a sutured wound, one or two stitches should be removed. If pus escapes it is cultured. A broad-spectrum antibiotic is started.

Deep cellulitis

The skin and deep tissues feel hard. Antibiotics are started. If tenderness persists an incision is made, dividing the muscles layer by layer until pus is encountered.

Progressive synergistic gangrene

Sometimes, if a sutured abdominal or thoracic incision becomes infected, the infection extends rapidly and widely. It starts as a painful ulcer which spreads. Surrounding the ulcer is a zone of gangrene, and around that a red, painful area. This condition is called bacterial synergistic gangrene. The micro-organisms responsible for this condition are a micro-aerophilic streptococcus and a staphylococcus. The condition is seen more often in immunosuppressed and malnourished patients. The reason for its relentless spread is the deadly combination of infection, local ischemia (sometimes due to too tight sutures) and diminished host defences.

Treatment

This involves wide excision of the necrotic area. Multiple procedures are usually required. Penicillin etc. are given for the staphylococcus, and metronidazole for other opportunistic anaerobes. The mortality rate of the condition is fairly high.

Section

2

GENITOURINARY TRACT

Chapter

30 KIDNEY AND URETER

INVESTIGATION OF THE URINARY TRACT

A wealth of information about the urinary tract can be obtained by different laboratory, imaging and endoscopic techniques.

Laboratory tests

Urine examination

A great deal urine of information can be derived from a simple urine examination employing microscopy and biochemical tests, and its value should not be underestimated. The presence, or rise in the level of, each type of chemical or cell indicates an abnormality.

Renal function tests

Depending upon the state of hydration, the normal kidney can produce both markedly concentrated and very dilute urine. Using this information a simple test can be devised to assess renal function, as follows: fluid is withheld for 12 hours overnight, and the specific gravity of the first morning specimen is tested. If it is 1.025 or greater the renal function is good. One litre of water is now given by mouth. If the kidney function is good, within four hours the specific gravity should be as low as 1.002. This easy-to-perform test is greatly under-utilized, due to non-application of basic concepts of renal function.

Blood urea and serum creatinine levels

The levels of blood urea and serum creatinine reflect renal function. However, these levels are raised only when considerable reduction in kidney function has taken place. The normal blood urea level is 15 to 40mg/dL(2.5 to 6.5mmol/l). The normal level of creatinine in the serum is 0.5–0.9mg/dl; this is a more sensitive test of renal function than blood urea, which can be raised even due to severe dehydration.

Imaging

Radiology

Preparation

When taking plain x-rays of the abdomen, the purpose of preparation for each one of the following radiographic techniques is the same: to ensure that the number of shadows due to intestinal gas is minimal. For this purpose food is withheld overnight, and laxative tablets given on the evening before.

Plain x-ray

Soft tissue shadows of the kidneys can be detected on a good x-ray film. The outline of the psoas muscle is also visible; it becomes hazy in a case of perinephric abscess due to inflammatory edema of the parts. The majority of urinary calculi are radio-opaque and therefore show up on plain x-ray.

Intravenous urogram

Food is withheld overnight and sodium diatrizoate solution is injected intravenously. The important properties of this dye are that it is radiopaque and is excreted and concentrated in the urine. Thus in a few minutes it outlines the renal pelvis and the ureters. As the dye accumulates in the bladder this viscus is also shown up. Not only does this test indicate the renal function on each side, it also shows the location of the kidneys, and the presence of lesions like bifid pelvis, hydronephrosis, and filling defects due to papillomas or radiolucent stones. At the same time intravenous urography is useful for studying the detailed anatomy of the pelvicalyceal system before embarking upon operations like pyeloplasty. In recent years the importance of intravenous urography has greatly diminished, because most of the information provided by it can be obtained by ultrasonography. However, ultrasound does not tell us anything about the function of the kidneys.

The iodinated contrast media used in pyelography may be associated with minor and sometimes major adverse reactions; they should be used with caution and with preparation to deal with any major adverse reactions. Some of the reactions like laryngeal edema and bronchospasm are anaphylactic in nature and can be prevented by pretreatment with steroids and antihistamines. Further, the incidence of these reactions can be reduced by using low-osmolar contrast agents.

Retrograde pyelography

A cystoscope is passed into the bladder. A ureteric catheter is now passed up into the ureter under vision. A radio-opaque dye is injected up the catheter to outline the pelvis and ureter. The test is useful in cases where the kidney function is poor, specially when accurate anatomical information about the renal pelvis is required for planning the operation of pyeloplasty in a case of hydronephrosis.

Renal arteriography

A radiopaque dye is injected into the aorta above the level of the renal arteries. This is commonly done through a catheter passed up from the femoral artery (*retrograde arteriography*). However, it can also be done through a needle passed into the aorta just above the renal arteries (*translumbar arteriography*). In *selective renal arteriography* a hooked catheter is passed up from the femoral artery, and the hook is guided into the renal artery to outline the renal vasculature on that side.

Cystography

The bladder is filled with a radiopaque dye and x-rays taken. Distortions of the outline of the bladder as well as filling defects due to tumors and radiolucent stones are well shown up by this technique.

A *micturating cystogram* gives more useful information. After filling the bladder with dye the patient is asked to void, and while he is doing so he is screened under the x-ray tube. One looks particularly for the presence of reflux up the ureters, and for the function of the bladder neck. X-ray pictures are also taken.

Urethrography

The urethra can be imaged in antegrade fashion with a micturating cystogram or by retrograde injection of radiopaque fluid. The antegrade technique is useful to detect lesions of the posterior urethra like posterior urethral valves. Retrograde urethrography is required to outline the anterior urethra. By this technique valuable information about the presence and length of a urethral stricture is obtained. Urethral dilatation and diverticulum formation above a stricture is also shown up. A radiopaque dye is injected into the urethra and x-rays taken from an oblique angle, in order to avoid foreshortening of the posterior urethra.

The lower end of a stricture can be shown up through a urethroscope, but only urethrography can indicate the length of the stricture and the condition of the urethra above it.

Ultrasonography

Ultrasonography has nearly replaced intravenous urography as one of the most important investigations for the urinary tract. It can tell us about the location and the different dimensions of the kidneys, the thickness of their cortices, any dilatation of the pelves and calyces, any stone in the pelvis, and any abnormality of the ureter, and can give us similar information about the bladder. However, unlike intravenous urography it cannot tell us anything about the function of the kidneys. Renal ultrasound is useful in distinguishing cystic from solid lesions. Bladder sonography is useful in detection of calculi, tumors and residual volume. Sonography of the testis is used to differentiate between inflammatory conditions and testicular torsion.

Doppler sonography can be used for evaluation of renal vessels.

Computerized tomography (CT scan)

Like ultrasonography, a CT scan provides us with images of sections through the body. However, these sections are all taken at right angles to the long axis of the body. Therefore they are more reproducible, and comprise a more accurate and complete record. Again, as each of the different tissues has a different and defined density in the CT scan, it is easier to distinguish the one from the other on the basis of a CT scan report. As against this must be mentioned the ability of the ultrasound probe to be tilted and thus provide a perspective from many different angles. Ultrasonography is very much cheaper than a CT scan, and much more widely available.

Spiral/helical CT produces thinner sections with high resolution. With the help of a computer workstation, a high quality three-dimentional image can be created. It also saves much time due to continuity in the taking of the pictures.

Positron Emission Tomography (PET)—CT scan detects changes in the body's metabolism caused by abnormal cells. It is useful for accurate detection and localization of a variety of cancers at an early stage.

Magnetic resonance imaging (MRI)

This is particularly valuable in the investigation of masses in the adrenal, uterus and adnexa, and the staging of cancers of the kidney, bladder, prostate and uterus. MR urography produces urogram-like images without the need for contrast material. This is particularly useful in situations where contrast material is contraindicated.

Isotope renogram

Radionuclide renal studies are used to assess renal perfusion and various aspects of renal function and structure. The information gained depends on which radiopharmaceutical is used. Currently, three types of isotope renograms are commonly used, namely:

- Technetium-99m-dimercaptosuccinic acid (DMSA).
- Technetium-99m-diethylenetriamine pentaacetic acid (DTPA),
- Technetium-99m-mercaptoacetyltriglycine (MAG-3). The required isotope is injected intravenously and the radioactivity recorded by Gamma camera and analysed by computer.

The findings are as follows:

- In a *normal* kidney radioactivity on the Gamma camera rapidly reaches a high peak, and within 10 to 15 minutes most of it has disappeared due to the isotope having been excreted in the urine.
- In *acute urinary obstruction* a high peak is attained rapidly, but the isotope cannot be excreted so the level remains high. In *renal artery stenosis* a low peak is followed by rapid excretion.
- When the kidney function is *impaired* the peak is low, and excretion also takes place slowly.

This study is thus very useful in distinguishing between different types of dysfunction of the kidneys.

Further:

- DMSA has a prolonged transit time through the renal cortex and can be used to define renal masses. It is mostly bound to the renal tubular cells and is used for detection of cortical lesions such as scars, pyelonephritis and renal masses.
- DTPA (Technetium 99 d-t-pentaacetic acid) is entirely excreted by glomerular filtration and is used to measure relative renal perfusion and glomerular filtration rate. It is also used to evaluate obstruction in the renal tract.
- MAG-3 is a relatively new agent. Because of superior imaging and lower radiation doses it is now frequently used for renal perfusion and drainage studies.

Endoscopy

Urethroscopy and cystoscopy

With cystourethroscopes the interior of the urethra and bladder can be visualized, and a diverticulum, a stone, a ureterocele, and an enlarged prostate can all be seen. Flexible cystoscopes allow the procedure to be carried out under local anesthesia.

Ureteroscopy

The interior of the ureter and of the renal pelvis can be visualized through a *ureteroscope* and a *nephroscope* respectively. Ureteroscopes comes in sizes 7 through 12 French. The larger sizes require dilatation of the ureteric orifice by an angioplasty type of balloon.

Endoscopes give us very direct and first-hand information about the interior of the urethra, bladder and ureter. Bleeding points can be identified, tumors localized and biopsied, and stones and strictures treated.

CONGENITAL ANOMALIES OF THE KIDNEY AND URETER

About congenital anomalies in general. Sometimes a baby is born with an organ either missing or imperfectly formed. It is then not an easy matter to create an exact replica. The reasons are not far to seek. Nature takes a period of nine months working round the clock to produce and perfect each organ in the mother's womb; the surgeon has only an hour or two in the operation theatre. Again, as nature works at the molecular level, her tools of the trade are infinitely more sophisticated than those of the surgeon. It should not surprise anyone, therefore, if the organs constructed by the surgeon, usually from adjacent but different tissues, are sometimes not as perfect in form or in function as those created by nature. This fact should be clearly explained to the baby's parents in advance of the surgery, to avoid raising hopes of a perfect result and subsequent disappointment.

Absent kidney

About once in 2,000 persons one kidney may be absent, so that pyelography demonstrates only one kidney and cystoscopy shows one ureteric orifice.

Ectopic kidney

An ectopic kidney occurs once in 1,000 cases, when the kidney is arrested during its normal ascent, usually at the pelvic brim. If such an abnormally placed kidney becomes the seat of a pathological process, the diagnosis is difficult, and may be missed. An ectopic kidney lying in the pelvis in a female patient may cause obstructed labour.

Horse-shoe kidney

This has an incidence of 1 in 400. The kidneys and ureters develop from the mesonephros and metanephros. Each ureteral bud arises from the mesonephric duct

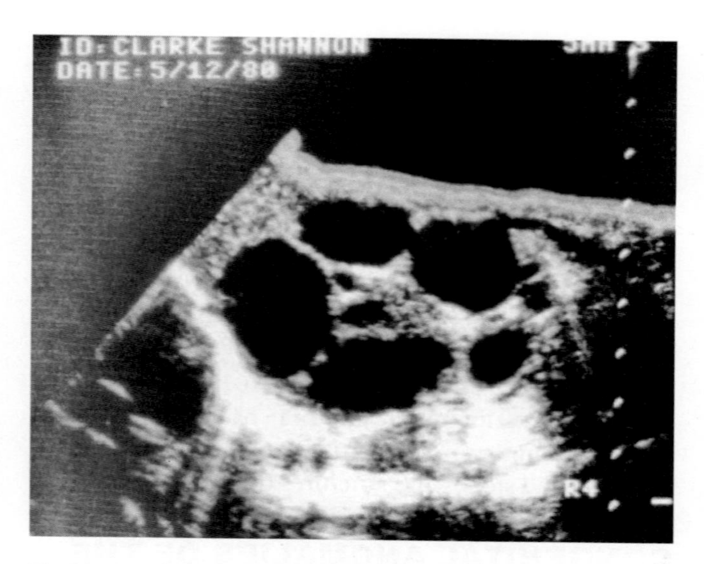

Fig.30.1 Ultrasound scan of congenital cystic kidney

of the same side, and penetrates the metanephros. The mesonephros contributes the ureters, pelves, calyces and collecting tubules; the metanephros supplies the nephrons. If the lower medial portions of the two kidney anlages get fused together, the result is a horse-shoe kidney. Such a kidney fails to ascend all the way to its adult position, and therefore lies at a lower level than normal. The bridge joining the lower poles lies in front of the 4th lumbar vertebra. Stasis of urine occurs due to two factors. Firstly, as the lower poles of the kidneys are joined together, the pelves face upwards rather than downwards, so that drainage is impaired. Secondly, the ureters are kinked as they pass over the isthmus.

Clinical features

These are due to stasis of urine. Infection, stone formation and tuberculosis can all occur. A firm, immobile mass below the umbilicus can be a horse-shoe kidney. However, the diagnosis can be confirmed only by ultrasonography or intravenous urography. With urography the lowermost calyx can be seen to be pointing medially. At the same time the ureters curve outwards in the upper part of their course.

Treatment

In the past the isthmus of a horse-shoe kidney was divided to improve drainage. Nowadays this is not considered to be necessary, and surgery is carried out only if indicated by the development of hydronephrosis or a calculus.

Crossed ectopia

Crossed ectopia or unilateral fusion of the kidneys is rare. If both pelves face medially the result is a unilateral long kidney. If the pelvis of the crossed kidney faces laterally, an S-shaped kidney results.

Congenital cystic kidneys

In this condition the kidneys are greatly enlarged, and are riddled with cysts of varying sizes. The condition is inherited as an autosomal dominant, so the risk of transmitting the disease to the offspring is fairly high, and this fact should be mentioned during genetic counselling.

Clinical features

The disease rarely manifests itself before adult life, and is slightly more common in women. If both kidneys are large and nodular, the diagnosis is most likely congenital cystic kidneys. Most of the renal parenchyma is replaced by the cysts. As such, the urine secreted by these diseased kidneys is of a poor quality, having a low specific gravity. There may be a dull ache in the loin, probably from tension inside one of the cysts. A cyst may rupture producing hematuria, but the most common complication encountered is pyelonephritis. The majority of adults with this condition suffer from hypertension. In later years chronic renal failure supervenes, with anorexia, headache, dyspepsia and anemia. In the past very few patients used to survive beyond the fifth decade.

Diagnosis

The diagnosis is easily made by ultrasonography, which shows up the cysts to good advantage (Fig.30.1).

Treatment

In order to avoid burdening the poorly functioning kidneys, the patient should take a low-protein diet, and to prevent anemia he should take iron. If infection occurs it should be treated appropriately. If the different cysts are punctured, renal function is improved somewhat; this can be done percutaneously under ultrasound control. When renal failure supervenes it is managed by bilateral nephrectomy and renal transplantation.

Other types of cystic kidneys

Infantile polycystic disease

This disease is rare. The kidneys are large and may obstruct labour.

Unilateral multicystic disease

This presents as a mass in the flank, and after making sure that the other kidney is present and functioning well, it should be treated by nephrectomy.

Solitary renal cyst

This may have a congenital origin, but its appearance in adult life suggests that it is acquired. It may produce a symptomless swelling, or be associated with loin pain.

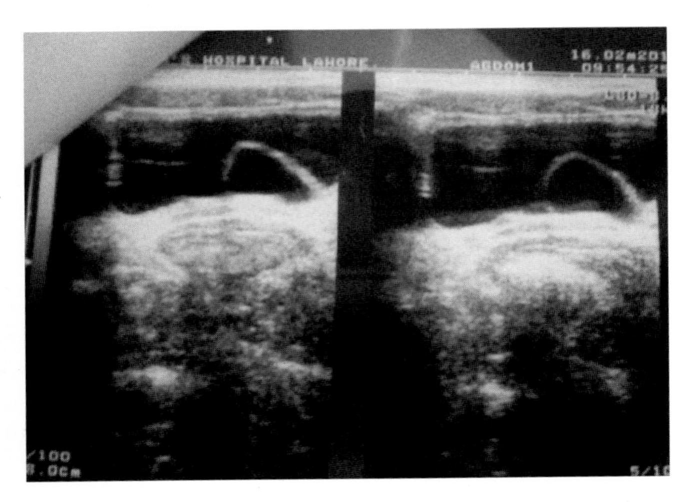

Fig.30.2 A ureterocele projecting into the urinary bladder

These days such a cyst is often found incidentally during an ultrasound examination for a different condition. If on aspiration the cyst contains clear fluid and no malignant cells, it may be watched. However, it should be kept under regular observation by ultrasound examinations. If it enlarges it is best operated upon and the needful done according to the situation found at operation.

Aberrant renal artery

Sometimes in a case of hydronephrosis the lowermost branch of the renal artery appears to be the cause, as it crosses over the pelviureteric junction (PUJ). In actual fact, however, in most cases the PUJ is already obstructed, and the artery merely accentuates the obstruction as the pelvis prolapses forwards over it. In such a case the artery may need to be divided to relieve the obstruction. However, it often supplies a large part of the kidney and cannot be sacrificed. In that case a dismembering type of pyeloplasty needs to be done, i.e. one in which the pelviureteric junction is divided across, the cut end of the ureter enlarged by slitting it open for some distance, and the pelvis and ureter re-anastomosed in front of the aberrant artery, so that the vessel need not be divided.

Duplication of the renal pelvis

In this condition the upper pelvis is the smaller one, and drains the upper major calyx. The lower pelvis drains the middle and lower major calyces. A double pelvis is more prone to develop the complications of stone formation, infection or hydronephrosis than a normal pelvis, because each of the two pelves, and specially the upper one, is smaller and narrower than the normal pelvis. If stones damage one calyx, that part of the kidney may have to be removed in a partial nephrectomy.

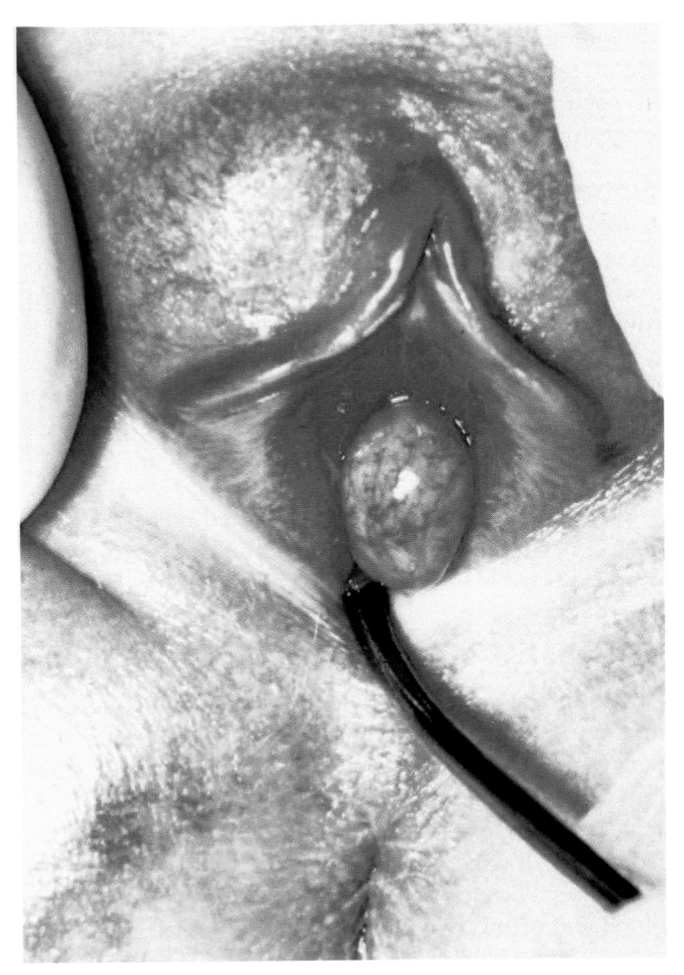

Fig.30.3 Ureterocele prolapsing into urethra and presenting at vulva

Duplication of a ureter

In this condition the two ureters usually join up in the lower third of their course. In other cases both open separately into the bladder. In that case the ureter draining the upper pelvis crosses its fellow and opens below it into the bladder.

Ectopic ureteric orifice

This is clinically important only if the orifice lies below the bladder sphincter, because in that case it results in incontinence of urine. It may not be easy to spot the opening at urethroscopy. If the urine is clear the ideal treatment is to reimplant this ureter into the bladder. On the other hand if repeated infections arise, the part of the kidney draining through this ureter should be removed by a partial nephrectomy.

Retrocaval ureter

In this condition the right ureter passes behind the inferior vena cava instead of lying to the right side of it. Sometimes, due to the distortion of its course and the pressure of the cava the ureter becomes obstructed. In such a case it should be divided across and re-anastomosed in front of the cava.

Ureterocele

A ureterocele arises when there is congenital stenosis of a ureteric orifice. The intramural part of the ureter dilates into a cyst. The condition is usually not recognized till adult life. During cystoscopy the cyst is seen to enlarge with each efflux of urine, after which it slowly collapses (Fig.30.2). In females occasionally a ureterocele prolapses into the urethra and presents at the vulva (Fig.30.3).

Treatment

Endoscopic incision is the preferred method of treatment of a ureterocele; it is incised in its inferior part with a needle electrode to relieve obstruction.

INJURIES TO THE KIDNEY

The kidney is one of the commonly injured abdominal organs. Renal injury is broadly classified as blunt or penetrating. A kidney may be injured by a blow to the loin or from in front, or by being crushed during a road accident. The extent of the injury varies a good deal, from a small subcapsular hematoma to a complete tear extending from the capsule to the pelvis. In such a case blood and urine collect in the retroperitoneal area.

Renal injuries are categorized into five grades by the American Association for the Surgery of Trauma (Table 30.1): This renal injury scaling system helps to standardize different groups of patients, select appropriate therapy, and predict results of therapy.

Table 30.1 Grading of renal trauma (American Association for the Surgery of Trauma)

Grade	Description
I	Contusion or stable subcapsular hematoma; no laceration.
II	Superfical laceration <1cm deep, not extending into pelvis; stable perirenal hematoma.
III	Laceration >1cm, not extending into pelvis; no urine extravasation.
IV	Laceration extends to renal pelvis. Injury to main renal artery or vein with contained hemorrhage.
V	Shattered kidney. Avulsion of renal hilum.

Clinical features

There is usually pain and tenderness in the loin. A few hours after the accident hematuria may be seen, sometimes accompanied by clot colic. If the injury is severe, hypotension may occur and abdominal distension may appear after about forty-eight hours due to paralytic ileus from involvement of the splanchnic nerves. If a large perirenal hematoma forms, the contour of the loin may become convex.

Investigations

CT with contrast or intravenous urography indicates the severity of renal injury and shows a normal contralateral kidney. CT provides superior anatomical details regarding the extent of renal laceration, the magnitude of perinephric hematoma or urinoma, and the presence of associated abdominal injuries.

Treatment

If the contrast CT/IVU show moderate degree of renal injury, conservative treatment is carried out. The great majority of blunt injuries to the kidney settle down with conservative management. The patient should rest in bed until hematuria has been absent for a few days. Morphine is given for analgesia and sedation. The pulse and blood pressure are recorded every hour. A sample of each specimen of urine should be kept, to watch the progress of the hematuria. Blood should be grouped and cross-matched, so as to be available in case of continuing hemorrhage. With such management hematuria often diminishes, pain and muscle guard decrease, and the pulse becomes normal.

Operation becomes necessary in a few patients. The indications for operation are the following:

- If there is continuing blood loss.
- If a gross swelling develops in the loin.
- If selective renal angiography shows renal artery thrombosis.

Renal trauma may result from penetrating injuries such as stab and gunshot wounds of the abdomen. The extent of renal injury tends to be less predictable and of greater severity. In these patients, as a laparotomy is generally required for associated abdominal injuries, renal exploration may also be carried out.

Operation

In general, in cases of renal trauma the kidney is best approached from in front, through a midline incision. Other viscera are first examined for evidence of injury. The peritoneum overlying the aorta is next incised and a vascular clamp applied to the renal artery; control of the renal pedicle allows the renal bed to be explored without excessive bleeding.

The kidney is now exposed by incising the peritoneum in the paracolic gutter and retracting the colon medially. Small tears in the kidney can be sutured over a piece of detached muscle. If the tears involve only one pole of the kidney a partial nephrectomy can be performed. If the kidney has multiple lacerations or the kidney pedicle is damaged, nephrectomy should be carried out.

Injury to the ureter

The ureter is commonly injured by gunshot or stab wounds, when primary repair is best. The lumen of the ureter being narrow, a circular anastomosis tends to stenose due to contraction of the fibrous tissue. To prevent this, each end of the ureter is slit down the side a short distance ('spatulated') to enlarge the opening. When the ends are now joined together, stenosis is avoided.

Injury to the lower end of the ureter occurs from time to time during *difficult pelvic surgical procedures* or the operation of hysterectomy, at the site where it crosses obliquely in front of the vaginal fornix to reach the bladder. Commonly the operator is a gynaecologist:

- If a urologist is available, it is best to immediately reimplant the ureter into the bladder.
- If, on the other hand, the gynaecologist has to deal with the situation unaided, the best he can usually do is to tie a ureteric catheter or other fine tube into the ureter and bring its end outside. He can then request a urologist to repair the ureter:
  - If the lower end of the ureter has been divided during hysterectomy it can be reimplanted into the bladder.
  - If, as happens rarely, the damage has taken place during oophorectomy, the divided ends of the ureter have to be anastomosed together.

Sometimes the ureteric injury is not recognized during operation. These patients may later present with symptoms like abdominal pain, fever, mass or urinary leakage from the wound. Diagnosis is made by an IVP or a CT scan. Exploration is indicated, and debridement, drainage of urinoma and repair of the ureter carried out.

In a situation where a longer segment of the *distal* ureter is damaged, a bladder flap may be constructed to bridge the gap and the ureter implanted into the flap.

HYDRONEPHROSIS

A hydronephrosis is an aseptic dilatation of the kidney due to a partial obstruction to the outflow of urine. If the pelvis is intrarenal, more damage is caused to the kidney by its dilatation than if it is extrarenal. In either case in advanced hydronephrosis the kidney may be reduced to a mere fibrous sac (Fig.30.4 a and b). Usually it takes years before this stage is reached.

Hydronephrosis may be unilateral or bilateral:

Unilateral hydronephrosis

When hydronephrosis is present on only one side the cause must lie in the ureter of that side, because if it was located at a lower level, i.e. in the bladder or the urethra, the pelvic dilatation would have been bilateral. The obstruction is commonly located at the pelvi-ureteric junction, but sometimes at a lower level.

Pelvi-ureteric junction obstruction

When the obstruction is at the pelvi-ureteric junction (PUJ), the cause usually lies in the wall of the ureter, but is not visible externally. It may be:

- Congenital stenosis.
- Physiological narrowing of the PUJ.
- An aberrant renal artery.

Aberrant renal artery.

If an inferior branch of the renal artery happened to be crossing in front of the PUJ and a hydronephrosis developed, in the past it was thought that this was an abnormally placed vessel (an aberrant artery), and that it had produced the hydronephrosis by obstructing the outflow of urine from the pelvis. We know now that in most of these cases the cause of the hydronephrosis is an intrinsic PUJ obstruction, and the dilated pelvis is merely bulging forwards over this normally placed vessel.

Obstruction at a lower level in the ureter

Here the cause may lie in the lumen of the ureter, in its wall, or outside the ureter:

- *Intraluminal.*

A stone in the ureter may produce hydronephrosis by causing partial or intermittent obstruction.

- *Intramural.*
  - A *congenital small ureteric orifice* may result both in a ureterocele (cystic dilatation of the intramural ureter), and hydronephrosis.
  - *Stricture* of the ureter may arise in a case of tuberculosis, or after damage to the ureter during a pelvic operation, usually hysterectomy.
  - A *neoplasm* of the ureter, or a tumor of the bladder involving the ureteric orifice, may be the cause of the obstruction.

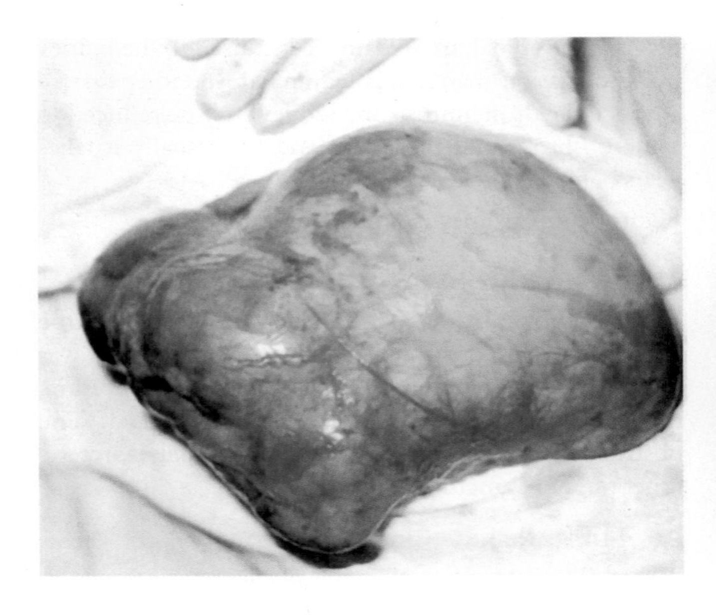

a

Fig.30.4 (a) Nephrectomy for advanced hydronephrosis

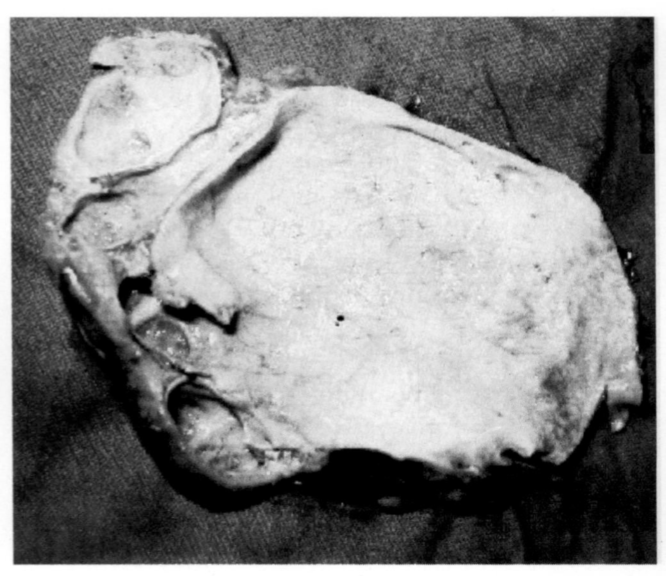

b

Fig.30.4 (b) Specimen slit open, showing hugely dilated kidney and completely destroyed renal parenchyma

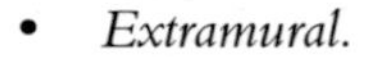

- *Extramural.*

The ureter may be involved by a growth arising in a neighbouring organ, e.g. carcinoma of the cervix, rectum or prostate.

Clinical features

Usually the patient complains only of a dull ache or a sense of weight in the loin, which may be aggravated by excessive fluid intake. An enlarged kidney may be palpated. On the other hand sometimes there may only be attacks of renal colic, without a palpable kidney.

Bilateral hydronephrosis

Bilateral hydronephrosis may be caused by any of the conditions mentioned above if they occur on both sides. However, much more commonly it is the result of some form of obstruction to the urethra. The conditions which may result in bilateral hydronephrosis include the following:

- *Congenital.*
  - o Congenital valves of the posterior urethra.
  - o Congenital contracture of the bladder neck.
  - o Phimosis.
- *Acquired.*
  - o Stricture of the urethra, either traumatic or gonorrhoeal.
  - o Enlargement of the prostate, usually benign but occasionally malignant.
  - o Carcinoma of the cervix or rectum involving both ureters.
  - o Carcinoma of the bladder involving the ureteric orifices.

Clinical features

Bilateral hydronephrosis commonly presents with symptoms of uremia, i.e. polyuria with resultant thirst, along with loss of appetite. There may only be a dull ache in the loins.

During *pregnancy* some dilatation of the ureters and renal pelves occurs, and becomes maximum by the fifth or sixth month. After delivery the situation returns to normal within a few weeks. It is due to the hormone progesterone producing atony of the ureters. In the dilated, atonic ureters urine does not drain freely and infection often results.

Investigations

Ultrasound

Confirmation of the diagnosis of hydronephrosis can be obtained by an *ultrasound scan*, which shows up the dilated pelvis and calyces as black cavities. The dimensions of the pelvis and the thickness of the cortex should be measured and recorded for comparison with future scans.

Intravenous urography

This is nowadays utilized mainly for assessing the functional state of each kidney (Fig.30.5). It should be noted that if the hydronephrosis is at an advanced stage, the 15 and 30 minute films will not be of much use, as the kidney function will be too poor for any excretion of the dye to take place so early. In such a case pictures should be taken at increasing intervals until the excretion of the dye is demonstrated. The length of time which elapses before sufficient dye is excreted for visualization gives a rough idea of kidney function on each side; the longer the time period the worse the state of kidney function.

Radio-isotope renogram

This test assesses the function of each kidney, and detects significant obstruction. DTPA and MAG-3 renal scans are commonly used for this purpose. The relative differential functions of each kidney are measured and the rapidity of clearance of the radioisotope from the collecting system calculated. Retention of radioactivity in the collecting system indicates significant obstruction.

Treatment

If the hydronephrosis is of a slight degree no treatment may be required. However, repeated ultrasound scans at yearly intervals are advised in order to monitor the progress of the condition. If on repeated ultrasound scans the dilatation is increasing, operation is usually the best course. Other indications for operation include repeated attacks of colic and recurrent bouts of infection. In bilateral cases when the cause lies in the bladder or urethra it should be removed; the hydronephrosis will then regress.

Operation

At operation the aim should be conservation of renal tissue. Nephrectomy should be performed only if the renal parenchyma has been mostly destroyed. In case of bilateral hydronephrosis, the underlying cause needs to be treated.

Anderson-Hynes pyeloplasty

If surgery is required for pelvi-ureteric junction (PUJ) obstruction, the most common procedure employed is the Anderson-Hynes operation. In this procedure the excess part of the pelvis is removed along with the pelvi-ureteric junction. The upper part of the remaining pelvis is now closed. The upper end of the ureter is slit down the side in order to enlarge its opening, and it is anastomosed to the lower part of the pelvis.

In other types of pyeloplasty the PUJ is not disconnected, but a flap is turned down from the pelvis to widen the pelvi-ureteric junction and improve drainage from the pelvis. The advantage of the Anderson-Hynes operation lies in the fact that it can be applied to every case, including cases where an artery is passing across the PUJ. In the other operations the artery would have to be divided, and this could result in ischemic infarction in the part of the kidney supplied.

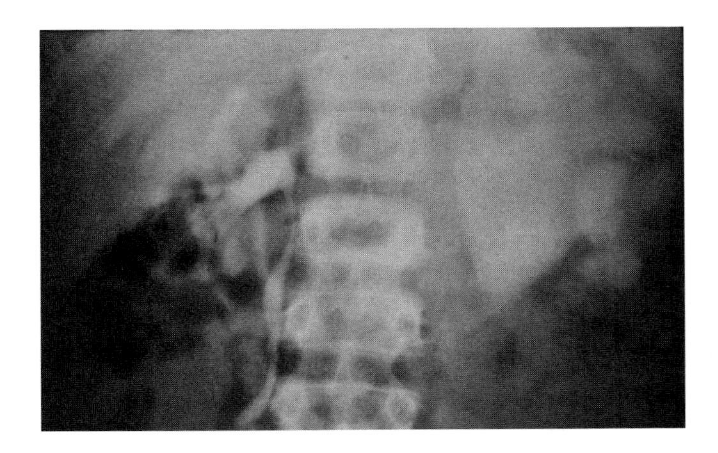

Fig.30.5 Intravenous pyelogram showing left-sided hydronephrosis

Surgery on the fetus

If severe bilateral hydronephrosis develops in the fetus, the fetal urine output is low, with resultant oligohydramnios. The cramped space in the uterus leads to pulmonary hypoplasia, which may be life-threatening:

- If the lungs are mature, immediate delivery and decompression of the hydronephrosis should be carried out.
- If the lungs are immature, the decompression can now be performed even in utero by insertion of specially designed shunts between the fetal urinary bladder and the amniotic cavity (vesico-amniotic shunts).

RENAL CALCULUS

Stone formation in the kidneys is a fairly common event. In the 'stone belt' of the world, which stretches across North Africa, Arabia and the southern parts of Iran, Pakistan and Rajasthan, the condition is extremely common. Whether this is due to the hot and dry climate of these areas resulting in underhydration, and leading to precipitation of crystals in the concentrated urine, is not certain.

Etiology

Urinary calculi develop as a result of excessive excretion of calcium, oxalate, uric acid or cystine:

- *Hypercalciuria* may be:
  - o Idiopathic.
  - o Due to increased intestinal absorption of calcium (in hyperparathyroidism).
  - o Due to decreased renal reabsorption of calcium (calcium leak).
  - o Due to prolonged recumbency (e.g. in paraplegia) where bone reabsorption is increased.
- *Hyperoxaluria* may occur as a result of increased intestinal absorption of oxalate after ileal resection or colon bypass surgery.
- *Uric acid* stones are associated with hyperuricosuria, and may occur without a raised level of uric acid in the blood.
- *Cystinuria* results from a disorder of cystine metabolism.
- Magnesium ammonium phosphate stones occur due to the combined presence of obstruction (or a foreign body).
- Urinary calculi are also seen in patients with sarcoidosis.

However, in the above-mentioned regions of the world where urinary stones are endemic, in most cases none of the above causes can be found.

Varieties of urinary calculi

About 80% of all urinary calculi are composed of calcium oxalate. The other common types of stones include the following: magnesium ammonium phosphate (15%), uric acid (4%), and cystine (1%).

Oxalate stones

The surface of a calcium oxalate stone is rough. The sharp projections damage the mucosa of the renal pelvis, so that hematuria results. Altered blood may be deposited on the surface of the stone, rendering it black in colour. An oxalate stone produces a dense shadow on x-ray. It is very hard, and on section it is laminated concentrically. 'Envelope-shaped' oxalate crystals are seen in the urine.

Phosphate stones

These usually contain calcium magnesium phosphate. They are smooth and dirty white. If the urine is alkaline they enlarge rapidly and may fill the renal calyces, taking on their shape (Fig.30.6). The surface of phosphate stones is smooth, so that they cause less pain and hematuria than oxalate stones. They are radiopaque, but less dense on x-ray than oxalate stones.

Uric acid and urate stones

These are yellow or brown in colour, and are smooth and hard. They are not opaque to x-rays. However, most of them contain a mixture of calcium oxalate, so that they show up on plain x-rays. Urate stones are more soft, and are commonly seen in children. In some persons there is greatly diminished resorption of cystine from the renal tubules, and excessive quantities of cystine are excreted in the urine; in such patients cystine stones can form. They are soft, and pink or yellow in colour. They may assume a cast of the renal pelvis. They are radiopaque due to the sulphur they contain.

Xanthine and *indigo* calculi are very rare.

Clinical features

Most cases of calculi present between the ages of thirty and fifty years. Males are slightly more often affected than females. There may be no symptoms, specially in the case of the more smooth phosphate stones. In such cases uremia may be the first indication of the presence of the stones.

Pain is the presenting and most important symptom in most cases. It can be of two kinds, fixed renal pain and ureteric colic:

Fixed renal pain occurs when a stone is lying in the renal pelvis. It is located in the renal angle, or occasionally in the hypochondrium. It is usually made worse by movement.

Ureteric colic is a very severe pain, which radiates from the loin to the groin. It comes suddenly and the patient rolls about in agony. If the stone is in the intramural part of the ureter there may be painful straining, followed by the passage of a few drops of blood-stained urine. This is called strangury.

During the attack of renal colic there is tenderness over the renal angle---*Murphy's renal punch*. At the same time, the kidney may be tender on bimanual palpation, which is an important clinical method of examination of the kidney. If the stone leads to the development of a hydronephrosis or a pyonephrosis the kidney may become palpable.

Hematuria is not normally a leading symptom. Occasionally, small quantities of blood may render the urine smoky in colour. Small amounts of pus may also be found in the urine.

Investigations

Ultrasound examination

This shows up every calculus, whereas x-rays show up only those stones which are radiopaque. Ultrasonography indicates the location and the dimensions of the kidney, the thickness of the cortex, the presence and the degree of any dilatation of the calyces and pelvis, and the number and sizes of stones in the pelves and ureters.

Plain x-ray

Plain x-ray should be taken after an overnight fast and after emptying the bowel by a laxative, otherwise the shadows of gas and minerals in the intestines obscure the picture.

The appearance of a kidney stone can be mimicked by:

- A calcified mesenteric lymph node.
- A gallstone.
- A phlebolith.
- A calcified lesion in the kidney.

Gallstones and mesenteric lymph nodes lie anteriorly, and a lateral radiograph can be taken, which will show that they are located anterior to the bodies of the vertebrae.

Intravenous urography

Intravenous urography helps in confirming that the opacity due to a stone is intrarenal, and in showing in which part of the kidney it is situated. At the same time it reveals the function of both kidneys. A non-opaque stone may also be shown up as a filling defect in the pelvis. At times, it is not possible to localize these radiolucent calculi on intravenous urography. In this situation, non-contrast spiral CT is invaluable.

TREATMENT OF RENAL CALCULI

The treatment of kidney stones resolves itself into the relief of renal colic and the removal of the calculi. For the relief of pain morphine, in a dose of 15mg subcutaneously, and an antiprostaglandin agent diclofenac in a dose of 50mg i.m., are effective.

Methods of removal of stones

Classically, stones in the kidneys were removed by open operation. These have been mostly replaced by minimally invasive methods including extracorporeal shock wave lithotripsy (ESWL), percutaneous nephrostolithotomy *(PCNL)* and ureterorenoscopy. For the last two decades these procedures are being used with increasing frequency, so that today only a small percentage of all cases are removed by open operation. The modern methods are first described, followed by the older open methods.

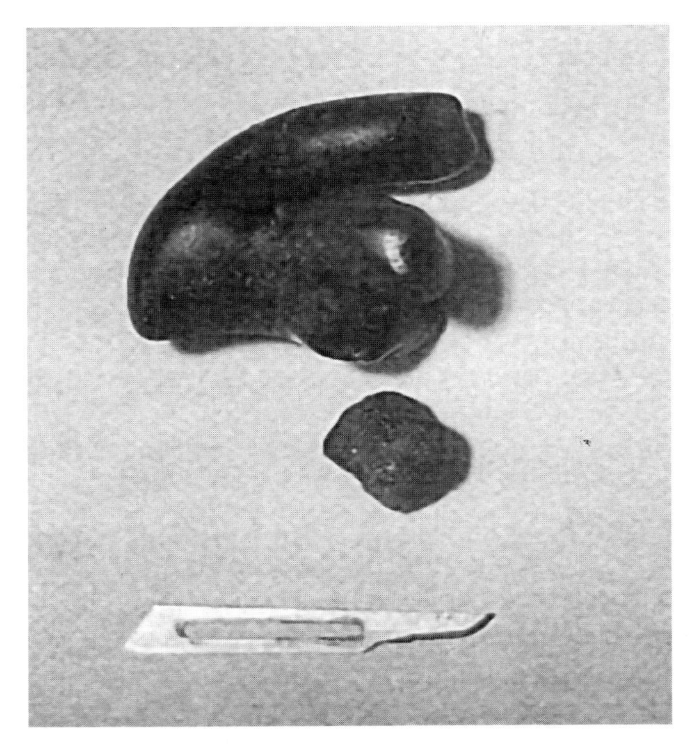

Fig.30.6 Stone taking the shape of the renal pelvis and black in colour due to altered blood on its surface. Note the smaller stone which lay in the lower calyx.

Modern methods

Extracorporeal shock wave lithotripsy

If high energy shock waves (electrohydraulic, acoustic or piezoelectric) are concentrated onto a crystalline stone in the kidney, it disintegrates into small particles, which are then passed out with the urine. In this method the waves are focussed onto the stone with the aid of fluoroscopy or ultrasound. After being broken down, the small bits pass out with some colic.

Advantage

ESWL has revolutionized the treatment of urinary calculi. The *advantage* of this method is that the kidney does not have to be exposed at open operation. As such, the pain and the problems associated with a major wound in the loin, e.g. infection, hematoma formation, etc., are avoided.

Disadvantages

However, there are also important *drawbacks* to the method. Whereas in the case of open operation all the stones and pieces of gravel are removed completely and with certainty, with lithotripsy the gravel is left in the urinary tract to pass out. Specially if the stone was a large one, this mass of gravel can produce its own problems, the more important ones being obstruction and resulting infection. Oxalic and phosphate stones disintegrate well; cystine stones, being harder, are less easy to fragment. Also, generally speaking, small stones are more suitable for treatment by ultrasound lithotripsy than the larger ones.

Small pieces of fragmented calculi can collect in, and obstruct, the distal ureter, like sand occluding a straw. This condition is called *steinstrasse* ('stone street'). In such a situation a *double-pigtail* catheter is usually passed through a cystoscope up into the ureter to allow drainage by the side of the gravel, so that the kidney is not obstructed and the stones have time to pass out. In order to avoid dislodgement, one 'pigtail' of the catheter is left in the renal pelvis and the other in the bladder. Finally, sometimes impacted stones need to be removed endoscopically.

Percutaneous nephrostolithotomy (PCNL)

In this method a trocar needle is passed under x-ray visualization from the loin into the pelvis of the kidney. A guide wire is passed through the trocar which is withdrawn. A series of dilators is now passed over the guide wire to dilate the track, so that a 28 to 30F sheath can be placed through the parenchyma into the collecting system. Through this sheath fibreoptic telescopes can be passed into the renal pelvis and the stones visualized. If these are small they are extracted as a whole; if large they can be broken up with an ultrasonic, electrohydrolic, pneumatic or laser lithotripter. The fragments can either be removed or they are excreted with the urine. This technique is used for calculi more than 2.5cm in diameter and those that do not respond to extracorporeal shock wave lithotripsy.

By the same technique a nephrostomy catheter can be placed in the renal pelvis for decompression of an obstructed collecting system.

Ureterorenoscopy

In the case of ureteric stones a rigid ureteroscope or in case of calyceal stones a flexible ureterorenoscope of size 9 to 12 French, is passed up the urethra, bladder and ureter to the level of the stone. If the stone is small enough to be extracted intact, a stone basket or grasping forceps can be used for its removal. If it requires fragmentation before removal, ultrasonic or laser lithotripsy can be employed for this purpose.

The laser fibre is passed through the operating port of a ureteroscope. The small fibre size, accuracy and safety allow successful ureteral stone fragmentation with minimal invasiveness. The laser pulses are given at low energy levels. At the same time the particular wavelength is absorbed selectively by the stone and minimally by the tissues. This is therefore a safe and effective method of stone fragmentation.

Older open methods

Exposure

Position

The patient is placed on a four-piece table in the lateral position, with the affected side uppermost. The opposite lower limb is flexed, the limb of the same side being extended. The trunk is held in this position by a strap passing over the pelvis. The table is 'broken' opposite the patient's waist to open out the lumbar region and increase the space between the ribs and iliac crest.

Incisions

The nerves of the lateral abdominal wall run obliquely, from above downwards and forwards. Therefore, in order to avoid damaging them, most incisions in this area are made in the same direction.

Morris's incision

This incision, which is the most popular, starts at the renal angle and runs downwards and forwards to a point about 3cm above and medial to the anterior superior iliac spine. The external oblique is split along the direction of its fibres. The internal oblique and transversus muscles are then divided in the same line. The fascia of Gerota is now opened. Blunt dissection of the perirenal fat allows the kidney to be mobilized and delivered into the wound. It may be mentioned that the smaller stones in the pelvis can be removed without mobilizing the kidney, thus minimizing the dissection.

Drainage

After most operations on the kidneys a drain is placed inside the perirenal fascia, in order to allow egress to any urine which may leak from the pelvis. It is led out through a separate stab incision to allow the main wound to heal uninterruptedly.

Closure

The fascia of Gerota is closed by a few interrupted sutures of catgut. Each layer of muscles is sutured separately, using either polyglactin or monofilament polypropylene.

Procedures on the kidney

The different open operations for removal of renal stones include pyelolithotomy, nephrolithotomy, partial nephrectomy and nephrectomy.

Pyelolithotomy

This is the most common open operation carried out on the kidney for the removal of calculi. The posterior wall of the pelvis is cleared of its surrounding fat. The pelvis is now incised along its long axis. The stone is removed with a suitable forceps. If a small stone is lying in a calyx and the neck of the calyx is wide enough, the stone can be removed by a forceps introduced through the pelvis. A bougie is now passed down the ureter in order to demonstrate free passage, and to detect any stone lying lower down. The pelvis is flushed with saline. In the case of multiple stones it is a great advantage if, at this stage, the kidney is delivered outside the wound and x-rayed, to detect any small stones still remaining in the various calyces, so that they can also be removed. The pelvis is finally closed with interrupted sutures of fine plain catgut.

Nephrolithotomy

If a stone is lying in a calyx and cannot be removed via the pelvis due to the narrowness of the neck of the calyx, it can be removed by making a small incision in the renal parenchyma directly onto the stone. Interrupted catgut stitches passed through the kidney substance and tied over a piece of muscle, to avoid them cutting through, help hemostasis.

Partial nephrectomy

If a stone is lying in the lowermost calyx, and the calyx is dilated and damaged so that it does not drain very well, it is necessary to remove the calyx in order to prevent the reformation of the stone. Now, it is self-evident that if the calyx is to be removed, the lower pole of the kidney must be excised. Thus it comes about that a stone in the lowermost calyx is often treated by a lower polar partial nephrectomy.

Nephrectomy

This operation is indicated if stones have destroyed most of the renal substance, and the other kidney has been proven by intravenous urography or radioisotope renogram to be functioning normally.

Treatment of bilateral renal calculi

Bilateral kidney stones are about eight times less common than unilateral ones. However, when they do occur they should be taken more seriously, because they can obstruct both ureters simultaneously, producing anuria. Usually the kidney with the better function is operated upon first, and the other side is dealt with a few weeks later. The idea is, by operation on the first side, to get the patient into as good a position as possible before tackling the other side.

URETERIC CALCULI

Site of pain

Colic due to a stone in the *upper third* of the ureter spreads from the loin to the groin.

When the stone enters the *lower ureter* the colic commences anteriorly at a lower level, and the pain may be referred to the testis in the male and the labia in the female. The testis becomes retracted due to spasm of the cremaster muscle.

When a stone lies in the *intramural* part of the ureter, it produces pain referred to the tip of the penis, and strangury.

If the stone becomes *impacted* in the ureter the colic passes off and is replaced by a dull pain, along with backache due to distension of the pelvis.

Some *hematuria* may be caused by a stone in the ureter; more commonly the blood can be detected only by microscopic examination. Abdominal examination is usually negative, although sometimes there may be tenderness over a part of the course of the ureter.

Investigations

Radiography

Plain x-ray

This may show a stone as an elongated shadow in the line of the ureter. More commonly, however, the stone is not visible on x-ray, either because it is very small or because the overlying gas in the intestines obscures its shadow.

Other shadows mimicking stones:

- In the region of the upper ureter a *calcified mesenteric lymph node* may lie along the line of the ureter and cause confusion; however, the shadow of a calcified lymph node is usually stippled in appearance.
- In the lower part a *phlebolith* in one of the veins in the pelvis may do likewise, but most phleboliths are circular rather than oval.

Intravenous urogram (IVU)

If an IVU is obtained during an attack of ureteric colic there is normally no excretion, or delayed excretion, on the affected side. If an x-ray is taken the day after the injection, the ureter may be outlined down to the level of the obstruction. If an IVU taken during an attack of pain shows normal excretion on the affected side, this means the patient is not suffering from ureteric colic.

Noncontrast spiral CT scan

This is the imaging modality of choice in patients with renal or ureteric colic. It is rapid and avoids the use of a contrast material. It is also invaluable in detecting radiolucent ureteric calculi.

Cystoscopy

A stone may be seen projecting from a ureteric orifice. If the stone is impacted in the lower part of the ureter, petechial hemorrhages may be seen around the ureteric opening.

Treatment

Treatment of a stone in the ureter resolves itself into management of the colic, and removal of the stone.

Treatment of the colic

A good drug for the relief of pain is morphine, in a dose of 15mg subcutaneously. The anti-prostaglandin drug diclofenac in a dose of 50mg i.m. or i.v. has also been found to be very effective.

Removal of the stone

One half of all ureteric calculi pass spontaneously, the other half require intervention. Generally, stones smaller than 80mm can be allowed to pass spontaneously if they are not causing pain, obstruction or infection. However, an asymptomatic, non-obstructing stone more than 50mm wide that has stayed in one position for more than three months has very little chance of spontaneous passage and should be removed.

Methods of removal

The methods of removal of a ureteric stone include extracorporeal short wave lithotripsy, endoscopic fragmentation, basket extraction and surgery.

In the case of stones in the lower third of the ureter a *Dormia basket* may be used to extract the stone if it is small (Fig.30.7). This is a basket-like arrangement of wires at the tip of a fine ureteric catheter (introduced through a cystoscope), which can be opened to trap the stone, so that the stone and the catheter can be withdrawn together.

A stone may be stuck at the ureteric orifice, which is the narrowest part of the ureter. In such a case this orifice can be enlarged by a *meatotomy*. However, this procedure is sometimes followed by urinary reflux, and therefore should be avoided if possible. These days a ureteric stone can be visualized through a *ureteroscope* and removed by the use of a Dormia basket under vision.

Operative treatment

Since the introduction of the endoscopic and lithotriptic management of ureteric calculi, the occasions on which open operation is required for a ureteric stone are few. Such is usually the situation if the stone is large or impacted, or if extracorporeal shock wave lithotripsy and an experienced endoscopist are not available.

Incisions

For a stone in the *upper two-thirds* of the ureter the incision is made along a line drawn from the renal angle to a point a few cm above the mid-inguinal point. For stones in the upper 1/3rd of the ureter the upper part of this line is incised, for the middle 1/3rd the lower part. All the three muscles are divided along this line, although in slim individuals the muscles may be divided in the line of their fibres. The peritoneum is displaced medially by gauze dissection and the ureter is found adhering to it. The stone is milked a short distance upwards, the ureter incised and the stone extracted. The incision in the ureter is closed by 4/0 plain catgut *or vicryl*, a drain placed and the wound closed in layers.

In the case of a stone in *the lower third* of the ureter a subumbilical midline incision is commonly employed.

INFECTIONS OF THE KIDNEY

There are three possible routes by which infection can reach the kidneys. These are the hematogenous, the lymphatic and the ascending routes. The great majority of urinary infections arrive via the ascending pathway:

- *Hematogenous* spread from infected tonsils, carious teeth or skin infections, specially boils and carbuncles, occasionally occurs.
- *Lymphatic spread* upwards from the bladder or bowel to the kidney is probably exceedingly rare.
- *Ascending route*. Ascent of bacteria along the lumen of the ureter is by far the most common method of spread of infection to the kidney. In the male the length of the urethra and the antibacterial properties of the prostatic secretions are effective barriers to invasion by this route. In contrast in females the urethra is very short and periurethral contamination with pathogenic bacteria, including fecal flora, is common. This explains why females have a higher incidence of urinary tract infections than males. Sexual intercourse can also force bacteria into the bladder, explaining the frequency of cystitis following shortly after marriage (honeymoon pelvis).

In many patients an *obstructive lesion* is responsible for repeated infections, due to stagnation of urine. In a few others the primary focus of infection may lie in the genital tract. By far the most common organisms responsible for urinary tract infections are E. coli and other gram-negative bacilli, specially Proteus. Apart from these, Streptococcus fecalis and staphylococci also occur from time to time.

PYELONEPHRITIS

In renal infection, apart from the pelvis the parenchyma is always involved; therefore it is more correct to call the condition pyelonephritis rather than pyelitis. On section of the kidney there may be yellow streaks of pus radiating from the medulla into the cortex.

ACUTE PYELONEPHRITIS

Etiology

Infections commonly ascend up the urinary tract via the urethra.

In children

- Urinary infections are very much more common in girls because of the shortness of their urethra, so that perineal bacteria can ascend to the bladder easily.
- They are common in both sexes because of:
    - The shortness of the oblique intramural segment of the urethra, so that vesicoureteric reflux is common and leads to infection.
    - The common occurrence of congenital anomalies of the urinary tract producing obstruction, and usually requiring operative relief.

It should be remembered that urinary tract infection in childhood may be overlooked, as there may be no symptoms referable to the urinary tract. Therefore one should be on the lookout for it in a child who fails to thrive or has a high temperature with rigors; the urine should be examined in such cases for pus cells.

In women

Similarly, in adults most urinary infections develop *in women* because of:

- A short urethra.
- Bruising of the urethra during sexual intercourse ('honeymoon pelvis').
- Further, in females pyelonephritis is more common during pregnancy than in the general population. This is usually attributed to relaxation of smooth muscles, including the ureteric smooth muscle, during pregnancy. This results in stasis of urine and infection.

Due to obstruction

Ascending infection is potentiated by any obstructive process, e.g. due to prostatic hypertrophy, stricture, stone or bladder tumor. *Quite often such infection is precipitated by the passage of a catheter,* therefore full aseptic precautions should be taken during the procedure.

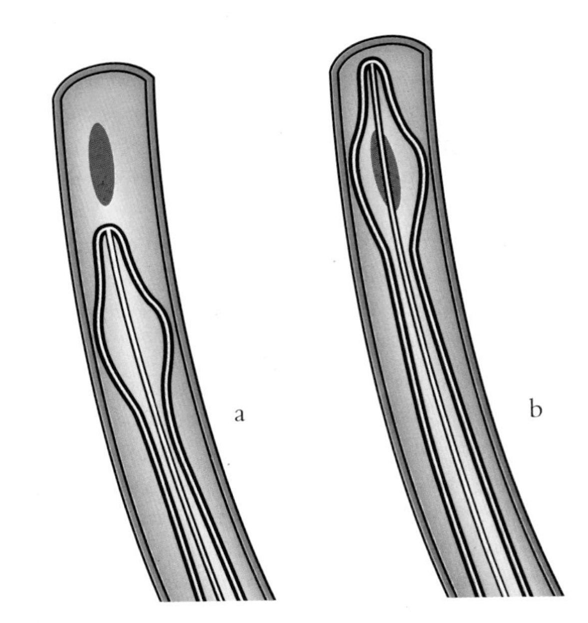

Fig.30.7 Dormia basket extraction of stone ureter

Clinical features

The illness starts suddenly with a rigor and vomiting. There is severe pain in the loin. The temperature rises, and is swinging in type. Cystitis develops, and leads to frequency of micturition. There is scalding pain on passing urine. The loin and the hypochondrium are tender. *If the infection is bilateral and severe, symptoms of uremia may be present.* The urine is scanty and concentrated. If a centrifuged deposit is examined under the microscope, it is loaded with pus cells and bacteria.

Differential diagnosis

If the symptoms and signs are atypical the condition may be confused with acute appendicitis, acute cholecystitis or pneumonia. In pyelonephritis the pain does not start from the midline; this helps distinguish it from appendicitis. Intravenous urography will show no shadow, or a hazy shadow, of the renal pelvis on the affected side.

Ultrasound examination

This shows the kidney grossly swollen with the pelvis full of pus and sloughs (Fig.30.8 a). The second picture taken after 3 months' treatment with antibiotics shows that the sloughs and pus have been cleared and the gross anatomy of the kidney restored (Fig.30.8 b).

Treatment

If treatment is to be successful it must be started early and continued for a sufficiently long time; *brief courses of antibiotics allow the organisms to become resistant to them*, so that the treatment fails to eradicate the infection. After the course of treatment has been completed, follow-up with repeated cultures and white cell counts of the urine is necessary to ensure that the condition has been cured. Intravenous pyelography to exclude the presence of abnormalities in the urinary tract is an essential part of the follow-up of the case.

Before any antibiotics are started a mid-stream specimen of urine *must* be taken and sent for culture and tests of the sensitivity of the organisms to antibiotics. After the specimen has been obtained, a broad-spectrum antibacterial e.g. ampicillin or co-trimoxazole, should be started pending the results of the tests. When these arrive, the antibiotic may have to be changed.

For *pain* an antispasmodic e.g. hyoscine, and an analgesic, e.g. paracetamol or metamizole, should be prescribed. Morphine or pethidine may sometimes be required. Bed rest is an important part of the treatment.

In E. coli infections the urine is acid. In these cases *alkalinization* of the urine, using powders containing potassium citrate and sodium bicarbonate, helps not only in relieving symptoms but also in inhibiting the growth of the organisms by changing the pH of the urine.

The patient should drink large quantities of fluids. If vomiting and dehydration occur, intravenous fluids may be required. When a course of an antibiotic has been started, the urine should be cultured about four and seven days later, to find out what effect the antibiotic is having. The antibiotic should be continued for at least three weeks.

Surgery

If a congenital abnormality is found which is causing obstruction, and after the infection has been eradicated by antiotics, surgery will be required, as otherwise the infection will continue to recur.

If, in a child with vesicoureteric reflux, conservative measures fail and renal scarring results, they are dealt with by:

- Submucosal injections of Macroplastique in jelly form around the ureteric orifice to narrow the patulous orifice.
- Alternatively, reimplantation of the ureter into the bladder is carried out, to put an end to the reflux by creating an oblique tunnel for the ureter through the bladder wall.

Choice of antibacterial agent

No one agent is the drug of choice for all cases. Equally effective alternate choices of antibiotic therapy include the following: Ampicillin or amoxicillin, cephalexin or cephradine, and nitrofurantoin. Co-trimoxazole is another useful addition to this list of drugs.

The use of these drugs is often associated with side effects. At the same time compliance with the doctor's instructions is often quite poor. Therefore the rate of treatment failure is quite high, upto 15%.

Gram-negative bacteremia

In gram-negative bacteremia the urinary tract often provides the portal of entry. Frequently the bacteremia follows instrumentation in the presence of pre-existing urinary infection that has been ineffectively treated. The patient experiences a shaking chill followed by high fever, peripheral vasodilatation and hypotension. The organisms are frequently resistant to the usual drugs and require large doses of parenterally administered antibiotics.

Bactericidal drugs

Drugs that are bactericidal are preferred, to prevent liberation of additional quantities of endotoxin by the multiplying bacteria. An aminoglycoside such as gentamicin, tobramycin, or amikacin, and amoxil or a similar drug in combination have proved effective. Vancomycin can be used as prophylaxis or therapy for staphylococcal infections. Drug dosage is carefully regulated according to renal function.

CHRONIC PYELONEPHRITIS

Repeated bacterial infections of the kidney cause chronic renal insufficiency. However, when such a case is investigated, underlying urinary tract disease is nearly always found, e.g. vesicoureteral reflux, stone or stricture. Most of the damage is caused to the renal tubules which are atrophic, dilated and sometimes cystic. In contrast, the glomeruli retain their structure till late in the disease. The histologic picture is non-specific: inflammatory changes, associated with fibrosis and scarring.

Clinical features

Chronic pyelonephritis produces few symptoms until it ends up in renal insufficiency, and then the symptoms are similar to those of any other form of chronic renal failure. Similarly, the physical findings are few. However, if the disease is the end result of many episodes of acute pyelonephritis, intermittent symptoms of fever, flank pain and dysuria may have occurred in the past.

Laboratory findings

Microscopic study of the urine is nonspecific. There may be an increased number of leucocytes, but their presence in the urine does not prove the existence of upper urinary tract infection. Bacteriuria alone is also not diagnostic of chronic pyelonephritis, and conversely, patients who have chronic pyelonephritis may have negative urine cultures.

X-rays show loss of cortical thickness, blunting of calyces, contracture, cortical scars with an irregular contour, and decreased excretion of contrast material. In the absence of stones, obstruction and tuberculosis, and without a history of ingestion of analgesics, chronic pyelonephritis is virtually the only disease that produces a localized scar over a deformed calyx. Ultrasound examination shows up blunted calyces with thinning of the overlying cortex, and aids in diagnosis.

Management

The management of chronic pyelonephritis should be directed towards:

- Treating infections if present.
- Preventing future infections.
- Monitoring and preserving renal function.

Investigations should be carried out to detect the underlying cause, which can usually be found. In advanced cases diminishing renal function may require recurrent hemodialysis. Transplantation of a kidney from a donor or a cadaver may be possible.

PYONEPHROSIS

In this condition the kidney is reduced to a sac containing pus and urine. A pyonephrosis can result from the following:

- Infection in a hydronephrosis: in such a case the wall of the sac often consists of a thin shell of fibrous tissue, with very few remnants of renal substance.
- Infection in a case of renal calculus (calculus pyonephrosis).
- Acute pyelonephritis.

Clinical features

There is fever, anemia, and a tender swelling in the loin. If the pyenophrosis is open, cystitis may result, producing frequency and dysuria; if it is closed the fever may be quite high, with a swinging temperature.

Investigations

Ultrasound

Ultrasound examination shows the enlarged kidney containing fluid with echoes, i.e. turbid fluid. If the cause is a stone it is visualized, with an acoustic shadow underneath.

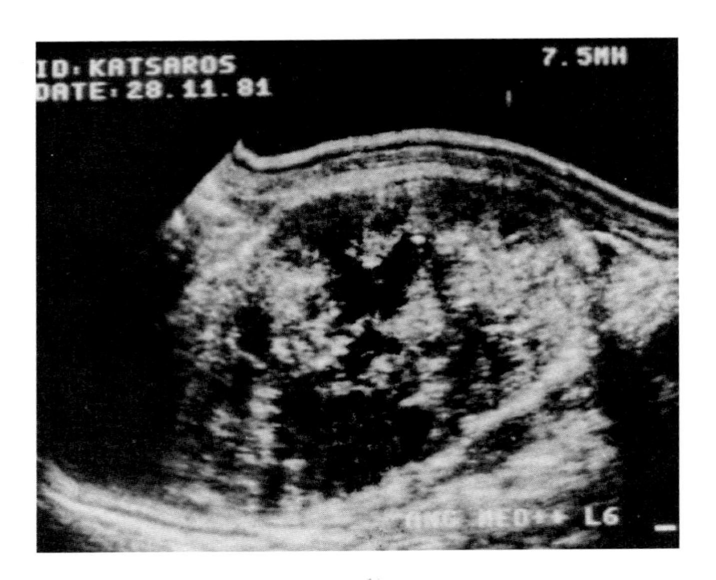

a

b

Fig.30.8 (a) Acute pyelonephritis. The pelvis is full of sloughs, pus and edema fluid. (b) After three months of chemotherapy; the sloughs and pus have been cleared and the gross anatomy of the kidney restored.

Plain x-ray

This also shows up most stones.

Intravenous urography

This shows absence of excretion of dye on the affected side.

Cystoscopy

In open pyonephrosis this may show efflux of pus from the ureter on the affected side.

ESR

If in a case with a renal swelling, kidney function on the affected side is absent as shown by the intravenous pyelogram, the differential diagnosis includes hydronephrosis and pyonephrosis. To distinguish between the two conditions, ESR plays an important part; in hydronephrosis it is normal, in pyonephrosis it is markedly raised.

Management

The appropriate antibiotics should be administered through the intravenous route for maximum effect. At the same time immediate drainage of the kidney must be carried out. This can take the form of either percutaneous or open nephrostomy. When the case has stabilized, either appropriate corrective surgery or nephrectomy should be carried out. Nephrectomy is indicated when obstruction is known to have destroyed most of the renal substance, and function on the other side is good. Corrective surgery can be undertaken if a remediable obstruction is found, and the kidney substance is in a good state of preservation.

Perinephric abscess

A perinephric abscess consists of a collection of pus in the perinephric space due to rupture of an acute cortical abscess into this space. Patients with pyonephrosis are very susceptible to the formation of a perinephric abscess. In a few patients such an abscess arises due to hematogenous spread, usually from sites of skin infection.

The *clinical presentation* of perinephric abscess is similar to that of pyelonephritis, but the symptoms come on more gradually. A mass in the flank can be felt in about half the cases.

Laboratory findings include leucocytosis, raised serum creatinine, and pyuria in about 75% of cases.

Pyelonephritis usually responds to appropriate antibiotic therapy in four or five days, while perinephric abscess does not. Therefore, if the condition does not resolve within that period, perinephric abscess should be suspected.

On plain x-ray the psoas border is not visible, being obscured due to the inflammatory edema. There may be a scoliosis towards the affected side due to spasm of the muscles. CT scan shows the perinephric collection of pus.

Treatment

Tube drainage under ultrasound guidance should be instituted, the pus sent for culture and sensitivity tests, and antibiotics commenced. If this fails to clear the infection, open drainage should be carried out through a lumbar incision and any pockets of pus opened. A large drain should be placed in the perinephric space and the wound closed around it. On receipt of the culture report the antibiotics may have to be changed.

TUBERCULOSIS OF THE KIDNEY

Pathology

Tuberculosis of the urinary tract cannot arise except as a blood-borne infection. However, the distant focus from which the infection arrives at the kidney is normally not demonstrable. Microscopic lesions gradually enlarge and discharge pus and tubercle bacilli along the tubules, producing ulceration of the pyramid.

The progress of the disease is slow. In the early stages *tubercle bacilluria* may be the only evidence of tuberculosis. However, it should be taken seriously and treated with the appropriate drugs. With the passage of time tuberculosis may produce one of the following lesions in the kidney:

- A *caseous mass* may form in the cortex.
- This may rupture into the pelvis, discharging its contents and resulting in the formation of a *cavity* in communication with the pelvis.
- Alternatively, it may rupture into the perinephric space leading to a *perinephric abscess*.
- A stricture may form at the pelviureteric junction, leading to *hydronephrosis*.
- Secondary infection, usually with E. coli, may supervene, leading to the development of a *pyonephrosis*. The whole kidney may become a mass of caseous material.
- Finally, in generalized *military tuberculosis* the kidney may also be involved.
- Untreated, the disease spreads along the ureter to give rise to tuberculous *cystitis*.
- In the male it can also spread to the seminal vesicles and the *epididymis*.

Clinical features

Tuberculosis of the kidney occurs most commonly between the ages of twenty and forty, men being twice as often affected as women. The earliest symptom is increased *frequency* of micturition, both by day and night.

At the same time there may be *suprapubic pain* and *terminal hematuria*. These symptoms are due to tuberculous cystitis. In a few cases there may be *painless hematuria*, the blood coming from an ulcer situated on a renal papilla. In most other cases the blood is only detected on microscopic examination.

There is usually slight *loss of weight* and some evening rise of temperature.

On examination the kidney is usually not enlarged to such an extent as to be palpable. The prostate, seminal vesicles, vasa deferentia, and epididymes should always be examined for evidence of tuberculous involvement, which usually takes the form of one or more nodules in these structures.

Investigations

An early morning specimen of *urine* should be examined. It should be centrifuged and the sediment stained with *Ziehl-Neelsen's stain* for acid-fast bacilli.

At the same time *guinea-pig inoculation* and *Lowenstein-Jensen (LJ) culture* should be carried out. Staining for acid-fast bacilli is usually negative, while LJ culture and guinea-pig inoculation are positive in a high percentage of cases.

Plain x-ray may show calcification in healing foci, either in the form of specks or as broad dense areas. A *chest x-ray* should be taken to rule out pulmonary tuberculosis.

In early cases *intravenous urography* may show absence or irregularity of a calyx. When a calyx is completely obstructed an abscess may form, which displaces adjacent calyces. The fibrosed ureter is shortened, and is therefore more straight than a normal ureter. If cystitis develops the bladder becomes more rounded due to spasm.

On *cystoscopy* the earliest change takes the form of edema around the ureteric orifice followed by the development of tubercles, and later ulcers, in the area. In long-standing cases as the ureter becomes shortened, its orifice remains open—the *golf-hole ureter*. In advanced disease the capacity of the bladder gradually diminishes.

Treatment

Anti-tuberculosis therapy is carried out. If the full course of medicines is given there is a high cure rate, with few recurrences. In certain situations operation may become necessary:

- If very advanced disease is present, nephroureterectomy may be carried out.
- For hydronephrosis, pyeloplasty may be employed.
- If a caseous mass is present in the renal cortex it may be deroofed (cavernostomy) and evacuated.

NEOPLASMS OF THE KIDNEY

Benign neoplasms are very rare. Adenomas usually produce no symptoms and are found incidentally at autopsy. Angiomas can produce hematuria.

Malignant neoplasms occur commonly either in infancy and early childhood, or after the age of forty. The common renal malignancy of childhood is Wilms' tumor. In adult life hypernephroma (*Renal cell carcinoma)* occurs commonly, and transitional cell carcinoma of the renal pelvis is seen from time to time.

NEPHROBLASTOMA (WILMS' TUMOR)

Nephroblastoma (Wilms' tumor) is the most common intra-abdominal tumor of children. The incidence is 1/10,000 live births. The peak incidence is between 2 and 4 years; very few cases occur after the age of 7. In about 5% of patients, both kidneys are affected. An interesting feature of this tumor is that growths arising below the age of one year have a much better prognosis.

Etiology

Knudson has explained the development of nephroblastoma on the basis of his two-hit hypothesis, namely that two separate factors act to cause the disease:

- A tumor suppressor gene is normally present on chromosome 11; this is lost ('first-hit').
- This then allows tumor development in the presence of any predisposing factor; this constitutes the 'second-hit'.

Pathology

On *section* the tumor is greyish or pinkish white in colour. As regards consistency, the slower growing tumors are firm, whereas rapidly growing tumors are soft. This is in fact a general rule among most tumors, of whichever organ.

Microscopically the tumor is unusual in having both epithelial and connective tissue elements; most other tumors have either the one or the other type.

Histological markers of a poor *prognosis* include :

- Extreme cellular pleomorphism (anaplasia).
- Presence of sarcomatous changes.

Tumors with these characteristics are termed UH (unfavourable histology), while those without anaplasia and sarcomatous changes are called FH (favourable histology). Whereas the relapse-free survival rates in UH tumors are only about 30%, the same rates for FH tumors are as high as 75%. Therefore the histopathology

Table 30.1 Modified NWTSG staging of nephroblastoma

Stage I	Tumor limited to kidney
Stage II	Tumor extends beyond capsule but completely excised
Stage III	Local spread of tumor in abdomen
Stage IV	Deposits in brain, lung or liver
Stage V	Bilateral renal involvement

report is an important part of the data on which the estimate of prognosis is based.

Staging

Staging by the National Wilms' Tumor Staging Group (NWTSG) is shown in (Table 30.1).

Clinical features

Swelling

The infant is nearly always brought because the mother noticed a swelling in the abdomen, which has been enlarging rapidly. Along with this the general health deteriorates. On examination the swelling is found to be filling most of the abdomen; however, it can usually be shown that the tumor is arising from one side. This tumor usually grows within a capsule, pushing the rest of the kidney aside.

Fever

A number of patients run a slight temperature, which subsides when the tumor is removed.

Hematuria

Normally there is no blood in the urine, as the tumor is away from the pelvis. Hematuria is a bad sign, as it shows the tumor has burst through its capsule into the renal pelvis.

Certain *anomalies* may occasionally be associated with Wilms' tumor:

- Aniridia.
- Hemihypertrophy.
- Deformities of the external genitalia.

Metastases

Wilm's tumor metastasizes early by the *bloodstream* to the lungs, and less commonly to the liver and bones. Lymphatic dissemination is a great deal less common.

Investigations

Ultrasound examination

This is first carried out, and confirms that a solid mass arises from the kidney. The other kidney is examined, the liver checked for secondaries, and the renal vein imaged to exclude venous tumor extension.

Intravenous urography

This shows the kidney displaced upwards or downwards by the tumor, with the calyces stretched out on the surface of the mass; it also indicates renal function.

Chest x-ray

This may show cannon ball secondaries in the lungs.

CT scan or MRI

These are very useful in providing information regarding tumor extension, status of the contralateral kidney, presence of regional lymphadenopathy and invasion of the inferior vena cava (IVC) by the tumor.

Radioisotope skeletal scan

This shows up any bony metastases.

Blood count

A blood count and biochemical profile are also performed.

Differential diagnosis

The only swelling with which a Wilms' tumor can be confused is a neuroblastoma:

- If x-rays show secondaries in the bones, this favours the diagnosis of neuroblastoma.
- Higher frequency of calcifications is observed in neuroblastomas.
- Neuroblastomas usually cross the midline and encase the abdominal aorta and inferior vena cava.
- Neuroblastomas produce various tumor markers such as vanillylmandelic acid (VMA).

Treatment

The treatment of a nephroblastoma consists of urgent nephrectomy followed by chemotherapy and radiotherapy. In contrast to renal cell carcinoma, radiotherapy and chemotherapy have much to offer after nephrectomy for nephroblastoma. During recent decades survival has improved dramatically due to improved surgical techniques as well as refinements in radiotherapy and chemotherapy.

Nephrectomy

Radical nephrectomy is carried out, through an anterior transperitoneal approach for better access to the renal vessels. It entails removal *en bloc* of Gerota's fascia (with its contents: kidney, adrenal and perinephric fat) along with the upper ureter and renal vessels. This en bloc removal is carried out because it has been shown that spread into the perinephric fat worsens the prognosis.

In *bilateral tumors* a radical nephrectomy is carried out on the side of the larger tumor, with partial nephrectomy on the other side. In these cases a *renal hyperperfusion syndrome* develops after operation, and can lead to chronic deterioration in renal function. This effect has stimulated a renal-sparing approach to surgery, particularly as effective chemotherapy is becoming available.

Extensive *lymphadenectomy* is not advised, but lymph node sampling probably improves staging. If *venous tumor thrombus* is found, it may recede after preoperative chemotherapy. If the tumor thrombus extends to the heart cardiopulmonary bypass may be required for its removal.

Chemotherapy and radiotherapy

Postoperative adjuvant chemotherapy and radiotherapy have dramatically improved the survival in these patients. A combination of radiotherapy and chemotherapy maximizes benefits and minimizes side effects. Again, combination chemotherapy is more effective than single agents, vincristine, actinomycin D and doxorubicin being commonly employed.

However, the preoperative use of these therapies has been decried on two grounds:

1. Staging is more accurate in the untreated patient.
2. Upto 8% children prove, after nephrectomy, to be suffering from some other condition.

However, preoperative chemotherapy is indicated in selected groups of patients. These include:

- Inoperable tumors.
- Tumor in a single kidney.
- Bilateral tumors.
- Extension of tumor into the inferior vena cava.

Recurrence

Recurrence after treatment is difficult to manage, and a multidisciplinary approach is best. Ifosfamide, cisplatin and etoposide are all effective and are used. The prognosis after nephrectomy, chemotherapy and radiotherapy is much better under the age of 1 year; under this age 80% infants survive five years, over it only 30%.

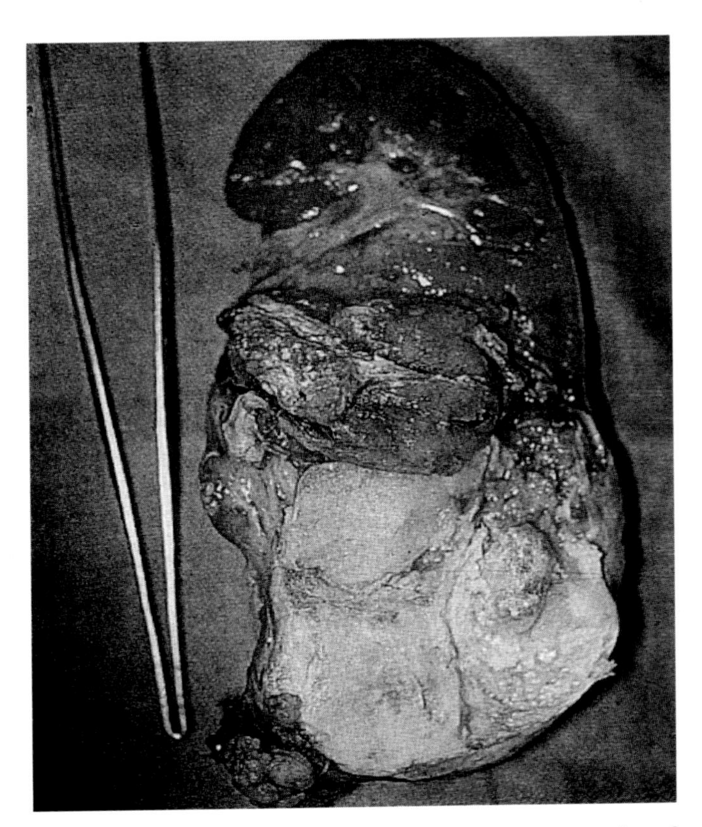

Fig.30.9 Renal carcinoma occupying one pole of kidney, as is usual

RENAL CELL CARCINOMA

Pathology

This is an adenocarcinoma and is the most common neoplasm of the kidney in adults. It is usually rounded in shape, and occupies one or the other pole of the kidney (Fig.30.9). On section it is commonly yellow due to the fat content, often with hemorrhagic areas. Fibrous septa divide it into lobules. In the larger tumors the cells at the centre, being away from the blood supply, often undergo necrosis.

Microscopy

Microscopically, solid alveoli of cubical or polyhedral clear cells are seen, with deeply staining small rounded nuclei and abundant cytoplasm. There are numerous blood vessels, whose walls appear to be made up of tumor cells at places.

Spread

As the tumor enlarges it tends to grow into the renal veins. From the veins tumor emboli can lodge in the lungs to produce cannon-ball secondaries. The other common sites for metastases are the bones. At the same

Table 30.2 TNM classification for renal cell carcinoma

T-PRIMARY TUMOUR	
T0:	No evidence of primary tumor
T1:	Tumor < 7cm limited to kidney
T2:	Tumor > 7cm limited to kidney
T3:	Tumor extends into perinephric tissue but not beyond Gerota's fascia
T4:	Tumor extends beyond Gerota's fascia
N-REGIONAL LYMPH NODES	
N0:	No regional lymph node metastasis
N1:	Metastasis in a single lymph node
N2:	Metastasis in more than one lymph node
M-DISTANT METASTASIS	
M0:	No distant metastasis
M1:	Distant metastasis

time spread by lymphatics occurs, first to the lymph nodes in the hilum of the kidney and from there to the para-aortic nodes.

Clinical features

Men are twice as often affected by renal cell carcinoma as women. The earliest sign is *hematuria*, which is usually intermittent. If the blood gets coagulated during its passage through the ureter it may produce *colic*. In other cases there may simply be a dull pain in the loin. Occasionally the patient comes with the complaint of a *swelling*. Unusual presentations include:

- The rapid development of a *varicocele* due to blockage of the left spermatic vein by tumor cells.
- Moderate *fever* due to absorption of blood and necrotic material.
- A *spontaneous fracture* due to a bone secondary.
- Cough or *hemoptysis* due to secondaries in the lungs.

Finally, an increasing number of tumors is being detected *incidentally* because of the increasing use of CT and ultrasound scans.

Paraneoplastic syndromes

Renal cell carcinoma is associated with a variety of paraneoplastic syndromes in about 10–40% of patients. These include:

- Polycythemia.
- Hypercalcemia.
- Hypertension.
- Hepatic dysfunction.

Diagnosis

The presence of any of the above clinical manifestations may cause a clinician to suspect renal malignancy and to begin investigations:

Ultrasound scan

If an ultrasound scan is now carried out, it shows whether the lesion is solid or cystic. If it is a *cyst* it can usually be left alone, but its progress should be monitored repeatedly by ultrasound scans, and in case of enlargement it should be aspirated for cytological examination. If the mass is *solid* the liver, renal vein and inferior vena cava should be examined to exclude the presence of hepatic metastases and spread via the renal vein.

CT or MRI

Finally, a *CT* scan (Fig.30.10) or *MRI* confirms that the mass is solid and may give some indication of its nature and extent, which helps greatly in staging.

Spiral CT with 3-dimentional reconstruction

This can help a surgeon plan surgery.

Biopsy

Imaging usually provides enough information for diagnosis, so biopsy is sometimes not done.

Venacavagraphy

If there is doubt about spread via the renal vein, a vena cavography should be carried out.

Chest x-ray

This should always be taken to show up or rule out lung secondaries.

Isotope bone scan

This should be carried out, as it shows up bone metastases. If it is positive, the sites of metastases should be examined by radiography for details concerning the metastases.

Staging

The Tumor-Node-Metastasis (TNM) system is currently used (Table 30.2). Clinical staging depends primarily on the CT scan.

Treatment

Nephrectomy

If metastases are not present, the treatment of renal cell carcinoma is nephrectomy. Even if metastases are present, nephrectomy may still be performed to control local symptoms such as pain or hematuria. In order to provide for removal wide of the tumor, the perinephric fat is excised with the kidney. This operation is called *radical nephrectomy*. However, there is no evidence that radical nephrectomy confers a survival advantage compared to simple nephrectomy.

Manipulation of the kidney or its veins during the operation can result in dislodgement of tumor emboli. To prevent this eventuality, the renal pedicle should be ligated first. The abdominal approach is best for accomplishing this.

Removal of para-aortic nodes has been advocated; however, there is no evidence to confirm a survival advantage of this more extensive procedure.

Upto 10% of patients have a vena caval tumor thrombus. If no metastases are present, removal of the thrombus can be followed by prolonged survival.

Partial nephrectomy may be employed in the following situations:

- In a solitary kidney.
- With bilateral tumors.
- In cases where the tumor has been detected incidentally by radiology, and is quite small in size.

Embolization

In cases with advanced disease and a symptomatic primary tumor, embolization relieves symptoms with less morbidity than that associated with nephrectomy. At the same time, it can reduce the vascularity of very large tumors before surgery. The renal artery can be occluded by a variety of materials introduced via a percutaneous arterial catheter.

Radiotherapy

This does not improve survival, whether given pre-or postoperatively. However, it can relieve the pain of bone metastases.

Treatment of metastases

Renal cell carcinoma is unusual in that resection of solitary metastases (specially pulmonary or cerebral) can be followed on occasion by long-term survival. Radiotherapy relieves pain due to skeletal metastases in most patients, and internal fixation can stabilize long bones affected by metastatic disease.

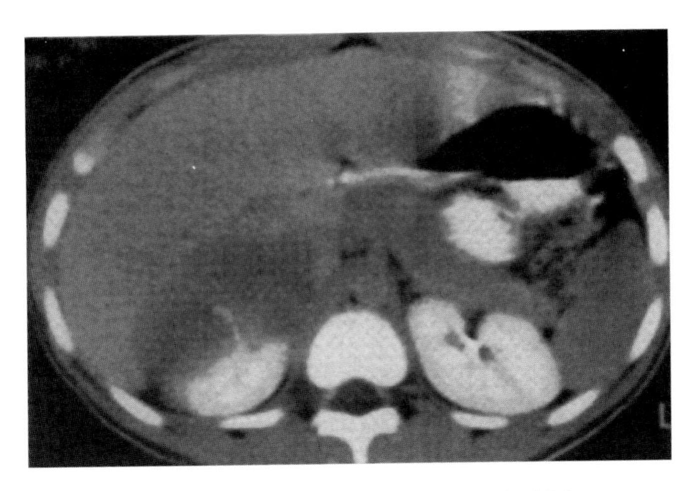

Fig.30.10 CT scan: Renal carcinoma right kidney

No *cytotoxic agent* used either alone or in combination has shown more than a 10% response rate.

Immunotherapy

For metastatic renal cell carcinoma both interferons and interleukins have been used. Interferons have produced remissions in 13% of patients for about 8 months. Interleukins are lymphokines produced by T lymphocytes which enhance the killing of tumor cells. Interleukin-2 has elicited remissions in 20% patients for about three years. The two types of agents have also been combined with additive effects.

Adoptive immunotherapy

This is the latest approach. It involves administration of cells which have antitumor activity. Initial reports have been encouraging.

Newer biologic agents

Currently various antiangiogenic agents (Sunitinib) and inhibitors of tyrosine kinase and other cell cycle activators (Temsirolimus) have demonstrated prolonged survival in advanced renal cell cancer.

Prognosis

This depends upon:

- Histological type.
- Presence of local extension into the renal vein, perinephric tissues and lymph nodes.
- Distant metastases.

The overall survival rate for renal tumors is about 50% for 5 years and 33% for 10 years. Stage-wise 5 year survivals are approximately as follows:

- Stage I found incidentally, 85%.
- Stage I, 65%.

- Stage II, 55%.
- Stage III 40%.

This shows the importance of early diagnosis.

PAPILLOMA OF THE PELVIS

Papillomas of the renal pelvis are transitional cell tumors, which resemble bladder papillomas but are less common. They tend to invade the kidney and become malignant. Multiple tumors of the ureter and the bladder can arise due to seeding.

Clinical features

These tumors present with hematuria, which may continue for weeks. The kidney is usually not palpable. Clot colic may occur.

Investigations

The *urine* shows red cells, and may show exfoliated malignant cells.

Ultrasonography and *CT scan* show a soft tissue mass in the renal pelvis.

On *intravenous urography* a filling defect is seen in the pelvis.

Treatment

Papillomas of the renal pelvis are treated by nephroureterectomy. The excision of the ureter should extend downwards to include the intramural ureter along with the ureteric orifice, to minimize the chances of leaving behind tumor implants.

Squamous-celled carcinoma of the renal pelvis

This tumor is rare. It is usually preceded by leukoplakia, and in most cases a stone is present; these factors result in metaplasia of the transitional epithelium of the renal pelvis to squamous, predisposing the patient to the development of squamous-celled carcinoma. Symptoms are vague, so that the diagnosis is often missed. As the diagnosis is often made at a late stage, the prognosis is poor.

Operative steps of nephrectomy

The patient is placed on the table in the lateral position with the affected side uppermost. The leg on the affected side is fully extended, the other leg which lies underneath in this position is flexed at the hip and the knee. The patient is held in this position by a strap which passes over the pelvis, and is fixed at either side to the edges of the table. An arm rest supports the upper arm, so that it does not lie on the chest and embarrass respiration.

Morris's incision is the one most commonly employed to expose the kidney. It commences at the renal angle and runs forwards and downwards towards the anterior superior iliac spine. All muscle layers are divided in the line of the incision. If this is made with the use of a cutting diathermy current, it saves a good deal of both blood and time.

Alternatively, the incision is made over the 12th rib which is resected subperiosteally avoiding the pleura. This allows the incision to be made at a higher level, providing for better exposure of the kidney. The perinephric fascia is now opened and the perinephric fat dissected away from the kidney all round, using mostly blunt dissection. The blood vessels at the hilum are exposed, ligated individually and divided, and the kidney removed. The wound in closed in layers, leaving a suction drain in place.

Chapter

31 URINARY BLADDER

Cystoscopy

In the diagnosis and management of diseases affecting the urinary bladder, cystoscopy plays a critical role. Many conditions can only be diagnosed by direct visualization of the bladder mucosa, e.g. sources of bleeding, inflammatory lesions and bladder trabeculation. Tumors can be visualized as well as biopsied; they can also be resected through the working element of a cystoscope.

Conventional cystoscopes are rigid and vary from 15 to 24 French in size. They have fibreoptic illumination which allows better visualization.

Flexible cystoscopes:

- Result in less discomfort and potential urethral trauma, especially in male patients.
- Provide visualization in all directions.
- Make the lithotomy position unnecessary; the examination can be carried out in the supine position.

EXSTROPHY OF THE BLADDER

Exstrophy of the bladder arises due to incomplete development of the infraumbilical part of the abdominal wall and of the anterior wall of the bladder. It arises once in 50,000 births with a male to female ratio of 3:1. Intra-abdominal pressure causes the posterior bladder wall to bulge out through the defect. The trigone is seen at the lower part, with spurts of urine being discharged from the ureteric orifices (Fig.31.1). The exposed bladder mucosa tends to become chronically inflamed. When the bladder wall is reduced backwards the edge of the abdominal wall defect can be felt. Umbilical and inguinal hernias may be present.

The rami of the pubic bones are widely separated and the pelvic ring is 'open', affecting the gait. On the other hand in those females who become pregnant this separation of the pubes facilitates delivery. In the male child epispadias is present, and the penis is shorter and broader than normal.

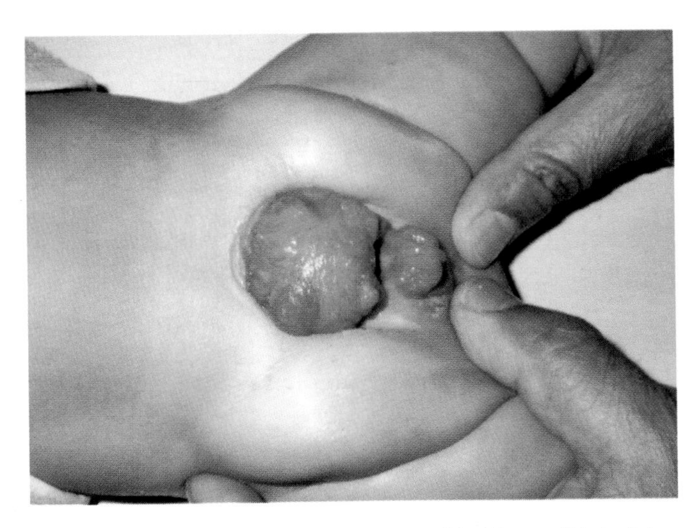

Fig.31.1 Exstrophy of the bladder. The bladder wall is bulging forwards due to pressure of the abdominal contents. Note the accompanying epispadias

The unfortunate patient smells of urine and remains wet all the time. He suffers repeated urinary infections, and untreated, most such patients die of renal failure before the age of thirty.

Treatment

Past practices

In the past ectopia vesicae was treated by *diversion of urine*. This was achieved by one of the following two methods:

Uretersigoidostomy

The classical method was ureterosigmoidostomy, i.e. implantation of both ureters into the sigmoid colon. The patient passed a mixture of urine and feces per anum. He was no longer wet or foul smelling. However, most patients did not live beyond their teens or twenties due to:

- The urine refluxing up the ureter to cause recurrent urinary infections.

- Excessive absorption of chloride ions by the colonic mucosa produced hyperchloraemic acidosis.

Isolated loop of terminal ileum

Later, in order to avoid hyperchloraemic acidosis, surgeons started diverting the urine to an *isolated loop of terminal ileum*, which was opened out in the right iliac fossa. Because disposable ileostomy bags become available about this time, this method become more popular than ureterosigmoidostomy. However, the life-long care of an ileal-loop diversion is no easy matter.

Recent methods

Recently, the prevalent methods of treatment have been the following

Reconstruction of the bladder in three stages

- Closure of the bladder and abdominal wall is carried out in the neonatal period. The pubic symphysis is brought together in the midline and the bladder neck placed behind it.
- This is followed by repair of the epispadias at the age of 12–18 months, the urethral groove being closed to make a tube.
- Finally, at the age of 4–5 years, bladder neck reconstruction is carried out for continence.

Results

Despite treatment by multistaged procedures, less than half the infants achieve full continence.

Mitrofanoff procedure

In those patients who fail to achieve continence and are unwilling to self-catheterize through the regular urethra, the vermiform appendix is detached from the cecum, leaving its blood supply intact. One end of the appendix is connected to the bladder, the other to the abdominal wall (Fig.31.2), intermittent catheterizations being carried out through its lumen—the Mitrofanoff method.

Although results in recent series are a great deal better than in the past, exstrophy of the bladder remains one of the unsolved problems in surgery, posing a challenge to surgeons of the future.

RUPTURE OF THE BLADDER

The bladder may be ruptured in its intraperitoneal or extraperitoneal portion.

Intraperitoneal rupture

This may be caused by:

- A blow on a fully distended bladder.
- Gunshot and stab wounds.
- Passage of instruments.
- Diathermy coagulation and resection of bladder tumors.

Following the trauma there is sudden severe pain in the hypogastrium, with shock. However, soon the pain gets diminished due to wide distribution of the urine in the peritoneal cavity. If the quantity of urine is large, shifting dullness may be found. The abdomen distends due to paralytic ileus and is rigid with the development of peritonitis. Because the bladder is collapsed after rupture, the patient has no desire to pass urine, and there is no dullness in the suprapubic region.

Extraperitoneal rupture

This occurs after:

- Instrumentation.
- Tumor resection.
- Penetrating wounds.
- Fracture of the pelvis with penetration by bone spicules.

It cannot be differentiated from rupture of the posterior urethra, so it is discussed along with it.

Diagnosis

The diagnosis of rupture of the bladder may be confirmed by passing a catheter and injecting a radio-opaque dye. X-rays taken will show leakage of urine outside the bladder.

Treatment

If rupture of the bladder is strongly suspected, operation should be carried out at once. A midline subumbilical incision is commonly used. The edges of the tear in the bladder wall are trimmed and repaired by two layers of absorbable stitches, and a wide-bore catheter is left in the bladder, to be removed after about a week. Early operation is followed by a low morbidity and mortality rate.

Bladder injury during childbirth

The bladder may be injured during childbirth. The most common example of obstetric injury to the bladder is that which occurs in *neglected obstructed labour*. In this condition there is pressure necrosis of the anterior wall of the upper part of the vagina and the contiguous wall of the bladder due to prolonged and unrelieved pressure of the baby's head, and a vesico-vaginal fistula results.

This is a most distressing condition for the poor sufferer, with urine constantly dribbling from the vagina so that she is wet and foul-smelling all the time. The fistula requires very skilful repair of the walls of the vagina and bladder in layers. The incidence of vesico-vaginal fistula can be reduced only by better obstetric care.

Foreign bodies in the bladder

These are not common.

- Hairpins and similar assorted objects have been found in the bladder, which in most cases have been introduced during urethral masturbation.
- Occasionally a piece of tubing may be left behind after cystostomy.

The foreign body may result in infection, perforation of the bladder or stone formation.

Treatment. A small foreign body can be removed endoscopically using an operating cystoscope; a larger one requires an open suprabupic operation.

RETENTION OF URINE

Retention of urine may be acute or chronic.

Acute retention

Etiology

The most common causes of acute retention include:

In the male:

- Prostatic obstruction.
- Urethral stricture.
- Rupture of the urethra.
- Phimosis.

In the female:

- Retroverted gravid uterus.
- Bladder neck obstruction.

In both sexes:

- Acute urethritis.
- Fecal impaction in the rectum.
- Spinal anesthesia or spinal cord injury.
- Blood clot in the bladder.

Clinical features

The patient is unable to micturate, although he has not passed urine for several hours. If the patient is slim the distended bladder may be seen, otherwise it can be palpated as a slightly tender swelling above the pubic symphysis which is dull to percussion. As the bladder muscle contracts, spasms of acute pain occur from time to time.

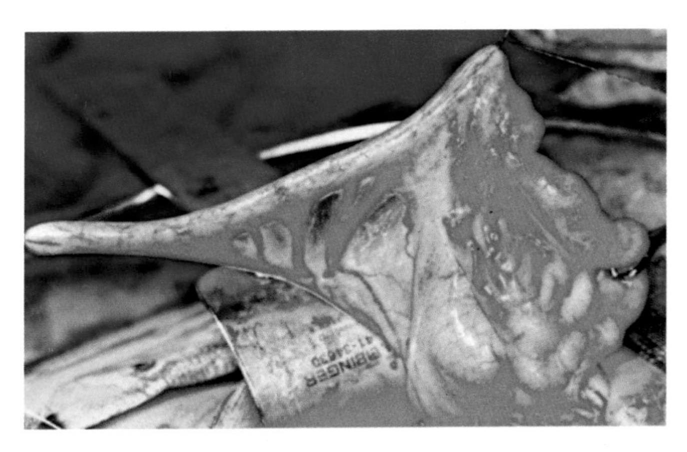

Fig.31.2 Mitrofanoff procedure. To provide a suprapubic fistula for self-catheterization, the vermiform appendix is detached from the cecum, leaving its blood supply intact. One end of the appendix is connected to the bladder, the other to the abdominal wall, intermittent catheterizations being carried out through its lumen.

Examination

On inspection a tight phimosis, or in the case of a circumcised patient a meatal stricture, may be seen. On palpation along the urethra on the ventral aspect of the penis, an area of induration due to a stricture or a calculus in the urethra may be felt.

Digital rectal examination may reveal an enlarged prostate. In order to exclude a neurogenic cause, the reflexes in the lower limbs and sensations in the perineum must be tested as a routine in all cases.

Treatment

Conservative

If a patient presents with acute retention of urine he must be admitted and made comfortable. A few cases will pass urine just like that; most will require more active measures. A *sedative* injection and sitting in a tub or basin of hot water will sufficiently relax the sphincters in a few patients so that urine can pass.

Catheter

If the above measures are unsuccessful, a catheter will have to be passed into the bladder to evacuate the urine. This should be carried out under full aseptic precautions, i.e. mask, sterile gloves, cleansing of the genitalia with an antiseptic, use of a sterile catheter, etc. In the absence of a stricture the catheter should pass easily.

The common conditions in which the catheter will not pass are two:

- If the middle lobe of the *prostate* is enlarged it may obstruct the passage of the catheter. In that case a coude' catheter, i.e. one with a bent tip, will usually pass. Alternatively a suprapubic catheter can be passed or if the patient is fit, an immediate prostatectomy may be carried out.

- In the case of *stricture* the catheter will be held up. Only a filiform bougie will be able to pass. These are fine bougies made of gum elastic. When one filiform has been made to pass, a series of follower bougies can be screwed onto it and the stricture dilated. A small catheter can now be passed and left indwelling.

Suprapubic puncture

If after two or three attempts the catheterization is still unsuccessful, the urine may be evacuated by suprapubic puncture, e.g. with a lumbar puncture needle.

Suprapubic catheterization

Alternatively, a catheter is inserted into the bladder through a 1.5cm incision made under local anesthesia about 2cm below the point where the bladder wall starts receding. The fibres of the linea alba are divided. The catheter on its introducer is passed until it meets the resistance of the muscle wall of the distended bladder. It is passed into the bladder with a short, sharp thrust downwards and backwards. The introducer is removed. The catheter is passed onwards and secured to the skin with a stitch (suprapubic catheterization).

Chronic retention

Chronic retention comes on gradually and the bladder distends slowly; therefore the distension of the bladder is painless. If the blood urea is above 70mg/dl, the bladder should be decompressed very slowly, as bleeding can sometimes start from the rapid decompression of a chronically distended, inflamed bladder mucosa.

THE BLADDER IN SPINAL INJURIES

Immediately after a spinal cord injury spinal shock occurs, from which the bladder may take weeks to recover. The detrusor muscle is paralysed, so that the bladder distends and overflow incontinence results. In the stagnant urine infection takes place, which gradually damages the kidney so much over a period of time as to end up in renal failure.

In order to assess the extent of the neurological damage the following examinations are performed:

- The level of *sensory* and *motor* loss is charted, in order to find out the upper level of the neurological lesion. It may be mentioned that sacral segments S2, 3 and 4, which contain the bladder outflow, lie at the level of the T12 and L1 vertebrae. If the sensory loss below this level is total, recovery is unlikely. On the other hand if the lesion is incomplete, some recovery of bladder function may take place.
- The *bulbo-cavernosus* and *anal* reflexes are tested. If these are present it indicates that the sacral cord is intact, and a reflex or automatic bladder will ultimately emerge. If the reflexes are absent and perineal sensation is lost, recovery is unlikely and the bladder will behave in an autonomous fashion.

Assessment after three months

A full assessment of the bladder function is carried out at the end of three months after injury:

- Lesions *above cord segment D10.* These result in an upper motor neurone type lesion. All bladder reflexes are intact, but the bladder is separated from higher control and inhibition. Irregular detrusor contractions with spasm of the external sphincter produce the condition called detrusor sphincter dyssynergia. The intravesical pressure is chronically raised, so that the upper urinary tract suffers from back-pressure effects. Hydronephrosis may result, ultimately ending up in renal failure.
- Lesions *involving segments D11 to L2.* These involve the sympathetic outflow; the result is an upper motor neurone type of lesion, with the additional loss of sympathetic afferents and sensory efferents from the bladder.
- Damage to the *sacral centre S2, 3, 4 and cauda equina lesions.* This type of damage results essentially in a lower motor neurone bladder. The detrusor is paralysed due to injury to the parasympathetic outflow. Abdominal straining and manual pressure on the bladder can produce emptying. If D11 and 12 segments are intact, sensations through the hypogastric nerves enable the patient to know when the bladder is getting full. Alternatively, intermittent catheterization may be employed.

INCONTINENCE OF URINE

Etiology

The common causes of incontinence in men differ from those seen in women:

- In the *male.* In men *chronic retention with overflow* is a very common cause of incontinence. This may be secondary to benign prostatic hypertrophy, hypertrophy of the bladder neck, or a urethral stricture. There is a long history of hesitancy (difficulty in initiating urination) with a poor stream, along with 'dribbling incontinence' at night. The bladder is usually visibly distended, and is palpable as a painless suprapubic swelling.

- In the *female*. In women the most common cause of leakage of urine is stress incontinence i.e. the involuntary loss of urine associated with an elevation of intra-abdominal pressure. The patient complains of leakage of urine when she laughs, coughs, sneezes, or even changes posture.

  Physical examination shows that the bladder is not distended. If a finger is placed on either side of the urethra and pushed upwards to support the pelvic floor, urinary incontinence is prevented (*Bonney's test*).

  The most probable cause of stress incontinence is hypermobility of the urethro-vesical junction which results in failure of transmission of increases in pressure equally to urethra and bladder.

Treatment

Minor degrees of stress incontinence can be controlled by *alpha adrenergic drugs* which tone up the bladder neck muscle. *Faradic stimulation* and exercises of the pelvic floor also help greatly.

Surgery

However, sometimes the bladder has herniated backwards through the damaged anterior wall of the vagina (cystocele). In such a case surgical repair of the vaginal wall (*anterior colporrhaphy*) is required. At the same time the neck of the bladder is slung up to the pubis by sutures.

Alternatively many surgical procedures like tape or sling insertions can be performed to support the urethra and prevent its hypermobility.

Other causes of incontinence (common to both sexes)

These include the following conditions:

- *Congenital*. An ectopic ureteric orifice below the level of the sphincter.
- *Trauma*. Injury to the urethra during pelvic surgery or from fracture of the pelvis.
- *Neurogenic*. Spinal cord injury, multiple sclerosis, cerebral vascular accident, and Parkinson's disease.
- *Psychogenic*. Hysteria and depression may be accompanied by incontinence of urine.
- *Infection*. Urge incontinence can be induced because of urinary tract infections.

VESICAL CALCULUS

A stone in the bladder is common at two ages: in childhood and in old age.

In children

Etiology

- In the poorer countries, where protein deficiency leads to endemic metabolic bladder stone disease, bladder stone is very common.
- Elsewhere in the world, bladder stone in children is quite uncommon and occurs due to the same causes as in adults, i.e. obstruction, infection or a foreign body (urinary catheter).

Clinical features

The child with a stone in his bladder suffers pain during micturition, and pulls on his penis. Terminal hematuria may be seen.

Diagnosis

Before the advent of x-rays the method of detecting a bladder stone consisted of the passage of a metallic bladder sound and feeling and hearing the click resulting from its contact with the stone. Today ultrasonography is used to show up the stone.

Treatment

Classically, the stone was dealt with by crushing it between the jaws of a 'blind' lithotripter, the fragments being washed out by a Bigelow evacuator. These days optical and electrohydraulic lithotrites are used, as well as an ultrasound probe or Holmium laser.

In old age

In old men the obstructive lesion responsible for a vesical calculus is usually an enlarged prostate. The stone is dealt with at the same time as the lesion causing it.

Small stones can be fragmented during a transurethral procedure by using the electrohydraulic or pneumatic lithotripter (Fig.31.3) to fracture it. Stone-crushing forceps can then be used to fragment the stone to pieces that may be irrigated from the bladder.

Large stones are more difficult to fragment and extract transurethrally and are best dealt with by suprapubic cystotomy. In such a case bladder outlet obstruction may be dealt with by simultaneous removal of the prostate. Alternatively, a suprapubic tube may be left indwelling and a transurethral resection of the prostate carried out as a secondary procedure.

DIVERTICULUM OF THE BLADDER

A bladder diverticulum is an outpouching of the mucosa through the muscle wall of the bladder. If the protrusion passes outwards only through the inner muscular layers of the wall it should be called a saccule.

Etiology

The most common *cause* of a diverticulum is an *obstructing lesion* at the bladder neck; examples of the same include:

- Congenital valves of the posterior urethra.
- Bladder neck contracture.
- Urethral stricture.
- Benign prostatic enlargement.

A *congenital diverticulum* occurs occasionally. In this variety, there is no vesical neck obstruction. Congenital diverticulae have muscle in their walls, whereas acquired diverticulae lack vesical musculature and comprise of bladder mucosa only which is protruded by the normal increase in intravesical pressure during micturition through a weakness in the bladder wall.

The most common site for a diverticulum is near a ureteric orifice, usually above and lateral to it. The diverticulum is lined by mucosa and its wall is formed of fibrous tissue. When it enlarges it may compress the ureter. Alternatively, it may incorporate the ureter into its floor, so that vesico-ureteric reflux develops.

Clinical features

Most patients are males above the age of 50. The patient usually presents with symptoms of the *bladder neck obstruction* which caused the diverticulum.

However, sometimes a patient reports with a urinary tract *infection*, or a *calculus*, which has arisen due to the diverticulum.

In many cases *hematuria* is a leading symptom. The blood comes from the mucosal lining of the diverticulum, which is inflamed due to the stagnation of urine in its lumen.

In occasional cases *micturition occurs twice*, the second act being due to urine from the diverticulum.

Complications

These include the following:

- Hydronephrosis may develop due to compression of the ureter by the diverticulum.
- A carcinoma may arise in a small number of cases.

Diagnosis

Diverticula are usually discovered incidentally by *cystoscopy* or *ultrasound*. The orifice of the diverticulum may appear as a dark round hole. On the other hand a saccule, being shallow, is well illuminated.

Treatment

A diverticulum requires operation only for complications. If it is small and bladder neck obstruction has been dealt with by prostatic resection, the diverticulum need not be removed. During removal of a diverticulum a ureteric catheter is passed up the ureter on the affected side in order to avoid damage to it during dissection.

URINARY FISTULAE

A urinary fistula is an abnormal communication between any part of the urinary tract and the skin or some other internal hollow organ. If a fistula refuses to heal, this may be due to one of the following conditions:

- Distal obstruction.
- A foreign body.
- A chronic infection, e.g. tuberculosis.

Causes of fistulae

Urinary fistulae may be congenital or acquired:

Congenital fistulae

The common types of congenital urinary fistulae include patent urachus and anorectal anomalies:

- ***Patent urachus.***

The urachus is a canal in the fetus which connects the urinary bladder with the allantois. Normally it closes down and is replaced by a fibrous cord—the median umbilical ligament. Occasionally it persists in its patent form. A patent urachus does not leak, because the contractions of the bladder start from the apex, where the urachus is attached to the umbilicus, and pass down the organ. The urachus reveals itself usually in middle age, and then only if bladder neck obstruction from some cause arises. In such a case there may be leakage of urine from the umbilicus.

Treatment

The bladder neck obstruction is dealt with. If leakage still persists, the urachus is excised and the bladder closed.

- ***Anorectal anomalies.***

In some cases of anorectal anomalies a fistula may be present between the rectum and the urethra, or the vagina in the female.

Treatment

In the newborn the fecal stream is diverted by a colostomy. Later, when the rectum is mobilized and brought down to the perineum, the fistula is also closed. Alternatively, the fistula can be closed in the newborn during the operation of *posterior sagittal anorectoplasty*.

Acquired fistulae

- ***Traumatic urinary fistula.***

The common causes of this condition are the following:

  - o Penetrating wounds.
  - o Unrecognized division of ureter or bladder during surgery.
  - o Avascular necrosis following radiotherapy for malignant disease.

- ***Vesico-vaginal fistula.***

This is always a distressing condition because of uncontrolled leakage of urine, which causes ammoniacal dermatitis of the inner thighs with maceration of the skin. Some of its common causes are the following:

  - o This fistula may develop due to injury to the bladder during *hysterectomy*.
  - o In *carcinoma of the cervix* a vesico-vaginal fistula may develop due to ulceration of the carcinoma into the bladder or after radiotherapy to this lesion.
  - o In areas with inadequate obstetric facilities this is a curse on women from the poorer sections of society.

CYSTITIS

Etiology

Infection can reach the urinary bladder via different routes:

- Most commonly, bacteria ascend to the bladder via the urethra.
- Obstruction at the bladder neck may result in infection in the stagnant urine.
- Finally, infection may reach the bladder via the hematogenous route, from infected tonsils, carious teeth etc.

The most common organism involved is *E. coli,* others being Proteus, *Strep. fecalis* and staphylococci.

Clinical features

There is marked frequency of micturition during the day and at night. Lack of sleep produces exhaustion. Pain may be severe in the hypogastrium, or the penis or labia. Pyuria is always present, and the urine may be blood-stained. On examination there is tenderness over the suprapubic region. A midstream urine specimen should be examined microscopically and also cultured.

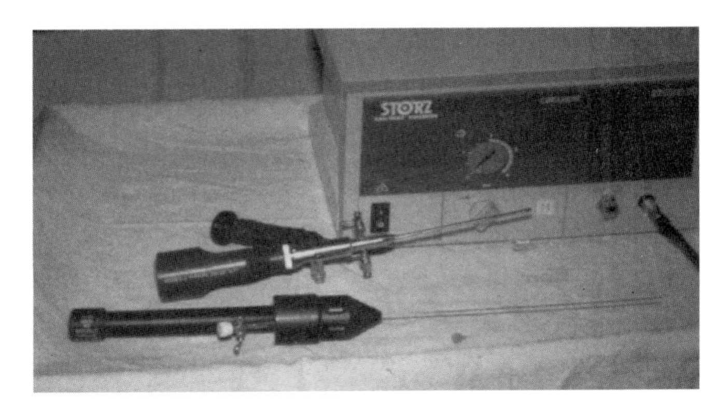

Fig.31.3 Pneumatic lithotripter; the lithotripter probe is passed through the endoscope to fragment the calculus

Treatment

Treatment with a chemotherapeutic agent should be commenced as soon as the urine has been sent for culture. While awaiting the culture and sensitivity reports, nitrofurantoin, 50mg q.i.d. may be started. If the infection recurs, the case must be investigated further to detect the underlying cause; however in men even one episode merits investigation.

Tuberculous cystitis

Tuberculous cystitis is always secondary to renal tuberculosis. Cystoscopy shows tubercles around one ureteric orifice. In long-standing cases there is much fibrosis, and the *capacity of the bladder is reduced* resulting in greatly increased frequency of micturition.

Treatment

The treatment of tuberculous cystitis is by antituberculosis drugs.

Ileocystoplasty

If the bladder is greatly contracted, the marked frequency can be alleviated by ileocystoplasty. In this operation a segment of small intestine is isolated, its lumen is opened along the antimesenteric border, and it is sutured as a patch to the opened dome of the bladder to enlarge its cavity.

BILHARZIASIS OF THE BLADDER

This disease is prevalent in the valley of the Nile, and is also found in some neighbouring Arab countries.

Life cycle

Bilharziasis is caused by a trematode called Schistosoma hematobium. It is acquired while standing in infected water. The embryos in the water cause infestation of the human being by penetrating the skin of the feet. They reach the liver through the blood-stream, where they mature into adult worms. From the liver they travel down the portal vein and the inferior mesenteric vein against the flow of blood. They cross the portal-systemic anastomotic channels at the lower end of the esophagus and reach the plexus of veins in the urinary bladder.

Eggs are shed in the urine. On reaching fresh water the miracidium emerges from the egg. It penetrates into a snail, reaches its liver, and leads to the development of daughter cysts. These are liberated on the death of the snail. They shed large numbers of embryos into the water, thus completing the life cycle.

Clinical features

When the embryos penetrate the skin urticaria develops. After a few weeks high temperature with eosinophilia occurs. Finally, when ova are shed in the urine intermittent painless hematuria results, which is the classic symptom.

Investigations

The ovum is recognized in the urine without staining, under the low-powered microscope.

Cystoscopy may show pseudo-tubercles, nodules, 'sandy patches', ulcers or papillomas, and in neglected long-standing cases carcinomas, mainly squamous-celled.

Treatment

This is by niridazole, or by compounds containing antimony, repeated courses being required. Bilharzial papillomas and carcinomas of the bladder require surgical treatment.

TUMORS OF THE URINARY BLADDER

Tumors of the bladder are moderately common, the vast majority being malignant. Males are affected about three times more often than females. Most patients are elderly, 75% being over 60 years.

Etiology

- In 1895 Rehn was the first to show a relationship between a chemical agent and cancer. He reported cases of *bladder cancer* in a German *dye* factory manufacturing *aniline, one of the aromatic amines.* However, it was not until the 1950s that the risk from aromatic amines was clearly established. These dyes were formerly used in the paint, dyestuffs, rubber and chemical industries, but in the advanced countries none have been used since the 1960s.
- Smoking an average of 15 *cigarettes* a day doubles the risk of cancer of the bladder, so that 40% of the patients are smokers.
- Chronic over-ingestion of *analgesics* containing phenacetin.
- Pelvic *irradiation*.
- *Bilharziasis*, 80% of cases in Egypt being due to this cause.

Multiple genetic events appear to be involved including activation of oncogenes and inactivation or loss of tumor suppressor genes. Loss of genetic material on chromosome 9, and deletion of chromosome 11p and 17p have been described in patients with bladder cancer.

Pathology

In the bladder the most common sites of occurrence of tumors are the lateral walls and the trigone. The overwhelming majority of bladder tumors arise in the mucous membrane:

Benign urothelial tumors

These are extremely rare.

Malignant tumors

These are of three histological types:

- ***Transitional cell carcinomas* (95%)**

  These are morphologically of three types:

  - *Papillary* tumors (70%) tend to be pedunculated and grow into the bladder lumen. They are usually superficial and well differentiated.
  - *Solid* tumors (20%) are sessile with ulceration, necrosis and calcification. They tend to be invasive lesions and are usually less well differentiated than papillary lesions.
  - *Carcinomas in situ* appear as flat, red, velvety patches in the bladder and may be difficult to distinguish from chronic infection. Histologically they are poorly differentiated. Most cases show malignant cells on cytological examination of the urine.

- ***Squamous tumors.***

  These account for only 1% of urothelial tumors. They are usually caused by chronic irritation of the bladder, from a calculus or an indwelling catheter. In Egypt these tumors constitute 80% of bladder cancers. They arise in patches of the bladder which have undergone squamous metaplasia as a result of infestation with *S. hematobium*. These bilharzial tumors are nodular lesions, are usually well differentiated, and carry a low risk of lymph node or distant metastases.

- ***Adenocarcinomas.***

  These are extremely rare.

Grading

Bladder tumors are *graded* into well-differentiated, moderately differentiated and poorly differentiated tumors according to the degree of cellular anaplasia; however, of late moderately differentiated tumors are no longer reported pathologically. There is a strong correlation between tumor grade and stage.

Prognosis

The important factors in prognosis include:

- Tumor stage.
- Tumor grade.
- Vascular invasion.
- Presence of associated carcinoma in situ.

However, some tumors remain localized whereas others that appear identical recur or become invasive.

Factors that result in a poor prognosis include:

- A high proliferative rate.
- Aneuploidy.
- Loss of expression of tumor suppressor genes.

Spread

So long as the tumor is confined to the mucous membrane or muscle coat, distant metastases are uncommon. Once it has infiltrated into the perivesical fat, it spreads to the iliac and para-aortic lymph nodes. It can also spread via the blood-stream to the lungs, liver and bones.

Clinical features

The first symptom is *intermittent painless hematuria*. With the passage of time the intervals between the episodes of hematuria become shorter, and the bleeding more profuse. The anemia may become so severe as to necessitate blood transfusion.

Other patients may present with recurrent urinary tract *infections* or sterile pyuria.

An obstructed ureter may result in *pain* in the loin. Similarly, infiltration of a nerve may cause pain referred to the perineum, the groins or thighs.

The tumor may be detected *incidentally*, either during cystoscopy or on routine 'dip-stick' testing for hematuria: 10 % of these patients will have a bladder cancer.

Investigations

The clinical problem is usually of unexplained hematuria.

Urinalysis

A urine sample is obtained for culture and for examination for malignant cells.

Urinary cytology

This is specially helpful if carcinoma *in situ* is suspected. In such cases 90% of specimens will be positive; in well-differentiated tumors only 50%.

New tests

To overcome the shortcomings of urinary cytology such as low sensitivity for low-grade superficial tumors, several new tests have been developed. These tests can:

- Detect cancer specific proteins in the urine (BTA/NMP22[1]).
- Augment cytology by identifying:
  - Cell surface markers.
  - Cytogenetic markers in the nucleus.

These tests can play a role in initial diagnosis and follow-up.

Intravenous urogram/CT urogram

This may show a filling defect within the bladder; however, its primary purpose is to exclude a source of bleeding in the upper urinary tract.

Cystoscopy

This is carried out under local anesthesia. A papilloma shows delicate villi which sway about in the fluid. On the other hand in the case of a more malignant papilloma both the stalk and the villi are more thick and short. Nodules may be present around the growth.

Biopsy

At cystoscopy a *biopsy* of the tumor should always be carried out.

Ultrasound

Abdominal ultrasound shows up papillary tumors larger than 1cm in diameter.

Staging

If histological examination shows the tumor to be *superficial*, no further staging is required.

With invasive cancers it is necessary to distinguish between localized extension and advanced pelvic or disseminated disease.

A modified UICC (TNM) staging system for bladder cancer is given in (Table 31.1). For this purpose CT scan or MRI is better than bimanual examination, which often understages these tumors.

1 NMP22: Nuclear Matrix Protein no. 22

Table 31.1 Modified UICC (TNM) staging system for bladder cancer

Tis		Carcinoma in situ
Ta		Does not cross lamina propria
T1		Extends beyond lamina but does not infiltrate muscle
T2		Invades muscle layer
	2a	Involves the inner half
	2b	Involves the outer half
T3		Invades extravesical tissues
	3a	Microscopic involvement
	3b	Macroscopic involvement
T4		Fixed to pelvic viscera
	4a	Adjacent viscera like prostate, vagina or uterus
	4b	Pelvic side wall or abdominal wall
N0		No nodes
N1		Single node – 2cm
N2		Single node > 2.5cm or multiple – 5cm
N3		Nodes > 5cm
M0		No metastases
M1		Metastases

Treatment

Surgery

All patients with bladder tumors should first undergo *transurethral resection (TUR)* of the tumor under general or local anesthesia. Separate samples of the tumor and its muscle base should be sent to the laboratory to help in the detection of muscle invasion. CT scan or MRI should be done both before and after the resection, as the further management depends upon the grade and stage.

Carcinoma in situ

All macroscopic disease should be resected first. With localized disease this is all that is required; with widespread disease this should be followed by intravesical instillations of Bacillus Calmette-Guerin (BCG) weekly for six weeks, and can be repeated. This treatment is highly effective. On the other hand systemic chemotherapy and radiotherapy are quite ineffective in treating carcinoma in situ.

Non-muscle invasive tumors

Here, TUR should be followed by intravesical therapy with mitomycin C. This should be followed by regular check cystoscopies.

Muscle invasive tumors

This carries a poor prognosis in advanced stages with 5-year survivals of 50%.

In all the above three types of case if the tumor fails to respond or relapses after treatment, further treatment can be offered.

Radical cystectomy and pelvic lymphadenectomy

This is now the standard treatment for T2-T3 tumors without secondary spread, and of carcinoma in situ that has not responded to Bacille Calmette-Guerin. Bone scan and CT scan of the chest should be done preoperatively to exclude metastases.

Urinary diversion

Traditionally, the ureters are reimplanted into an ileal segment, which is used as a *urinary conduit* to an abdominal wall stoma. Urine drains continuously and is collected in a bag attached to the skin around the stoma.

Continent urinary diversion

A continent urinary diversion can be utilized. An intra-abdominal pouch is fashioned from ileum (the Koch pouch), and can be catheterized intermittently by the patient through the abdominal stoma.

Neobladder

In this technique, after cystectomy a pouch of ileum, into which the ureters have been implanted, is sutured to the internal urethral meatus. The patient is continent because the external urinary sphincter is preserved. He can either void spontaneously by using the Valsalva manoeuvre[1], or catheterize the pouch intermittently via the urethra.

Finally, open surgical removal of the cancer must be totally avoided.

Chemotherapy

The poor results of radiotherapy are explained by the presence of unrecognized distant disease at the time of the initial treatment.

Neo-adjuvant chemotherapy

Accordingly, urologists are turning increasingly towards chemotherapy, where the recent introduction of multi-agent regimens has brought fresh hope. Methotrexate, vinblastine, adriamycin and cisplatin (M-VAC) have shown good results. Such treatment *prior* to cystectomy (neo-adjuvant chemotherapy) can 'down-stage' the

1 Valsalva maneuver: breathing out against a closed glottis, by closing the mouth and pinching the nose.

tumor in most cases, and make it more easily dealt with by surgery.

A newer combination of cisplatin and gemcitabine has shown similar results with lower toxicity and improved tolerability.

The treatment of *disseminated disease* is palliative, as median survival is only six months. Multi-agent therapy can increase the survival time, but the already debilitated patient has to face significant morbidity.

Treatment of recurrences

If a tumor recurs after a course of transurethral resections, it should be dealt with by intravesical chemotherapy with mitomycin C or BCG. Depending on the stage, grade and type of tumor further treatments in the form of radiotherapy or cystectomy can be offered. However before major interventions are planned it should be ensured that:

- There is no evidence of spread of the disease.
- The patient is fit for the operation.

Chapter

32 PROSTATE

BENIGN PROSTATIC HYPERPLASIA

Benign prostatic hyperplasia is a very common condition. It occurs usually above the age of fifty, and especially after 60. Over 50% of males above the age of fifty have various degrees of bladder outlet obstruction secondary to benign prostatic hyperplasia. The cause is unknown; the most popular theory considers it as due to a relatively greater quantity of estrogens compared to the male hormone, as the quantity of the latter diminishes with advancing age.

Pathology

Both the glandular and connective tissue elements undergo hyperplasia, especially in the submucous area. These form nodular enlargements in each lateral lobe, and compress the outer part of each lobe into a false capsule. When the hyperplasia affects the subcervical area a 'middle lobe' develops, and projects upwards into the bladder. In such a case urine remains in this post-prostatic pouch after micturition, and calculi can form in it.

The urethra becomes stretched and elongated by the enlarging prostate, and is compressed from the sides into an antero-posterior slit. The bladder hypertrophies to overcome the obstruction; if the obstruction is unrelieved it ultimately undergoes atony and becomes a passive bag. Gradually, due to back pressure, hydroureter and hydronephrosis develop. Reflux may occur into the dilated ureters and result in damage to the kidneys. Ascending infection may produce pyelonephritis.

Clinical features

Frequency

This is usually the first symptom. In the beginning it is noticed only at night; later it occurs during the day as well. The following factors contribute towards its development:

- Stretching of the sensitive bladder neck epithelium by the intravesical enlargement of the prostate.
- Increasing amounts of residual urine, so that the bladder refills early and the patient has to void repeatedly.
- Cystitis, by irritating the bladder mucosa.
- Finally, due to prolonged back pressure the distal tubules lose their ability to reabsorb water and salt and polyuria results, so that large volumes of urine have to be expelled, leading to even more frequent voiding.

Difficulty in micturition

This is the next most frequent symptom. The patient has to wait for micturition to commence. Straining makes matters worse, whereas on the contrary in cases of stricture of the urethra straining facilitates micturition. The stream is thin and weak, with dribbling at the end. Cystitis and acute retention of urine result in pain in the hypogastrium. A dull pain in the loins may indicate the development of hydronephrosis.

Acute retention of urine

This may be the symptom which brings the patient to the doctor, and often results from postponement of micturition so that the bladder is overstretched.

Chronic retention

If the retention of urine is chronic, the gradual stretching of the bladder is painless and the distended bladder passes unnoticed. The only symptom is dribbling, which occurs due to overflow from the full bladder.

Hematuria

This may occasionally occur due to rupture of a prostatic vein from congestion. Finally, the patient may present with symptoms due to renal failure, e.g. anorexia, hiccups, vomiting, thirst and drowsiness.

The international prostate symptom score

This is a useful index for measuring the severity of symptoms of benign hyperplasia of the prostate.

The patient is asked:

Over the last one month how often have you:

- had a sensation of incomplete emptying of the bladder?
- had to urinate again within two hours?
- stopped and started several times during micturition?
- found it difficult to postpone micturition?
- had a weak urinary stream?
- had to strain to begin urination?
- had to get up during the night to micturate (on average)?

If the answer to any question is 'not at all', the score is zero; if almost always, the score is 5. Intermediate replies get appropriate marks.

Symptom severity score

The severity of symptoms is determined as follows:

Score	Severity
1–7	Mild
8–19	Moderate
20–35	Severe

Clinical examination

During the clinical examination the *tongue* should be inspected for the presence of dryness, and the external meatus for stenosis. The *hypogastrium* should be palpated to detect bladder distension, and the *renal areas* for tenderness which may be present due to hydronephrosis.

Rectal examination

This is carried out. In benign hyperplasia the lobes of the prostate are found to be increased in size, smooth, convex and elastic. When pressure is exerted a slight degree of mobility of the gland is noted. Hardness and fixity of the gland suggest a carcinoma.

Nervous system

This is examined to exclude a neurological lesion, e.g. spinal tumor or tuberculosis. For this purpose testing for the knee and ankle jerks, and for sensation in the lower limbs, is generally sufficient.

Investigations

The *urine* is examined for the presence of infection and is cultured.

The *blood* is examined for the white cell count, urea and creatinine levels as well as PSA (prostate specific antigen).

A *plain x-ray* of the abdomen may show calculi in the urinary tract and sclerotic metastases in the pelvis and lumbar spine in case the enlargement is due to carcinoma.

Urinary flow rate

As urinary symptoms are unreliable, it is useful to have objective information. The most useful is the urinary flow rate, in which the patient is asked to void into a machine from a 'comfortably full' bladder, and the flow is converted into a graph tracing. A maximum flow rate of less than 10ml/second from a voided volume of more than 200ml strongly suggests obstruction.

Ultrasound examination

Ultrasonography is carried out over the hypogastrium.

Transurethal ultrasound (TRUS)

At the same time, ultrasonography is performed using a transrectal probe. These two methods together provide an effective, reliable and non-invasive method of assessing the size of the prostate, the volume of the residual urine, and the size of the bladder.

Evaluation of the upper urinary tract is indicated if hematuria is present.

Intravenous urography

This is used less often, but can show a filling defect due to a benign prostatic hyperplasia (Fig.32.1 a and b).

Cystourethroscopy

This should always be carried out before a prostatectomy to detect a urethral stricture, a carcinoma, bladder pathology etc.

TREATMENT

The aim of treatment of benign prostatic hyperplasia is to improve the quality of life by removing outflow obstruction and restoring comfortable micturition. Because the disease is not associated with any risk of mortality, the patient's preference should be the dominant factor in the decision. Symptomatic patients should be given the option of immediate treatment or watchful waiting. Treatment options include drug therapy and surgical techniques.

Drug therapies

- A-*blockers* like *tamsulosin* and *terazosin* relax the smooth muscle of the bladder neck; they thus improve micturition. Postural hypotension is a significant side effect. Young patients with small prostates derive the greatest benefit.
- *Androgen withdrawal*. Androgens are necessary in the development of prostatic hyperplasia. Androgen

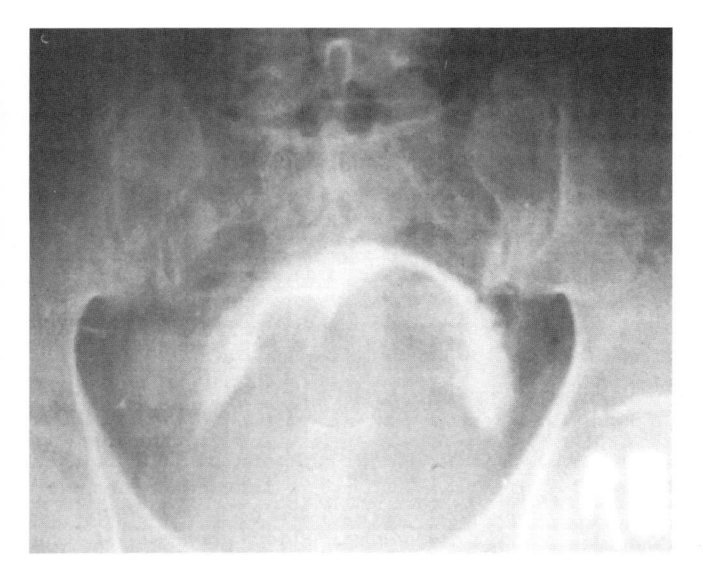

a

Fig.32.1 a Cystogram showing very gross benign prostatic hyperplasia

withdrawal therefore causes regression of this condition; however, loss of libido and potency make this course of action unattractive. Testosterone has marked effect on secondary sex characters; on the other hand, dihydrotestosterone stimulates hyperplasia of the prostate. The enzyme 5 alpha-reductase converts testosterone into dihydrotestosterone. *Finasteride* inhibits this enzyme and results in reduced production of dihydrotestosterone; it thus helps reduce the size of the prostate. After 6 months of administration of finasteride the size of the prostate is reduced by about 20 percent.

Patients with mild to moderate symptoms can employ drug therapy, and a number of them will not require operative treatment.

Indications for operation

Dysuria

As mentioned above, the mere presence of an enlarged prostate is not an indication for operation, because many old people have prostatic enlargement without any symptoms. Again, mild symptoms do not warrant surgery. However, increasing difficulty in micturition, with delay in starting the act and a poor stream, or very marked frequency which upsets the patient's life routine, are situations where prostatectomy is advised.

Acute retention

If acute urinary retention is present it has to be treated by catheterization. If acute retention recurs after catheterization, *prostatectomy* should be carried out.

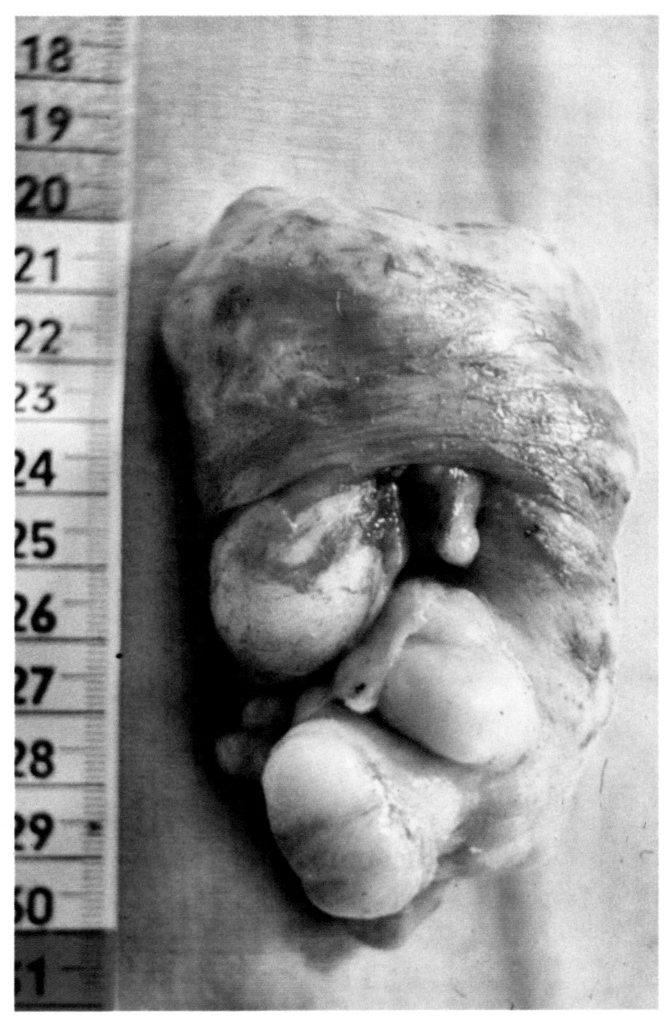

b

Fig.32.1 b. 10cm long prostate removed at suprapubic prostatectomy

Chronic retention

In the case of chronic retention, if the serum creatinine is normal and there is no infection prostatectomy can be carried out without preliminary catheter drainage. If uremia is present decompression of the bladder is essential, to be followed in due course by prostatectomy. Such cases are also dehydrated, and intravenous fluid replacement should be carried out.

Complications

The development of stones, diverticula, infection or persistent hematuria indicates the necessity of surgical treatment.

The operations available

The prostate may be approached:

- Transurethrally.
- Transvesically.
- Retropubically.
- Via the perineum.

Perineal prostatectomy has been long abandoned due to the high incidence of incontinence and fistula formation. Further, transurethral resection has all but replaced the older methods of open prostatectomy.

Minimally invasive techniques

Finally, minimally invasive surgical procedures have been introduced, including:

- Transurethral incision and ultrasonic aspiration of the prostate.
- Cryosurgery.
- Prostatic stents.
- Laser prostatectomy.

Except for the first method, their final position has yet to be established.

Description of methods

Transurethral resection and the newer methods are described first, to be followed by the older methods of transvesical and retropubic prostatectomy.

Newer methods

Transurethral prostatectomy

Fibreoptic resectoscopes with the rigid lenses of Professor Harold Hopkins have greatly facilitated transurethral resection. Strips of tissue are cut from the bladder neck down to the level of the verumontanum using a high frequency diathermy current. Accurate hemostasis can be achieved. Damage to the external sphincter is avoided by staying above the verumontanum. The strips of tissue are removed from the bladder by using a bulb evacuator. A 3-way Foley is left indwelling for constant irrigation.

This method has all but replaced the older methods of prostatectomy, mainly because the necessity of incising the abdominal wall and the bladder is dispensed with. In this way abdominal pain and paralytic ileus are prevented, the patient can get out of bed earlier, and convalescence is greatly expedited. However, the method requires sophisticated equipment and specialized training. Therefore the transvesical and retropubic methods still have a place in certain parts of the world.

Minimally invasive methods

Hyperthermia

Heat can be selectively delivered to the prostate by microwave probes placed in the prostatic urethra. Several sessions are required. However, there is very little improvement in minimal flow rate.

Laser prostatectomy

The laser probe directly touches and vaporizes the prostatic tissue, the result being the immediate removal of obstructing tissue in a manner similar to transurethral prostatectomy.

Long-term follow up has not shown significant benefit over the standard methods..

Prostatic stents

Short tubes made of titanium or a superalloy are available for use in patients who are not fit for anesthesia.

Older methods

Transvesical prostatectomy

Classically, the method of prostatectomy had been through the transvesical route, mainly because it could be carried out without very specialized training or equipment. The bladder may be opened through a midline incision. Alternatively, a Pfannensteil's incision may be employed. This is made transversely just above the pubis, being convex downwards. The rectus sheath is divided in the line of the incision and the upper flap raised upwards. The rectus muscles are now separated in the midline.

The peritoneum is displaced upwards, and the bladder opened. A finger is passed into the urethra and pushes forwards, separating the lateral lobes; it is then worked between the adenoma and the false capsule all round. The urethra is divided with a curved scissors, and the adenoma removed. Hamostasis is achieved by diathermy or suture ligation.

In *Freyer's* technique the bladder is drained by a stout tube. In *Harris's* method the prostatic arteries are suture-ligated at 5 and 7 O'clock at the bladder neck, using his boomerang needle.

The bladder is then closed, a 3-way Foley catheter being left in place for continuous irrigation. For the first day or two after operation constant irrigation of the bladder is carried out till the fluid returned becomes pale pink.

Retropubic prostatectomy

This method is superior to transvesical prostatectomy as the bladder muscle is not incised and therefore the return of bladder voiding is more prompt. At the same time, hemostasis is achieved under vision.

The prevesical space is opened through a Pfannensteil's incision. A self-retaining retractor is placed in position and the bladder retracted upwards by its third blade. The anterior capsule of the prostate is incised by diathermy transversely about 1cm below the bladder neck. The prostatic adenoma is enucleated with the finger or by the use of a curved scissors, which also divides the urethra. A wedge is removed from the posterior bladder neck to prevent a stricture. Hemostasis is obtained by diathermy under vision, an indwelling 3-way Foley catheter is placed and the prostatic capsule closed.

Complications of prostatectomy

Hemorrhage

This is the most important complication after prostatectomy through any route. Clot retention is signaled by a distended bladder and a catheter that does not drain. The bladder should be washed out by a syringe.

Secondary hemorrhage occurs during the second week, and may be associated with infection. If clots are present they have to be washed out, and an antibiotic should be started.

Infection

This can occur, and should be treated with an appropriate antibiotic. If prostatectomy is to be carried out on a patient who has had an indwelling catheter for a prolonged period of time, parenteral antibiotics should be administered as a prophylactic measure.

Incontinence

The internal sphincter at the bladder neck is put out of action by every type of prostatectomy. However, if incontinence occurs it means the external sphincter has also been damaged; its treatment is quite difficult.

Stricture

This may occur at the bladder neck or at the external meatus. At the meatus it may be due to an excessively large catheter left indwelling for a long period.

Osteitis pubis

This is a rare but distressing complication of open prostatectomy.

Complications of transurethral prostatectomy

The following can occur:

- *Water intoxication*, from absorption of excessive amounts of irrigating fluid.
- *Perforation of the prostatic capsule*.

It should be remembered that after every type of prostatectomy retrograde ejaculation of the semen into the bladder occurs, rendering the patient infertile.

Distant complications of prostatectomy

Pulmonary atelectasis, pneumonia, and deep vein thrombosis can all occur, so that early ambulation is important. Myocardial infarction can also be precipitated.

Catheterization

A catheter should be passed into the urinary bladder only by a doctor or a trained nurse. Catheterization should only be carried out under full aseptic precautions i.e. mask, sterile gloves, sterile sheets etc. The glans or labia should be cleansed with a suitable antiseptic. Even so, a sterile catheter is best passed with a non-touch technique, i.e., being held with a sterile forceps. In an adult, the size of the catheter should not be larger than about 16 F, as it only increases the chance of urethritis and stricture formation. 7 to 10ml of fluid in the balloon is enough to help retain the catheter in place; with larger volumes bladder spasms may be caused by the detrusor contracting to expel the balloon.

Closed system drainage bag

The catheter should be connected to a closed system drainage bag. This bag should be emptied only by opening the outlet at its bottom, the connection with the catheter being left undisturbed, as otherwise infection can be introduced. These points are stressed because careless technique can result in infection which, in the presence of stagnation and reduced general resistance of the patient, can run riot in the urinary tract.

Bladder neck stenosis

This condition may be due to congenital muscular hypertrophy, in which case it occurs in children. Alternatively, it may arise from fibrosis around the bladder neck, when it is seen during middle age.

Clinical features

There may be difficulty in micturition or repeated urinary infections. A distended bladder may be visible or palpable. Reflux of bladder urine into the ureters may cause loin pain and pyelonephritis. A bladder diverticulum may develop due to raised bladder pressure, or a hernia may arise due to straining.

Treatment

Adrenergic alpha blockers, e.g. tamsulosin can be useful by producing relaxation of the bladder neck. In other cases bougie dilatation of the bladder neck may work.

If these measures fail transurethral resection or simple incision of the bladder neck is effective.

CARCINOMA OF THE PROSTATE

Carcinoma of the prostate is the most common malignancy in men above the age of sixty-five years, the median age at clinical diagnosis being 72 years. However, the condition is very much less common than benign prostatic enlargement. The tumor arises in the external group of glands, so it can develop even after 'prostatectomy' for benign hyperplasia.

95% of the tumors are adenocarcinomas, the remaining few being transitional cell carcinomas, either as extension from a bladder tumor or arising in the prostate from its own transitional epithelium.

Risk factors

Prostate cancer is more common in the Western countries than in the East. It is endocrine-dependent and requires testosterone to grow; thus it never occurs in eunuchs. High fat intake and other factors are associated with high prostate cancer rates. Finally, first-degree relatives have an eight-fold increased risk of developing prostatic cancer.

Grading

Gleason's system of grading is the most popular. It assigns a grade of 1 to 5 depending on degree of differentiation, gland formation, and the relation of cancer cells to stroma.

Flow cytometry

The use of flow cytometry to determine DNA ploidy is an important prognostic tool. Cells with an abnormal number of chromosomes have a higher risk of progression and recurrence. On the other hand patients with diploid untreated, localized disease have a 90% 6-year survival rate.

Tumor volume

Apart from grade, the strongest predictor of tumor progression and metastases is tumor volume.

Spread

The fascia of Denonvilliers prevents backward growth, therefore the tumor usually spreads *upwards*, where it may involve the lower ends of the ureters, leading to anuria.

Blood spread

This occurs to *bones*, particularly the pelvis and the lower lumbar vertebrae, probably due to connections between the prostatic and pelvic veins.

Lymphatic spread

- Primary lymphatic spread occurs to both the internal and external iliac lymph nodes.
- The secondary field includes inguinal, common iliac and para-aortic nodes.

Staging

The American Urological System of staging is given in Table 32.1.

Clinical features

Most sufferers are old men. The disease may present in various forms:

- A *hard nodule* may be felt in the prostate during rectal examination for dysuria.
- *Tissue* removed at prostatectomy may show features of malignancy on microscopic examination.
- The patient may present with *pain* in the lower back or sciatica.
- Bilateral *sciatica* in an old man is especially significant.
- A *bleeding tendency* may occur due to destruction of bone marrow from metastases.

Diagnosis

This requires careful digital rectal examination, followed by laboratory and imaging procedures, and biopsy.

Digital rectal examination

Signs of malignancy include asymmetry of the gland, induration and hard nodule formation. More than half the tumors detected in this way have spread beyond the prostate. The method has its limitations:

- A third of cancers less than 1.5cm in size are missed.
- Further, only the peripheral zone is accessible to digital rectal examination, so that tumors confined to the central zone will be missed.

Laboratory tests

Prostatic specific antigen (PSA)

The discovery of prostatic specific antigen has revolutionized the early detection as well as the monitoring of prostate cancer. This glycoprotein serine protease liquefies coagulated semen and is 100 per cent specific to the prostate. Both benign and malignant prostate cells produce PSA, but malignant cells produce about 15 times more per gram of tissue. Moderate elevation may therefore be due to a benign gland, but seldom with high levels. Normal PSA levels are age-related and rise with advancing age. Levels outside the normal range should be investigated with prostatic biopsy. As a general rule, men above 80 years of age should not undergo PSA testing.

Utility of the test

- The PSA level is directly proportional to the *stage* of the prostate cancer; 95% of patients with a PSA level below 10 ng/ml have disease confined to the prostate.
- At the same time, PSA is the best test for *monitoring therapy* of prostate cancer; following radical prostatectomy persistently elevated levels indicate residual or metastatic disease.

Other laboratory tests

If metastases are present:

- Tests for hemoglobin, white cells and platelets are carried out, as any of these can be deficient due to replacement of the red marrow by the malignant deposits.
- Serum creatinine should be estimated to rule out back pressure effects on the kidneys.
- Liver function tests to rule out replacement of liver tissue by metastases.

Bone scan

Nuclear bone imaging is the best technique for detecting bone metastases, which produce 'hot spots' in the areas of the red marrow i.e. the axial skeleton. The false negative rate is only 2%.

If hot spots are shown, they should be examined by radiography, which shows osteosclerotic secondaries in the pelvis and lumbar vertebrae if present.

Transrectal ultrasound (TRUS)

This gives detailed images of prostatic anatomy. However, only one-third of hypoechoic lesions are cancer; at the same time upto 40% of prostatic cancers are isoechoic and therefore missed. The functions of transrectal ultrasound are:

- To *guide a biopsy needle* to a suspicious nodule.
- To perform ten spaced biopsies for mapping the extent of the cancer.

Computed tomography

CT scan can show prostatic size and contour, but is not very accurate in assessing extra-capsular spread. It is used primarily to assess enlargement of *lymph nodes* and predict nodal metastases. The use of CT for staging prostate cancers has decreased since the availability of prostatic specific antigen.

Table 32.1 American Urological Association classification of cancer of the prostate

Stage A	Clinically unsuspected tumor found on pathological examination of TURP specimen.
Stage B	Confined within capsule:
	B1: Involving one lobe, less than 2cm.
	B2: Involving one lobe, more than 2cm.
	B3: Involving both lobes.
Stage C	Extension beyond capsule.
	C1: Minimal extension.
	C2: Bulky extension.
Stage D	Metastatic disease.

Magnetic resonance imaging

This gives better images of the prostate and seminal vesicles than CT and can differentiate malignant nodules, but often understages capsular invasion. The use of endorectal coils may improve its quality.

Prostatic biopsy

With spring-loaded biopsy guns and ultrasound guidance, transrectal biopsy is simple and safe, and can be performed on an outpatient basis without general anesthetic.

Treatment

For localized disease

If the investigations listed above indicate localized disease, the treatment options include observation alone, external beam radiotherapy and radical prostatectomy.

Observation alone

In some cases, the risk of progression of the cancer in the patient's lifetime is so slight that no intervention is warranted. This applies to men over 80 years of age with localized disease and men over 60 with stage A1 disease, i.e. clinically unsuspected tumor found on transurethral resection of the prostate, with 3 or fewer foci in specimen.

Radiation

- *External beam radiotherapy.* In patients with positive margins after radical prostatectomy, external beam radiotherapy can reduce local recurrence rates from 30 to 5 per cent, but survival rates are not improved.
- *Targeted radiotherapy.*

With the help of three-dimentional imaging, targeted radiotherapy is delivered to the prostate. This is an effective treatment for stage A, B and C prostatic cancer. Standard therapy consists of 5000 cGy over five weeks to the pelvis with a further prostate boost of 2000 over two weeks. Local control is achieved in 80 to 90 per cent of cases.

Complications occur in about 10% of patients and include impotence, strictures, proctitis and small bowel fistula.

- *Brachytherapy.*

  Accurate implantation of radioactive seeds in the prostate can be undertaken under the guidance of transurethral ultrasound (TRUS) and computer software. Brachytherapy can be administered alone or, in high-risk patients, in combination with external beam radiation.

Surgery

Radical prostatectomy

This implies complete surgical removal of the prostate and seminal vesicles. The operation was associated with a very high complication rate in the past. However, detailed studies of the neuroanatomy of the region were carried out, and the retropubic approach modified to spare the neurovascular bundles responsible for erection. This improved both the continence and positive margin rates considerably.

Survival after surgery for localized disease is as follows:

- At 5 years 80 %.
- At 10 years 70 %.

Ten to fifteen per cent patients encounter local recurrence.

Surgery versus radiation

In patients with localized disease, the results achieved with radical prostatectomy and external beam radiotherapy are similar. The best course to follow is as follows:

- For patients with an expected life-span of less than 5 years (i.e. those more than 80 years old), observation is advised.
- In those with a 5 to 10 year expected life span, external beam therapy gives results similar to surgery with less morbidity.
- For patients under 70 with an expected life-span of more than 15 years, surgery is best, because radiotherapy is often followed by persistent elevation of prostatic specific antigen.

Hormonal therapy

About 80% of patients with metastatic prostate cancer have a measurable response to endocrine therapy, with a mean duration of response of 2 to 3 years. The eventual progression of disease is due to growth of androgen-independent cell populations.

The pituitarty-gonadal axis can be manipulated at different levels to induce androgen deprivation:

Orchiectomy

Bilateral orchiectomy is simple and safe, and produces castrate levels of hormones within a few hours. General, regional or local anesthesia may be used. The side effects include gynecomastia, impotence and hot flushes.

Subcapsular orchidectomy

If a normal appearing scrotum is important to the patient, the orchiectomy may be carried out by the subcapsular method (preserving the tunica albuginea), or a synthetic testicular prosthesis may be implanted.

Estrogens

Exogenous estrogen blocks androgen metabolism at many levels, i.e. the pituitary, the testis, and the tumor. Unfortunately, at doses necessary to produce castrate testosterone levels (3–5mg/day), diethylstilboestrol is associated with increased cardiovascular complications and deaths. Smaller doses e.g. 1 to 2mg daily do not produce these side-effects, but then they do not reliably produce castrate levels either. Although diethylstilboestrol has been supplanted by newer drugs, it is the least expensive therapy, and very low doses are being studied in trials of combination therapy.

Luteinizing hormone releasing hormone (LHRH) analogues

Administration of LHRH analogues causes a rise in testosterone levels, but this level drops to castrate levels within two weeks. The clinical effect is equivalent to orchiectomy or stilboestrol. LHRH analogues are available as daily subcutaneous injections, a nasal spray, or a monthly and three monthly depot injection.

Antiandrogens

Pure antiandrogens such as flutamide and biclutamide block the binding of testosterone and dihydrotestosterone to the androgen receptor. Side effects include gynecomastia, flushing and diarrhea.

Total androgen blockade

This consists of a combination of orchiectomy or LHRH analogues with an antiandrogen; patients with low disease burden and good performance status benefit most from this method of treatment.

Other complications of metastatic disease

These include:

Spinal cord compression

This is well palliated by both radiation and surgical decompressive laminectomy.

Ureteric obstruction

Local extension can impinge on the trigone and produce obstructive uropathy. Antegrade or retrograde stenting is the procedure of choice.

Bone pain

In case of intractable pain, local radiotherapy and/or oral prednisone may be considered in addition to analgesia.

PROSTATITIS

Acute prostatitis

Acute prostatitis is moderately common. The usual organisms are *Esch. coli* and the pyogenic cocci. The infection may be hematogenous or from the urinary tract. There may be fever with rigors and dysuria. The initial part of urine, on standing, may show threads. Perineal heaviness and pain on defecation may be felt. The prostate is tender on palpation.

Treatment is by antibiotics, which should be given in adequate doses and for several weeks.

Chronic prostatitis

Chronic prostatitis usually results from inadequate treatment of acute prostatitis. The organisms are the same as in acute prostatitis, along with trichomonas and chlamydia. In improperly treated cases fibrosis occurs and the prostate becomes shrunken in size.

Clinical features

There may be pain in the perineum or in the lower part of the back, extending down the legs. Mild intermittent fever or premature ejaculations may be the presenting symptoms. The gland may feel normal. The prostatic fluid, obtained by prostatic massage, may show pus cells and bacteria. Urethroscopy may show the inflamed prostatic urethra.

Treatment

Treatment is by antibiotics, after sensitivity testing. If trichomonas is present, metronidazole is used.

Chapter

33 URETHRA AND PENIS

CONGENITAL ANOMALIES

Congenital urethral obstruction

In males the urethra can be divided into anterior and posterior parts. The posterior part includes the prostatic and membranous urethra while the anterior part consists of the bulbous and penile urethra. Obstruction can occur anywhere in the urethra from the bladder neck to the external urinary meatus.

Etiology

A wide range of congenital anomalies may be the underlying cause in infants. These include posterior urethral valves, anterior urethral valves, urethral diverticula, congenital meatal stenosis, urethral polyp and urethral atresia.

Posterior urethral valves

Posterior urethral valves are the most common cause of lower urinary tract obstruction in infants. They consist of two membranes which arise from either side of the verumontanum and fuse in the midline anteriorly.

Secondary pathology

The valves result in mechanical obstruction in the urethra, leading to secondary pathological changes in the proximal urinary tract. The proximal urethra, bladder, ureters and kidneys are affected by the back-pressure in that order. The posterior urethra gets elongated and dilated. The urinary bladder becomes hypertrophied and stiff resulting in high intravesical pressure. The back pressure results in ureteral dilatation, hydronephrosis and eventually renal failure.

Presentation

Congenital obstructive uropathies present with a wide variety of symptoms ranging from minor voiding problems to conditions incompatible with life such as overt renal failure and respiratory distress. They generally present with dysuria, weak urinary stream and retention of urine.

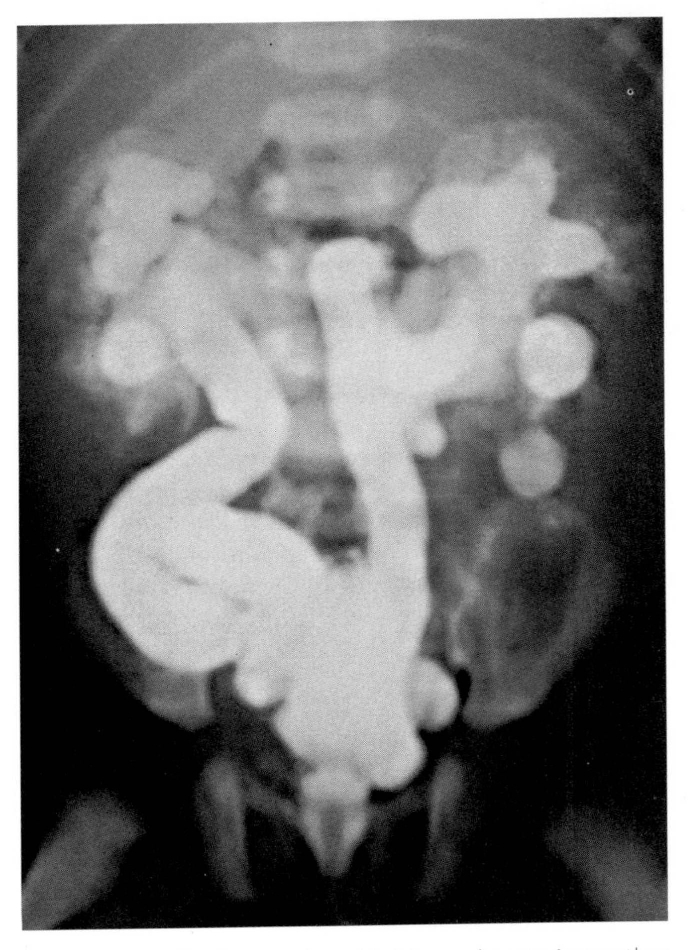

Fig.33.1 Renal pelves, ureters, bladder and posterior urethra grossly dilated due to obstruction by congenital posterior urethral valves

Diagnosis

Ultrasound demonstrates a thick-walled distended urinary bladder, with unilateral or bilateral dilatation of the ureters and kidneys. Micturating cystourethrogram (Fig.33.1) findings include hugely dilated posterior urethra, hypertrophied bladder and unilateral or bilateral vesico-ureteric reflux

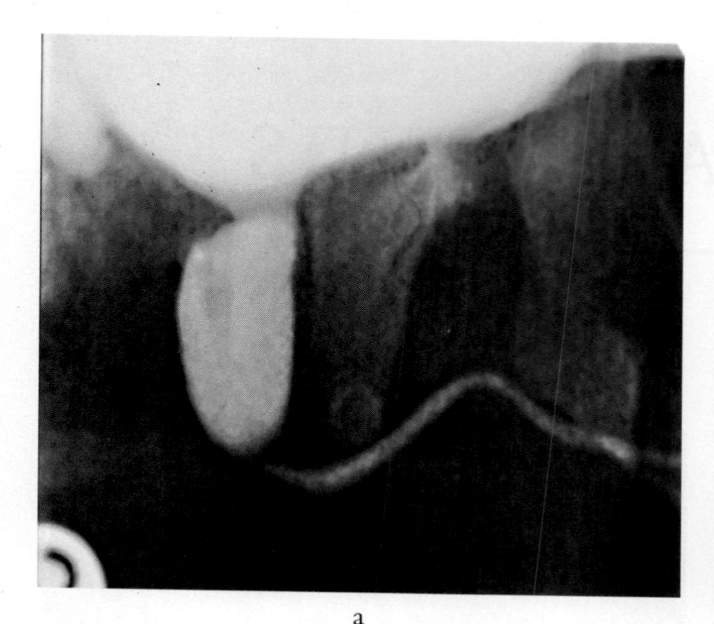

a

Fig.33.2 (a) Micturiting cystogram showing dilated posterior urethra due to congenital posterior utrethral valves, and very fine line of urine in anterior urethra

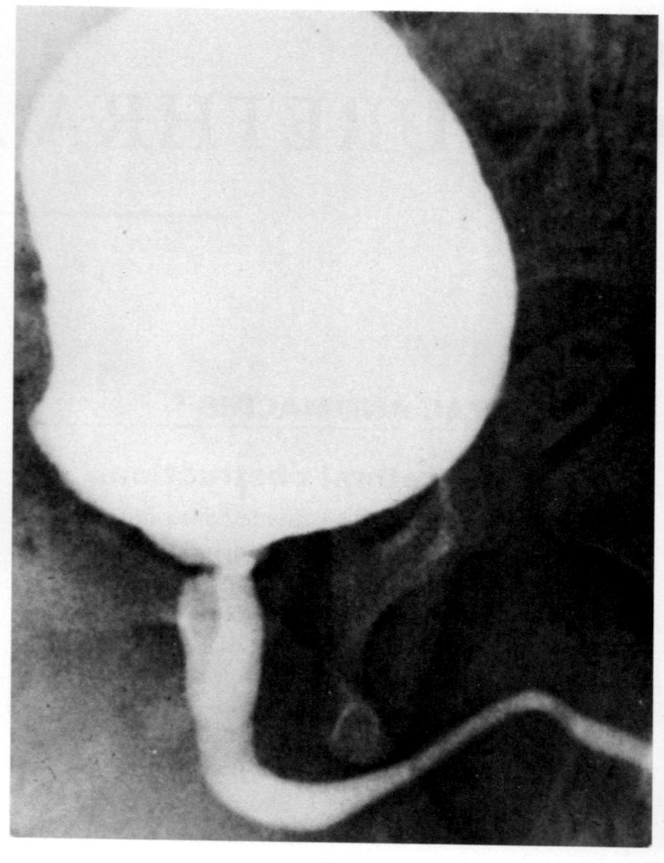

b

Fig.33.2 (b) After transurethral resection of the urethral valves. The postgerior urethra is no longer dilated and urine is flowing freely.

Treatment

The initial resuscitation includes catheterization, and management of electrolyte imbalance, septicemia and acidosis. After the patient is stabilized, the obstruction is relieved by resection of the valves through a pediatric resectoscope (Figs. 2 a and b). A few advanced cases may develop end-stage renal failure and require renal transplantation.

HYPOSPADIAS

Hypospadias is the most common congenital anomaly of the urethra, occurring once in every 350 male infants. The external meatus is located at some point on the under surface of the penis or in the perineum.

Classification

Hypospadias is classified according to the location of the urethral meatus (Table 33.1). In glandular hypospadias (Fig.33.3) the penis is straight. In all other types of hypospadias the penile shaft is curved downwards (chordee) (Fig.33.4), and the urethra and corpus spongiosum are absent distal to the external meatus. The inferior aspect of the prepuce is poorly developed.

The patient passes urine without any problem, but during adult life both sexual function and fertility are interfered with, except in glandular hypospadias. If the penis is curved markedly it is impossible to insert it into the vagina. If the urethral meatus is at the root of the penis the sperms are not deposited into the vagina on ejaculation. Fig.33.5 shows a perineal hypospadias.

Treatment

The aims of treatment in most cases are two: to straighten the penis and to carry the meatal opening to the tip of the penis. Both these aims have to do with proper coitus and placement of sperms in the depth of the vagina, otherwise as just mentioned, as far as micturition is concerned most of these children have no problem. Only rarely is the meatus narrow, when a simple meatotomy suffices.

Operations

Various surgical procedures have been described to correct hypospadias. The choice of the surgical procedure depends on the following factors:

- Location and size of the meatus.
- Presence, degree and location of chordee.
- Presence or absence of urethral plate distal to the meatus.
- Amount of the dorsal prepucial skin.

Table 33.1 Classsification of hypospadias

Name	Location of meatus
ANTERIOR HYPOSPADIAS	
Glandular	Ventral surface of the glans
Coronal	Coronal sulcus
Anterior penile	Distal third of the shaft of penis
MIDDLE HYPOSPADIAS	
Middle penile	Middle third of the shaft
POSTERIOR HYPOSPADIAS	
Posterior penile	Posterior third of the shaft
Penoscrotal	Base of the shaft in front of the scrotum
Scrotal	The scrotum
Perineal	Behind the scrotum

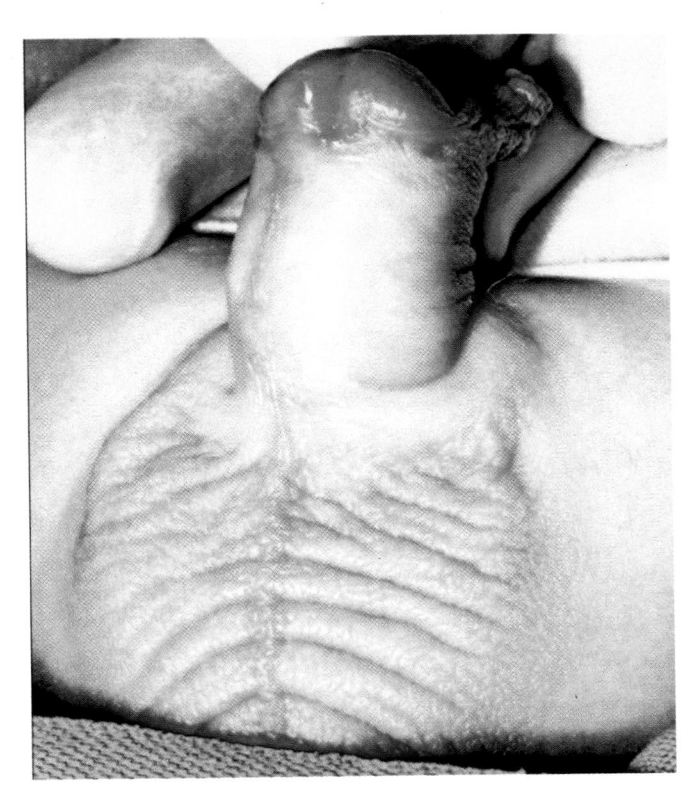

Fig.33.3 Glandular hypospadias. This is the only variety of hypospadias in which the penile shaft is straight.

In the *milder* forms, i.e. glandular and coronal hypospadias, small flaps from the under surface of the penis are adequate; they can be shifted as one-stage operations. If a good urethral plate is present distal to the meatus, it can be simply tubularized.

In the *severe* forms of hypospadias:

- In the past surgical correction used to be carried out in two stages. In the first stage the fibrous tissue on the ventral aspect of the penis was excised, allowing the penile shaft to straighten, i.e. correcting the chordee. In the second stage a skin tube was made from the ectopic meatus to the tip of the glans. The first stage was usually carried out at the age of about two, and the second stage at around four years of age.
- During recent decades the whole correction is carried out in one stage. The skin around the whole penile shaft is elevated and the fibrous tissue distal to the ectopic meatus excised, thus straightening the penis. The gap between the meatus and the tip of the glans is now filled by making a urethral tube by one of the following methods:
    - If the gap is moderate in length, a *preputial island flap* is used. A quadrangular flap is marked out of the delicate skin of the inner side of the prepuce. The subcutaneous tissue of the penis, with its contained vessels, is dissected in such a manner as to make a pedicle for the flap. This flap is now swung to the ventral side of the penis, sutured into a tube and used to make the urethra.
    - If the gap is very long, as in peno-scrotal hypospadias, a *bladder mucosal graft* is used as follows: The prevesical space is opened and the bladder muscle incised. A generous area of bladder mucosa is dissected free and removed; it is used as a free graft to make the urethral tube.
    - Recenty, *buccal mucosal graft* has been successfully used. The graft is harvested from either the cheek or the lip and used to reconstruct the urethra. This obviates the need for taking a graft from the urinary bladder.

During the operations on the penis the infiltration of 1 in 200,000 adrenaline into the subcutaneous tissues greatly reduces bleeding and facilitates the procedures.

Hypospadias surgery is extremely delicate work. It should be carried out only if one has the proper training and the temperament, otherwise more harm is done than good.

Epispadias

Epispadias is very rare, the urethra opening on the dorsum of the penis (Fig.33.6). Epispadias often coexists with bladder exstrophy.

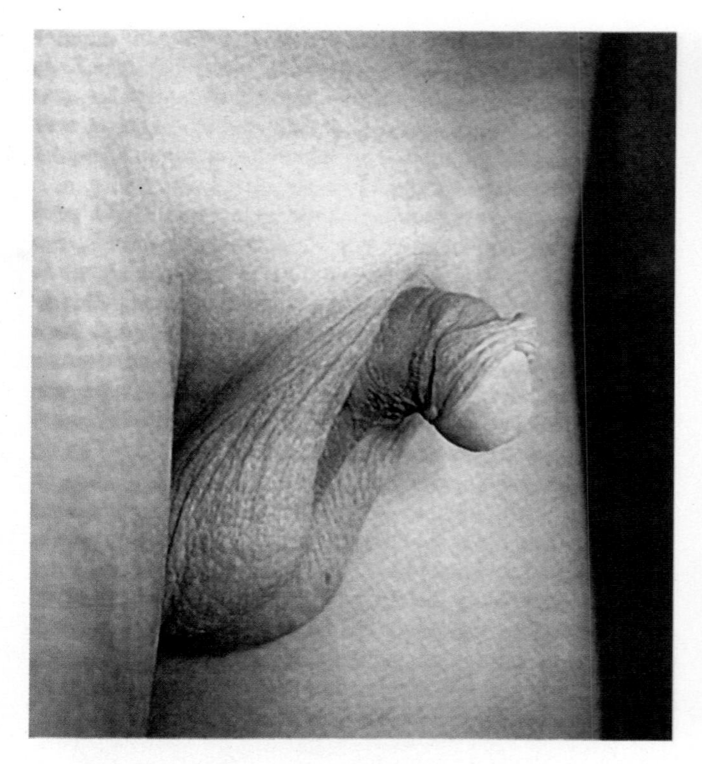

Fig.33.4 Middle penile hypospadias. The shaft of the penis is curved downwards (chordee).

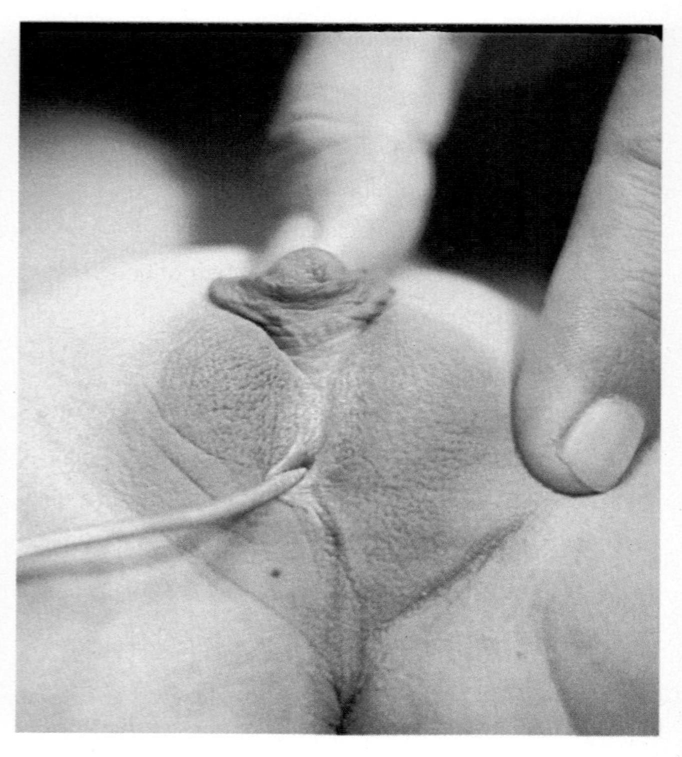

Fig.33.5 Perineal hypospadias, the orifice lying behind the split scrotal sacs, with a bougie in the urethra.

RUPTURE OF THE URETHRA

Rupture of the urethra occurs commonly at two sites: the bulbous urethra and the membranous urethra. At either site it may be complete, i.e. a transection, or incomplete, i.e. a partial tear.

Mechanism of injury and clinical features

Bulbous urethra

Rupture of the bulbous urethra is the more common accident. Nearly always it occurs due to a fall astride a projecting object, commonly either the cross-bar of a bicycle or a loose manhole cover. Another important cause of such an injury is urethral instrumentation. The patient presents with bleeding from the urethra, a painful hematoma in the perineum, and retention of urine.

Membranous urethra

Rupture of the *membranous* urethra in males occurs most commonly in association with fracture of the bony pelvis, usually due to a motor vehicle accident. A few cases occur due to falls from heights, industrial crushing injuries, and sporting accidents. The bone disruption produces a shearing force, the prostate and the puboprostatic ligaments being pulled in one direction, the membranous urethra and the urogenital diaphragm in the other.

The injury should be suspected in any patient with a pelvic fracture. Rectal examination will show the prostate to be in a higher position than normal. This 'high riding prostate' is the result of disruption of the urethra, with the prostate elevated from its normal position by a pelvic hematoma.

Urethrography

When a patient presents in the above manner it is important to find out whether the urethra has been ruptured and if so whether the tear is partial or complete. For this purpose a *retrograde urethrogram* should be carried out. A number 12F Foley catheter is passed into the urethra so that the balloon lies just inside the external meatus. About 1ml of saline is injected into the balloon to seat it in the fossa navicularis. The patient's pelvis is now rotated to an approximately 30^0 oblique position. About 25ml of 25% contrast medium is injected into the urethra, and an x-ray taken. The oblique position is best for demonstrating the entire anterior and posterior urethra; in the anteroposterior view the bulbous urethra is foreshortened and the areas of extravasation overlap the urethra, making the interpretation of the x-rays difficult.

The action taken depends upon the findings at urethrography:

- If the x-ray shows a normal urethrogram it means the urethra is not ruptured but merely contused. In such a case the catheter should be advanced into the bladder and cystography performed to rule out a bladder rupture.
- If the urethrogram shows extravasation of the dye but the urethra is in continuity and contrast material goes freely into the bladder, there is a partial rupture of the urethra.
- If extravasation is demonstrated and *urethral continuity is lost*, a complete urethral rupture is present.

Treatment

Urethral contusion

If the urethrogram is normal and a contusion without rupture is diagnosed, no special treatment is required. The patient is usually able to void normally and his hematoma clears promptly.

Partial rupture

If on urethrography there is minimal extravasation and partial urethral continuity, a catheter should be placed in the bladder for a few days to allow the tear to heal.

Complete rupture

If the urethrogram shows a complete rupture, whether of the bulbous or the membranous urethra, most surgeons these days place a suprapubic tube into the bladder. This is left in place for about six months.

Delayed repair

After the six month's delay, staged reconstructive procedures are employed. This time lag allows the extent of the stricture to declare itself and periurethral induration to subside. On the other hand patients dealt with by immediate repair have a much higher incidence of re-stricture, impotence and incontinence.

Extravasation of urine

Extravasation of urine takes place in neglected cases of rupture of the bladder or urethra.

Deep extravasation

This follows extraperitoneal rupture of the bladder or intrapelvic rupture of the (membranous) urethra. Urine extravasates in the layers of the pelvic fascia and in the retroperitoneal tissues. In these cases it is necessary to drain the prevesical space and to perform suprapubic cystostomy. Later, the treatment is as described above for rupture of the bladder and urethra.

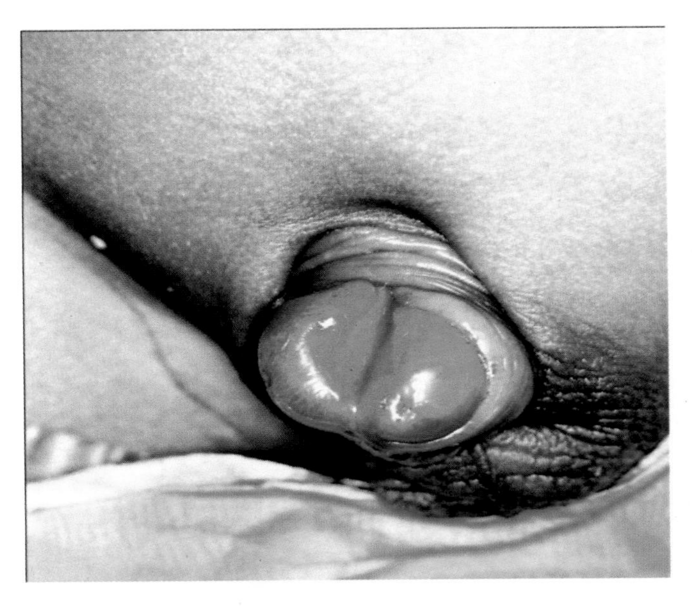

Fig.33.6 Glandular epispadias

Superficial extravasation

This takes place after rupture of the bulbous urethra. The membranous layer of superficial fascia (Colles' fascia) is attached to the triangular ligament at the midperineal point, to the ischiopubic rami and just below the inguinal ligament. Therefore, the urine cannot extend down the thighs; it collects in the subcutaneous tissues of the scrotum, penis and abdominal wall (Fig.33.7). Urgent operation is essential to eliminate spreading cellulitis and the resulting sepsis. Multiple incisions are made in the skin and superficial fascia, and antibiotics are administered. The subsequent management is by delayed (secondary) repair of the urethra.

URETHRITIS

The most common organism involved in urethritis is the gonococcus, the others being *Chlamydia trachomatis*, staphylococci, streptococci and *Trichomonas vaginalis*.

Gonococcal urethritis

The gonococcus (Neisseria gonorrhoeae) is a Gram-negative diplococcus which affects the anterior urethra in the male, and the urethra and cervix in the female. After sexual intercourse with an infected partner symptoms commence after two to ten days. At first there is discomfort on micturition, often progressing to a scalding pain. A urethral discharge appears, being seropurulent at first, then becoming purulent. In chronic cases there may be only a slight morning discharge, or slight staining of the underclothes. In some cases there

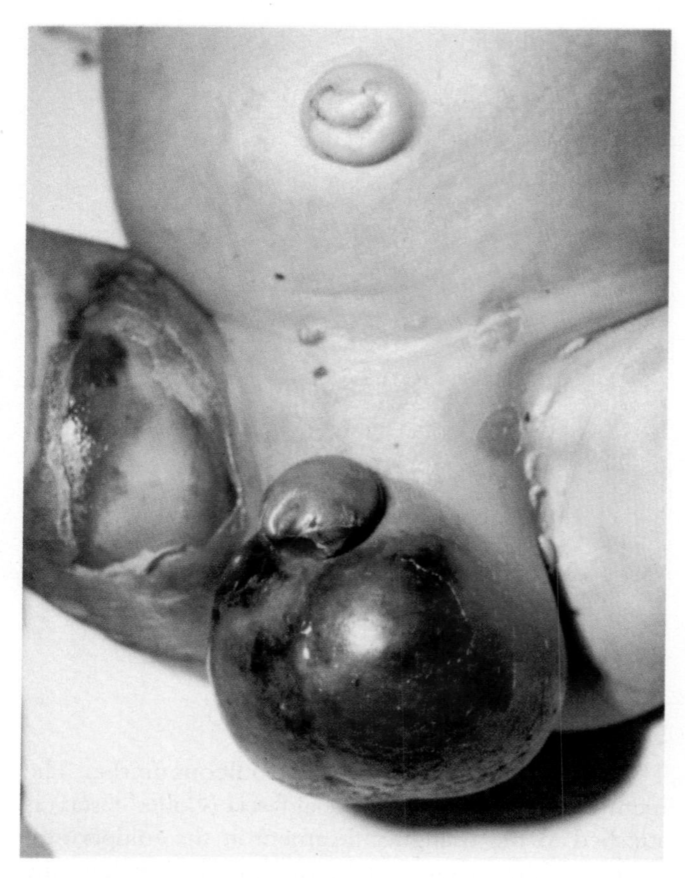

Fig.33.7 Superficial extravasation of urine. The scrotum is swollen from urine, with its skin gangrenous from ischemia due to stretching. The penis is buried in the scrotum. The attachment of Scarpa's fascia below the inguinal ligament is preventing the urine from spreading to the right thigh.

may be no symptoms at all. These are the most dangerous cases from the point of view of spread of infection to others, because the patient does not seek treatment and remains infective.

Diagnosis

Collection of discharge

A specimen of urethral discharge should be obtained from the distal urethra using calcium alginate urethral swabs inserted at least 2cm into the urethra and rotated gently. The swabs should be rolled over the slide rather than streaked, otherwise the cellular morphology may be distorted.
PCR tests are used on the discharge or on urine.

Treatment

Ceftrioxane is generally prescribed due to the gonococci having become resistant to the antibiotics in common usage.

Non-gonococcal urethritis

Patients suffering from non-gonococcal urethritis generally belong to higher socio-economic classes than those with gonococcal urethritis. However, this cannot help in the diagnosis of an individual case. Again, in general symptoms are more severe in gonorrhoea. The most common organisms responsible for non-gonococcal urethritis are chlamydiae, which are small bacteria, but like viruses they are obligatory intracellular parasites.

The drug of choice for *Chlamydia trachomatis* is oxytetracycline hydrochloride. Given in a dose of 500mg by mouth four times a day for seven days, it is highly effective. If the patient is pregnant erythromycin is preferable. It is given in the same dose and for the same duration as oxytetracycline.

Trichomonas vaginalis

This is a flagellated protozoan parasite. Its significance as a cause of genitourinary tract disease in men is controversial. It has been associated with urethritis, prostatitis, epididymitis and infertility. Routine tests for trichomoniasis are not indicated for all men with non-gonococcal urethritis. However, there are groups of men with non-gonococcal urethritis who merit investigation for trichomoniasis. These include:

- Patients whose disease has failed to respond to antibiotics, including tetracyclines.
- Men with long-standing symptoms.
- Men whose sexual partners have symptoms or signs suggesting trichomoniasis.

Treatment

Metronidazole is the drug of choice for the treatment of trichomoniasis, in a dose of 250mg by mouth, three times daily for seven days; this results in cure rates of about 95%. However, recently *T. vaginalis* organisms resistant to high levels of metronidazole have been isolated.

Complications of urethritis

Urethritis can be followed by one or more serious complications, specially epididymitis and urethral stricture.

URETHRAL STRICTURE

Urethral strictures may arise due to the following:

- Trauma.
- Inflammation, e.g. gonorrhoea.
- Instruments, e.g. indwelling catheters.

- Operations, e.g. prostatectomy.
- A few strictures are congenital lesions.

Clinical features

As a stricture develops the stream of urine becomes progressively *narrower*, so that micturition takes a longer time to be completed. Immediately after micturition *dribbling* may occur; this is due to urine trickling from the dilated urethra above the stricture.

Increased *frequency* may be seen. This is because of incomplete evacuation, so that the bladder fills up again quickly. *Cystitis* resulting from stagnation of urine may also contribute to the frequency.

The stricture may be palpable as an induration in the wall of the urethra. The back-pressure effects of urethral stricture produce dilatation of the bladder, the ureters and the kidneys.

Investigations

Urethroscopy

This allows a very definite and accurate diagnosis. False passages may also be seen, being the result of inexpert use of bougies.

Urethrography

Whereas urethroscopy can show only the lower end of a stricture, urethrography indicates not only the presence of a stricture but also its length, as the dye goes up through it to outline its upper extent (Fig.33.8). Any urethral diverticulum is also shown up.

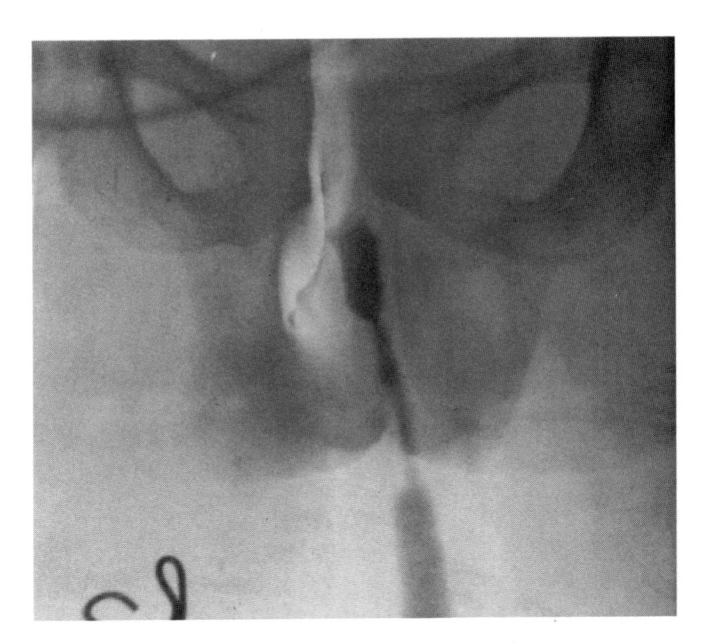

Fig.33.8 Urethrogram showing long stricture posterior perineal part of urethra.

Treatment

A urethral stricture is dealt with either by dilatation or operation.

Dilatation

Classically the treatment of a stricture consisted of repeated dilatations for many years, and sometimes for life, causing the patient a great deal of misery. They are normally carried out under local anesthesia using lignocaine gel. The bougies must be used with extreme gentleness and care to avoid making a false passage.

However, the dilatations of the past have been mostly displaced by internal urethrotomy or urethroplasty. They may still be useful with the elderly and in strictures following radical prostatectomy.

Operative treatment

This depends on the length of the stricture:

- If it is *very short* it can be divided through a urethroscope using an *internal urethrotome or laser* under direct vision. A follow-up urethroscopy can be performed at about three months, and the procedure repeated if necessary.
- A *short* stricture can be dealt with by excision and reanastomosis of the ends that are spatulated to avoid re-stricture.
- Urethroplasty. If the stricture is a *long* one it cannot be dealt with by excision and reanastomosis. In such a case, after excising the strictured urethra, a free graft of the buccal mucosa is utilized to replace the urethral tube.

Phimosis and paraphimosis

Phimosis

In phimosis the preputial orifice is abnormally small. The most common cause of this condition is congenital narrowing of the opening, the other important cause being inflammation of the lining of the prepuce.

When the patient passes urine the prepuce balloons out, and a thin stream of urine comes out. Due to difficulty in the passage of urine the bladder empties incompletely, i.e. residual urine results. Due to further back pressure hydroureter and hydronephrosis follows.

Paraphimosis

Paraphimosis results when a tight prepuce is retracted but cannot be returned. It acts as a venous tourniquet proximal to the glans, which becomes greatly swollen causing much pain and dysuria.

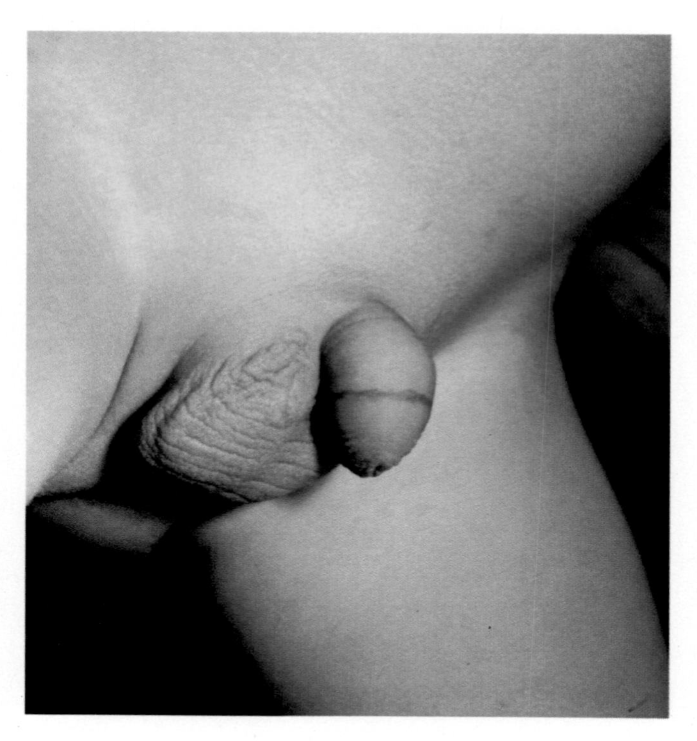

Fig.33.9 Before circumcision the line of incision on the prepuce has been marked on the penis with a pen to avoid cutting away too much skin.

Treatment

The treatment of phimosis is circumcision. In the case of paraphimosis the urgent requirement is for the relief of the constriction. As the tissues are grossly edematous the best line of action is simply to divide the constricting band by a short incision on its dorsal aspect. This allows the edema to subside, and circumcision can be performed at a convenient date a week or two later.

CIRCUMCISION

Circumcision has been practised around the world for thousands of years. Among Jews and Muslims it is carried out as a religious ritual, among other communities only if indicated on medical grounds, as in paraphimosis or for problems of hygiene.

Technique

In any circumcision at any age the line of the skin incision should first be marked by a pen to avoid removing too much skin (Fig.33.9).

Clamp device circumcision

This technique is used in newborns. The two devices commonly employed include: the Plastibell and the Gomco clamp.

Plastibell

The foreskin is freed of adhesions and a dorsal slit made in the prepuce. The Plastibell is placed over the glans. The foreskin is ligated over the groove of the bell and the prepuce is cut away. The ring separates in a few days.

Gomco clamp

In this method the circular steel clamp crushes the two layers of the preputial skin together, sealing them and also ensuring hemostasis. The redundant prepuce is cut away.

Open method

In adolescents and adults the open technique is decidedly the safest, to avoid injury to the urethral orifice. The line of the incision is marked by a pen. A circumferential incision is made in the skin along this line. The prepuce is slit dorsally in the midline. The inner lining of the resulting two flaps is now cut away leaving a 5mm margin, and the cut edges of the skin and the inner lining sutured together. Only bipolar diathermy must be used for hemostasis, to avoid thrombosis of veins at the base of the penis.

CARCINOMA OF THE PENIS

Etiology

Carcinoma of the penis is caused by chronic irritation of the glans and prepuce by smegma. This is proved by its widely varying incidence in different communities, dependent upon their practice regarding circumcision. Thus Jews practice circumcision at birth; among them carcinoma of the penis is virtually unknown. Muslims circumcise their children during infancy; among them this neoplasm is very rare. Most other communities do not circumcise their boys routinely, and penile carcinoma occurs regularly in their men.

Other risk factors include leukoplakia of the glans and penile warts due to papilloma virus.

Pathology

Carcinoma of the penis is a squamous cell carcinoma. There are two pathological types of this tumor. The first or infiltrating type often commences in an area of leukoplakia. The second type is the papilliferous variety; this usually develops in a pre-existing papilloma. The tumor grows slowly. It spreads to the inguinal, and then to the iliac lymph nodes. Distant metastases are infrequent. It is classified into four stages as in (Table 33.2).

Table 33.2 Stages of carcinoma of the penis

Stage I	Confined to the skin
Stage II	Involving corpus spongiosum or cavernosum
Stage III	Invading the urethra
Stage IV	Involving adjacent structures; occasionally, distant metastases

Clinical features

Although most patients are middle-aged, a fair number are below the age of 40. Mild irritation and discharge of pus may be followed by a blood-stained foul discharge. There is usually no pain. If untreated, the whole glans becomes a fungating, foul-smelling mass. Biopsy should be carried out to confirm the diagnosis.

Treatment

Primary tumor

Here the mainstay of treatment is surgical excision. Tumors of the glans require amputation of the glans, those with more spread need partial penile amputation. Advanced tumors are dealt with by total amputation of the penis with a perineal urethrostomy.

Lymph nodes

First a 3-week course of antibiotics is given; this causes any enlargement due to infection to subside. In the case of palpable nodes, if ultrasound-guided fine needle biopsy confirms the diagnosis, block dissection of both groins is carried out. If no nodes are palpable, for T2 or larger tumors block dissection should be performed. If pelvic nodes are enlarged on CT scan, they may require radiation or excision.

Prognosis

With tumors confined to the penis, 5-year survival rates are about 80%; with nodes involved, close to 40%.

Chapter

34 TESTIS AND SCROTUM

UNDESCENDED TESTIS

The testis originates on the posterior abdominal wall. It descends into the inguinal canal during the ninth month of fetal life, and should be fully descended in the full-term infant. If in the newborn infant the testis cannot be palpated in the scrotum the various possibilities are the following:

- **Retractile.** The testis may be retractile. This means that although the testis is normally descended, due to an overactive cremasteric reflex it retracts up into the inguinal area. The child should be examined in a relaxed atmosphere, preferably in the mother's lap, and if the weather is cold the hands should be warmed. An effort should be made to 'milk' the testis down into the scrotum. If the effort is successful it shows that the testis is normally descended and only retracts up from time to time.

  Treatment. A retractile testis needs no treatment. The parents should be reassured that no operation is necessary, and that gradually as the weight of the testis increases it will constantly hang down low in the scrotum.

- **Ectopic.** The testis may be ectopic. Such a testis has descended normally through the inguinal canal. However, its further descent into the scrotum is prevented as follows: normally the gubernaculum guides the testis downwards. It has many tails, but the strongest of these is the one which attaches it to the bottom of the scrotum. In the case of an ectopic testis one of the other tails is more thick, and pulls it down in its own direction. Thus it may come to lie at the perineum (Fig.34.1), pubic area or femoral triangle. Therefore, if the testis is missing from the scrotum and cannot be milked down from above, it should be looked for at those sites.

  Treatment. The ectopic testis should be mobilized at operation and placed in the scrotum, where it should be fixed by placing it in a dartos pouch as described below.

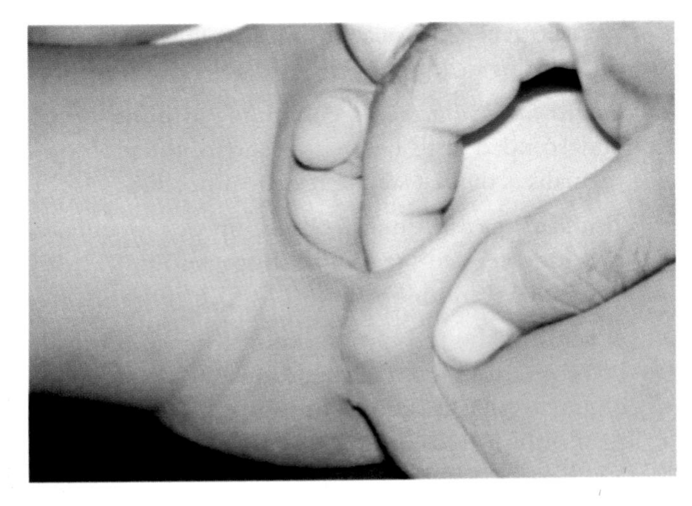

Fig.34.1 An ectopic left testis located in the perineum

- **Undescended.** The testis may be undescended. In such a case it cannot be 'milked' down, nor can it be felt at any of the above-named ectopic sites but it shall be present along the normal line of descent. It is rarely that such a testis is absent. In the vast majority of cases it is incompletely descended, and lies in the inguinal canal or just above the internal inguinal ring. In the majority of cases a hernia sac is also present.

Harmful effects of incomplete descent on the testis

- Although the testis develops in the abdomen it requires, for its normal growth and function, a temperature a few degrees lower than that prevailing inside the abdominal cavity.

  Upto the age of 18 months, the incompletely descended testis differs little in its microscopic appearance from a normal testis. After that time, due to the higher temperature of its environment, its development becomes retarded. Microscopic examination shows a reduced number of germ cells, atrophy and loss of seminiferous tubules, and gradual loss of spermatogenesis.

At puberty the incompletely descended testis is quite flabby and small, the eipthelial elements are immature, and by the age of sixteen irreversible changes have occurred in the germinal epithelium. Its power of spermatogenesis is negligible. Its internal secretory activity is also somewhat reduced, but in spite of this the secondary sex characters of the patient develop normally.

- If an undescended testis is allowed to remain indefinitely in the abdomen, the chances of its developing a *malignancy* during adult life are increased about 10 times over the general population. This 10-folds increase in risk remains so despite corrective surgery.
- *Indirect inguinal hernia* is commonly associated with undescended testis because closure of the processus vaginalis is the last step in testicular descent.
- *Testicular torsion* may occur more frequently in undescended testis because normal scrotal attachments are absent.
- A testis in the scrotum is mobile, hence relatively protected from blunt *trauma*. However, a testis in the inguinal canal is subject to injury by compression against the pubic bone.
- An empty hemiscrotum can cause adverse *psychologic* effects on a boy's body image and self esteem.

Ideally an imperfectly descended tesies should be brought down satisfactorily into the scrotum *within the first two years* of the child's life for it to function properly.

Treatment

An undescended testis should be operated upon and brought down into the scrotum. If the baby presents at birth it is usual to wait for about one year before carrying out orchidopexy, as it sometimes descends spontaneously during this period. If by the age of one year the testis has not descended into the scrotum, it is unlikely to come down at a later date, and operation should be carried out.

Current recommendations are that orchidopexy for an undescended testis should be performed between the age of 12–18 months. This practice is based on the evidence that histological damage occurs to the undescended testis after 18 months and that spontaneous descent does not occur beyond the first year of life. After the age of 3, the child becomes more and more concerned with his body image. If the undescended testis is left untreated, such children have been found to suffer from psychological symptoms and disorders such as indecision, fear, depression, etc.

Operation

- ***Orchidopexy.*** The inguinal canal is opened. Any hernia sac is ligated and excised. The spermatic vessels are gently dissected as they lie retroperitoneally on the posterior abdominal wall, to enable them to lengthen. The inferior epigastric artery and veins are ligated and divided, to allow the spermatic cord and the vas to follow a more straight course to the scrotum and thus gain length. These manoeuvres usually allow the testis to be brought down into the scrotum. It is then fixed there by making a pouch for it between the skin and the dartos muscle (*'dartos pouch'*), to prevent it from retracting upwards after the operation.
- If the testicular vessels are so short that the testis cannot be brought down fully, one of the following courses may be adopted:
    - ***Two-stage orchidopexy.*** The testis is brought down as far as possible, and is anchored with a non-absorbable suture. After a year or more, further mobilization is carried out.
    - ***Fowler-Stephen orchidopexy.*** The testicular vessels are divided, and the testis brought down into the scrotum (Fowler-Stephen procedure). The testis is usually adequately supplied through the arteries of the vas and the cremaster muscle. However, it should be clearly understood by all concerned that *a certain number of testes undergo atrophy after this operation.* To reduce the incidence of such atrophy, the vessels may be divided first, and the orchidopexy carried out after some time. This procedure is most suited to an intra-abdominal testis with its very short vessels.
    - ***Microvascular autotransplantation.*** The abnormally short testicular vessels may be divided at the lower pole of the kidney and anastomosed to the origins of the inferior epigastric artery and vein by the use of microvascular techniques, thus gaining very valuable length.
    - ***Orchidectomy.*** If the undescended testis is completely atrophic or the patient has presented after puberty and the other testis is normal, orchidectomy is carried out to prevent the development of malignancy, which arises a great deal more commonly in the undescended testis than in the normally placed organ.

Bilateral cryptorichidism

If only one testis is undescended, the cause is likely to be a mechanical block to descent, and has to be treated by operation; it is unlikely to be hormonal deficiency,

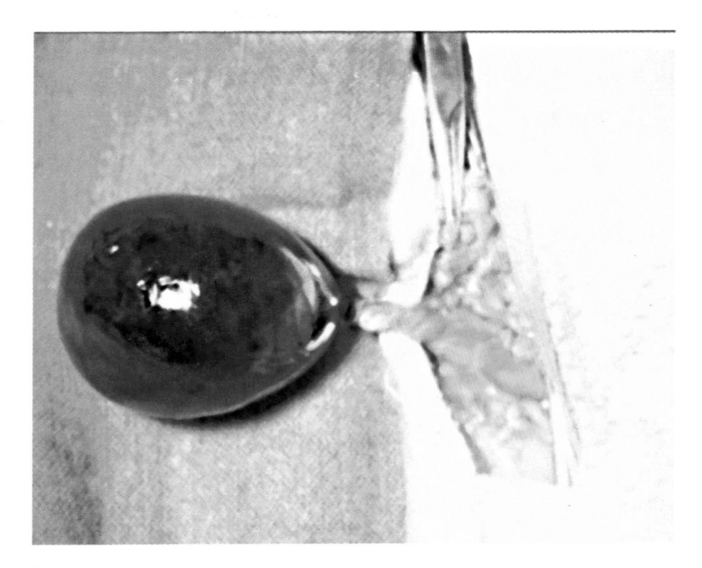

Fig.34.2 Torsion testis

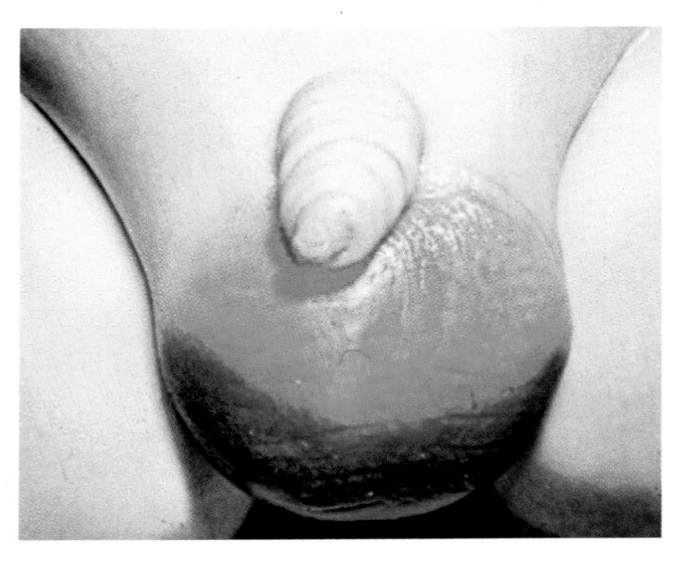

Fig.34.3 Torsion testis

because if that was the case the other testis would also be undescended. On the other hand if both testis are incompletely descended it is more likely that a deficiency of hormones is responsible. Therefore biweekly injections of chorionic gonadotrophin, extracted from the placenta, are given for six to eight weeks. Longer courses are not employed, otherwise secondary sex characters may develop prematurely. If hormonal treatment fails to bring the testes down, after waiting for a few months they must be brought down by operation, carried out either together or one side after the other.

Non-palpable testis

A non-palpable testis may be either located intra-abdominally, or it may be absent. A testis is absent either because of testicular agenesis or testicular atrophy secondary to testicular torsion in utero ('vanished testis'). Surgery for a non-palpable testis has two goals:

- Diagnostic, to identify whether a testis is present or absent.
- Therapeutic; if the testis is found, to carry out orchidopexy.

Diagnostic laparoscopy

This is the most definite way to locate an abdominal testis. If the facility is not available, a CT or MRI scan may be obtained, although their yield is not optimal.

Therapeutic options

Various options for an intra-abdominal testis include:

- Fowler-Stephen orchidopexy.
- Microvascular autotransplantation.
- Laparoscopic single stage orchidopexy.
- Laparoscopic staged Fowler-Stephen orchidopexy.
- Testicular remnant ('nubbin') orchidectomy.

Testicular prosthesis

If orchidectomy is performed for an atrophic testis, or if a testis is absent, a testicular prosthesis may be placed in the scrotum to avoid the psychological impact of an empty scrotum.

TORSION OF THE TESTIS

Occasionally a testis undergoes torsion around its longitudinal axis (Fig.34.2). A painful swelling develops (Fig.34.3), and if left untreated the testis undergoes infarction (Fig.34.4) followed by atrophy. Torsion does not occur in a normal testis. In cases in which torsion occurs, either the tunica vaginalis extends to a high level so that the testis hangs within the tunica, or the testis is separated from the epididymis and twists around the mesentery joining it to the epididymis.

Clinical features

Torsion commonly occurs between the ages of ten and twenty five years; it is also seen during infancy. There is sudden agonizing pain in the groin with vomiting. If the testis is incompletely descended and lying in the groin the painful swelling may be mistaken for a strangulated inguinal hernia. Torsion of the fully descended testis has to be distinguished from acute epididymo-orchitis. The testes may have a horizontal lie within the scrotum. Elevation of the testis usually relieves the pain in epididymitis but increases it in torsion.

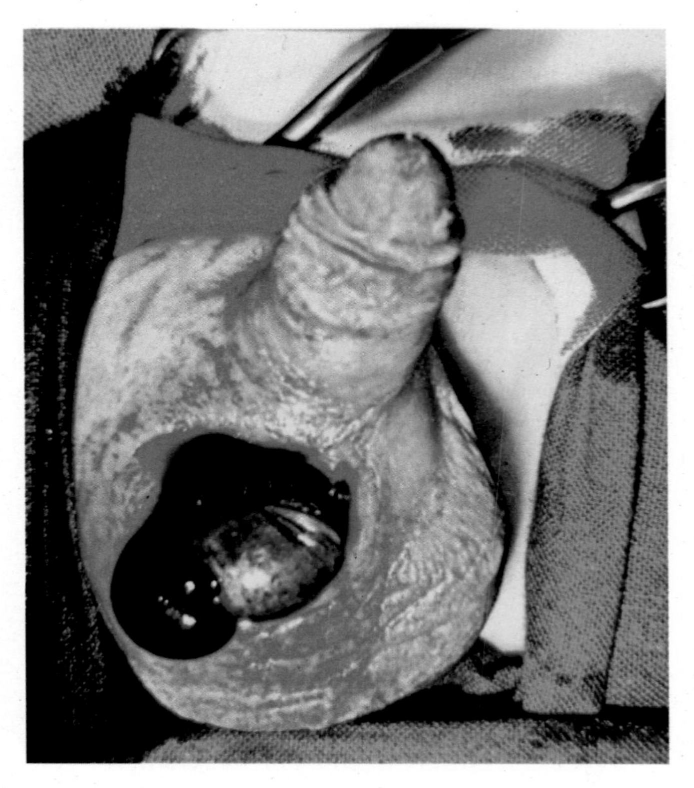

Fig.34.4 Gangrenous testis delivered at operation, resulting from a neglected case of torsion

In case of doubt, diagnostic studies such as the following can distinguish between torsion and epididymitis:

- *Colour Doppler sonography.*
- *Nuclear scan testicular flow studies.*

However, if torsion is strongly suspected, time should not be wasted in such investigations and surgical exploration should be carried out urgently.

Treatment

Management should be on clinical grounds. If there is any suspicion of torsion, immediate surgical exploration of the scrotum should be carried out. After detorsion the testis is fixed in position by placing it in a dartos pouch, i.e. between the dartos and the scrotal skin. The opposite testis should also be fixed at the same time, as the anatomical variation responsible for the torsion is likely to be bilateral.

VARICOCELE

In some young adults the veins of the pampiniform plexus become varicose; this condition is called a varicocele. The left side is affected in 95% of cases (Fig.34.5). Occasionally a varicocele occurs in middle age, due to obstruction of the left testicular vein by the growth of a renal carcinoma along the left renal vein. In such a case the kidneys must be investigated.

Clinical features

A varicocele may produce no symptoms, but in some cases the patient experiences a dragging pain on the affected side. Due to its increased weight, the scrotum hangs lower than normal and on palpation the dilated, tortuous veins feel like worms in a bag. The testes may be slightly smaller than the opposite side, due to a minor degree of atrophy. When the patient lies down the veins empty in lower grades of varicocele. However, a varicocele which is due to a renal carcinoma does not empty on lying down.

Many men suffering from varicocele are subfertile. This is because of the fact that due to venous congestion and the excessive volume of blood in the parts the temperature in the scrotum is raised. The ideal temperature for spermatogenesis is a few degrees lower than that prevailing in the internal organs. This rise in temperature reduces the sperm count and motility and reduces fertility. After a successful operation for this condition both these values improve.

Treatment

An asymptomatic varicocele requires no treatment. For discomfort, embolization of the testicular veins can be first employed. If the varicocele recurs, inguinal or suprainguinal ligation of the testicular veins is carried out. This procedure can also be done laparoscopically. After this operation the sperm count and the conception rate both show improvement, although recurrence occurs in some cases.

HYDROCELE

A hydrocele is the collection of serous fluid in some part of the processus vaginalis. It may be congenital or acquired:

Congenital

A hydrocele may be a congenital lesion, due to persistence of a part of the processus vaginalis. It presents during the neonatal period or infancy, and may take one of three forms:

- ***Congenital hydrocele***: The processus vaginalis persists in its entirety, its upper end remaining open to the peritoneal cavity (Fig.34.6a). In most cases this opening is very small so a hernia does not develop. For the same reason such a hydrocele cannot be emptied by squeezing it. However, when the patient is recumbent while asleep, the hydrocele empties gradually during the night so that it is smaller in the

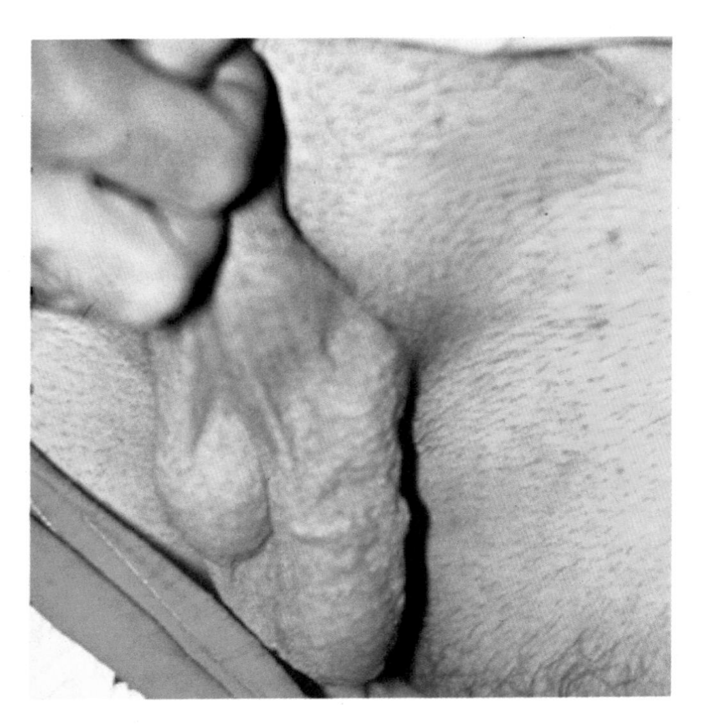

Fig.34.5 Varicocele. The lesion is on the left side, as is found in the vast majority of cases.

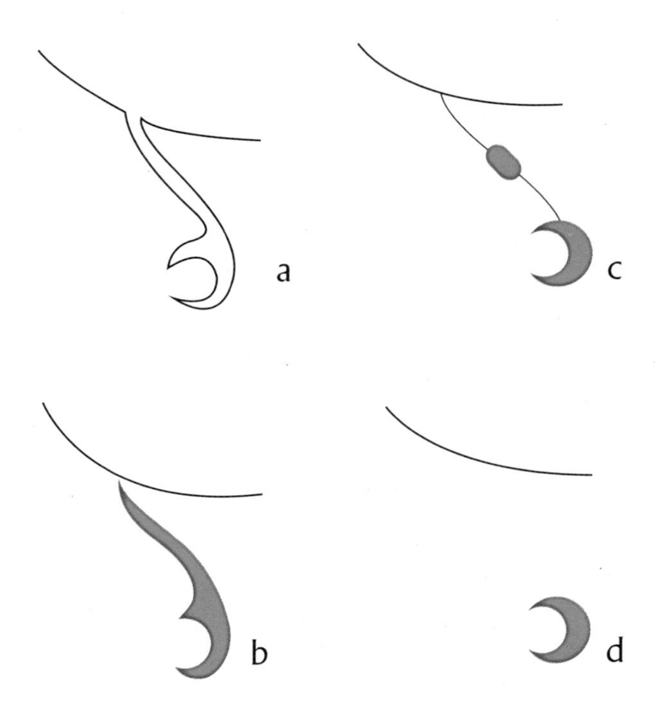

Fig.34.6 Hydroceles (a) congenital (b)infantile (c) encysted (d) vaginal

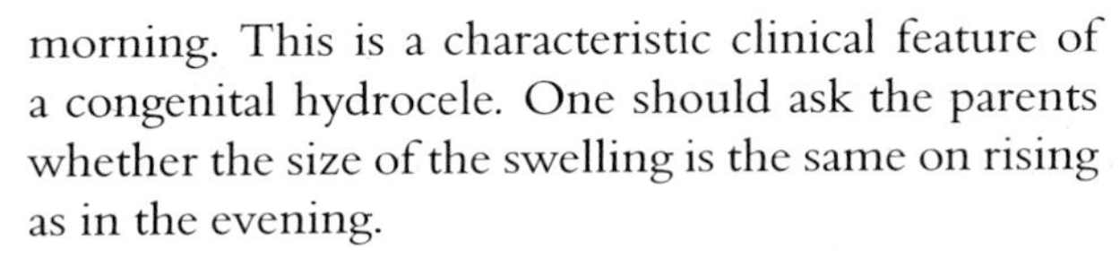

morning. This is a characteristic clinical feature of a congenital hydrocele. One should ask the parents whether the size of the swelling is the same on rising as in the evening.

- ***Infantile hydrocele***. Here also the whole of the processus vaginalis persists, but its upper end is closed (Fig.34.6b). The size of this type of hydrocele remains constant irrespective of the time of the day.
- ***Encysted hydrocele of the cord.*** Here the middle portion of the processus vaginalis persists while both the upper and lower portions become obliterated, so that a smooth oval cystic swelling results (Fig.34.6c). If gentle traction is applied to the testis the swelling moves downwards and becomes less mobile, confirming the diagnosis. Unlike the first two varieties an encysted hydrocele does not always present soon after birth but may appear later due to collection of fluid in the pre-existing sac. Because the infant skin is quite thin, these hydroceles are usually *brilliantly transilluminant.*

Acquired

Later in life a hydrocele may be acquired, when it may be either primary (idiopathic) or secondary. As it consists of a collection of fluid in the tunica vaginalis it is called a vaginal hydrocele:

- *Primary vaginal hydrocele (Fig.34.6d).* This is the hydrocele which occurs in adults, and is commonly seen in middle-aged men. Its cause is not known but is considered to be lymphatic obstruction. The only complaint of the patient is the swelling, therefore he sometimes allows it to become very large before seeking relief. On examination the swelling is fluctuant and transilluminant. Unlike an inguinal hernia which comes down into the scrotum from above, in a hydrocele it is possible to 'get above the swelling' at the root of the scrotum. In actual practice this means that if the testes is held in the hand, with the index finger behind the root of the scrotum and the thumb in front of it, the two can be made to meet above the swelling. Unlike the congenital types of hydrocele the primary vaginal variety is always confined to the tunica vaginalis.
- *Secondary hydrocele.* This is merely an effusion into the tunica vaginalis resulting from certain diseases of the testis, of which the common ones include:
    - o Acute epididymo-orchitis.
    - o Chronic (usually tuberculous) epididymo-orchitis.
    - o Malignant tumors of the testes.
    - o Trauma.

Such a hydrocele rarely attains a large size, so the testis and epididymis can usually be palpated through it.

Ultrasound examination

If a clinician uses the relevant clinical methods, i.e. palpation, percussion, fluctuation, and transillumination properly, he does not need the help of an ultrasound examination to find out whether a hydrocele is present or not, and whether it is primary or secondary. However in a doubtful case an ultrasound examination helps elucidate the situation. It is to be hoped that the advent of diagnostic methods like ultrasound will not result in clinicians losing interest in the classical clinical methods, which can provide the same information immediately, without any cost, and anywhere.

Treatment

Congenital hydrocele

In congenital and infantile hydroceles the processus vaginalis commonly becomes obliterated over a period of 12 to 18 months. Therefore it is usual not to operate upon a hydrocele during the first two years of life unless a hernia cannot be excluded with certainty. After the age of two, if the hydrocele has not resolved it should be operated upon. The operation of choice for congenital hydroceles is high ligation of the processus vaginalis, as for inguinal hernia. The distal part of the sac is laid open but no attempt is made to remove it. Reaccumulation of fluid in the distal sac is rare.

Primary vaginal hydrocele

If left untreated a vaginal hydrocele may continue to enlarge. It may be the seat of hemorrhage or infection, and sometimes calcification occurs in its wall. In the days before surgery became safe, this hydrocele of adults was treated by repeated tapping. The sac used to refill, and over a number of years the wall became thick and less translucent, so that aspirations became more difficult. Today there is little justification for treating a hydrocele by tapping, except in patients with coexisting severe medical conditions.

Lord's operation

The treatment of a vaginal hydrocele is by operation, the most popular procedure being Lord's operation, especially when the sac is thin-walled. An incision is made through the skin and the coverings of the testis including the tunica vaginalis, so that the hydrocele sac is opened. A series of fine catgut sutures are placed radially all round from the cut edge of the tunica to the vicinity of the testis. When these sutures are tied the whole hydrocele sac gets imbricated into a narrow fringe around the testis. The secretory surface is thus greatly reduced.

Because very little dissection of tissues is required, only a moderate degree of edema occurs and the post-operative course is smooth. In any case the patient should be warned that some edema will result.

An alternative procedure for hydrocele is *Jaboulay's operation,* in which the sac is everted and its flaps stitched together behind the testis.

Secondary hydrocele

The treatment of a secondary hydrocele is the treatment of the underlying condition responsible for it, e.g. tuberculosis, tumor, etc.

EPIDIDYMO-ORCHITIS

Epididymitis nearly always arises due to spread of infection from the urinary tract. Further, such an infection very commonly spreads to the testis, so that the condition is more accurately termed an epididymo-orchitis.

Acute epididymo-orchitis

Acute epididymo-orchitis:

- Follows non-gonorrhoeal urethritis more commonly than gonorrhoea.
- It can also follow any form of urethral instrumentation, e.g. catheterization, bougienage, cystoscopy, etc.

The initial symptoms are those of acute prostatitis. When epididymitis supervenes there is severe pain in the testis and groin, along with fever. The scrotal skin becomes red and edematous. The swelling of the epididymis may soften and discharge pus. Resolution of the swelling may take many weeks.

Treatment

Strict bed rest is the first essential part of treatment. More pain is felt in the scrotum if it hangs down, therefore scrotal support should be provided. Urine is sent for culture, and doxycycline or ciprofloxacin are started. When the culture report arrives the antibiotic may have to be changed. Antibiotics are continued for two weeks or more, as necessary. If pus forms drainage must be carried out.

Chronic epididymo-orchitis.

Non-tuberculous

This results from unresolved epididymo-orchitis. There is discomfort and the epididymis is thickened. For treatment, the same antibiotics are used as for the acute condition, but for four weeks.

Tuberculous

This accounts for nearly 90% of cases of chronic epididymo-orchitis; the infection has usually spread to the epididymis from the urinary tract. The onset is nearly always gradual. Commonly a single nodule is noticed in the epididymis.

Diagnosis

In every case the urine and serum must be examined for tubercle bacilli by Lowenstein-Jensen culture and guinea-pig inoculation.

Imaging

Imaging of the urinary tract and chest x-ray should be performed to rule out pulmonary and renal tuberculosis respectively. Culture of the semen may sometimes help diagnose a case.

Treatment

If a primary lesion is found in the urinary tract or lungs, its treatment should take priority, and the epididymitis will also resolve. If there is no sign of resolution within about three months of antituberculosis treatment, the drug regimen may be changed. However, if there is still no improvement, epididymectomy or orchidectomy should be carried out, but the course of antituberculosis drugs is continued for its full recommended duration.

MALIGNANT NEOPLASMS OF THE TESTIS

About 99% of tumors of the testis are malignant. Of these, the common ones are seminoma and teratoma. These together constitute about 80% of cancers of the testicle. Combined seminoma and teratoma accounts for another 10%. The remaining few neoplasms include interstitial tumors, lymphomas, etc.

Age incidence

A teratoma occurs at a younger age than a seminoma; the peak of its incidence is seen in the third decade, that of seminomas in the fourth decade. An imperfectly descended testis is about 10 times more prone to become malignant than a normally placed one.

Pathology

Most testicular tumors arise from the germ cells. They are often characterized by two types of primitive cells, the trophoblast and the yolk-sac cells. When trophoblast is present b-human chorionic gonadotrophin (b-HCG) is produced; when yolk-sac cells are present, alpha-fetoprotein is formed. These two substances act as tumor markers for these neoplasms.

Seminoma

A seminoma arises from the mediastinum of the testis. The testis is firm and smooth, and on section it is homogenous and pink or cream in colour. In rapidly growing seminomas areas of necrosis may be present. Histologically, rounded cells with clear cytoplasm and large rounded nuclei are seen, the cells being arranged in sheets. Infiltration by lymphocytes suggests a good host reaction and better prognosis. Seminomas spread mostly to lymph nodes, blood spread being rare.

Teratoma

These tumors arise in the rete testis from totipotent cells and therefore elements of ectoderm, mesoderm and endoderm are usually represented, although one of these commonly predominates. This tumor may attain a very large size. The cut section is yellowish in colour, and shows cystic spaces containing gelatinous fluid. Cartilaginous nodules may be present.

The *histological types* of teratoma graded in order of increasing malignancy include:

- Differentiated.
- Intermediate.
- Anaplastic.
- Trophoblastic.

The anaplastic type may show elevated levels of alpha-fetoprotein, while in the trophoblastic type raised levels of human chorionic gonadotrophins may be seen. As mentioned above, as the presence of these hormones in the serum helps to indicate the presence of these tumors, they are tumor markers.

Mixed cytology

Although classically testicular tumors have been classified as above, it is becoming clear that different malignant tissues are often present in a single tumor, which is partly seminoma and partly teratoma, and the behaviour of the tumor depends on how much of each type of tissue is present. The presence of yolk sac or trophoblastic tissue in a tumor is associated with a worse prognosis than the presence of differentiated tissue.

Interstitial cell tumors

These are rare tumors that arise either from the Leydig or Sertoli cells. The former type masculinize the patient, the latter causes feminization.

Clinical features

Presenting symptoms

- Commonly, the patient presents with a *painless swelling*, with a sense of heaviness. Unfortunately, upto one-third of testicular tumors are misdiagnosed on the first clinical assessment. The common errors in diagnosis arise from the presence of pain or hydrocele or a history of trauma. It should be remembered that pain may result from hemorrhage into the tumor, a hydrocele often accompanies a neoplasm, and the 'trauma' may have merely focussed attention on the tumor.

- The presenting symptoms may be due only to *metastases*, e.g. chest pain, dyspnoea and hemoptysis with pulmonary metastases.

Rate of growth

The rate of growth of tumors of the testis varies greatly. Occasionally a teratoma may have been present for two or three years. On the other hand metastases from a highly malignant tumor may kill the patient within a few weeks (hurricane type of tumor). Similarly, a rapidly growing tumor may be mistaken for a case of epididymo-orchitis.

Examination

On examination the testis is enlarged, firm and smooth. Testicular sensation is lost very early. However, the testis should not be squeezed firmly, as this may result in dissemination of cells. A secondary hydrocele is present in a few cases.

The cord may be thickened due to hypertrophy of the cremaster, which results from the excessive work this muscle has to do to support the heavy testes.

The *abdomen* should be palpated to detect enlarged para-aortic lymph nodes just above the umbilicus; grossly enlarged para-aortic lymph nodes may be painful. The *liver* is palpated to find out if it is enlarged. The *left supraclavicular region* is examined, as spread via the thoracic duct may lead to enlargement of a lymph node at that site.

Staging

Cancers of the testis can be classified into four stages, depending upon the extent of spread (Table 34.1).

Note: Stage II is further subdivided into a, b and c depending upon whether the nodes are less than 2cm, 2 to 5cm or more than 5cm in diameter.

Investigations

Imaging

Ultrasound often supports the clinical diagnosis by showing that the mass is solid. *Abdominal ultrasound* and *CT scan* demonstrate the spread of a testicular tumor.

An *x-ray chest* shows any metastases in the lungs, which are common in the case of teratomas.

Table 34.1 Stages of carcinoma of testis

Stage	Description
Stage I:	Lesion in testis only.
Stage II:	Nodes involved below diaphragm.
Stage III:	Nodes involved above diaphragm.
Stage IV:	Pulmonary, hepatic or distant metastases.

Tumor markers

The levels of HCG, AFP and LDH are determined. When raised, they are used to follow the response to the treatment. They are repeated after orchidectomy to assess the completeness of the tumor removal.

Treatment

Successful management of testicular tumors demands careful clinical examination, a high index of suspicion and prompt inguinal exploration if the diagnosis is suggested by the physical findings; the typical testicular tumor feels stony hard and heavy.

Orchiectomy

The primary treatment of choice for tumors of the testis is orchiectomy. This is carried out through a high inguinal incision. Soft clamps are applied over the spermatic cord in the inguinal canal to prevent venous dissemination of cancer cells, and the testicle is mobilized for inspection and frozen section biopsy, if necessary. If the diagnosis of testicular tumor is confirmed the testis is removed along with the entire spermatic cord.

Further management

Further management depends upon the results of the investigations and the histopathology report.

Seminomas

Seminomas are very radio-sensitive tumors.

- In stages I and II excellent results are obtained by irradiation.
- In stages III and IV on the other hand, chemotherapy is employed. The commonly used regimen consists of bleomycin, etoposide and cisplatin. These are toxic agents which require close supervision. Gastrointestinal, bone marrow, and skin toxic effects are common.

If a seminoma has negative markers and no detectable metastases, orchidectomy should be followed by radiotherapy of 3000 cGy to the retroperitoneal lymph nodes; however, newer modalities of follow-up and treatment are now also available.

Survival rate following this is almost 100 percent.

Non-seminomatous germ cell tumors (NSGCTs)

In the recent past the treatment of teratomas used to be by orchidectomy with radiotherapy or retroperitoneal node dissection. The radiotherapy and node dissection have now been replaced by platinum-based combination chemotherapy using bleomycin, etiposide and cis-platinum. After adequate chemotherapy the patients are re-staged; if persistent bulky disease is present this is resected surgically. The course to be followed after orchidectomy is determined as follows:

In stage I disease:

- If tumor markers i.e. AFP and HCG are negative, no treatment should be given but a close follow-up instituted.
- If the markers are positive the patient should be treated with chemotherapy until they become negative.

In stage II, III and IV disease:

- Four to six cycles of chemotherapy are given.
- After this if the markers return to normal but a mass persists, surgical excision of the residual disease should be carried out.

Prognosis

Seminomas

In cases without metastases as many as 95–100% patients survive five years. If metastases are present the figure drops to 75%.

Teratomas

In stages 1 and 2, 85% survive for five years; in stages 3 and 4, only 60%.

Choriocarcinoma

Most patients with choriocarcinomas are dead within two years despite intensive therapy.

Section

3

MUSCULOSKELETAL SYSTEM

Chapter

35 FRACTURES AND DISLOCATIONS

This chapter describes the general principles of management of fractures and dislocations; individual injuries to the limbs are detailed in the next chapter.

Definitions

A ***fracture*** is defined as a break in the continuity of a bone produced by forces that exceed the ultimate strength of a bone. The relative position of the distal segment to the proximal is called *displacement* and the relative tilt is called *angulation.*

A ***dislocation*** consists of a displacement, in relation to each other, of the bone ends taking part in a joint. A complete loss of contact between two articular surfaces is called *dislocation*, while a partial loss of contact between articular surfaces is called *subluxation*.

A ***sprain*** is the stretch or tear of a ligament

A ***strain*** is injury to a tendon or muscle.

When a fracture is sustained, a major soft tissue injury usually accompanies it. The surgeon must be familiar with the soft tissues, e.g. nerves and blood vessels, adjacent to a fracture and must look out for damage to them. If the fracture has resulted from violent trauma, the surgeon must examine the patient thoroughly for injuries to other organs. At the same time he should remember that multiple fractures, even when closed, can cause shock from internal hemorrhage.

MECHANISM AND CLASSIFICATION OF FRACTURES

Bone is relatively brittle, yet it has sufficient strength and resilience to withstand considerable stress. Fractures result from:

- A single traumatic incident.
- Repetitive stress.
- Abnormal weakening of a bone (pathological fracture).

A direct force usually produces a transverse fracture i.e. simple fracture. A more severe trauma or crush results in multiple pieces of the bone called a comminuted fracture.

Open and closed fractures

When the fracture hematoma communicates with the external or internal environment, this is called an **open** fracture. When no such wound is present the fracture is classified as closed. *This distinction is very important.* Open fractures are likely to be contaminated with pyogenic bacteria, and this can result in bone infection. Therefore their treatment is much more detailed than that of closed fractures.

Types of fractures

Forces applied in different directions result in different types of fractures:

- A bending force applied to a long bone usually produces a *transverse* or *oblique* fracture line.
- In *oblique* fractures the fracture line is at some angle to the transverse plane of the bone.
- A direct blow or crushing force often produces a *comminuted* open fracture, along with severe soft tissue injury.
- A torsion (twisting) force applied to bone produces a *spiral* fracture. The mechanism of a spiral fracture can be demonstrated by holding a piece of chalk between the two hands and twisting it; the cut ends have the same shape as the bone suffering a spiral fracture.
- A compression force applied along the long axis of a bone results in an *impacted* fracture at the junction between the metaphysis and diaphysis; the cortical bone of the diaphysis gets impacted into the cancellous bone of the metaphysis.
- Finally, violent muscle contraction may produce an *avulsion* of a portion of bone where a tendon is attached.

Pathological fracture

If the bone is weakened by some condition it may break after a trivial injury. Such a fracture is called a pathological fracture:

- The most common cause of a pathological fracture is a secondary tumor deposit from a carcinoma. Other causes include:
- Senile osteoporosis of the elderly.
- Infection.
- Metabolic bone-wasting diseases.
- Finally, healthy bone may fracture with repeated minor trauma. Such fractures are called *stress* or *fatigue* fractures; the most common example is a fracture of the second metatarsal after a long march, where moderate stress repeated thousands of times ultimately breaks the bone.

Signs of a fracture

These are the following:

- There is severe *pain* at the fracture site.
- The patient is *unable to use* the part.
- The site of the fracture is *tender*.
- Within a few hours *swelling* and bruising appear.
- If the bone ends are displaced, *deformity* is present.
- *Abnormal movement* can be elicited at the fracture site.
- *Crepitus* can also be elicited. This is a grating sensation when the bone ends are moved against each other. However, both crepitus and abnormal movement cause much pain. Therefore they should not be elicited.

Associated problems

The clinician should not focus his attention only on the break in the bone. He should be aware that fractures in general, and major and multiple fractures in particular, can be accompanied by widespread effects:

- Locally, the injury has often damaged different soft tissues.
- Systemically, compounds released fom the injured site can produce serious effects on different organ systems.

Systemic effects of skeletal injuries

Fractures may produce major systemic efects:

- Major skeletal injuries may be acompanied by massive bleeding, accumulation of extravascular fluid, and hypovolemic shock. Fractures of the femur or pelvis result in loss of 500to 1000ml of fluid into the tissues.
- *Fat embolism*. Fat and other substances released from the injured site may result in impaired lung function in the *'fat embolism syndrome'*.
- Multiple fractures continue to bleed and accumulate fluid. They cause pain and generate systemically active mediators that predispose to gut disorders, a sepsis-like state, and the *multiple organ dysfunction syndrome*, with a high mortality rate.

Local effects

Fractures sometimes cause significant local effects:

Immobility

- Fractures imposing *immobility* increase the risk of deep vein thrombosis, with potential for life-threatening pulmonary embolism and chronic venous insufficiency.
- Fractures heal slowly, sometimes taking months before full function can be allowed.
- *Prolonged bed rest* required in major fractures of the axial skeleton results in disuse osteoporosis, joint stiffness, pressure sores, as well as cardio-respiratory deconditioning and psychological stresses.

If surgical stabilization can allow use of the injured part, it helps.

Vascular injuries

Vascular injuries accompanying fractures may cause hemorrhage, ischemia or both, and the examiner must look for pallor, coldness, empty veins, paraesthesias, paralysis, and pain persisting after fracture immobilization.

Arterial injuries threatening ischemia require immediate repair. This should be followed by distal fasciotomies, because post-ischemic swelling produces compartment syndromes and the nerves passing through the zone of injury may be damaged.

Multiple injuries

Cases with multiple injuries require x-rays of the cervical spine, chest and pelvis; and may need CT scan of the skull, diagnostic peritoneal lavage or abdominal CT, and bladder catheterization.

Examination

Evaluation of the limb must be thorough, with examination for swelling, wounds, deformity, instability and ischemia.

X-rays

These should be taken as required; *they should include the joint above and below* the suspected fracture.

Compartment syndrome

A compartment syndrome is a condition in which accumulating fluid and/or external compression creates high pressure within a closed fascial space, reducing perfusion of the tissues within that compartment below a level necessary for viability. This is one of the most serious complications of trauma to a limb.

Muscle groups in the extremities are bound by tough, unyielding fascial envelopes called compartments. If muscle swelling occurs due to fractures, bleeding, surgery or blunt trauma, interstitial fluid pressure rises to a level greater than that of the draining veins. A vicious circle is established, with increasing capillary leakage and increasing pressure. Loss of capillary bed perfusion causes local muscle and nerve ischemia even though arterial flow is continuing and pulses are palpable.

Volkmann's ischemic contracture

This is the end state of neglected acute compartment syndrome with irreversible muscle necrosis leading to ischemic contractures, paralyzed and shortened muscles and impaired sensation producing severe disability. Unconscious patients, and those with peripheral nerve injuries, are particularly at risk as they are insensitive to the ischemic pain.

Clinical signs of compartment syndrome include:

- Pain that is greater than expected from the primary clinical problem, such as a fracture or contusion.
- Pain on passive stretch of involved muscles.
- Swollen and tense compartment on palpation.

Intracompartmental pressure

Raised tissue pressure is the primary event in acute compartment syndrome; thus, changes in intracompartmental pressure (ICP) will *precede* the clinical symptoms and signs. If the diagnosis is in question, ICP can be measured by different methods including electronic pressure monitors; this permits observation rather than fasciotomy in doubtful cases.

If ICP is higher than 30mm Hg below the mean arterial pressure, compartmental perfusion is impaired and fasciotomy should be carried out. Any associated fracture is at the same time stabilized with external or internal fixation, and wound closure postponed until the swelling has subsided.

Radiography

If a fracture is suspected, the injured part must be x-rayed. While taking the x-rays the following points must be kept in mind:

- The whole bone must be x-rayed in two planes at right angles to each other *including the joint above and the joint below the injured area*. Only thus can one be sure of not missing a fracture.
- In certain fractures, e.g. of the scaphoid bone, an oblique view must also be taken.
- In a hairline fracture of the scaphoid the fracture line may not be visible on the first x-ray. Radiographs must be repeated on subsequent occasions, when the fracture sometimes shows up.
- Stress views can be obtained in doubtful cases.
- CT scan should be used in comminuted fractures and intra-articular fractures.

STAGES OF HEALING OF A FRACTURE

The process of fracture repair varies according to the type of the bone involved and the amount of movement at the fracture site. In a tubular bone in the absence of rigid fixation, healing proceeds in five stages:

- ***Tissue destruction and hematoma formation.*** As the vessels are torn, a hematoma forms around and in the fracture. The fracture ends undergo necrosis for a millimeter or two due to deprivation of blood supply.
- ***Inflammation and cellular proliferation.*** Within 8 hours of the fracture there is an acute inflammatory reaction with proliferation of cells under the periosteum and within the breached medullary canal. The ends of the fragments are surrounded by cellular tissue, which bridges the fracture site. The clotted hematoma is slowly absorbed and fine new capillaries grow in the area.
- ***Callus formation.*** The proliferating cells are potentially chrondrogenic and osteogenic, and under a favorable environment they start producing bone and cartilage. Osteoclasts derived from the blood cells mop up dead bone. The thick cellular mass, with its island of immature bone and cartilage, forms the *callus* or splint on the periosteal and endosteal surfaces:
    - o The bone formed initially at the periphery of the callus by intramembranous bone formation is the *hard* callus.
    - o The *soft* callus forms in the central regions with low oxygen tension and consists primarily of cartilage and fibrous tissue.

  Bone gradually replaces the cartilage through the process of endochondral ossification, enlarging the hard callus and increasing the stability of the fracture fragments. This process continues until new bone bridges the fracture site, reestablishing continuity between the cortical bone ends. This entire process is dependent on:

- o Age.
- o Local vascularity.
- o Nutritional status.
- o Growth factors.
- o Hormones.
- o Type of fixation.

- ***Consolidation.*** Mineralization of the fracture callus now proceeds apace. As this happens, the bone ends gradually become enveloped in a fusiform mass of callus containing increasing amounts of woven bone.

  The increasing mineral content is closely associated with increasing stiffness of the fracture callus. Stability of the fracture fragments progressively increases because of the internal and external callus formation, and eventually clinical union occurs and the fracture site becomes stable and pain-free.

  Radiographic union often occurs later than *clinical union*, when x-rays show bone trabeculae or cortical bone crossing the fracture site. However, even at this stage healing is not complete. The immature fracture callus is weaker than normal bone, and it only gains full strength during remodelling.

- ***Remodelling.*** During the final stages of repair, remodelling of the repair tissue begins with replacement of woven bone by lamellar bone and resorption of unwanted callus. Fracture remodelling continues for years after clinical and radiographic union, with osteoclastic resorption of superfluous or poorly placed trabeculae, and formation of new struts of bone along lines of stress. However, in adults slight internal and external irregularity persists indefinitely.

Healing without callus

If the fracture is *perfectly reduced and rigidly immobilized*, e.g. in internal fixation by a plate or an intramedullary nail, callus formation does not occur. Instead, capillaries invade the bone and grow across it to unite with each other. Cells derived from these capillaries remove dead bone and lay down new bone so that a living cortex is directly remade. This process is called *primary bone healing*. This process is unlike healing by callus. It is not visible radiologically, and it takes months rather than weeks to be completed.

Biological healing

Clinical and experimental studies have shown that callus is the response to movement at the fracture site. It serves to stabilize the fragments as rapidly as possible—a necessary precondition for bridging by bone. This phenomenon is seen in closed static nailing of the long bones.

The time taken for union. This depends on the age of the patient, the limb involved, the direction of the fracture line etc:

- Fractures in adults take twice as long to unite as fractures in children, as growth and repair are more active in the latter.
- Lower limb fractures take twice as long to unite as upper limb fractures.
- Oblique or spiral fractures heal more quickly than transverse fractures, because in the former types the fractured surface is greater in area.
- Open fractures unite very slowly.

Disturbances of normal healing in bones

- Healing of fractures may be delayed (delayed union).
- It may take place in malalignment (malunion).
- It may not take place at all (non-union).

Delayed union and non-union

Delayed union

If a fracture is not united by such time as it is expected to heal, i.e. it displays tenderness and abnormal movement at the fracture site, it is said to display delayed union. The callus may be invisible on x-ray, or may not fully bridge the fracture site.

Clinical signs of delayed union include:

- Persistent pain.
- Tenderness.
- Motion at the fracture site.

Radiographic hallmarks of delayed union include:

- Persistence of the fracture line.
- Hypertrophic callus with a persistent fracture line.
- Minimal or no callus production.

A fracture displaying delayed union may continue to heal until it finally unites.

Non-union

In this condition the healing process stops before union has occurred. Non-union is generally established when a minimum of nine months has elapsed since injury and the fracture shows no visible signs of healing for 3 months. Abnormal movement persists, and on x-ray the fracture line remains visible permanently.

Pseudarthrosis

In other cases movement at the fracture site is so persistent that cartilage is laid down between the fractured ends. A cleft develops between the layers of cartilage covering each fracture fragment. Cells at the periphery of the cleft develop into synovial cells, producing a false joint (pseudarthrosis).

The causes of delayed union and non-union

A number of factors may interfere with healing of fractured bones:

- *Excessive movement* at the fracture site may produce delayed union because the callus is being constantly 're-fractured' by the movement occurring in the healing tissue.
- *Infection* of the fracture hematoma in an open fracture upsets the healing process.
- A *poor blood supply* at the fracture site delays healing because the invasion of the hematoma by blood vessels is slow or absent. Therefore, osteoblasts are slow to appear in the fracture hematoma. In fracture of the neck of the femur the vessels ascending the neck to the femoral head may be ruptured by the fracture. In such cases union fails to take place, because the blood supply of the head is lost.
- *Excessive periosteal stripping* leads to decreased blood supply at the fracture site and may contribute to delayed union and non-union.
- *Interposition of soft tissues*, e.g. muscle, between the fracture fragments. The soft tissue physically separates the fractured ends, so it is impossible for them to unite.
- *Systemic disease* e.g. uremia, diabetes mellitus, chronic liver disease may interfere with healing generally.
- *Drugs*. Certain drugs like steroids, non-steroidal anti-inflammatory agents (NSAIDs), methotrexate etc. are associated with delayed union and non-union.
- *Patient factors*. Too early weight-bearing, lack of proper physiotherapy, excessive alcohol intake, smoking, etc. can lead to non-union.

Malunion

A malunited fracture is one that has healed with the fragments in a non-anatomical position. For example, a long bone may unite with significant angulation at the fracture site, or with over-riding of the fragments. This occurs due to imperfect reduction or loss of reduction during the healing period and usually results in impaired function. Besides, the deformity is cosmetically unattractive.

Treatment of non-union and mal-union

In the first instance the *cause* of the non-union or mal-union has to be treated. Local causes like infection, soft tissue loss, and local neuro-vascular deficit are addressed.

Similarly, *systemic illnesses* like diabetes mellitus, chronic liver disease, anemia, hypoproteinemia etc. are corrected.

Surgical options for non-union include rigid internal fixation with or without bone grafting. The bone graft can be taken from the iliac bones and recently allografts are being used. Rigid internal fixation can be provided with intramedullary interlocking nails and dynamic compression plates.

Proper counselling of the patients is mandatory to address the *patient factors* involved.

Impairment of function after union

Adhesions

If adhesions form between the fracture site and the overlying muscles; the latter when stimulated cannot glide over the bone and contract, so that movement at the adjacent joints is limited and the effectiveness and force of the muscles is reduced.

Sudeck's atrophy

(Reflex sympathetic dystrophy) Normally some osteoporosis occurs after a fracture. Occasionally this may be grossly exaggerated, with pain and joint stiffness. This syndrome is called Sudeck's atrophy. It may be due to extreme reluctance of the patient to use the limb after removal of splintage, or from another cause. No specific treatment is available. The patient is encouraged to use the limb under the supervision of a physiotherapist.

THE TREATMENT OF FRACTURES

The management of a fracture is best considered under two headings: general management of the patient, and local management of the fracture.

General management of the patient

The general management of the patient starts in the accident and emergency department according to the Advanced Trauma Life Support (ATLS) protocols. This includes general care of the patient with a fracture and includes:

- Measures to deal with the pain and blood loss caused by the fracture.
- Care of any associated injuries.
- Emergency splinting of the fractures.

Pain

A good deal of pain occurs in most fractures, and must be relieved. This can be done by splinting, and by analgesics such as pethidine and morphine. At the same time, in certain situations a nerve block may be used for analgesia, for example epidural anesthesia for rib or hip fractures. For lesser grades of pain paracetamol may suffice.

Blood loss

In all fractures some blood is lost. Fractures of the long bones and open fractures may present with hypovolemic shock. For example a patient with a fracture of the femur may lose *over two liters of blood* into the thigh muscles without much swelling. Such blood loss produces shock and must be replaced. At the same time, the use of inflatable pneumatic trousers (Military anti-shock trousers or MAST) for transport may help maintain blood pressure and decrease ongoing blood loss in these cases.

Associated injuries

Fractures of the *pelvis* can cause injury to the *bladder* or *urethra*. These injuries must be looked for, so that they are not missed. Their care is described in the appropriate chapters.

Fractures of the long bones may cause injury to neighboring *nerves* and *vessels*. The injured extremity should be evaluated rapidly for neurovascular compromise, soft tissue injuries, and joint instability. Peripheral pulse and capillary refill are evaluated and motor and sensory examinations carried out to the extent of the patient's ability to cooperate. All findings must be carefully documented for comparison with any later changes.

Emergency splinting of fractures

After the neurovascular examination is completed and soft tissue trauma or wounds evaluated, fractured extremities should be splinted to minimize further injury using a *plaster-of Paris or fibre-glass slab,* specially if the patient has to be transported to a hospital for reduction of his fracture. Such a slab is the best kind of splint, as it moulds itself to the contours of the body while being applied, and is therefore both effective and comfortable. In case of non-availability air splints, splints made of wood or Kramer wire, or even pillows can be used, to stabilize the extremity. A fracture of the humerus can be splinted with a sling. Femur fractures are best splinted in a Thomas splint with skin traction.

MANAGEMENT OF THE FRACTURE

The aims of treatment of a fracture are three: reduction, immobilization and rehabilitation. The fracture, if displaced, must be reduced as accurately as possible *(reduction).* It must then be held in place for as long as is required for it to unite *(immobilization).* In the meantime the soft tissues, specially the muscles in the area, must be exercised as far as possible, in order to prevent their atrophy through disuse *(rehabilitation).*

REDUCTION

This means restoring the bones to their normal anatomical position. Reduction, when required, can be accomplished by closed manipulation or open operation.

Closed reduction

This has the great advantage that the skin remains intact and there is no chance of the fracture becoming infected. Therefore, whenever possible, closed reduction is to be preferred.

Anesthesia

General anesthesia is commonly used. This not only makes the procedure painless but also relaxes the muscles so that the manipulation becomes easier (manus = hand; manipulation = to move something by the use of the hands).

Local blocks

If general anesthesia cannot be used or is not available:

- The fracture hematoma may be infiltrated with a local anesthetic*:* the *hematoma block.*
- The local anesthetic may be used intravenously distal to a tourniquet (intravenous regional anesthesia), *the Bier's Block.*

Manipulation

Having anaesthetized the patient or the part, the bone ends are manipulated to restore the normal anatomy. The actual movements required for the reduction of common fractures are described in the following chapter. However, in general the surgeon seeks to reverse the mechanical events which caused the fracture. Nowadays fluoroscopes and image intensifiers are used for help in achieving accurate closed reductions.

Open reduction

Open reduction has to be employed under the following circumstances:

- If closed reduction fails in bringing the fracture fragments into a satisfactory and acceptable position.
- If the reduction is lost subsequently during the healing period.

- Where it is common knowledge that closed reduction cannot succeed in its objective. Some examples follow:
  - o If soft tissues are interposed between the bone fragments.
  - o If the surgeon cannot obtain any purchase on one of the two fracture fragments, as in a fracture through the anatomical neck of the humerus accompanied by dislocation of the head of the humerus.
  - o In fractures around joints in which there are several small fragments whose accurate replacement is essential for normal joint function. Examples include certain fracture-dislocations around the ankle and depressed fractures of the tibial condyles.

IMMOBILIZATION

The aims of immobilization are two:

- To maintain correct alignment of the bones while healing is taking place.
- To prevent movement of one fragment over the other. This is extremely important if union is to take place. If movement occurs at the fracture site the delicate granulation tissue or early callus is broken, and healing has to start again from the beginning. In fact if such movement occurs repeatedly, delayed union or even non-union may result.

Methods of immobilization

Immobilization may be provided externally or internally:

External fixation may be provided by:

- Splints.
- Casts.
- Braces.
- Traction.
- External fixators.

Internal fixation is commonly provided by the use of:

- Intramedullary implants—intramedullary nails (reamed and unreamed) and rush nails.
- Onlay implants—dynamic compression plate (DCP), low contact DCP and locking compression plates (LCP).
- Tension band wires.
- K-wires.

External fixation

- ***Splints*** are usually made of wood or plaster of Paris (Fig.35.1a). In a first-aid situation an appropriately-sized piece of wood or other stiff material, even a folded newspaper, may be used as a temporary splint; it is bandaged to the side of the broken limb. This method has been replaced nowadays with the newer commercially available splints. Nowadays, splints are available in different sizes and shapes.

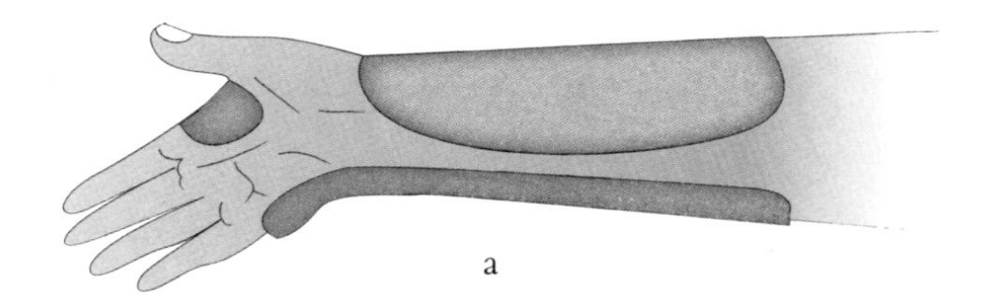

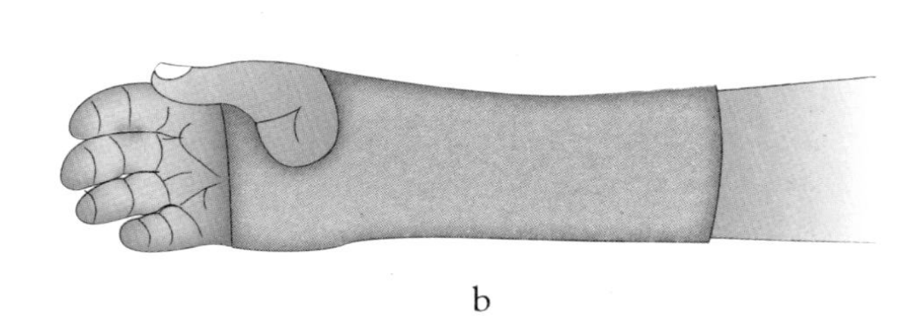

Fig.35.1 (a) plaster slab, (b) plaster cast.

- ***Casts.*** The goal of a cast is semi-rigid immobilization (Fig.35.1b). In fractures, considerable swelling often occurs due to the accompanying soft tissue injury. As a cast is closed all round the limb, the swelling can raise the tissue pressure to high levels. This can compress arteries and nerves and result in paralysis and/or ischemia. It is therefore a good idea to split the cast on one side through its entire length *(bivalve the cast)*. The skin should be exposed throughout, to ensure that no strand of cast material continues to constrict the limb.

Classically, *plaster of Paris* has been used to apply the cast. Recently, *fiberglass* casts are used for the same purpose. Fiberglass is more rigid, water-resistant and lighter than plaster of Paris. Cotton padding is applied over the skin before the application of a cast. The bandages are available in different widths suitable for different bones e.g. 6 inches width for tibia and 4 inches width for forearm bones. The casts should generally be applied in the position of function of the joint. While applying casts great care must be observed, as disastrous complications may result from the cast.

The usual *complications associated with casts* include:

- o Loss of reduction.
- o Pressure necrosis of skin.

- o Cuts during the cast removal.
- o *Compartment sysndrome*. In this condition, in a patient with a cast, a swollen muscle in a tight fascial compartment can undergo necrosis due to loss of blood supply. Where there is danger of developing this complication, bivalving the cast, as explained above, will reduce the pressure on the limb. If compartment syndrome is suspected after cast application, it is better to remove the cast along with the cotton padding.

- ***Bracing***. This consists of a 1/8-inch thick moldable plastic material applied directly over the fractured part. This method of treatment is used for those fractures which can be treated by closed non-operative methods, for example undisplaced fractures of the foot. The method consists of a compression dressing followed by short casts for a few weeks.
- ***Traction***. This allows constant controlled force for initial stabilization of long bone fractures and aids in reduction during operative procedures. The option for skeletal versus skin traction depends on the case:
  - o With *skin traction* a maximum of 5kg of traction should be used, as more weight especially in elderly patients is associated with the skin getting irritated or peeled off.
  - o Where traction is to be used for longer duration and greater fragment control is required, *skeletal traction* in the form of a wire or Steinman pin is preferred. Weight up to 20% of the body weight can be applied through skeletal traction. Some sort of local anesthesia is needed for pin insertion. Common examples are tibial skeletal traction, femoral skeletal traction, balanced traction and halo traction.
- ***External fixators***. External fixation systems in current clinical use (Fig.35.2a) can be categorized according to the type of bone anchorage used. This is accomplished :
  - o Either by using *threaded pins*, which are screwed into the bone.
  - o Or by drilling small-diameter transfixion wires through the bone and then placing the wires under tension to maintain the position of the bone bone fragments. In this method a minimum of three pins are passed into the long bone above, and a similar number below the fracture site. Shafts of the pins close to their outer ends are attached to a steel bar. The fracture is now reduced under anaesthasia and the joints between the pins and the bar tightened. In this way the bone ends are rigidly and accurately held against each other for the required number of weeks until they unite. Fixators are
    - ▪ Linear (AO), and
    - ▪ Circular (Illizorov) in configuration.

Internal fixation

This is normally provided after exposing the bones at a surgical operation, which may be required for a fracture in the following situations:

- If reduction is impossible by closed means. This may be due to the fact that:
  - o Soft tissues e.g. muscles are interposed between the bone fragments, and need to be extracted at open operation to allow the bone ends to be brought together.
  - o One of the two fracture fragments cannot be manipulated, e.g. in fracture of the neck of the humerus with dislocation of the shoulder.
- If it is impossible to maintain reduction by external splintage. This is commonly seen in fractures of the neck of the femur.
- In non-union.
- In pathological fractures.
- In poly-trauma cases as part of treatment all fractures are fixed.
- If it is hazardous to the patient to maintain reduction by closed methods. Thus in inter-trochanteric fracture of the femur the fracture can be immobilized by traction. However, this requires prolonged immobilization in bed. In elderly patients this may produce bedsores, hypostatic pneumonia, or deep vein thrombosis which may lead to pulmonary embolism and death. Therefore this fracture in the elderly is best treated by open reduction and internal fixation, so that the patient can be immediately mobilized.

METHODS OF INTERNAL FIXATION

A number of methods are available to the surgeon to deal with different situations:

Intramedullary fixation techniques

A variety of implants is available for intramedullary fixation of fractures. This method of treatment is based on the principles of biological union. Closed nailing techniques are being used in modern orthopedics. Options for intramedullary fixation are interlocking nails, flexible nails and rush nails.

- ***Interlocking intramedullary nails*** are being used as the gold standard implants for long bone fractures these days. These implants provide axial alignment as well as rotational control. They can be used as static and dynamic nails depending upon the geometry of the fracture. They come as reamed and unreamed nails, the former being hollow and the latter solid nails. Examples of intramedullary nails are Trigen nails and Russell-Taylor nails.
- ***Flexible nails.*** These are being increasingly used in pediatric patients and patients with open physeal plates. Examples are Enders nails and FINS.
- ***Rush nails.*** These are like thick K-wires and are used for closed or open fractures of forearm bones.

Onlay implants

These implants are used on the surface of the bone and are based on primary bone healing. There are several varieties of the plates. Examples include plates and screws, (Fig.35.2b), dynamic compression plates, and locking compression plates.

Dynamic compression plates are based on the principle of compression at the fracture site. The screws are placed eccentrically which produces compression at the fracture site. In fractures of forearm bones a minimum of six cortices above and below are engaged, in the tibia and the humerus a minimum of eight are needed for rigid fixation.

The ***dynamic hip screw*** and ***dynamic compression screws*** are examples of implants where the lag screw is passed into the neck or the condyles of the femur and a plate of definite angle is attached with the screw and fixed with the bone with screws.

Some fractures are fixed with screws only, for example medial malleolus fracture and fracture neck of femur. The screws provide the compression across the fracture.

Tension band wiring

In this method of internal fixation, K-wires are passed across the fracture site and these are then secured with circlage wires in a figure-of-eight loop. This is based on the principle that the movement of the joint will provide the compression across the fracture. Fracture of olecranon and patella are common examples which are fixed with tension band wiring.

K-wires

Some fractures are internally fixed with K-wires. This technique is mostly used in pediatric fractures, for example supracondylar fracture of the humerus. The fixation is not rigid, so some sort of external support like back slab is applied to the limb postoperatively.

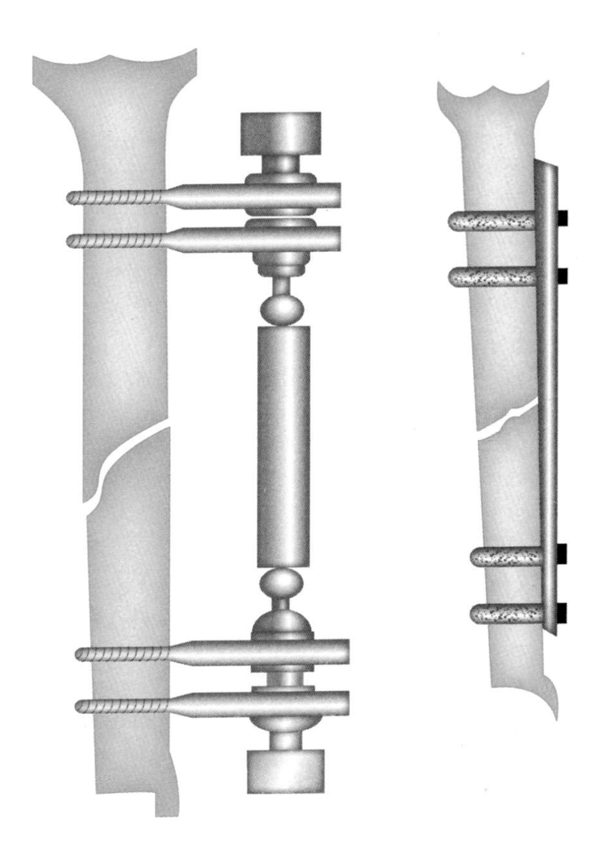

Fig.35.2 Treatment of fracture of a long bone by: (a) use of external fixator (b) onlay bone plating

PROSTHESES

Prostheses are being used increasingly these days in traumatic and elective situations:

- Some intra-articular fractures are severely comminuted and primary internal fixation is not possible. In such circumstances the fractured part is replaced with prosthetic material. Common examples include:
  - o Comminuted fractures of radial head and neck in young individuals.
  - o Displaced fractures of neck of femur.
  - o Comminuted fractures of proximal humerus in the elderly.
- In certain situations the joint congruity and movements at joints are restricted due to degenerative and pathological processes like:
  - o Rheumatoid arthritis.
  - o Osteoarthritis.
  - o Infections.

  - o Post-traumatic and drug-induced avascular necrosis.

  The whole joint is then replaced.

- Prostheses can also be used as a part of reconstructive surgery for primary or secondary tumors around a joint. There are different varieties of prostheses which are being used in modern day arthroplasty, like surface replacement, unipolar replacement, bipolar replacement and total joint replacement:
  - o *Surface replacement.* In relatively young patients, when one side of the joint is destroyed by a pathological process but sufficient bone stock is preserved and the other part is normal, surface replacement is done on the affected site. The common example is surface replacement in hip surgery.
  - o *Unipolar replacement.* In elderly patients after trauma, some fractures are not reconstructable primarily; in such situations unipolar replacement is done, as in the Austin Moore prosthesis after fracture neck of femur in the elderly.
  - o *Bipolar replacements.* These are considered better than unipolar replacements and are being increasingly used these days. These implants carry the benefit of decreased surgical trauma to the patient during the future total joint replacement as only one side of the joint has to be replaced.
  - o *Total joint replacements.* These are being used in elderly patients after trauma with good ambulatory status preoperatively, and in elective situations where the joint has been destroyed by the pathological process. Example are total hip, knee and shoulder replacements.

Cemented and uncemented replacements

Joint replacements may be carried out with or without the use of cement:

- *Uncemented* replacements are used in elderly patients with sufficient bone stock, and in young patients where the joint is being replaced as a consequence of a pathological process. These are based on the 'press-fit' placement principle; you press the prosthesis onto the denuded surface after removing the diseased or injured part, and it fits snugly.
- *Cemented* replacement is carried out on elderly patients with poor bone stock and in revision surgeries after uncemented joint replacement. In this process a minimum thickness of 3mm bone cement is used between the implant and the bone.

OPEN FRACTURES

Open fractures, acute dislocations and cauda equina syndrome are considered orthopedic emergencies. The incidence of open fractures has increased over the past few decades and their treatment has always been a challenge for orthopedic surgeons.

Common *mechanisms* of open fractures include:

- Road traffic accidents.
- Gunshot wounds.
- Suicide bombs.
- War injuries.
- Blast injuries.
- Farm yard injuries.
- Falls from a height.

Open fractures are associated with soft tissue injuries and bleeding wounds. There may be massive contamination with soil, along with organic and inorganic matter. Soft tissues and muscles may be lost. As far as the bone itself is concerned, its periosteum may be stripped, and there may be massive comminution and loss of bone.

Classification

Several classification systems are used for open fractures, of which the *Gustilo and Anderson classification* is the most popular. It is based on:

- Size of the wound.
- Soft tissue injury.
- Contamination.
- Fracture pattern.
- Energy of impact i.e. low and high energy trauma.

Types

The types of open fractures and their characteristics are shown in (Table 35.1).

Management

This is carried out according to the ATLS protocols:

- The *neuro-vascular status* of the limb is documented.
- *Compartment syndrome* is looked for.
- Tissue *cultures* are requested for culture and sensitivity.
- The wound is *washed* in the emergency room and all dead tissues and foreign material removed.
- A first generation cephalosporin with aminoglycoside or second generation cephalosporin is started. In penicillin-sensitive patients quinolones can be started.

- *Tetanus* prophylaxis is given according to the vaccination history.
- Adequate *debridement* is then carried out, the dead tissue with a rim of healthy tissue being removed, and the fracture surface curetted to remove foreign material.
- Finally, the wound is *washed again* with plenty of saline. Depending upon the type of injury, internal or external fixation is now carried out.
- The wound can be closed primarily or delayed primary closure can be carried out; in larger wounds with soft tissue loss, skin grafts and flaps are utilized.

Wounds sustained during war *are almost always left open*, because a soldier with a wound may have to be evacuated over long distances to the base hospital. During the journey it may be impossible to provide sufficiently close supervision and treatment to the wound. If the wound has been sutured and becomes infected, the pus would not find an exit. The raised pressure in the tissues would drive the septic material into the veins, producing sepsis which is dangerous and could prove fatal. If on the other hand the wound is left open, any pus which forms drains freely onto the surface, so that there is little risk of septic absorption.

REHABILITATION

Rehabilitation should commence immediately after reduction and immobilization. In fact *psychological rehabilitation* should proceed from the moment the injury is sustained, by means of words of explanation and reassurance.

Physiotherapy

Exercise under the supervision of a physiotherapist plays a very important part in rehabilitation.

Therapeutic exercises can be categorized into static or dynamic exercises.

- ***Static*** exercises are isometric exercises in which no observable movement occurs, *the muscle acting against resistance*.
- ***Dynamic*** exercises may be either active or passive:
  - ***Active exercise*** occurs when voluntary contraction of muscles produces movement without the application of additional external resistance. These exercises are of two types:
    - Active *range of motion exercises* include those movements within the available range of motion. They are performed to maintain motion.
    - In active *stretching exercises* the athlete utilizes voluntary efforts to move beyond the restricted range of motion. These are designed to increase motion.
  - ***Passive exercises***. In passive exercises the different motions include: distraction, compression, rolling, etc. They are employed in patients who are not capable of producing these motions with voluntary muscle activation, and therefore a *physical therapist* uses this manual technique to increase joint play.

Table 35.1. Types and characteristics of open fractures

Type	Wound size	Soft tissue injury, contamination	Comminution
I	< 1cm	Minimal Nil	
II	Upto 10cm	Moderate	Moderate
III	* Any size	Severe	Massive

*Type III includes all farmyard injuries, railroad accidents, segmental fractures, shotgun injuries.

As far as the physical aspects of rehabilitation are concerned, *those joints in the limb which are not immobilized should be put through their full range of movement daily from the beginning,* so that they do not stiffen. For example in Colles' fracture which occurs in old people the shoulder and elbow can become stiff very quickly. Therefore the hand should be placed behind the head (full abduction and external rotation at the shoulder) and behind the back (full adduction and internal rotation) at least once every day.

Injuries to articular cartilage

Because cartilage lacks blood vessels, it cannot respond to cell damage with inflammation. However, injuries that disrupt subchondral bone as well as the overlying cartilage initiate the fracture healing process, and the repair tissue from bone will fill an articular cartilage defect. Cartilage healing then follows the sequence of inflammation, repair and remodeling like that seen in bone or dense fibrous tissue. Unlike these tissues, the repair tissue that fills cartilage defects from subchondral bone initially differentiates toward articular cartilage rather than toward dense fibrous tissue or bone.

Exposure of cartilage to air by traumatic or surgical disruption of the joint capsule and synovial membrane can alter cartilage matrix composition by stimulating degradation of proteoglycans or suppressing synthesis

Table 35.2 Grades of ligamentous injuries

Type I	Stretch, but no disruption of fibres.
Type II	Tear of some fibres.
Type III	Complete discontinuity of the ligament.

of proteoglycans. A decrease in matrix proteoglycans concentration decreases cartilage stiffness and makes the tissue more vulnerable to damage from impact. Prompt restoration of the synovial environment by closure of the synovial membrane will allow chondrocytes to repair the damage to the macromolecular framework of the matrix, and the tissue may regain its normal composition and function. On the other hand, prolonged exposure of the articular surface to air can desiccate the tissue and kill chondrocytes.

It is not clear what duration of exposure causes irreversible damage. The available evidence, based on animal experiments, suggests that damage to the matrix macromolecular framework occurs with any disruption of the synovial membrane, but clinical experience suggests that permanent or progressive damage in human joints rarely occurs following temporary disruption of the synovial cavity. Furthermore, cartilage can be restored to its normal condition if:

- The loss of matrix proteoglycans does not exceed the amount the cells can replenish.
- A sufficient number of chondrocytes remain viable.
- The collagenous meshwork of the matrix remains intact.

Injuries to ligaments

Bony injuries to the limbs are often accompanied by ligamentous injuries. In addition, a ligament injury can occur independently as a primary injury to a joint; these are referred to as sprains. Ligament injuries are graded as in Table 35.2.

Ligaments heal by progressive scar formation and contracture, and recent studies indicate that if gross instability is not present, repair is improved by early motion.

Treatment

Type I and II injuries are treated by immobilization or protected motion.

Treatment of type III injuries varies from non-intervention (as in type III acromioclavicular separation) to immediate surgical reconstruction (as for a torn anterior cruciate ligament in a professional athlete).

The operation for a ruptured cruciate ligament is quite ingenious. The ligament is replaced by the middle 1cm of the ligamentum patellae. At each end of the ligamentum patellae a block of bone is taken, from the femur and the tibia respectively, so that bone joins up with bone. A tunnel is drilled through the appropriate condyle of each bone in the correct direction. The ligament with a block of bone at either end is passed through the tunnel. Screws are driven in between the bone blocks and the condyles to secure the blocks in position. Fixation of the new ligament in a taut position is assured, so that movements can be allowed immediately to prevent any tendency to stiffness or disuse atrophy.

PEDIATRIC ORTHOPEDICS

Anatomy

Pediatric bone has a higher water content and lower mineral content per unit volume than adult bone. Therefore it is less brittle than adult bone. The physis (growth plate) is a cartilaginous plate that varies in thickness depending on age and location. It is frequently weaker than bone in torsion, shear, and bending, predisposing the child to injury through this delicate area. The periosteum in a child is a thick fibrous structure (up to several millimeters) that covers the entire bone except the articular ends.

Principles

The general principles for management in children are similar to those in adults, and the emergency management starts according to the Advanced Trauma Life Support (ATLS) protocols. There is need to pay special attention to the mechanism of injury, as the patient might not be able to narrate the incident clearly. Pain tolerance is poor in children as compared to adults. Similarly special care is needed to document the neuro-vascular status of the patient and any development of compartment syndrome periodically. Sometimes it becomes difficult to decide whether a crack is a fracture or the physeal plate. In such a case x-ray of the opposite normal limb should be carried out. CT scan and MRI are needed to evaluate intra-articular fractures.

Management

Conservative

Most pediatric fractures can be managed conservatively with the aid of splints, casting, traction and bracing. Moreover, owing to the better potential for regeneration, the acceptability criterion is wider as compared to adult trauma.

Operative

Indications for operative intervention include fractures that are:

- Intra-articular and displaced.
- Associated with vascular injury.
- Associated with compartment syndrome.
- Inherently unstable.

The battered baby syndrome

The term 'battered baby' is used for a young child who is deliberately and often repetitively injured at the hands of a parent or other adult. The child is usually under the age of two years and unable to give a history, and the parent takes advantage of this fact. The injuries commonly consist of abrasions, bruises, and fractures of ribs, skull or long bones. Suspicion should be raised if the injuries do not fit in with the history given by the parent. Suggestive findings include a history of mechanism of injury that is inconsistent with the fracture pattern, and multiple fractures, bruises and/or cigarette burns in various stages of healing.

The child should be admitted to hospital immediately to protect it, while the social worker investigates the case, to arrive at a diagnosis and to suggest measures to prevent repetition of the abuse.

Chapter

36 INJURIES TO THE LIMBS

Upper limb

The upper limb is a single functional unit, the active part being the hand. The arm has no function other than to carry the hand this way and that, to place it in the desired position where it can perform its functions of grip etc. If the hand is no more, the arm has no function to perform. The real active parts of the hand are the thumb and fingers. Therefore, injuries to the thumb and fingers have an importance quite out of proportion to their size.

PECTORAL GIRDLE

Acromio-clavicular dislocation

This injury commonly occurs from a violent downward blow on the point of the adducted shoulder, the force being transmitted through the humeral head into the acromio-clavicular joint, commonly in contact sports. Chronic injuries are associated with degenerative changes and are seen in people involved in athletic activities, weight lifting, and in those working with jack-hammers and heavy vibrating tools. The injury is graded into five types:

- Type I: Acute sprain.
- Type II: Acromio-clavicular ligament is torn.
- Type III: Acromio-clavicular and coraco-clavicular ligaments are torn and the clavicle is visibly elevated.
- Type IV, V and VI: The clavicle is displaced posteriorly, inferiorly and beneath the coracoid respectively.

The characteristic anatomic feature is downward sag of the shoulder and arm. The inner end of the clavicle produces a prominence. X-rays are taken with the patient holding a 5kg weight alternatively in both hands to differentiate between type II and III injuries where the subluxation is accentuated.

Management. Type I, II and III fractures are managed conservatively in a polysling. Type III fracture in young active patients and type IV and V fractures are managed by surgery.

Fracture of the clavicle

Fracture of the clavicle is a common injury. The usual mechanisms are falls on the outstretched hand or on the point of the shoulder, and direct blows on the bone. Other mechanisms include bicycling and skiing. Most fractures occur in the middle-third of the bone. The lateral fragment is displaced downwards by the weight of the limb; the medial fragment is held up by the sternomastoid muscle.

X-rays

These fractures are easily visualized with an antero-posterior radiograph of the chest, but suspected medial-third fractures are mostly seen on CT scan chest. For the lateral-third fractures sometimes oblique and axillary views are required to identify the local disrupted anatomy associated with the fractures. In suspected clavicle fractures, injuries to the lung, pleura, ribs, brachial plexus and upper limb vessels must be ruled out.

Management

Medial and middle-third fractures are managed conservatively in a broad arm sling for 4 to 6 weeks. A figure-of-eight bandage is only rarely required. Surgery may be required for lateral-third fractures with significant displacement of the fragments. Surgery is also indicated:

- For bilateral fractures.
- For open fractures.
- For fractures associated with neuro-vascular compromise.
- For cosmetic reasons.

Fracture of the body of the scapula

Comminuted stellate fractures occur in the body of the scapula from direct violence as in motor vehicle accidents.

Scapular fractures rarely cause symptoms and usually heal uneventfully. The arm should simply be rested in a sling until pain subsides enough to allow mobilization of the shoulder. The following types of fractures are treated surgically:

- Displaced scapular neck fractures.
- Capsular neck fractures associated with clavicle fractures.
- Markedly displaced fractures of the glenoid cavity.

Fractures of the ribs usually occur at the same time, and should be treated appropriately.

THE SHOULDER

Dislocation of the shoulder

This is the most common dislocation in man. The most common mechanism is indirect trauma to the upper extremity with the shoulder in abduction, extension, and external rotation.

Commonly the head of the humerus dislocates forwards from the shoulder joint so as to lie beneath the coracoid process to produce a subcoracoid anterior dislocation. Rarely, the humerus dislocates posteriorly, usually due to convulsions or electrical shock. Very uncommonly it subluxates vertically downwards.

Clinical features

Subcoracoid dislocation

The clinical findings in a subcoracoid dislocation are typical. The outer aspect of the shoulder is flattened, the arm is held in a position of slight abduction and external rotation. The patient is not able to move the shoulder due to muscular spasm. There is squaring of the shoulder owing to a relative prominence of the acromion, a relative hollow beneath the acromion posteriorly, and a palpable mass anteriorly. Similarly there is loss of deltoid contour. There might be sensory loss in the 'regimental batch' area on the arm.

X-ray

On x-ray *the glenoid cavity is empty* and the head of the humerus is seen to be lying below the coracoid.

Posterior dislocation

The rare posterior dislocation is less easily diagnosed because the clinical appearance of the shoulder is essentially normal. Also, on x-ray the head of the humerus is not displaced medially to any great extent. Special x-ray views called 'axillary views' are required to show up this dislocation.

Treatment

If the patient is given a general anesthetic relaxing the muscles, reduction of a dislocated shoulder is easy.

Kocher's method

This method is generally employed. Traction is applied to the humerus with the elbow flexed to 90 degrees which is then externally rotated to 75 degrees, in order to stretch and abolish the spasm of the subscapularis muscle. Traction is now maintained and the elbow brought across the body to fully adduct the shoulder. The patient's hand is next brought to his opposite shoulder so as to rotate the shoulder internally. During this final rotation reduction is felt to occur and the contour of the shoulder returns to normal.

Other methods to relocate the shoulder are *Stimson's technique* and the *Hippocratic method*. Post-reduction antero-posterior and trans-scapular x-rays are essential.

Post-reduction care

The arm is kept in a sling and bandaged to the side of the trunk for three weeks. After this the shoulder is gradually mobilized, *but avoiding external rotation in abduction*. In the elderly, exercises are started sooner to prevent stiffness.

Recurrent dislocation

After reduction most dislocations of the shoulder heal and cause no further disability. However, occasionally the shoulder becomes unstable and repeatedly dislocates after trivial violence. The instability could be due to trauma to the labrum or capsule, or it may be atraumatic. This causes considerable disability and requires relief.

MRI or arthroscopy can help surgical planning by identifying tears of the anterior labrum, which cause persistent disability.

Treatment

- For *traumatic instability* operation is the only satisfactory method of treatment. The operation may be carried out arthroscopically or through open surgical exposure. Surgical options include the *Bankart procedure*, in which the labrum and capsule are reattached to the anterior part of the glenoid using sutures through bone.
- *Atraumatic instability* (instability without a preceding dislocation) is usually managed conservatively; surgical options include repair of the anterior labrum and capsulorrhaphy.

THE HUMERUS

Fracture of the neck of the humerus

Fracture of the surgical neck is a common injury in adults with osteoporosis, specially elderly females, due to a fall on the outstretched hand, while in children the anatomical neck is involved. The patient complains of pain in the shoulder and cannot move the joint. Neer classified these fractures into six types:

- Type I through IV are fractures with one, two, three and four parts respectively.
- Type V is fracture-dislocation of the shoulder.
- Type VI is associated with articular surface fractures.

Treatment

This depends on the type of injury:

- Simple undisplaced fractures of the surgical neck are dealt with by rest in a polysling for two to three weeks, followed by gentle passive exercises.
- Fractures of the anatomical neck are treated in a similar manner.
- The treatment of fracture of the anatomical neck combined with dislocation of the shoulder is difficult, and open operation is required, a hemiarthoplasty being generally carried out.

For Neer's different fracture types:

- Two-part fractures are managed conservatively.
- Three-part fractures are generally fixed.
- Four-part fractures are treated by prosthetic replacement of the head of the humerus.

The shoulder becomes stiff after these injuries; this improves over the next few months but some stiffness may remain.

Fracture of the shaft of the humerus

The shaft of the humerus is usually fractured in the middle third:

- From an indirect twisting force, which causes a spiral fracture.
- From direct violence, resulting in a transverse or comminuted fracture.

This fracture occurs in adults. There may be no displacement, or marked angulation or overlapping may result.

The proximal half of the humerus is also a common site for pathological fracture from carcinomatous metastases.

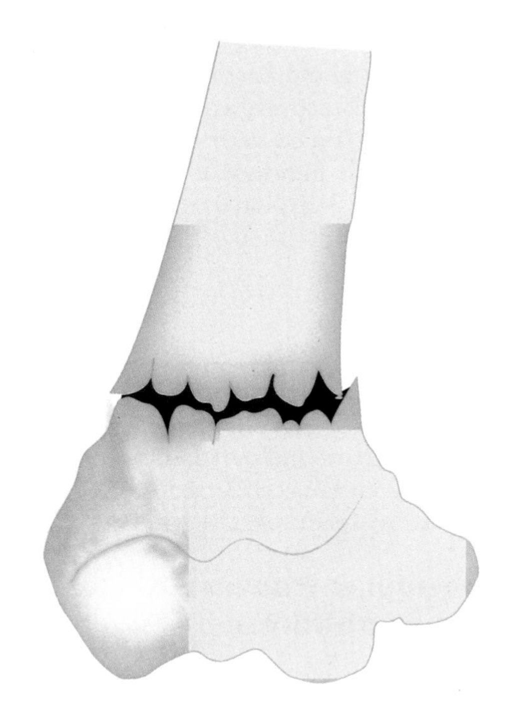

Treatment

Reduction of these fractures is often not necessary since gravity acting on the arm exerts steady traction which tends to correct any angulation that may occur. Support of the arm with a hanging arm cast allowing the elbow to hang free for three weeks may be sufficient. Alternatively a plaster slab is applied which runs from the acromion down the lateral side of the arm, below the elbow and up the medial side of the arm. Immobilization is maintained for about 3 weeks, during which period the hand is kept mobile. For the next 3 weeks the arm is removed daily from the sling to exercise the shoulder.

If satisfactory reduction cannot be achieved or maintained, surgical treatment with compression plating or intramedullary nailing is appropriate. Surgery is indicated for:

- Open fractures.
- Pathological fractures.
- Intra-articular and segmental fractures.
- Patients with polytrauma.

Radial nerve injury

This occurs in a mid-shaft fracture of the humerus, being usually a neurapraxia or axonotmesis, with an excellent prognosis. If recovery does not take place within 3 weeks electromyography should be carried out to determine whether subclinical recovery is occurring. Meanwhile physical therapy is started with the help of a cock-up splint. Exploration is indicated if such recovery is not evident. The nerve is explored and primary repair or cable graft is carried out. If repair is not possible, tendon transfer is instituted.

THE ELBOW

The elbow very often becomes stiff following an injury. The cause of this stiffness is not known; it is thought to be adhesions in and around the joint capsule. Soon after injury the joint should be protected. After 2 or 3 weeks movements are gradually encouraged.

Supracondylar fracture of the humerus in children

This is one of the most common and serious fractures of childhood (Fig.36.1). It should always be regarded as potentially dangerous because of the risk of injury to the brachial artery. The fracture occurs through a fall on the outstretched hand. The deformity is mostly the same, the lower fragment being displaced backward and tilted backwards.

Clinical features

The elbow swells markedly and this obscures the other physical signs. However, the olecranon and the two epicondyles can be palpated; they are found to be normally related to each other. On the other hand in posterior dislocation of the elbow the olecranon lies abnormally posterior to the epicondyles. This distinguishes the two conditions.

The most important point to keep in mind is the possibility of the blood supply to the forearm being interrupted due to this injury. This may happen at the time of the injury if the brachial artery is contused or lacerated by the proximal fragment of the humerus. The radial pulse will not be palpable. More commonly the radial pulse is present at the time of the injury, but is obliterated by swelling and by flexion of the elbow after reduction. Therefore the radial pulse must be repeatedly palpated during the first two days after injury.

Supracondylar fractures are classified as flexion and extension types. Extension type fractures are classified by Gartland into three types:

- Type I: Undisplaced fractures.
- Type II: Fractures through the anterior cortex only.
- Type III: Fully displaced fractures.

Treatment

Type I and stable Type II fractures are treated with a posterior splint with 90 degrees of flexion. All patients should be observed closely following immobilization.

Displaced i.e. Type III fractures have classically been treated by closed manipulation and immobilization in as much flexion as tolerated without circulatory embarrassment. Currently, however, *percutaneous pinning under fluoroscopic guidance* has become the most popular method for type III and unstable type II fractures, as it allows the achievement of more anatomical reduction. Postoperatively the limb is kept in a posterior splint for three weeks. If there is evidence of impaired circulation or compartment syndrome, immediate brachial artery exploration and forearm fasciotomies must be carried out to restore the blood supply and tissue perfusion. The pins and plaster are removed at 3 to 4 weeks and active exercises started.

Supracondylar fracture of the humerus in adults

Most of these fractures result from a simple fall in middle-aged and elderly women in which the elbow is either struck directly or is axially loaded in a fall onto the outstretched hand. In younger individuals, motor vehicle and sporting accidents are the more common causes.

Antero-posterior and lateral x-rays are required for these fractures, and in case of comminution CT scan of the elbow is needed. These fractures are treated by surgical fixation with plates and screws. Immobilization is continued for 3 to 4 weeks followed by range-of-motion exercises.

Dislocation of the elbow

This is usually caused by a heavy fall on the outstretched hand with the elbow slightly flexed, or a direct force on the posterior forearm in the flexed position. The dislocation can be postrolateral, anterior, medial and lateral. Posterolateral dislocation is the commonest, the ulna and radius being displaced backward, or backwards and laterally, in relation to the humerus (Fig.36.2). The patient cannot move the elbow, which lies in a position of slight flexion. *The point of the olecranon can be felt to be abnormally posterior to the humeral epicondyles.* This distinguishes posterior dislocation of the elbow from supracondylar fracture. Anteroposterior and lateral x-rays of the elbow show the dislocation.

Treatment

The dislocation should be reduced as soon as possible. The patient is given a general anesthetic to relax the muscles. It is then easy to reduce the dislocation by

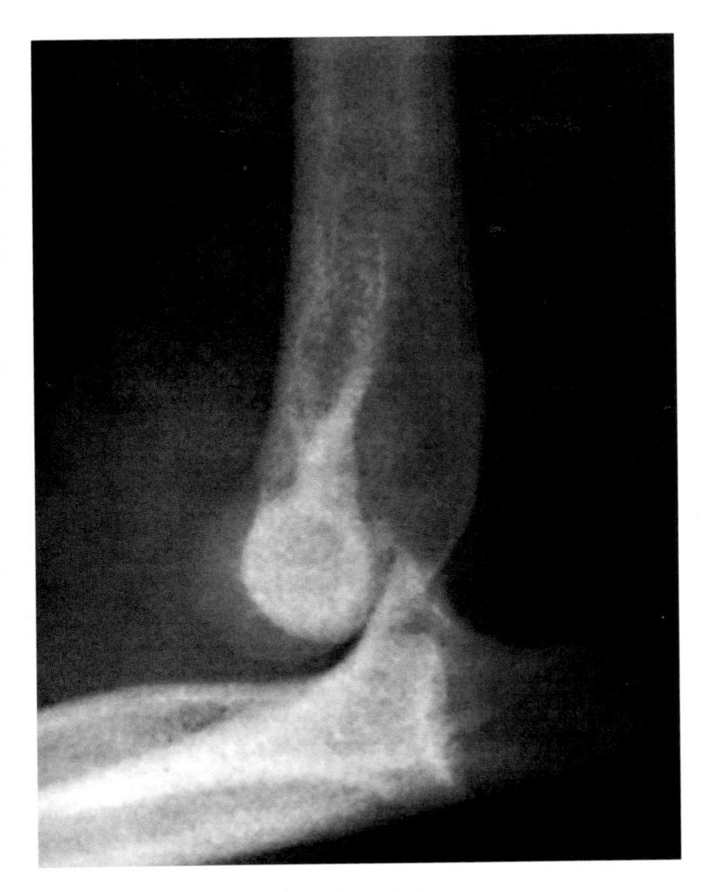

Fig.36.2 Posterior dislocation of elbow

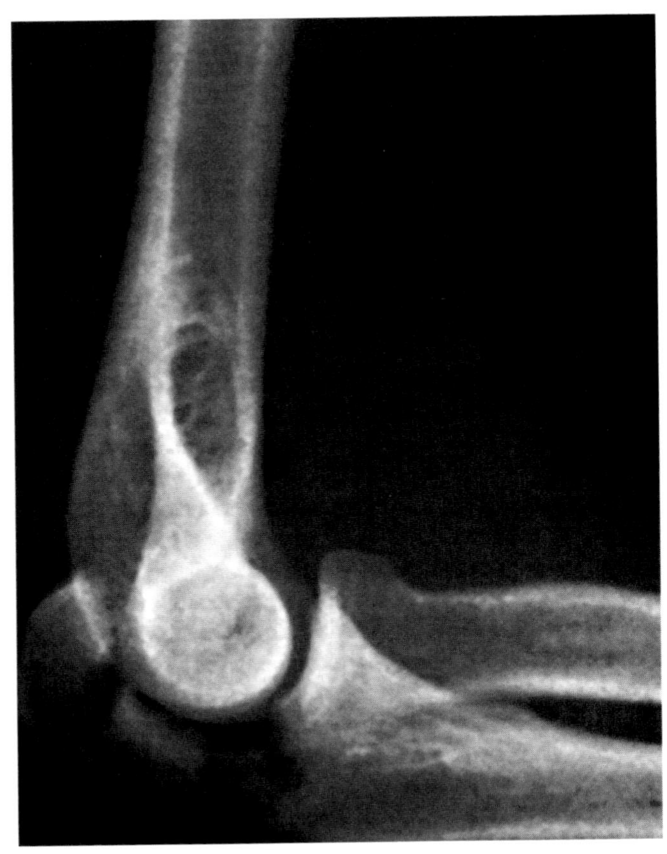

Fig.36.3 Fracture of olecranon

applying traction in the long axis of the slightly flexed ulna, while pressure is applied behind the olecranon. Once reduced the elbow can be put through a full range of movements and varus and valgus instability is assessed. The elbow is now rested in a plaster slab in 90 degrees of flexion for three weeks before exercises are begun. If the elbow cannot be held in a reduced position, redislocates before post-reduction radiography, or dislocates later in spite of splint immobilization, the dislocation is deemed unstable, and operative treatment is carried out.

Fracture-dislocation of the elbow

In severe trauma posterior dislocation of the elbow may be accompanied by fracture of the coronoid process and of the radial head. These are much less stable injuries than simple posterior dislocations. Good results have been reported with repair of the coronoid or anterior capsule, repair or replacement of the radial head, and lateral collateral ligament repair. If the radial head is not reconstructable, then it can be excised and replaced with a prosthetic one to avoid later instability of the elbow.

Fracture of the olecranon

A fall on the point of the elbow or direct trauma to the olecranon typically results in a comminuted olecranon fracture (Fig.36.3). Alternatively, a fall onto the outstretched upper extremity accompanied by a strong, sudden contraction of the triceps results in a transverse or oblique fracture. A combination of these may produce displaced, comminuted fractures. These fractures are classified by Mayo into three types:

- Type I: Undisplaced fractures.
- Type II: Displaced stable fractures.
- Type III: Displaced fractures associated with ulno-humoral instability.

Treatment

Non-displaced fractures and displaced fractures in the elderly are treated conservatively; otherwise all olecranon fractures are treated surgically. Surgical options include tension band wiring, plates and screws and lag screws. Following sound internal fixation early movement of the elbow should be commenced.

Fracture of the head of the radius

This fracture occurs due to a fall on the outstretched hand with the elbow extended and forearm pronated. The neck of the bone may be fractured, or alternatively a fragment may be split off from the head. There may be only some painful limitation of movement with tenderness over the head of the radius. The injury is shown on x-ray, and may be any one of three types:

- Type I: Non-displaced fractures.
- Type II: Displaced fractures.
- Type III: Comminuted fractures.

Treatment

Type I fractures can be treated conservatively, the elbow being immobilized for three weeks in a plaster slab. For type II fractures if there is block of elbow movement or more than 2mm displacement, surgery is advocated.

The treatment of type III fractures is surgical; if the radial head is non-constructable, it should be excised and replaced with a prosthetic head, to prevent proximal migration of the radius.

In children

In children the fracture usually involves the neck of the radius. If the head is displaced, closed reduction should be tried. However, if this fails, open reduction is carried out. The head of the radius is not removed in children, because it results in arrest of growth at the proximal end of the radius. This causes severe shortening of the radius and produces progressive derangement at the elbow and the radioulnar joints.

The shafts of the radius and ulna

Fracture of one bone without angulation

This may occur due to a direct blow to the forearm. Undisplaced fractures with stable proximal and distal joints can be treated conservatively in plaster. The fracture requires immobilization in an above-elbow plaster for six weeks in an adult, and three weeks in a child. Most single bone *displaced* fractures are treated surgically.

Fractures of both forearm bones

These fractures usually occur at approximately the same level, and are caused by a direct blow. Occasionally the bones may be fractured by torsion of the forearm; in this case the fractures are oblique and are placed at different levels in the two bones. These fractures often produce severe displacement which is very difficult to correct without open operation. Displacement is usually more severe in adults; children often suffer no more than a greenstick fracture with minor angulation. In severe trauma the excessive swelling of muscles within tight fascial compartments may cause muscle ischemia (compartment syndrome), which may require urgent fasciotomy to release the affected muscle groups. Untreated, this can lead to Volkmann's ischemic contracture.

Treatment

Supination and pronation involve rotation of the radius around the ulna. This movement requires precise reduction, as it is adversely affected by even slight angulation at the fracture site; and accurate reduction is best achieved by open reduction and plate fixation.

Dynamic compression

Internal fixation is carried out with dynamic compression plates and screws. These plates have eccentrically placed holes that allow compression together of the fractured ends as the screws are tightened.

Intramedullary implants

Alternatively these fractures can be fixed with intramedullary implants. After operation early mobilization helps recovery of function.

In children

In a child an acceptable reduction can sometimes be obtained by closed manipulation but if not, the fractures are treated by internal fixation using thin intramedullary pins, because such fine pins do not interfere with growth of the bones.

Fracture-dislocations of the forearm bones

These take one of two forms:

Monteggia fracture-dislocation

This consists of a fracture of the proximal third of the ulna and dislocation of the radial head. The usual case is due to a blow on the back of the upper forearm; the force breaks the ulna with anterior angulation, and dislocates the head of the radius forwards. All Monteggia fractures are treated surgically.

Galleazi fracture-dislocation

This consists of a fracture of the distal third of radius and dislocation of the inferior radioulnar joint. These fractures are treated surgically with plates and screws.

The presence of a displaced fracture of one forearm bone should alert the clinician to the possibility that the superior or inferior radioulnar joint is also dislocated.

The general rule, that fracture of the shaft of a long bone demands an x-ray not only of the bone itself but also of the proximal and distal joints, is nowhere more true than in these fractures.

THE DISTAL RADIUS AND ULNA

Colles' fracture

This is a fracture of the distal end of the radius produced by a fall onto the palm of the outstretched hand. It is most common after the age of 45. Above this age it is the most common of all fractures especially in females, due to the frequency of osteoporosis in post-menopausal women. The fracture occurs about 2cm above the wrist joint. The lower fragment is displaced laterally and backwards, and is tilted backwards. Therefore the articular surface, instead of pointing downwards and slightly forwards, is directed downwards and backwards. At the same time the lower fragment is impacted into the upper. Quite often the styloid process of the ulna is detached from its origin by the pull of the medial collateral ligament.

Clinical features

Just above the wrist there is a prominence at the back caused by the posterior displacement of the lower fragment. This appearance is given the name of *dinner-fork deformity*. The fracture site is tender. The radial styloid no longer lies at a lower level than the ulnar styloid; the two styloid processes are nearly at the same level.

Treatment

The fracture is reduced by manipulation and immobilized with a plaster or fibre-glass slab. This is completed after 24 hours, when any swelling has subsided, to form a plaster cast. The wrist is immobilized in palmar flexion and ulnar deviation. The plaster extends from the distal palmar crease to just below the elbow for six weeks. While the limb is in plaster the patient is encouraged to use the hand freely for everyday activities, and exercises of the fingers, elbow and shoulder are carried out. Physiotherapy prevents stifness of joints. At the same time the patient is instructed to place her hand behind the head and behind the back at least once daily to prevent stiffness of the shoulder. This is necessary because in the age group in which Colles' fracture is common, joint stiffness occurs very commonly after immobilization.

Complications

Most cases have full recovery of function. However, the following complications occur from time to time:

- *Mal-union*. To detect this, x-ray should be carried out 10 days after reduction. If redisplacement has occurred the fragments should be manipulated again into position and fixed by pins.
- *Stiffness* of the fingers or shoulder from disuse. To prevent stiffness, exercises of the fingers and shoulder should be carried out both in the plaster and after removal of the plaster, as explained above.
- *Carpal tunnel syndrome*. If the diagnosis is confirmed after nerve conduction studies, the flexor retinaculum should be divided.
- *Reflex sympathetic dystrophy* of the bones of the wrist and hand.

Smith's fracture

This is the reverse of Colles' fracture, the distal fragment being displaced anteriorly rather than posteriorly. It is uncommon. After reduction it is immobilized in an above-elbow plaster cast for six weeks in supination and slight dorsiflexion.

THE HAND

The carpus

Any of the wrist bones may be injured, but by far the most common injury is fracture of the scaphoid, followed by dislocation of the lunate.

Fracture of the scaphoid

This injury occurs commonly in young adults from a fall on the outstretched hand that imposes a force of dorsiflexion, ulnar deviation, and intercarpal supination. There is pain in the wrist, but function may be nearly normal. There is tenderness over the anatomical snuff-box. Physical signs suggest a sprained wrist.

Provocative tests include:

- *The scaphoid lift test*. Reproduction of pain with dorsal-volar shifting of the scaphoid.
- *The Watson test*. As the wrist is moved from ulnar to radial deviation with compression of the tuberosity, there is dorsal displacement of the scaphoid accompanied by pain.

The most common fracture is through the waist of the scaphoid. As the blood supply of the scaphoid is through its proximal pole, the rate of non-union is high in fracture through the waist. X-rays (which should include a 17-degree oblique view) may sometimes not show the fracture, because no displacement occurs at the fracture site.

Treatment

- For *stable and undisplaced* fractures of the distal third and through the tuberosity of scaphoid seen on x-ray, a plaster cast should be applied to include proximally from the base of thumb nail and extending from the proximal palmar crease to just below the elbow. This is kept in place for about eight weeks.

- *For hair-line fracture.* Sometimes when a wrist is sprained a fracture of the scaphoid may be present but not visible on x-ray, because of the hair-line nature of the fracture line. In such a case a 'scaphoid' type of plaster, as described above, should be applied. After two weeks the plaster is removed and another x-ray taken. If a fracture was present, by this time some resorption of bone will have taken place at the fracture site so that the injury will be obvious on the x-ray. The plaster should now be reapplied and kept on for eight to twelve weeks.
- *For displaced and unstable fractures.* Here surgery is the preferred treatment. Avascular necrosis may occur and lead to osteoarthritis of the wrist. If non-union occurs one can accept the un-united fracture if the patient is having a sedentary life style, otherwise internal fixation of the fracture with bone grafting is done.

Dislocation of the lunate

When a person falls on the outstretched hand with the wrist in hyperextension, the lunate may be squeezed out from between the capitate bone and the radius. It comes to lie in front of the wrist bones, with its concave surface forwards, and is best visualized on lateral x-rays. In difficult cases *CT, MRI or technetium bone scan* is used to identify the dislocation. The lunate may compress the median nerve in the carpal tunnel and produce anesthesia in the lateral three and a half digits and motor paralysis in the distribution of the nerve.

Treatment

Reduction by manipulation is attempted under general anesthesia. Strong traction is first applied to the hand. The wrist is hyper-extended and direct pressure applied over the displaced bone, when it may pop into position. A plaster is applied for four weeks. If unsuccessful, open reduction through a palmar approach is carried out with ligamentous repair and pin fixation. The blood supply of the displaced lunate is greatly reduced because most of its soft-tissue attachments are torn. If the median nerve is compressed it should be immediately released. At operation the lunate is reduced and the flexor retinaculum divided to prevent compression of the nerve.

The metacarpals

Fractures of the metacarpals

Axial load or injuries are frequently sustained during ball sports or sudden reaches made during everyday activities, such as to catch a falling object; these cause shearing articular fractures or metaphyseal compression fractures. Fractures of the diaphysis and joint dislocations usually require a bending component in the mechanism of injury, which can occur when the hand is trapped by an object and is unable to move with the rest of the arm. Finally, individual digits can be caught in furniture or workplace equipment to sustain torsional injury, resulting in spiral fractures.

Treatment

An aluminium splint is applied with the finger in the position of function, i.e. the metacarpophalangeal joint in full flexion and the interphalangeal joints in extension, the splint being kept on for three weeks. Alternatively a Buddy slab can be applied. When pain disappears, mobilization is started. If forward angulation of the neck is excessive, percutaneous pinning is necessary to maintain acceptable reduction.

Thumb metacarpal fractures

These injuries are caused by a blow to the tip of the thumb. The common type is Bennett's fracture, which is an intra-articular chip fracture.

Treatment. Minimally displaced fractures can be treated by closed reduction and a plaster cast to include the thumb. Because of the inherent instability of the fracture the most common method of treatment involves closed reduction with percutaneous or open reduction and K-wire fixation.

The fingers

Dislocations of the metacarpophalangeal joints

When the dislocation is incomplete, reduction by manipulation is easy. When complete, with the head of the metacarpal displaced volarward and the base of the phalanx dorsalward, the major obstruction preventing reduction is the displaced volar fibro-cartilaginous plate lying dorsal to the metacarpal head. Manipulation alone is successful in up to 50% of cases; the remainder require open reduction.

Fractures of the proximal and middle phalanges

Nondisplaced phalanx fractures are treated by splinting in a position of function (metacarpophalangeal joints flexed 70 degrees and interphalangeal joints in slight flexion). Malleable aluminium splints are used, with foam padding held in place by adhesive tape.

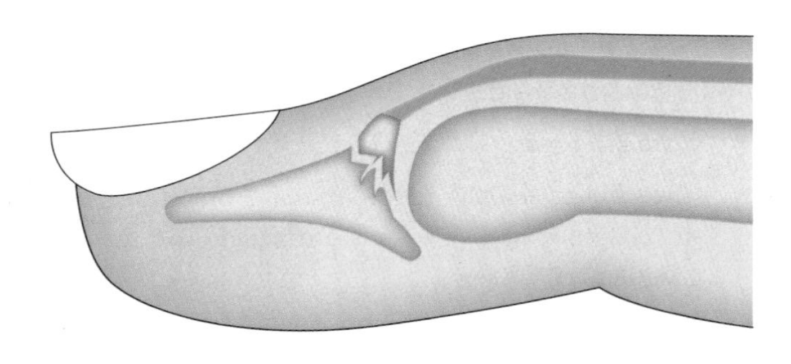

Fig.36.4 Mallet finger.

Displaced fractures require manipulative reduction prior to splinting.

Unstable fractures are treated with open reduction and fixation with wires.

Fracture of the terminal phalanx

The terminal phalanx is commonly fractured by a crushing injury. The pulp is also usually crushed. Often there are associated injuries of the nail and nail bed, which may be more of a problem and are commonly neglected. The skin may be lacerated so that the fracture is open. If the wound does not heal satisfactorily the finger-tip becomes permanently tender. The patient does not use the finger, which therefore gradually becomes stiff.

Treatment

Any wound should be cleansed to prevent infection. If a subungual hematoma is present it is drained; this gives considerable relief from pain. Nail bed lacerations should be repaired with fine absorbable sutures. The fracture is now splinted with a protective aluminium splint for three weeks keeping the proximal interphalangeal joint free. Angulated fractures should be reduced and, if unstable, pinned with a K-wire before splinting.

Mallet finger

In this injury the terminal slip of the extensor tendon to the distal phalanx becomes avulsed, usually taking a small fragment of bone with it (Fig.36.4). It is caused by sudden forced flexion of the terminal phalanx while the extensor of the finger is contracting. There is localized pain and swelling. The patient is unable to extend the terminal phalanx, which remains in a position of 30 degrees flexion.

Treatment remains controversial. Some recommend no operative treatment for all mallet fingers (including those with a significant articular fracture and joint subluxation), with full-time extension splinting for 6 to 8 weeks. Others recommend surgery for displaced dorsal base fractures comprising >25% of the articular surface.

Lower Limb

The functions of the lower limb are locomotion and weight bearing, and both legs function together as a single unit. Stiffness of one lower limb produces a limp and interferes with the function of both legs. The foot is not as important as the hand. Even after amputation of a part of the foot e.g. in tarso-metatarsal amputation, or of the whole foot as in Syme's amputation, the function of the lower limb can be carried out to a reasonable extent by the use of a prosthesis. Not so in the hand; amputation of the hand is really equivalent to amputation of the arm.

THE PELVIS

Fractures of the iliac crest

These fractures are of little significance, and should be treated like severe soft tissue injuries. Bed rest is advised for a week or two till pain subsides.

Fractures of the pelvic ring

These injuries can occur after low-energy trauma leading to individual bone fractures, or high-energy trauma leading to pelvic ring fractures:

- *Low-energy injuries* may result from sudden muscular contractions in young athletes that cause an avulsion injury or a straddle-type injury.
- *High-energy injuries* typically result from a motor vehicle or motorcycle accident or falls from heights.

Classification

Pelvic fractures are classified according to the mechanism of injury into antero-posterior compression, lateral compression, vertical shear and combination injuries.

Anteroposterior compression injury

This is usually caused by *frontal collision* and results in pubic rami fracture. The anterior sacroiliac ligaments are partially torn and the symphysis pubis is disrupted – the so-called open book injury.

The *treatment* of the fracture depends on the displacement

of pubic bones: if this is less than 2cm, conservative treatment is indicated; if more than 2cm, external or internal fixation is done.

Lateral compression injury

In this type of injury *side-to-side compression of the pelvis* causes the ring to buckle and break. This is usually caused by falls from heights or road traffic accidents. There are fractures of the pubic rami on one or both sides anteriorly and fracture of sacrum or ilium posteriorly. In severely displaced posterior fractures the pelvis becomes unstable. In fractures with more than 1.5cm leg length discrepancy open reduction is required, otherwise the stable injuries are managed conservatively.

Vertical compression injury

This occurs when someone falls from a height on one leg. The innominate bone on that side is displaced vertically, fracturing the pubic rami and disrupting the sacroiliac region on the same side. These injuries are much more difficult to manage requiring internal or external fixation, but without very beneficial results.

Associated injuries

Blood from injured vessels and fracture surfaces may collect in the tissues; if sufficient in quantity it may produce hemodynamic instability. It is therefore recommended that initial management should be instituted according to ATLS protocols, followed by emphasis on the pelvic injuries.

It is very important to note that a fracture of the pelvis may itself produce considerable internal hemorrhage and injury to the viscera---the male urethra, the bladder, and rarely the rectum and vagina. Blood loss should be replaced.

Management

In case of massive hemorrhage from the pelvic fracture some emergency procedures like Military Anti-Shock Trousers (MAST), a pelvic binder, and in dire cases angiographic embolization of the bleeding point may be needed.

In fractures of the *pubic rami* rupture of the urethra may be present. If the patient passes urine, extravasation will occur in the perineum. Therefore he is asked not to pass urine, and urethrography is carried out under full aseptic precautions. A rectal examination is carried out to exclude the rare perforation of the rectum by a fragment of bone.

Open pelvic fracture

An open pelvic fracture is defined as a pelvic fracture with a direct communication between the fracture site and a vaginal, perineal, rectal or skin laceration. Such fractures used to have a very high mortality rate, e.g. 40 %, most deaths resulting from hemorrhage and sepsis. This has been reduced considerably by the following measures:

- *Control of sepsis.*
- *Control of hemorrhage* before massive blood loss leads to coagulopathy, i.e. disseminated intravascular coagulation.

  Bleeding is controlled by various measures:

  - Direct ligation.
  - Bilateral ligation of internal iliac arteries, to reduce the blood supply to the pelvic bones and viscera.
  - Transcatheter embolization of bleeding points.
  - Application of an external fixator after reduction of the fracture; this reduces blood loss from the cancellous bone.
- *Pneumatic anti-shock trousers* (which compress the legs to prevent pooling in these parts) help improve the circulation.

  Most of the hemorrhage in cases of pelvic injury is from fracture surfaces and venous lesions. For its control, it is best to tamponade the low-pressure retroperitoneal bleeding by splinting the pelvis and to provide blood transfusions, sometimes in massive amounts.
- If the *rectum* is injured, not only should the fecal stream be diverted by a sigmoid colostomy, but also the feces present in the rectum at the time of the operation should be irrigated out.

Imaging

Generally x-rays in AP, lateral, pelvic inlet and pelvic outlet views are needed. CT scan is also required in most of the fractures to delineate the local bony and soft tissue injuries.

Treatment

- Stable undisplaced fractures and fractures of pubic symphysis with less than 2.5cm displacement are treated conservatively.
- Unstable injuries like pubic diastases of more than 2.5cm, unilateral sacro-iliac disruptions and bilateral posterior unstable disruptions are managed surgically.

THE HIP

Dislocation of the hip

Anatomy

The hip is a ball-and-socket joint with stability conferred by bony and ligamentous restraints, as well as the congruity of the femoral head with the acetabulum. The acetabulum is formed from the confluence of the ischium, ilium, and pubis at the triradiate cartilage. Forty percent of the femoral head is covered by the bony acetabulum at any position of hip motion. The effect of the labrum is to deepen the acetabulum and increase the stability of the joint.

Posterior dislocation

The hip may be dislocated posteriorly which is most common, or alternatively it may dislocate anteriorly or inferiorly (obturator). Posterior dislocation takes place when the hip is flexed and adducted, because in this position the head of the femur is covered by capsule rather than bone. Thus a force applied in the long axis of the femur may dislocate the head over the posterior lip of the acetabulum, which may also be fractured. For example, when a front seat passenger in a car is thrown forwards and the knee strikes the dashboard, a posterior dislocation can result. The head of the femur escapes into the sciatic notch where rarely the sciatic nerve may be damaged. The leg is held flexed, abducted and medially rotated. The patient may present in a state of shock due injuries to other organs like head, chest and abdomen sustained during massive trauma.

The classic appearance of an individual with a posterior hip dislocation is a patient in severe pain with the hip in a position of flexion, internal rotation, and adduction.

Posterior dislocation is classified into five types:

- Posterior dislocation with minor chip of acetabulum.
- Dislocation with single large fragment of acetabulum.
- Acetabulum comminuted.
- Floor of acetabulum fractured.
- Associated femoral head fracture.

Anterior dislocation

If force is applied to an abducted hip an anterior dislocation can result. In patients with an anterior dislocation the hip is held in marked external rotation with mild flexion and abduction.

X-ray

This confirms the dislocation and any associated fracture.

Treatment

Urgent reduction is attempted in the emergency department. The patient is given general anesthesia and a muscle relaxant. He is transferred on a canvas stretcher to the floor. The hip and knee are each bent to 90 degrees. The head of the femur now lies behind the acetabulum and needs to be lifted by pulling the thigh vertically upwards. Once reduced, the hip is again flexed to 90 degrees and gentle force applied backwards to check the stability. Immediate CT is done to rule out any intra-articular fragment. Other methods of reduction include Stimson gravity technique and Bigelow technique.

After reduction skin traction is used for 4 weeks. For the next four weeks walking is allowed on crutches. Full weight-bearing is allowed in six to eight weeks. In a number of cases post-traumatic arthritis develops 10 to 30 years after injury.

Central acetabular fracture-dislocation

This is caused by a blow on the greater trochanter which drives the head of the femur through the floor of the acetabulum.

Treatment consists of applying lateral and longitudinal traction on the head of the femur to bring it into its normal position. It is achieved by passing a trochanteric screw and a transverse proximal tibial pin. In young active patients restoration of an anatomic acetabulum reduces the likelihood of post-traumatic arthritis. Generally, the operation is delayed for about a week until the patient is stabilized, because immediate surgery can be associated with significant blood loss.

Postoperative complications

These include:

- Thromboembolic complications.
- Hip stiffness.
- Late osteonecrosis of acetabular fragments or femoral head.

Operative treatment of acetabular fractures requires particular skill. If an experienced surgeon is not available, the patient should be transferred to another centre, or non-operative treatment employed.

THE FEMUR

Fractures of the femur are common injuries, and can be classified as follows:

- Fractures of the proximal femur.
    - Femoral neck fractures.
    - Intertrochanteric and subtrochanteric fractures.

- Femoral shaft fractures.
- Supracondylar fractures.

Fractures of the proximal femur

These are common in persons above the age of 60, in whom generalized osteoporosis makes the bones increasingly fragile. The incidence continues to rise as the number of the elderly increases due to better medical care. The causative injury is often slight, usually a fall or stumble. Before the advent of internal fixation for these fractures patients were treated with traction in bed for weeks, and mortality rates were very high; although modern methods of management have improved the situation significantly, they are still quite high. These fractures occur much less commonly in young adults or children, and then from high-energy trauma such as motor vehicle accidents.

Femoral neck fractures

These fractures may be subcapital or midcervical (Fig.36.5 a and b). The patient complains of pain in the groin or thigh and is unable to bear weight on the extremity. The leg appears shortened and externally rotated, and any attempt at motion causes severe pain. Ecchymosis may be seen behind the greater trochanter. The fractures are classified into four types by Garden:

Type I.	Unicortical fracture.
Type II.	Undisplaced fracture.
Type III.	Partially displaced fracture.
Type IV.	Fully displaced fracture.

Undisplaced fractures may be difficult to diagnose and initial x-rays may be negative. Some patients with undisplaced fractures have surprisingly little pain and are even able to bear weight. If a patient has unexplained bone pain and negative x-rays after a fall, an MRI or CT scan readily demonstrates a fracture if present.

Osteonecrosis

Because the femoral head is covered all round with cartilage which has no blood vessels, its blood supply comes in mostly through the neck. A fracture of the neck disrupts these blood vessels, so that osteonecrosis and non-union are common.

Treatment

In young patients

In young active patients fractures of the neck of the femur are generally reduced under an image intensifier and fixed with a cannulated screw.

In the elderly

- Undisplaced fractures (Type I and II) are treated by fixation with cannulated screws.
- Displaced fractures (Type III and IV) are managed by cemented excision and replacement of the femoral head.
- In case of pre-existing arthritis of the hip joint, total hip replacement is advocated.

Even medically ill patients can usually tolerate internal fixation, especially if carried out percutaneously with multiple pins under local anesthesia.

Timing

Internal fixation should be carried out as early as possible. However, the elderly patient must be medically stabilized first.

Intertrochanteric and subtrochanteric fractures

- Intertrochanteric fractures are usually osteoporotic fractures (Fig.36.5 c).
- Subtrochanteric fractures are commonly pathological fractures.

Patients present with inability to bear weight, shortening, external rotation of the leg, and swelling or ecchymosis about the hip.

Treatment

- Intertrochanteric fractures are fixed with a dynamic hip screw and plate.
- Subtrochanteric fractures are dealt with by dynamic compression screws to allow early mobilization and prevent thrombo-embolism.

Results

In intertrochanteric fractures the blood supply to the femoral head is not disrupted, therefore osteonecrosis and non-union are uncommon. However, subtrochanteric fractures have a significant incidence of delayed union and non-union.

Prevention of thromboembolism

In the elderly patient with a fracture of the proximal femur, prophylactic measures should be employed before and after operation to avoid thromboembolic disease:

- Low-dose aspirin.
- Antiembolism stockings.
- Rapid mobilization with sitting in a chair within 24 hours if possible.

Fractures of the shaft of the femur

Fractures of the shaft of the femur occur at any age. They occur usually due to severe violence, e.g. from a road accident. The limb is unstable, with rotational deformity, shortening, and pain on motion. There is usually marked displacement with angulation and overlap, and muscles may be interposed between the fragments. As is the case of the humerus, the upper half of the femur is a common site for pathological fracture due to *metastatic* tumors.

Nerve damage

Damage to the *sciatic* nerve or *femoral* artery may be present, therefore neurovascular examination is essential. If signs of distal ischemia are present, arteriography should be carried out.

Blood loss

Considerable blood loss, often more than two liters, may take place into the muscles of the thigh. This blood must be replaced. At the same time, the use of inflatable pneumatic trousers for transport may help maintain blood pressure and decrease blood loss in these cases.

Classification

These fractures are classified into four types:

Type I:	Minimal or no comminution of both fragments.
Type II:	Less than 50% of cortices comminuted.
Type III:	50–100% cortical comminution.
Type IV:	Circumferential comminution.

Treatment

The aims of treatment are three:

- The *alignment* of the femur must be restored.
- The *length* must be restored.
- Stiffness of the knee must be prevented.

These can be achieved by either conservative treatment or internal fixation.

Conservative treatment (traction)

Shortening due to over-riding is produced by the pull of the powerful thigh muscles. This pull must be neutralized. Currently, in adults operative management is the rule; closed management for femoral shaft fractures is limited to patients with such significant medical conditions that operative management is contraindicated; it is also advocated in children under the age of 8 years.

The methods of applying traction include the following:

- Sliding traction in a Bohler-Braun splint (Fig.36.6).
- Fixed tration in a Thomas splint (Fig.36.7).

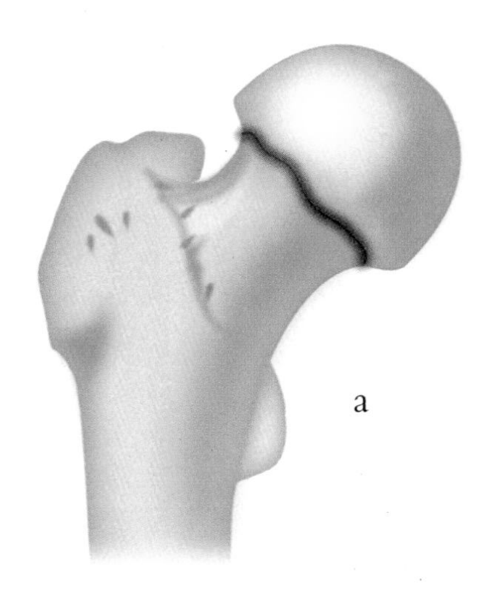

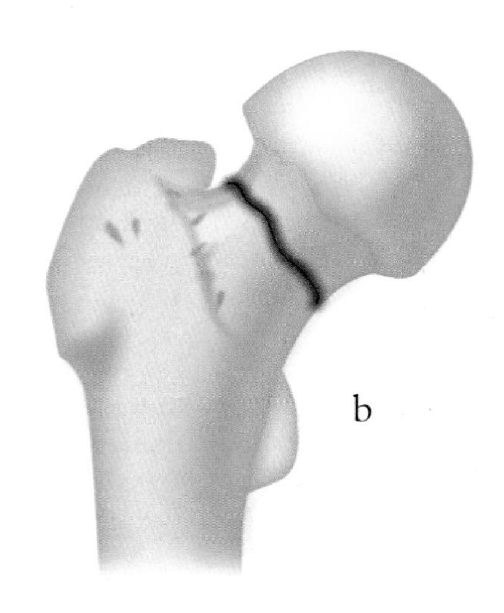

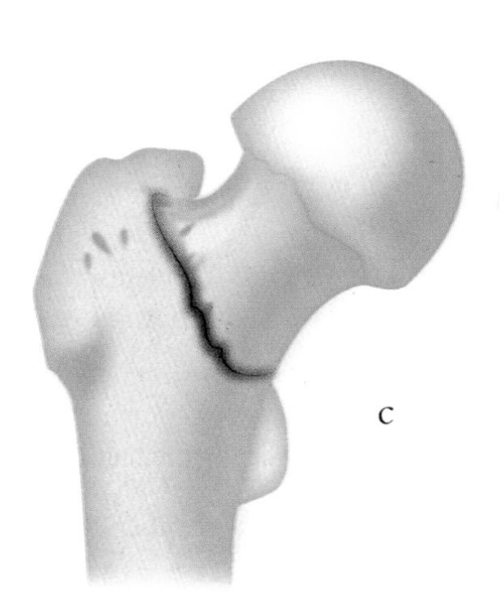

Fig.36.5 Fractures of neck of femur: a. subcapital b. midcervical c. intertrochanteric

- In infants adhesive plaster strips are applied to the medial and lateral sides of each leg, and the legs are slung up on an overhead bar.

Internal fixation

This is the preferred method of treatment for a femoral shaft fracture in adults; moreover, intramedullary implants and biological healing are gaining popularity over onlay implants like plates. The options for femoral shaft fractures include:

- Antegrade nailing.
- Retrograde nailing.
- Compression plating.
- External fixators.

Modern interlocking nails allow multiple screws to be driven across the femur both proximally and distally; thus both rotation and lengthening is prevented.

Infection rates with internal fixation are low, of the order of 0.5 to 1 percent. Therefore, there is an increasing tendency to treat fractures of the femur by internal fixation. *This is of special benefit in the elderly*, who do not take to prolonged immobilization kindly. At the same time, up to 1.5cm of shortening is acceptable, as this amount is concealed by pelvic tilt.

Knee stiffness

Stiffness of the knee is a common complication of fractures of the femoral shaft due to scarring in the thigh muscles and adhesion formation in the joint. Mobilization is achieved by physiotherapy, with first passive and later active exercises.

Treatment of femoral shaft fractures in children

In children treatment is advocated according to the age of the patient:

- From birth up to six months a pelvic harness is used.
- Upto 24 months an immediate spica cast is employed.
- Between 2 to 5 years traction for a few days is followed by spica cast.
- Between 6 and 11 years flexible intra-medullary nails and compression plates are generally used.
- From 12 years to maturity femoral fractures are fixed like adult patients. However, before the closure of the physis flexible nails are preferred.

Supracondylar and intracondylar fractures of the femur

These fractures present a special problem because the gastrocnemius flexes the distal fragment, producing posterior angulation at the fracture site. This is very difficult to control conservatively, and the fracture is best treated by internal fixation using a blade plate, dynamic compression screw and supracondylar nail.

Fractures of the tibial plateau

These occur from varus or valgus forces.

- In *young* individuals, motor vehicle accidents account for the majority of these fractures. Because of their strong, rigid bones, the patients typically develop split fractures and have a higher rate of associated ligamentous disruption.
- *Elderly* patients with osteopenic bone may experience these fractures after a simple fall. Due to the decreased strength and rigidity of their bones, they sustain depression fractures and have a lower rate of ligamentous injury.

Imaging

Anter-posterior, lateral and oblique radiographs are required to see these fractures. A CT scan is usually obtained to see a clear picture of the local area involved.

Concealed hemorrhage

These fractures lie in close approximation to the trifurcation of the popliteal artery. Therefore, they may be associated with massive concealed hemorrhage, and close supervision is needed to rule out the compartment syndrome.

Treatment

- Patients with less than 10mm joint line depression can be treated *conservatively*, with immobilization in a cast or brace and protected weight bearing, especially if the patient:
    - o Is over 50 years of age.
    - o Is not very active.
    - o Has osteoporosis.
    - o Has medical contraindications to operation.
- Young active patients with more than 10mm joint line depression are candidates for *surgical treatment*, which consists of elevation of depressed articular surfaces, bone grafting if necessary, and internal fixation with plates and screws. Ruptured collateral ligaments are also repaired.

Postoperatively, continuous passive motion aids in recovery of range of motion, and protected weight bearing is allowed for 8 to 12 weeks in a brace.

The patella

Fractures of the patella

These may be caused by direct or indirect violence, the latter being the more common:

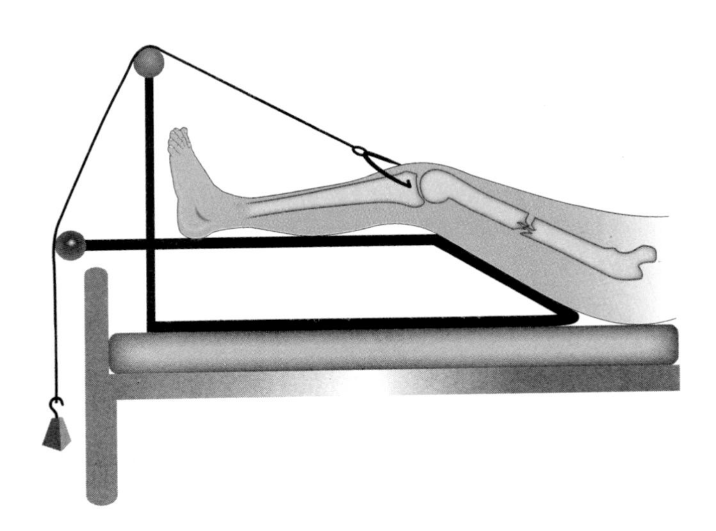

Fig.36.6 Bohler-Braun splint

Indirect violence

This commonly takes place when a person slips on one foot. To save him from falling, the quadriceps muscle on the opposite side contracts violently, resulting in a clean break of the patella into an upper and a lower fragment:

- If the prepatellar expansion of the quadriceps is *not ruptured,* the two fragments of the patella remain undisplaced. Such a fracture is detected as a crack on lateral x-ray of the knee (Fig.36.8). The patient can extend his knee, but only with pain.

  Treatment is by immobilization of the knee in a plaster cylinder for six weeks combined with isometric quadriceps exercises. This is followed by mobilization of the knee.

- If the prepatellar quadriceps expansion as well as the patellar retinacula are *ruptured* the fragments are widely separated. (Fig.36.9) The gap is palpable on examination, and obvious on x-ray. The joint fills with blood and clot. Without operation the proximal fragment of the bone remains retracted, the gap fills with scar tissue, and repair takes place with lengthening of the tendon and permanent limitation of active extension.

  Surgical treatment is therefore required:

  - o If the fracture is comminuted, the smaller fragments are excised and the patellar or quadriceps tendon attached to the larger fragment using wires or non-absorbable sutures through drill holes.
  - o For transverse fractures the fragments are brought together by tension band wiring, including a figure-of-eight wire. If fixation is not stable then the knee is immobilized in a cylinder cast in extension.

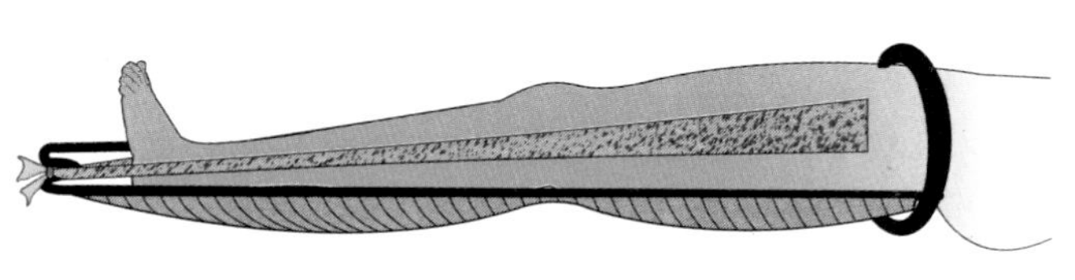

Fig.36.7 Thomas splint

- If extreme comminution is present, the patella is excised and the retinacula repaired.

Direct blow

A direct blow on the patella also usually produces a comminuted fracture. It is impossible to restore a perfectly smooth articular surface, so osteoarthritis results. These fractures should therefore be treated by *removal of the patella*. After this operation powerful active extension of the knee is possible, but there may be some loss of flexion. Graduated isometric exercises in a plaster cast are followed by isotonic exercises.

THE KNEE

Dislocation of the knee

Dislocation of the knee takes place in two situations:

- *High-energy*. A motor vehicle accident with a dashboard injury involves axial loading to a flexed knee.
- *Low-energy.* This includes athletic injuries and falls:
  - o Hyperextension leads to anterior dislocation.
  - o Flexion plus posterior force leads to posterior dislocation (dashboard injury).

Associated injuries include fractures of the femur, acetabulum, and tibial plateau. Knee dislocation may be anterior, posterior, medial, lateral and rotational. The dislocation is usually associated with severe distortion of the local anatomy.

Need for immediate reduction

A knee dislocation is a potentially limb-threatening condition. Because of the high incidence of neurovascular compromise, *immediate reduction is recommended before radiographic evaluation.*

Following reduction, anteroposterior (AP) and lateral

views of the knee should be obtained to assess the reduction and evaluate associated injuries. Widened knee joint spaces may indicate soft tissue interposition and the need for open reduction. After reduction special attention is paid to distal pulses and ligamentous instability. After relocation, if pulses are not palpable and ankle-brachial index (the ratio of the blood pressure in the lower legs to the blood pressure in the arms) is less then 0.9, immediate surgical exploration of the arteries is indicated.

Injuries to ligaments

Injuries to the ligaments of the knee joint are common among athletes. Clinical examination provides useful clues to diagnosis. X-rays are usually normal, but MRI helps define the extent of the injury.

Collateral ligaments

Medial collateral ligament (MCL)

A blow on the lateral side of the knee while the patient is standing abducts the tibia on the femur and places stress on the medial collateral ligament. The classic example of this type of injury is seen when the bumper of a car hits the outer side of a pedestrian's knee:

- With minor violence only a few fibres of the ligament are torn, but the ligament itself remains intact.
- If the blow is more severe the ligament is ruptured.
- An even stronger forced abduction may rupture one or both cruciate ligaments.

If the medial collateral and cruciate ligaments are ruptured the tibia becomes completely unstable on the femur. Pain and valgus stress in 30 degrees of flexion is diagnostic of MCL injury.

Treatment

Most MCL tears are managed conservatively in a hinged knee brace. MCL grade III tears associated with anterior or posterior cruciate ligament rupture are treated surgically.

Lateral collateral ligament (LCL)

This ligament is injured much less often than the medial, because very few blows fall on the knee from the inner side. Varus stress in 30 degrees of flexion is indicative of LCL injury.

Isolated injuries are managed conservatively, while grade III tears associated with anterior or posterior cruciate rupture are managed surgically.

An exact description of the injury helps distinguish the one lesion from the other:

- Gross swelling within an hour or two indicates hemarthrosis.
- Swelling arising slowly over a period of 24 hours means an effusion and points to a less severe injury.

Localized tenderness may be elicited over an injured collateral ligament.

Pain

- If a ligament has been sprained but not ruptured, stressing the ligament causes pain.
- If the ligament is ruptured the knee may be too painful to elicit abnormal movement.

The joint should be examined under anesthesia. The tibia in full extension is abducted and then adducted, and any abnormal movement compared with that in the other knee. If excessive movement is present it means that the appropriate collateral ligament is ruptured.

Cruciate ligaments

Injuries to these ligaments depend upon the line of stress in the accident:

- If the front seat passenger of a car is thrown forwards and the front of his tibia hits the dash-board the posterior cruciate ligament may be ruptured.
- If the knee is forcibly hyperextended a rupture of the anterior cruciate ligament may occur.

In order to test the cruciate ligaments the knee is flexed to a right angle.

- The upper end of the tibia is now drawn forwards. Normally the anterior cruciate ligament prevents this movement; if this displacement can take place it means the ligament is ruptured.
- Similarly, if abnormal backward displacement can occur, it indicates that the posterior cruciate ligament is torn.

Imaging

A stress x-ray of the knee will show up the tilting of the tibia over the femur.

MRI shows up the rupture of a cruciate ligament.

Treatment

Anterior cruciate ligament

The treatment decision should be based on age, activity level, instability and associated injuries. Generally anterior cruciate ligament injury associated with grade-three MCL or LCL injury is an absolute indication for reconstruction of the anterior cruciate ligament. Young individuals with higher activity level and those involved

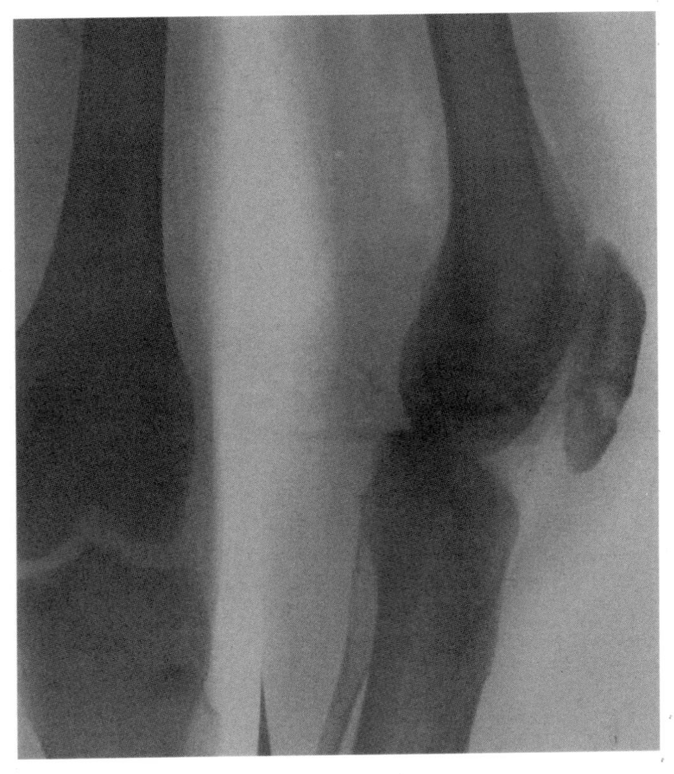

Fig.36.8 Transverse fracture of patella due to pull of quadriceps femoris. The lateral patellar retinacula are not torn, so the two patellar fragments are not separated.

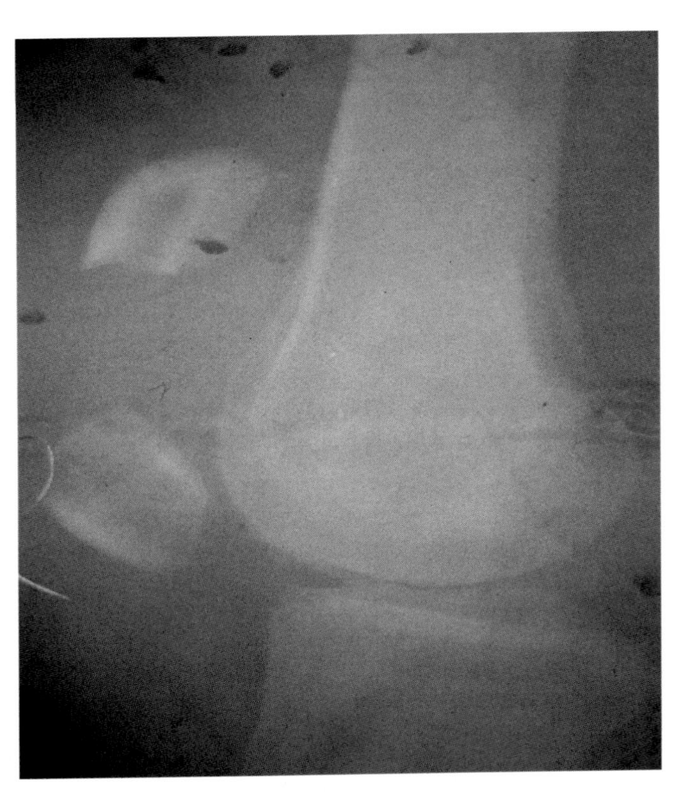

Fig.36.9. Transverse fracture of patella. Lateral patellar retinacula are torn, so the quadriceps femoris has pulled the two patellar fragments wide apart.

in moderate and strenuous activity are treated with ACL reconstruction. The ACL is reconstructed with a graft consisting of a hamstring tendon, or by a bone-patellar tendon-bone graft.

Posterior cruciate ligament (PCL).

This injury is usually a result of a dashboard injury in a road traffic accident. Alternatively, trauma on the flexed knee from behind with the foot plantar flexed may lead to PCL injury. The posterior drawer test is most sensitive for this injury. With the knee flexed to a right angle the upper end of the tibia is pushed backwards; if this is possible, the test is positive.

Treatment

Most PCL injuries are managed conservatively. PCL tears associated with grade III MCL or LCL tears are treated surgically, and patients in whom rehabilitation has failed are also offered surgical repair.

Injuries to the menisci

These are the most common injuries to the knee that require surgery. The medial meniscus is torn approximately three times more often than the lateral meniscus. In young individuals sports-related injuries are seen more often, whereas in the elderly degenerative tears are more common. Meniscal tears are classified according to their position (anterior, middle, posterior) and according to their shape and appearance (bucket-handle and parrot-like tears).

Clinical findings

After a twisting injury the patient falls, and has pain and tenderness at the anteromedial aspect of the knee. He cannot straighten the joint fully. The next day the whole joint is swollen. In about two weeks the swelling lessens and he resumes his activities.

'Locking of the knee'

In some cases, at the time of the injury the torn portion of the meniscus may become interposed between the tibial and femoral condyles and prevent full extension of the knee. Such a mechanical block to flexion or extension is called 'locking'. Because of pain and limitation of movement it may not be noticed that the joint is locked. As the effusion settles, the displaced meniscus may itself return to its original position so as to unlock the joint. In other cases it may require manipulative reduction. Many months after a return to apparent normalcy the knee may still be prone to locking and giving way.

Imaging

There are no specific features on plain x-ray, but meniscal tears can be demonstrated by MRI, arthrography or arthroscopy:

In *arthrography* air is injected into the knee. This separates the meniscus from the tibial and femoral condyles, so that it shows up better.

In *arthroscopy* the interior of the knee is examined through an endoscope (arthroscope) introduced through a small incision.

However, *MRI* scans provide accurate diagnosis of all types of internal derangements of the knee, including meniscal tears, osteochondral injuries and cruciate ligament tears, and have virtually replaced arthrography and arthroscopy.

Treatment

Meniscal repair

Peripheral longitudinal tears and those in conjunction with ACL tears should be surgically repaired.

Partial meniscectomy

Tears that are not repairable, and complex radial and degenerative tears along with bucket-handle tears, are treated by partial meniscectomy carried out arthroscopically.

THE TIBIA

Fractures of the tibia may be divided into fractures of the condyles, the shaft, and the distal end of the tibia (i.e. ankle fractures).

Fractures of the tibial condyles

These have much in common with fractures of the femoral condyles, and have been discussed with them above.

Fractures of the shafts of the tibia and fibula

These are the most common long bone fractures. The tibia being subcutaneous along most of its length, tibial fractures are often short of soft tissue coverage. As most of the fractures are high-trauma during motor vehicle accidents, the incidence of open fractures is always high in tibial shaft fractures.

Mechanism and displacement

Fractures of the tibia and fibula occur from direct or indirect violence:

Direct trauma

This is mostly due to road traffic accidents and leads to transverse, comminuted, displaced fractures. The incidence of soft tissue injury is high. Direct trauma occurs in two forms:

- *Penetrating.*

  The pattern of injury is variable. Fractures may result from:

  - Low-velocity missiles (handguns).
  - High-velocity mechanisms (shotguns, assault weapons).
  - Vehicle accidents.

- *Bending.* This results in three-or four-point (ski boot) injuries. The fractures are short oblique or transverse, with a possible butterfly fragment. Crush injury can occur. Highly comminuted or segmental patterns are associated with extensive soft tissue compromise. Compartment syndrome must be ruled out.

Indirect trauma

- *Torsional mechanisms.* These are caused by twisting with the foot fixed, and falls from low heights. These fractures are spiral, generally non-displaced, and have minimal comminution and little soft-tissue damage (Fig.36.9).
- *Stress fracture.* These injuries occur due to overuse of the limb.

In military recruits, these injuries most commonly occur at the metaphyseal/diaphyseal junction, with sclerosis being most marked at the postero-medial cortex.

In ballet dancers, these fractures most commonly occur in the middle third of the tibial shaft; they are insidious in onset and are overuse injuries. Radiographic findings may be delayed for several weeks.

Clinical evaluation of fractures

The neuro-vascular status of the limb must be assessed before and after the reduction of the fracture in the emergency room. High-energy trauma may lead to blister formation which is a contraindication to early surgery. Compartment syndrome must be ruled out. Tibial shaft fractures are commonly associated with ligamentous injury to the knee.

Imaging

Plain antero-posterior and lateral x-rays suffice. In case doubt exists, oblique and stress views can be obtained. All x-rays must include the joint above and below to rule out any intra-articular extension of the fracture.

For stress fractures, Technetium bone scan and MRI are needed.

Treatment

Conservative treatment

Most closed tibial shaft fractures can be treated with manipulation and cast.

Trafton's criteria

Fractures that satisfy these criteria can be left as such and immobilized in a long leg cast:

- More than 50% cortical contact.
- Less than 10 degrees of varus/valgus and anterior/posterior angulations.
- Less than 10 degrees of rotation deformity.
- Less than 1.5cm shortening.

A long leg cast is applied and after 4–6 weeks it can be reduced to a patella-bearing cast.

Operative treatment

Nowadays intra-medullary fixation is preferred in long bone fractures. Surgical options include dynamic compression plates and screws, and external fixators. In undisplaced tibial shaft fractures with an intact fibula, conservative treatment with early weight-bearing may be employed. However, some authorities prefer primary nailing of such fractures.

Open fractures

These high energy fractures are accompanied by severe soft tissue injury and contamination. Their initial management is according to the ATLS protocols. They are classified as follows:

- Type I: Less than 1cm wound, minimal soft tissue injury and contamination, low energy transverse and short oblique fractures.
- Type II: Wound up to 10cm, moderate soft tissue injury and contamination, low energy oblique fractures, minimal comminution.
- Type III: Severe soft tissue injury and contamination, high-energy fractures, massive comminution, segmental fractures.

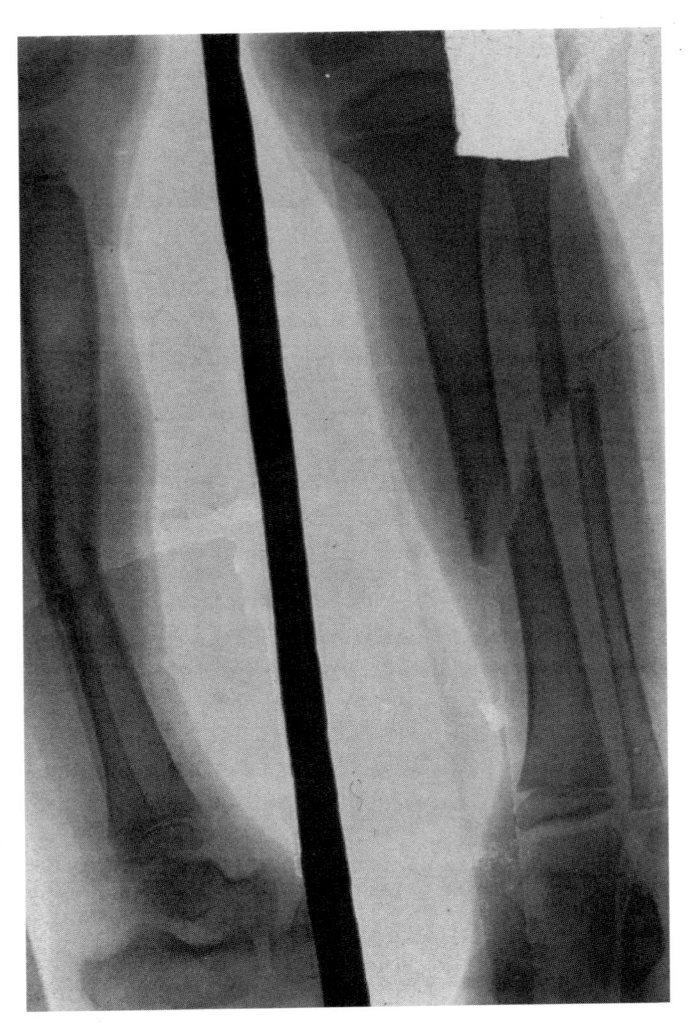

Fig.36.10 Spiral fractures of tibia and fibula from a twisting force

THE ANKLE

Fractures of the ankle

Mechanism and patterns

Pattern

The pattern of ankle injury depends on many factors, including:

- The patient's age and bone quality.
- Position of the foot at the time of the injury.
- Magnitude, direction, and rate of the force; whether a rotational or axial force acts on the joint.

Classification

These fractures are classified into the following types:

- Type A: Fractures *below* the level of the syndesmosis.

- Type B: Fractures *at* the level of the syndesmosis.
- Type C: Fractures *above* the syndesmosis.

Treatment

This depends upon the site and extent of the injury:

Fractures

- *Conservative treatment.* This is indicated for:
  - Nondisplaced, stable fractures with an intact syndesmosis.
  - Displaced fractures for which stable anatomic reduction is achieved.
  - Multiple trauma patients in whom operative treatment is contraindicated because of the condition of the patient or the limb.
- *Surgical fixation.* This is needed f or:
  - Open fractures.
  - Unstable fractures.
  - Fractures having failed to achieve or maintain closed reduction.
  - Fractures that require abnormal foot positioning to maintain reduction (e.g., extreme plantar flexion).

Injuries to ligaments

Lateral ligament

- A *sprain* of the lateral ligament should be treated by compression bandaging for two weeks using a crepe bandage. The ankle is mobilized within the limits of pain.
- A *rupture* of the lateral ligament should be protected by a below-knee plaster for not less than six weeks. If it is treated as a simple sprain, with early exercises and activity, the torn ligament may fail to heal and recurrent subluxation of the ankle may occur. Some surgeons prefer to suture the torn capsule and ligaments at operation to ensure that the torn ends of the ligament are correctly apposed. After operation the ankle is protected in plaster for six weeks.

Inferior tibio-fibular ligament

Rupture of this ligament is best treated by internal fixation using a screw passed through the fibula into the tibia. Plaster-of-Paris is applied for six weeks.

Medial ligament

Injuries to the medial ligament complex occur in eversion or abduction and are much less common.

THE FOOT

Fractures of the calcaneum

Most of these fractures result during a fall from a considerable height onto the heel, from the force of the body weight transmitted down along the long axis of the tibia. Thus both heels may be injured at the same time. In many of the more severe cases there is also a compression fracture of a thoracic or lumbar vertebral body. The subtalar joint is damaged, causing marked restriction of inversion and eversion, leaving the foot stiff.

In road traffic accidents a fracture of the calcaneum may result when the accelerator or brake pedal impacts the plantar surface of the foot. A twisting force may cause extra-articular fracture of the calcaneum. These fractures are mostly seen on plain AP, lateral, and axial views. CT scan is used in comminuted fractures.

Treatment

Conservative

This is indicated in:

- Undisplaced fractures.
- Fractures in cases where surgery is contraindicated, like severe peripheral vascular disease or insulin-dependent diabetes.
- Fractures with blistering and massive prolonged edema, large open wounds, or life-threatening injuries.

Non-operative treatment consists of a supportive splint to allow dissipation of the initial fracture hematoma. This is followed by the use of:

- An elastic compression stocking to minimize dependent edema.
- A prefabricated fracture boot locked in neutral flexion to prevent an equinus contracture.
- Early range-of-motion exercises at the subtalar and ankle joint; non-weight-bearing restrictions are maintained for approximately 10 to 12 weeks, until radiographic union.

Surgical

Operative treatment is indicated for:

- Displaced intra-articular fractures.
- Fracture-dislocations.
- Selected open fractures.
- Displaced fractures of the tuberosity of the calcaneum.

Fractures of the talus

These are most commonly associated with a motor vehicle accident or a fall from a height with hyperdorsiflexion of the ankle. The *neck* of the talus fractures as it hits the anterior margin of the tibia. The talus is vulnerable because of its peculiar blood supply. When its body is markedly displaced, osteonecrosis rates can be upto 100% and lead to osteoarthritis.

AP, lateral and Canale views[1] along with CT scan are generally needed for these fractures.

Treatment

Undisplaced fractures and minimally displaced fractures of the talus that achieve anatomical reduction are managed in a short leg cast for six weeks. Most displaced fractures are treated surgically.

Fractures of the metatarsals

These fractures are caused usually by a heavy weight falling on the dorsum of the foot. Sometimes the soft tissues of the foot are also severely crushed. In such a case the metatarsals unite but the foot remains thickened, stiff and painful:

- If the medial and lateral column of the foot is maintained then conservative treatment is advocated.
- In case of severe displacement and loss of either of the columns, and in open fractures, operative treatment is indicated.

Special attention is paid to the soft tissue injuries as most of these fractures are open.

Treatment

Undisplaced fractures are treated in a well-padded cast. In displaced fractures with more than 2mm tarso-metatarsal displacement, operative treatment is indicated. The medial column is fixed with screw and the lateral column with K-wires.

Jone's fracture

Avulsion of the styloid process distal to the cancellous tuberosity of the 5th metatarsal, called Jone's fracture, is a minor injury. The process is avulsed by the pull of the peroneus brevis contracting during forced inversion of the foot. The foot should not be immobilized. Only adhesive strapping is applied to support the foot and control swelling.

Fractures of the phalanges

These commonly occur when a phalanx is struck by a dropped object, or is struck against an object. Treatment consists of restoring alignment, taping the digit to an adjacent digit, and pain relief.

---

1 Canale view: Place foot on x-ray plate with foot in maximum plantar flexion and internally rotated 15^0

Chapter

37 DISEASES OF BONES AND JOINTS

CONGENITAL DISEASES OF BONES AND JOINTS

Congenital diseases of bones and joints include developmental anomalies and dysplasias:

- In developmental anomalies the abnormal growth occurs in utero and is static at birth. Any changes after that time are only secondary.
- In dysplasias abnormal growth occurs both in utero and after birth.

Some congenital diseases are genetic in origin, while others are due to disturbances in the intrauterine environment. For the majority the etiology is unknown.

DEVELOPMENTAL ANOMALIES

Developmental dysplasia of the hip (DDH)

This is a condition in which there is inadequate development of the hip with impaired ossification of the lateral acetabular epiphysis. There are several factors involved in the etiology of DDH:

- Female gender.
- Shallow acetabulae.
- Breech presentation.
- First baby.
- Oligohydramnios.

Unstable hips occur in about 8 per 1,000 live births.

Pathology

As the femoral head starts to be displaced from its central position, this exerts pressure on the lateral acetabular epiphysis, causing ossification and growth to be delayed. Spontaneous normalization is no longer possible by this stage. As the displacement progresses, the femoral head comes out of the acetabulum, usually in a craniodorsal direction. The acetabulum is secondarily filled with fatty and connective tissue.

If the femoral head has left the acetabulum, shortening of the iliopsoas muscle will occur. The tendon, which is located right next to and partially fused with, the hip capsule, becomes an obstacle to reduction.

The elevated position of the femoral head causes shortening of the leg. At the same time, the abductors (particularly the gluteus medius and minimus muscles) and the hip extensors (gluteus maximus) are shortened and weakened. This leads, on the one hand, to a flexion contracture of the hip and, on the other, to inability to stabilize the pelvis when standing on one leg. The consequence is an abnormal pelvic tilt that is compensated by hyperlordosis of the lumbar spine.

If the ossification deficit is only slight, the displacement of the femoral head does not occur, and the acetabular dysplasia may heal up spontaneously during subsequent growth as ossification catches up. There remains the risk, however, that the joint abnormality may become exacerbated during the pubertal growth spurt.

Diagnosis

Developmental dysplasia of the hip may be diagnosed at birth, or later.

DDH at birth

The condition can be diagnosed clinically at birth with the help of the following signs:

Skin folds

On inspection there may be pronounced asymmetry of the skin folds on the affected side in case of unilateral disease.

Galaezzi sign

A positive Galaezzi sign may be seen. This is performed by holding the feet together and flexing both knees. It is demonstrated by foreshortening of the femur on the affected side.

Examination in abduction

In this test, with the baby supine and from a position of 90° flexion, the hips are simultaneously abducted and externally rotated. While the hips of a healthy neonate can almost always be abducted down to the examination table, in dislocation or subluxation of the hip, abduction is inhibited on the affected side.

Ortolani test

With the baby supine and the hips flexed and abducted, the examiner's index and middle finger push the greater trochanter forwards. A clunk indicates reduction and suggests developmental dysplasia of the hip.

Imaging

Ultrasound

Morin index

Ultrasound examination is used as a screening tool in the population at risk. It is ideally employed between the fourth and the sixth weeks of life. The Morin index is calculated, which is the percentage of the head covered by the acetabulum. A Morin index less than 50% is suggestive of DDH.

X-rays

After the introduction of ultrasonography this method of diagnosis in not being recommended in the neonate, as the femoral head starts to ossify as late as at one year of age.

An anteroposterior x-ray of the pelvis is needed. A horizontal *Hilgenreiner line* passes through both triradiate cartilages, and a *Perkin line* is drawn from the lateral edge of the acetabular roof, perpendicular to the Hilgenreiner line, and crosses across the Hilgenreiner line to form four quadrants. Normally the center of the femoral head is in the lower inner quadrant. In the early stages of a dislocation, the center is shifted to the lower outer quadrant and, in a high dislocation, to the upper outer quadrant.

Treatment

First six months

- If the hip is *dislocatable*, it is observed for three weeks; if it is now stable, no treatment is given but supervision is continued for six months.
- If at three weeks the hip is *unstable*, treatment is started.
- If the hip is *dislocated*, then after relocation, the treatment is started immediately.

The rules of this treatment are:

- The hip must be properly reduced.
- Extreme position must be avoided.
- The hip should be able to move.

The common options are: abduction splint, Pavlic harness, and Von Rosen splint.

6–18 Months

If despite the treatment the hip is unstable or the child presents initially at this age, the hip is first reduced and is then held in this position till the acetabulum develops normally. Stable and concentric reduction is checked clinically, radiologically and with arthrography.

Splintage

In stable concentric hips, a spica is applied for six weeks. The Pavlic harness is applied for another four months. Concentric reduction and normal acetabular development is checked regularly during this period.

If the hip is not reducible or the reduction is not concentric, open reduction is carried out. The psoas tendon is divided and the thick ligament teres-limbus is removed. The hip is reduced and a spica applied.

18 months–4 years

By this time, closed reduction is impossible, and open reduction is carried out. The hip is kept in spica for three months followed by splintage for another three months.

After 4 years

At this stage treatment is difficult. Generally, open reduction with primary femoral shortening and pelvic osteotomy is carried out.

Club foot (talipes equino-varus)

[talus = ankle; pes = foot; equino=horse]

In this condition the fore-foot is plantar flexed and inverted at birth. It occurs in 1 out of 800 children, and is bilateral in up to 50% cases.

The disease is more common in males as compared to females. There are several possible mechanisms thought to be responsible for this disease, for example a genetic defect in the form of arrested development, and neural tube defects due to its occurrence in myelomeningocele.

Pathological anatomy

The neck of the talus points downwards and medially, whereas the body is rotated slightly outward in relation to both the calcaneum and the ankle mortise. The posterior part of the calcaneum is held close to the fibula by a tight calcaneo-fibular ligament, and is tilted into equinus and varus; it is also medially rotated beneath the ankle. The navicular bone and the entire forefoot are shifted medially and rotated into supination. The skin and soft tissue along the medial border of the foot are also under-developed.

Clinical features

The foot is turned and twisted inward so that the sole faces posteromedially. The calf muscles are atrophied and the foot is short. The ankle is in equinus, heel in varus, middle foot in cavus and forefoot in adduction and supination.

X-rays

Radiographic assessment is made on an antero-posterior film by measuring the *talocalcaneal angle*, a line drawn along the long axis of the talus on the medial side, and another line along the long axis of calcaneum on the lateral side. The normal angle is 30–55°. The talocalcaneal angle is also measured in the lateral view, which normally is 25–50°. Similarly, the tibio-calcaneal angle is measured which normally is 10–40° in stress lateral views.

Treatment

The aim of the treatment of club foot is a plantigrade, supple foot that will function normally. Conservative treatment is begun early, usually on the first day of life. This is done by *serial casting of the foot*, i.e. application of a new cast every 3 weeks, for 9 to 12 weeks. The order of correction is as follows: first the forefoot adduction is corrected; secondly the heel varus and finally the equinus deformity is corrected.

Operative treatment

This is reserved for non-responsive patients. The popular options are:

- Turco's procedure of postero-medial release.
- McKay's procedure of posteromedial and posterolateral releases.

If the patient presents after the age of five years, bony procedures are also done along with soft tissue releases. After the age of 12 years the surgical option is triple arthrodesis.

Congenital anomalies of the hand

These include:

- Failure of formation of parts.
- Failure of separation, e.g. syndactyly.
- Duplication, e.g. polydactyly.
- Overgrowth and undergrowth.
- Congenital constriction band.

Phocomelia

(Gr. *phoke* seal + *melos* limb). In this condition the arm is missing and the hand is suspended from the body near the shoulder; the hand is usually deformed and contains only three or four digits. Certain drugs, e.g. thalidomide, may interfere with the development of the fetus and produce phocomelia. Treatment of these patients generally is conservative.

Syndactyly

Syndactyly, or "webbed fingers," is caused by failure of the fingers to separate during embryological development. It is the most common congenital anomaly of the hand, with an occurrence of one per 2,000 births.

- In *complete* syndactyly the fingers are joined right upto the fingertips.
- In *incomplete* syndactyly they are joined only in the proximal part.
- In *complex* syndactyly bones are also joined together.

Surgical reconstruction is best carried out before the child is of school age. The surgical operation includes three steps:

- Separation of the digits.
- Reconstruction of the commissure.
- Resurfacing of the intervening borders of the digits by skin grafts.

DYSPLASIAS

Osteogenesis imperfecta (Brittle bone disease)

This disorder occurs with an incidence of 1 in 20,000. There is abnormal synthesis of type I collagen with resultant abnormalities in bones, teeth, ligaments, sclera and skin.

Clinical features

These depend on the severity of the disease. There is generalized osteopenia and a tendency of increased fractures after minor trauma. There is florid formation of callus, which remains pliable for a long time and ultimately results in non-union. There are generalized deformities of the long bones and kyphoscoliotic deformities with compressed fractures of the spine.

The skin is thin and loose, and there is hypermobility of the joints and ligaments. The colur of the sclera ranges from blue to grey. The teeth may be discoloured and carious, and dentinogenesis imperfecta (crumbling teeth) may be present. The severity of the disease varies from the mild to the fatal.

Management

Mostly symptomatic treatment is given. Fractures can be prevented by braces and orthopedic appliances. When they occur, they are managed conservatively. When severe deformities are present, multiple osteotomies may be needed.

Multiple exostoses (Diaphyseal aclasis)

An exostosis is the formation of new bone on the surface of a bone. This is a hereditary dominant disorder, associated with appearance of multiple hard lumps at the ends of long bones along the apophyseal border. In the lower limb, these exostoses appear around the knee, and in the upper limb along the scapula and ulna. The patient usually presents with multiple hard lumps, pain and sometimes pressure symptoms on the local or regional neuro-vascular bundle.

X-ray

On x-ray the long bone metaphyses are broad and poorly modeled, with sessile or pedunclated exostoses arising from the cortices. A mottled appearance around the lump is indicative of calcification of the cartilage cap.

Treatment

Generally no treatment is needed. The exostosis is excised if it causes hindrance in movement, pain, pressure effects or for cosmetic reasons. The excised tissue must be sent for histopathology. Sudden increase in size and constant enlargement after physeal closure are signs of malignancy. There is a 1–2% incidence of chondrosarcoma in these patients.

Torticollis

This term is used when the chin is twisted upward and towards the opposite side of the pathology. Torticollis may be congenital or acquired.

Congenital torticollis

The sternomastoid muscle is believed to experience ischemia in utero or during birth. It becomes fibrous and fails to elongate as the child grows, consequently deformity develops. During the first few weeks of life a lump--a 'sternomastoid tumor'--appears in the muscle which gradually disappears. This lump can be easily distinguished from other neck swellings in the newborn by demonstrating by palpation that the *upper and lower poles of the swelling are continuous with the sternomastoid muscle.*

Over the next few weeks the lump disappears. The damaged muscle is replaced by fibrous tissue, which contracts over a period of time. The result is that when the neck grows the sternomastoid fails to grow with it. Due to the shortness of the sternomastoid the head is pulled down on the side of the lesion and rotates towards the opposite side. In severe cases the muscle stands out like a cord (Fig.37.1). If left untreated it leads to gross asymmetry of the face, which is a serious matter. The visual mechanisms also grow in an asymmetrical manner.

Treatment

To release the contracture, surgical division of the muscle is required. This is carried out through a transverse skin crease incision. Braces are usually given for a few weeks postoperatively and stretching exercises are then started. An ocular consultation should be sought both pre-and post-operatively.

Acquired torticollis

Childhood torticollis may be due to:

- Trauma.
- Ocular dysfunction.
- Infection (abscess, lmyphadenitis, tuberculosis, tonsillitis).
- Atlanto-axial rotatory displacement.

Sometimes the torticollis is due simply to spasm of the neck muscles.

DISORDERS OF THE GROWING SKELETON

Disorders which affect the epiphyseal plate or epiphysis are peculiar to the growing skeleton. They may take the form of disturbances of growth and osteochondritis.

Disturbances of growth

If growth on one side of a limb proceeds faster than on the other, the limb becomes curved, being convex on the side of the more rapid growth. Unequal growth in the leg produces bow-leg or knock-knee. In the spine it probably produces 'idiopathic' scoliosis.

Knock-knee and bow-leg

At the end of growth, the knees are normally in $5–7^0$ of valgus. Any deviation from this is regarded as a deformity, which may be due to:

- Metabolic disorders.
- Trauma.
- Infection.
- Tumor.
- Renal osteodystrophy.

During the early period of growth around the age of four years, the knees are in physiological valgus. If after the age of 10 years, in knock-knee the intermalleolar distance is more than 8cm, or in bow-leg the intercondylar distance more than 6cm, operative treatment is considered.

Treatment

Before the closure of the physes

Stapling of the physis on one or the other side of the knee can be done to restrict growth on that side and allow correction of the deformity. Staples are removed once there is slight over-correction of the deformity.

After maturity

Valgus knees are corrected by supracondylar osteotomy.

Scoliosis

This is the apparent lateral curvature of the spine; it actually is a triplanar deformity with lateral, antero-posterior and rotational elements.

The types of scoliosis include:

- Congenital.
- Idiopathic.
- Neuromuscular.
- Postural.
- Pulmonary.
- Various other factors, like trauma, infections and tumors.

Congenital scoliosis

This generally occurs due to failure of formation or failure of segmentation of the bony vertebral column as follows:

- Failures of *formation*, e.g. wedge vertebra and hemi-vertebra.
- Failures of *segmentation*, e.g. block vertebra and unilateral segmentation bar.

These commonly develop during the fifth and sixth weeks of intra-uterine life. On *physical examination*, club foot and atrophy of muscles is seen. The reflexes must be assessed. MRI is usually needed to rule out diastematomyelia and tethered cord syndrome. *Surgery* is generally required for these patients.

Idiopathic scoliosis

This is the commonest type of scoliosis. It may occur in infants, juveniles and adolescents. Most curves below 20^0 resolve spontaneously or remain unchanged. Curves more than 20^0 need supervision for progression.

Treatment

Conservative

This is reserved for skeletally immature patients with curves less than 45^0. In high thoracic curves a Milwaukee brace is given; in low thoracic curves a Boston brace is applied.

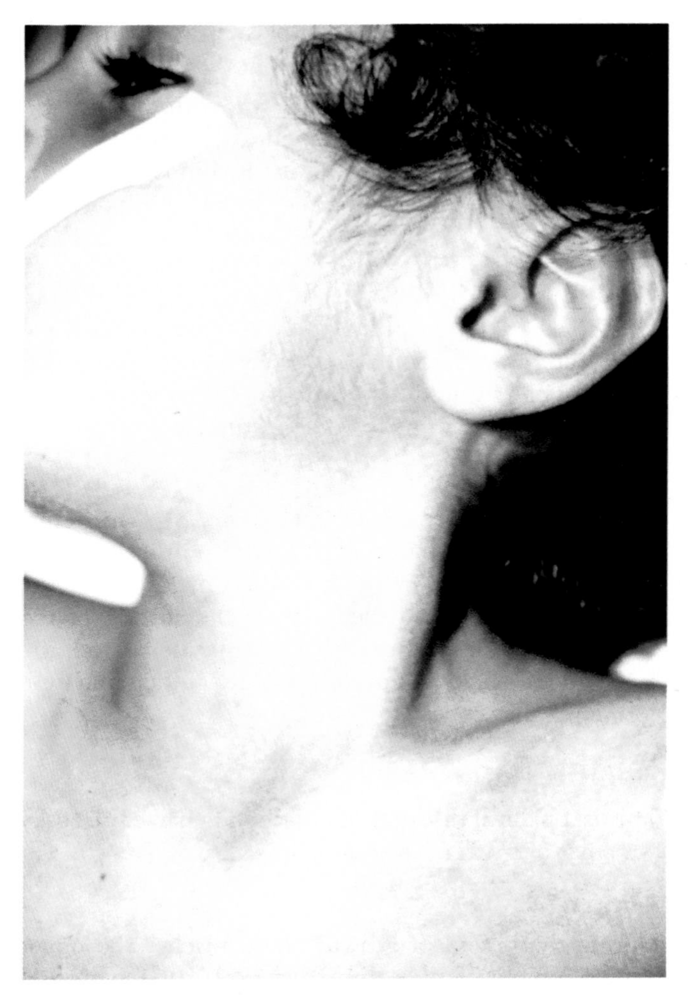

Fig.37.1 Congenital torticollis. The fibrosed, shortened sternomastoid muscle is standing out like a cord.

Surgical

This is meant for curves more than 45^0 in skeletally immature patients and 50^0 in skeletally mature curves. The surgical option consists of vertebral fusion of the following varieties:

- Anterior fusion.
- Posterior fusion.
- Combined anterior and posterior fusion.

In young skeletally immature patients Harrington rods and Luque rods can be used. Each Luque rod runs up one side of the spinous processes, and is anchored to bones on the way.

Neuromuscular scoliosis

Polio and cerebral palsy are the common causes of neuromuscular scoliosis. The scoliosis is due to muscle imbalance. Scoliosis in cerebral palsy is associated with considerable pain.

Initially these patients are *managed* with braces and supports, the aim being to maintain stable sitting of the patients. Surgery is carried out in situations where it is expected that the curve will progress once the braces are removed.

Postural scoliosis

This affects children of school age. There is a simple curve without rotation of the vertebrae. It is due to bad posture while sitting at school desks. *Treatment* consists of gymnastics and training in good posture.

Pulmonary scoliosis

Fibrotic disease of one lung or pleura, e.g. empyema, may result in contraction of the chest wall on that side and cause scoliosis. *Treatment* consists of removing the thick layer of fibrosed pleura from the surface of the lung *(decortication)* at thoracotomy. This allows both the lung and the chest wall to expand fully, at the same time correcting the scoliosis.

Perthes disease

This is a painful disorder of childhood characterized by avascular necrosis of the femoral head.

Pathology

During the period of growth blood reaches the upper femoral epiphysis only through vessels passing around the periphery of the epiphyseal plate. It seems that some factor interferes with this blood supply and produces avascular necrosis of the ossification centre of the epiphysis.

Clinical features

The disease affects children between 5 and 10 years of age, mostly boys. Some cases are bilateral. There is pain in the front of the thigh and knee and the child limps. On examination there is restriction of abduction and internal rotation, first due to muscle spasm and later due to flattening and deformity of the femoral head.

X-ray findings

The ossific nucleus of the femoral head is smaller than on the other side. The hip joint space is increased due to effusion.

The femoral head is divided into three pillars by lines at the medial and lateral edges of the sequestrum:

- Group A cases have normal height of the lateral pillar.
- Group B cases have partial collapse.
- Group C cases have severe collapse, of the lateral pillar.

Patients in groups B and C who are more than nine years of age have a poor prognosis.

Treatment

This aims at containing the diseased epiphysis within the acetabulum until reossification is complete; this affords the best chance of obtaining a spherical head. It may require the patient to walk with the hip in a position of abduction.

Children under 6 years

- Group A and B need symptomatic treatment.
- Group C patients need an abduction brace.

Children 6–8 years old

- Group A and B need abduction brace with or without osteotomy.
- In group C the outcome will not improve irrespective of the treatment offered.

Children 9 years and above

An operative procedure with containment of the hip is needed; postoperatively a walking abduction brace is used for the duration of healing (12 to 18 months).

The *outcome* depends upon:

- Stage of the disease.
- Final sphericity of the head.
- Congruity of the head with the acetabulum.

Degenerative arthritis can present in the fourth to sixth decades.

GENERALIZED DISEASES OF BONE

Paget's disease

This is a chronic and progressive metabolic disease of abnormal bone remodeling. There is enlargement and thickening of the bone, but the internal architecture is abnormal and the bone is unusually brittle. There is a marked increase in osteoclastic and osteoblastic activity; these processes run continuously in adjacent areas and on both endosteal and periosteal surfaces, so the bone increases in thickness but it is structurally weak and easily deformed. The disease may be localized to one bone or generalized.

Paget's disease is unusual before the age of 55 years. After 55 years the incidence is 3–4%, and after 80 years 10%.

The *complications* associated with this disease include:

- Pathological fractures.
- Osteoarthritis.
- Nerve and spinal cord compression.
- Hypocalcemia in bed-ridden patients.
- High output cardiac failure due to arteriovenous fistulae in the affected highly vascular bone.

Clinical features

Most patients are asymptomatic and the disease is diagnosed accidently on x-rays requested for some other disorder. A few patients present with pain and discomfort. Primary presentation of the disease is due to deformities of the bone or pathological fractures. The limbs look bent—*osteitis deformans*—and feel thick and the skin is unusually warm.

The skull may enlarge and the skull base may be flattened (*platybasia*). Involvement of the spine leads to kyphoscoliosis and spinal cord or nerve root compression. Cranial nerve involvement leads to impaired vision, facial palsy, trigeminal neuralgia and deafness. Deafness can also be due to otosclerosis.

Diagnosis

The *x-ray* picture is most of the time classical for Paget's disease. The bones are thick, sclerotic and with coarse trabeculations. Sometimes fine cracks develop on the convex surface of the long bone.

Laboratory

Serum calcium and phosphate are normal but alkaline phosphatase level is increased. 24-hour urinary excretion of pyridinoline is increased along with increased level of urinary hydroxyproline.

Management

General indications for treatment include:

- Persistent bone pain.
- Repeated fractures.
- Neurological complications.
- High output cardiac failure.
- Hypocalcemia due to immobilization.

Surgery

This is reserved for:

- Pathological fractures.
- Spinal decompression.
- Nerve entrapment.
- Joint replacement in severe arthritis.

For some months before and after major bone surgery, where there is risk of excessive hemorrhage, drugs that decrease the bone turnover are given, e.g. calcitonin and bisphosphonates.

Osteoporosis

This is defined as a decrease in the bone mass more than 2.5 standard deviations (SD) below the average for premenopausal women in the relevant population group. It is a metabolic disorder associated with qualitative loss of bone. The bone is fully mineralized but is abnormally porous and its strength is less than normal for a person of that age and sex.

There can be increased bone resorption, decreased bone formation or both. Osteoporosis may be:

- *Regional* (localized to a bone or group of bones).
- *Generalized.*

It may be:

- *Primary* where there is no obvious cause.
- *Secondary* due to some endocrine, metabolic or neoplastic disorder.

Primary osteoporosis

This is divided into two types: postmenopausal and senile osteoporosis.

Postmenopausal osteoporosis

This is a high-turnover type of osteoporosis, and is due to withdrawal of estrogen at the menopause, which leads to unrestrained osteoclastic activity.

The *risk factors* include:

- Family history.
- Anorexia nervosa.
- Early onset menopause.
- Dietary insufficiency.
- Increased alcohol intake and smoking.
- Chronic lack of exercise.

It presents with vertebral compression fractures and low-energy fractures of the distal radius (Colles' type).

Diagnosis

This is based on bone mineral density assessment by DEXA Scan. Other diagnostic options include dual photon absorptiometry, quantitative CT and Singh's Index.

Treatment

The options include:

- *Hormone* replacement therapy. This is associated with increased risk of bleeding and of uterine and breast cancer.

- High doses of *calcium* and *vitamin D*; calcium is given in a dose of 1500mg/day and vitamin D over 800 units/day.
- Bisphosphonates.
- Calcitonin.
- Fluoride.

Senile osteoporosis

This occurs due to steady loss of bone mass after the age of 75, and affects females and males in a ratio of 2:1. These patients generally present with hip fractures after trivial trauma.

Treatment is generally the same as in type 1 osteoporosis.

Secondary osteoporosis

The common causes include:

- Immobilization.
- Chronic alcoholism.
- Hypercorticism.
- Prolonged use of glucocorticoids.
- Gonadal hormone deficiency.

Vitamin D deficiency

Deficiency of vitamin D may arise during childhood, when it produces the condition called rickets. If deficiency arises during adult life it results in osteomalacia.

Rickets

In this condition there is inadequate mineralization of the bone throughout the skeleton. In children the defect lies in the zone of provisional calcification. The adult presentation of the disease is called *osteomalacia*. The disorder is broadly divided into three types: vitamin D deficiency, renal tubular defects and renal osteodystrophy:

Vitamin D deficiency

This may be due to:

- Dietary insufficiency.
- Malabsorption.
- Phosphate deficiency.
- Crohn's disease.

The laboratory parameters show low or normal calcium, low phosphate, high PTH and low vitamin D levels. It is *treated* by high doses of vitamin D (up to 5000 i.u. daily).

Renal tubular defects

Vitamin D-dependent rickets type I and II are common examples of this condition.

- In type I disorder, there is a defect in renal 25-(OH)-vitamin D 1 alpha-hydroxylase, so there is lack of conversion of 1-hydroxy to di-hydroxy cholecalciferol.
- In type II disease, the defect is in the intracellular receptors for 1–25-(OH) 2 vitamin D3.

Treatment

The treatment of nutritional rickets is by supplementation with high doses of vitamin D 3,000 i.u. daily (normal daily requirement 400 i.u.). Calcium supplementation enhances the rate of healing. For persistent deformities correction is delayed until the underlying metabolic defect has resolved, at which time osteotomies can be performed.

Renal osteodystrophy

In end-stage renal disease, the damaged kidney excretes smaller quantities of phosphate. The resulting hyperphosphataemia causes hypocalcemia and results in osteomalacia, osteoporosis and osteosclerosis—the features of renal osteodystrophy.

Treatment consists of calcium and vitamin D supplementation, restriction of dietary phosphate, phosphate binders like calcium carbonate, and hemodialysis/renal transplantation.

Osteomalacia

In adults deficiency of vitamin D affects the bones of the pelvis, and they are rendered quite soft. This condition is called osteomalacia (*malacia* = softness). The causes include:

- Nutritional deficiency.
- Malabsorption.
- Anticonvulsant therapy.
- Hepatic and renal disorders.

The condition is *much more common in females*, and usually develops to its full extent during lactation, due to the drain on the calcium stores in the blood. The body weight pushes the sacral promontory downwards. Similarly the femoral heads push the acetabula upwards. This results in a triradiate pelvis and greatly narrows the pelvic outlet. The narrow pelvic outlet may result in obstructed labor.

Treatment

Vitamin D is *administered*, usually in the form of vitamin D3 intramuscularly or orally. Two to four doses of 200,000 i.u. are given at intervals of 1 month until the deficiency is made good. The serum D_3 is repeatedly determined to avoid over-dosage. Early bone deformities can be dealt with by splintage. Severe deformities may require division of the bone (osteotomy) for correction.

Gout

This is a disorder of purine metabolism characterized by hyperuricemia, deposition of monosodium urate monohydrate crystals in joints and peri-articular tissues, and recurrent attacks of acute synovitis. Late changes include cartilage degeneration, uric acid urolithiasis and renal dysfunction. There is abnormality in the nucleic acid and purine metabolism. Urate crystals are deposited in minute clumps in connective tissue, including articular cartilage. The commonest sites are the small joints of the hands and feet. After minor trauma, these crystals are dispersed in the joint cavity, where they start the inflammatory reaction. With the passage of time, urate deposits may be built up in the joints, periarticular tissues, tendons and bursae.

Gout may be:

- *Primary* where there is no obvious cause.
- *Secondary* due to prolonged hyperuricemia from acquired disorders such as:
  - o Myeloproliferative diseases.
  - o Renal dysfunction.

Clinical features

The patient presents with an acute attack of severe pain, typically in the metatarsophalyngeal joint of the big toe. The attack lasts for one to two weeks. The joints feel hot and tender and resemble acute cellulitis.

Diagosis

A serum *uric acid* level more than two standard deviations above the mean is helpful in establishing the diagnosis.

The true diagnosis is established by characteristic *negatively birefringent urate crystals* in the synovial fluid.

On *x-ray* characteristic punched-out cysts or deep erosions in the para-articular bone ends, known as *tophi*, appear; these excavations are larger and slightly further from the joint margin than in rheumatoid erosions.

Treatment

The acute attack is managed by:

- *Rest* and non-steroid anti-inflammatory drugs (NSAIDs).
- Avoidance of *alcohol* and *diuretics.*
- *Uricosuric drugs* like probenecid and sulfinpyrazone can be used if the renal function is normal.
- *Allopurinol*, a xanthine oxidase inhibitor, is usually preferred. But these drugs should not be started during an acute attack.

DISEASES OF MUSCLES, TENDONS AND FASCIAE

Tennis elbow

In this condition the patient complains of pain in the elbow, specially when he uses the hand and therefore contracts the wrist and finger extensors. The lesion in this condition is lateral epicondylitis. This can result from activities that require repetitive pronation and supination of the forearm with the elbow bent.

Microscopic findings

Lateral epicondylitis is initiated as a micro tear, most often within the origin of the extensor carpi radialis brevis. This shows immature reparative tissue that resembles angiofibroblastic hyperplasia.

Diagnosis

The diagnosis of tennis elbow is made by demonstrating that discomfort is localized to the origin of the extensor carpi radialis brevis. Tenderness is present over the lateral epicondyle approximately 5mm distal and anterior to the midpoint of the condyle. Pain usually is exacerbated when grasping objects, by forearm supination, and by resisted wrist dorsiflexion.

Imaging

Plain radiographs usually are negative; occasionally calcific tendinitis may be present. MRI shows tendon thickening with increased T1 and T2 signals.

Treatment

Non-operative treatment is successful in 95% of patients with tennis elbow, and includes rest, ice, steroid injections, and physical therapy with ultrasound, friction massage, stretching and strengthening exercises.

Numerous surgical procedures have been described for the treatment of tennis elbow. Currently, a rather limited approach is favoured, which consists of exposure of the diseased extensor carpi radialis brevis origin, resection of degenerated tissue, and direct repair of muscle to bone.

Supraspinatus tendinitis

In this condition pain is felt in the shoulder, especially on abduction and rotation, and localized tenderness is present over the insertion of the supraspinatus tendon, usually between 30 and 50 years of age.

Acute pain may follow deposition of calcium hydroxyapatite crystals, usually in the supraspinatus tendon slightly medial to its insertion. It is thought that local ischemia leads to fibro-cartilaginous metaplasia and deposition of crystals by the chondrocytes. Symptoms are due to florid vascular reaction which produces swelling and tension in the tendon.

Symptoms

Aching pain is felt after overuse which increases in severity rising to an agonizing climax. After a few days the pain subsides and the shoulder returns to normal function. Sometimes the recovery is very slow and the patient may end up with adhesive capsulitis. It should be remembered that *whenever the shoulder is painful from any cause it rapidly becomes stiff because of disuse.*

Treatment

Initially, a polysling is given with non-steroidal anti-inflammatory medication. In severe cases a single injection of corticosteroid (methylprednisolone) is given with local anesthetic (lignocaine 1%) in the hypervascular area. In resistant cases, surgery is carried out.

Stenosing tenosynovitis

Stenosing tenosynovitis of the abductor pollicis longus and extensor pollicis brevis tendons occurs typically in adults 30 to 50 years old. Women are affected six to ten times more frequently than men. The cause is almost always related to overuse, either in the home or at work, or is associated with rheumatoid arthritis.

The presenting *symptoms* usually are pain and tenderness at the radial styloid process. Sometimes a thickening of the fibrous sheath is palpable.

Finkelstein test

This test is usually positive: on grasping the patient's thumb and quickly bending the hand ulnarward, the pain over the styloid tip is excruciating. However, the test is not diagnostic; the patient's history and occupation, the radiographs, and other physical findings also must be considered.

Treatment

Conservative treatment, consisting of rest on a splint and the injection of a steroid preparation, is most successful within the first six weeks after onset. If this fails, the retinaculum overlying the tendons may have to be divided.

Carpal tunnel syndrome

Carpal tunnel syndrome (tardy median palsy) is the result of compression of the median nerve within the carpal tunnel. Paraesthesia over the sensory distribution of the median nerve, i.e. the lateral three and a half fingers, is the most frequent presentation; it occurs more often in women and frequently causes the patient to awaken several hours after falling asleep, with burning and numbness of the hand that is relieved by exercise.

Physical signs

- The *Tinel sign* may be shown in most patients by percussing the median nerve at the wrist.
- *Phalen test.* Acute flexion of the wrist for 60 seconds in some patients, or strenuous use of the hand, increases the paraesthesias.
- Application of a *blood pressure cuff* on the upper arm sufficient to produce venous distension may initiate the symptoms.

Treatment

Carpal tunnel syndrome can be divided into early, intermediate, advanced, and acute stages:

- Patients with early carpal tunnel syndrome and mild symptoms respond to night splints and steroid injection.
- If signs and symptoms are persistent and progressive, especially if they include thenar atrophy, division of the deep transverse carpal ligament is indicated.

The results of surgery are good in most instances, and benefits seem to last in most patients. Some degree of atrophy of the median-nerve-innervated thenar muscles has been reported in about half of the patients treated by operation.

Dupuytren's contracture

Dupuytren's contracture is a proliferative fibroplasia of the subcutaneous palmar tissue occurring in the form of nodules and cords that may result in secondary progressive and irreversible flexion contractures of the finger joints. Dupuytren's contracture occurs 10 times more frequently in men than in women, in their 40s to 60s.

Treatment

In the absence of contractures, treatment is not indicated because nodules and cords usually are painless. Rarely is the presence of a palmar nodule alone an indication for surgery, unless sufficient discomfort, pitting, and maceration occur. Patients with slowly progressing, non-disabling contractures should be examined periodically, about every six months.

Surgical treatment

This is technically easier when joint contractures are smaller. Ideally, patients are operated on when their disease is mature and quiescent, and the tendency for surgical trauma to accentuate the disease process is less. If surgical intervention is carried out in the proliferative stage, stiffening and increase in flexion contractures may occur. Nonetheless, contractures that are disabling may warrant surgery.

Surgical procedures commonly used in treating Dupuytren's contracture include:

- Subcutaneous fasciotomy.
- Partial or complete fasciectomy, with or without skin grafting.

Ganglion

A ganglion is a localized, tense, cystic swelling containing clear gelatinous fluid. It usually overlies and communicates with the capsule of a joint. The origin of ganglia is uncertain. They are mostly seen on the dorsum of the wrist (Fig.37.2). The patient presents with a painless lump, though there is slight ache and weakness. The swelling does not move with the tendon. If a ganglion does not resolve spontaneously, excision is carried out.

Chronic bursitis

Chronic bursitis is the result of repeated pressure or injury to various bursae, e.g. prepatellar bursa (housemaid's knee), olecranon bursa etc. A semimembranosus bursa often communicates with the knee joint. In that case it may enlarge when there is effusion in the joint, e.g. in osteoarthrosis. It is then called a *Baker's cyst.*

PARALYSIS OF MUSCLES

There are two important results of paralysis of muscles:

- *Loss of function*. This is due to failure of the affected muscles. An important effect is loss of joint stability.
- *Liability to deformity*:
  - o In the *adult* this is not a serious problem. The non-paralyzed muscles are liable to develop contracture, but this can be controlled by passive movements and by splintage.
  - o In the *child* the problem is much more serious because growth is disturbed. The non-paralysed muscles become short, so the joints become fixed in the direction of the active muscles. Secondary bony deformities develop, and cause even greater fixation of the joint. It should be remembered that in a totally paralysed limb no deformity develops, because there is no muscle imbalance to distort it.

The management of paralysis

The aims of treatment of a case with paralysis are three:

- *Elimination of deformity*. In the adult, passive movements and splints are able to prevent deformity.

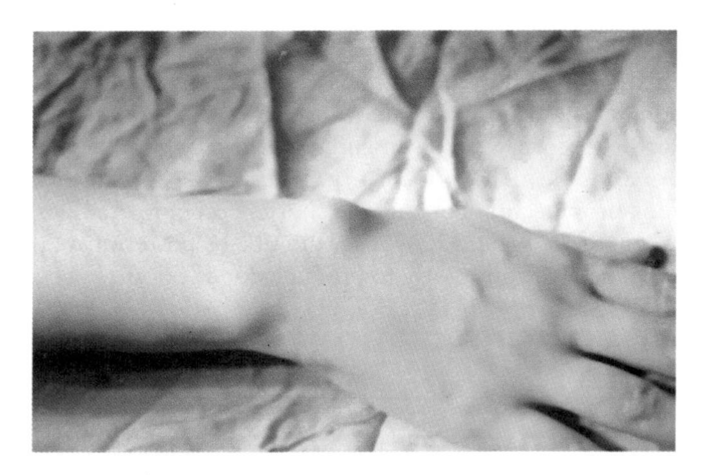

Fig.37.2 Ganglion wrist. Hemispherical swelling on

  In the child this is not enough, and the contracted tendons of the unopposed muscles have also to be divided.
- *Prevention of recurrent deformity*. For this purpose it is necessary to restore muscle balance across the joint. Either the paralyzed muscle group is reinforced, or the non-paralyzed muscles are weakened:
  - o The paralysed group is usually reinforced by *tendon transfer*. The tendon of a normally acting muscle is divided and inserted into a new site so that its mode of action is altered. Often it acts in place of its antagonists.
  - o The non-paralysed muscle group may be weakened by *tenotomy* or by *lengthening* of its tendon.
- *Restoration of joint stability and function*. Joint stability may be restored by tendon transfer. If this is impracticable or fails, in the adult arthrodesis (fusion of the joint) is usually carried out. In children external splintage is the only solution until they are old enough for arthrodesis.

Poliomyelitis

Poliomyelitis is an acute febrile illness due to a neurotropic virus. It produces irregularly distributed flaccid paralysis by damaging the anterior horn cells. It has been eliminated from most parts of the world by universal immunization at birth; unfortunately it still exists in a few countries. The paralysis and wasting are nearly always asymmetrical, affecting particularly the lower limbs, and the spine and trunk muscles. There is no sensory loss.

Management

In the early and recovery phases the paralyzed limb is splinted to minimize deformity. After two years no further recovery can occur and reconstruction can begin. For example in the foot due to paralysis of the dorsiflexors foot-drop occurs. For this the shortened tendo-Achilles is lengthened (Fig.37.3). Also, the tibialis posterior may be transferred anteriorly to produce dorsiflexion.

INFECTIONS OF BONES AND JOINTS

ACUTE OSTEOMYELITIS

Before the days of antibiotics, acute osteomyelitis used to be a serious and sometimes fatal condition. Nowadays it can be dealt with satisfactorily if detected in time.

Etiology

The vast majority of cases of acute osteomyelitis are due to bacteria, the infection being blood-borne. In some cases the primary focus may be evident in the form of a boil, but quite often there is no obvious cause. It is thought that lowered general resistance of the patient and local trauma predispose to this condition, but there is no proof of this. The usual organism is *Staphylococcus aureus*; Group A streptococcus and *H. influenza* are the next most common organisms. Acute osteomyelitis occurs mostly during the period of skeletal growth, the peak incidence being during childhood. Males are affected more often than females.

Pathology

The disease nearly always begins in the metaphysis. During childhood the epiphyseal cartilage acts as a barrier, so arthritis does not occur as a complication of osteomyelitis.

The infective process moves towards the surface, producing thrombosis of the vessels and leading to avascular necrosis of bone in the process. Finally, the exudates lift up the periosteum, causing severe pain. The pus under the periosteum is under tension, so the patient rapidly develops signs due to the toxic absorption. The pus tracks around the bone, stripping the periosteum and interrupting the periosteal vessels. Thus progressively larger areas of the cortex lose their blood supply, i.e. become infarcted. Untreated, the pus finally perforates the periosteum and tracks through the muscles to discharge as a sinus on the skin.

The dead piece of bone is called a *sequestrum*. The new bone around it which is laid down by the periosteum is called the *involucrum*. The openings in the involucrum through which pus is discharged are called *cloacae*.

Clinical features

The onset of acute osteomyelitis is usually sudden, with marked toxicity. The pain rapidly increases in severity. The child keeps the limb motionless. The temperature is often markedly raised. Local tenderness is the essential physical sign. It usually comes on before the swelling. If in a child the maximum tenderness is over the metaphysis of a long bone it should be presumed to be due to acute osteomyelitis until proved otherwise.

The adjacent joint may contain an effusion, raising the possibility of suppurative arthritis. However, some movement of the joint is possible in osteomyelitis, whereas in septic arthritis absolutely no movement is possible.

Diagnosis

The history must be taken very carefully. A history of trauma may divert attention from osteomyelitis.

Example

A young girl was brought to a hospital with a history of a fall, with pain and tenderness in the thigh. X-ray showed no fracture. A diagnosis of soft tissue injury was made, and a firm crepe bandage applied. Next day the child was taken elsewhere in severe endotoxic shock, with pyemia and septic thrombosis of the inferior vena cava, as shown by veins running upwards on the sides of the trunk. The thigh was swollen with pus (Fig.37.4 a and b).

It was obvious that the history of injury had misled the clinician. Because osteomyelitis was not suspected, she was not placed on any antibiotics. Further, the firm bandaging (meant to give support to the 'soft tissue injury') may have forced the pus into the veins and caused pyemia. In spite of immediate drainage of pus and every possible intensive treatment the child died.

Remember that *if your initial enquiries set you on the wrong diagnostic track, no power on earth can bring you back on the correct path.* The consequences can be as tragic as in this case.

Exogenous osteomyelitis

This is most often the result of a compound fracture. *Symptoms are usually less severe,* because some drainage is available via the wound through which the micro-organisms entered. On the blood examination, there will be raised total leukocyte count, and neutrophils will be predominant in the differential count. ESR will be raised and C-reactive protein (CRP) will be raised markedly.

Differential diagnosis

Conditions which can mimic osteomyelitis include Ewing's sarcoma, rheumatic fever and leukemia.

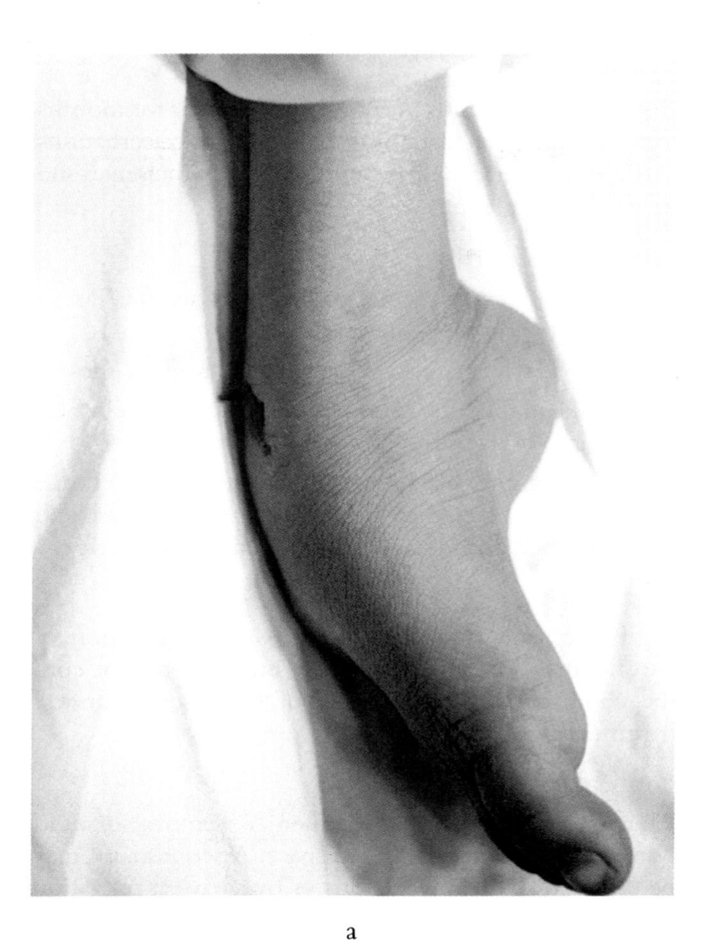

a

Fig.37.3 (a) Shortened gastocnemius muscle from its unopposed action due to post-polio paralysis of ankle dorsiflexors

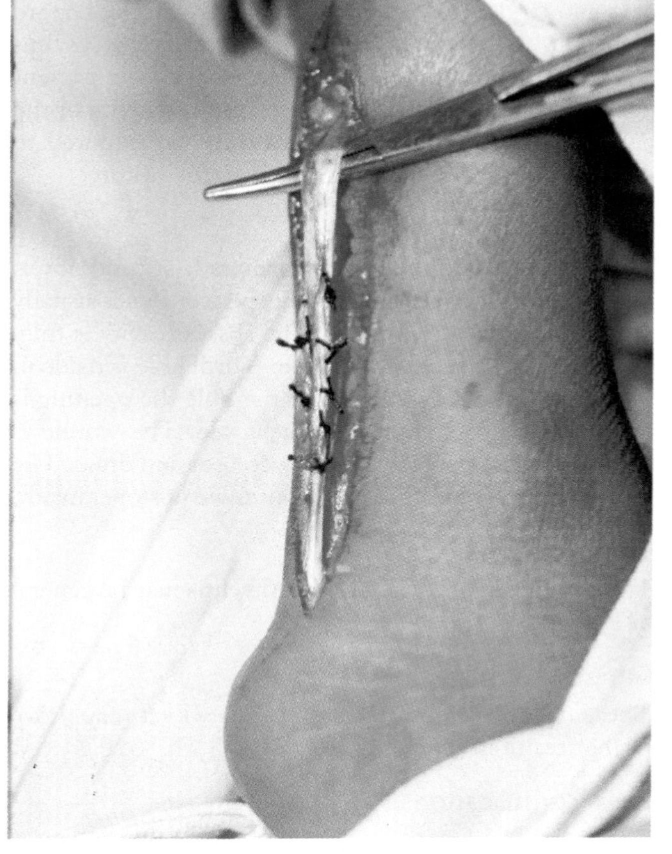

b

Fig.37.3 (b) Lengthening of the tendo-Achilles

Imaging

MRI

This has proved very sensitive and specific in establishing the early diagnosis.

Tri-phasic bone scans[1]

These are helpful in acute cases.

X-ray

For the first week or more, x-ray of the bone is normal. However, in two or three weeks new bone can be seen deposited under the elevated periosteum. At this time some rarefaction of bone due to local hyperemia may also be visible.

1 The three-phase bone scan detects different types of pathology in the bone. After injection of the Technetium-99m, the three phases are recorded between the first few seconds and three hours. The first phase shows perfusion to a lesion; cellulitis is detected in this phase. Moderate to severe pathology shows up in the first two phases, chronic pathology in the third.

Treatment of acute osteomyelitis

The child is admitted to hospital and the limb splinted. Toxic patients require intravenous fluids and electrolytes. If the patient is seen within 48 hours of onset, antibiotics are immediately started. However, before they are commenced blood should be taken for culture. If antibiotics are started within 48 hours of onset, the area of disease can be sterilized and complete resolution of infection occurs. If not, the condition becomes chronic and poses a long-term problem.

Antibiotics are administered parenterally. As most cases are due to *Staphylococcus aureus*, cloxacillin is commenced along with an aminoglycoside. In patients allergic to penicillin, clindamycin may be used or quinolones can be started. In infants *Hemophilus influenzae* is often the cause, and ampicillin is used. If the case fails to respond, chloramphenicol may be substituted.

If the patient is seen 48 hours or more after the onset, pus may be present requiring drainage. If the temperature settles down to normal within two to three days and tenderness gradually disappears, antibiotics are sufficient. If, however, the temperature subsides but does not become normal, it means that pus is present or the antibiotic is inappropriate to the sensitivity of the organism. In either case the area must be explored to drain any pus and obtain the organism for culture.

Operation

This is carried out under general anaesthasia. Incision is made over the tender area and deepened. Pus is usually found under the periosteum. The abscess cavity is fully opened and pus taken for culture. A drill hole is made in the bone. If pus flows out from the hole the opening is enlarged until free drainage is achieved. The wound is either left wide open or closed over a suction drain. The limb is splinted and antibiotics continued postoperatively.

Complications

The complications of acute osteomyelitis may be general or local.

General complications

These include septicemia and pyemia which may prove fatal or result in metastatic abscesses.

Local complications

These include the following:

- Suppurative arthritis, if the epiphyseal line is intra-articular.
- Spontaneous fracture.
- Chronic osteomyelitis.

Chronic osteomyelitis

Acute osteomyelitis may pass into chronic osteomyelitis if it is not treated early or is treated inadequately, so that infected bone dies to become a sequestrum. It may take one of two forms:

- Acute hematogenous osteomyelitis leaves behind a large sequestrum.
- A *Brodie's abscess* may form. In this case the disease is localized, resulting in a chronic abscess within the bone. Pus and granulation tissue are surrounded by sclerotic bone. It may follow a pyogenic septicemia, leaving a bone abscess which may remain dormant for years; or it may be seen in a patient who in the past had osteomyelitis in a different bone. It becomes painful from time to time. Examination shows tenderness and thickening of the bone. X-ray shows a band of sclerosis around a radiolucent area.
- Amyloidosis may follow long-standing chronic osteomyelitis.

Clinical features

Chronic osteomyelitis may remain quiescent for months or years. However, from time to time acute exacerbations occur with fever, local pain and swelling, which may end up in discharge of pus.

Imaging

An x-ray may reveal a sequestrum in a cavity. A CT scan can also show up the sequestra.

The reasons why such an abscess fails to heal are these:

- Unlike in the soft tissues, the abscess cannot close by collapse of its walls.
- Infection provokes the formation of dense bone around it, so that white cells, antibodies and antibiotics cannot reach the contents of the cavity.

Treatment

Antibiotics and splintage can help an exacerbation of chronic osteomyelitis to subside, but they cannot cure the condition. For eradication of the disease surgical treatment is required.

Surgical treatment

The purpose of surgical treatment is removal of dead bone and elimination of dead space. A sequestrum may be detected by probing a sinus or by x-ray. At operation the sequestrum is approached by removing the overlying portion of the involucrum. If a cavity is present the overhanging walls are removed with an osteotome until it is *saucerized*, i.e. made to look like a saucer, which is a broad and shallow vessel.

A Brodie's abscess should be treated by laying open and curetting the cavity under antibiotic cover.

The best after-care consists of *leaving the wound completely open* i.e. unsutured, and treating it with irrigation and dressings. This allows the wound to fill with granulations and then finally epithelialize. However, some surgeons prefer to close the wound by suture and irrigate it constantly with antibiotic solutions. With this regimen the wound may sometimes refuse to heal; therefore, if this course is followed, postoperative supervision must be very watchful.

Acute suppurative arthritis

Etiology

Acute suppurative arthritis may occur due to one of the following:

- A penetrating wound or a compound fracture involving the joint.
- Blood-borne infection, the common organisms being streptococcus, staphylococcus and pneumococcus.

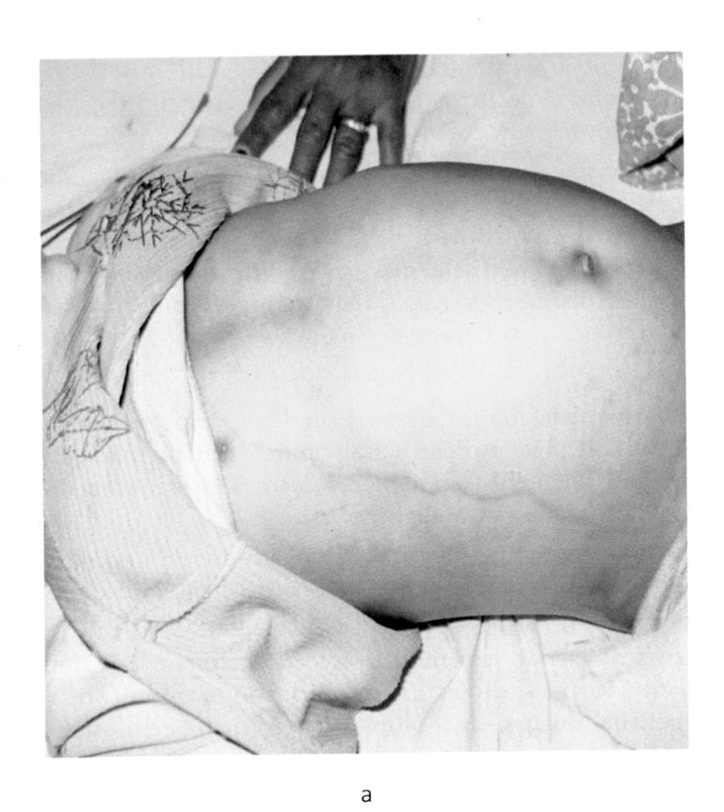

a

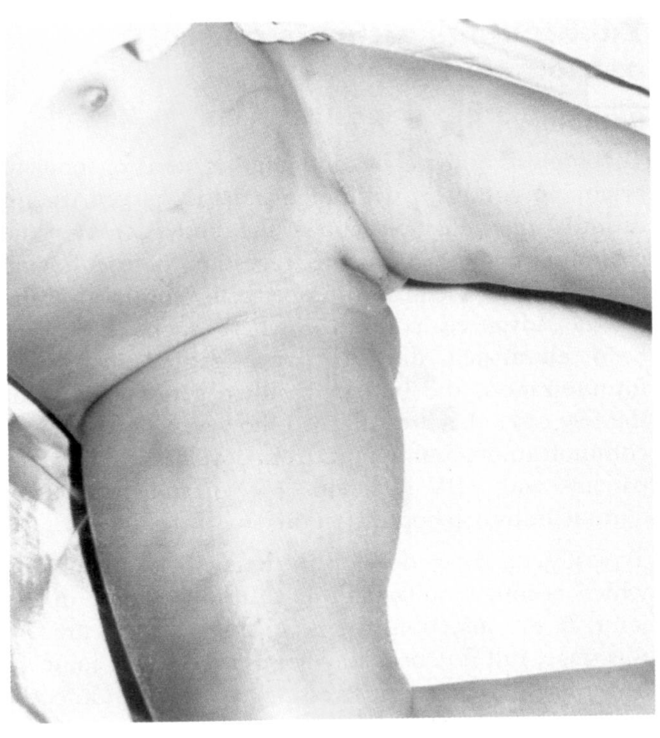

b

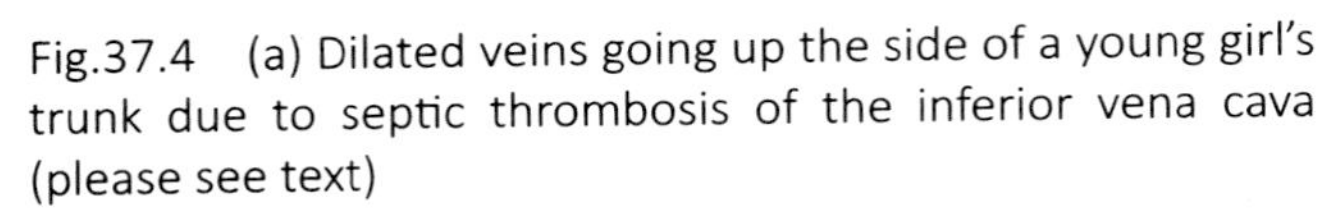

Fig.37.4 (a) Dilated veins going up the side of a young girl's trunk due to septic thrombosis of the inferior vena cava (please see text)

Fig.37.4 (b) Thigh swollen with pus due to acute osteomyelitis

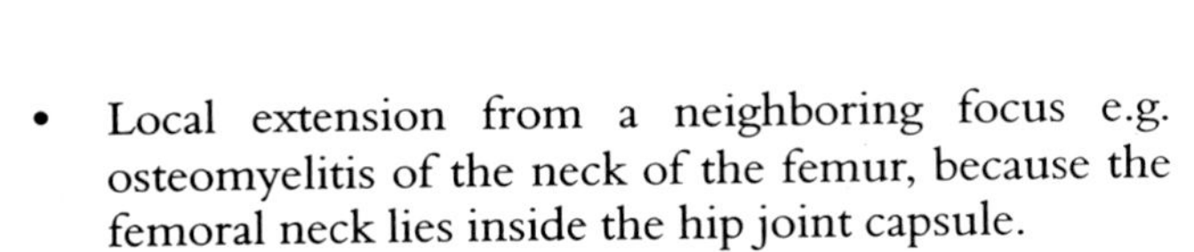

- Local extension from a neighboring focus e.g. osteomyelitis of the neck of the femur, because the femoral neck lies inside the hip joint capsule.

Staphylococcus aureus and hemolytic streptococcus are the two most common organisms that cause pyogenic arthritis, apart from gonococcal and coliform organisms and *Hemophilus influenza* (in children). Septic arthritis is more common in debilitated patients or those undergoing steroid therapy or immunosuppressant therapy.

Clinical features

There is steadily increasing pain and malaise. The patient tends to avoid movement of the joint, and is severely toxic with a raised temperature and pulse rate. On palpation the joint is hot and tender. Movements are prevented by muscle spasm and are extremely painful.

X-rays

These reveal effusion with increased joint space. In more advanced infections erosions and joint space narrowing may be seen.

Diagnosis

This is by *aspiration* of the joint with culture, Gram staining and analysis of the synovial fluid, along with biopsy of tissue. The presence of organisms and an elevated white cell count in the fluid may be diagnostic; the count may range from 20,000 to 30,000, with up to 90% of neutrophils.

Treatment

Medical

Antibiotics are started with coverage for *S. aureus* (cephalosporin), streptococci (cephalosporin or a penicillin), and in children *H. influenza* (ampicillin). When the culture report arrives the antibiotic may have to be changed. Antibiotics are given intravenously for two weeks, followed by oral administration for four weeks.

Surgical

The joint is drained by an open washout. If the joint is destroyed, resection arthroplasty is carried out. Patients who undergo drainage improve more rapidly and surely.

At a later stage arthodesis or rarely joint replacement arthroplasty may be carried out, but only after infection has been totally eradicated.

Tuberculous arthritis and osteomyelitis

Pathology

Tuberculosis of the bones and joints is hematogenous in origin. In countries without mandatory pasteurization of milk the infection enters the body through the gastrointestinal tract due to ingestion of the bovine strain of the bacillus in imperfectly sterilized milk. In the advanced countries, where tuberculosis has been eliminated due to pasteurization and BCG immunization, the human bacillus is responsible for the few cases that are still seen; however, the disease is common among immigrants from developing countries, patients with HIV infection (AIDS), and patients on chronic immunosuppression therapy.

Typically, tubercles develop in the synovial membrane which becomes bulky, and an effusion collects in the joint. If the infection can be diagnosed and cured at this stage, full function may be restored to the joint. If, however, the disease progresses, hypertrophic infected synovium (pannus) gradually covers the cartilage surface and erodes the subchondral bone, destroying the cartilage as well. Healing leaves a fibrous ankylosis. Free mobility of a joint depends upon the presence of articular cartilage; when this is destroyed, loss of mobility is bound to occur.

The most common site in the skeleton is the spine. At the same time the disease may start in any synovial joint, specially a joint with extensive synovial membranes e.g. the hip or knee.

Spine

In the spine the diagnosis is rarely made until the bodies of two neighboring vertebrae are involved. If treatment is delayed an abscess forms and the vertebral bodies collapse. The pus may track long distances; for example pus arising from a lumbar vertebra may track inside the psoas muscle sheath to present in the groin.

Vertebral collapse produces a forward angulation of the spine--a *kyphosis*. Pressure from the pus and from angulation of the spine may damage the spinal cord and produce paraplegia.

Clinical features

Symptoms

These arise from the diseased joint and from the systemic effects of the disease. Usually the first symptom is *pain* in the joint which is often more severe at night. The pain gets worse, and increasing stiffness comes on. The stiffness is due to bone destruction and muscle spasm. There is *swelling* of the joint, which is made more prominent by the wasting of the associated muscles. As the bone is destroyed the joint dislocates and the *local deformity* becomes obvious.

In the *spinal column*, because of its deep location, the swelling is not visible until a good deal of pus has collected, and stiffness may be slight and go unnoticed. Therefore a mild ache may be the only symptom of this serious disease. *Systemically* the patient feels unwell, weak and feverish, and may have 'night sweats'.

Signs

In superficial joints the *synovial thickening* and *effusion* may be visible. The muscles acting on the joint are markedly *wasted*. The joint is moderately *tender*. The skin over the joint is not red, only slightly warm.

In the spine the only physical sign in early disease is *tenderness* on percussion of the spinous processes. Later, a *kyphus* may be seen and an abscess may be visible in the groin.

In really poor patients the infection even today runs riot. (Fig.37.6) shows a young girl from a village. She is pouring out pus at multiple sites from tuberculosis of various bones and lymph nodes. It is a pity that in this day and age, when man is reaching up to the moon and mars, there should be people suffering misery like this. A small fraction of the trillions spent on the arms race could eradicate tuberculosis from the whole world.

Laboratory findings

The white cell count is high, with a lymphocytosis.

The polymerase chain reaction (PCR) is very sensitive and specific for tuberculosis.

The erythrocyte sedimentation rate *(ESR)* is slower to rise and remains high for longer after subsidence of the inflammation; it is therefore nowadays used less often.

X-ray findings

The earliest changes are soft tissue swelling and distension of the capsule by effusion. Later, destruction of the articular cartilage causes narrowing of the joint space. Bone destruction is seen as areas of osteolysis. Extensive destruction of joint surfaces causes deformity. As healing takes place, the areas of necrosis are seen to be surrounded by osteosclerosis. The appearance may be that of a cyst surrounded by sclerotic bone. A chest x-ray is always taken and may or may not show active tuberculosis.

Diagnosis

This depends on recovery of organisms from the joint. Joint aspiration and/or biopsy are essential, with demonstration of acid-fast bacilli on smears, or positive cultures. If aspiration is not diagnostic open synovial biopsy is necessary.

Differential diagnosis

Tuberculous arthritis must be differentiated from rheumatoid arthritis occurring in a single joint, and from septic arthritis. In the spinal column the differential diagnosis is from pyogenic osteomyelitis, ankylosing spondylitis, prolapsed disc, and tumors.

Treatment

This consists of antibiotic therapy, symptomatic treatment of the affected joint, and if necessary, surgical debridement.

General supportive measures include rest and proper caloric and protein intake.

Patients are started on *antituberculous chemotherapy*. The treatment is highly successful if initiated before necrosis and abscess formation has taken place. If pus is present, it is aspirated for culture and sensitivity before the drugs are started. 4-drug therapy is commenced, with pyrazinamide, rifampicin, isoniazid, and ethambutol. If liver enzymes rise above twice their upper normal limits, pyrazinamide and/or rifampicin may have to be discontinued. In any case, after 2–3 months only two drugs are continued, for a total of 6–9 months. If the first two drugs are stopped before time, the remaining two have to be continued for a longer period.

Surgery

Involved joints should be immobilized by traction or splinting.

The *synovial stage* of the disease can be arrested by antibiotics alone, so surgery is not required. However, if the synovial membrane is markedly inflamed and thickened, synovectomy may be helpful.

If an *abscess* has formed it is evacuated after about a month of antibiotic therapy. The bone ends can then be brought into apposition and immobilized in a cast, and sound arthrodesis usually takes place. If subchondral bone is involved or the joint fails to respond to the drugs, surgical debridement is indicated.

In *joints with severe destruction* arthrodesis is the treatment of choice.

If the disease has been inactive for over 10 years total joint arthroplasty can be considered.

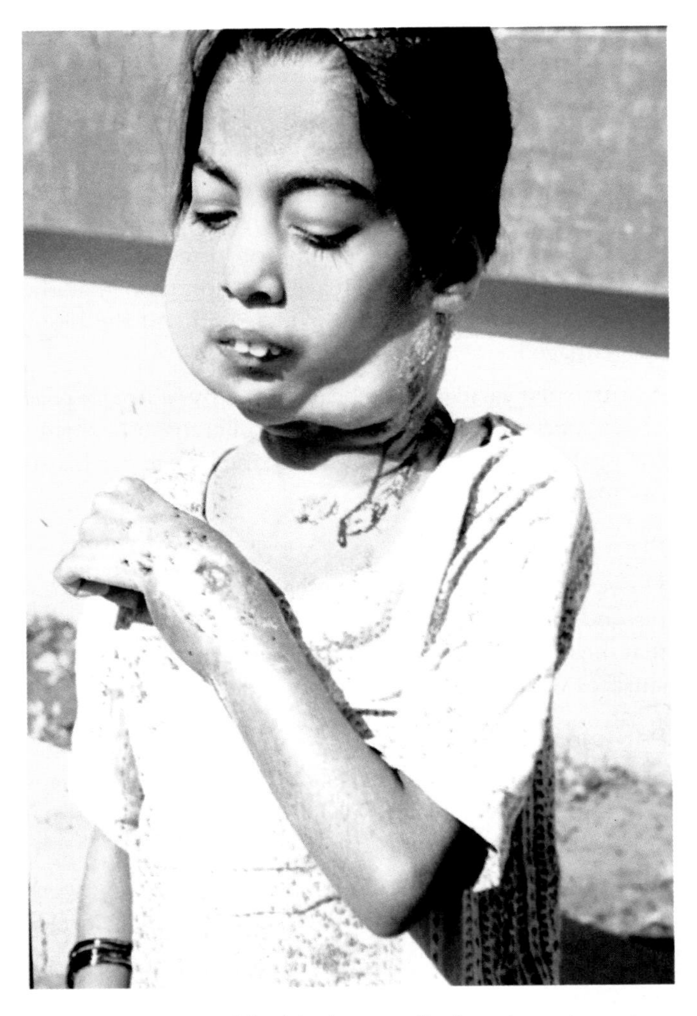

Fig.37.6 Young girl with sinuses discharging tuberculous pus from the jaw, neck, wrist, etc.

RHEUMATIC DISEASES

Osteoarthrosis

Osteoarthrosis is a term used to describe degenerative changes in synovial joints. It is a very common condition in middle age. Usually it is primary. However, sometimes it may be secondary to an injury to the joint during childhood or youth.

Etiology

Articular cartilage is designed to bear loads and stresses. If the loads applied to the joint increase, or the same loads are applied through unusually small areas because the joint surfaces no longer match each other, this equilibrium is disturbed, because the applied stresses increase in severity. The equilibrium is also disturbed if the disease damages the cartilage so that it is no longer strong and smooth. Thus osteoarthrosis can occur in any joint whose mechanics have been disturbed.

Secondary osteoarthrosis

When osteoarthrosis develops after a preisposing event it may be called secondary osteoarthrosis. The predisposing factors either damage cartilage or reduce the contact area in the joint. Thus:

- *Injuries to articular cartilage* may render the joint liable to develop osteoarthrosis over the next few years.
- *Diseases which make the joint surfaces irregular* e.g. Perthes disease or slipped femoral epiphysis, predispose the patient to the development of osteoarthrosis by reducing the contact area in the joint, so that the pressure on the cartilage is increased and the tissue damaged.
- Articular cartilage may be damaged by *bacterial or other enzymes*, e.g. in septic arthritis, tuberculous arthritis, or rheumatoid arthritis, and secondary osteoarthrosis may result.

Primary ostoarthrosis

However, *the great majority* of cases of osteoarthrosis at the hip and knee are *idiopathic* and are called primary. It is felt that these are mostly due to anatomical variations in joint surfaces which produce high local contact pressures.

Pathology

- The first change consists of loss of proteoglycans (highly glycosylated proteins) in the territorial matrix of the chondrocytes.
- Swelling and fragmentation of the collagen network of the cartilage occurs, so that its articular surface becomes rough (*fibrillation*).
- This process extends deeper until bone is exposed, a condition which is called *ulceration*. Scarring and fibrosis of the capsule occur, with loss of range of motion.
- At the same time, new bone formation occurs at the periphery of the joint, producing outgrowths which are called *osteophytes*.

Where the cartilage is destroyed the subchondral bone becomes sclerosed. The subchondral bone may degenerate with formation of cysts. These cysts may collapse; this deforms the bony articular surfaces, and at the same time loose pieces of bone are separated.

Clinical features

Symptoms

The first symptom is pain on exercise or at night. It gets more severe as the joint is used, especially in the weight-bearing joints. Pain is also felt when the joint is first moved after a period of immobility. Pain may wake up the patient several times during the night. With the passage of time the joint loses some of its range of movements. In the joints of the lower limb pain and stiffness produce a limp. As the disease progresses the stiffness becomes increasingly severe until all movement at the joint is lost. The joint may become stiff in a position which is functionally useless. If more than one joint is involved the patient may be crippled and forced to use a wheelchair.

Signs

There may be some swelling of the joint due to effusion. Movement in certain directions may be restricted. If the hand is placed over the joint as it moves, a sensation of grating may be felt; this is called *crepitus*, and is due to the irregularity of the bony surfaces rubbing against each other.

X-ray

The x-ray findings are characteristic. The normal joint space in an x-ray is due to the thickness of two articular cartilages. As this cartilage gets thinner, the joint space diminishes. Bony changes next become evident: sclerosis of subchondral bone, cyst formation and osteophytes. Finally the bone collapses.

Vs rheumatoid arthritis

The great deal of bone formation distinguishes this condition from rheumatoid arthritis in which bone loss is the important finding.

Treatment

Therapeutic measures for osteoarthrosis include the following:

- Modification of activities to avoid excessive strain on the joint.
- Anti-inflammatory analgesic drugs.
- Currently, glucosamine and chondroitin sulfates are being used with promising results.
- Intra-articular injections of hyaluronic acid derivatives are also considered beneficial in restoring the congruity of the articular cartilage.
- Weight loss to reduce the burden on the lower limb joints.
- Range of motion exercises to minimize contractures.
- Walking aids such as a stick.

Osteoarthrosis tends to be very slowly progressive and symptoms can be satisfactorily managed for many years. However, when symptoms become intolerable surgical intervention may be indicated.

Surgical treatment

Some of the operations used in osteoarthrosis are the following:

- Arthroscopic debridement and lavage of the joint is being done with encouraging results.
- If one condyle of the tibia is damaged, the knee develops an angular deformity concave in that direction, and weight-bearing becomes malaligned. The alignment can be restored to normal by a *wedge osteotomy*.
- If it is felt that the damage to the joint has become too extensive for osteotomy to be useful, the joint must be either replaced by an artificial joint (*replacement arthroplasty*) or stiffened (*arthrodesis*):

Replacement arthroplasty

Total hip replacement has been used for primary and secondary osteoarthrosis as well as rheumatoid arthritis. Up to 90% implants survive upwards of 10 years. The major problems consist of loosening of the bone-cement interface and infection. For this reason uncemented porous prosthetic designs have been introduced that allow bony ingrowth to provide permanent stability.

With a successful operation pain is abolished and the joint rendered mobile and stable. But if the prosthesis becomes loose or infected the preoperative disability returns and may then be difficult or impossible to relieve.

The chances of loosening or infection are greater if the prosthesis has to stay in for a long time. Therefore, although prosthesis is good treatment for a patient over sixty years of age, its use should be postponed in the young as far as possible, because of their longer expected life span.

Arthrodesis

Failure rates of total hip replacement are higher in young active patients. At the same time, because of their longer life expectancy, the risk of long-term failure is also greater. Therefore arthrodesis, i.e. fusion of the femur to the hip bone, is more often employed in those under the age of 40.

Rheumatoid arthritis

Pathology

Rheumatoid arthritis is a systemic disease; however, its major manifestations are in the joints. The cause of rheumatoid arthritis is unknown. The most popular theory considers the disease to be immune in nature.

Unlike osteoarthrosis, the disease affects all the supporting structures of the joint, including synovium, tendons, tendon sheaths and bursal tissues.

The hypertrophied synovium (pannus) creeps over the articular surface, destroying the cartilage. At the joint margins the inflamed synovium induces osteoclastic bone resorption and creates periarticular erosions. The bone becomes osteoporotic from a combination of:

- Hyperemia.
- Immobility due to pain.
- Increased osteoclastic activity due to inflammatory cytokines.

The ligaments and joint capsule become lax, allowing subluxation of the joint. Ultimately the process in a particular joint can become burnt out, with subsidence of the infection and ankylosis of the joint.

Systemic manifestations of the disease include pericarditis with valvular involvement, granulomas in the lungs, and uveitis.

Clinical features

Symptoms

Women are more commonly affected by rheumatoid arthritis than men. The disease may commence any time in adult life, or in childhood. According to the diagnostic criteria of the American Rheumatism Association, a diagnosis of rheumatoid arthritis can be made if the patient has five of the following features for more than six weeks:

- Morning stiffness.
- Pain on motion in at least one joint.
- Swelling in at least one joint (soft tissue thickening or fluid).
- Swelling of at least one other joint.
- Poor mucin precipitate from synovial fluid.
- Characteristic histological changes in synovium.
- Characteristic histological changes in nodules.

The disease usually affects more than one joint, and often starts in the small joints of the hands or feet. Later, all the movable joints in the body may be involved together, or one after the other. Each involved joint becomes painful, stiff and swollen. It may remain so for a couple of months, then settle down for many months. The patient feels unwell, and may have low grade fever.

Signs

The inflamed joint shows marked synovial thickening, and typical deformities develop. Limitation of movement, muscle wasting and deformity gradually develop, so as to cripple the patient. The most characteristic deformity in rheumatoid arthritis consists of subluxation at the metacarpophalangeal joints.

X-ray

The findings include joint space narrowing, periarticular erosions, soft tissue swelling and osteopenia. Gradually, the destruction of bone and stretching of the capsule allows the joint to subluxate and finally dislocate. The active disease may remit, leaving the articular cartilage destroyed. This joint may now progressively develop osteoarthrotic changes, and the x-ray may look like that from a case of osteoarthrosis.

Laboratory findings

The ESR is markedly raised, specially in longstanding cases.

An abnormal immunoglobulin known as the *rheumatoid factor* may be demonstrated in the blood by the Latex or Rose Waaler tests. However, this factor is found in some healthy individuals and in many chronic infections, and is not always present in rheumatoid arthritis. Therefore, its presence is not diagnostic. It may be mentioned that in osteoarthrosis, on the other hand, the blood picture is entirely normal and there is no systemic disturbance.

Treatment

This involves a team effort of the rheumatologist, orthopedic surgeon, physical therapist, occupational therapist, and social worker. The aim of treatment is to halt progression of the disease, restore or maintain function, and relieve pain.

Medical treatment

The drugs employed include:

- Analgesics (aspirin, codeine).
- Mild anti-inflammatory analgesics (ibuprofen, naproxen).
- Strong anti-inflammatory/analgesics (phenylbutazone, indomethacin).
- Drugs that modify the immune response (gold salts, penicillamine).

Corticosteroids are usually reserved for acute exacerbations or life-threatening situations such as vasculitis.

Orthopedic management

The aim should be to maintain muscle strength and range of motion of joints, and to avoid deforming forces. Symptomatic joints should be protected with splints or walking aids. If symptoms persist despite medical treatment, surgery may be required and can take one of many forms:

- *Synovectomy*:
  - o *Surgical synovectomy* slows the progression of the disease. In the knee arthroscopic synovectomy can be undertaken and provides results similar to those obtained by arthrotomy.
  - o *Radiation synovectomy* using intraarticular injection of a short-half-life isotope such as dysprosium-165 ferric hydroxide, also produces comparable results.
  - o Finally, *synovectomy by external beam irradiation* has been employed with some success in early cases.
- *Replacement arthroplasty*. In the hip with disabling pain and stiffness, and the knee with instability due to collateral ligament laxity, total replacement arthroplasty is preferred over synovectomy.
- In the ankle, *arthrodesis* gives better results.
- *Other* operations include:
  - o Release of a carpal tunnel syndrome.
  - o Silicone replacement arthroplasties, to restore mobility to the metacarpophalangeal joints.

Ankylosing spondylitis

Ankylosing spondylitis is one of the groups of seronegative spondyloarthropathies. The condition is more common in men. It is a serious illness which makes the patient a cripple. There is calcification and later ossification of the ligaments of joints of the axial skeleton, which results in complete bony ankylosis.

The tissue antigen HLA-B27 occurs in nearly all patients with ankylosing spondylitis, but only in a small percentage of the normal population. Thus tissue typing can help in diagnosis, but it is not clear how this genetic factor predisposes to the disease.

The joints most affected include the sacroiliac and costal joints, and the joints of the hips, the spine (ascending from the lumbar level), and the shoulders. The spine is not only ankylosed but also becomes increasingly concave forwards, so that the patient is bent down and cannot look forwards. Patients in whom the thoracic cage is ankylosed and the spine flexed may die of pulmonary infection, because of stagnation of secretions due to severe reduction in their vital capacity.

Investigations

The ESR is high. *This test should always be carried out in young adults with persistent low backache.* X-rays show obliteration of the sacro-iliac joints and ossification in the spinal ligaments (bamboo spine).

Treatment

There is no specific treatment. However, nonsteroidal anti-inflammatory drugs (NSAIDs) help relieve pain. Slow-release indomethacin (75mg at night) is often the best choice.

An *exercise* programme is essential to maintain movement, relieve symptoms and prevent deformity. Exercises should be carried out at least twice daily. In addition, patients should be encouraged to take part in whatever sport they like.

Surgery plays little part, but total hip replacement arthroplasty is occasionally required.

TUMORS OF BONES

Tumors of bones are named after the predominant type of tissue formed by the tumor. Benign tumors take the suffix '-oma', and malignant tumors '-sarcoma'. For example, benign and malignant tumors arising from cartilage are called chondroma and chondrosarcoma respectively, those from fibrous tissue fibroma and fibrosarcoma, and so on.

Common features of bone tumors

Bone tumors present with pain, a lump, a tender area, or a pathological fracture. The diagnosis depends upon the clinical features, x-ray appearances and histology.

A *genetic basis* for some bone tumors is suggested by:

- The increased incidence of bone sarcomas in cases of hereditary multiple exostoses, osteogenesis imperfecta, enchondromas, Paget's disease, familial cancer syndromes, etc.
- Reports of an increased frequency of osteosarcomas in siblings and cousins of patients with osteosarcoma.

Clinically, a benign tumor presents as a mass; a malignant growth often presents with pain or a pathological fracture. On x-ray two features particularly suggest malignancy:

- An ill-defined osteolytic lesion in the bone.
- Evidence that the tumor has penetrated the periosteum and invaded the soft tissues.

Biopsy

Before treatment *biopsy* is essential, and open biopsy was considered preferable in the past. However with the availability of trained cytologists, suction needle biopsy has dispensed with the need of open biopsy. Needle biopsy can also be used in tumors of the spine.

SPECIFIC BONE TUMORS

Osteoid osteoma

This is a small, sessile, benign tumor of the bone. Most patients present with severe night pain which is relieved with analgesics. The size of the tumor is less than 1.5cm; if the size is more than this, then it is termed an osteoblastoma. Common sites are proximal femur, diaphyseal tibia and spine.

CT scan, MRI and bone scan normally establish the diagnosis.

The tumor is treated with NSAIDs and removal of the nidus with a rim of normal tissue.

Osteosarcoma

This is a highly malignant tumor that occurs most commonly in the second and third decades of life, in the metaphyseal region of long bones, especially those of the leg. Paget's disease predisposes to a sarcoma, usually an osteosarcoma; these tumors develop in old age because Paget's disease occurs in the elderly.

The tumor contains small pleomorphic spindle cells which destroy bone, producing an osteolytic lesion with ill-defined edges on x-ray. It also lays down abnormal bone of irregular structure. Patients *present* with pain and a mass or swelling (Fig.37.7).

Spread occurs via the blood-stream to produce secondary tumors in the lung, and evaluation of the chest by CT scan is necessary.

X-ray

If the tumor has lifted the periosteum, neoplastic bone gets deposited as spicules of bone radiating from the shaft to give a '*sunray appearance*'. As the periosteum is lifted by the tumor, new bone may be formed subperiosteally. On x-ray this bone appears as a triangle (*Codman's triangle*).

Bone scan

This is carried out to rule out bone metastases.

CT/MRI

CT or preferably MRI of the region is performed for surgical planning.

Treatment

Chemotherapy

Osteosarcoma is not particularly sensitive to radiation, but does respond well to *combination chemotherapy* including methotrexate.

Surgery

Usually, after 6–8 weeks of preoperative chemotherapy, definitive surgical excision is carried out. This may be in the form of:

- Limb-preserving excision or.
- Limb-ablative amputation.

If the limb is saved, resected bone can be replaced by prosthesis or allografting. The removed tissue is examined to see if it has responded to chemotherapy. If it has shown a response, the same chemotherapeutic regimen is continued; if not, a different regimen is instituted.

Radiotherapy

Radiotherapy, whether preoperative or postoperative, has not been found to be of any use. However, it has some effect on secondaries. Results of combination chemotherapy with resection are better than even radical surgical amputation without adjuvant chemotherapy. Preoperative intra-arterial chemotherapy and radiation have also been tried instead of neoadjuvant chemotherapy, and results are comparable.

Citrovorum factor rescue

An interesting mechanism is utilized to make methotrexate fully effective. Methotrexate is effective against osteosarcoma cells only in large doses. However, such a dose would result in unacceptable toxicity to normal cells. This is where citrovorum factor comes in; this is an antidote to methotrexate, but only normal cells possess the cell membrane transport system which can enable them to utilize it to save them. When large doses of methotrexate are given along with citrovorum factor, the latter protects ('rescues') the normal cells, while the tumor cells are destroyed by the methotrexate. The phenomenon is called citrovorum factor rescue.

Cartilaginous tumors

Osteochondroma

An osteochondroma almost certainly arises due to localized disturbance of growth of the bone at an epiphysis. A portion of epiphyseal cartilage gets left behind in the periosteum of the metaphysis. The cartilage cap proliferates, endochondral ossification occurs in it, and the osteochondroma grows. As the bone grows, gradually the epiphysis shifts away from the tumor. Therefore, the tumor is found at some distance from the epiphysis. The growth of an osteochondroma ceases with the completion of bone growth. Excision is curative if all the cartilage is removed.

Chondroma

This tumor is a lobulated mass of cartilage. It occurs most commonly in the metacarpals, phalanges and metatarsals.

A chondroma may arise in the medulla (enchondroma). In such cases the bone is thinned by the tumor and pathological fracture may occur.

In other cases the tumor may be on the surface of the bone (ecchondroma).

The tumors may be solitary or multiple. In multiple tumors malignant change sometimes occurs.

Treatment

The usual treatment is curettage and bone grafting. The most serious concern is the possibility of malignant degeneration, and careful sampling at the time of biopsy is required to exclude the possibility of chondrosarcoma.

Chondrosarcoma

This tumor affects a broad age range (20 to 60 years). The pelvis, femur, tibia and other long bones are usually involved, and lesions closer to the axial skeleton are more likely to be malignant.

The *treatment* of a chondrosarcoma is by excision or amputation, because it is radio-resistant. Commonly it arises in the hip bone or scapula, as mentioned above. In that case it has to be treated by hind-quarter or fore-quarter amputation respectively.

Fibrous lesions

Fibroma

Small intracortical fibrous lesions are common incidental findings on x-ray in the metaphysis of long bones in children.

Fibrosarcoma

This tumor contains spindle-shaped fibroblasts. It may arise in bone or soft tissue. These tumors metastasize through the blood to the lungs. The 5-year survival rate is about 30%.

Fibrosarcoma is *treated* by early amputation, or in the trunk by wide block resection. The tumor is moderately radiosensitive, and adjuvant chemotherapy can be effective in improving survival rates.

Cystic lesions

Solitary bone cyst

These lesions occur in children in the metaphyses of long bones, commonly the humerus or femur. They are painless and can present with a pathological fracture as the initial manifestation of the disease. The cysts show on x-rays as osteolytic defects. As the skeleton matures, the cysts tend to gradually disappear. In young children partial or complete healing can be obtained by a series of three intraosseous injections of methylprednisolone. Cysts in older children are best treated by curettage and bone grafting.

Aneurysmal bone cyst

These cysts occur usually in the ends of long bones. They form expanding osteolytic lesions containing bloody fluid. Pathological fracture can occur through the cyst, and callus formation after such a fracture may obliterate it. The tumor is composed of fibrous tissue, vascular spaces, giant cells, and reactive bone. Local resection and bone grafting is the preferred treatment.

Round cell tumors

Ewing's sarcoma

This is a highly malignant bone tumor of children aged 5 to 15 years, arising usually in the middle of a long bone. X-rays show layers of subperiosteal new bone (onion-skin appearance). A painful hot swelling appears with irregular fever. Therefore the condition has to be distinguished from acute osteomyelitis. A soft tissue variant of this neoplasm, primary neuroectodermal tumor (PNET), occurs as well. On immuno-histochemical examination it exhibits neural differentiation.

Other tumors

Giant cell tumor (Osteoclastoma)

This tumor is seen most commonly in young adults, in the epiphyseal regions of long bones, especially around the knee. It contains undifferentiated spindle cells and multinucleated giant cells.

A giant cell tumor is osteolytic. It expands and thins the bone, sometimes resulting in a pathological fracture. Remnants of the original bone run across the cavity produced by the tumor. Thus it has a *soap-bubble appearance* on x-ray.

Although usually benign, a malignant variant sometimes occurs, and even the benign lesions show local aggressive behavior and a tendency to recur after surgical treatment.

Treatment

Curettage is followed by recurrence in 25 to 50 percent of cases. Therefore:

- *Wide resection* is usually carried out.

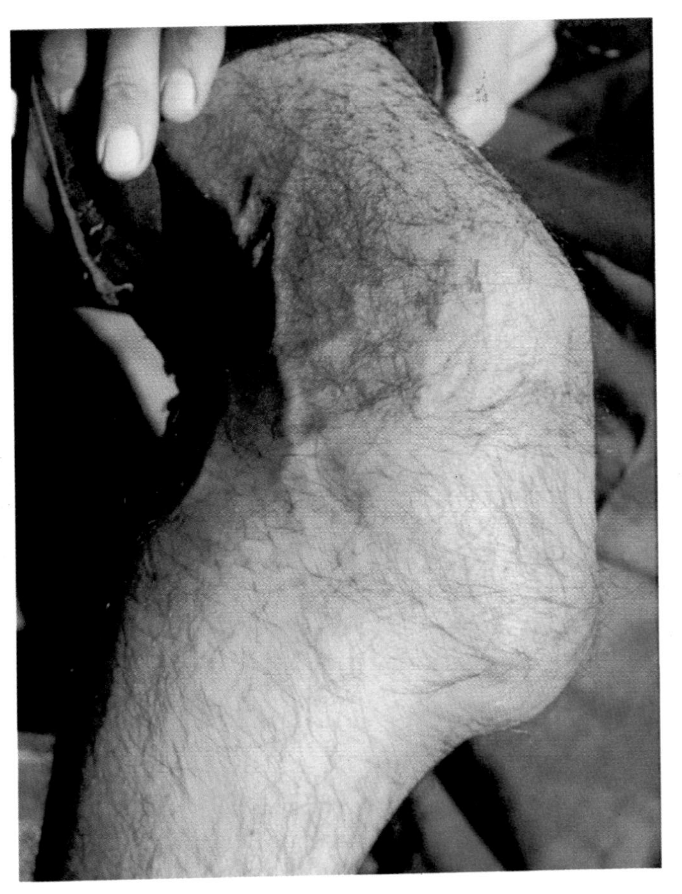

Fig.37.7 Osteosarcoma of upper end of tibia. Note the dilated veins over the tumor indicating increased vascularity.

- Alternatively, the cavity left after curetting is filled with methyl methacrylate cement. During polymerization of the cement, heat is generated which kills tissue within several millimeters of the margin in bone. In the long run the cement can cause degeneration in the articular cartilage. It is therefore usually removed after about two years and the cavity filled by bone grafting. The cavity may be electrocoagulated circumferentially to prevent the recurrence of tumor.

Secondary tumors in bone

The majority of secondary tumors in bone arise from carcinomas of the breast or prostate. A fair number arise from the bronchus, kidney, uterus and thyroid. The majority are osteolytic. A few, mostly from the prostate, are osteosclerotic.

Treatment consists of a combination of analgesics, radiotherapy, and internal fixation in anticipation of pathological fractures.

DISEASES AFFECTING THE HAND AND FOOT

The hand

Infections

Hand infections occur most often in manual workers and housewives. The infecting organism is most commonly *Staph. aureus*, besides *Strep. pyogenes* and gram-negative bacilli. Early detection of pus is important. Inflammatory edema commonly occurs, especially on the dorsum of the hand, because most of the lymphatics travel on the dorsum. The fibrinous exudate is followed by a degree of fibrosis, which is an important cause of stiffness of the hand.

Types of infection

Infections may take place around or under the nail; in the terminal pulp space, web space, or palmar space; or in the synovial sheaths of the flexor tendons.

Paronychia

Acute paronychia

This is the most common infection of the hand. It lies under the skin around the margin of the nail (Fig.37.8). Common organisms are *Staphylococcus aureus* and *Streptococcus hemolyticus*.

Antibiotics given early may abort the infection. If pus has formed it must be let out. The eponychium is stripped gently and completely from the base of the nail. If pus has extended under the nail the undermined portion of nail is trimmed away.

Chronic paronychia

The onset of chronic paronychia is slow, and the history dates back many months. The infection may be caused by bacteria or fungi. If the infection is bacterial, antibiotics are ineffective, but freely opening up the infected area helps. If fungi are responsible, anti-fungal remedies e.g. nystatin ointment can be tried.

Apical subungual infection

This infection arises from a prick or splinter under the nail. A small bead of pus forms at the edge of the nail. A V-shaped segment is removed from the free edge of the nail and the pus evacuated.

Infection of the terminal pulp space

This is the second most common infection of the hand. Bacteria usually enter through a prick. The pulp space is closed at its proximal end by a septum of deep fascia. Through the fat of the pulp run the terminal branches of the digital artery. When pus collects in this closed space, its pressure may cause thrombosis of the artery and lead to avascular necrosis of the terminal phalanx.

Clinical features

Dull pain and swelling are the first symptoms. The pain is worse when the hand is dependent, because the venous engorgement of dependency further raises the interstitial tissue pressure, which is already elevated due to the inflammatory edema. When pus forms there is throbbing pain. The regional lymph nodes may be enlarged and tender. If the pulp feels hard, pus is present.

Treatment

In the very early stage when there is no localization, large doses of antibiotics may cause resolution. Once pus is present immediate drainage is necessary. A short incision is made over the point of maximum tenderness.

Infection of the web space

In this condition the web is swollen and the adjacent fingers separated. Untreated, the pus can track into an adjacent web space, and also along the proximal segments of the adjacent fingers. A transverse incision is made and the pus evacuated.

Deep palmar abscess

This type of abscess lies under the palmar fascia. It is a serious but fortunately rare infection of the hand. The fingers are held flexed, because this position relaxes the palmar fascia. There is gross edema of the dorsum of the hand because the lymphatics draining the hand lie on the dorsum, and lymphangitis occurs. It is drained by a transverse incision along a flexion crease.

Acute suppurative tenosynovitis

Infection into a flexor tendon sheath is commonly introduced by a needle prick. The whole sheath may be involved rapidly. The organism is *Staph. aureus* or *Strep. hemolyticus*.

Signs

The classical signs are four:

- The whole finger is swollen.
- There is tenderness over the sheath.
- There is uniform swelling.
- The finger is flexed, with pain on extension.

Spread

The sheath of the thumb extends up to the forearm as the radial bursa. Again, the little finger sheath joins up with the ulnar bursa, which surrounds the tendons of all the fingers in the palm. Therefore infection from these two digits may extend up to the hand or, in the case of the thumb, even the forearm.

Treatment

Full doses of cloxacillin are given. The hand and forearm are placed in the position of rest, splinted and elevated. Splinting gives rest to the part, and elevation helps in drainage of the edema fluid. Unless rapid improvement occurs, incision and drainage is carried out. Transverse incisions are given both at the distal palmar crease and the distal digital crease (i.e. the upper and lower ends of the sheath) to drain pus. Using a fine catheter, the whole length of the sheath is irrigated with antibiotic solution.

Complications of hand infections

Suppuration may continue, and require re-exploration. A stiff digit may result.

It should be remembered that in some professions a stiff finger is a very serious disability; in such cases amputation of the useless digit may be preferable. However, one should not be in a hurry to suggest this to the patient; rather one should let him ask for it himself, if he feels it is necessary.

In the case of the *thumb* one must save all that is possible even though it may be stiff, because the thumb alone is almost equal to all the fingers due to its very important role in the grip. While holding any object the thumb is normally on one side, while all the fingers combined are on the other.

Principles of treatment of hand infections

Antibiotic therapy

This is started immediately. Cloxacillin and ampicillin can be used first. When culture reports are received, the antibiotic may be changed.

If pus has formed one must not depend on antibiotics. Drainage must be carried out at once.

Postoperative care

After operation the hand is placed in the position of rest, which is the one assumed while holding a cricket ball. A light plaster-of-Paris slab, moulded to fit the palm and forearm, is applied. The forearm is suspended in a sling as high as possible to lessen edema. In all cases rest is insisted upon. When the acute phase has passed, gentle voluntary movements are encouraged.

After-treatment

Adequate after-treatment is necessary, with physiotherapy to restore mobility.

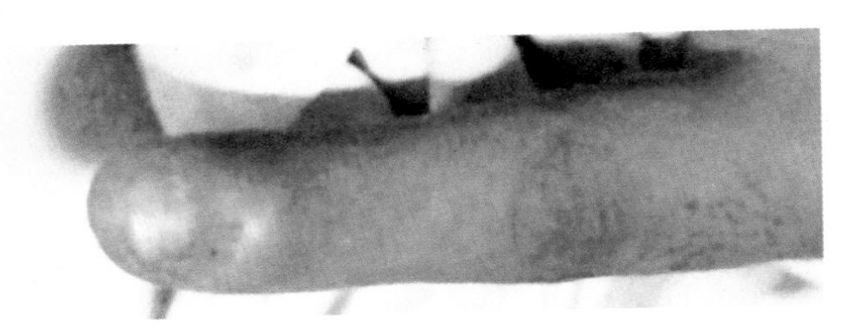

Fig.37.8 Paronychia. Pus under the nail-fold of the index finger

Hand injuries

Serious injuries of the hand cause a great deal of disability.

Evaluation of the injury

Careful examination of the injured hand is essential in order to find out the extent of damage to arteries, nerves, tendons, bones and joints. Because of the pain and swelling all the clinical methods cannot be easily employed, but the maximum possible information should be obtained. Injuries to the hand cause a great deal of disability. They can be classified into the following types:

- *Tidy injuries.* These are due to sharp agents, e.g. glass, knives etc. The cuts are clean and incised. Tendons, nerves and blood vessels may be divided.
- *Untidy injuries.* These injuries are commonly due to industrial accidents. The skin wound is irregular. There may be one or more fractures (Fig.2.2).
- *Indeterminate injuries.*

Examples of indeterminate injuries include severe crush or burn. It is impossible to know the full extent of the injury immediately. One must wait for a week or two to see what remains. Only then is excision of dead tissue carried out, followed by repair. It is essential to get skin cover after excising all dead tissue. If feasible, the skin is sutured. If not, a free graft or a flap may be used. One should not carry out primary repair of nerves or tendons in these injuries.

Principles of technique in hand surgery

Hand surgery requires meticulous attention to detail:

- A *bloodless field* is essential for accurate surgery, so a tourniquet is used.
- As a tourniquet has to be used, the patient is more comfortable under a *general anesthetic*.
- If local anesthesia is used, adrenaline must not be used with the local anesthetic agent in the fingers, as it may cause spasm of the digital artery and result in avascular necrosis of the digit.

- Careful *wound toilet* is essential. All dirt and debris must be removed.
- All *dead tissues* must be excised.
- *Absolute hemostasis* is essential, because a hematoma may result in infection and spoil an otherwise excellent result.
- *Antibiotics* and *tetanus toxoid* are employed.
- In the postoperative period *elevation* and *immobilization* is essential, to give rest and to drain the edema fluid. The hand is splinted in the position of function, in which the metacarpophalangeal joints are flexed, while the interphalangeal joints are extended.
- In tidy injuries even digital *nerves* may be repaired. This kind of work requires the use of microsurgical techniques, with magnification of the operative field.

The foot

Flat-foot

At birth the foot is flat. The normal arch of the foot is acquired when the infant stands up. It is maintained by the shape of the bones of the foot, by their ligaments, and by the action of the muscles. Flat-foot in adult life may be due to persistence of the infant shape, or to collapse of the arches which had developed. Flat-foot may not be the cause of the pain in the foot; soldiers with flat feet often do not complain of any pain in their feet.

Flexible flat foot

This deformity can be corrected passively. It is normal in toddlers and disappears as the medial arch is fully developed. Sometimes it is due to excessively lax ligaments.

Rigid flat foot

This deformity cannot be corrected passively. It may be due to tarsal coalition (fusion of two tarsal bones), inflammatory joint disease or neurological disorder.

X-rays are done to see tarsal coalition.

Idiopathic flat-foot

This is the most common form of flat-foot in the adult. It is seen most often in people who stand for a long time e.g. hairdressers. The medial longitudinal arch collapses, causing pain in the medial part of the sole of the foot. Local tenderness may be found in this area. If these ligaments are stretched by dorsiflexion of the foot, pain occurs. At a later stage the foot is painless, but the gait is awkward and inelastic.

Treatment

This is required only if there is pain. Rest is prescribed. Arch supports help relieve the pain. In severe cases a change of occupation to a sedentary job is advised.

Ingrowing toe-nail

An ingrowing toe-nail is commonly seen in the big toe, from encasing the feet in tight shoes and by cutting the toe-nails short and convex. One edge of the nail (usually the lateral edge) curls inwards, and gets buried in the groove in which it lies. Granulations develop and chronic infection persists (Fig.37.9).

Treatment

Conservative methods succeed in early cases. Tight shoes are avoided, the nail is cut straight, and hot sitz baths help the inflammation to resolve. If these measures fail operation is carried out.

Operation

The part of the nail-bed which lies under the proximal part of the nail is thick and white. This, the 'germinal matrix', is the area from which growth of the nail takes place, and which must be removed for cure. Only about one-fourth of the germinal matrix on the affected side *(shown shaded in Fig.37.10)* has to be removed; the remaining three-fourths of the nail continues to grow as before. The operation is carried out under local anesthesia. The germinal matrix can also be destroyed chemically by applying a drop of phenol. In resistant cases the whole of the nail and nail bed may have to be removed.

Madura foot

This is a chronic granulomatous disease found mostly in tropical countries, notably in India and Africa. It is usually caused by a filamentous organism *(Nocardia madurae)* which resembles actinomyces and is found in road dust. The foot is grossly thickened, nodular and hard, with multiple sinuses. The infection may burrow deeply and numerous cavities develop in the bones. Secondary infection usually occurs, with deterioration of the condition (Fig.12.2).

Treatment

Long courses of amikacine and co-trimoxazole are administered. When the inflammatory masses shrink, they can be surgically excised.

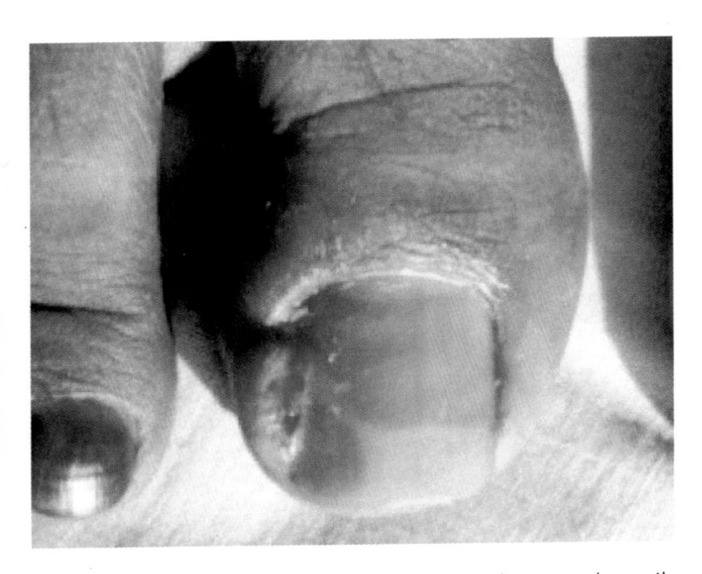

Fig.37.9 Ingrowing toe-nail. The nail has dug into the nail-fold and produced sepsis and granulation tissue.

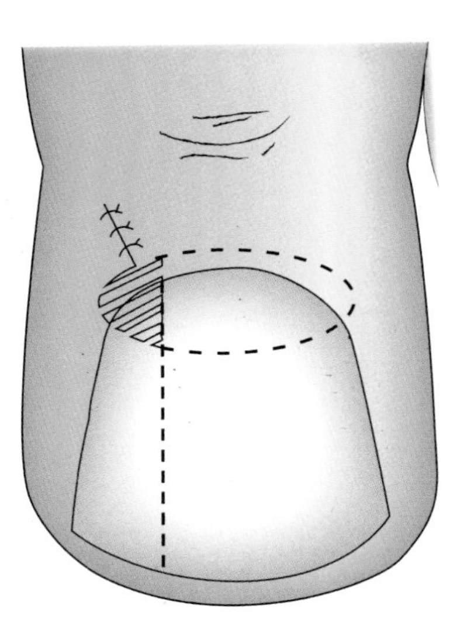

Fig.37.10 Operation on ingrowing toe-nail. Only the shaded area of the nail-bed needs to be removed; the remainder of the nail-bed and nail continue to grow as before

Section

4

THORAX

Chapter

38 BREAST

BENIGN BREAST DISEASE

Congenital anomalies

Extramammary breast tissue

This is occasionally found, commonly in the axilla (Fig.38.1). It usually makes its appearance in adult life, when stimulated by pregnancy or lactation. The treatment of choice is excision of these supernumerary structures.

Supernumerary nipples

The millk line is an ectodermal thickening stretching from the mid-clavicle to the groin. In some mammals many nipples develop on the milk lines; in women normally only one develops on either side.

The most common anomaly of the breast is the presence of additional nipples on the milk line. These are called supernumerary nipples, and should be removed by operation not only for cosmetic reasons, but also because any abnormal structure is more liable to undergo malignant change than a normally developed organ.

Absent nipple

One or both nipples may rarely be *absent*. Occasionally, a nipple fails to evert following birth, and remains inverted or retracted throughout life. A problem arises when the mother tries to breast-feed her baby.

Acquired conditions

Infantile mastitis

Placental estrogen may produce a swelling of the breast in the newborn. The condition is called infantile mastitis. It is self-limiting, but may occasionally lead to cellulitis.

Precocious puberty

Adrenal cortical and ovarian tumors may produce precocious puberty, in which breast hypertrophy may be the earliest sign of the presence of the underlying endocrine disorder.

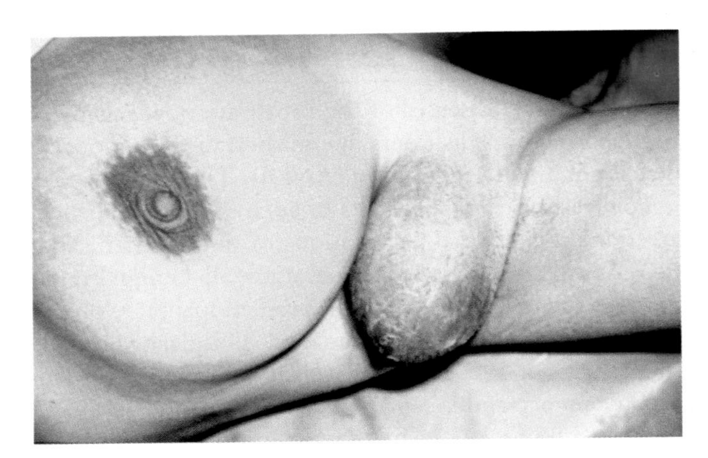

Fig.38.1 Accessory breast axilla

Gynecomastia

Gynecomastia is the development of a female type breast in a male. It is usually unilateral, and occurs in young men.

Unilateral gynecomastia

Unilateral gynecomastia (Fig.38.2) is not due to hormonal dysfunction, because if such was the case both breasts would have enlarged. Thus it is the target organ, i.e. the breast on the affected side, which is excessively responsive to a normal level of hormones in the blood.

Bilateral gynecomastia

This, on the other hand:

- May have a *hormonal* cause. It is common in hepatic cirrhosis, where there are high levels of circulating estrogens. It is also seen after estrogen administration for prostatic cancer.
- *Some drugs* used for cardiovascular diseases like spironolactone, methyldopa and calcium channel blockers can produce gynecomastia.
- Other drugs leading to breast development include cimetidine, diazepam and tricyclic antidepressants.

Treatment. It is not normally necessary to be concerned about malignancy in a case of gynecomastia. However, this mass often produces a good deal of psychological stress in the otherwise healthy young man, and is best removed. If the lump is quite small, subcutaneous mastectomy can be carried out through a circumareolar incision, leaving no residual scar; if it is too large for this approach, a curved submammary incision can be used. In older men the mass is often irregular, and a biopsy is required to rule out a carcinoma.

ABERRATIONS OF NORMAL DEVELOPMENT AND INVOLUTION

Many so-called diseases of the breast are now regarded more correctly as disorders due to aberrations of normal development and involution (ANDI). The term disease is now reserved for disorders of such severity that they are frankly abnormal. Aberrations of development and involution can account for most, if not all, benign breast disorders. For example, most premenopausal women experience breast discomfort and nodularity before menstruation. For most, this is little more than an inconvenience and is regarded as a normal physiological process. In 2 to 3 percent of women the symptoms are more severe and they are referred to a breast clinic with 'cyclical mastalgia'. In the past most such women were described as suffering from 'fibrocystic disease' although often there is little evidence of either fibrosis or cyst formation.

Symptoms of benign breast disease

The following symptoms may be associated with the presence of conditions listed under each symptom.

Breast pain

Pain is the most common reason for referral to a breast clinic. The patients fall into two clear-cut groups: those whose symptoms are related to the menstrual cycle (cyclical mastalgia) and those where there is no such correlation (non-cyclical mastalgia).

Cyclical mastalgia

This is much the more common type of pain. The discomfort lasts for a varying period of time prior to menstruation; this is therefore a condition of premenopausal women. The pain is usually bilateral, and is felt in the upper outer quadrants. There are no mammographic or pathological characteristics of cyclical mastalgia.

Symptoms of this condition correlate with the menstrual cycle, therefore the cause must be hormonal. The following factors have been considered important by different researchers:

- Excess of estrogens.
- Abnormal prolactin production.
- Inadequate intake of essential fatty acids.

Management

Most patients require reassurance only, specially to the effect that no neoplasia is present. For the few patients who experience pain in spite of reassurance, drug therapy is required:

- Excess of estrogens can be countered by the anti-estrogen tamoxifen in a dose of 10mg daily.
- Danazol (200–400mg daily) acts as an antigonadotrophin.
- Abnormal prolactin levels can be lowered by the prolactin lowering agent, bromocriptine (5mg daily).

Each of these drugs, however, is associated with considerable side effects.

Non-cyclical mastalgia

This tends to be more chronic, unilateral and located in the medial quadrants of the breasts. Analgesics should be prescribed.

Sclerosing adenosis

This constitutes one of the causes of non-cyclical mastalgia. Microscopically, proliferation of terminal duct lobules and myoepithelial cells is seen, along with stromal fibrosis. Macroscopically, sclerosing adenosis may have a star-shaped appearance and may calcify; it may thus mimic carcinoma both clinically and radiologically.

Other causes of non-cyclical mastalgia include:

- Cancer.
- Previous biopsy for benign disease.
- In the elderly, referred root pain from cervical spondylosis.

Breast lumps

Fibroadenoma

Fibroadenoma is a common, well-circumscribed lesion of the breast that tends to occur in young women or girls. The peak incidence is between 21 and 25 years of age. The lump is movable, smooth, painless, lobulated, and without any fixation to the overlying skin. The mobility of the mass is a characteristic feature of fibroadenoma; it is so freely movable that it is called a *breast mouse.* Microscopically, fibroadenomas are of two types, intracanalicular and pericancalicular. The former is smaller and firmer, whereas the latter tends to grow to a large size.

Fibroadenomas are *treated* by excision and biopsy because of their continued growth and the need to be certain of the diagnosis.

Giant fibroadenoma

A giant fibroadenoma grows rapidly, sometimes to a very large size. The microscopic appearance is the same as in the common fibroadenoma. The treatment consists of enucleation through a cosmetic incision.

Phyllodes tumor

These tumors occur in premenopausal women. They have the features of a common fibroadenoma but can grow rapidly to a large size to involve much of the breast. The skin may be stretched over the lesion but is not actually involved by the tumor. Axillary node metastases are rare, and this helps distinguish this tumor from carcinoma. It would be very rare to see a carcinoma totally replacing the breast tissue where both the skin and the axillary glands were not involved; such a situation is seen in a phyllodes tumor.

If axillary lymphadenopathy occurs, it indicates an extremely aggressive form of the disease. The neoplasm may outgrow its blood supply and areas of necrosis may occur.

Treatment

Normally, phyllodes tumors can be removed with a 1cm margin. Very large tumors require wider excision; those with aggressive histology require total mastectomy.

Cyclical nodularity

This condition presents with a lump the size of which varies with the menstrual cycle. Examination shows a diffuse nodular swelling that may be slightly tender. The change usually resolves with the next menstrual cycle. If it does not, aspiration cytology or biopsy is indicated. If malignancy can be excluded, patients with this condition can simply be reassured, but follow-up is essential.

Breast cysts

These are quite common. They can be regarded as aberrations of normal lobular physiology. They are commonly seen in perimenopausal women. They commonly appear suddenly. Before this, the cyst has existed in a flaccid state; accumulation of an excess of fluid makes it tense and brings it to the patient's notice. The lump possesses some mobility, but not as much as that of a fibroadenoma. Diagnosis is straightforward, and aspiration of the cyst confirms it.

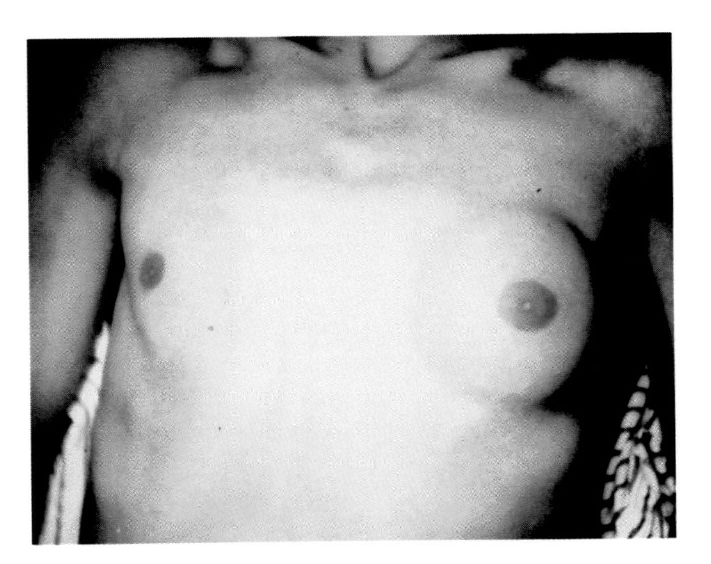

Fig.38.2 Unilateral gynecomastia.

Breast cysts are treated by aspiration. However, the fluid must be microscopically examined for neoplastic cells. *Again, if the aspirate is blood-stained or the fluid collects again, the cyst should be excised.* Thus if a cyst is treated by aspiration, it must be followed up properly.

A clinician, on mere physical examination, should never indicate to his patient that this cyst is benign; that can be shown only on histology or cytology.

Galactocele

If during lactation a duct gets distended with milk and desquamated epithelial cells, a galactocele is the result. It usually lies under the areola, and can often be emptied by pressure. It should be excised, because it can become infected. Also, it can calcify and be confused with a malignant lesion.

Fat necrosis

If a firm or hard lump has developed in the breast, and has not enlarged since it appeared, it can be an area of fat necrosis. It usually follows trauma, which exposes the fat to calcium, leading to the formation of calcium soaps. It may be impossible to distinguish it from carcinoma on clinical examination or even on mammography. Skin retraction, irregular edges, and fine stippled calcification may all be present. Usually a history of trauma can be obtained. The fat may liquefy to produce a cyst, but the longer-standing cases are scarred and contracted. Excision biopsy is the treatment of choice, so that the diagnosis is beyond any doubt.

Acute mastitis and breast abscess

Breast infections can be divided into two types:

Lactational abscesses

These are the result of infection by *Staphylococcus aureus* and develop:

- At the commencement of breast feeding due to a cracked nipple.
- At weaning due to engorgement from incomplete drainage of breast milk.

If seen before frank suppuration, antibiotic treatment alone is sometimes successful. Many cases are due to penicillinase-producing staphylococci; therefore a second-line penicillin or a cephalosporin should be employed.

Treatment

If pus has formed drainage is necessary. The incision should be placed in the dependent part of the abscess to allow drainage of pus under the influence of gravity. The wound is left open and packed loosely with antibiotic-soaked ribbon gauze. However, primary closure under antibiotic cover has also been practiced.

Non-lactational abscesses

These arise in the periareolar area in cases of duct ectasia, due to stagnation of the contents of a dilated duct. This condition is also called chronic mastitis. The infecting organisms are a mixture of bacteroides and anaerobic streptococci.

Treatment is carried out on lines similar to those employed for lactational abscesses, the antibiotics commonly used being metronidazole and flucloxacillin. Definitive treatment requires excision of the dilated duct when the condition has become quiescent.

Acute mastitis should ideally be prevented. During breastfeeding strict nipple hygiene should be adhered to, and any cracks or inflamed areas promptly treated. If some redness develops, an ice-pack gives relief, and a breast pump prevents stasis and intraductal growth of bacteria.

Chronic breast abscess

A chronic abscess is rare. It can look like a carcinoma, though it is often due to *tuberculosis*. The lesion is not warm and is not tender. Sinuses can develop in old-standing cases. Diagnosis can only be made by biopsy. Treatment requires adequate drainage.

A chronic abscess may also result from *inadequately drained mastitis*. The induration and edema can make it look like a carcinoma. Wide local drainage with careful biopsy to rule out malignancy is required.

Intraduct papilloma

These benign lesions of the lactiferous ducts occur beneath the areola. The most common symptom is a bloody nipple discharge. They often cannot be palpated, being soft and small; they have to be located by milking the duct in which they lie, so as to express blood from the nipple. If a patient presents with a small palpable mass under the areola and a bloody nipple discharge, there is a 95% chance that she has an intraductal papilloma. When no mass can be felt, a deep-lying carcinoma with invasion of a duct must be looked for.

Intraductal papillomas should be *treated* by excision of the duct as a wedge resection:

- If a mass can be felt, the area around it should be excised as a wedge.
- If no mass can be felt, the duct from which blood can be expressed should be probed, and an incision made along the probe until the papilloma is identified. The portion of the duct bearing the papilloma is then removed (Microdochotomy).

In either case the tissue is sent for histopathology to ensure that the lesion is benign.

Risk of cancer in benign breast disease

Benign breast disease in general is not associated with increased risk of carcinoma, except for conditions with epithelial hyperplasia/atypia and papillomatosis.

CARCINOMA OF THE BREAST

Breast carcinoma is the most common form of cancer in women, and is one of the leading causes of death in women above the age of 30. In the Western world the incidence varies between 1 in 8 women in high prevelance areas i.e. USA and Western Europe, to 1 in 16 women in regions with a low prevalence.

Risk factors

Although the cause of breast cancer remains unknown, certain risk factors can be enumerated:

Sex. Breast cancer is 100 times more common in women than in men. Thus sex is an important risk factor for this cancer, although it is often forgotten as such.

Social class. The greatest mortality rate is seen in the highest socio-economic class. It is thought that dietary factors and obesity affect the solubility of fat-soluble estrogens.

Age. Breast cancer is almost unknown before puberty and is very rare under the age of twenty. From then onwards the incidence keeps rising till old age.

Age at menarche and menopause. Women whose menarche occurs before the age of 12 are at twice the risk of those starting menstruation after this date. Similarly, women whose menopause comes after the age of 50 years run twice the risk of those who stop menstruating before the age of 45.

Family history. If a first-degree relative has suffered from this condition, the risk is increased two-fold; if a second-degree relative, then 1.5 times.

Nulliparity removes a protective effect against breast cancer; thus single and nulliparous women have a 1.5 times higher risk than parous women.

Obesity. Obese women run a nearly two-fold increased risk.

Previous breast cancer. The relative risk of developing a second breast cancer 20 years after the first is 1.5.

Irradiation. Atomic bomb survivors from Nagasaki and Hiroshima, and women who have had multiple chest x-rays for treatment of pulmonary tuberculosis, have a higher incidence of breast cancer.

Genetic correlation

Some inherited breast cancers (approx 5%) are associated with mutation of a gene i.e. BRCA 1 [BRCA stands for BReast CAncer]. This mutation and some others i.e. BRCA 2 are associated with early onset breast cancer as well as ovarian cancer. These days genetic testing is available for women at high risk.

Pathology

Carcinoma of the breast can arise from the nipple, the ducts, or the lobules.

Paget's disease (1%)

This is a carcinoma of the ducts of the nipple. It commences as a weeping eczema of the nipple, and may so remain for many years, until ultimately an underlying mass develops. Therefore, any eczematoid lesion of the nipple in a female which persists for more than a few weeks should be biopsied to exclude the possibility of Paget's disease. At the same time, this condition should also be distinguished from a frank tumor that is simply eroding the skin of the nipple. The prognosis is better than for the average carcinoma of the breast if treated by mastectomy and axillary clearance.

Ductal carcinoma

- *In situ(5%)*. This is a preinvasive form of breast cancer. It is confined to the duct system and does not invade the basement membrane or the surrounding tissues. Comedo and papillary forms are the most common and both are associated with multicentric disease. The abbreviation DCIS is in common use for this tumor.
- *Invasive*. These tumors can be subdivided into the following types:
    - o *Infiltrating ductal carcinoma with productive fibrosis*, not otherwise specified, i.e. *scirrhous carcinoma* (65%). This tumor presents typically in a perimenopausal or postmenopausal woman as a solitary, non-tender, firm, ill-defined mass. The tumor possesses a poorly defined border. The cut surface shows a star-shaped tumor with a chalky-white streak, so that it cuts like an unripe pear. The cells are arranged in single rows that occupy irregular cleft spaces between collagen bundles ('Indian filing'). These tumors account for two-thirds of all invasive mammary cancers, and have a relatively poor prognosis. However, factors such as tumor size and axillary node involvement are of more prognostic importance than histological features alone.
    - o *Medullary carcinoma* (6%). These are soft, well-circumscribed, bulky tumors with smooth contours. There is intense infiltration of the stroma with small lymphocytes. They are often large, yet axillary involvement and distant spread are late. This diagnosis indicates a favourable prognosis, the overall 5 year survival rate being as high as 85 to 90%.
    - o *Papillary carcinoma* (2%). These tumors are also well-circumscribed. They demonstrate the formation of papillae, and are associated with a good prognosis.
    - o *Mucinous (mucoid) carcinoma* (2%). This consists of masses of jelly-like material, with small clumps of tumor cells lying in a sea of mucoid material. The prognosis is better than for the average carcinoma.
    - o *Inflammatory carcinoma*. This is a clinical label applied to a very aggressive and lethal form of breast carcinoma which is not related to any specific cell type. The lymphatics are blocked with malignant cells, so that the breast is red, hot, swollen and painful. The surface veins and axillary nodes are also full of cancer cells. This tumor is usually seen postpartum in younger women with the full breasts of lactation. The prognosis is grave, and treatment is usually unable to control the disease.

Table 38.1 TNM system for staging of breast cancer

T	(primary tumor)
TIS	Carcinoma in situ.
TO	No demonstrable tumor in breast.
T1	Tumor 2cm or less; skin not involved or involved locally in Paget's disease.
T2	Tumor 2 to 5cm.
T3	Tumor greater than 5cm.
T4	Tumor any size with any of the following: skin infiltration, ulceration, peau d'orange, attachment to pectoral muscle or chest wall.
N	(regional lymph nodes)
NO	No palpable axillary nodes.
N1	Palpable, movable, axillary nodes.
	N1a: metastasis not suspected.
	N1b: metastasis suspected.
	N2 Palpable, fixed, axillary nodes.
	N3 Supra or infraclavicular nodes; edema arm.
M	(distant metastases)
MO	No distant metastases.
M1	Clinical or x-ray evidence of distant metastases; skin involvement beyond the breast.

Lobular carcinoma

- **In situ**. This is a preinvasive form of breast cancer, possessing the potential for becoming invasive. It is usually discovered by chance. It has no mammographic features and is usually found on biopsy performed for other reasons.
- **Invasive** (10%). This tumor is characterized by the 'Indian filing' of invading malignant cells, and shows a *tendency to occur bilaterally*.

Clinical staging

By clinical staging the surgeon makes an attempt to identify the extent of the malignant lesion. Not only does clinical staging of cancer provide a reasonably accurate indication of prognosis, but it *also serves as the primary method for comparing different techniques of treatment*.

TNM system of staging

The TNM system of staging has achieved universal acceptance, not only in the case of breast cancer but also in many other types of cancer. It is based on clinical examination for the tumor (T), regional lymph nodes (N), and distant metastasis (M). The TNM system in respect of the breast is shown in (Table 38.1).

Staging sheet and diagram

The actual staging is carried out as in (Table 38.2). In the case of every patient with breast cancer a staging sheet as well as a diagram for locating the mass within the breast should be completed and kept as a part of the hospital record. It provides an accurate description for anyone examining the patient on follow-up visits. It also makes it possible to compare one's work with that carried out anywhere else, or to collaborate with an institution at home or abroad.

Diagnosis

The evaluation of a breast for any symptom should be carried out by a triple-assessment including the following:

- Clinical examination.
- Mammography or ultrasonography as indicated.
- Needle biopsy (FNAC or Core needle).

The most common initial evidence of breast cancer is a *lump* in the breast, usually painless and discovered by the patient herself. A painful breast mass, a nipple discharge and a retracted nipple are all much less common as presenting signs than a painless lump. Other less common accompanying complaints are skin puckering, breast enlargement and arm edema. Occasionally systemic metastases to the bones, axilla, supraclavicular area or lungs produce the initial symptoms or signs of disease.

Generally, breast cancer tends to spread quite early by both lymphatic and hematogenous routes and with widespread metastases.

However, a few cases remain locally invasive for years, without showing evidence of distant spread.

Even when the most experienced clinicians examine a breast and give their opinion about the presence or absence of cancer, they are correct only 70% of the time. Therefore any discrete lump or mass in the breast must be considered as possibly a carcinoma.

About 50% of breast cancers are found in the upper outer quadrant of the breast, the remainder arising in the other quadrants and the areolar region. Tumors do not usually become palpable until they are greater than 1cm. in diameter. It has been calculated that it takes approximately 5 years for a tumor to reach this size from the single cell stage. *Thus it is easy to understand why distant metastases have so often taken place before the tumor is detected by the patient or the surgeon.*

Mammography

Mammography is an x-ray examination of the breast. It requires special techniques, an x-ray film designed for examining soft tissues, and a radiologist skilled in interpreting the x-ray images of the breast. The classic features of breast cancer on mammography include:

- Tissue asymmetry.
- Mass effect.
- Density with irregular margins.
- *Stippled calcification* (Fig.38.3 a).
- Skin thickening.
- Nipple inversion.

A combination of mass effect and microcalcification is the most reliable evidence.

The *sensitivity* of mammography varies between 60–90% depending on age, breast density, tumor size and location. Hence a 10% false negative rate is usually mentioned in most reports.

Mammography is specially useful in the following situations:

- In screening procedures, specially in high-risk populations, e.g. patients with previous breast cancer or with relatives having breast cancer.
- When a mass is palpable in the breast but the diagnosis is uncertain: fine calcification, irregular borders, and variable density of the lesion suggest a malignant lesion. However, it should be remembered that only 50 % of cancers show calcification on mammography. Therefore, the absence of calcification does not rule out malignancy.
- In a large fatty breast, when the patient has symptoms but no lump is palpated; in such breasts tumors cannot easily be felt, but the mammogram is most accurate in the fatty breast.
- Preoperative mammography also acts as a baseline for radiological evaluation of the breast in the years after the initial mammogram.
- In the follow-up of women who are treated by breast conservation.

It should be remembered that mammography can detect some tumors which cannot be found in any other way. The 5 year survival rate for tumors found in this manner may be as high as 90%.

Ultrasonography

Ultrasound clearly differentiates a cystic from a solid mass. Further, it shows variegated density and lobulated margins of a malignant mass (Fig.38.3 b). However, it is unsatisfactory for diagnosing early breast cancers because of its inability to detect microcalcification, or to discriminate lesions smaller than 5mm.

Table 38.2 TNM criteria for actual staging

Stage	Tumor	Nodes	Metastases
I	T1	NO or N1a	MO
II	TO	N1b N1b	MO
	T1	NO	
	T2	N1a	
		N1b	
III	Any T3	Any N	MO
	Any T4	Any N	
	Any T	N2 or N3	
IV	Any T	Any N	M1

Color doppler

If color Doppler shows increased local vascularity, (Fig.38.3 c), this is quite typical of malignancy.

Biopsy

It should be a general rule that *no patient should be subjected to a mastectomy for cancer until and unless histological proof of the presence of cancer has been obtained.* This can be done only by some form of biopsy.

This may take the form of fine needle aspiration, core biopsy or open surgical biopsy and frozen section.

- **Fine needle aspiration cytology (FNAC)** (Fig.38.3 d). This has the advantage of being an outpatient procedure and producing immediate results. However, it requires expert and specialized interpretation by a cytopathologist. At the same time the method has its limitations:
  - o The *false-negative* rate is about 10% due to missing the tumor at the time of aspiration or from failing to aspirate a particularly hard scirrhous carcinoma.
  - o The *false-positive* rate is about 2%, due to confusion with an excessively cellular fibroadenoma or the effects of pregnancy, lactation or hormone therapy on normal breast tissue.
  - o Aspiration cytology cannot differentiate between *in-situ* and invasive cancer.
- **Core biopsy**. Core biopsy using a Trucut type needle can be employed as an outpatient procedure under local anesthesia.

It offers the advantage that it provides a histological rather than a cytological specimen. It can be carried out by a stereotactic method under mammographic control. However it is liable to miss small cirrhotic tumors.

- **Open surgical biopsy.** This is occasionally required in patients who are clinically suspected to have cancer yet in whom fine needle aspiration cytology or core biopsy fails to demonstrate malignant disease. It is best performed under general anesthesia, the patient being discharged home the same day. The definitive operation if indicated is carried out a few days later after discussion of the different treatment options with the patient; this delay in operation has no effect on the recurrence or survival rates.

Technique

Every open biopsy of the breast for a suspected malignancy should include a small piece of *skin* in the specimen, to see if it is involved. The submitted tumor tissue should also be tested for the presence of *hormone receptors*. Lines of tension in the skin of the breast (*Langer's lines*) are generally concentric with the nipple, and incisions that parallel these lines result in fine scars. At the same time incisions for biopsy should be kept within the boundaries of potential incisions for mastectomy that may be required for definitive treatment. If possible, the skin incision should be placed in the circumareolar position, because it is more cosmetic, the scar being invisible. If the lesion is small total excision is carried out, but in the case of a large lesion an incisional biopsy is taken.

Frozen section

Frozen section examination of an excised specimen at the time of the definitive operation was very popular at one time. However, it is not as often employed today:

- Because of the wider availability of fine needle aspiration cytology.
- Because the patient being anaesthetized is unable to discuss various treatment options with the surgeon in the light of the pathological findings.

Evaluation

Once the diagnosis of breast cancer has been made, the patient should have chest x-ray, hemoglobin, blood count, electrolytes and liver function tests. The value of other more sophisticated tests is open to doubt:

- As far as *scintiscans* are concerned, there is a very low incidence (about 1%) of true positive bone scans in operable cancer.
- There is an even lower positive yield with liver and brain scanning.

However, patients with clinical stage III disease and those with symptoms suggesting metastases should undergo further investigation, the bones being scanned by scintigraphy and the liver by ultrasonography.

TREATMENT OF CANCER OF THE BREAST

The treatment of breast cancer requires a multidisciplinary approach, with co-operation between surgeons, radiotherapists, medical oncologists and pathologists, along with counsellors and breast care nurses.

A number of breast cancers have metastasized before the patient presents for treatment; therefore the treatment of breast cancer resolves itself into two parts: the eradication of local disease, and the control of distant metastases.

- For the eradication of *local disease* the mainstays of treatment include:
    - o The different surgical operations available for removal of the cancer.
    - o Radiotherapy.
- For *metastases* the methods of management include:
    - o Cytotoxic chemotherapy.
    - o Radiotherapy.
- Finally, *hormonal manipulation* can be used both against local and metastatic disease.

Surgical treatment

The main objective of surgery is adequate locoregional control. Surgical treatment has to deal with disease both in the axilla and the breast.

The breast

Cancer of the breast is often multicentric in origin, and this constitutes a strong argument in favour of complete removal of the breast in all cases. However, this concept is challenged by advocates of conservative surgery.

The axilla

It is very desirable that histological proof be obtained of the presence or absence of *metastatic disease in the axilla*. This is important for two reasons:

- It allows accurate staging of the cancer into stage I or II and enables a more definite prognosis to be given.
- It enables the exact number of affected lymph nodes to be determined, which has great significance. If three or less than three nodes are affected the

Fig.38.3 Step-by-step use of imaging methods for a breast lesion in a patient

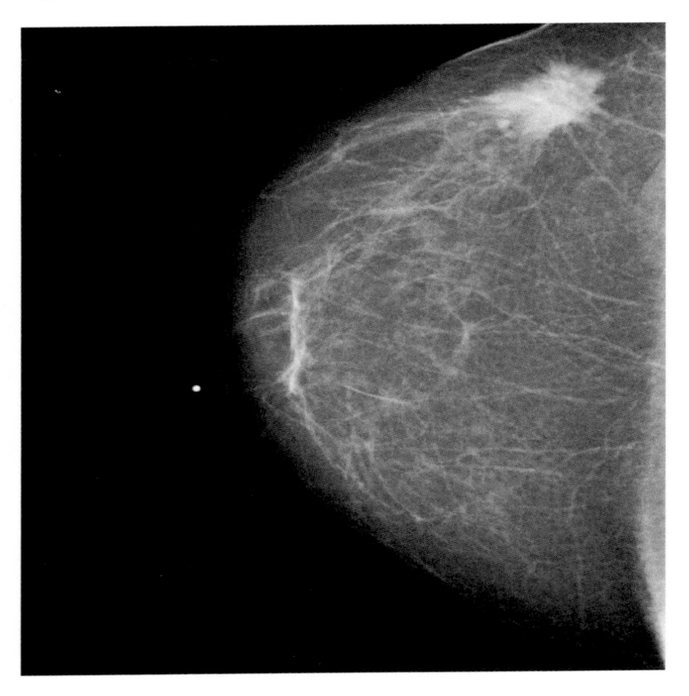

(a)Mammography showing carcinoma in an otherwise featureless fatty breast

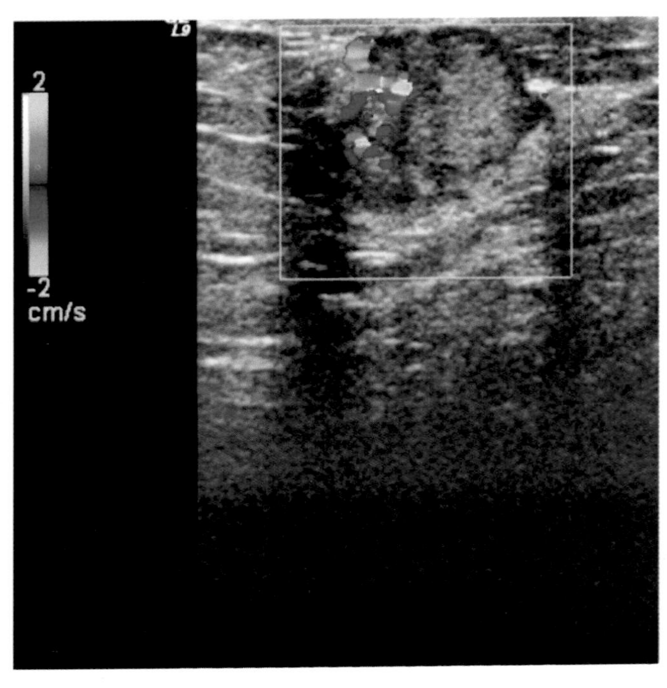

(c) Increased vascularity on colour Doppler. Findings in a,b,c are fairly typical of malignancy. [Note, on the left side, colour scale going up from blue through red to yellow.]

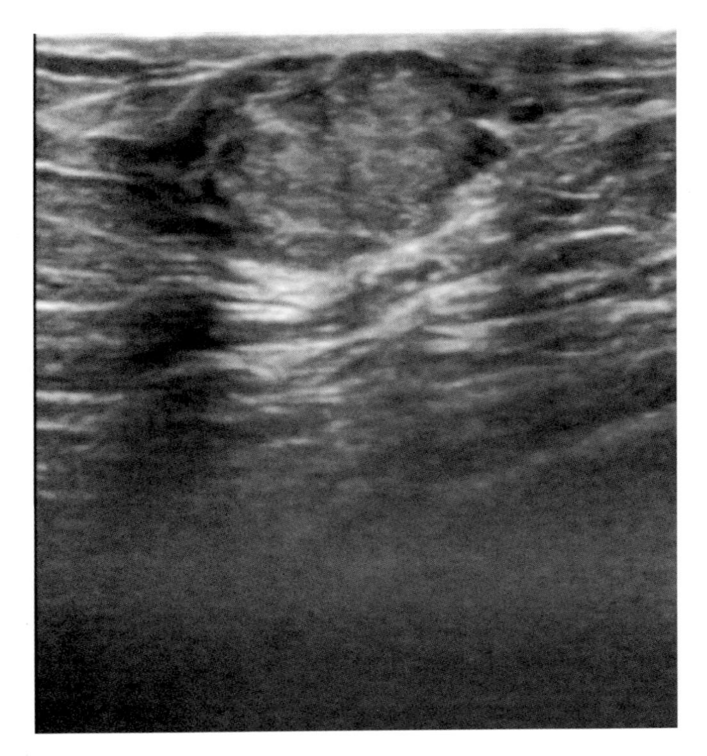

(b) On ultrasound, solid lesion with variegated density and lobulated margins

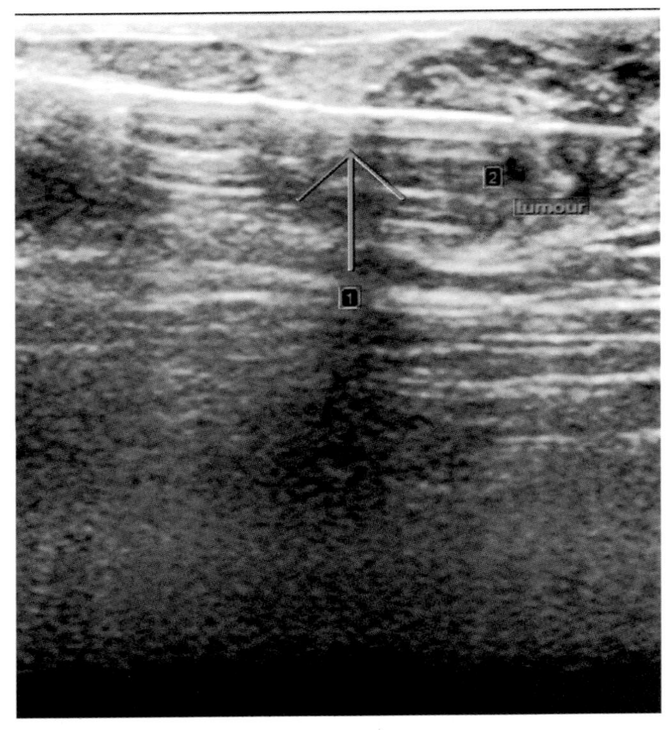

(d) Percutaneous needle biopsy under ultrasound guidance; the needle is seen going across the field and into the tumor (green arrow). **Histology confirmed invasive ductal carcinoma.**

prognosis is good. On the other hand, if four or more nodes contain tumor, the prognosis is much worse. Therefore, dissection or sampling of the axilla is an important part of any complete operation for breast cancer.

As far as the actual extent of dissection of the axilla is concerned, it has been argued that axillary clearance, which sometimes results in lymphedema of the arm, needlessly overtreats the 50% patients with negative axillary nodes. Hence sampling is carried out more often then clearance.

Sentinel node biopsy

The first one or two regional lymph nodes—the 'sentinel' nodes—draining the tumor area are the earliest seat of metastasis to the axilla. A sentinel node is localized by injecting patent blue dye or radioisotope in and around the tumor and following the dye by dissection till the node. If on frozen section the node is negative for metastases, the axilla is free of tumor in 97% of cases, and axillary clearance can be avoided.

Procedures employed

In the surgical treatment of breast cancer, the breast and the axillary contents are removed wholly or in part.

For ease of understanding:

A. The procedures available for the breast and the axilla will be first listed separately.
B. We shall next examine their various combinations.
C. Finally we will consider the choice of combinations for different cases.

Operations

On the breast

- *Total mastectomy*. The whole of the breast is removed, including the nipple and areola as well as the skin over the protuberant breast.
- *'Conservative' operations,* namely *quadrantectomy* and *segmentectomy*. Quadrantectomy involves removal of the whole quadrant in which the tumor is located. Either term implies removal of the tumor with an adequate margin of normal tissue i.e. 1cm.

On the axilla

- *Axillary clearance*. The contents of the axilla i.e. fat and lymph nodes are removed, staying medial to the axillary vein to spare the lymphatics draining the upper limb.
- *Axillary sampling*. The nodes of the anterior chain are 'sampled'.
- *Axillary lymphangiography*, followed by removal of only those nodes found to contain tumor (sentinel node). This technique is designed to save uninvolved nodes.

Combinations in common use

These include the following:

- *Total mastectomy and axillary sampling*. (i.e. sentinel node biopsy by frozen section).
- *Total mastectomy and axillary clearance* (i.e. modified radical mastectomy).

  Note: In the original radical mastectomy the pectoralis major was also removed. This operation has been abandoned, as its results have been found to be equivalent to those of modified radical mastectomy.
- *Quadrantectomy, Axillary Dissection and Radiation Therapy* (Q.U.A.R.T.). In this procedure the quadrant of the breast bearing the tumor is excised and axillary dissection carried out. This is followed by radiation of the breast.

The choice of the combination

- *Tumors larger than 2–3cm* are best treated by mastectomy and axillary clearance, which has long been described as the 'gold standard' operation. This method is suitable for all tumors, but tumors larger than 2cm should definitely be provided with the benefit of removal of the entire breast.
- *Tumors smaller than 2cm* can be treated by partial mastectomy i.e. 'segmentectomy' or 'quadrantectomy' (plus axillary procedure), *provided only if radiotherapy and follow-up of a high standard are available, and provided the margins of the removed tissue are shown to be free of tumor.*

Contraindications to breast conservation

Even so, the following constitute contraindications to breast conservation:

- Tumors larger than 3cm.
- Tumors which are located centrally.
- Bilateral and multifocal tumors.
- Poorly differentiated tumors.
- Breasts showing Paget's disease of the nipple.
- If the patient prefers to be treated by total mastectomy.

Note: Recently, in the case of tumors less than 3cm in size, *quadrantectomy, axillary dissection and radiatiotherapy* to the breast has been tried. The five year survival figures have been reported to be similar to those after modified radical mastectomy. International trends favour a reduction in radical procedures. *However, this regime also requires high standards of pathological classification, radiotherapy, chemotherapy, and follow-up.*

Breast conservation

The psychological effects on women of the mutilation caused by total mastectomy have led to this technique being employed for the smaller tumors. This involves wide excision of the primary with at least 1cm safe margins and axillary dissection (sentinel node biopsy or clearance), followed by radiation to the breast. Breast conservation is indicated for tumors 3cm or less in size depending upon breast size.

However, it may be stated here that surgery for breast cancer can leave psychological effects either way. Women who undergo mastectomy are concerned about the effect on their looks; those who have conservative operations worry about the chances of recurrence.

Technique of modified radical mastectomy (Patey)

The breast and axillary contents are dissected en bloc. The excised mass consists of:

- The whole breast.
- The skin overlying the protuberant breast along with nipple and areola.
- All the fat, fascia and lymph nodes of the axilla.

While dissecting the axilla, the pectoralis minor may be divided for better access. The surgeon remains medial to the axillary vein. Thus he avoids damage to the upper limb lymphatics accompanying the vein, and prevents the development of lymphedema of the arm.

Suction drainage

Drainage with continuous suction is achieved by connecting the non-collapsible drain with:

- A glass bottle in which vacuum has been created by evacuating the air with a sucker, or.
- A collapsible plastic bottle from which air has been evacuated by compression and which, as it springs open, creates a negative pressure.

This step greatly expedites healing by preventing accumulation of exudate under the flaps. Apart from mastectomy, this method can be used wherever the possibility of accumulation of fluid under skin flaps exists.

It may be mentioned that a recently suggested alternative approach avoids drainage and actively encourages the collection of serous fluid as a 'seroma'. This exudate gets organized and fibrosed; it is supposed to partly fill the cavity left behind by the mastectomy and provide a fuller contour. However, suction drainage appears less likely to be followed by complications.

If a wide area of skin has been sacrificed, it may not be possible to approximate the skin edges. A deficiency is left which should be treated by immediate split-skin grafting. When the wound has healed, movements of the arm are encouraged to prevent stiffness of the shoulder.

Breast reconstruction

The mutilation produced by mastectomy can be minimized by breast reconstruction, which should be offered specially to premenopausal women. It may be performed at the time of the mastectomy or delayed for 3–6 months after the operation. The advantage of a few months' delay is this: a reconstructed breast generally cannot match the original, and therefore immediate reconstruction results in unfavourable comparison by the patient. With delayed reconstruction the patient will compare favourably the reconstructed breast with the mastectomy.

Breast reconstruction may be carried out by:

- Implanting a *silicone prosthesis* of the breast under the pectoral muscles.
- Employing a *latissimus dorsi myocutaneous* ***flap***: In this operation the latissimus is divided from its origin and, along with an overlying ellipse of skin, is tunnelled forwards to be spread out and sutured over the pectoral region. The ellipse of skin ensures that there is no shortage of skin after removal of the breast and its overlying skin.
- The more recent innovation, which gives a better cosmetic result, employs a myocutaneous flap of *rectus abdominis* muscle supplied by the superior epigastric artery and with an overlying ellipse of skin.
- Finally, the areola can be constructed by grafting a disc of skin from the upper medial thigh, and the nipple by taking a segment from the opposite nipple.

Adjuvant therapy for breast cancer

[*Adjuvant:* that which reinforces or enhances the action of a treatment]. Fewer than 50% of women treated surgically for apparently curable lesions are alive 10 years later. This liability to early spread made it necessary to look for adjuncts to the treatment of breast cancer in the hope of altering potential metastatic disease. Three types of adjunctive therapy have been developed: radiotherapy, chemotherapy and hormone alteration.

- ***Adjuvant radiotherapy.***

Both preoperative and postoperative radiotherapy have failed to alter survival rates. However, post operative radiotherapy has had some effect on local recurrences.

- ***Adjuvant chemotherapy.***

The use of chemotherapy as an adjunct to primary treatment of breast cancer is *one of the most important advances in cancer care.* This fact can be properly appreciated only if it is remembered that, until the 1950's, nothing could be done for the distant micrometastases that had taken place before diagnosis in nearly half the patients with breast cancer. Since that time, an increasingly bright picture of the situation has been emerging.

Combination chemotherapy

Although chemotherapy was started with one drug, it was soon found that when two or more drugs were used in combination, the therapeutic effects were cumulative but the side effects were not.

Three-drug regimen

This was obviously a great advantage of the method of multiple-drug therapy (combination chemotherapy). Today, a three-drug combination of methotrexate, cytoxan and 5-fluorouracil (CMF) is commonly used, 6 three-weekly cycles with these drugs being employed.

Five-drug regimen

Further, vincristine and prednisolone are often combined with the above three drugs in the form of a five-drug regimen, when the results are even better. This kind of combination chemothrerapy is employed in the following groups of patients:

- In women aged less than 50 years:
  - In node-positive patients: Useful in all cases.
  - In node-negative patients: May be of value.
- In women aged more than 50:
  - In hormone-receptor-negative patients, due to doubts about efficacy of tamoxifen.
  - In women with one to three positive axillary nodes, the 5-year relapse-free survival rate is as high as 88%, compared with 50% in the group where no adjuvant chemotherapy has been used. Unlike tamoxifen, combination chemotherapy is more effective before the age of 50. Before this age, it reduces mortality at the end of five years by 34 %, after this age by only 18 %. Unfortunately, chemotherapy is often accompanied by serious sequelae, e.g. myelosuppression with leucopenia and anemia, as well as alopecia.

Neo-adjuvant chemotherapy

When three cycles of chemotherapy are given before surgery the regimen is called neo-adjuvant.

Comparison between radiotherapy and chemotherapy

For many decades radiotherapy was the standard adjuvant therapy after radical mastectomy if the axillary nodes were found to contain tumor. It was later found that *multiple drug chemotherapy given after operation gives superior results*; therefore it is now used more often than radiotherapy.

This superiority of multiple drug therapy over radiotherapy is not entirely unexpected. The only way radiotherapy could possibly affect metastatic disease could be by whole body irradiation; however, this is known to be associated with an extremely high morbidity. Fortunately, *because the side effects of the different drugs used in multi-drug therapy do not cumulate*, multi-drug chemotherapy achieves control of metastases with a significantly lower level of morbidity.

Adjuvant hormonal therapy

The response of breast cancer to hormones is dependent on the presence in the cancer cells of hormone receptors. If these receptors are present it indicates a more differentiated tumor. Such neoplasms respond to all forms of therapy better than receptor-negative tumors:

- If both estrogen receptors (ER) and progesterone receptors (PR) are present, 80% of tumors will respond to hormonal manipulation.
- Tumors that are both ER and PR-negative respond in only 10% of cases.

It follows therefore that when a breast tumor is removed it should be sent not only for histological examination *but also for detecting the presence of hormone receptors.*

The different forms of hormonal manipulation include the following:

- **Antiestrogens.** Tamoxifen is an antiestrogen which acts by blocking estrogen receptor sites. The oral dose for best reslts is 20mg. per day. Tamoxifen is more effective over the age of 50; above this age, it reduces the risk of recurrence at the end of 5 years by 18 %, below it by only 4 %. Side effects are minimal.
- **Aromatase inhibitors.** Aromatase is the enzyme that synthesizes estrogen. Aromatase inhibitors are thus anti-estrogens and serve as second-line hormone therapy. They are indicated for post-menopausal women who respond and later relapse after tamoxifen. As aromatase inhibitors have been shown to be as effective as tamoxifen but with less

severe side effects, they are sometimes used as first-line hormonal therapy in hormone-receptor-positive patients.

For advanced breast cancer in post-menopausal women, aromatase inhibitors are used in those patients who fail to respond to tamoxifen. Examples of aromatase inhibitors include letrozole and anastrazole.

Note: In the past the operations available for hormone manipulation included oophorectomy, adrenalectomy and hypophysectomy. The latter two had particularly severe side effects. *They have been abandoned* due to the success of the various oral agents. Adjuvant hormone therapy achieves medical oophorectomy by knocking out the ovaries.

Treatment of recurrent breast cancer

Recurrent cancer of the breast may take the form of local recurrences or wide dissemination:

For local recurrences

Radiation is a very useful agent. Examples of such local lesions include subcutaneous nodules and bony metastases (Fig.38.4).

Operation may also be useful for small local lesions, but only if margins clear of tumor can be obtained. The patient with local recurrence is investigated for distant metastases (bones, lungs).

For distant metastases

The important problem in recurrent cancer is usually wide dissemination. The treatment of choice here consists of the use of hormone therapy and/or chemotherapy. The initial choice out of the above two methods is easy: it depends upon whether or not the tumor is hormonally sensitive; this can be determined by testing for the presence of hormone receptors. As mentioned before, 80% of patients with breast cancers which are both ER and PR-positive respond to hormonal manipulation. Thus if the patient's hormone receptor status is positive, she should be treated by hormonal manipulation; if she is receptor-negative, chemotherapy should be used.

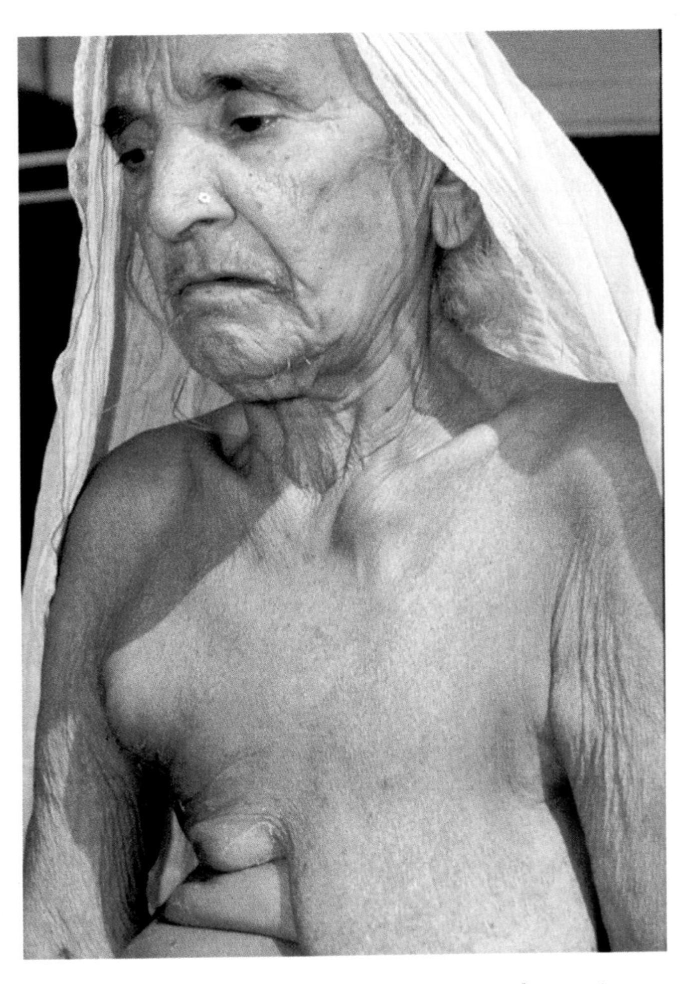

Fig.38.4 The patient had right mastectomy for carcinoma some years ago. The inner end of the left clavicle is enlarged due to a metastasis.

Special situations

Locally advanced disease (stage III)

The management of these tumors has given disappointing results because of poor local control and subsequent metastatic disease, resulting in an overall survival rate of only 20%. The different approaches are as follows:

- ***Neo-adjuvant chemotherapy***, to 'downstage' the tumor prior to surgery or irradiation: not only does the tumor shrink and become more amenable to surgery, but also chemotherapy is delivered to potential micrometastases immediately after diagnosis. The results of this method are promising.
- ***Adjuvant chemotherapy***: This improves the disease-free survival rate.
- ***High-dose radiotherapy*** has given results similar to those with radical mastectomy. Local recurrences can be reduced by surgically debulking the tumor, or by giving even higher doses of radiation by an interstitial implant.

The elderly

In the elderly, tumors are slow-growing, usually estrogen-receptor positive with a good prognosis, and can be treated with the anti-estrogen tamoxifen alone. However, as the cosmetic compulsion to retain the breast is less strong at this age, it is best to add mastectomy, tamoxifen alone being reserved for the very frail.

Pregnancy

The use of radiotherapy during pregnancy is inadvisable; therefore total mastectomy is used more often than quadrantectomy and segmental resection. Hormone treatment is not often employed, as most tumors are hormone receptor negative. On a diagnosis of breast cancer, pregnancy should be avoided till the time for most recurrences, i.e. about three years, has passed.

Lactation

The tumor should be treated on standard lines, lactation being suppressed by bromocriptine.

Ductal carcinoma in situ

The best treatment is a mastectomy, not only for extensive disease but even for the screen-detected smaller tumors.

Metastatic breast cancer

Treatment aims at alleviating symptoms and prolonging survival. Investigations aim at determining the full extent of the disease, and should include examination of the primary and regional nodes, chest x-ray, abdominal ultrasound, and bone scintigraphy.

In general, palliation of metastatic breast cancer can only be carried out by systemic therapy. The exceptions, where local treatment is employed, consist of radiotherapy for painful bony deposits and internal fixation for pathological fractures.

Because of fewer side effects, hormonal treatment is the preferred systemic method, but its application is limited by the fact that receptor-positive tumors are fewer in number. Tamoxifen and anastrazole are used first. When resistance to these is encountered, other drugs take their place.

Chemotherapy is more effective in younger patients and in rapidly growing tumors. The therapy does not prolong life, but symptoms are controlled and the quality of life improved.

Prognosis

Five and 10 year survival figures for patients with breast cancer are shown in Table 38.3.

The following point to a poor prognosis:

- Young age.
- Rapid growth of the tumor.
- Poor differentiation.
- Lymphatic permeation.
- Blood vessel invasion.

Survival of breast cancer cases

Table 38.3 shows the fibe and 10 year survival figures of patients of breast carcinomas treated at a cancer hospital in Pakistan.

Table 38.3: Five and 10 year survival figures at Shaukat Khanum Memorial Cancer Hospital (SKMCH), Lahore, Pakistan*.

Stage	5-year survival more than	10-year survival more than
1	92%	76%
2	82%	59%
3	72%	43%
4	15	?

As the figures amply show, early diagnosis and treatment provide rich dividends.

It may be noted that SKMCH is a dedicated cancer facility following up to date practices. These figures may not reflect the position across the country.

*Jamshed A. et al. IJC_431_12R4.

Chapter

39 THORAX

Tests of lung function

In the pulmonary alveoli blood and expired air exchange oxygen and carbon dioxide across the alveolar membrane. Any severe disturbance of this mechanism may lead to changes in the level of the blood gases. *Blood* O_2, CO_2 *and pH* determinations measure adequacy of lung function. *Chest expansion, vital capacity* and *forced expiratory volume* measure the patient's ability to ventilate.

Lung scanning

The movement of air in the tracheobronchial tree can be measured by lung scanning after *inhaling* radioactive xenon. If the same radioactive xenon is given *intravenously*, lung scanning can measure the flow of blood in the pulmonary vasculature. In this way the relationship between ventilation and perfusion *(ventilation/perfusion ratio)* can be worked out:

- If an area of lung is ventilated but not perfused, e.g. in pulmonary embolism, a part of the tidal volume is wasted. The larger such an area of lung the more dangerous the situation.
- If on the other hand a part of the lung is perfused but not ventilated e.g. in collapse of a lobe, the lobe acts as a right-to-left shunt, supplying deoxygenated blood to the arterial system. If the shunt is large cyanosis may result.

Pulmonary angiography

An outline of the pulmonary vessels can be obtained with radiopaque diatrizoate injected into the right ventricle (pulmonary angiography). Both pulmonary angiography and lung scanning help in the diagnosis of pulmonary embolism.

CHEST INJURIES

In civilian practice chest injuries consist either of stab and bullet wounds, or are sustained during road accidents. In war they are quite common. There are two main varieties of chest injuries, namely pentrating wounds and crush injuries, though both types may be present in the same patient.

Penetrating chest wounds

Stab wounds

Stab wounds are most commonly found on the left side of the front of the chest, the knife being in the assailant's right hand. If the knife penetrates the heart these wounds are associated with a high mortality rate. If it punctures only the lung they are relatively benign, causing only a moderate-sized hemothorax.

Missile wounds

Missile wounds are much more commonly fatal, because they often go through-and-through, and thus can cause damage to a larger number of structures. Low or high velocity bullets may be used:

Low velocity

Most civilian gunshot wounds occur with low velocity. Such missiles core out a hole through the body and damage only those tissues with which they come in direct contact. They cause death if they:

- gamage vital structures or.
- cause exsanguinating hemorrhage.

Because of its low kinetic energy the path taken by a hand-gun bullet through the body can be deflected by bone or even parenchymal organs such as the liver.

High velocity

On the other hand wounds due to high-velocity rifle bullets and bomb fragments produce extensive tissue damage by cavitation and shock waves. Energy from the bullet is dissipated into the surrounding tissues which are violently accelerated forwards and outwards. For a split-second this creates a large cavity about 30 times the size of the missile. The cavity has a subatmospheric pressure and is open at both entrance and exit holes. It then collapses sucking air, debris and bacteria into the wound and producing a large volume of devitalized and contaminated tissue. The mediastinal structures, the diaphragm and the abdominal organs may be damaged. A *thoracotomy* may be required in order to assess the extent of damage and undertake repair.

Extent of damage

Damage is directly proportional to the density of the tissue. Liver, spleen and muscle are damaged to a greater extent than tissues like lung which mainly consist of air. The destruction is also inversely proportional to the number of elastic fibres present; skin and lung are resistant whereas rigid bone is shattered.

Thoraco-abdominal wounds

A stab or bullet wound of the lower chest may penetrate the diaphragm and damage intra-abdominal organs. The main indications for exploration are signs of persistent bleeding or the likelihood of the perforation of a hollow viscus. The best route for exposure is through the thorax, because it allows correction of the thoracic injuries while providing adequate exposure of the upper abdomen through the diaphragm.

Crush injuries of the chest

These are common in road accidents. There may be bruising of the chest wall, rib fractures, a stove-in chest, a flail chest, lung contusion, or rupture of the aorta or myocardium.

Fractures of the ribs

Ribs may get broken either from direct violence or when the chest is crushed.

- When each rib is broken at only one point and the *number of broken ribs is small*, the problem is usually a simple one, requiring only rest and analgesics, or at most strapping.
- When some ribs are broken both anteriorly and posteriorly, a *flail segment* of chest wall results which is dangerous because of paradoxical respiration as explained below.
- If a *large number of ribs*, e.g. eight or ten, are broken, even if each one is broken at only one point, a critical situation can arise. Firstly, a single rib fracture can result in a blood loss of 150ml. Multiple fractures may cause substantial blood loss into the chest wall and pleural cavity. Secondly, because of the fractures the chest cannot expand properly, a problem which is made worse by the considerable pain which results. Secretions therefore get retained, further reducing vital capacity and setting the stage for the development of hypostatic pneumonia. This is even more likely in the case of elderly persons with their reduced vital capacity and diminished ability to fight infections.
- In a head-on car crash if the driver is not wearing a safety belt the *steering column* and wheel can hit the front of his chest and produce extensive damage. A fracture-dislocation of the upper end of the sternum occurs, with bilateral fractures of the ribs at their anterior ends. This can also cause paradoxical respiration and pose a danger to life.

Stove-in chest

In a stove-in chest a segment of the chest wall is pushed in and kept there by the surrounding ribs coming over it, reducing the volume of the underlying lung. It reduces the vital capacity, but does not produce as big a disorder of ventilation as flail chest.

Flail chest

A short flail chest is more dangerous. In this condition a segment of chest wall becomes loose due to fractures of a few ribs both in front of and behind it. When the chest expands during inspiration and a negative pressure is created, this loose segment instead of moving out is sucked in and prevents expansion of the lung, seriously interfering with ventilation.

The function of the other lung is also interfered with:

- During inspiration, due to expansion of the chest wall on the uninjured side, that lung expands properly and the pressure inside it becomes negative. Normally, air from outside would have filled this partial vacuum with inspired air. However, the pressure inside the lung on the injured side does not become negative as explained above. Therefore during inspiration air flows from the injured side to the healthy lung instead of being sucked into the injured side.
- Similarly, during expiration this same air flows back into the injured lung due to the pressure inside the normal lung being higher. Thus air in the two lungs keeps moving to-and-fro, preventing air from outside from coming in.

Therefore it will be seen that due to the severe physiological disorder produced by it, even a small flail segment of chest wall can produce a dangerous degree of hypoxia.

The serious interference with ventilation results in rapid shallow respirations with cyanosis, tachycardia and hypotension. Respiration is noisy from tracheo-bronchial secretions. Cerebral hypoxia produces confusion and restlessness, and this is followed by unconsciousness in severe cases.

Treatment

The treatment of flail chest is carried out as follows:

- The paradoxical movements due to a flail chest can be controlled by intermittent positive pressure ventilation (IPPV).
- However, if it is desired to avoid the danger of ventilator-associated pneumonia, oxygen can be given along with opiate analgesia, and supplemented by physiotherapy; only if this fails to stabilize the situation should recourse be had to IPPV.
- At the same time, operation to stabilize the chest wall may be required in severe chest injury

Blood and air in the pleural cavity

Traumatic hemothorax

In most chest injuries some blood collects in the pleural cavity. The source of the bleeding may be the chest wall, the lung, or the heart and great vessels. Due to constant churning of the blood from the respiratory movements, it becomes defibrinated and therefore does not clot. This is fortunate, because it is easier to remove liquid blood from the chest cavity (by aspiration) rather than to evacuate clotted blood. Bleeding is usually moderate, and should be dealt with by daily aspirations. If accumulation is progressive, indicating a persisting source of blood loss, a thoracotomy may be required to control the bleeding.

Aspiration of the pleural cavity (thoracentesis)

This is carried out most conveniently using a 3-way stopcock connected with the aspiration needle. When the valve is turned in one direction, fluid can be aspirated into the syringe. The valve is next turned in the other direction, and fluid flows into a tubing which carries it to a kidney-tray. The great advantage of the use of this simple implement lies in the fact that at no time does the system have to be disconnected, so that the system remains closed and the chances of infection or of introduction of air into the pleural cavity are minimized.

Traumatic pneumothorax

In many forms of trauma air enters the pleural cavity, usually with blood as well (hemopneumothorax). It may reach the pleural cavity through a wound in the chest wall. More commonly it leaks from the damaged lung.

Tension pneumothorax

If the leak in the lung is valvular, at every inspiration air leaks into the pleural cavity, but cannot return to the lung during expiration. A considerable quantity of air thus accumulates in the pleura, producing complete collapse of the lung and displacing the mediastinum to the opposite side (tension pneumothorax). This is a very serious condition and threatens life. If, after trauma to the chest, the patient is in respiratory distress with the intercostal spaces bulging on one side of the chest along with a tympanitic note, and the trachea shifted to the opposite side, a tension pneumothorax is present. This condition is readily apparent on clinical examination and one should not wait for x-ray confirmation.

The best immediate *treatment* consists of water-seal drainage:

- A needle inserted through the chest wall will confirm the diagnosis because of the hissing sound of the air being expelled, but is useless therapeutically.
- A short scalpel incision will relieve tension and restore both ventilation and venous return.
- An intercostal drain can then be inserted through the same short incision with aseptic precautions and closed drainage provided.

Surgical emphysema

If the parietal pleura is damaged air may leak into the subcutaneous tissues and cause surgical emphysema. If this air is leaking from a peripheral part of the lung it soon becomes absorbed, and is not of much consequence. On the other hand, if a major bronchus has been ruptured, the air leaks under considerable pressure. The emphysema may spread to the whole trunk and neck, and produce asphyxia by compression of the trachea.

In such cases *tracheostomy* helps, by acting as a safety valve and relieving the pressure in the major bronchi.

If the benefit resulting from tracheostomy is not sufficient, thoracotomy and repair of the bronchus has to be carried out.

Contusion and laceration of the lung

In most cases of moderate and severe chest trauma the lung is injured. Contusion produces consolidation, but usually resolves spontaneously. Laceration permits the leakage of blood and air into the pleural cavity. Major lacerations produce persistent collapse of the lung and leakage of air, and should be repaired at thoracotomy. The damaged lung often becomes secondarily infected. This can be prevented by chemotherapy, bronchial aspiration and physiotherapy.

Examination

The damage must be carefully assessed. The chest wall is examined for paradoxical movement (multiple rib fractures), depression (stove-in chest), or sucking wounds. The position of the trachea and apex beat, along with a tympanitic or dull note over the affected lung, may indicate the presence of a pneumothorax, a hemothorax or massive collapse of the lung. An immediate chest x-ray is essential for accurate diagnosis.

Treatment of chest injuries

Advances in transportation have provided an opportunity to sustain life in patients who previously would have died.

Helicopter retrieval

In the advanced countries helicopter retrieval with resuscitation en route by positive pressure ventilation, external cardiac massage, and blood volume replacement are employed for patients with major trauma. Even in the under-developed countries the concept is catching on.

Patients reaching hospital can survive

More than 80 percent of all patients with ruptured aorta, trachea or bronchus die rapidly at the site of injury. Those who reach hospital are a self-selected group who should survive with appropriate treatment. Once in hospital, resuscitative measures are best carried out with caution and in an unhurried manner, because most survivors have reached an impaired but balanced respiratory and hemodynamic status compatible with life.

If ventilation can be maintained at an adequate level, the rib fractures heal and the crisis is tided over.

Improving ventilation

Treatment is aimed at improving ventilation by the following means, as dictated by the situation:

Relief of pain

Pain is relieved with repeated small doses of morphine or other analgesic, or intercostal block. The intercostal nerves may be blocked by injecting a small amount of local anesthetic near the posterior part of each nerve. This is a good way of abolishing pain for a few hours, because relief from pain is obtained without sedation, which is a side effect of many potent analgesics, and which depresses respiration.

Removal of secretions

- If pain is relieved it may become possible for the patient to bring up his *tracheobronchial secretions* by coughing.
- If this is still not possible, the sputum may be sucked out through a *bronchoscope*.
- If secretions still persist, suction through an *endotracheal tube* or after performing a *tracheostomy* may be required. A tracheostomy transforms the condition of a seriously ill patient:
  - It permits very effective suction of secretions.
  - It eliminates the dead space of the pharynx and reduces the work of respiration.

Removal of blood or air

Blood and air are removed from the pleural cavity by aspiration, if their quantity is enough to compress the lung. If the blood or air reaccumulates rapidly, an indwelling tube or a thoracotomy may become necessary. A sucking wound should be immediately sealed with a pad of cloth or cotton until definitive surgical repair can be carried out. As mentioned above, tension pneumothorax can be confirmed in an emergency by plunging an aspirating needle into the chest which allows the air under tension to escape. However, to release the tension a scalpel incision is required. A catheter can next be introduced and connected to a water seal or electric suction apparatus.

Oxygen

Oxygen is usually required, and *blood transfusion* and *fluid replacement* may be needed.

Shock lung

In a fairly high percentage of patients who have sustained major trauma, shock lung or post-traumatic respiratory failure develops.

The mechanism of production of this condition is as follows:

- Severe trauma produces extensive intravascular coagulation.
- This leads to micro-thromboembolism of the smaller lung vessels.
- Consolidation of the lung produces severe depression of gas exchange.
- Lung compliance is markedly decreased, and impairs ventilation.

Similar changes are seen after septicemia, massive blood or fluid infusions, and after heart-lung by pass.

Treatment is urgent. An endotracheal tube should be passed and positive pressure ventilation carried out. Steroids are given in large doses. Antibiotics and intravenous fluids are given as indicated.

DISEASES OF THE CHEST WALL

Thoracic outlet syndrome

The thoracic outlet is the space through which the subclavian artery, vein and brachial plexus pass from the neck into the upper extremity. It is bounded by the clavicle, the chest wall and the scalene muscles. Occasionally, a rib arises from the seventh cervical vertebra, either on one or both sides. Such a 'cervical' rib is seen in 0.5% of individuals.

Cervical rib

Pathology

- There may be a complete rib.
- The anterior part of the rib may be a fibrous cord.
- The rib may end blindly.
- There may be a fibrous band in the insertion of the scalenus anterior.

Obstruction of the subclavian artery and vein, or pressure on the brachial plexus, may occur in the thoracic outlet. Distal to this constricted segment, a section of the artery gets dilated due to turbulence of the blood flow which causes lateral stresses on the wall of the artery, leading to the formation of an aneurysm.

Small emboli

In the dilated area a thrombus may form, part of which may become detached as an embolus. If showers of small emboli settle in the digital arteries, ischemic episodes occur, which may superficially resemble Raynaud's phenomenon. However, whereas in Raynaud's phenomenon all the fingers of *both* hands are involved, here only one hand is affected.

Clinical features

Symptoms

These may be neurological or vascular, and in most cases one or the other type predominates.

Neurological

Neurological symptoms and signs result from stretching or compression of the lower roots of the brachial plexus. Pain and paraesthesias in the fingers, hand or arm, and muscular weakness and wasting are common..

Vascular

Vascular symptoms and signs are due to pressure on the subclavian artery and are strictly unilateral. They may vary from recurrent minor episodes of digital ischemia to sudden massive ischemia of the whole limb.

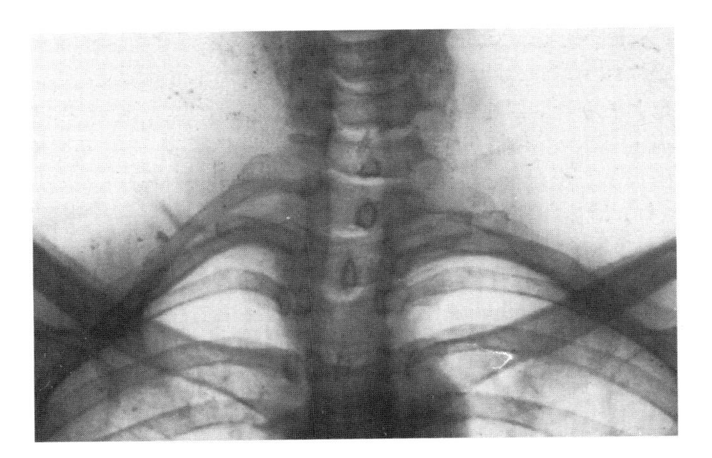

Fig.39.1 Right-sided cervical rib arising from 7th cervical vertebra and inserted into 1st rib

Signs

A cervical rib or other bony abnormality may be visible or palpable just above the clavicle. There may be a palpable thrill and bruit over the artery. The distal pulses may be reduced or absent, and the blood pressure in the affected arm may be lower than on the normal side.

Investigations

X-rays of the neck, shoulder and thoracic outlet should be taken. MRI is useful, as it can identify the brachial plexus and demonstrate the angulation of the lower trunk of the plexus over a fibrous band. If vascular involvement is suspected aortic arch angiography should be carried out. Patients presenting with venous obstruction require phlebography. However, clinical assessment remains the most important factor in diagnosis and choice of treatment.

Treatment

If a patient has *only neurological symptoms* he usually derives benefit from correction of faulty posture, with shoulder girdle strengthening exercises. As the scapula now rides high, the angulation of the lower trunk of the brachial plexus is reduced, and symptoms are relieved. In the few cases where surgical treatment is required, resection of the cervical rib is the recommended procedure, although in many cases division of the scalenus anterior may be sufficient.

If *vascular symptoms* are predominent, the need for surgical treatment is urgent. The aims of the operation are:

- To remove the compressing structure.
- To repair the subclavian artery.
- To restore the distal circulation by removing emboli and propagated thrombus.

However, this work should be done only by those with special interest and experience in this condition.

A cervical rib which is not causing symptoms should generally be left alone. Finally, neurological symptoms may be produced not only by a cervical rib but also by a normal first rib, specially in a weak and slim person, and more particularly in middle age due to sagging down of the shoulders; all that is needed is exercise of the shoulders to elevate the scapula and eliminate the droop of the shoulder.

Funnel chest (pectus excavatum)

In this deformity there is a depression of the body of the sternum and the xiphoid process, with backward curving of the costal cartilages and adjacent parts of the ribs. When severe, this deformity leads to greatly reduced ventilation, and predisposes to respiratory infections. Similarly, the venae cavae and the heart are distorted out of shape, so that cardiovascular disturbances are common.

Treatment

If symptoms are severe the deformity has to be corrected by operation. The 3rd to 7th costal cartilages on both sides are resected subperiosteally. At the sternal angle the anterior cortex of the sternum is divided transversely. The lower end of the body of the sternum is lifted forwards and a stainless steel strut placed transversely behind it and over the ribs to maintain the sternum in an elevated position. The long-term functional and cosmetic results of this operation are good.

Kyphoscoliosis

If fibrosis develops in one pleural cavity due to empyema, etc., the resulting contracture shortens that side of the chest. The spinal column bends forwards and to the affected side, i.e. a kyphoscoliosis develops.

Decortication

Vigorous exercises can do much to prevent deformity. However, if the cause of the deformity is extensive fibrosis, the whole thick layer of fibrous tissue in the pleural cavity has to be removed to allow the lung to expand. This removal is called decortication and is carried out at a thoracotomy. If the correct plane of cleavage between the fibrous tissue and the pleura can be found, the operation is not as tedious or bloody as might be imagined.

Cold abscess

The common cause of a cold abscess of the chest wall is tuberculous intercostal lymphadenitis. Other less frequent causes include tuberculosis of the spine, ribs and sternum. In neglected cases the abscess ruptures, producing a persistent discharging sinus. An abscess has to be distinguished from a lipoma and an empyema necessitatis. Treatment consists of a full course of antituberculosis drugs, with repeated aspirations of the pus.

Empyema necessitates

An empyema necessitatis arises when a neglected empyema perforates the chest wall and presents as a subcutaneous collection of pus. If the tract is direct it demonstrates a cough impulse; if it is tortuous it does not. X-ray of the chest shows up the empyema. Treatment is aimed at the empyema, which should be aspirated and the pus cultured; the empyema is then drained. The superficial abscess will probably disappear. If it does not do so, it may require separate drainage.

DISEASES OF THE PLEURA

Pneumothorax

When air is present in the pleural cavity the condition is called pneumothorax. It may reach the pleural cavity in one of the following ways:

- It may enter after trauma to the chest *(traumatic pneumothorax).*
- It may be introduced deliberately *(artificial pneumothorax).*
- It may appear without any obvious exciting cause *(spontaneous pneumothorax).*

Diagnosis

The *physical signs* of a pneumothorax include a hyper-resonant note on percussion and absent breath sounds.

X-rays show translucency on the affected side with absence of lung markings; the margin of the collapsed lung is visible.

Spontaneous pneumothorax

The common causes of this condition are the following:

- Tuberculosis.
- Emphysematous bulla.
- Solitary lung cyst.
- Honeycomb lung.
- Idiopathic.

If a small subpleural *tuberculous* cavity ruptures, air leaks into the pleural cavity resulting in a pneumothorax. There is usually infection and irritation of the pleura, resulting in the appearance of fluid in the pleural cavity and some fever. Treatment is that of the underlying tuberculous lesion.

A *non-tuberculous* spontaneous pneumothorax is rarely associated with fever or fluid formation. In a few cases an underlying lesion e.g. an emphysematous bulla, a lung cyst, or a honeycomb lung may be demonstrated.

Treatment

If the patient comes during the first attack and there is no underlying cause, the air may be allowed to get absorbed, or occasional aspirations may be carried out. If the air fails to be absorbed or collects again, investigation by tomography, C.T. scan or thoracoscopy should be carried out, and the needful done.

Hemothorax

The conditions in which blood can collect in the pleural cavity include trauma, thoracic operations, new growths and leaking aneurysms, but some cases apparently arise spontaneously. The respiratory and cardiac movements defibrinate the blood so that it remains fluid. Blood irritates the pleura, producing pain and shock, and exciting the formation of an effusion. The signs are those of fluid in the pleura, and the diagnosis is confirmed by aspiration with a needle.

Treatment

Pain should be relieved and major blood loss corrected. The blood should be aspirated using a 3-way stopcock or other device so that air cannot enter. Aspirations are carried out daily until no more blood is obtained and the x-rays appear clear. Vigorous breathing exercises are supervised from the beginning.

If the aspirating needle fails to remove blood it indicates that the hemothorax has clotted. In such a case streptokinase may be injected and aspiration again tried after 24 hours. However, usually such an effort is unsuccessful, and if the clot is large thoracotomy with evacuation of clot and 'decortication' of the lung is required, to prevent development of fibrous contracture of the chest wall and lung.

Empyema

An empyema is a suppurative infection confined to a natural anatomical space by normal epithelial boundaries. A thoracic empyema is a localized collection of pus in the pleural cavity. When the word empyema is used alone, a thoracic empyema is meant.

Etiology

An empyema is always secondary to infection in an adjacent organ. Examples include the following:

- Lung:
  - o Pneumonia.
  - o Lung abscess.
  - o Tuberculosis.
  - o Bronchiectasis.
  - o New growth.
- Esophagus:
  - o Perforation.
  - o Carcinoma.
- Chest wall:
  - o Wounds.
  - o Osteomyelitis of ribs.
- Abdomen.
  - o Subphrenic abscess.
- Postoperative.
  - o After thoracotomy.

Pathology

The most common cause of an empyema used to be pneumonia in the underlying lung. In the antibiotic era, empyema has become a less frequent complication of pneumonia, and the bacteriological spectrum has shifted from Pneumococcus and Streptococcus to Staphylococcus, Streptococcus and gram-negative organisms. Anaerobic organisms are also isolated from a significant proportion of cases. Multiple isolates, often mixed anaerobes and aerobes, occur in approximately 25% of cases.

'Frozen chest'

With inflammation and exudation, fibrin is deposited on the surface of the pleura, causing fusion of the lung to the chest wall at the periphery of the area. The granulation tissue is soon converted into a plaque of fibrous tissue. As this contracts, the ribs are drawn together and fixed, the diaphragm is raised and immobilized, and the mediastinum is drawn towards the affected side. The end-result of a severe chronic empyema is a fixed and contracted chest wall with a functionless lung.

Clinical features

Empyema should be suspected in a patient with fever and a pleural effusion on x-ray. Aspiration with Gram staining and culture of the fluid confirms the diagnosis and guides selection of antibiotics. The gross appearance of the fluid is usually diagnostic, though some seropurulent effusions are sterile.

most common hospital procedure for Americans over the age of 65 years.

Under x-ray fluoroscopy, a catheter is guided to the heart and the tip is manipulated to engage the ostium of the coronary artery. Pressure is measured at the tip of the catheter and angiograms (angios) are obtained while hand-injections are made of iodinated contrast material through the catheter. Mostly non-ionic contrast (Ioperomide) is used, as it is less arrhythmogenic as well as safer in patients suffering from kidney disease.

Coronary angiography

The patient lies down on the cardiac catheterization table with the image intensifier and camera above the chest and the x-ray tube below the table. The camera can be made to pivot towards the left and right of the patient. These are known as the left anterior oblique and right anterior oblique views respectively.

The camera is also able to pivot towards (cranial) and away (caudal) from the patient's head. The camera takes cineangiographic images as the ostium of the coronary artery is engaged and contrast material is injected to opacify the artery. Online fluoroscopy also allows visualization of the coronaries at any time without having to take pictures. Fluoroscopy is used to position the table and camera and during "test" injection of contrast.

The severity or degree of stenosis is measured in the cardiac cath lab by comparing the area of narrowing to an adjacent normal segment, as a percentage reduction.

Indications

Coronary angiography (Left heart cath) is indicated in:

- Precordial chest pain.
- Recurrent chest pain after coronary interventions.
- Prior myocardial infarction.
- Recurrent chest pain after artery bypass grafting.

Contraindications of coronary angiography

- Sensitivity to contrast material.
- Hemodynamically unstable patient.
- Renal insufficiency (creatinine > 1.5mg/dl).
- INR more than 1.5.
- Hemoglobin less than 10mg/dl.

Right heart catheterization

If a catheter is placed in the right femoral vein to measure pressures of the right side of the heart, the procedure is called right heart catheterization. It may be used:

- In *congenital* heart disease.
- In heart failure or hypotension, constrictive pericarditis, valvular heart disease, or ruptured ventricular septal defect.
- To measure cardiac output before therapeutic procedures.

Multidetector computed tomography (MDCT)

64-slice multidetector computed tomography (MDCT) allows us to non-invasively characterize the atherosclerotic lesions and define luminal and vessel wall alterations alike. The technique has been demonstrated to have a high diagnostic accuracy as compared with invasive coronary angiography.

With the introduction of 64-slice MDCT systems, improved temporal and spatial resolution as well as substantially shorter scan times have led to improved image quality throughout the entire coronary tree. The 256-slice scanners are even more advanced.

MDCT angiograms are analysed on a three-dimensional workstation using a combination of axial images, multiplanar reconstruction, cross sectional views and 3D volume rendered images.

Indications of MDCT

- Chest pain with probability of coronary disease.
- Prior infarction.
- Dysrhythmias.

Electrophysiological study

Sometimes an electrophysiological study is conducted before placing an implantable cardioverter/defibrillator to determine which device is best, and afterwards to monitor the success of the treatment.

Cardiac output measurement

The basic function of the heart is to provide blood to the tissues. Therefore, the ultimate index of function of the heart is the volume of blood pumped by it per minute i.e. the cardiac output. This requires measurement of the arterial and venous oxygen content, and tissue oxygen consumption.

This is done with a Swan-Ganz catheter as described above under right-heart catheterization.

Importance of measurement of cardiac output

The cardiac output measures the left ventricular function, which affects the risk of operation; therefore the preoperative measurement of cardiac output has considerable clinical significance.

BASIC TECHNIQUES IN CARDIAC SURGERY

Cardiac surgery is different from other types of surgery

The heart is different from other organs. If one wishes to operate upon the bones or the joints, the intestines or the thyroid, one has only to expose that organ and the surgical procedure can commence. The same is not true in the case of the heart.

In order for life to go on, the heart must continue to pump blood to all parts of the body. But if an operation like removal and replacement of a heart valve has to be carried out, the heart obviously has to remain motionless for a considerable period of time. How is life to continue during this period ?

The function of the heart is to circulate the blood first through the lungs so that it can be oxygenated, and then through the whole body so that the oxygen can reach all organs, and CO_2 and other waste products can be removed. If this function of the heart, i.e. to circulate the blood through a 'lung' and then through the body, could be taken over for a certain period, the heart could be kept motionless and operated upon, without any harmful effects on the body. The heart-lung machines perform precisely this function.

Heart lung machines

These vary a lot, but the principle underlying them all is the same. Each consists of a *pump* (the replacement for the heart) and an *oxygenator* (the 'lung'). Blood returning from the body is withdrawn from the right atrium by the pump, passed through the oxygenator, and pumped into the aorta fully oxygenated. Thus although the blood is diverted from the heart and lungs, it is supplied to the body in a well-oxygenated form.

Heart-lung machines provide the surgeon with periods for intracardiac surgery of two or three hours with safety, so that even complicated anomalies can be effectively treated. The oxygenator also contains a heat exchanger which helps lower the temperature of the patient during surgery.

As the blood interfaces with tubes and an artificial membrane, this could lead to an activation of the clotting mechanism. To prevent such an eventuality, the patient is anticoagulated with heparin.

Operations on the heart

Operations on the heart can be carried out in one of two ways:

Closed heart operations

In these the heart and lungs continue to function while the operations are carried out. Closed mitral commissurotomy was the first operation to be carried out on the heart, and for some time was the only cardiac surgical operation performed routinely.

At the same time, operations carried out on the main vessels outside the heart or the pericardium *(extracardiac operations)* do not require a bypass.

Open heart operations

In these operations the heart is stopped and its function is taken over by the 'Heart Lung Machine' and the 'Membrane Oxygenator', as outlined above.

Technique

Most major open cardiac operations e.g. coronary bypass, valve replacements, etc. are performed through a midline sternotomy incision. The pericardium is opened. The patient is heparinized. A plastic cannula is passed into the aorta through a purse-string suture. Similarly the right atrium is cannulated. The cannulae are connected to the heart-lung machine. Thus during the whole operation the responsibility of oxygenating the blood and supplying it to the body is taken over by the heart-lung machine.

When the operation is completed the patient is weaned from cardiopulmonary bypass after achieving normothermia. Protamine is given to neutralize the heparin. The cannulae are removed. During heart-lung bypass the efficiency of the extracorporeal circulation is constantly monitored by measuring the arterial blood pressure, arterial blood gases and electrolytes, and the urinary output.

Myocardial preservation

During operations on the heart the surgeon requires a motionless and relaxed heart for the duration of the operation. During this period the heart muscle needs to be protected from damage due to anoxia. This can be achieved by reducing the metabolic needs of the myocardium by:

- Arresting the heart.
- Reducing the myocardial temperature.

Methods of myocardial preservation

There are many ways of myocardial preservation during surgery and this depends upon the surgeon's preference:

- *Hypothermic fibrillating heart.*
- *Moderate hypothermia with intermittent fibrillation.*

In this method the patient is put on cardiopulmonary bypass and cooled to 25–30⁰ C. The aorta is clamped intermittently for 10–15 minutes in which the myocardium is hypothermic. After 15 minutes the clamp is removed and the heart is reperfused.

- *Drug-mediated myocardial protection.*

This is achieved by beta-adrenergic receptor-blocking and calcium-channel blocking agents.

- *Cardioplegia (Multidose)*

This method gives the best results for myocardial preservation during cardiac surgery with an arrested still heart. The solutions used contain high doses of potassium in addition to buffers. They induce diastolic arrest when infused into the coronary arteries. The solution is mixed with blood or crystalloid solution (Ringer's lactate). It can be delivered in blood at normal blood temperature and in crystalloid solution. This is infused every 20 minutes. The initial dose is 10ml/kg followed by 5ml/kg every 20 minutes.

Cardiolplegia in addition to hypothermia (28⁰ C) reduces the myocardial metabolism and myocardial oxygen consumption.

Hypothermia

The higher the temperature of the various tissues the greater their metabolic demands. It follows that by cooling the tissues their metabolic needs can be greatly reduced, enabling them to survive short periods of total deprivation of oxygen or longer periods of partial deprivation. This can be achieved during the operation by using a hypothermia unit. In general the temperature for most acquired heart diseases is lowered to 28–30⁰ C. In complex congenital anomalies and infants, this can be lowered even further and the heart lung machine switched off for a short period; this is known as 'Total circulatory arrest'.

CONDITIONS AMENABLE TO CARDIAC SURGICAL TREATMENT

These include congenital and acquired conditions affecting the heart.

CONGENITAL HEART DISEASE

A congenital cardiac abnormality occurs about six times in every 1,000 live births. Many anomalies are quite severe, so that they are incompatible with life without early inerevention. Even in babies who survive beyond infancy, life expectancy is greatly reduced, so that surgical correction is desirable in nearly every case.

The anomalies can be divided into those with a normal arterial oxygen saturation *(acyanotic cases)* and those with reduced saturation *(cyanotic cases).*

Acyanotic congenital heart disease

Acyanotic congenital cardiac defects have left to right shunts and present with increased pulmonary blood flow. The common conditions belonging to this group include patent ductus arteriosus, coarctation of the aorta, and atrial and ventricular septal defects.

Patent ductus arteriosus (PDA)

This is a common anomaly. The ductus connects the left pulmonary artery with the aorta, and blood flows from the high-pressure aorta into the pulmonary artery. The systolic blood pressure is high and the diastolic low, producing a collapsing or water-hammer pulse. The pulmonary vessels are dilated, and on x-ray screening their pulsations are increased ('hilar dance'). The additional circulation of blood through the lungs and the left heart results in left ventricular dilatation. Some cases with small to moderate patent ductus arteriosus may remain asymtomatic until the second decade of life. Those with a large duct present with cardiac failure early.

The *symptoms* are of pulmonary overcirculation and include dyspnoea, feeding intolerance, failure to thrive/ retardation of growth and repeated chest infections. A typical continuous machinery murmur is audible to the left of the sternum.

The important *complications* of patent ductus arteriosus include bacterial endocarditis, cardiac failure and early death.

Treatment

A small-sized duct can sometimes close spontaneously during the first few months. Surgical ligation via left thoracotomy is the gold standard treatment of PDA.

- In a *premature* neonate ibuprofen (an anti-prostaglandin) can be tried, to induce spontaneous closure.
- A persistent duct in a *full-term* neonate however will require closure, especially if moderate or large-sized.
- In an appropriately sized baby, usually greater than 10kg, percutaneous closure via angiography, using PDA occluding devices (e. g. an Amplatzer device), is now an option.

Coarctation of the aorta

This malformation consists of a localized severe stenosis of the aortic arch, located usually just distal to the origin of the left subclavian artery. It can occur alone or in association with other anomalies, especially VSD (10%).

Clinical features

Symptoms depend on the severity of the coarctation and the age at presentation.

In neonate

Severe, critical coarctation can present *in a neonate* as severe left ventricular (LV) failure due to the LV pressure load and with poor distal perfusion; this manifests itself as ashen-grey cold extremities, with a poor urine output and acidosis.

In this setting prostaglandin infusion is life-saving, distal perfusion being re-established by reopening the PDA. The patient can thereby be stabilized and then taken to the operation theatre for repair of the coarctation.

Later in life

Long-standing coarctation produces:

- Hypertension *above* it with headache, irritability, and throbbing and pulsations in the head and neck. Due to the severe hypertension there may be left ventricular failure and/or intracranial hemorrhage. The carotid and subclavian arteries pulsate markedly. Collateral vessels can be seen over the scapular regions.
- *Below* the constriction there is hypotension, with cold legs and intermittent claudication. The pulses in the lower limbs are weak or absent. Untreated, very few patients used to survive beyond the age of forty-five, as they died of hypertension.

Diagnosis

Echocardiography establishes the diagnosis. On x-ray there is left ventricular enlargement, a prominent ascending aorta and notching of the ribs from the enlarged intercostal vessels.

Cardiac catheterization and *angiography* delineate the anatomy and measure the size of the isthmus. *CT Angiography/MRI* can demonstrate the precise anatomy.

Treatment

The presence of coarctation is an indication for surgical intervention:

- In *neonates and infants* surgical repair with end-to-end anastomosis is carried out. Subclavian flap or patch aortoplasty can also be considered.
- In *older children, adolescents or adults* percutaneous balloon dilatation, with a stent placed to maintain the dilatation, is commonly employed.
- In *adults* interposition grafts can also be considered.

The overall mortality rate is less than 1 percent. Delayed treatment can lead to persistent hypertension despite relief of coarctation; therefore *early intervention* is advised. Relief of symptoms normally occurs after timely intervention.

Atrial septal defect (ASD)

This is a common congenital cardiac defect. When the septum between the atria is defective blood flows from the left to the right atrium (L-R shunt), so that the right side of the heart and the lungs are overfilled.

Different types exist:

- The commonest type is the secundum ASD.
- Sinus venosus ASDs are associated with partial anomalous pulmonary venous connections.
- Primum ASDs are endocardial cushion defects associated with a cleft mitral valve.

Symptoms always appear by middle age, if not earlier. They are usually due to pulmonary over-circulation. The classic finding of a secundum ASD is that of a wide fixed splitting of the second heart sound. Increased flow can also produce a pulmonary systolic murmur.

Diagnosis

Echocardiography establishes the diagnosis.

The pulmonary arteries are sometimes actively pulsatile on fluoroscopy *(hilar dance).*

Treatment

- Some small defects can close during the first year of life.
- Those that persist should be closed if hemodynamically significant.
- Simple secundum ASDs can be closed percutaneously or by surgery, while other forms of ASD all require surgery.

The ideal time for ASD closure is before school-going age. The operative mortality approaches zero in centres familiar with the operation.

Ventricular septal defect

This is one of the most common of congenital cardiac anomalies. It also occurs as part of more complex anomalies. The defect allows the passage of blood from the left to the right ventricle so that there is pulmonary over-circulation with pulmonary plethora and hypertension.

Symptoms include failure to thrive, poor feeding, and recurrent chest infections. This is a serious lesion and the defect requires early repair, usually in infancy.

Risk factors include:

- Young age (less than three months).
- Multiple defects.
- Established pulmonary hypertension.

Classification is based on location. The commonest form is perimembranous VSDs. Muscular and perimembranous VSDs can close spontaneously and need to be followed closely by a pediatric cardiologist.

Management

This consists of surgical closure. In case of multiple VSDs, or if complete repair is contraindicated, palliation is carried out with a PA band. In this procedure a band is placed around the base of the pulmonary artery to reduce the excessive flow of blood into the pulmonary artery and prevent pulmonary hypertension.

Delayed treatment can lead to fixed pulmonary vascular disease, reversal of shunt and inoperability—*Eisenmenger's syndrome.*

Cyanotic congenital heart disease

In all these anomalies there is central cyanosis due to an intracardiac shunt from right to left.

Tetralogy of fallot

This is the most common of the cyanotic conditions. There is an anteriorly malaligned ventricular septal defect that is positioned so that the aorta over-rides the septum and there is pulmonary annular/valvular narrowing. This leads to RV infundibular hypertrophy. High right-sided pressures therefore lead to R-L shunting.

The patient is classically undersized with central cyanosis and finger-clubbing. There is a systolic thrill and murmur in the pulmonary area. Untreated, many of the severe cases used to die during infancy; the less severe cases survived into adult life. Before the invention of the heart-lung machine this condition was uniformly fatal.

Treatment

Blalock invented his very ingenious operation to deal with this condition. He anastomosed the left subclavian artery to the left pulmonary artery, to improve pulmonary blood flow---the Blalock-Taussig shunt. This palliated many patients, and a modified BT shunt is still used to palliate patients who cannot be completely repaired. However, nowadays the Tetralogy of Fallot is corrected completely, early in life, using cardiopulmonary bypass.

Transposition of the great vessels

This is the commonest congenital cyanotic disease of the neonate. In this condition the aorta arises from the right ventricle, and the pulmonary artery from the left. The baby is severely cyanosed. In fact life is only possible if mixing occurs at some level, i.e. there is either an atrial or ventricular septal defect or a patent ductus arteriosus. If intervention is not carried out early, the disease carries a high mortality, with a 50% mortality in neonates and 90% dying in infancy.

Treatment

The ideal surgical management is the Jatene procedure, an arterial switch operation performed on a neonate. The aorta and pulmonary artery are detached from their roots and reattached to the opposite root, the pulmonary root becoming the new aortic root, and the aortic root becoming the new pulmonary root. The coronary arteries are transplanted from the aorta (new pulmonary artery) to the pulmonary artery (new aorta).

ACQUIRED HEART DISEASE

The common acquired heart lesions requiring surgical treatment include valvular heart disease (mitral and aortic valve disease), heart block and ischemic heart disease.

Mitral valve disease

Mitral stenosis commonly follows rheumatic carditis, most patients being in their third or fourth decades. Symptoms include:

- Tiredness and cold feet due to a low cardiac output.
- Dyspnoea and hemoptysis due to pulmonary hypertension.
- An enlarged liver, distended neck veins, ascites and edema due to right ventricular failure.

A clot dislodged from the left atrium may produce systemic embolism.

Radiology, echocardiography, cardiac catheterization and angiocardiography help in defining the extent of the disease.

Treatment

Operation is advised in any patient who is being inconvenienced by symptoms which cannot be controlled medically. If active rheumatism, a septic focus, atrial fibrillation or congestive failure are present these should be treated before operation is undertaken.

Percutaneous mitral commisurotomy (PTMC)

Closed mitral commisurotomy was one of the earliest and best cardiac operations. Good results were obtained in suitable cases. This operation has now been largely given up as in pliable and suitable valves percutaneous mitral commisurotomy is preferred.

Severely stenotic and calcified valves are not suitable for PTMC. In such cases, a valve replacement is the operation of choice. In suitable patients with mitral regurgitation, a mitral valve repair can be attempted which is supported by a prosthetic ring.

Valve repair in advanced rheumatic valves carries poor long-term results as compared to repairs for degenerative valve disease. Pre-operative preparation requires a period of bed rest, restriction of fluids and salt, diuretics and breathing exercises.

Aortic valve disease

At the aortic valve, stenosis or regurgitation may be present. Symptoms are due to insufficient blood reaching the systemic circulation and consist of syncope, angina and dyspnoea of effort. The murmur in stenosis is heard in systole only, in regurgitation it is both systolic and diastolic. The pulse pressure is low in stenosis, high in regurgitation. The condition is a serious one, and reduces life expectancy greatly.

Treatment

In adults, all defective valves require replacement. However:

- In neonates and children, a stenotic aortic valve can be treated by *percutaneous aortic balloon valvotomy*.
- In high risk elderly and frail patients, *transcatheter aortic valve implantation* is an attractive alternative to a standard aortic valve replacement.

Mechanical valves are in general use. The use of *tissue valves* is restricted to:

- Patients who cannot use anticoagulants.
- Patients above the age of 70, due to their higher incidence of failure in younger patients.

Tricuspid valve disease

Like the mitral and aortic valves, the tricuspid valve can also be affected by rheumatic fever. The most common lesion is regurgitation which presents with an elevated JVP, enlarged pulsatile liver, ascites and ankle edema. Tricuspid stenosis is relatively rare but occurs in advanced tricuspid valve disease. This valve when affected is repaired with good results.

Different types of valves

Prosthetic valves

These can be divided into two groups: tissue (bioprosthetic) and mechanical valves:

Tissue valves

These are mainly porcine valves mounted on a stent. They have excellent hemodynamics and are least thrombogenic i.e. they only require anticoagulation for 3 months and then this can be discontinued. The *disadvantage* of tissue valves is that in young patients with rheumatic fever they have a limited life and early structural valve degeneration sets in within 5–7 years which will require a reoperation.

Mechanical valves

These valves have a longer life and excellent hemodynamics. Modern mechanical valves are bi-leaflet, made of a pyrolytic carbon disc, an orifice ring and a polyester fiber cuff (St. Jude). This valve along with other mechanical valves mainly used in the past (ball and cage and tilting single disc) require lifelong anticoagulation with warfarin sodium as they are thrombogenic. The level of anticoagulation is monitored by measuring the INR (international normalized ratio) which is kept at 2.5–3.5. There is a risk of having a thromboembolic event if the INR is below the desired level or a fatal bleed if it goes above the desired level.

Heart block

The most common cause of heart block is degeneration of the conduction tissue in old age, the other causes being congenital cardiac lesions and ischemic heart disease. The atrial impulse fails to stimulate the ventricles due to interference with conduction in the bundle of His. The ventricles beat independently, at the rate of 25 to 50 per minute. If the rate is very slow the low cardiac output may lead to heart failure. A sudden slowing of the rate may produce syncope.

Treatment

Sympathomimetic drugs can increase the rate, but the response becomes less with continued use. If the slow pulse rate needs correction, artificial pacemakers are used.

Artificial pacemakers

In a common version of artificial cardiac pacemaker, the device is inserted in the left shoulder area where an incision is made below the clavicle creating a small pocket into which the pacemaker is housed. The lead is fed into the heart through a large vein using a fluoroscope to monitor the progress of lead insertion.

When the pacemaker does not detect a heart beat within a normal beat-to-beat time period, it stimulates the ventricle with a low voltage pulse. This activity of sensing and stimulating is pursued on a beat by beat basis.

ISCHEMIC HEART DISEASE

Atherosclerosis of the coronary arteries is a very common cause of death in adult males. The atheroma produces narrowing of the arteries, which if severe enough produces pain, i.e. angina. If the occlusion is total, necrosis of the myocardium (infarction) takes place. There are two main branches, the left and the right, and six to eight sub-branches, which can become occluded and need to be bypassed.

The atheromatous plaques usually obstruct the first few centimetres of the coronary artery. This segment can be bypassed by:

- A pedicled arterial conduit (internal thoracic artery).
- A vein graft between the aorta and the distal part of the coronary artery. However, before this can be done the exact location of the plaque must be determined by coronary angiography.

Patients with symptomatic ischemic heart disease will require some form of intervention. This could be in the form of:

- Coronary angioplasty and stenting, or.
- Coronary Artery Bypass Grafting (CABG).

Treatment

Coronary angioplasty

This can be done at the time of coronary angiography in one sitting. Arteries with lesions suitable for angioplasty are dilated with balloon catheters which are passed from the femoral arteries, up the aorta, and into the coronary arteries. The balloon is positioned across an area of stenosis in the artery and distended to dilate the stenotic segment. Short stenoses can be dealt with by this technique. Once dilated, a stent is placed to ensure the longevity of this dilatation.

A variety of stents are available, which include:

- Bare metal stents.
- Drug eluting stents; these continue to discharge the appropriate drug.

The technique is called percutaneous transluminal angioplasty.

Caution

Occasionally, serious complications can arise, so the procedure should be employed only if cardiac surgical help is immediately available. In about 4% of cases the procedure fails in its objective, and emergency coronary artery bypass is required, which generally proves effective

Coronary artery bypass grafting (CABG)

In certain conditions like left main-stem stenosis or left anterior desending artery (LAD) stenosis, angioplasty is not recommended, so the treatment of choice is CABG. These days CABG carries a mortality of 1–3 %, with good long-term results and freedom from re-intervention. A coronary artery bypass graft can be performed either by using the cardiopulmonary bypass and arrested heart, or on a beating heart without cardiopulmonary bypass.

The conduits available for CABG are arterial (internal mammary arteries, radial artery and gastroepiploeic artery) and venous (the long saphenous vein).

Arterial conduits give the best long-term results. Thus, left internal mammary artery (LIMA) to LAD anastomosis has a >90% 8 years' patency. Venous conduits have a 70 % 5–7 year patency.

'Beating heart surgery'

In this method a median sternotomy is performed and the patient heparinized. The left internal thoracic artery (LITA) and long saphenous vein are harvested. The target vessel is then stabilized using a heart stabilizer Octopus (Medtronic). LITA is anastomosed to the LAD, and saphenous vein to the other target vessels. The heparin is reversed and the wound closed after achieving hemostasis. This method is gaining popularity as the patient is saved from the deleterious effects of the cardiopulmonary bypass.

DISEASES OF THE PERICARDIUM

Cardiac tamponade

If fluid accumulates in the pericardial sac it compresses the heart and prevents diastolic filling. This causes a rise in the venous pressure and a fall in the cardiac output. If this happens rapidly, e.g. after an injury or after cardiac surgery it may produce shock, and if untreated may prove fatal. The area of cardiac dullness is enlarged and the heart sounds are weak. The jugular venous pressure is raised and there may be a paradoxical pulse, i.e. the pulse is weaker on inspiration. An echocardiogram is the most effective and accurate investigation in pericardial disease. Aspiration of the fluid should be immediately carried out.

Aspiration of the pericardium. A short-bevelled needle should be used. It is introduced along the left side of the xiphisternum upwards and backwards, with the needle at an angle of 45^0 to the skin. This site avoids the pleura. It is less likely to damage the coronary vessels, and is more likely to encounter fluid which gravitates between the heart and the diaphragm.

Constrictive pericarditis

In this condition the pericardium is greatly thickened, fibrosed and calcified, and this inelastic casing prevents diastolic filling and systolic emptying. Historically, the condition was attributed to tuberculosis, but infection, trauma and idiopathic causes are now more common. Venous congestion is shown by the engorged neck veins, enlarged liver, ascites and edema of the ankles.

The blood pressure is low and the pulse volume small. X-ray screening shows decreased cardiac pulsation and pericardial calcification. The diagnosis can be confirmed by echocardiography. The only effective treatment is surgical removal of the constricting pericardium. This allows the heart to fill and empty normally.

CARDIOVASCULAR MONITORING AND POSTOPERATIVE CARE

Cardiovascular monitoring

The aims of perioperative cardiovascular monitoring are to detect potentially dangerous hemodynamic changes, to direct treatment, and to assess its effects. Routine monitoring during and after cardiac surgery includes:

- *Clinical* monitoring.
- *Continuous* electronic monitoring: electrocardiogram, arterial pressure, central venous pressure, and pulse oximetry.
- *Intermittent* measurements of urine output, blood gases, and the core-peripheral temperature gradient also provide useful information about the cardiovascular system.

It is essential to maintain normal levels of blood gases, by ventilation if necessary.

Warm hands and feet

Cardiac output can be roughly estimated by finding out whether perfusion of the skin and the kidneys is satisfactory, i.e. by recording the skin temperature and the urinary output. *In all branches of surgery, warm hands and feet and a good volume of urine are simple but important signs that the patient is progressing satisfactorily.*

Postoperative cardiac intensive care

This aims at the maintenance and optimization of tissue perfusion and oxygenation and, if necessary, prompt treatment of complications.

High dependency area

Patients are nursed in a high dependency area with the same monitoring facilities as in the operation theatre and with access to blood gas and electrolyte analysis. The area should be close to the operation theatre and there should be adequate space for equipment and for the performance of emergency surgical procedures. A *one-to-one nurse to patient ratio* is essential until the patient is hemodynamically stable and extubated.

Heart transplantation

This is discussed in chapter 15 on transplantation.

Section

5

VASCULAR SYSTEM

Chapter

41 ARTERIES

Disease of the arteries may take one of three forms: occlusion, dilatation and arteritis:

- The lumen of the artery may be *occluded* by atheroma, thrombosis, embolism etc.
- The artery may be *dilated* due to degeneration of its wall, leading to an aneurysm.
- Finally, the wall of the artery may be the seat of *inflammation*.

ARTERIAL OCCLUSION

Arterial occlusion may be partial (i.e. stenosis), or complete. Both types of occlusion are caused most often by atherosclerosis, the other common causes being embolism and trauma. The severity of the symptoms produced by occlusion depends upon whether alternative routes of blood flow, in the form of collaterals, are available.

Clinical features of arterial occlusion in the limbs

A limb with an occluded artery is usually painful, pale, paralysed and pulseless.

Pain

This may take one of two forms, intermittent claudication and rest pain.

- *Intermittent claudication*. When the patient starts to walk there is no pain. After he has walked a few steps cramping pain appears, most often in the calf but sometimes in the thigh or buttock. If he now stands still the pain is relieved. The distance a patient can walk before pain comes on is called the *claudication distance*. As a rough guide, this distance is inversely proportional to the severity of arterial occlusion, i.e. if the distance is short it means the degree of occlusion is severe.
- Rest pain is severe pain felt in the foot even at rest. It is usually worse at night, and is aggravated by elevating the foot.

Pallor

Ischemic limbs look pale, specially on elevation. When the limb is lowered from the bed it becomes blue; this is due to venous congestion, and indicates sluggishness of any remaining circulation. Bright red spots may also be seen; these are due to extravasation of blood from the capillaries.

Paralysis

Ischemic limbs are often paralysed and without sensation. These are both bad signs, and indicate a poor prognosis.

Pulselessness

If a main artery is occluded, the arterial pulsations below that level are absent. If good collaterals are present the pulses may be palpable, but are greatly diminished in volume. If a patient has symptoms of arterial disease the following arteries must be palpated for the presence of pulsation:

- Radials.
- Carotids.
- Abdominal aorta.
- Femorals.
- Popliteals.
- Posterior tibials.
- Dorsalis pedis.

Temperature

Severely ischemic feet are cold to the touch.

Ulcers and gangrene

In severe arterial insufficiency ulcers may form on or between the toes, or elsewhere on the feet. When gangrene sets in, the affected patch of skin becomes black and dry. If rest pain, cyanosis, edema and hyperaesthesia are present with or without ulcers, the situation is described as pregangrene.

Murmurs

If an artery is narrowed, blood flowing through it produces turbulence, which results in a systolic murmur being audible over the vessel. A complete vascular examination should include auscultation of the following arteries:

- Subclavians.
- Carotids.
- Abdominal aorta.
- Femorals.

A continuous machinery murmur over an artery indicates the presence of an arteriovenous fistula.

Atheromatous plaques

Atheromatous narrowing or occlusion are commonly found at the following sites:

- Aortic bifurcation.
- Iliac arteries.
- Femoro-popliteal segment.
- Distal arteries.

Double blocks result in more severe ischemia.

INVESTIGATIONS FOR ARTERIAL OCCLUSION

Numerous tests need to be carried out on patients suffering from arterial diseases. Most patients suffering from pathological processes affecting the arteries tend to be elderly; therefore, metabolic and age-related diseases, e.g. diabetes, hypertension, myocardial ischemia and bronchitis should be excluded.

Blood tests

Tests to detect abnormalities in the blood, e.g. hyperlipidemia, polycythemia, and thrombocythemia, should be carried out, besides the C-reactive protein and white cell count.

Plain x-rays

These show up calcification in arteries.

Blood flow

Three basic parameters are analyzed in the study of peripheral vascular disease: pressure, volume and velocity of the blood flow.

Pressure

Normally, large arteries produce little resistance to blood flow, so that there is almost no pressure gradient between the aorta and the small arteries of the foot. Narrowing due to atheromatous plaques produces increased resistance and a pressure drop across the stenosis. This pressure drop develops even before total flow to the limb is reduced and therefore provides a very sensitive index for assessing the presence of significant arterial disease.

Ankle: brachial index

A blood pressure cuff is applied to the calf above the ankle. As a stethoscope cannot hear the sounds, a Doppler sensor is used. The normal ankle systolic pressure is about 10mm Hg higher than the brachial systolic pressure. Thus the ankle : brachial index is normally greater than 1.0, and a value below 0.9 indicates the presence of hemodynamically significant arterial narrowing. A value below 0.5 suggests rest pain and below 0.3 indicates imminent necrosis.

Foot ulcers may be due to:

- Ischemia.
- Neuropathy.

If an ischemic etiology is confirmed by non-invasive tests, the probability of successful healing of the lesion can also be predicted. An ulcer in a patient with an ankle pressure of 30 to 40mm Hg is not likely to heal unless a vascular bypass can improve the perfusion pressure in the foot. Toe pressure measurements are even more accurate in predicting the probability of successful ulcer healing.

Volume

An air-filled plethysmograph is used to measure the changes in volume of the limb during a cardiac cycle.

Velocity

Doppler studies

Continuous wave Doppler studies provide direct information about the arterial disease. An ultrasound signal is beamed at an artery. The reflected beam is picked up by a receiver. Its frequency is changed due to its passage through moving blood. The change of frequency is converted into sound, and the loudness of this sound over the concerned artery indicates the volume of blood flowing through it. The *Doppler blood flow detector* is a very useful instrument. To provide an objective record the signal can be converted into a waveform which is recorded on a strip chart.

Distal bypass grafts may fail for a variety of reasons. Postoperative surveillance allows the failing graft to be identified before occlusion occurs.

Duplex scanning

This provides both:

- *B-mode imaging* which defines anatomical complications of the graft, and.

- *Doppler velocity* measurements which identify a low-flow state before thrombosis actually occurs.

A low-flow state exists when the peak systolic flow velocity is less than 45cm/second. An abnormal B-mode scan or velocity measurement should be followed up with an arteriogram to assess the graft for possible revision.

Transcutaneous oxygen tension measurement

This provides a measure of the adequacy of the arterial oxygen supply to the tissues. An oxygen-sensing electrode is placed on the skin. The oxygen tension is measured at the foot, the calf and the thigh, with a reference electrode placed over the chest.

The normal value in the lower limb is around 55mm Hg. Comparing the value at the lower limb with that at the chest yields an index, which should normally be 0.9. Severe peripheral vascular disease produces significant changes in the oxygen tension measured at the foot.

The study is therefore valuable in assessing a patient's risk of limb or tissue loss, and in differentiating ischemic rest pain from neuropathic pain. Values of less than 20mm Hg are usually obtained in patients with rest pain and ischemic ulcers. If ischemic pain is confirmed, the patient is at a high risk for ishaemic loss of tissue or limb, and should be evaluated for a vascular bypass procedure.

Ultrasound (B-mode)

These images provide information about the diameters of the various vessels at different levels, and are very valuable adjuncts of velocity measurements, as explained above.

Angiography

In this technique a radiopaque dye is injected into an artery and x-rays taken. These show the dye in the vessel and show up any stenosis, occlusion or dilatation. In most cases the dye is placed into some part of the aorta, from where it flows into the different arteries and is photographed. The catheter is introduced usually via the *femoral* artery.

Indications

- To show up arterial disease.
- To show up characteristic arrangements of the feeding vessels of different malignant tumors for diagnosis of such lesions.

Complications

These include:

- Thrombosis,
- Hematoma.
- False aneurysm formation.
- Arterial dissection.
- Allergic reaction.

Because of these hazards, this test is now reserved for cases where surgery is contemplated.

Digital subtraction angiography

This investigative method has been developed to avoid the hazards of arterial catheters, and is now the standard technique. First a plain x-ray of the part to be examined is taken. A radiopaque dye is now injected intravenously and further radiographs taken. Using digital techniques employing a computer, the x-ray densities of the first film (due to the non-vascular shadows) are subtracted from the image containing the contrast medium. This greatly enhances the outline of the artery. Reasonably good views of the arteries can be obtained using this method, although the image is inferior to that obtained by conventional arteriography. Improvements of these images are in fact making invasive angiography obsolete with further advances in imaging techniques.

MANAGEMENT OF CHRONIC ARTERIAL OCCLUSION

Most patients suffering from intermittent claudication derive benefit from general advice and medical treatment, others require surgical measures.

General advice

- If the patient suffers from diabetes or hypertension these conditions should be kept under control meticulously.
- Smoking must be given up completely, specially in Buerger's disease, as it makes the patient's condition much worse.
- Exercise should be taken regularly within the limits of pain; this helps in the development of the collateral circulation.

Diet

There are two types of lipoproteins in the serum, those containing cholesterol and those rich in triglycerides. The serum should be tested. If the former type are increased, a low cholesterol diet is prescribed; if the latter, weight reduction should be stressed.

Medical treatment

Half a tablet of aspirin is prescribed daily, as it has an anti-adhesive effect on the platelets. Rest pain will require relief by analgesics such as paracetamol or diclofenac. Oral vasodilators may be tried, but are of doubtful value.

Care of the feet

Soft and comfortable socks should be worn. The toe-nails should be trimmed very carefully, avoiding damage to the adjacent skin, specially in diabetic patients, because the sites of such trauma may act as starting points for the development of gangrene.

Buerger's exercises

If the head of the bed is elevated (Buerger's position), the circulation to the feet is increased. The same is the effect of Buerger's exercises (raise the limb for 2 minutes, lower it for 2 minutes, repeat the cycle about a dozen times). This routine should be carried out daily for a few weeks.

Lumbar sympathectomy

Both surgical and chemical sympathectomy are now outdated and obsolete.

ARTERIAL OCCLUSION IN THE LOWER LIMBS

In atherosclerosis affecting the arteries of the lower limb, surgery has a definite role to play.

Indications for operation

- *Rest pain* is an absolute indication for surgery, provided the distal vessels are patent and the patient fit for operation.
- *Claudication* is a relative indication for operation. If the patient can modify his activity so that claudication is prevented, operation may be avoided.
- If *ischemic ulcers* do not respond to treatment, reconstructive surgery may be advised to prevent limb amputation.
- In arterial occlusion due to an *embolus* urgent embolectomy is indicated to save the limb.

OPERATIONS FOR DISEASE AT DIFFERENT SITES

Aorto-iliac artery stenosis

This condition can be treated by one of the following operations:

- An *aortofemoral bypass* is the method of choice. A synthetic arterial graft is anastomosed above to the aorta and below to the femoral artery, bypassing the stenosed segment.
- An *iliac endarterectomy* can also be used, but the long-term results are not so good. In this operation the artery is opened, the atheromatous plaques removed, and the wound in the artery sutured, using a vein patch over the wound to prevent stenosis.
- If the patient is not fit for major surgery *transluminal balloon angioplasty* may be employed. Under local anesthesia a guide wire is negotiated through the stenosis. A balloon catheter is now introduced into the femoral artery and passed up to lie across the stenosis. It is inflated with contrast medium to a pressure of 5 to 10 atmospheres, which is maintained for about 15 seconds. Inflation of the balloon produces fissures in the atheromatous plaques, thus dilating the stenosed part. An endothelial lining gradually develops over these fissures, so that the lumen of the artery is enlarged. Re-stenosis is more common after balloon angioplasty than after reconstructive surgery, but the angioplasty can be repeated if necessary. This procedure is very successful in the ilac and femoropopliteal segments.

Femoral and profunda artery stenosis

This condition responds well to operation provided the vessels above and below the block are normal. A femoro-popliteal bypass graft is commonly used. The patient's own long saphenous vein gives the best results; in order to be used successfully, its direction has to be reversed after removal, so that its valves do not obstruct the downward flow of blood.

Profundoplasty

If, along with atherosclerosis in the femoral artery, there is also stenosis at the origin of the profunda femoris, which is otherwise normal, profundoplasty is a useful operation to carry out. The incision in the femoral artery is extended along the profunda until normal artery is found. Atheroma is now removed and the opening closed, with a vein patch to prevent narrowing of the vessel.

Arteries below the popliteal

In these vessels direct arterial procedures are unrewarding. The lumen of these vessels is small. Therefore the flow of blood here is poor, and this results in a high rate of graft failure.

Results of operation

When reconstructive surgery is carried out for aorto-iliac disease the results are excellent. However, if femoro-popliteal occlusion develops at a later stage, the outcome may be compromised. Surgery for femoro-popliteal disease is less useful, the success rate at the end of 5 years being only about 50%.

ACUTE ARTERIAL OCCLUSION

Acute occlusion of the arterial supply to a limb represents an emergency. If an extensive collateral circulation is not present, irreversible ischemic changes begin about 6 hours after the event. Sudden occlusion of an artery may result either from trauma or embolism.

Occlusion due to trauma

Blunt trauma to an artery may affect it in one of the following ways:

- Bruising due to blunt trauma may cause roughening of the intima so that *thrombosis* occurs, resulting in occlusion.
- The intima may become detached from the underlying muscle, and the resulting *sub-intimal hematoma* may occlude the artery.
- During a long march the muscles in the unyielding *anterior fascial compartment* of the leg may be so swollen as to compress the anterior tibial artery and cause both distal ischemia and the crush syndrome. The treatment is urgent fasciotomy to release the compression of the artery.

Management

When a limb has been injured its examination must always include palpation of the pulses. If the pulses are absent and the limb is pale and cold, arterial occlusion should be strongly suspected. In such a situation the artery must be immediately exposed:

- If the artery is found to be lacerated the affected part may be resected and an end-to-end anastomosis carried out, or a vein graft employed.
- If the artery is bruised it may be in spasm. In that case 4% lignocaine solution should be applied locally to overcome the spasm.
- If the pulse still does not return, the artery should be opened and the thrombosis or subintimal hematoma dealt with, usually by resection of the involved segment of the artery.

Embolic occlusion

An embolus is a body that is foreign to the bloodstream and which may get lodged in a vessel and cause obstruction. Emboli may consist of blood clot, air or fat. The most common emboli are made of blood clot. The most frequent site of origin of the blood clot is the roughened intima over necrosed cardiac muscle, in a case of myocardial infarction. Other sites include places where the blood flow is relatively sluggish. Examples include the left atrium in the case of mitral stenosis, and the cavity of a large aneurysm.

Sites of lodgement of emboli

Emboli can get lodged in any part of the body, producing ischemia of the part. Emboli may be arterial or venous.

Arterial emboli

- The most common sites of lodgement of arterial emboli are the *lower limbs*, due to the straightness of the arteries leading to them. There is pain, pallor, pulselessness and paresis.
- *Cerebral* embolism commonly leads to hemiplegia, and embolism into the *retinal* artery leads to blindness.
- In *mesenteric* arterial embolism gangrene of the small intestine may follow.

Clinical features

In its clinical presentation, embolic occlusion differs from the thrombotic occlusion which complicates atherosclerosis. In thrombosis there is a preceding history of claudication, which is lacking in embolism. On the other hand in embolic occlusion a source of the emboli can be found, and paralysis occurs within 4 to six hours of the onset of pain; both these features are missing in thrombosis.

In a patient who has not had pain in the limb previously, severe pain suddenly develops and the limb becomes cold with mottled blue and white patches. Movement of the toes and touch sensation are lost. The distal pulses are absent, but the femoral pulse may be more forceful, due to the embolic occlusion immediately distal to it.

Clinical findings suggestive of an embolic cause include cardiac arrhythmia, myocardial ischemia and valvular disease, and the absence of features predisposing to atherosclerosis. The presence of normal pulses on the contralateral side is strongly indicative of an embolic source.

Treatment

If a case of embolism is left untreated, stasis of blood occurs both proximal and distal to the embolus, and this results in thrombosis which spreads in both directions. This extension can be prevented by immediately starting an infusion of 5,000 to 10,000 units of *heparin* until the embolus can be removed by operation. At the same time, the severe ischemic pain requires relief by *analgesics*.

Embolectomy

The treatment of choice in a patient with embolism in a limb artery is urgent *embolectomy* within a few hours. This may be carried out under local or general anesthesia, depending on the location of the clot.

The artery is exposed and held up with tapes. As soon as a longitudinal incision is made into the artery, the thrombus begins to extrude and is removed, together with the embolus. As bleeding occurs arterial clamps are applied. A Fogarty catheter is now passed, in turn upwards and downwards, until it reaches beyond the clot. It is a fine catheter with a balloon at the tip. The balloon is inflated and the catheter withdrawn slowly, bringing out the clot. The process is repeated a few times until brisk bleeding commences, indicating that all clot has been evacuated. The arteriotomy is now closed.

Postoperatively anticoagulant therapy is continued. Prevention of further emboli requires treatment of the cause. If that is not possible, long-term anticoagulant therapy with warfarin is started.

Therapeutic embolization

Different materials may be injected into visceral arteries belonging to the following tracts, to occlude their lumen:

- Gastrointestinal.
- Respirarory.
- Urinary.
- Gynaecological.

This may be done for the following purposes:

- To arrest hemorrhage.
- To treat arteriovenous malformations.
- To suppress the growth of advanced tumors.

Commonly gelfoam and metal coils are used.

GANGRENE

Definitions

- *Gangrene* is defined as death with putrefaction of macroscopic portions of tissue.
- *Necrosis* indicates the death of individual cells or groups of cells.
- A *sequestrum* is a dead piece of bone.
- A *slough* is a piece of dead soft tissue e.g. fascia, tendon or skin.

The classic presentation of gangrene is seen when the condition affects the distal part of a limb. However, certain viscera may also be affected by gangrene, notably the appendix, the small intestine, and occasionally the gallbladder.

Causes

Gangrene may result from one of many pathological processes:

- *Ischemia*. This may be secondary to one of the following conditions:
    - o Atherosclerosis, with thrombosis on an atheromatous plaque.
    - o Embolism, the clot having come from the left atrium in atrial fibrillation, or the left ventricle in coronary thrombosis.
    - o Diabetes, the contributing pathological processes being arteritis and neuropathy.
    - o Thromboangiitis obliterans (Buerger's disease).
    - o Raynaud's disease and ergotism, due to repeated arterial spasm.
    - o Inadvertent intra-arterial injection of drugs, specially thiopentone and cytotoxic drugs.
- *Infections*. The common example consists of gas gangrene.
- *Trauma*.
    - o Direct trauma: examples include pressure sores and the constriction groove of strangulated intestine.
    - o Indirect trauma e.g. gangrene of the hand due to compression of the brachial artery by the lower end of a fractured humeral shaft in a supracondylar fracture.
- *Physical agents*. Examples include burns due to heat, boiling liquids, chemicals, electricity and irradiation.

Clinical appearance

The gangrenous part is cold and motionless. Arterial pulsation, capillary response to pressure and sensation are all absent. The colour changes due to ischemia take place as follows:

- At first there is pallor.
- Later, there may be dusky grey or purple discoloration due to the pooling of blood in the part.
- Finally, the colour changes to a greenish or brownish black, due to the disintegration of hemoglobin and formation of iron sulphide.

Types of gangrene

Gangrene may be either dry or moist, depending on whether the occlusion of the circulation occurs gradually or suddenly.

Dry gangrene

In atherosclerosis the reduction of blood supply takes place slowly over a period of weeks or months due to gradually increasing narrowing of the arterial lumen by atheromatous plaques. If this happens in an exposed part, e.g. a limb, the parts dry up before the stage of necrosis supervenes. The dryness discourages the growth of bacteria, so that putrefaction does not occur, and there is no foul smell. The part is dry, wrinkled, and black due to the iron sulfide produced by the breakdown of hemoglobin.

Dry gangrene of the skin can also result after extravasation into the subcutaneous fat of a drug meant for intramuscular injection. (Fig.41.1).

Moist gangrene

This results if, at the time when ischemia occurs, the part is moist. In such cases putrefaction of the tissue proteins takes place and anaerobic infection sets in, producing a foul smell. Examples of this are seen in the following conditions:

- When an artery is suddenly occluded, as by a ligature or due to an embolus.
- When venous obstruction is present along with arterial occlusion.
- In diabetes, because of the increased likelihood of infection in diabetic tissues.
- Whenever gangrene occurs in an internal organ, e.g. in acute appendicitis and strangulated bowel, because the viscera are always moist.

When seen in a limb, the affected part becomes swollen and discoloured, and the epidermis is raised in blebs. If infection is by gas-producing organisms, crepitus may be felt on palpation.

If gangrene remains untreated it may get circumscribed or spread in extent. The outcome depends upon the adequacy of the circulation in the areas adjacent to the gangrenous part.

Line of demarcation

At the distal limit of the living part a layer of granulation tissue develops, which is marked on the surface by a band of hyperemia. The granulations extend into the dead tissue until those which have penetrated farthest are unable to obtain enough nourishment. At this level the skin and deeper tissues break down, so that an ulcer forms all round the limb. This is the line of demarcation between the gangrenous and healthy tissue.

In *dry* gangrene if the blood supply to the living tissues is adequate the line of demarcation develops within a few days (Fig.41.2), and separation of the gangrenous part takes place with the minimum of infection. When bone is also involved, separation takes longer than when soft tissues alone are affected.

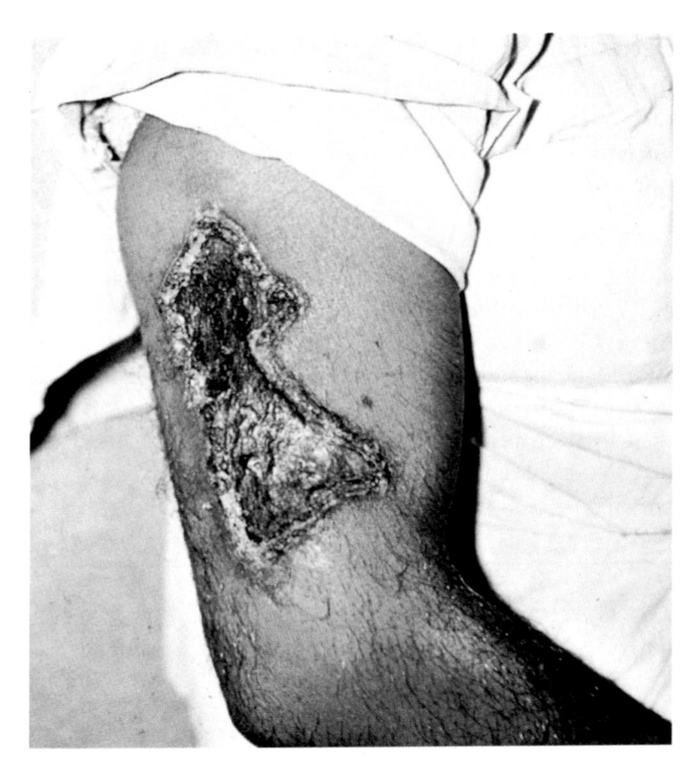

Fig.41.1 Dry gangrene skin of the arm from a subcutaneous injection of a drug meant for intramuscular use

In *moist* gangrene the conditions are more favourable for the growth of bacteria. Therefore, more infection and suppuration takes place, and the line of demarcation develops at a higher level than in dry gangrene, so that more of the limb is lost. Therefore every effort should be made to convert moist gangrene into the dry type.

Spread of gangrene

The moist type of gangrene may spread upwards, either as a whole or in the form of black patches of skin at a higher level than the gangrenous part. Infection may also spread upwards. If a clear line of demarcation does not form, a local amputation runs the risk of leaving gangrenous tissues behind. To avoid this possibility, in the case of the lower limb an above-knee amputation may have to be carried out.

Treatment

As far as possible one should try to save the limb in cases of gangrene. In arterial disease if the blood supply above the gangrenous area is good, or if a poor blood supply can be improved, a conservative excision may be successful and an amputation avoided. Methods of improving the blood supply include direct arterial surgery. If the limb is badly crushed, or the patient is suffering from gas gangrene or rapidly spreading gangrene, amputation has to be carried out to save his life.

General treatment

In embolic gangrene the patient may need treatment for cardiac failure, atrial fibrillation and anemia. Diabetes, if present, must be controlled. Pain should be relieved by non-narcotic drugs.

Local treatment

The limb should be kept exposed to encourage dryness, and cool to reduce the metabolic rate and the need of the tissues for oxygen. The pressure areas, e.g. the heel, should be protected by foam pads etc., to prevent the development of fresh patches of gangrene. Where an area of skin becomes hardened, it may need to be lifted, in order to release underlying pus.

SPECIAL VARIETIES OF GANGRENE

Diabetic gangrene

Three factors contribute to the development of diabetic gangrene:

- The peripheral neuritis of diabetes results in trophic changes.
- Atheroma of the arteries results in ischemia.
- An excess of sugar in the tissues lowers their resistance to infection.

The *neuropathy* produces a harmful effect in two ways:

- Impaired sensation results in neglect of minor injuries so that damage to the tissues becomes more widespread.
- At the same time the muscular involvement leads to deformities in the foot, so that the pressure on the metatarsal heads increases. This leads to the development of callosities, which act as sites of entry for infection. Infections affect the relatively avascular structures like tendons and fasciae to a greater extent than structures which are more richly supplied with blood, such as muscles. Through the tissue planes the infection can rapidly spread upwards.

In *diabetic gangrene* major arterial disease is usually absent, so that the dorsalis pedis and posterior tibial pulses are palpable, and intermittent claudication and rest pain are absent. Any pus is examined, and the blood and urine are tested to detect the presence and severity of diabetes.

Treatment

The diabetic state should be brought under control by diet and drugs. Gangrene is managed along the usual lines. If no major arterial obstruction is present, the effort should be to save as much of the limb as possible. If infection spreads upwards rapidly, free drainage of the area with removal of sloughs must be carried out. If this is done, rapid healing often follows.

Traumatic gangrene

This may be due to direct or indirect trauma.

Direct traumatic gangrene

The most common example of this type of gangrene is a bedsore, besides the ulcers resulting from the pressure of splints or plasters.

Bedsores

These most commonly develop in a patient who is bedridden, specially if he has suffered injury or disease of the spinal cord. Thus the most important factors in the development of bedsores are:

- *Pressure.*
- *Loss of the trophic influence* of nerves.
- *Moisture.* This increases the rate of extension of a bedsore.
- *Anemia* and malnutrition. If the patient is also anemic or malnourished, not only is the tendency to develop bedsores increased, but any sores that form tend to spread more rapidly.

Common sites

The most common sites for the development of bedsores are over the:

- Sacrum.
- Greater trochanter.
- Heels.

Prevention

While looking after bedridden patients, the prevention of bedsores requires extremely vigilant nursing:

- An air mattress, with alternating cells inflated and emptied by an electric pump, is employed. In this way constant pressure on any area of the skin is prevented. Such a mattress helps considerably in preventing bedsores.
- The bedsheets must be kept free of all wrinkles.
- Sweat, urine or feces must not be allowed to collect over the skin, as these cause maceration of the skin which helps a bedsore spread.
- The posture must be changed two-hourly.

If bedsores actually form treatment is difficult, hence the very great importance of prevention.

Treatment

All the measures mentioned above under prevention must be continued. As far as the management of the bedsores is concerned:

- If there is pent up pus, it should be evacuated.
- Small quantities of slough can be treated by Eusol solution; large sloughs require surgical removal.
- Edematous granulations can be made more firm and pink by magnesium sulphate glycerine paste, which withdraws water by its hygroscopic effect.
- In an otherwise healthy patient excision of dead tissues can be followed up by shifting a skin flap to cover the raw area.

Indirect traumatic gangrene

This occurs due to occlusion of an artery from one of the following causes:

- *Pressure*, e.g. from a broken bone in a fracture.
- *Thrombosis*, e.g. following injury.
- *Ligation* of a main artery.

If the collateral circulation is adequate, gangrene might still not occur after the above incidents.

Treatment

The cause of the arterial occlusion should be dealt with. If the gangrene is dry, a line of demarcation indicates the level above which the tissues are viable, and amputation is carried out above that level. On the other hand moist gangrene spreads rapidly, and amputation is required to save the patient's life.

Frostbite

This occurs due to exposure to cold. The vessel wall is damaged with edema, blistering, and finally gangrene. The part should be warmed gradually to body temperature, being wrapped in cotton wool. Warm drinks, analgesics and if necessary paravertebral injection of the sympathetic chain may be employed.

Thiopentone

Thiopentone, meant for administration into the basilic vein in the antecubital fossa, may by mistake be injected into the brachial artery. The aspiration of bright red blood, and a cry of agony from the patient during the injection, will indicate to the clinician that a faulty injection has been made.

The needle should not be removed, and 5ml of 1% *lignocaine* should be injected in order to abolish the vascular spasm, followed by dilute *heparin* solution. *Low molecular weight dextran* should be given intravenously, to make the blood less viscous. If no improvement occurs, the artery should be exposed and any clots flushed out.

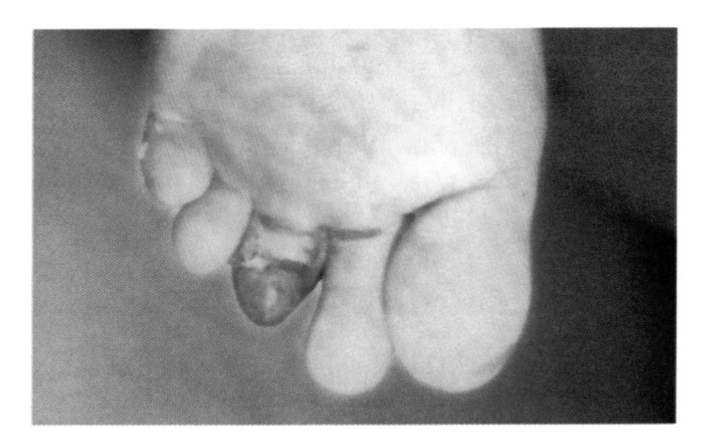

Fig.41.2 Dry gangrene distal half of middle toe. A clear line of demarcation is visible.

AMPUTATIONS

Indications

An amputation is indicated when a limb or a part of it is:

- ***Dead*** i.e. gangrene is present. This may be due to occlusion of:
  - Major vessels, e.g. from atherosclerosis or embolism.
  - Peripheral vessels, e.g. in diabetes, Buerger's disease, Raynaud's disease, intra-arterial thiopentone injection, etc.
- ***Dangerous.*** This is the situation in:
  - Both moist gangrene and gas gangrene. The danger to life arises from the absorption of the potent toxins of the clostridia or other anaerobic bacteria. Amputation is required as a life-saving measure.
  - The part may also be a danger to life if it is the seat of:
    - A malignant tumor e.g. an osteosarcoma.
    - An arteriovenous fistula which cannot be dealt with surgically and which has resulted in heart failure.
- ***A total loss.*** Some examples of this include the following:
  - When a limb is the seat of multiple severe lacerations and fractures, perhaps with partial amputation, due to a bomb-blast injury or a road accident.

- o If severe contractures or paralysis, usually after polio, make the limb impossible to use, and interfere rather than help with locomotion.
- o If, in a patient with an ischemic foot, severe rest pain makes life miserable. In such a situation amputation improves the quality of life.

Consent

It should be remembered that before an amputation is carried out, *informed and written consent* of the patient must be obtained. This should be a routine before any operation, but specially before an amputation.

Amputations at different levels

Amputations may be classified into minor and major amputations

Minor (distal) amputations

These are commonly carried out:

- Either after *injury*, e.g. to a finger or toe, or in a patient with small vessel disease (diabetes or Buerger's disease), where gangrene of the toes occurs but the blood supply to the surrounding tissues is good. In such a case a local amputation can be followed by healing.
- In *diabetes*, infection plays a major part in the pathological process. Because of the infection the wound has to be left open. At the same time the infection tends to spread up the tendon sheaths. For these reasons the excision of a metatarsal bone ('ray' excision) is often recommended. This opens up the tissue planes, with better drainage of pus.
- *Trans-metatarsal amputation*. This can be utilized in Buerger's disease if more than one toe is affected by gangrene. This operation is carried out employing a long plantar flap, so that the suture line is on the dorsal side, away from the weight-bearing area.

Major amputations

Above-knee and below-knee amputations

The most common major amputations employed in the lower limb are the below-knee and the above knee amputations. The advantages of the one are the disadvantages of the other:

- In major vessel disease the *above-knee amputation* provides an absolute guarantee of sound healing of the stump due to the abundant blood supply available from the big muscles of the thigh. However, the function of the artificial limb is not as good as in a below-knee amputation.
- A *below-knee amputation* provides a lesser certainty of sound healing of the stump. However, should the stump heal the ultimate function of the limb is of a higher quality.

In the past, in cases of major vessel disease, twice as many above-knee amputations were performed as below-knee. However, during recent years this ratio has been reversed, partly because arterial surgery is now available to improve the blood supply to the limb.

Flaps containing muscles

If muscles, which have a rich blood supply, could be raised as a part of the flap which is to be used to cover the bony stump, the chances of healing of the wound would be increased. In this connection:

- In the case of the *above-knee* amputation because big muscles are present all round the stump, equal anterior and posterior flaps are commonly employed.
- In the *below-knee* amputation thick muscles are available only in the calf. Therefore a single long posterior flap is used.

Through-knee amputation

In through-knee amputation a long anterior flap is preferred. The patellar tendon is sutured to the hamstrings so that, acting from below, both the rectus femoris and the hamstrings help in stabilizing the hip joint in the erect posture.

Syme's amputation

In a Syme's amputation the lower ends of the tibia and fibula are sawn across just above the line of the ankle joint. The stump is covered by a posterior flap consisting of the skin of the heel with its underlying thick pad of fibrofatty tissue for weight-bearing.

Points of technique in anaputation

- The main artery and vein supplying the limb are individually ligated, to avoid the development of an arteriovenous fistula.
- The nerves are gently drawn down, cut with a sharp knife and allowed to retract upwards, so that the stump neuroma which inevitably forms should be away from pressure.
- The bone is cut with a saw and any splinters removed, to avoid the formation of spurs.
- Muscles are stitched together over the bone, by means of sutures which incorporate the deep fascia.
- Absolute hemostasis is ensured; however, suction drains are used, to prevent the collection of serum or blood.

Postoperative care of an amputation

Dressing

A gauze and cotton wool dressing, held in place by a very carefully applied firm bandage, is employed. The dressing may be left undisturbed till the time for removal of the stitches, unless excessive pain or fever indicate the development of infection.

Prosthesis

An amputation is a demoralizing operation. The modern tendency, therefore is to fit a prosthesis *immediately*. In this connection the recently introduced inflatable prostheses are extremely useful. With such a prosthesis a lower limb amputee can get on his feet the day after the operation. This goes a long way in reducing the severity of the acute depression which he is otherwise likely to experience.

Exercises

In the past, exercises of the stump were an important part of rehabilitation, and prepared the stump for the prosthesis. Nowadays, with the prosthesis immediately applied to the stump, mobilization automatically provides exercises for the stump muscles, preventing the development of disuse atrophy and contractures.

Complications

Some of the complications of an amputation, which must be guarded against, are the following:

- Reactionary hemorrhage.
- Hematoma formation.
- Infection.
- Sequestrum formation.
- Wound dehiscence.
- Gangrene of the flaps.
- At a later stage, an adherent scar.

Phantom limb

Sometimes a patient remarks that he can feel the amputated limb, and that it is painful (phantom limb). The surgeon should reassure the patient that these symptoms will spontaneously disappear in due course.

ANEURYSMS

An aneurysm is a sac formed by the dilatation of the wall of an artery, a vein, or the heart.

Types of aneurysms

An arterial aneurysm may be true or false.

True aneurysms

A true aneurysm contains all the three layers of the arterial wall in its sac, and is most all often due to atherosclerosis. It may be fusiform or saccular:

- A *fusiform aneurysm* is spindle-shaped, the stretching process affecting the entire circumference of the artery.
- In a *saccular* aneurysm only a part of the circumference of the arterial wall is stretched, so that an eccentric localized sac results.

False aneurysms

A false aneurysm usually arises after a lateral tear in the wall of an artery. The hematoma which collects by the side of the artery gradually develops a cavity which is surrounded by a wall of fibrous tissue and communicates with the lumen of the artery. In its external appearance it resembles a saccular aneurysm. However, unlike the latter its sac contains none of the layers of the arterial wall.

A *dissecting* aneurysm results from hemorrhage which causes longitudinal splitting of the arterial wall, producing a tear in the intima and establishing communication with the lumen. When it affects the thoracic aorta, the dissection may spread down into the abdomen and involve the ostia of the renal arteries. The resulting ischemia of the kidneys may cause anuria.

Symptoms

These may be produced by an aneurysm when it:

- *Expands*, compressing adjacent structures, e.g. the esophagus, producing dysphagia.
- *Ruptures*, producing severe hemorrhage.
- Gets *thrombosed*; for example if a popliteal aneurysm gets thrombosed, gangrene of the foot can result.
- *Releases emboli*; for example, emboli from an aortic aneurysm can produce ischemia of the toes.

Signs

Along the course of an artery is seen a swelling, which exhibits expansile pulsation. A thrill may be palpable, and a bruit heard on auscultation. Proximal pressure causes the pulsation to become less marked; when the pressure is released the force of the pulsation is restored.

Neighbouring structures may be affected by the pressure of the aneurysm:

- If veins are compressed distal edema may result.
- Compression of nerves may produce impaired sensation.

- Compression of the esophagus may cause dysphagia.
- Dyspnoea may result from pressure on the trachea.

Differential diagnosis

A large tumor lying over the abdominal aorta may pulsate like an aneurysm. However, firstly the pulsation can be shown to be transmitted rather than expansile; secondly, if the patient assumes the knee-elbow position the tumor falls away from the aorta and the pulsation ceases.

If an abscess in the axilla or groin is about to be incised, one should make sure that it does not pulsate, i.e. it is not an aneurysm, otherwise incision could be followed by torrential hemorrhage. Finally, a highly vascular tumor like an osteogenic sarcoma may pulsate and cause confusion.

Investigations

The swelling should be investigated by ultrasound examination, CT scan or MRI to confirm the diagnosis of aneurysm. Finally, arteriography should be carried out to define the runoff bed.

Abdominal aortic aneursysm

An aneurysm of the abdominal aorta may be an incidental finding or may be symptomatic, and its treatment differs accordingly:

- *Asymptomatic aneurysm*. If an abdominal aortic aneurysm is not producing symptoms, its recommended treatment depends upon its size. If its diameter is greater than 55mm on ultrasonography, its chances of rutpure are high, and it should be operated upon; if less than 55mm, it should be treated conservatively. However, in the latter case regular ultrasonographic assessment will be required.
- *Symptomatic aneurysm*. Most patients with abdominal aortic aneurysms which are producing symptoms will be dead within one year if left without surgery; most who are operated upon will live. Therefore operation should be carried out in these cases.

Procedure

Classically, abdominal aortic aneurysm has been treated by *open* surgical repair. However, repair using an *endovascular prosthesis* is now an established procedure and, compared to open repair, has a lower mortality during the 6 years following the operation.

Complications of repair

- Myoardial infarction and lower lobe atelectasis may occur.
- Because of clamping of the abdominal aorta above and below an aneurysm during its open repair, the blood supply to the kidney, colon or spinal cord may be jeopardized, resulting in renal failure, ischemic colitis, or paraplegia respectively.
- In endovascular repair the graft may migrate or become infected.

Arteriovenous fistula

An arteriovenous fistula:

- May be a congenital malformation.
- May result from a penetrating wound of an artery and its accompanying vein.
- May be created artificially in the forearm of a patient undergoing hemodialysis, so that the catheters in the artery and vein can be connected to the hemodialysis machine.

Effect on the vein

The high pressure arterial blood flowing into the vein makes it dilated, tortuous and thick-walled ('arterialized').

Effect on the circulation

In the presence of the fistula the arterial blood, instead of coursing through the capillary bed, follows the easier path and leaks directly into the vein in large quantities, greatly enhancing the venous return. This in turn increases both the cardiac output and the pulse rate. Left ventricular enlargement and cardiac failure follow if the fistula is a large one.

Effect of location of the AV fistula

- A congenital fistula in the *distal* part of a limb in a child results in overgrowth of the limb due to the increased circulation.
- Conversely, a fistula in the *proximal* part of a limb may lead to the formation of non-healing ulcers due to relative ischemia from short-circuiting of the blood through the fistula.

Clinical features

A *pulsatile* swelling is seen, over which a thrill can be palpated and a continuous (machinery) murmur auscultated. The *veins* around the area of the fistula are dilated, as they are helping to carry away the excessive amounts of blood. If *pressure* is applied to the artery proximal to the fistula the swelling diminishes in size, the thrill and the murmur disappear, and the pulse rate and pulse pressure fall to their normal levels (Nicoladoni's sign).

Imaging

Duplex scanning (grayscale ultrasound plus colour Doppler) and/or angiography confirms the presence of the lesion.

Treatment

- Some *congenital arteriovenous malformations* are so small that they require no treatment. Others may be so large and extensive that removal is hazardous. These cases can sometimes be successfully treated by embolization after selective catheterization.

  Embolization. A catheter with a bent tip is passed into the parent artery. The tip is introduced into the origin of the artery supplying the AV fistula. Plastic microspheres are injected into the artery; they occlude the lumen of the vessel and result in thrombosis of the vessels constituting the fistula.
- *Acquired AV fistulae* tend to be progressive, and therefore often require surgery. The vessels are separated. If possible they should be repaired by suture. If this is not feasible, the vein as well as the artery have to be ligated both above and below the lesion (quadruple ligation). Alternatively, vascular continuity may be restored by vein or Dacron grafting.

ARTERITIS AND VASOSPASTIC CONDITIONS

Thromboangiitis obliterans (Buerger's disease)

In this condition inflammatory changes occur in the walls of small and medium-sized arteries and veins, leading to thrombosis and occlusion of the affected vessels. The plantar, tibial, and sometimes the radial arteries are commonly affected, usually in a young male below the age of 30 years. *The patient is nearly always a smoker*; the condition does not occur in women or in non-smokers. The symptoms and signs are those which are commonly seen in occlusive arterial disease. On microscopy inflammatory changes are seen in the arterial walls leading to thrombosis. Dry gangrene usually affects the toes, occasionally the fingers.

Treatment

The patient *must stop smoking immediately and permanently*; a reduction in the number of cigarettes smoked is not enough to prevent the progression of the disease. Surgery on the affected arteries is not possible due to their small size. If an artery is occluded it may be dealt with as for atherosclerosis. However, the case often ends up in amputations of digits.

RAYNAUD'S SYNDROME

The term Raynaud's syndrome refers to a group of disorders in which:

- Intermittent vasopasm occurs in the arterioles of the hands or feet, usually following exposure to cold, so that the fingers become *blanched*.
- As the blood flow is greatly reduced, metabolites accumulate in the capillaries. Due to the effect of these metabolites the capillaries dilate and become filled with blood which is rapidly de-oxygenated, the part becoming *blue*.
- Finally the arterioles relax, oxygenated blood courses through the parts, and the hands become *red*, with a burning sensation.

Thus the condition is recognized by the change of colour from white, through blue, to red.

This symptom-comlex may be primary, when no other condition can be identified after appropriate investigation, or it may be secondary to a wide variety of underlying disorders:

Primary

Raynaud's disease.

Secondary

Collagen diseases, e.g. disseminated lupus erythematosus, rheumatoid arthritis.

Arteriosclerosis.

Thromboangiitis obliterans.

Cold injury (e.g. frostbite).

Use of vibrating hand tools.

Polycythaemia vera.

Ergot poisoning.

Primary Raynaud's syndrome (Raynaud's disease)

This occurs mostly in young women, and affects the upper limb more often than the lower. Many patients with mild to moderate cold sensitivity are not disturbed by their symptoms enough to seek medical advice. It should be remembered that *primary Raynaud's syndrome is almost always a bilateral condition*. If the symptoms are unilateral the cause is much more likely to be an embolus in a digital artery, either from a subclavian artery compressed by a cervical rib, or from an atheromatous plaque in a proximal artery.

Treatment

Only protection from cold can prevent attacks. Calcium antagonists provide some relief. In winter electrically heated gloves afford defense against the cold. Sympathectomy at best provides short-lived relief and is obsolete.

Secondary raynaud's syndrome

This results in a greater severity of digital ischemia than the primary form, and patients are more likely to seek medical advice.

Diagnosis

The diagnosis of Raynaud's syndrome depends upon the history of colour changes on exposure to cold. Pain in the digits is not a usual feature but may occur, particularly in the secondary variety where there is digital vessel occlusion and a significant amount of tissue damage, leading to ulceration and gangrene. Such ischemic damage is extremely rare in the primary form of Raynaud's syndrome where the attacks are related solely to vasospasm and there is no obstructive element.

Different *causes* of the secondary disorder must be looked for. History-taking should include enquiry into the use of vibrating tools and ingestion of drugs, specially ergotamine. A history of heavy smoking in a male may suggest thromboangiitis obliterans. During physical examination the clinician must look for painful, swollen joints to rule out rheumatoid arthritis and systemic lupus erythematosus; a subclavian bruit to exclude thoracic outlet obstruction; and absent peripheral pulses to eliminate atherosclerosis.

Investigations

These should include x-ray of the thoracic outlet to show the presence of a cervical rib, and x-rays of the hands to show the joint disruption characteristic of rheumatoid arthritis. Blood tests should include ESR, rheumatoid factor, antinuclear factor, anti-DNA antibody, electrophoresis, cryoglobulins, and cold agglutinin assays.

Treatment

General measures

No curative treatment is available for Raynaud's syndrome and the aim is palliation by reduction in the frequency and severity of the attacks. Reassurance that the condition is generally benign is important, specially in primary Raynaud's syndrome where progression to digital ischemia is extremely rare. Most patients can achieve worthwhile improvement by avoidance of cold by the use of electrically heated or thick woollen gloves in cold weather, and by giving up smoking. For the few patients who continue to have frequent or severe attacks, drugs provide some relief.

Drugs

Nifedipine is a calcium channel blocking agent. It is given by mouth and produces a reduction in vascular tone with vasodilatation. Side effects are common and include headache, flushing, peripheral edema and blurred vision.

Chapter

42 VEINS

The most important disease processes affecting the veins are two: varicosity and thrombosis.

VARICOSE VEINS

A varicose vein is one which is dilated, lengthened and tortuous. The change is brought about by increased pressure in the lumen of the vein, which stretches the vein wall. Stretching in the transverse axis is seen as dilatation of the vein. When the vein wall stretches in the longitudinal direction its ends remain at the same fixed points, therefore it has to become tortuous in order to accommodate its additional length. Thus the vein becomes both dilated and tortuous.

What causes the increased pressure in the lumen of the vein? The etiology differs according to the site and underlying pathology. Veins in the submucosa of the lower end of the esophagus become varicose (esophageal varices) because of increased pressure in the portal venous system, due to cirrhosis, etc. Veins in the lower limbs become varicose when their valves becomes functionless (incompetent). Such an incompetent valve is commonly located at the termination of the long saphenous vein, sometimes at a site lower down the limb.

VARICOSE VEINS IN THE LOWER LIMBS

In European and American communities varicose veins of the legs are an extremely common condition. Not so in many of the Eastern countries, where this condition is uncommon. The most likely explanation is that the inhabitants of the latter have better veins.

Etiology

- *Primary*. The most common lesion leading to the development of varicose veins in the legs is a functionless (incompetent) valve. Such cases constitute the *vast majority* of cases.
- *Secondary* varicose veins are predisposed to by:
  - Any cause of venous obstruction, e.g.:
    - Tumor.
    - Pregnancy.
    - Thrombosis of the deep veins.
  - In children and adolescents varicose veins may be due to:
    - Congenital arteriovenous fistula.
    - Extensive cavernous hemangioma.

Pathology of primary varicose veins

In the upright position in the normal limb, with each muscle contraction blood in the deep veins is pumped upwards and prevented from returning by the valves in the veins. When this happens, the pressure in the deep veins is reduced. This allows blood in the superficial veins to empty into the deep veins, ready to be pumped upwards with the next muscular contraction. The valves in the superficial veins ensure that only a short segment between each pair of valves can empty through the corresponding perforating veins and widespread transfer of blood from superficial to deep veins is prevented. However, if there is extensive incompetence in the superficial valves, it is possible for blood to spill over from deep veins at a high level, down the superficial veins, and finally to enter the deep veins at a low level every time these veins fall slack after muscle contraction. This is how primary varicose veins develop.

With such a retrograde circuit based on an incompetent long or short saphenous vein, its upper end provides the source, its main stem and branches form the pathway of incompetence, and one or more perforating veins are the re-entry points. This state is usually curable by removal of the source and the pathway of incompetence, but enlarged re-entry points (the perforators) that allow back flow may also need to be closed off.

The main valves affected are located at the following sites:

- The termination of the long saphenous into the femoral vein.

- The termination of the short saphenous into the popliteal vein.
- The mid-thigh.
- On either side of the tibia and fibula where there are communications *(perforators)* passing through openings in the deep fascia above the ankle.

Symptoms

The most common complaint is of a tired and aching sensation in the leg, specially the calf, towards the evening. There may be itching of the skin over the varices. In longstanding cases a 'varicose ulcer' may form along the course of the long saphenous vein over the medial malleolus.

Examination

The varicosities are most commonly distributed along the course of the long saphenous vein (Fig.42.1); the short saphenous vein is affected less often. The upper end of the long saphenous vein may be varicose (saphena varix). Telangectasia (small dilated vessels near the surface of the skin) may be present. There may be some ankle edema.

Location

- Varicosities on the medial thigh and calf suggest incompetence of the long saphenous vein.
- Those at the posterolateral calf suggest short saphenous incompetence.
- Veins at the anterolateral thigh suggest involvement of the anterolateral tributary of the long saphenous vein.

Investigation

Tourniquet tests have now been given up entirely.

Duplex ultrasonography

This is the gold standard of investigation for varicose veins today. It utilizes a grayscale to visualize the structure of the vein, and a colour Doppler to visualize the flow of blood. It helps to determine:

- Locations of incompetent saphenous junctions.
- Reflux in the saphenous veins.
- Locations of incompetent perforators.

Management

Patients with asymptomatic varicose veins should be reassured. Active treatment is required for patients with bleeding, edema, eczema or venous ulcer.

Compression therapy

Below-knee stockings exerting different degrees of pressure are available and provide relief, but are not very popular. They should be applied skillfully, otherwise they can be harmful by producing a tourniquet effect.

Ultrasound-guided foam sclerotherapy

Under ultrasound guidance a detergent, generally sodium tetradecylsulphate, is injected in the form of a foam into all the affected veins. The sites of injection are marked and cannulated, the leg is elevated to empty the veins, and injections made. This is immediately followed by compression bandaging, the bandages being left in place for a week to ten days. After this, elastic stockings are worn for another few weeks.

The chemical destroys the endothelial cells resulting in thrombosis followed by fibrosis, and ultimately obliteration of the lumen of the vein. Side effects are common. Symptoms are improved but a number of cases recur.

Endovenous laser ablation

A laser fibre is inserted into a vein through a catheter. As the catheter is withdrawn, the tip of the laser fibre applies heat to the vein. This causes the blood to clot, ultimately ablating the vein by fibrosis. This method is suited to most cases.

Radiofrequency ablation

A bipolar endovascular catheter generates heat to ablate the vein.

Complications

With endovenous methods a small percentage of patients suffer modest complications.

Surgical treatment

The operation is generally carried out under general anesthesia.

Ligation and stripping

The basic principle of the operative treatment of varicose veins is the ligation and division of those veins into which the high-pressure leak from the deep venous system has primarily occurred, and removal of the trunk and its dilated tributaries by stripping.

The different operations include:

- Saphenofemoral flush ligation and long saphenous stripping.
- Saphenopopliteal flush ligation and short saphenous stripping.

Note: despite numerous trials, ligation of perforators has not borne out its early promise.

Preserving the saphenous veins

Care must be taken not to damage or destroy normal competent saphenous veins, because they may be needed for coronary bypass operations for coronary occlusion in the future.

Complications of varicose veins

These include the following:

Thrombophlebitis of a vein, which is red and tender. Elastic bandages are applied over foam rubber pads, and the patient allowed to go about.

Eczema may occur because the patient scratches the skin which itches. An ointment containing hydrocortisone, or one containing zinc oxide and coal tar, is used.

Hemorrhage. A varicose vein may rupture and bleed furiously. The patient may not be aware of the simple fact that blood will continue to flow under pressure if he remains standing, or sitting with the legs hanging from a chair. He must be told to lie down at once. The bleeding point is pressed upon and the hemorrhage will promptly stop. A firm bandage should now be applied over a sterile gauze pad. To aid hemostasis further, the leg may be elevated over one or two pillows, but only after the bleeding point has been firmly bandaged, to avoid air embolism.

Venous ulcer

(Gravitational ulcer, Varicose ulcer). These ulcers are chronic, tend to recur, and cause considerable disability. They follow either varicose veins or deep vein thrombosis. The cause in either case is venous stasis, which results in local anoxia and edema. Signs of venous insufficiency are usually present, along with dermatitis, with brown discoloration, thickening of skin and edema.

Site of venous ulcer

The site of occurrence of a venous ulcer is quite constant; it nearly always lies on the anteromedial surface of the tibia just above the medial malleolus. In this condition syphilis must be excluded by serological tests, and atherosclerotic ischemia by checking the peripheral pulses. If these cannot be felt because of edema, the Doppler ultrasound may be employed. Malignant change may occur in a long-standing ulcer (Marjolin's ulcer).

Pathophysiology

The pathophysiology is not fully understood. In the normal person during walking, the contractions of the calf muscles pump blood in a cephalad direction in the

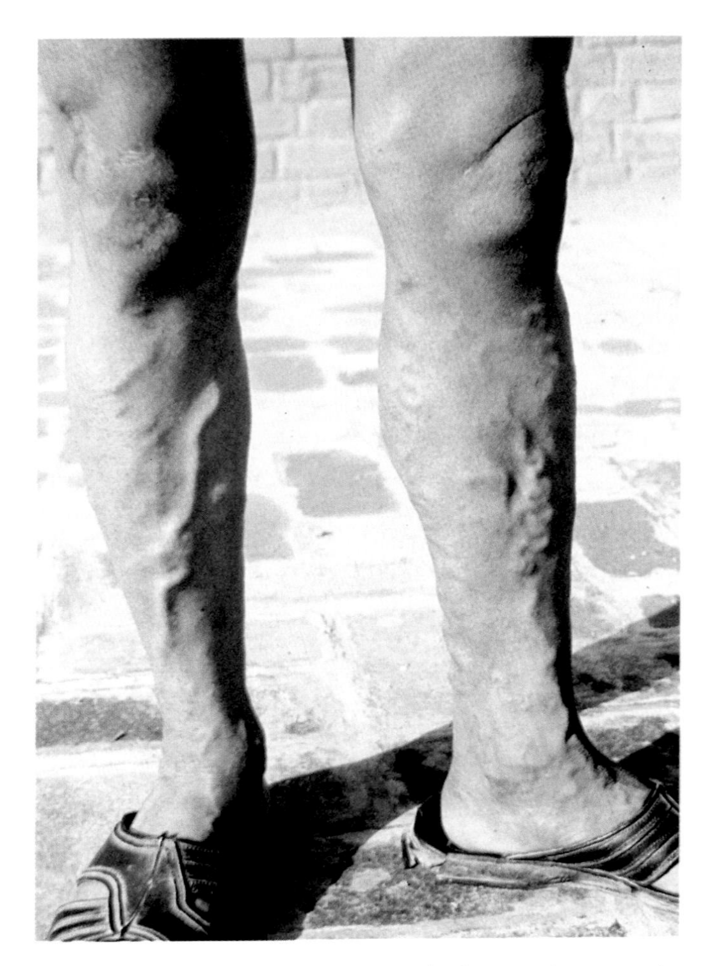

Fig.42.1 Bilateral varicose veins of the long saphenous vein systems

deep system. In a patient with incompetent perforator valves, the high venous pressure in the deep veins is transmitted to the superficial venous system, and causes extravasation of plasma and blood cells. In time the subcutaneous tissue becomes firm, with a leathery feel.

Venous ulcers resulting from varicose veins heal promptly after ambulatory treatment or ligation operations. On the other hand post-thrombotic ulcers tend to be refractory to treatment, and require bed-rest and skin grafting.

The bisgaard method

This method of treatment of venous ulcers is very useful. The limb is elevated. Massage, alongwith passive and active movements, is now carried out. A firm elastic bandage is next applied from the base of the toes to the knee and the patient encouraged to walk. Movements in walking alternatively stretch and relax the bandage and produce a venous pumping effect.

For the treatment of incompetent perforators, *subfascial*

ligation, i.e. ligation under the deep fascia, has been mostly abandoned.

THROMBOSIS

Apart from varicosities, the most important pathological change affecting veins is thrombosis.

Etiology

The main factors responsible for producing thrombosis are three *(Virchow's triad)*:

- Changes in the *vessel wall.*
- Diminished rate of *blood flow.*
- Increased *coagulability* of blood.

Risk factors

Several conditions increase the risk of thromboembolism:

- Age.
- Obesity.
- Immobility.
- Pregnancy and high-dose estrogens.
- Malignancy.
- Heart failure.
- Trauma and surgery.

In most of these conditions stasis is a factor.

Pathological effects

The pathological effects of thrombosis include the following:

- *Locally*, the clot may get dissolved and the vein become recanalized. Alternatively, the clot may organize into fibrous tissue. If the thrombus is infected an abscess may form, or pyemia may occur due to systemic spread of the infection. In the pelvic veins a clot sometimes calcifies, leaving behind a small circular radiopaque shadow, which to the beginner may look like a stone in the lower end of the ureter.
- *Distally*. If the vein remains blocked a collateral circulation soon opens up, as shown by the appearance of tortuous superficial veins.
- *Proximally*:
  - o The clot may extend into the larger veins, where a portion of the thrombus may become detached, get lodged in a branch of the pulmonary artery, and produce pulmonary infarction.
  - o If an infected thrombus, e.g. from septic thrombosed hemorrhoids, gets lodged in the portal vein it may result in the formation of abscesses in the liver (pylephlebitis).

Thrombosis in the superficial veins is commonly accompanied by inflammation (thrombophlebitis), while in the deep veins it usually occurs without it (phlebothrombosis).

Superficial venous thrombosis. (Thrombophlebitis)

This can occur in one of the following situations:

- A grossly varicose vein.
- A vein cannulated for infusion.
- Occult malignant neoplasms.
- Local trauma.
- Polycythaemia.
- Thrombo-angiitis obliterans.

At the site of the vein a painful, red and tender cord is found. When thrombophlebitis occurs below the knee it is usually self-limiting; the risk of thromboembolism is minimal and anticoagulation is not needed. When thrombophlebitis extends above the knee embolization may occur; such patients should be closely observed for cephalad progression of thrombus. *Treatment* consists of bed rest and a crepe bandage. Aspirin relieves pain, and also helps by reducing the coagulability of the blood. If an abscess forms it must be drained.

Deep vein thrombosis (Phlebothrombosis)

Deep vein thrombosis is serious because the thrombus is much more likely to embolize to the lungs. Half the patients who develop embolism have no symptoms of deep vein disease. Deep vein thrombosis follows any condition where:

- The intima of the vein is damaged, e.g. in trauma.
- The circulation of the blood is sluggish, e.g. after a major operation or during a debilitating illness.
- The blood is rendered more coagulable e.g. after an operation. Postoperative thrombosis is common:
  - o In middle-aged and elderly persons.
  - o In the obese.
  - o After operations on the hip and those carried out for malignancies.

If more than one factor is at work, the chances of thrombosis are greatly increased.

The thrombosis often starts in a tributary of a main vein, where the circulation is sluggish. When it extends proximally to reach the main vein the faster bloodstream may break off a portion, which lodges in the pulmonary vasculature as a pulmonary embolus. The most common deep veins affected by phlebothrombosis are the pelvic and calf veins.

'White leg' and 'blue leg'

If a length of deep femoral vein gets thrombosed, edema and painful venous congestion in the lower limb results:

- If the lymphatics are also inflamed, a more pronounced and persistent swelling results (*phlegmasia alba dolens* or *'white leg'*).
- If extensive thrombosis of the iliac and pelvic veins occurs, infarction may affect parts of the lower limb. (*phlegmasia caerulea dolens* or *`blue leg'*).

Diagnosis

Clinical

Phlebothrombosis may cause no symptoms, except for some pain in the affected calf. A slight fever may raise suspicion. Homan's sign, in which forceful dosifexion of the ankle encounters resistance of the calf muscles, should not be elicited as it is not specific.

Laboratory

For thrombosis

D-dimer is a fibrin degradation product. Its concentration, determined by a blood test, helps diagnose thrombosis. A negative result virtually rules out thrombosis; a positive result means either thrombosis or other possible causes.

For embolism

The *Modified Wells score* is based on clinical features of deep vein thrombosis (DVT), heart rate, duration of immobilization etc. If the score is more than 4, pulmonary embolism (PE) is likely; if above 6, the patient has a high risk of PE.

Imaging

If the MWS is high, a *duplex compression ultrasound examination* is performed, deep veins of the leg being compressed; filling defects and a resistance to compression show up thrombosis.

Contrast venography is no longer used, as *MR venography* now provides as good an image.

Pulmonary embolism is diagnosed by *CT pulmonary angiography,* which shows up filling defects in the pulmonary arteries.

Management of deep vein thrombosis

Prevention

Candidates for surgery should be categorized as low, moderate and high risk:

- ***Low.*** Minor surgery, or major surgery below age 40, with no risk factors.
- ***Moderate.*** Major surgery, age above 40, or other risk factors.
- ***High.*** Extensive surgery and/or concomitant medical illness

In susceptible persons precautions against thrombosis must be taken before, during and after surgery. Patients in the moderate or high risk group should be considered for prophylaxis by anticoagulation.

Prophylactic methods

These include:

- Graduated elastic compression stockings.
- Subcutaneous low molecular weight dextran. This heparin can be given once a day.

Before operation. Women taking oral contraceptives are more prone to develop venous thrombosis after operation; before elective operations these should be stopped a month before surgery. If an elderly patient has been in hospital for lengthy investigations and has become immobile, he should be sent home for a few days for mobilization before readmission for surgery.

During operation. Specially during lengthy operations, the pressure of the table on the calf muscles can occlude the deep veins and render the flow of blood sluggish. To prevent this, the heels should be elevated on foam-rubber pads; at the end of the operation the legs should be elevated and massaged.

After operation. If the legs remain immobile after operation or the patient is dehydrated, the incidence of deep vein thrombosis is high. Massage and active leg movements should be prescribed and supervised, and dehydration corrected. The patient should get onto his feet as early as possible. Low dose heparin as described above is also useful. In highly susceptible individuals low molecular weight dextran may be used due to its property of inhibiting platelet adhesion; 500ml is given intravenously during the operation and 500ml during the following 24 hours.

Treatment

If deep vein thrombosis has developed the whole limb should be bandaged using crepe bandages, and bed rest advised until the local signs subside.

Anticoagulants should be used in full doses, heparin to start the course and warfarin to continue it. Anticoagulation prevents the propagation of the original thrombus and the development of new thrombi, while the existing thrombus is lysed by naturally occurring fibrinolysis. Intravenous heparin acts rapidly and its effects can be reversed promptly with protamine sulphate to minimize the possibility of bleeding complications.

Although anticoagulation is the treatment of choice, fibrinolytics such as streptokinase and recombinant tissue plasminogen activator have been evaluated. They can lyse upto 70% of thrombi, a feature that anticoagulants lack. However, complications are significant and the routine use of fibrinolytics has been prohibited by bleeding complications, specially in the postoperative setting.

Prevention of embolism

Pulmonary embolism may be prevented by placing one of several available inferior vena cava filters in position. This prevents any dislodged thrombus from getting into the right ventricle and pulmonary artery, and yet allows the flow of blood upwards through its interstices.

Air embolism

If a large volume of air enters the venous circulation, it can be very dangerous for the patient. When it reaches the right atrium the air is churned up. The foam enters the right ventricle and causes an air-lock in the pulmonary artery, which may cause right-sided heart failure. Some of the situations in which the air may enter the veins are the following:

- Air may be *sucked* into an open vein. This is most likely to happen during operations on the neck or axilla, where the negative pressure in the thorax helps suck the air into any large vein which may get opened.
- Air may reach the venous system after *insufflations* into the fallopian tubes or during illegal abortion.
- In the days when rigid bottles with air vents were used for intravenous infusions, air embolism was more common than with the collapsible bottles in use nowadays. If a rigid bottle has to be used, a float in the drip chamber, which plugs the outlet when the fluid falls to a low level, adds a measure of safety.

Treatment

Trendelenberg position

The operation table should be tilted so that the head is low – the Trendelenberg position. This encourages the air to pass into the veins in the lower half of the body, where it is relatively harmless. At the same time the patient should be turned onto his left side. In this position the air floats into the apex of the right ventricle, away from the origin of the pulmonary artery.

Aspiration

Air may be aspirated from the right ventricle by a needle passed upwards and backwards from below the left costal margin. Alternatively, the heart may be exposed for aspiration under direct vision.

Fat embolism syndrome

The fat embolism syndrome commonly follows extensive and multiple fractures, occurring in up to 5% of patients with combined pelvic and femoral fractures. Fat droplets activate platelet aggregation. The platelets being thus 'consumed', the patient suffers what is called a 'consumption coagulopathy'. At the same time fat in globules lodging in the lung is converted by lipase to free fatty acid that causes acute lung injury. Thus the patient presents with:

- Dyspnoea.
- Skin petechiae.
- Hypoxaemia.
- Thrombocytopenia.
- Falling hemoglobin.
- Fat globules in the urine.

Symptoms arise two or three days after injury and two types are recognized, the cerebral and the pulmonary, depending upon whether the chylomicrons aggregate maximally in the brain or the lung:

- In the *cerebral* type the patient is drowsy, restless, disoriented and later comatose.
- In the *pulmonary* type, there is increasing cyanosis with signs of right heart failure.

Ophthalmoscopy

If the condition is suspected, ophthalmoscopy should be carried out. Emboli in the retinal arteries may cause hemorrhages and `fluffy' exudate. Petechial hemorrhages are fairly common. The sputum and urine should be examined for the presence of fat globules.

Treatment is supportive and includes:

- Vasopressors.
- Inotropes.
- Mechanical ventilation.
- High-dose corticosteroids; these probably reduce platelet aggregation.
- Low molecular weight dextran; this reduces the viscosity of the blood.

Aspirin and heparin carry a significant risk of hemorrhage and are not recommended.

The whole subject of pulmonary embolism is discussed under 'postoperative pulmonary complications' in chapter 39.

Venous hemorrhage

If major veins are damaged by trauma or at operation in the neck, groin and specially the pelvis, bleeding can be torrential, and unless skillfully managed can kill the patient by exsanguination. Tight packing is the best immediate measure. With the packing in place the anesthetist obtains and transfuses sufficient blood for adequate volume replacement. The surgeon exposes veins both above and below the site of injury for control by vascular clamps, the simplest form of which consists of the commonly available small bull-dog clamps. Even if enough room is available for instituting such control, blood may still continue to flow furiously through numerous anastomosing channels, and often requires all the ingenuity that the surgeon can command.

Chapter

43 LYMPHATICS AND LYMPH NODES

Acute lymphangitis

Acute lymphangitis is said to be present when lymphatic vessels are acutely inflamed. This occurs when, from a focus of infection, bacteria spread proximally along these vessels. It is seen as red streaks in the skin along the course of the lymphatics.

Treatment consists of bed rest, elevation of the affected limb, and the use of intravenous antibiotics. Rapid resolution normally occurs. However, if pus forms it has to be drained. Recurrent attacks sometimes occur due to damage to lymphatics.

LYMPHEDEMA

Lymphedema is defined as the excessive accumulation of protein-rich interstitial fluid as a result of defective lymphatic drainage. The condition is subdivided into primary and secondary lymphedema, the latter being much more common.

Primary lymphedema

Cases of primary lymphedema are divided into those with hypoplastic and hyperplastic lymph vessels:

Hypoplastic cases

These constitute 90% of cases. The location of their hypoplasia may be:

- ***Distal***. These cases are seen in young women after puberty. They are mild and non-progressive.
- ***Proximal***. These occur equally between males and females, and have more extensive lymphedema.
- ***Proximal and distal***. These cases are also progressive.

Hyperplastic cases

These constitute only 10% of the cases. Lymphography shows dilated lymphatics and in the megalymphatic group the lymphatics have no valves.

Secondary lymphedema

- This is most often due to malignant disease metastatic to lymph nodes.
- Other causes include:
    - o Trauma.
    - o Venous disease.
    - o Infection, specially tuberculosis and filariasis.
    - o Inflammation, including rheumatoid arthritis and psoriasis.

If lymphedema appears after the age of 50, pelvic malignancy should be suspected and looked for.

Investigations

Lymphangiography

Contrast lymphangiography

The above findings can be confirmed by contrast lymphangiography, which also determines the type of lymphatic abnormality present by providing information on the presence of hypoplasia, megalymphatics and obstruction.

However, because of its difficult technique it has largely been given up as a routine procedure.

Isotope lymphangiography

This has mostly replaced the above procedure. Radioactive technetium-labelled colloid is injected into an interdigital web space in the foot. It is specifically taken up by lymphatics and allows the presence of lymphedema to be confirmed as an outpatient procedure. Normally, the colloid arrives at the groin within one hour. Gamma camera pictures provide information that the isotope is reaching the groin lymph nodes; later images may show a failure of progression, indicating proximal obstruction.

Ultrasound, CT and MRI

These can show enlarged lymph nodes, and guided biopsies of nodes can be taken if malignancy is suspected.

Needle or Tru-cut biopsies are preferable, since removal of large fibrotic nodes may worsen pre-existing lymphedema.

To rule out renal and hepatic causes, serum creatinine level and liver function tests should be obtained.

Treatment

Medical

Young women with distal hypoplasia can be managed by limb elevation, massage and elastic compression stockings. Stockings are poorly tolerated in warm climates and women tend to be conscious of their appearance. Antibiotics should be used for cellulitis, as well as prophylactically in low doses if the patient is troubled by repeated attacks.

Surgical

Surgery is appropriate for whole limb lymphedema that interferes with mobility or results in severe deformity. The lymphatic obstruction may be bypassed or the edematous subcutaneous tissues excised:

Lymphatic bypass

In a few patients in whom lymphangiography shows proximal lymphatic obstruction with normal distal lymphatics, the operation of *mesenteric bridge bypass* is quite ingenious. About 5cm of terminal ileum is isolated on its mesenteric pedicle. The gut segment is opened along its antimesenteric border and the mucosa stripped off. The isolated segment is brought down to the first normal group of lymph nodes below the level of the obstruction and sutured over them after they have been bivalved. Connections develop between the divided nodes and the submucosal plexus and lymph drains up the pedicle into the mesenteric lymph nodes. However this, and similar operations, have not borne out their early promise.

Reduction operations

These are employed in most cases:

Charles procedure. All diseased skin and waterlogged subcutaneous tissue are excised from the ankle to the knee, and split-skin grafts are used for coverage. It gives good results; however, the cosmetic appearance is not very satisfactory.

Homans operation. In this, the popular operation today, skin flaps are raised, the subcutaneous tissue excised, and the flaps trimmed and sutured back. The lateral and medial sides of the leg are operated upon with an interval of six months.

Filariasis

In parts of Africa, South America and India, filariasis is the most common cause of lymphedema. The worm enters the lymphatics and lodges in the lymph nodes where a severe fibrotic reaction causes obstruction to the lymphatic pathways which are grossly dilated. This results in severe swelling of the lower limbs called 'elephantiasis'.

Diagnosis is confirmed by finding microfilariae; as these enter the blood in large numbers at night, the blood sample should be taken at midnight. A strongly positive complement fixation test suggests active or past filariasis.

Treatment with diethylcarbamazine is very successful and destroys the microfilariae, but it cannot reverse established lymphedema; progression of the disease may, however, be slowed or prevented.

Lymphangioma

A cavernous lymphangioma (cystic hygroma) is seen in newborns as collections of lymphatic cysts in the neck or axilla. It is described in chapter 47 dealing with conditions of the neck.

LYMPHADENITIS

Acute lymphadenitis

Acute lymphadenitis results when a lymph node draining any area of infection becomes acutely inflamed. The node may suppurate and discharge pus. Treatment is on the usual lines for acute pyogenic infection, including incision and drainage where indicated.

Chronic lymphadenitis

Chronic lymphadenitis may be simple (pyogenic) or specific. The common type of specific lymphadenitis arises due to tuberculosis.

Chronic pyogenic lymphadenitis occurs if a persistent focus of infection is present in the area of the lymph node, e.g. recurrent tonsillitis, or multiple boils in the scalp or over the legs. Treatment requires eradication of the primary septic focus, when the lymph node enlargement subsides.

TUBERCULOUS LYMPHADENITIS

Tuberculous lymphadenitis is by far the most common form of chronic lymphadenitis. Although uncommon in the developed countries due to universal pasteurization of milk, it is still a major health problem in some parts of the world. It is common among children in regions where BCG inoculation is not universal. Lymph nodes of the neck are the most common site of this infection, the reason being that the orifices affording inlet to both the respiratory and alimentary tracts are located in this area, and a large number of lymph nodes guard these portals of entry. The infection is acquired either by contact with cases of open human tuberculosis, or by drinking infected milk.

Evidence of past disease may be seen in the mediastinal and mesenteric lymph nodes in the form of specks of calcification on routine x-rays of the chest and abdomen respectively. Tubercle bacilli reach the node via lymphatics, therefore most of the early tubercles are seen in the cortex. Microscopically lymphocytes, monocytes and giant cells are seen. If the disease spreads, many lymph nodes are affected.

When infection spreads out through the capsule, adjacent nodes may get *matted together,* and this feature helps distinguish tuberculosis from Hodgkin lymphoma and other causes of lymph node enlargement.

The inflamed nodes may break down to form caseous tuberculous pus, which may perforate the deep fascia and present as a fluctuant swelling on the surface. Finally, the skin may break down resulting in a sinus. When healing occurs, a good deal of scarring is produced; in cases with caseation calcification may also be seen.

Investigations

These fall into two categories, the general and the specific.

General

These are helpful but not diagnostic. The differential leucocyte count may show a lymphocytosis. The erythrocyte sedimentation rate (ESR) and CRP helps in following up the course of the disease.

The Mantoux reaction is a test of delayed hypersensitivity to tuberculin. Induration over an area of 10mm or more across is taken as a positive Mantoux test, and is seen in nearly 80% of the cases.

A chest x-ray helps in detecting healed pulmonary tuberculosis (fibrosis or calcification), or coexisting active pulmonary tuberculosis.

Specific

These are diagnostic of tuberculosis:

- *Bacteriological examination.*
  - o Slides are made from pus or lymph node imprints and stained with Ziehl Neelsen stains. The tubercle bacilli appear red.
  - o The only confirmatory proof of tuberculosis is the isolation of Mycobacterium tuberculosis from the pus or lymph node. Mycobacteria are cultured on Lowenstein-Jensen medium and examined weekly for eight weeks. Colonies usually appear in three to four weeks' time. By using a new medium, Middlebrook 7H12, mycobacteria can be isolated within nine days.
- *Histopathological examination.* This includes histopathology of the lymph nodes and of the walls of any cold abscess. Histopathology is diagnostic in 98% of cases. A granuloma characterized by epithelioid cells and giant cells of the Langhan's type, with central caseation and a peripheral rim of lymphocytes along with fibroblasts, is characteristic of tuberculosis.
- *Guinea pig inoculation.*
- *Biochemical tests* for different mycobacteria.
- *Serological tests*:
  - o Elisa.
  - o Radioimmunoassay.
  - o Flourescent antibody test.

Fine needle aspiration (FNA) is a useful tool for getting material for the diagnosis of tuberculous lymphadenitis. The diagnostic accuracy rate is 96%.

Treatment

The mainstay of treatment is drug therapy; surgery has a limited role to play in the treatment of this condition.

Drug therapy

As in the case of tuberculosis anywhere else in the body, lymph node tuberculosis is treated by multiple drug therapy. In the most popular regimen, the following four drugs are started together:

- Rifampicin 10mg/kg/day. The main adverse effect is hepatitis.
- Pyrazinamide (PZA) 20 to 30mg/kg/day; again hepatitis is an important side effect.
- Isoniazid (INH) 5mg/kg/day. There is a risk of peripheral neuropathy with this drug; to prevent this, pyridoxin 25mg/day is added.
- Ethambutol 15 to 20mg/kg/day. The main side effect is optic neuritis, and vision should be checked at frequent intervals.

All except the last one are bactericidal drugs.

The course is as follows:

All four medicines are given for two months, then rifampicin and INH for four months. Liver function tests are done. If the levels rise to twice the upper normal level, the first one (or two) medicines are stopped before time. In that case the other drugs have to be given for nine (or 12) months.

Response to treatment is assessed by examining the size of the lymph nodes and by determination of ESR/CRP.

Surgery

With the introduction of effective antituberculosis therapy, the role of surgery has become quite limited. Nowadays, surgery is most often needed for *excisional biopsy* of lymph nodes for diagnosis. The other indications for surgery include:

- Failure to respond to medical treatment.
- Persistent discharging sinus.
- Cold abscess not responding to medical treatment.

Post-BCG lymphadenitis

Occasionally the bacilli in a batch of BCG vaccine are not sufficiently attenuated, and a large number of infants develop lymphadenitis. When the inoculation is given over the deltoid, as is the common practice, one of the lymph nodes in the anterior (pectoral) group of lymph nodes enlarges. The node sometimes liquefies. The baby commonly remains well.

If the node is small it can be observed. If large, and specially if it has liquefied, single-drug therapy with isoniazid is considered legitimate. However, in the odd case in which spreading infection develops, multiple-drug therapy is required. Some workers have had better success with removal of the lymph node involved.

LYMPHOMAS

Lymphomas arise from the different types of lymphocytes (B cell, T cell or histiocyte). In common with other neoplasms, the less histologically differentiated they are, the more rapidly they grow. They can be divided into Hodgkin lymphoma and non-Hodgkin lymphomas.

HODGKIN LYMPHOMA

Hodgkin lymphoma, formerly known as Hodgkin's disease, is a cancer of the lymphatic system. It can occur wherever there is lymphoid tissue, and its cells can spread beyond the lymphatic system. As it progresses, it compromises the body's ability to fight infection. On section the nodes are pinkish grey in colour and rubbery in consistency. Unlike tubercular lymph nodes they remain discrete. The only exceptions to this rule are seen in some anaplastic forms of Hodgkin lymphoma. The spleen gets diffusely enlarged. Bone deposits occur in the bones with red marrow, specially the vertebral column and pelvis.

The WHO/REAL system classifies Hodgkin lymphoma (HL) into:

- Classical LH.
    - o Nodular sclerosis.
    - o Mixed cellularity.
    - o Lymphocyte-depletion.
    - o Lymphocyte-rich classical.
- Nodular lymphocyte-predominant.

Accurate subtyping leads to appropriate treatment and better outcome. Nodular sclerosis and lymphocyte-predominant are associated with the best prognosis, lymphocyte depletion with the worst.

Clinical features

Hodgkin lymphoma is more common in males. Two peaks of incidence occur, one in young adults and the other which becomes slowly more common with increasing age. A painless and progressive enlargement of the lymph nodes commences in the neck usually without, but sometimes with, constitutional symptoms e.g. malaise, fever and weight loss. Enlarged mediastinal nodes may obstruct the superior vena cava and produce marked congestion in the neck veins. A vertebra may collapse due to bony metastases and result in bone pain.

As stated above, the lymph nodes are discrete, except in late or anaplastic cases. The spleen and liver may be enlarged. Later, irregular fever often develops. When the disease becomes disseminated, anemia and pancytopenia may occur. The disease usually progresses quite slowly, but occasionally follows a rapid course.

Clinical staging

Clinical staging of Hodgkin lymphoma helps greatly in deciding upon the correct line of treatment. The condition is divided into four stages as shown in Table 43.2.

Investigations

When the disease is suspected a *chest x-ray* is ordered to exclude mediastinal node enlargement, and an *abdominal ultrasound* to detect involvement of the para-aortic lymph nodes, spleen and liver.

A *positron emission tomography (PET) scan* can be used to show small deposits that do not show on CT scanning. If a PET scan is not available, a Gallium scan may be used.

Fine needle aspiration of a lymph node in the neck is mandatory.

Flow cytometry[1] of the fine needle aspirate helps in diagnosis and classification of lymphomas.

Treatment

Patients with early disease (IA or IIA) are managed with radiation or chemotherapy, depending on age, sex and histological subtype.

Patients with later disease (III, IVA or IVB) are treated with combination chemotherapy alone.

Patients of any stage with a large mass in the chest are treated with combined chemotherapy and radiotherapy.

Chemotherapy

Chemotherapeutic agents are given in combination, as their clinical effects are summated but side effects are not. The two most popular regimens of therapy today utilize the following drug combinations:

- **ABVD.**

Adriamycin, Bleomycin, Vinblastin and Dacarbazine.

The course lasts six to eight months.

- **Stanford V.**

Doxorubicin, Vinblastine, Mechlorethamine,

Vincristine, Bleomycin, Etoposide and Prednisolone.

The course lasts three months.

Radiotherapy

In most cases external beam radiotherapy is used, and radiation given only to involved groups of glands, often along with chemotherapy. Thus radiotherapy may be administered only above, or only below, the diaphragm.

Side effects

These may be severe. Therefore, treatment must be very carefully planned, with regular blood counts.

Prognosis

Treatment has improved during recent decades. In a recent report the 5-year survival rate for those patients with a favorable prognosis was as high as 98%, while even that for patients with worse outlooks was above 85%.[2]

An international effort in 1998[3] identified seven prognostic factors that accurately predict the success rate of conventional treatment in patients with locally extensive or advanced stage Hodgkin lymphoma.

Table 43.2 The stages of Hodgkin lymphoma

Stage	Description
I	Confined to one lymph node group.
II	Affecting two or more lymph node areas, but on same side of the diaphragm.
III	Involving lymph nodes both above and below the diaphragm (the spleen is considered a lymph node).
IV	Spread beyond the lymph nodes, e.g. to bone marrow, liver .

Note: Each stage is further subdivided into subgroups A and B according to the absence or presence of associated generalized symptoms such as weight loss, fever, pruritus, anemia and bone pain.

The adverse prognostic factors include:

- Age $\geq$ 45 years.
- Stage IV disease.
- Hemoglobin $<$ 10.5 g/dl.
- Lymmphocyte count $<$ 600/μl.
- Male.
- Albumin $<$ 4.0 g/dl.
- White blood count $\geq$ 15,000/μl.

Freedom from progression (FFP) at five years for patients with zero factors is 84%, while for a patient with five or more factors it is 42%.

Surgery

With the development of highly effective chemotherapy and radiotherapy, there is a limited role for surgery in lymphomas. Biopsy examination is necessary for diagnosis and histological typing. Splenectomy in children carries the risk of overwhelming sepsis, most often due to encapsulated cocci (Streptococcus pneumoniae, Hemophilus infuenzae). If splenectomy is employed, long-term prophylactic antibiotics and pneumococcal vaccination should be given to these patients.

Re-staging laparotomy

Interestingly, while staging laparotomy is no longer employed, a 'restaging laparotomy' has been proposed, to accurately document residual or recurrent disease, because negative findings would spare the patient added toxic therapy without compromising his chances of survival.

1 Flow cytology is a laser method in which cells are suspended in fluid and counted and sorted by passing them in single file through an electronic detection apparatus.

2 Fermé C, et al (November 2007). "Chemotherapy plus involved-field radiation in early-stage Hodgkin's disease". NEJM 357 (19): 1916–27.

3 Hasenclever D. et al (1998), "A Prognostic Score For Advanced Hodgkin's Disease". NEJM 339 (21): 1506.

NON-HODGKIN LYMPHOMAS

Non-Hodgkin lymphomas (NHL) consist of a group of primary malignancies of lymphoreticular tissue. Most of them are monoclonal B-cell tumors. Any lymphoma that does not contain Reed-Sternberg cells is classified as non-Hodgkin lymphoma.

The clinical course of NHLs is more variable than that of Hodgkin lymphoma, the pattern of spread is irregular, and more patients have leukaemic features. They are classified into:

- Nodular (favourable).
- Diffuse (unfavourable) types.

However, non-Hodgkin lymphomas come in many forms, so that the WHO/REAL classification recognizes as many as 27 subtypes.

Clinical features

Non-Hodgkin lymphomas generally affect persons older than those suffering from Hodgkin lymphoma, the median age of onset being 50 years. In contrast to Hodgkin lympoma, only about two thirds of patients with NHL have asymptomatic lymphadenopathy; in the rest of the patients the onset of NHL occurs at a site other than a lymph node, commonly as an abdominal mass or a hepatic or splenic enlargement.

Constitutional symptoms such as fever, night sweats and weight loss are often present. Occasionally, the patient first presents as an *emergency* with superior vena caval syndrome, spinal cord compression, or ureteral obstruction from retroperitoneal node involvement.

Spread

In non-Hodgkin lymphoma the mode of spread is generally more unpredictable than in Hodgkin lymphoma, and most patients have disseminated disease when they present, because NHL can rapidly spread through the bloodstream to distal nodal and extranodal sites. This extranodal spread of NHL is comparable with the pattern of metastasis seen in carcinomas.

Treatment

As with Hodgkin lymphoma, chemotherapy and radiotherapy are the mainstays of treatment. Because most patients with NHL have disseminated disease at the time of presentation, chemotherapy has a greater role to play than radiotherapy or surgery.

Despite the large number of types of NHL, because of accurate subtyping the correct treatment is generally selected and the outcome is better. Overall, the prognosis is more favourable for the nodular than for the diffuse form of NHL.

Section

6

HEAD AND NECK, ENDOCRINES, ETC

have a life-threatening head injury are seldom seen by a neurosurgeon during the first critical minutes of medical care. This section is meant for those healthcare providers who are not neurosurgeons but who render emergency care to head-injured patients.

At the same time, patients with head injury are at many places looked after by general surgeons rather than neurosurgeons, therefore the general surgeon should have knowledge of the principles and practice in this field. Most patients do not require any neurosurgery but only medical and nursing measures. However, the surgeon must know when specialized investigations at a neurosurgical centre are required. At the same time, CT scan facilities are available at increasing numbers of hospitals. A general surgeon should be able to diagnose and evacuate an extradural hematoma if it appears on a CT scan.

Pathophysiology

Two major types of head injury are recognized:

Primary head injury

This is the initial impact of trauma to the brain. All degrees of brain injury result from displacement and distortion of the brain *at the time of impact*. At that moment a diffuse injury to the nerve cells occurs, which causes the immediate clinical picture of brain injury.

Secondary head injury

This is a complication of the primary head injury. The secondary changes include edema and intracranial hemorrhage, and these take time to develop. The rise in pressure resulting from the secondary changes produces deterioration in the level of the patient's consciousness a few hours after injury. On the other hand the clinical picture in the early stages results from the neuronal lesion alone. It should be remembered that the secondary changes are preventable.

Factors determining the severity of brain injury

Distortion of the brain

The brain has some mobility inside the skull because of the presence of cerebrospinal fluid around it. The severe distortion which results during injury may produce widespread damage to neurons, nerve fibres and blood vessels. This distortion causes sudden loss of consciousness. If it produces significant damage to nerve cells, persisting loss of consciousness and possibly focal neurological deficit may occur. The distortion may also damage the midbrain, the cells of which are responsible for normal consciousness by activating the cortex. Thus there may be prolonged unconsciousness without any evidence of injury to the skull.

Deceleration and acceleration

In most traffic accidents the moving head strikes a stationary object, e.g. the road. There is rapid *deceleration* of the skull. The brain continues to move and suffers distortion. On the other hand in cases of assault the stationary skull is struck by a moving object and rapidly *accelerates*.

Degrees of severity of brain injury

Injury to the brain may be classified, according to severity, into concussion, contusion and laceration:

Cerebral concussion

In cerebral concussion the damage is slight. There is only a brief physiological paralysis without structural damage. Transient unconsciousness occurs, followed by complete recovery.

Post-traumatic amnesia

The essential feature of concussion is amnesia for the blow; thus a patient who can clearly recollect the blow has no concussion. The length of time the patient is amnesic after the blow is called post-traumatic amnesia, and this is the best indicator of the severity of the concussion. Post-traumatic amnesia extends until the patient has continuous memory for who he is, what time it is, and where he is, i.e. 'for person, time and place'. Post-traumatic amnesia is constant and does not recede with time, unlike *retrograde amnesia*. The duration of amnesia also determines the prognosis of head-injured patients.

'Post-concussional syndrome'

Many patients suffer from this condition, consisting of headache, irritability, depression and vertigo. It is more common after minor concussion, probably because patients return to work too soon. A concussive blow must by definition be followed by full recovery. More severe injury can cause severe cerebral concussion which merges with permanent brain damage.

Cerebral contusion

In cerebral contusion there is more severe damage, including bruising of grey matter, edema, damage to nerve cells and fibres, and hemorrhage.

Cerebral laceration

In cerebral *laceration*, in addition to the above changes the brain surface is torn, with hemorrhage into the cerebrospinal fluid.

ACUTE INTRACRANIAL HEMATOMAS

As a result of the head injury, blood may collect outside the dura, underneath the dura, in the subarachnoid space or in the brain substance.

Acute extradural hematoma

Extradural hemorrhage commonly follows injury to the anterior branch of the middle meningeal artery, which occurs when a blow on the side of the head results in a fracture of the temporal bone. If a fracture in this area is seen on x-ray the patient must be admitted for observation. Blood passing outwards through the fracture line produces a swelling deep to the temporal muscle. If such a swelling is present, even a conscious patient must be admitted.

Clinical features. A moderate blow to the side of the head produces a short period of concussion—*the lucid interval.* During this time the blood is collecting inside the skull and also under the temporalis muscle. After a period of consciousness the patient becomes confused and irritable. Drowsiness follows confusion. The clot presses on the motor cortex producing first twitching and later paralysis of the face, the arm, and then the leg on the opposite side of the body, as the clot spreads upwards. The temporal lobe is pushed inwards and compresses the third nerve. This causes constriction and then dilatation of the pupil on the same side.

The brainstem gets displaced and the opposite crus is pushed against the rim of the tentorium producing hemiplegia, this time on the side of the hemorrhage. It should be remembered that the level of consciousness deteriorates only late, and then rapidly.

Finally, increasing pressure inside the skull forces the midbrain downwards, and impaction of a midbrain cone causes decerebrate rigidity and fixed dilatation of both pupils, when it is probably too late to do anything. It should also be remembered that the lucid interval does not always occur. If an extradural hematoma forms in a patient already unconscious from cerebral concussion, there is no lucid interval.

Acute subdural hematoma

If the skull is struck on the front or the back and the brain moves inside the skull the superior cerebral veins, which end in the superior sagittal sinus, may be ruptured where they cross the subdural space and produce a subdural hematoma. Most patients with subdural hematoma are unconscious right from the onset. The clinical features of subdural hematoma resemble those of extradural hematoma. However, there are differences. In the former, there is usually severe brain damage and persisting loss of consciousness without a lucid interval. In the elderly an acute subdural hematoma may follow a trivial injury. A CT scan is required for accurate diagnosis and surgery.

Acute intracerebral hematoma

This is uncommon. Usually cerebral laceration, contusion, edema and necrosis occur at the same time, compression being due to all these combined.

Secondary pathological changes

Apart from the trauma inflicted on the brain at the moment of impact, certain secondary pathological changes take place later, which may result in a further deterioration in the patient's condition. These changes include brain edema and respiratory failure.

Brain edema

The brain swells in response to any insult. The factors producing brain edema include the following:

- Hypotension or hypoxia can produce ischemia, resulting in cell death and consequent cytotoxic edema.
- Traumatic subarachnoid haemmorhage is the commonest cause of blocking the CSF pathways thus giving rise to hydrocephalus.
- Inappropriate secretion of antidiuretic hormone or the development of diabetic insipidus can alter fluid and electrolyte balance and aggravate cerebral edema.

The above changes separately or in combination can result in elevation of intracranial pressure.

Now, the cerebral perfusion pressure is the difference between mean arterial blood pressure and intracranial pressure. Thus, if the blood pressure remains unchanged, any rise in the intracranial pressure decreases the cerebral perfusion pressure; when the latter falls below 50mm Hg, cerebral perfusion is compromised. The resultant ischemia produces further brain edema. Thus a vicious circle is produced leading to increasing intracranial pressure, a deteriorating level of consciousness, and finally, irreversible damage to the brain.

If pressure in the supratentorial compartment continues to rise, the medial side of the temporal lobe herniates down through the tentorial opening and presses on the third cranial nerve. Also, it displaces the midbrain to the contralateral side, so that the opposite cerebral peduncle is indented by the free edge of the tentorium. Compression of the midbrain also blocks the flow of cerebrospinal fluid in the aqueduct which further raises the intracranial pressure. Thus the level of consciousness deteriorates, and on the same side as the compressing mass the pupil dilates and hemiparesis sets in.

Injury to the brain may occur either on the side of the blow to the head (coup), or on the opposite side (contrecoup).

Respiratory failure

Damage to the brain (and specially the brain stem) due to contusion, laceration, hematoma, or the resultant edema, may produce respiratory failure. This in turn causes more brain edema leading to irreversible changes. However, hyperventilation should not be employed, because this washes out CO_2, and a low pCO_2 reduces cerebral blood flow and produces ischemic damage.

Measures to minimize damage

These include the following:

- Because the brain is at risk from ischemic damage following injury, a normal cardiac output must be maintained.
- Hypotonic fluids should be avoided, because they may be drawn into the cerebral tissue and brain swelling increased.
- A rise in body temperature increases the metabolic demands of tissues and causes deterioration in the neurological state. In certain cases hypothermia may have to be employed to protect the brain from damage.

MANAGEMENT OF HEAD INJURY

Initial management

The attending doctor has four duties when faced with a case of head injury. These are known as the ABCD of head injury:

The **A**irway should be maintained.

Baseline observations should be made.

Complications should be anticipated.

Future action should be **D**etermined.

Airway

The most urgent and immediate duty is to clear and maintain the airway. Loose teeth, blood and vomit must be removed and the airway maintained by laying the patient semiprone, with the foot of the bed raised and an airway inserted. If the cough reflex is absent a cuffed endotracheal tube is required to prevent aspiration of saliva.

Baseline observations

Baseline observations must be made as soon as possible, so that any change of intracranial pressure can be appreciated. A careful history should be taken to ensure that conditions such as diabetic coma, subarachnoid hemorrhage or epilepsy have not caused the patient to fall, the head injury being a secondary event. The level of consciousness must be determined by the response of the patient to various stimuli defined by the *Glasgow Coma Scale* (Table 44.1). The lower the total of the score, the deeper the level of unconciousness and the severity of brain injury. *These parameters should be employed rather than ill-defined levels of consciousness* which mean different things to different people. If the patient is conscious, the length of amnesia before and after the accident must be assessed, as its duration is proportional to the severity of the head injury. The pulse, blood pressure, respiratory rate, temperature, and size and reaction of the pupils should be measured half-hourly.

Complications

Complications must be anticipated.

Determine future action

Future action must now be determined, about whether x-rays or CT scans are required, whether the patient needs to be admitted, and whether a neurosurgical consultation is called for.

Skull x-rays are required in the following situations:

- Loss of consciousness, or amnesia.
- Suspected fracture.
- CSF or blood from ear or nose.
- Neurological symptoms and signs.
- Difficulty in assessing the patient, e.g. if he is very young or drunk.

Anteroposterior and lateral *x-rays of the skull* are taken to show the site of a fissured or depressed fracture or lateral displacement of a calcified pineal gland. A lateral x-ray of the cervical spine is also essential. If the patient needs immediate intensive care, x-rays may be postponed.

The Glasgow coma scale may not accurately reflect the exact neurological status in:

- Children.
- Suspected base of skull fracture.
- CSF or blood from ear or nose.
- Neurological symptoms and signs masked if the patient is under the influence of alcohol.
- Difficulty in assessing the patient, e.g. if he is very young or drunk.

Admission

Admission is recommended in the following circumstances:

- Confusion or impaired level of consciousness.
- Skull fracture.
- Neurological symptoms and signs, e.g. headache, vomiting, seizures etc.
- Difficulty in assessing the patient.
- Difficult social or medical circumstances, e.g. no responsible adult with the patient.

In most cases overnight admission for observation is sufficient.

CT scan and neurological consultation

These are indicated in cases with:

- Skull fracture with confusion, focal neurological signs, or seizures.
- Depressed skull fracture.
- Penetrating fracture with leakage of CSF.
- Persistent confusion without skull fracture.
- Deterioration of level of consciousness.
- All patients with GCS below 9.

The most common cause of deterioration, shown by a declining level of consciousness, is raised intracranial pressure due to an intracranial hematoma, brain edema, or airway obstruction (which itself leads to brain edema).

Further course of action

The further course of action depends upon whether a CT scan is available or not:

A. CT scan is available

- If the CT scan is normal and physical examination shows no neurological deficit, the patient may be kept overnight or discharged. If he is allowed home, an accompanying person should be instructed to awaken the patient frequently over the next 24 hours to be certain that he remains arousable. Any deterioration in the level of consciousness should prompt re-evaluation.
- If the CT scan shows an *extradural* hematoma, urgent craniotomy is indicated. The journey to the neurosurgical centre can be hazardous, and the surgeon could decide to evacuate the hematoma before shifting the patient.

Evacuation of hematoma

If such a course is adopted, the appropriate side of the scalp is shaved. No local anesthetic is usually necessary.

Table 44.1 Glasgow Coma Scale (GCS)

The following parameters are recorded at regular intervals:

	Score
Eye opening	
None	1
To pain	2
To speech	3
Spontaneous	4
Verbal response	
None	1
Incomprehensible sounds	2
Inappropriate words	3
Confused	4
Orientated	5
Motor response	
None	1
Extends to pain	2
Flexes to pain	3
Withdraws to pain	4
Localizes pain	5
Obeys command	6
Total score	15

[*The Coma Score is the sum total of the sectional scores*]

Severe head injury	3–8
Moderate head injury	9–12
Minor head injury	13–15

A 5cm incision is made over the clot as shown by the CT scan; this is usually in the temporal region just above the zygomatic arch.The incision is made right down to bone. A mastoid retractor is now placed in position and will stop the scalp bleeding. The skull is just perforated using a perforator. This creates a conical hole and dark blood will ooze out. The hole is enlarged using a burr, when the hole becomes cylindrical and blood clot immediately bulges out. The clot is sucked away by a sucker which should, however, not be inserted into the cavity, as this can cause more bleeding as well as damage the brain. The patient can now be transferred to the neurosurgical service.

B. CT scan is not available

Here the decision about the best course of action will be more difficult. A feasible method would be to describe the findings of the history and physical examination to the neurosurgeon on the phone and seek his guidance according to the circumstances. The side of the hematoma may be decided by the shift of a calcified pineal gland on anteroposterior x-ray, the side of the first pupil to dilate or hemiparesis on the opposite side of the clot. The position of an exploratory burr hole is decided according to the site of the external injury and the site of the skull fracture. Exploratory burr holes can also be fashioned at the temporal, parietal and frontal regions in the absence of a CT scan. Ninety percent of hematomas are situated in these areas.

Postoperative management

After removal of any traumatic intracranial mass, the aim of management is to normalize the cerebral perfusion pressure and prevent secondary injury to the damaged brain. Intracranial pressure (ICP) monitoring may be indicated, specially in patients with marked depression or deterioration in neurological function. Because frequent examinations are not possible under general anesthesia, comatose patients who require emergency abdominal, thoracic or orthopedic surgery should also have ICP monitoring.

The following steps are also helpful:

- *Head elevation* facilitates venous drainage and reduces the intracranial pressure.
- *Sedation* reduces combative activity which elevates intracranial pressure.
- Prophylactic use of *anticonvulsants* prevents cerebral injury from seizures.
- Mild *dehdyration* protects the brain from insult due to fluid overload.
- *Prevention of hypotension* reduces the extension of ischemic injury. On the other hand aggressive treatment of hypertensive episodes reduces cerebral blood volume and causes further disruption of the blood-brain barrier.
- *Treatment of hyperthermia* avoids an increase in metabolic demands.

If intracranial pressure remains high despite these measures, mannitol (0.5 to 1.0 g/kg) can be used to reduce it. Mannitol is an osmotic diuretic which reduces brain swelling by drawing fluid from the extravascular spaces of the brain into the blood due to increase in the osmolality of the plasma.

The kidney function must be good. If diuresis does not occur, further administration is delayed. Furosemide (0.1mg/kg) can be used to supplement the action of mannitol; alone it is less effective.

Deep sedation with narcotics may be useful. Finally, there is no evidence that corticosteroids improve the outlook in severe head injury.

Nursing care

The nursing care of an unconscious patient is very detailed. Every physiological function of the body has to be supervised and aided:

- The eyes remain open, so they must be protected by bland ointments.
- A condom catheter obviates the necessity of passing a catheter into the bladder, yet the patient can be kept dry.
- Nasogastric tube feeding or intravenous infusions are necessary.
- Constipation develops, due to the small amount of residue which can be given to an unconscious patient in his diet; this requires management with enemas.
- The limb joints are put through their full range of movements daily, to prevent stiffness and contractures.
- If a tracheostomy has been performed, it requires to be taken care of; however, it is not often carried out, because an endotracheal tube may be used for upto a week.

FRACTURES OF THE SKULL

These are produced by two types of violence:

- Compression of the whole skull when it is distorted by hitting a hard, flat surface. This is the most common type of skull fracture.
- Local indentation, i.e. a depressed fracture.

Depressed fractures

A depressed fracture may result after a blow from two types of objects:

A large round object

A closed depression results (Fig.44.3). The brain is bruised but not penetrated. When the injury to the brain heals, the fibrous tissue in the scar may irritate the underlying brain and result in epilepsy. However, with this type of blow the chances of inciting epilepsy are low, being only about 4%.

A small round object

A compound depressed fracture results. The scalp is torn. The fractured bone lacerates the dura and brain. Infection may result. Epilepsy occurs in as many as 25% of these cases.

It may be noted that a hematoma in the scalp can simulate a depressed fracture, because clotted blood at the margin of the hematoma may feel like the edge of a depressed area. An x-ray may be required for differentiation.

Treatment

Operation is required if the fracture overlies the speech or motor areas, or if bone fragments have penetrated the dura mater. A flap of skull and overlying muscle is raised. The depressed bone is raised into position. The dura is opened. Bone fragments are carefully picked out. Removal of pulped brain is best carried out by irrigation with a stream of normal saline from a nozzle.

In the *newborn* pond shaped depressions may occur due to prolonged pressure of the head against the sacral promontory. Spontaneous elevation occurs within a few weeks, otherwise the fracture is elevated by making a small hole in the skull and hooking it up with an aneurysm needle introduced through the opening.

Compound fractures of the vault

These may be very severe, with escape of brain substance, and are commonly sustained as a result of high-speed motorcycle accidents. Crash helmets have helped reduce their incidence. Only skull x-rays give accurate information; probing of scalp wounds is dangerous. The x-ray should include the neck.

Fractures of the base of the skull

These are produced by compression of the skull with fissures radiating down from the vault. They become compound by opening into the middle ear, cribriform plate, or the different air sinuses.

Clinical features

The cranial contents i.e. cerebrospinal fluid or blood may escape from the ear or nose, and the cranial nerves may be damaged. Paralysis of nerves may occur immediately. If the paralysis recovers within a few weeks it suggests that it was due to compression from blood clot. If it does not recover, the cause was probably laceration of the nerve. If paralysis appears a few weeks after the injury, it means it has resulted from a scar or callus, and will not recover.

Epistaxis indicates the presence of a fracture of the cribriform plate. If the fracture extends into the roof of the orbit a *subconjunctival hemorrhage* results, the patch being wedge-shaped with the apex in front. Such a hemorrhage has to be distinguished from a 'black eye' resulting from a direct blow on the eye. In the case of a subconjunctival hemorrhage resulting from a fracture of the base of the skull, as the blood comes forwards from inside the orbit, the posterior limit of the hematoma cannot be seen (Fig.44.4); in the case of a black eye there is an area of white sclera behind it.

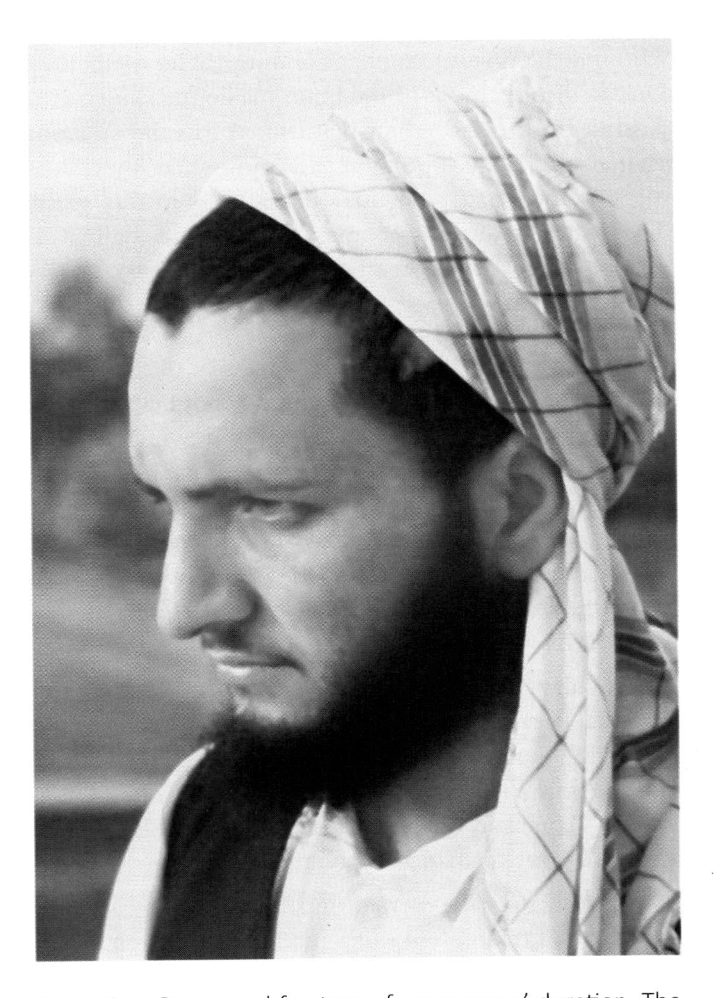

Fig.44.3 Depressed fracture of many years' duration. The fracture was caused by a large round object, so there was no penetration of the meninges by bony spicules. The patient had no neurological deficit.

Blood from the ear clots. If it does not, it is probable that it is mixed with cerebrospinal fluid, i.e. that a fracture into the roof of the middle ear is present.

Late effects of head injury

Chronic subdural 'hematoma'

Chronic subdural hematoma usually develops in an elderly person after a blow to the front or back of the head, who may be on anticoagulant or antiplatelet medicines. Due to displacement of the brain inside the skull, veins passing from the cerebral hemispheres to the superior sagittal sinus may rupture at the point where they cross the subdural space. A hematoma collects in this space. The fluid gradually becomes thinner and lighter in colour, and resembles cerebrospinal fluid (CSF).

Clinical features

Even a slight blow to the front or back of the skull may produce this lesion, so the patient may not have become unconscious at all, and this is a point which should be kept in mind. There is mental apathy going on to slowness of response to questions, and finally stupor. The stupor comes and goes, because the volume of the brain varies from time to time; the patient is inaccessible at times, but rouses to answer questions correctly though very slowly.

There may be no physical signs, specially in older patients, because by that age the brain shrinks in size, so that there is more room for the fluid to collect. There may be only an extensor plantar response on one or both sides. Changes in the size of the pupil occur late, when pressure-cone formation is about to occur.

A CT scan must be carried out if there is a reasonable suspicion of the presence of a subdural collection.

Treatment

Burr holes are made in the posterior parietal areas, when dirty ('machine oil') fluid gushes out. This is allowed to flow out, aided by lowering the head. The dura is left unsutured.

Post-traumatic epilepsy

The incidence of post-traumatic epilepsy varies from 2 to 26% in minor to severe head injury respectively.

Epilepsy occurring *soon after* injury does not indicate an intracranial hematoma. It is due to primary brain damage which may be slight and from which total recovery occurs. On the other hand *late* post-traumatic epilepsy indicates scarring in the cerebral cortex. In those patients who have suffered early epilepsy, and in major compound fractures with tears in the dura or intracranial hematomas, it is advisable to use anticonvulsant drugs prophylactically from 9 months upto 3 years.

The *outcome* after head injury depends on many factors. Predictors of a bad prognosis include increasing age, pre-existing illness, penetrating injury, delay in treatment and multiple trauma.

INTRACRANIAL ABSCESSES

Commonly, an intracranial abscess may be intracerebral or subdural; in the latter case it is called an empyema.

Intracerebral abscess

Etiology

A cerebral abscess may result from one of the following:

- *Implantation* from penetrating wounds: this is normally associated with a low mortality rate, because the organisms are usually derived from the skin and are not very virulent.
- *Metastases* from intrathoracic sepsis, specially subacute bacterial endocarditis, lung abscess, bronchiectasis or empyema. In these cases the septic embolus is lodged deep in the white matter close to the ventricle. Fatal septic ventriculitis can occur within a matter of days.
- *Local extension* due to septic thrombosis spreading from septic foci in the ear or frontal sinuses.
- Among patients with *compromised immunity*, either from an underlying illness such as HIV infection, or during pharmacological immunosuppression such as for organ transplantation.

Diagnosis

Evidence of infection at the above-mentioned sites in the chest and head and neck should be looked for. Fever and malaise may be followed by drowsiness and confusion, and later by localized weakness or seizures. Pyrexia is usually low-grade, with a moderate rise in the C-reactive protein. Later, along with signs of raised intracranial pressure, there may be localizing signs depending upon the site of the abscess.

Imaging

CT scan with contrast is the initial imaging method of choice. It demonstrates a well-defined ring-enhancing mass (enhancing with contrast) with a thin smooth wall. Diffusion-weighted MRI is valuable by indicating hypoxic edema.

Management

Urgent *surgical* drainage is the mainstay of treatment of a cerebral abscess. This can be carried out by needle aspiration through a burr hole. This should be repeated until no more pus is obtained. If aspiration fails because the capsule is too thick, craniotomy and excision of the abscess is necessary.

Broad-spectrum *antibiotics* are started intravenously. When the culture report arrives, they may be changed to those shown to be effective against the isolated organisms; they are later on given orally, for a total period of six weeks. Prophylactic anticonvulsants should be given to anticipate the common occurrence of seizures. The cause of the infection also requires treatment; this is often frontal sinus disease, middle ear infection, or congenital heart disease.

With early treatment, mortality is in single digits, if the abscess ruptures into a ventricle it is 80%; hence the importance of early diagnosis and treatment.

Subdural empyema

Infections of the frontal sinus or accessory air cells may result in septic thrombophlebitis of the superior sagittal sinus. From here, pus may reach the subdural space through the superior cerebral veins, resulting in a subdural abscess. In other cases open contamination of the subdural space takes place at operation or after trauma. Staphylococci, streptococci, and anaerobic cocci are commonly responsible. Once the subdural space is entered, infection can spread over the whole surface of the brain. The clinical features are similar to those of cerebral abscess and meningitis.

CT scan shows a hypodense subdural collection, with contrast enhancement at the margins, and some shift of the midline. Lumbar puncture should not be carried out because herniation can occur.

Treatment

The collection is drained through a craniotomy, at the same time relieving the raised intracranial pressure. If the pus is recent, burrhole drainage may suffice.

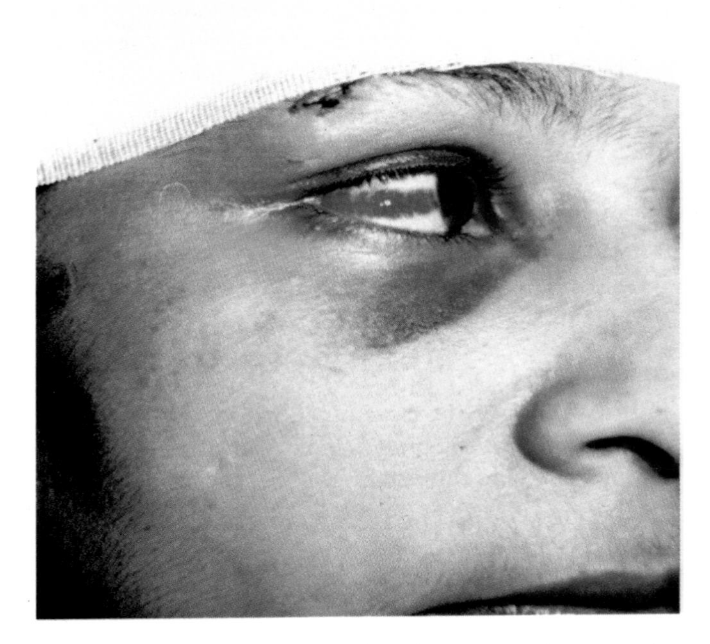

Fig.44.4 Fracture of base of skull. Note red blood under conjunctiva whose posterior limit cannot be seen, purple blood confined within orbital margin, and lacerated wound eyebrow covered by a bandage.

BRAIN TUMORS

Commonest tumors

The most common brain tumors are metastases. The common *primary* brain tumors are gliomas, meningiomas, pituitary adenomas and vestibular schwannomas.

The commonest *pediatric* brain tumors are medulloblastoma, ependymoma and cerebellar astrocytoma.

Clinical features

Every tumor has an *initial silent period*. If it is in a 'silent' area it will produce no symptoms until the intracranial pressure rises and headache and vomiting starts.

Intracranial tumors exert *both local and generalized effects* by their presence within a closed bony structure:

- *Local* effects of a tumor are either irritative or destructive. Irritation of adjacent cortex results in focal seizures, while compression of nearby brain tissue produces a focal neurological deficit.
- *Generalized* effects are produced by the raised intracranial pressure (ICP) due to the presence of the mass. The raised ICP may provide the only evidence of the presence of a tumor, or it may occur along with focal symptoms.

In *frontal* lobe tumors pressure symptoms occur late. *Temporal* and *parietal* lobe tumors obstruct the outflow from the corresponding ventricle, so symptoms may occur earlier. Similarly, *posterior fossa* tumors obstruct the flow of fluid from both ventricles, so that pressure symptoms arise very early. There is headache, vomiting, papilloedema, bradycardia and retarded cerebration. The vomiting of raised intracranial pressure is not preceded by nausea, and occurs without warning. Only 5–15% of patients with brain tumors present with epilepsy.

A few patients present only when cone formation is imminent. When the intracranial pressure inside a supratentorial compartment rises, the inner border of a cerebral hemisphere may be forced under the falx cerebri. The temporal lobe may be forced down into the tentorial opening. Further, the cerebellar tonsils may be pushed down into the foramen magnum. The pathways for cerebrospinal fluid absorption being blocked, the pressure rises abruptly. Signs of a threatened cone include violent paroxsymal headache, drowsiness, slow pulse and neck stiffness. Dilatation of one pupil is an urgent sign. Lumbar puncture must be avoided at this stage.

- *Meningeal irritation* may arise due to bleeding in, or malignant infiltration of, the subarachnoid space.
- *Other* signs may be present, e.g. a primary tumor elsewhere (lung or breast), or an endocrine disorder due to a pituitary tumor.

Investigations

History-taking, general examination in search of primary disease, and neurological examination must be carried out precisely and thoroughly.

X-rays

X-rays of the skull and chest, and ESR/CRP, are essential investigations in every case. The chest x-ray may show an unsuspected bronchial carcinoma as the primary tumor. On x-ray of the skull:

- Due to the *raised intracranial pressure*, the posterior clinoid processes may be eroded. At the same time, the pressure of tight convolutions on the inner table of the skull may produce a beaten-silver appearance.
- A bulky tumor in one supratentorial compartment may have caused lateral displacement of a *calcified pineal* body.
- Astrocytomas, angiomas, meningiomas, etc. may show characteristic *calcification*.

CT scan and MRI

These clearly show up a tumor when present. Meningiomas appear densely white. Gliomas are less dense. Astrocytoma cysts show as dark areas. Secondary tumors appear as multiple shadows. MRI and CT angiography have replaced carotid angiography.

General management

General management of brain tumors varies according to the clinical condition, associated symptoms, and the age of the patient.

Intracranial pressure

If the raised intracranial pressure is not urgently relieved, the outcome may be rapidly fatal. Severe headache and a deteriorating level of consciousness are ominous signs.

Intracranial pressure may be lowered by the following measures:

- *Mannitol* may be administered. Being an osmotic diuretic, it causes dehydration and thus extracts fluid from the CSF.
- *Dexamethasone* is most useful in those malignant gliomas and secondary tumors which have undergone necrosis. In these cases reduction of edema may restore a comatose patient to consciousness and eliminate the signs of paralysis. Regular administration of dexamethasone may prolong life. Dexamethasone also reduces the edema occurring during deep x-ray therapy.
- In case of supratentorial and posterior fossa tumors causing hydrocephalus, before operation the dilated ventricles may need either a ventriculo-peritoneal shunt or an emergency external ventricular drain. With supratentorial cysts or abscesses, the cavity of the cyst or abscess itself may be tapped.

Surgery

Surgery on the tumor itself can only be performed safely if the pressure is normal. To guard against postoperative epileptic fits, anticonvulsant therapy is started two days prior to surgery. At the same time, because of the risk of epileptic seizures the patient should not drive a vehicle for a period of one year after surgery for a supratentorial tumor.

Individual tumors

Gliomas

These account for over 50% of central nervous system tumors in adults, and most are supratentorial. They are divided into four histological grades. Grade 4 gliomas (glioblastoma multiforme) present with a history of a few weeks. They show a good initial response to steroids but carry a poor prognosis.

Treatment usually involves a combination of surgery and radiotherapy. In very large tumors surgical reduction of tumor mass is performed as a precursor to radiotherapy, which may take the form of:

- External beam irradiation (5000cGy over 5 weeks).
- Stereotactic focal irradiation using a linear accelerator.
- Cyber knife
- Proton beam.

Chemotherapy has limited application.

Meningiomas

Meningiomas are usually benign, but occasionally anaplastic varieties occur. They arise from the meninges and produce a mass effect from the tumor. They are best visualized by CT with contrast or MRI with gadolinium.

Treatment

Surgical resection

Meningiomas are best treated by resection, including the dura at the site of attachment of the tumor. In patients with large vascular tumors, preoperative transarterial embolization is employed; it helps reduce the blood supply and facilitates dissection. Careful preoperative preparation, microsurgical dissection and specialized postoperative care produce a very low operative mortality and morbidity. Very large meningiomas are best removed in stages.

Radiotherapy

Small tumors that are situated away from critical structures can be treated by radiotherapy.

Medulloblastomas

These are treated, after staging by MRI, by complete surgical excision followed by craniospinal irradiation. Combination chemotherapy provides a valuable adjunct. Despite aggressive surgery, radiotherapy and chemotherapy, patients treated for medulloblastoma have a survival rate of 65% at 7 years, falling to 40% at 10 years.

Vestibular schwannomas

These arise in the cerebellopontine angle and present with hearing loss, tinnitus and loss of balance.

Single metastasis

A metastatic tumor, if single and in an accessible site, can be excised with excellent symptomatic relief. Radiotherapy (3000cGy over 14 days) is used after such an excision, as well as for multiple metastases.

Tumors of the pituitary body

Tumors of the pituitary arise from one of the types of cells present in the organ. Thus they comprise three varieties of adenoma: chromophobe, acidophil and basophil. Apart from these, congenital tumors derived from Rathke's pouch are seen from time to time.

Chromophobe adenoma

This tumor commonly occurs in females between twenty and fifty years of age. It grows slowly over many years. It compresses the acidophil and basophil cells of the anterior pituitary, affecting the production of thyrotrophic and gonadotrophic hormones. The patient becomes fat and sluggish, and amenorrhoea sets in. Pressure by the enlarging tumor on the diaphragma sellae causes severe headache. The tumor then breaks through the diaphragm and presses on the decussating fibres of the optic chiasma causing bitemporal hemianopia. Finally, massive extension with raised intracranial pressure or epilepsy occurs.

Acidophil adenoma

This tumor is small in size. In children it causes gigantism, in adults acromegaly.

Basophil adenomas

These tumors are also small and produce Cushing's syndrome.

Prolactinoma

This is a benign tumor of the pituitary that produces a hormone called prolactin. Patients suffering from this tumor present with secondary amenorrhea and galactorrhea. Serum prolactin levels are usually high, 500ngm/dl.

Initial *management* is medical, and the most effective drug is bromocriptine, a dopamine agonist. It shrinks the tumor and brings prolactin levels to normal in 80% patients. However, if the patient does not respond, transphenoidal resection remains the best surgical procedure.

Diagnosis

The presence of most pituitary adenomas can be ascertained by MRI scanning. At the same time, tumors can be identified by an increase in the serum levels of the hormones produced by them, e.g. growth hormone, cortisol, and prolactin.

Differential diagnosis

Other lesions that may enlarge the pituitary fossa include craniopharyngiomas, meningiomas and metastatic tumors. All these lesions can produce hypopituitarism and visual loss, and the diagnosis is usually confirmed only at operation.

Treatment

Surgical

Most pituitary tumors can be successfully operated upon by the trans-sphenoidal route. The surgeon incises the septal mucosa in the nasal vestibule and approaches the sella turcica by a submucosal route along the nasal septum, reaching the pituitary fossa via the sphenoidal sinus. Even large tumors can be almost totally removed.

Medical

Medical management is possible for prolactinomas with bromocriptine, which inhibits prolactin secretion and reduces tumor size. Very ill patients with Cushing's syndrome who are not fit for surgery may be treated by agents that suppress cortisol synthesis, such as ketaconazole. However, the drug is not always well tolerated and is not the first line therapy for the ordinary patient with Cushing's disease.

Pituitary apoplexy

Pituitary apoplexy is bleeding into or ischemia of the pituitary gland, usually in the presence of a tumor of the pituitary, this is a clinical condition in which there is either haemmorhage or ischemia of the pituitary. Most of these patients present in a comatose condition. Immediate intensive care therapy, corticosteroids, and fluid and electrolyte replacement are required before transphenoidal surgical decompression.

HYDROCEPHALUS

Hydrocephalus implies an increase in the volume of CSF due to disturbance of production, flow or reabsorption of CSF. It may be congenital or acquired. If the ventricles communicate freely with the subarachnoid space the hydrocephalus is described as communicating; if they are sealed off at some point, it is non-communicating.

Congenital hydrocephalus

The most common cause of this condition is failure of development of arachnoid villi. A few cases are due to obstruction of the CSF pathway. This may be due to the Arnold-Chiari malformation, in which the roof of the fourth ventricle lies below the foramen magnum and there is obstruction of the exit foramina; or it may be due to congenital stenosis of the aqueduct of Sylvius.

Clinical features

The head may be enlarged before birth and produce obstructed labour. After birth rapid enlargement occurs. The fontanelles widen. The forehead bulges forward. The ventricles dilate enormously. The cortex is reduced to a mere shell, but remarkably, there are no motor symptoms. Intelligence may be preserved in spite of the enormous size of the head.

Hydrocephalus in children may be associated with spina bifida with spinal dysraphism. In spinal dysraphism the cord is tethered by a fibrous cord. During growth this fibrous cord exerts traction on the spinal cord, leading to a neurological deficit.

Acquired hydrocephalus

Non-communicating hydrocephalus

This occurs due to obstruction of the ventricles by tumor or inflammation.

Communicating hydrocephalus

- This usually follows inflammation and complicates meningitis.
- It may be due to blockage of the cisterns by organizing subarachnoid hemorrhage.

Diagnosis

To diagnose hydrocephalus some degree of ventricular enlargement must be demonstrated:

- During infancy, while the fontanelle is open, cranial *ultrasound* is useful for the detection of ventricular enlargement.
- In older patients *CT or MRI* are employed for the purpose.

The cause may be evident from the history, or from the presence of subarachnoid hemorrhage or meningitis. Further imaging may be required to identify a tumor.

Treatment

- If a tumor is the cause of the hydrocephalus it is removed if possible.
- ***Shunts***. For hydrocephalus due to other causes a shunting procedure is used:
  - o *Ventriculoperitoneal shunt*. The proximal end of a fine catheter is placed in the dilated lateral ventricle through a small drill hole in the skull. It is passed beneath the scalp, where it connects with a valve (Holter valve). A further tube is then passed under the skin and into the peritoneal cavity, which is entered through a small incision over the anterior abdomen.
  - o *Ventriculoatrial shunt*. Less commonly, the catheter is led via the neck veins into the right atrium. The valve allows flow of the fluid in only one direction, i.e. away from the ventricles.

These tubes are foreign bodies and liable to become infected and blocked. However, the ventriculoperitoneal and ventriculoatrial shunts are satisfactory treatment for hydrocephalus irrespective of its cause.

- ***Endoscopic third ventriculostomy***. This is useful in obstructive hydrocephalus due to aqueduct stenosis. A neuroendoscope is passed through the frontal horn of the lateral ventricle and through the foramen of Monro into the third ventricle. It pushes further to open the floor of the ventricle into the subarachnoid space, and is then removed. The third ventricle now drains freely into the subarachnoid space without the need of an implanted tubing with its risk of infection. However, the route sometimes becomes blocked; a shunt is then needed.

Acute hydrocephalus is an emergency as it can progress rapidly to dangerous levels. If a tumor is responsible it should be removed urgently, otherwise temporary ventricular drainage should be instituted.

Brain hemorrhage

Primary brain hemorrhage

The vast majority (90%) of these patients are hypertensive. The hemorrhage occurs because of a miliary aneurysm. Most of these hemorrhages are treated conservatively, only those with signs of raised intracranial pressure or focal signs being operated upon.

Subarachnoid hemorrhage

In 90% of cases subarachnoid hemorrahge occurs in non-hypertensive patients; however, if they are hypertensive, the prognosis is bad. The hemorrhage is usually secondary to rupture of aneurysms or arteriovenous malformations.

Aneurysms

Most (90%) of these aneurysms are on the anterior circulation (internal carotid, anterior cerebral or anterior communicating arteries). Only 10% are situated on the posterior circulation. Most of them occur between the ages of 35 and 55.

Arteriovenous malformations

These are developmental abnormalities in the vasculature of the brain, wherein plexuses of arteriovenous communications are formed. They commonly bleed during youth to produce neurological deficits depending on their location. They may be found incidentally during cerebral angiography for another condition; alternatively, attention may be drawn to them after a bleed.

Due to a blood pressure lower than in the arterial hemorrhages of stroke in old people, the bleeds are smaller, the neurological deficits more circumscribed, and recovery more likely. The likelihood of bleeding is reported between 2 and 6% per year, which amounts to a considerable figure during a lifetime. Therefore treatment is mandatory.

Investigations

CT angiography is the best method of investigation for localizing these lesions. However MRI scan is quite useful in diagnosing the mural nodule in arteriovenous malformations.

Management

If found incidentally, AVMs should be eradicated using one or more of the same methods as required after a bleed; these consist of:

- Endovascular embolization, to cause clotting and obliteration of the plexus from within. This works best in the smaller malformations. A catheter is inserted into the femoral artery and passed up the cerebral circulation to the aneurysm. Coils are pushed into the aneurysm, where they cause thrombosis.
- Microneurosurgery, to excise the plexus in toto and ligate its draining vein. This is suitable for the more superficial lesions and eliminates chances of re-bleed.
- Radiosurgery ('cyberknife'), a very advanced technique in which the robotic arm of a linear accelerator directs extremely fine beams of radiation from hundreds of directions, so that radiation to any point in the brain in minimal, yet the lesion gets a big dose within seconds. This ensures that:
  - Large doses of radiation to the surrounding brain matter are not delivered, almost completely avoiding the considerable side effects of conventional radiotherapy.
  - The treatment is completed in a single sitting instead of the weekly sittings of the past spread over months.

In certain patients a multimodality regime may be employed. Successful treatment reduces the chances of re-bleeds very greatly.

Parkinson's disease

This is a condition commonly seen in the elderly in which the neurons that produce dopamine in the substantia nigra, a part of the midbrain, start dying. The lack of dopamine leads to tremors, muscle rigidity and difficulty of gait.

Treatment

Medical treatment consists of the use of dopamine agonists. Surgically, deep brain stimulation has been introduced recently.

Deep brain stimulation (DBS)

In this technique 'brain pacemakers' are implanted, through drill holes in the skull at appropriate sites, into specific nuclei of the brain, for the treatment of Parkinson's disease and other disorders of movement. The lead wire is led to a battery which is placed subcutaneously in the chest of the patient. The target neurons get electrically stimulated to produce dopamine; this relieves the symptoms. However, being a new method, it requires long-term evaluation.

Chapter

45 SPINE, SPINAL CORD AND NERVES

Vertebral column

There are two main reasons for the importance of injuries to the vertebral column (the 'spine'). Firstly, this is the central part of the skeleton and deformity in this part has deleterious consequences for the patient. Secondly, injuries to the vertebral column are often associated with damage to the spinal cord, with paralysis of the limbs and/or the bladder.

DISLOCATIONS

True dislocations of the vertebral column are most common in the cervical region, where the surfaces of the articular processes lie nearly horizontally. In the dorsal and lumbar regions the vertical direction of the articular processes results in their being fractured.

During *hanging*, the atlas dislocates forwards over the axis. Either the odontoid process gets fractured or the transverse ligament of the atlas is ruptured, allowing forward displacement of the atlas. In this way the space in the vertebral canal is greatly reduced, the brain stem gets crushed, and death results from paralysis of the respiratory muscles.

During a *head injury* the base of the odontoid process may be cracked, and yet displacement may only occur after several days. If occipital pain persists after a head injury, x-ray of the odontoid process should be taken through the open mouth.

Dislocations of the *cervical vertebrae* commonly occur by falls on the head from a motorcycle or diving into shallow water, and affect the lower cervical spine due to its greater mobility. The inferior articular process of the upper vertebra is forced forwards over the upper margin of the superior process of the lower vertebra. If a facet on one side is dislocated forwards, a lateral x-ray shows a forward movement of nearly a quarter of the diameter of the vertebral body; if facets on both sides are dislocated, then over half the diameter. In the latter situation the narrowing of the vertebral canal causes serious neurological effects. Pain is felt in the neck and may be referred along a local nerve root due to pressure. Neck movements are restricted. Posterior tenderness is due to rupture of the interspinous ligament.

Treatment

If cervical spine injury is suspected, the neck should be protected by pillows on either side until x-rays have been taken. If dislocation is present, it should be reduced as soon as possible, but if there is evidence of cord involvement the situation constitutes an emergency.

Traction should be applied to the skull under local anesthesia, using skull tongs or a halo apparatus. The weights are increased under x-ray control upto 16kg. When the facets disengage, weights are reduced to about 4kg. If this fails, closed manipulation or open reduction will be required.

FRACTURES

Fractures and dislocations of the spine follow major trauma such as motor vehicle accidents or falls from a height. Seen from the standpoint of stability, the vertebral column is considered to be composed of three columns:

- The anterior column consists of the vertebral bodies, discs and longitudinal ligaments.
- The intermediate column contains the facet joints and their ligaments.
- The posterior column consists of the spinous processes and interspinous ligaments.

If all three columns are disrupted, the situation is extremely unstable. If on the other hand only one column is interrupted the spine may be regarded as stable.

Stable fractures

These do not interfere with the continuity of the spinal column. Examples include:

- Fractures of the *spinous and transverse processes*, which usually occur due to direct violence. Fractures of the transverse processes occur commonly in the lumbar region, where the corresponding kidney may also be injured.
- *Compression* fractures of the vertebral bodies. These usually occur due to a fall on the buttocks or the heels.
- Fractures of the *laminae or pedicles*. These may be accompanied by traumatic intraspinal hemorrhage *(hematomyelia)*. The bleeding may occur in the cord itself and cause flaccid paralysis by destroying the anterior horn cells; or it may occur outside the cord and cause root irritation.

Unstable fractures

Fracture-dislocations

These produce complete disruption of the vertebral column. There is rupture of the interspinous ligament, fracture or dislocation of the facet joints, and a fracture through the vertebral body. These injuries occur commonly at the dorsolumbar region, and only rarely in the neck. Damage to the spinal cord or cauda equina is seen in many cases. In most cases the injury occurs between T12 and L1, and classically from a flexion and rotation force, as in a motorcyclist thrown into the air and landing on one shoulder. The diagnosis is made on the basis of the history of flexion-rotation injury, the displacement, and the palpable gap between the spinous processes.

X-rays usually show a horizontal 'slice' fracture passing through the upper part of the vertebral body with forward displacement of the upper vertebra on the lower, along with increased space between the spinous processes at the affected level.

Treatment

Most unstable injuries in this region are accompanied by damage to the spinal cord and nerve roots. The T12/L1 interspace is level with the first sacral segment of the cord, so injury at this level can affect the cord only from the first sacral segment downwards. However, the lumbar nerve roots can also be damaged as they pass the lesion, so classically injury at this level consists of a lower motor neurone lesion of the lumbar segments along with an upper motor neurone lesion of the sacral segments.

Most of the damage is inflicted at the moment of injury. Therefore laminectomy for the purpose of general decompression is of no value; in fact, because it increases the instability of the spine, it is contraindicated. Prompt reduction of the dislocation is more effective in relieving pressure. If the displacement is minimal, alignment may be preserved by simple recumbency; if it is significant, open reduction with internal fixation is preferred.

Titanium cages

If the spine is unstable and needs fusion, titanium cages can be used. These are hollow metallic cylinders with screw-like threads on the surface, so that they can simply be screwed in place in the disc space. The walls of the cages are fenestrated and allow the bone to grow from the vertebral body through the cage and into the next vertebral body, thus fusing the metal and bone into a single mass. The cages offer excellent fixation, so most patients do not need post-operative back braces for support. The cages can be inserted through a minilaparotomy or through a posterior approach.

PROLAPSE OF INTERVERTEBRAL DISC

Each intervertebral disc consists of a central portion of spongy material, the nucleus pulposus, and a tough fibrous ring, the annulus fibrosus. During normal flexion of the spine the disc is deformed and bulges backwards slightly into the neural canal. If a strong flexion force occurs it ruptures the annulus. Portions of the annulus and nucleus escape into the spinal canal and compress the nerve roots. In four-fifths of cases the protrusion follows upon trauma due to a severe strain; in one-fifth it is degenerative.

Protrusions occur commonly in the most mobile portions of the spine. 80% occur in the lumbar region at L4/5 and L5/S1 levels, and 19% in the cervical region at C5/6 and C6/7 levels. Only 1% occur in the immobile dorsal spine. Most disc herniations are posterolateral because of the presence of the posterior longitudinal ligament in the midline, and consequently the symptoms are usually unilateral. They are uncommon in old people, probably because of age-dependent loss of water content and disc volume.

Lumbar disc protrusion

At first there is low back pain due to injury to the disc. Later, when nerve roots are compressed the pain radiates to the leg. There is root pain, increased on coughing, in the distribution of the affected nerve. Paraesthesias, tenderness in muscles, with sensory loss and motor weakness also occur. The most common roots involved are L5 and S1. Therefore the pain is usually in the back and side of the leg radiating to the sole of the foot, and is called *radicular pain*. Sensory loss occurs on the sole and outer side of the foot. The ankle jerk is lost.

Straight leg raising test

Attempts at passively raising the straight leg are painful due to stretching of the sciatic nerve (*Straight leg raising test*). The more severe the condition, the smaller the angle through which the straight leg can be raised without causing pain.

Other causes of radicular pain include:

- *Nerve root compression* by tumor, abscess or osteophyte.
- *Peripheral nerve compression* within the pelvis or gluteal area by tumor, abscess or hematoma.

Imaging

Plain x-rays

These cannot highlight soft tissue lesions; however, they are still used:

- To confirm or exclude other possibilities such as tumors, infections, fractures, etc.
- Inexpensively confirm the suspicion of the presence of a herniated disc. If a suspicion is strengthened by x-rays, *MRI* may be used to provide final confirmation.

MRI

This shows the soft tissues—spinal cord, nerve roots and surrounding areas—better than a CT scan, and its T2-weighted images provide the most conclusive evidence of a disc herniation.

Electromyogram and nerve conduction studies

These tests measure the electrical impulse along nerves and muscles. They indicate whether a nerve is damaged or is healing from a previous injury.

Treatment

- Two-thirds of the patients with simple sciatica settle with 6 to 8 weeks of *bed rest*.
- *Epidural steroid* injections may help a few.
- *Microdiscectomy*. For those in whom conservative treatment has failed, mirodiscectomy is the standard treatment. Through a 4cm incision the ligamentum flavum is incised. The prolapsed disc fragment is removed, the disc space cleared, and the wound closed.

Cauda equina syndrome

Some times a sudden prolapsed disc at the lumbosacral region gives rise to a syndrome characterized by saddle anesthesia (gluteal region), retention of urine and constipation or unilateral foot drop. This is an acute neurosurgical emergency and needs immediate surgery.

Cervical disc protrusions

These are relatively uncommon. In many cases the diagnosis is mistakenly made in cases of cervical spondylosis or referred pain from a cervical strain.

Cervical spondylosis

In old age the neck is not as supple and flexible as during youth. The difference is due to the presence of cervical spondylosis in the old person's spine. In this condition the intervertebral discs are degenerate. Also, osteophytes form at the postero-lateral corners of the vertebral bodies and project backwards into the intervertebral foramina. The condition may be symptomless or may cause neurological manifestations. Sudden strain on the spine may cause referred pain and muscle spasm in the occipital or post-auricular regions, along the trapezius, and between the scapulae.

Investigations

Because spondylosis as seen on x-rays is common and often asymptomatic, no investigation can substitute for a careful history and examination. Plain lateral x-rays, taken *in flexion and extension*, help in excluding other diseases as well as allowing assessment of the size of the vertebral canal and range of movement of cervical spine and intervertebral joints.

Treatment

Symptoms are relieved by wearing a collar, because it restricts movement. If they persist in a severe form, anterior cervical fusion is occasionally required. Compression of nerve roots may be caused by osteophytes in the intervertebral foramina. This may require excision of the back of these foramina by removal of the anterior half of the concerned articular facets (hemifacetectomy).

Spondylolisthesis

In this condition the body of the fifth (or occasionally fourth) lumbar vertebra gets separated from the laminae and spine due to a defect in the pedicles, remaining attached merely by thick fibrous tissue. The body slips forwards and carries with it the whole of the upper portion of the spine. The spinal canal is not narrowed, but root pressure can cause sciatica. There is long-standing low back pain.

Treatment

Rest and analgesics are required. A stiff corset may be needed in some patients. Surgical treatment is reserved for patients who:

- Fail conservative measures.
- Have disabling back pain.

- Have slips greater than 50 percent.
- Have multiple risk factors.

The most commonly used procedure is bilateral posterolateral fusion in situ, i.e. without attempting reduction of the slip.

Tumors of the vertebral column

Both *benign tumors* and *primary malignant neoplasms* are quite rare.

Secondary deposits are much more common. Most come from carcinoma of the breast or prostate.

A *neuroblastoma* of the sympathetic chain may protrude through an intervertebral foramen and compress the spinal cord. Severe local pain results. It later becomes girdle in type when the nerves get involved. The next stage is vertebral collapse and paraplegia, but deep x-ray therapy at the early stage may prevent it.

Secondaries from the prostate respond promptly to stilboesterol. Those from the breast regress with hormones or aminoglutethimide.

Spinal cord

SPINAL CORD INJURY

Traumatic injury to the spinal cord may result from vertebral fracture, fracture/subluxation, and penetrating injuries such as gunshot or stab wounds. The spinal cord gets injured due to one of the following types of lesion:

- Long-axis stretch causing concussion or rupture of nerve fibres and vessels within the cord, as seen in acute flexion injuries with severe compression fractures.
- The cord getting nipped between the lamina of the upper vertebra and the body of the lower vertebra, as commonly encountered in fracture-dislocations.

The spinal cord ends at the lower border of the body of the first lumbar vertebra, so injuries below this level damage only the cauda equina.

Injuries at different levels.

The effects produced by injuries at the various levels differ from each other:

- Injuries to the *neck* commonly cause dislocation. Here the neural canal is spacious, so cord injury may be slight or absent.
- The *dorsal* spine is strong and relatively immobile and can be broken only by major forces such as collapse of a roof. Displacement is marked and the space is limited, so cord injury usually results, and is severe.
- The *lumbar* spine is strong and has vertical articular processes. Therefore only major forces are able to break it and produce fracture-dislocations. The lumbar theca is spacious, so nerve injury may be absent or limited to a few roots of the cauda equina.

Different degrees of damage to the spinal cord

During injuries to the vertebral column the spinal cord may suffer concussion or partial or complete contusion.

Spinal concussion

When the vertebral column is acutely flexed the spinal cord gets stretched. This displaces the neurons and synapses so that synaptic conduction is disturbed. So all those functions which depend upon synaptic activity are lost below the level of the lesion:

- Each anterior horn cell receives hundreds of synapses. Stimuli passing through these maintain the *central excitatory state* which keeps the cell ready to respond for voluntary movement, muscle tone and reflex activity. Therefore, loss of the central excitatory state causes complete loss of all these three functions below the lesion, producing a flaccid paralysis and retention of urine.
- *Pain and temperature* sensation cross a synapse in the inferior sensory decussation and are therefore lost.
- *Joint position* sense ascends the posterior columns without a synapse, and is therefore preserved.

Recovery

- If the injury is merely spinal concussion, voluntary power and sensation return within one or two days.
- If concussion is superimposed on an underlying partial or complete cord injury, the stage of spinal shock is likely to be prolonged; the longer this stage, the less likely is recovery to occur.
- If a mass reflex appears, usually at three to six weeks, it indicates that no recovery is likely.

Partial or complete contusion of the cord.

This results from the cord being crushed between the lamina of the vertebra above and the body of the vertebra below. It produces a transverse zone of contusion and bruising. Oedema may cause a rise in the level of paralysis. Any damage inflicted on the cord is permanent.

Clinical features

Spinal fracture and cord injury should be suspected in patients with head injuries and multiple injuries. It is best to assume that the spine is unstable and immobilize the patient on a backboard with a hard cervical collar until careful examination has been made.

Clinical findings of spinal cord injury include spinal tenderness, weakness of the limbs, numbness or paraesthesia, respiratory embarrassment, and hypotension. Spinal root involvement produces sensory and motor impairment in the corresponding dermatome and myotome.

A *complete cord lesion* produces absence of reflexes, flaccidity, anesthesia, and autonomic paralysis below the level of the lesion. If the transection is above T5, hypotension occurs due to the loss of sympathetic vascular tone.

Spinal shock results immediately from *a long axis stretch* of the spinal cord. There is flaccid paralysis below the lesion and retention of urine.

In the early stages cord contusion can be diagnosed:

- If there is complete loss of all sensation below the lesion.
- If the level of sensory loss and paralysis rises after the injury.
- If the stage of spinal shock persists for more than forty-eight hours.

In cord contusion the *clinical course* falls into three stages:

- The stage of spinal shock.
- The stage of reflex activity.
- The stage of septic complications, including urinary tract infections and bedsores.

MANAGEMENT OF SPINAL CORD INJURIES

Prevention

Injury to the cervical spine is most common in contact sports such as rugby, football and wrestling, besides some non-contact sports like gymnastics, diving and horse-riding. In athletes, high-risk manoeuvres such as spear-headed tackling should be avoided. Strict adherence to rules prohibiting such dangerous moves reduce the incidence of quadruplegia by more than 70 percent. At the same time, helmets providing for protection of the head as well as the cervical spine should be used.

Treatment

The objectives of treatment are to correct spinal alignment, protect undamaged tissues, restore function to reversibly damaged neural tissues, and achieve permanent spinal stability. To achieve these, reduction and immobilization of a fracture/dislocation must receive top priority.

A: The stage of spinal shock

In the stage of spinal shock care is taken to avoid unnecessary movement or examination which might increase the cord damage.

First aid treatment

Cervical injuries are transported lying on the back with the head supported between pillows without flexion. Dorsal and lumbar fractures are transported with the patient face down. The patient should be turned onto a stretcher by *at least three persons controlling the head, trunk and pelvis,* to avoid torsion of the spine---'the log roll'. Sedation should be given to relieve pain and anxiety.

Examination

At the hospital the sensory level to pin-prick on the trunk is tested, in order to define the segmental level of the lesion, and to test whether the patient can recognize movement of the foot or knee. If he can, the case is one of concussion. If all sensations are lost, the outlook is grave. A lateral x-ray of the corresponding level of the vertebral column is taken without disturbing the patient. The utmost gentleness is necessary to prevent further injury to a partially damaged cord.

Reduction and immobilization

Cervical spine

Cervical spine injuries are managed as described under dislocations in the preceding section.

Dorsal spine

- Simple *wedge compression* fractures are very stable. Symptomatic treatment is given and early mobilization carried out.
- In *fracture-dislocations* the cord is often transected. The fracture is stable due partly to the support of the rib cage, and surgery is almost never indicated. Treatment is that of the paraplegia itself.

Lumbar spine

- If there is only minimal displacement, postural nursing is enough.
- If severe displacement is present open reduction is

required. The spine is next stabilized by plates bolted to the spinous processes.

- If there is no paraplegia the patient can be mobilized in a plaster jacket. If paraplegia is present plaster is avoided, as it results in pressure sores.

Indications for early operation

These include the following:

- A penetrating injury with or without a CSF leak.
- Inability to reduce the fracture/dislocation satisfactorily by closed methods.
- Severe compression of the spinal cord by an intraspinal mass shown by MRI.
- Neurological deterioration in a patient with an incomplete cord lesion initially.

Nursing

Air mattress

To prevent bedsores the patient is nursed on an air mattresss divided into cells. An electrical air pump fills and empties alternate cells every few minutes so that no part of the skin is under continuous pressure. Such an air mattress has revolutionized the care of the bedridden patient.

The skin is dried and powdered. The patient is turned every two hours to prevent local pressure. Laxatives or enemas are given to empty the bowels. Breathing exercises are instituted, because hypostatic pneumonia is a danger, specially if accessory muscles of respiration e.g. abdominal muscles are paralysed. Muscle contracture is prevented by massage and frequent passive movements of the limb.

Diet

A high-protein diet should be given to make good the loss of serum proteins from bedsores.

Bladder

In every case of cord injury retention of the urine is present in the initial stages. This may last from a few days to a few months in recoverable lesions. It is permanent in complete lesions. Most deaths after spinal injury are due to ascending infection from catheterization.

B: The return of reflex activity

If spinal shock does not recover even partly after 48 hours, partial or complete cord contusion is present. When spinal shock passes off, lower motor neurone paralysis persists in a few muscles corresponding to the level of the lesion, owing to crushing of the anterior horns at this level.

Partial cord lesions

These show spastic paralysis in extension with exaggerated reflexes and extensor plantar responses, and sometimes with uninhibited flexor spasms. Retention of urine may persist for upto one year.

Complete cord lesions

These are followed by spastic paralysis in flexion with gross flexor spasms and mass flexor reflexes of spinal automatism, which indicate complete lack of inhibition of spinal flexor reflex arcs. The slightest touch on the foot produces flexion of the ankle, knee and hip with evacuation of the bladder and rectum. The patient may misinterpret this as return of function. Actually it indicates that function will never recover.

Regional considerations

Cervical and thoracic spine

- In high cervical lesions all respiratory muscles are paralysed.
- If the fifth segment is injured the patient breathes only with the diaphragm, which is supplied mainly from the C4 segment.
- In lesions of C6 elbow flexion is present.
- Lesions at T1 produce paralysis of the small muscles of the hand and Horner's syndrome[1].

At lower levels a band of hyperaesthesia encircles the trunk one segment above the site of injury.

Lumbar spine

The *centre for the control of the bladder* lies opposite the 12th dorsal and first lumbar vertebrae.

- In complete cord lesions *above T10 segment* the bladder centre is intact and uninhibited; therefore, an automatic bladder develops; when the intravesical pressure rises, evacuation occurs. The patient has to wear a receptacle for urine in order to remain dry.
- Complete lesions *involving the bladder centre* produce paralysis of the detrusor supplied by the third and fourth sacral nerves. This results in permanent retention with overflow incontinence. However, since the upper abdominal muscles can be contracted voluntarily by the 7th to 10th dorsal segments, the patient can be taught to empty the bladder by straining, and by pressing his hands suprapubically, during the day. He must wear a receptacle at night. The care of the bladder is also discussed in the chapter on the urinary bladder.

---

1 Horner's syndrome: a small pupil, a drooping eyelid and decreased sweating on the affected side of the face, due to a tumor, spinal cord injury, etc.

The *centre for* ***defecation*** is located in the 1st and 2nd lumbar segments. Damage produces a patulous anus and incontinence.

Cauda equina

In cauda equina lesions the disabilities correspond to the nerves injured. Usually the sacral nerve roots are involved, resulting in anesthesia in the perineum and urinary retention.

Rehabilitation

The patient is confined to bed for two to three months until the spine stabilizes by bony healing. However, internal immobilization can cut short this time period. A great deal of progress in the care of paraplegics has been achieved due to work at the various paraplegic centres. The aims of treatment are the following:

- To keep the patient in the best possible physical condition by preventing the development of bedsores and urinary infections.
- To over-develop the muscles above the site of injury, so that these may move the pelvis.
- To move the splinted legs by movements of the pelvis.

Rehabilitation of muscle activities

Contractures are relieved by physiotherapy, tenotomy etc. If necessary the lower part of the completely isolated cord is destroyed by intrathecal alcohol to abolish mass reflexes and flexor spasm which would prevent walking.

Mobilization

- Rope climbing develops the muscles of the shoulder girdle.
- On parallel bars the patient learns to move his pelvis.
- Light aluminum splints are now fitted to the legs. Using sticks, the patient moves the pelvis from his shoulder. The splinted legs move with the pelvis.
- Thus the patient can walk slowly for a short distance to a wheelchair, in which he may move about. He can participate in occupations involving fine handicraft.

Bladder

In the treatment of a paraplegic, meticulous care of the bladder has a high priority. At the same time nursing of an extremely high standard is required, in order to prevent bedsores from developing. If the above steps are not taken, most paraplegics can die within a few years from ascending urinary infections, or due to septicemia from spreading bedsores.

Prognosis

If any cord function survives the initial injury, additional function usually returns if the cord and spine are protected from further injury. Patients with complete injury rarely recover function below the level of the lesion. Rehabilitation aims at self-care and readjustment of vocation. Life expectancy is reduced in paraplegics, and more specially in quadriplegics.

Cause of death

The causes of death in paraplegics include:

- Spinal shock.
- Respiratory failure from ascending edema if the lesion is near C5.
- Hypostatic pneumonia.
- Ascending urinary infections.
- Septicemia from unhealed bedsores.

SPINA BIFIDA

Embryology

During the second week of intrauterine life a longitudinal groove appears on the dorsum of the embryo. Its margins unite to form a tube from which the nervous system is developed. This tube of epiblast becomes separated from the surface by mesoblast. In each segment bars of cartilage appear on each side and fuse with each other to form the vertebral arches. If these arches fail to fuse spina bifida results. Its incidence is 0.1%.

The different types of spina bifida include the following:

Spina bifida occulta

In this variety the vertebral arches fail to fuse but the membranes do not protrude backwards. A patch of hair, a lipoma or a depression in the skin in the lumbosacral region are the only external evidence, called skin stigmata; they suggest that a spina bifida occulta exists. A fibrous band sometimes connects the skin to the membranes to produce a tethered cord. As the body grows, the spinal cord grows at a slower pace. This causes the band to pull on the membranes and nerve roots causing foot-drop, bed-wetting at night, bowel changes, or backache. A tethered spinal cord can present at any age with these symptoms and signs. The presence of a subcutaneous lipoma etc. is often noted before symptoms appear.

If the condition is suspected, an x-ray shows the gap between the laminae. Further evaluation should be carried out with MRI and CT scan.

Treatment

If tethering of the cord is demonstrated in a child, surgery

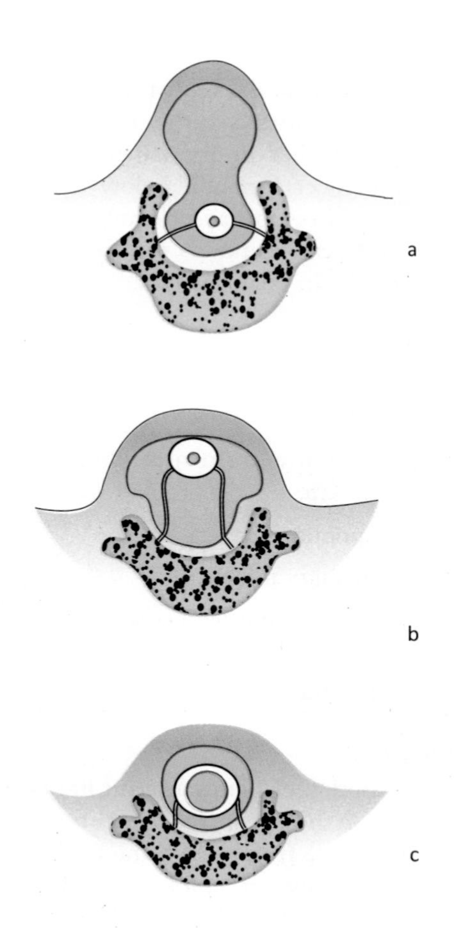

Fig.45.1 Different types of spina bifida (a) meningocele (b) meningomyelocele (c) syringomyelocele

to prevent deterioration is indicated *even if neurological symptoms are absent*. Any patient with symptoms requires urgent evaluation and treatment. If appropriately repaired in time, patients with occult spinal dysraphism show entirely normal development and function.

Meningocele

This is the most common form of spina bifida. A fluctuant and transilluminant swelling is seen in the midline of the back in the newborn (Fig.45.1a, 45.2). It is due to a protrusion of the meninges through the ununited vertebral laminae and soft tissues. It contains cerebrospinal fluid, and is in communication with the spinal theca.

Meningomyelocele

The normally developed cord or cauda equina lie in the sac (Fig.45.1 b). They may be adherent to the posterior aspect, and on transillumination are seen as a dark band in the midline. Interference with the spinal cord or nerves may occur, with bilateral talipes and trophic changes in the skin of the feet.

Syringomyelocele

Syringomyelocele is rare. In this condition the central canal of the cord is dilated (Fig.45.1 c).

Myelocele

In this, the most severe form of spina bifida, the neural groove lies open, and at its upper end the central canal discharges cerebrospinal fluid. Most cases are stillborn, or death occurs within a few days from meningitis.

Some cases of spina bifida develop hydrocephalus due to associated anomalies at a higher level.

Treatment

Operation for *meningocele* and *meningo-myelocele* is advised usually within a few days of birth, otherwise the sac may enlarge and ulcerate. The sac is opened and redundant membrane excised (in the case of myelomeningocele the membranes being separated from the underlying cord and cauda equina). The membranes are now repaired, and muscles and skin approximated over them.

Cases of *spina bifida* with gross paralysis require very detailed and meticulous care along the lines of the rehabilitation of cases suffering from traumatic paraplegia, and involving a huge expenditure on each patient during a lifetime.

TUMORS OF THE SPINAL CORD AND MEMBRANES

Spinal cord tumors can be divided into the following categories:

- *Extradural*, e.g. meningioma and neurofibroma.
- *Intradural*. These can be further subdivided into the following types:
  - o *Extramedullary* tumors, e.g. meningioma and neurofibroma.
  - o *Intramedullary* tumors: these consist of ependymomas which can be excised, and gliomas which cannot easily be removed.

Clinical features

- If the *posterior* nerve roots are involved, root pain and local sensory loss are the result.
- If the *anterior* horns are affected, wasting and loss of reflexes are found.
- Involvement of the *sensory tracts* leads to loss of sensations below the tumor.

- If the *pyramidal* tracts are destroyed, upper motor neurone paralysis is seen.
- Involvement of both pyramidal tracts leads to disturbed bladder function.

Extramedullary tumors

In these tumors root pain may be present for years before cord compression occurs:

- If the pain is referred to the *shoulder* and arms, it may be regarded as due to arthritis or neuritis.
- In the *chest* it may be labelled as angina pectoris.
- In the *abdomen* it may be thought to arise from the gallbladder or appendix, or from the pelvic organs.
- If the pain is increased on *coughing*, a spinal origin should be suspected. Finally, spastic paralysis sets in with a transverse level of sensory loss below the level of the tumor.

Intramedullary tumors

These extend over a length of the spinal cord, so they cause a wide belt of sensory loss and lower motor neurone paralysis. Root pain occurs late.

Cauda equina tumors

These produce root pain, sensory loss and lower motor neurone paralysis in the distribution of the sacral nerve roots.

Investigations

X-ray spine

This may show absorption of a pedicle or enlargement of an intervertebral foramen.

Lumbar puncture

This may show obstruction to the circulation of cerebrospinal fluid (CSF) by Queckenstedt's test: on compressing the internal jugular veins the pressure of the lumbar CSF does not rise.

Examination of the CSF

The fluid below a block becomes yellow and contains increased amounts of proteins.

CT scan and MRI

Both these investigations show up the presence of a spinal tumor to good advantage. They also help greatly in its differential diagnosis from other conditions.

CT and MRI have completely supplanted the older methods of investigations. However, in regions without CT scan or MRI, the previously employed methods, including cisternal myelography, may still have relevance.

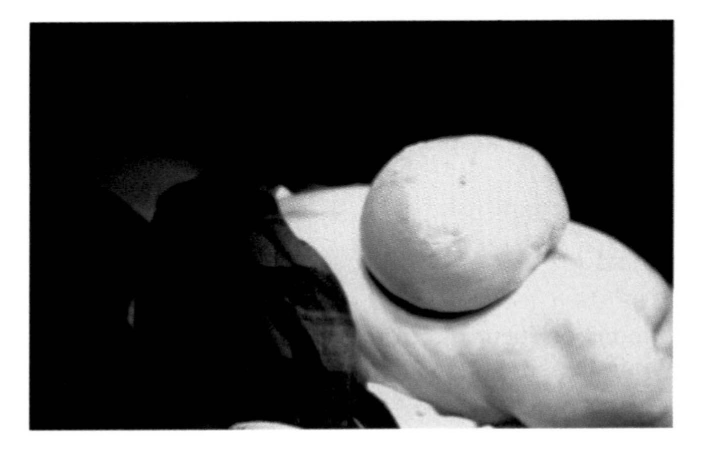

Fig.45.2 Large meningocele in newborn

Cisternal myelography

A needle is passed into the cisterna magna at the level of the 2nd cervical spine. 3ml of a radiopaque dye e.g. Myodil is injected. This gravitates down till it is arrested by the tumor, and x-rays are taken.

Treatment

The treatment of spinal tumors consists of exposing the concerned area of the spinal cord by laminectomy and excising the tumor.

Indications for laminectomy

Laminectomy is indicated for the following conditions:

- Spinal tumors.
- Trauma.
- Paraplegia due to Pott's disease.
- Chronic pain from malignant lymph nodes in the upper neck; the posterior nerve roots are divided.
- The pain of an irremovable new growth, the spinothalamic tracts being sectioned.

Nerves

CRANIAL NERVES

First

The first (olfactory) nerve may be injured by fractures of the cribriform plate causing partial or complete loss of smell on the affected side.

Second

The second (optic) nerve may be damaged by fractures involving the optic foramen, or by tumors or aneurysms. Primary optic atrophy with partial or complete blindness can occur. However the pupil contracts if the opposite retina is stimulated.

Third

The third (oculomotor) nerve is involved by tumors, trauma or aneurysm in the skull, sphenoidal fissure or orbit. Pressure on the nerve above the tentorium occurs when a midbrain pressure cone forms.

A partial lesion merely causes dilatation of the pupil. In a complete lesion there is also ptosis from paralysis of levator palpabrae superioris, and proptosis from paralysis of the majority of the ocular muscles. A lateral and downward squint occurs due to unopposed action of the external rectus and superior oblique muscles.

Fourth

The fourth (trochlear) nerve supplies the superior oblique, and is rarely involved alone.

Fifth

The fifth (trigeminal) nerve has three divisions.

Trigeminal neuralgia

In this condition sudden severe pain occurs in one or two divisions of the trigeminal nerve, commonly in a middle-aged or elderly person. The pain may be precipitated by exposure to cold, touch, eating, talking etc. Normally no cause can be found.

Treatment is started with drugs, carbamazepine being the most effective. If this fails treatment is by surgery.

The two standard surgical procedures for trigeminal neuralgia include:

- *Microvascular decompression*. Through a small incision and hole in the skull behind the ear and with an operating microscope, the surgeon spots the trigeminal nerve coming out of the brain stem. He mobilizes the artery compressing the trigeminal nerve root away from the nerve, and maintains the position by interposing inert Teflon felt between the vessel and the nerve.
- *Radiofrequency rhizotomy* (division of the root). This method of percutaneous rhizotomy requires an awake patient to describe the facial numbness produced by the radiofrequency lesion. The electrode is advanced to the Gasserian ganglion, its correct position tested with gentle electrical stimulation, and the electrode heated to produce a thermal injury.

  These methods give excellent (90%) pain relief.
- Recently these patients have been subjected to *gamma knife* with 26% pain relief.

Sixth

The sixth (abducent) nerve has a long intracranial course. It may be affected by fractures of the base of the skull or, along with other nerves, by lesions in the cavernous sinus, sphenoidal fissure or orbit. Internal squint results from paralysis of the external rectus.

Seventh

The seventh (facial) nerve may be involved at different sites:

- *Intracranial*. Lesions within the brain are supranuclear, nuclear or infranuclear.
  - o In *supranuclear* lesions the upper part of the face escapes, because those muscles have a bilateral innervation.
  - o In *nuclear* lesions the whole face, and the sixth nerve on the same side, are affected.
  - o In *infranuclear* lesions the auditory nerve is also commonly involved.
- *Cranial*. The intraosseous part of the facial nerve is affected by fracture of the base of the skull or middle ear disease. Paralysis may occur:
  - o Immediately after fracture, due to direct injury.
  - o Within a few days due to hemorrhage within the nerve sheath; in this case recovery is possible.
  - o After some weeks due to the pressure of callus, recovery is unlikely to occur.
- *Extracranial:*
  - o *Bell's palsy*. This is a herpetic neuritis of the facial nerve, and follows exposure to cold. The swelling of the nerve extends into the bony canal and compresses the nerve; it usually subsides before permanent damage has occurred, but in a few cases partial or complete paralysis persists.
  - o The branches of the facial nerve may be injured by broken windscreens or badly placed operation incisions.

The paralysed face is flat and expressionless. The eye cannot be closed. Corneal ulceration may follow due to exposure. Epiphora occurs due to drooping of the lower eyelid. The patient cannot whistle, and food collects between the gums and cheek.

Treatment. The angle of the mouth may be supported by small strips of adhesive strapping applied under tension.

Faradic stimulation and massage are prescribed. If recovery does not occur, the hypoglossal nerve may be anastomosed to the branches of the facial nerve.

Eighth

The eighth (auditory) nerve may be involved by middle fossa fractures or tumors.

Ninth

The ninth (glossopharyngeal) nerve may be injured in a fractured base of skull, with dysphagia due to paresis of the constrictor muscle.

Tenth

The tenth (vagus) nerve may be damaged in a fractured base of skull.

The *recurrent laryngeal nerve* may be damaged during *thyroidectomy,* and compressed due to infiltration by a carcinoma of the thyroid:

- *Partial* involvement affects the more sensitive abductor muscles only, so that if it is bilateral, asphyxia results and tracheostomy may be required.
- *Complete* involvement causes paralysis of both abductors and adductors, so the cord is held in the midway or cadaveric position. The opposite vocal cord increases its mobility, reaches across the midline and closes the glottis. The voice is adequate but monotonous.

Eleventh

The eleventh (accessory) nerve was commonly injured during removal of tuberculous lymph nodes in the neck. If the injury is recognized at operation, primary suture should be performed. With drug treatment of tuberculous nodes the injury is uncommon these days,

Twelfth

The twelfth (hypoglossal) nerve may be injured during removal of the submandibular salivary gland. Hemiatrophy occurs in the tongue, which is pushed towards the paralysed side on protrusion.

SPINAL NERVES

Injuries

In 1943, Seddon described three basic types of peripheral nerve injuries: neurapraxia, axonotmesis and neurotmesis.

Neurapraxia

This is a temporary interruption of conduction without loss of axonal continuity. In neurapraxia, there is a physiologic block of nerve conduction in the affected axons. This is the equivalent of concussion. Conduction in the intact nerve fibres is interrupted temporarily due to stretch or distortion, and without organic rupture. It is produced by minor stretch injuries. There is sensory loss, paraesthesiae and paresis for a few days. The fibres remain intact. The axons do not degenerate. When conduction returns, all functions return together within a few hours, and recovery is complete.

Treatment consists of splinting the limb in the position of relaxation of the paralysed muscle until recovery.

Axonotmesis

This involves loss of the relative continuity of the axon and its covering of myelin, but preservation of the connective tissue framework of the nerve, the epineurium and perineurium. Traction produces rupture of nerve fibres *within intact sheaths*. This may occur:

- During birth.
- By clutching for support while falling.
- By compression by tourniquets and splints.
- By incorrect posture on the operating table.

Wallerian degeneration occurs in the distal portions of the broken axons, leaving empty tubules. Slow recovery occurs by the downgrowth of axons into the distal tubules. Some nerve fibres are lost due to fibrosis in the tubules. However there is little maldistribution of fibres because the sheaths are intact. After a delay of nearly 10 days, axons proceed distally at the rate of approximately 1mm a day. When they reach their endings it takes three weeks for the end organs to become activated. As such muscles and skin areas farthest from the site of division are reinnervated last of all.

Clinical features

There is an initial picture of concussion with loss of sensation, tone, power, and reflex activity in the limb. This is followed by incomplete recovery. Numbness and paralysis persist only in those areas where fibres have actually been ruptured.

Secondary changes

Disuse results in impaired circulation, and the part becomes blue and cold. The nails are brittle and trophic changes occur due to minor unrecognized trauma. The paralysed muscles are overstretched by the unopposed action of antagonists. Periarticular adhesions fix the immobile joints in a contracted position.

Treatment

This is aimed at maintaining the nerves and joints in good working order while awaiting the arrival of down-growing axons:

- The part is protected by warm padding and splinted in the position of relaxation of paralysed groups.
- Muscle movement is maintained by regular galvanic stimulation of paralysed muscles.
- All joints are put through their full range of movements daily to prevent contractures.
- Moral support and encouragement is provided during the slow process of recovery.

If recovery fails to occur the nerve should be explored, when a perineural scar or an intraneural fibroma is usually found, and requires removal.

Neurotmesis

A peripheral nerve fiber contains an axon, myelin sheath (if in existence), their schwann cells, and the endoneurium. In neurotmesis there is a total severance or disruption of the entire nerve fiber. Neurotmesis may be partial or complete. It is commonly produced by penetrating wounds. It results in partial or complete division of nerve sheaths and fibres.

In the proximal portions of the divided axons retrograde degeneration occurs as high as the first node of Ranvier. The axons now subdivide to produce numerous end bulbs which grow downwards. But the gap between the nerve ends has by now been filled with organizing blood clot which acts as a barrier. Cells of the distal sheaths of Schwann sprout and grow proximally towards the proximal axons. In this way a very few axons find their way into distal tubules.

Extent of recovery

Even after accurate nerve suture the quality of regeneration is less perfect than in cases of axonotmesis, due to wastage and maldistribution of axons. The density of scar tissue is increased by local sepsis and inflammation, and by tension at the suture line. Maldistribution is greatest in the case of mixed motor and sensory nerves, e.g. the median and ulnar nerves at the wrist. The quality of recovery is best in purely motor nerves supplying large muscle groups e.g. the radial nerve.

Investigations

Nerve conduction studies and *MRI* scan are required to localize the lesion.

Treatment

This consists of fine and accurate suture in the absence of sepsis and tension, and placing the nerve in a suitable bed. If there is much loss of skin, plastic surgical operations to replace full-thickness skin must precede repair of nerve. In clean incised wounds immediate primary suture is best. In untidy contaminated wounds suture is postponed for about three weeks, because primary suture would require enlargement of the incision and this would spread infection. Secondly, in three weeks the nerve sheath becomes thick and easier to stitch.

Nerve suture

The two ends of the nerve are identified. The incision is prolonged to expose the nerve well above and below the seat of injury. The ends of the nerve are 'freshened' by a scalpel. Slices are removed until projecting fibres are seen and blood oozes from the cut surface. If necessary the ends are approximated by mobilization and posture. Sutures are inserted through the nerve sheath. Magnification is employed, and 7/0 to 9/0 polypropylene sutures are used, as they cause the least reaction.

If nerve suture is impossible due to loss of tissue, recourse may be had to:

- Nerve anastomosis.
- Nerve grafting.
- Tendon transplantation.
- Arthrodesis.
- Amputation, for persistent ulcers on the foot.

Tumors

Tumors of nerve sheaths

These tumors are made up essentially of myelin. Benign tumors include schwannomas (neurilemmomas) (Fig.45.3) and neurofibromas. Only about 1% of schwannomas become malignant.

INDIVIDUAL SPINAL NERVES

Injuries of the cervical plexus are uncommon and insignificant.

The *phrenic nerve* (C3, 4, 5) used to be crushed in the past to cause temporary paralysis of the diaphragm. The rise of the diaphragm reduced the size of the cavity in tuberculosis, which healed earlier. Drug treatment of tuberculosis has displaced this procedure.

NERVES OF THE UPPER LIMB

Brachial plexus lesions

Complete lesions of the brachial plexus are rare, because the severity of the trauma usually proves fatal. Incomplete lesions may be due to stabs or cuts. The main muscle groups are as follows:

C V — Deltoid, biceps and supinator.

C VI — Remaining muscles of shoulder, triceps and pronators.

C VII Extensors of fingers.

C VIII Flexors of wrist and fingers.

D I Small muscles of hand.

Upper brachial plexus lesion (Erb's paralysis)

This lesion occurs due to excessive depression of the shoulder in infants during a difficult delivery, and in adults after a fall on the shoulder. C5 and C6 are affected. The limb is internally rotated by the unopposed subscapularis. It hangs by the side, with the hand pronated. The function of the hand is preserved, therefore arthrodesis of the shoulder and elbow is useful.

Lower brachial plexus lesion (Klumpke's paralysis)

The lower nerve trunk or medial cord are injured by an unreduced dislocation of the humerus. When a falling person clutches at an object the nerve roots may be avulsed from the spinal cord. The first dorsal root is affected. The small muscles of the hand are wasted. Anesthesia affects the medial side of the hand.

Treatment consists of splinting the limb to relax the paralysed muscles. Physiotherapy should be continued for two years before recovery is assessed.

Circumflex nerve

This nerve winds around the uppermost part of the shaft of the humerus. It may be injured in fractures of the humerus. The deltoid is paralysed and wastes rapidly. Recovery commences in a few weeks if the cause of the compression is removed and the arm supported in right-angled abduction.

Nerve to the serratus anterior

This nerve is injured by a blow or an operation on the breast or chest wall. 'Winging' of the scapula results. Overhead abduction of the shoulder is not possible.

Radial nerve

This nerve may be injured in the *axilla* in a dislocation of the shoulder or after the use of crutches. The patient cannot extend the elbow, the wrist, or the fingers, and wrist drop occurs. Anesthesia is seen over the dorsum of the forearm and hand.

Injury in the *spiral groove* of the humerus may occur due to:

- Pressure of the arm on the edge of the operating table.
- Prolonged application of a tourniquet.
- Fracture of the shaft of the humerus.

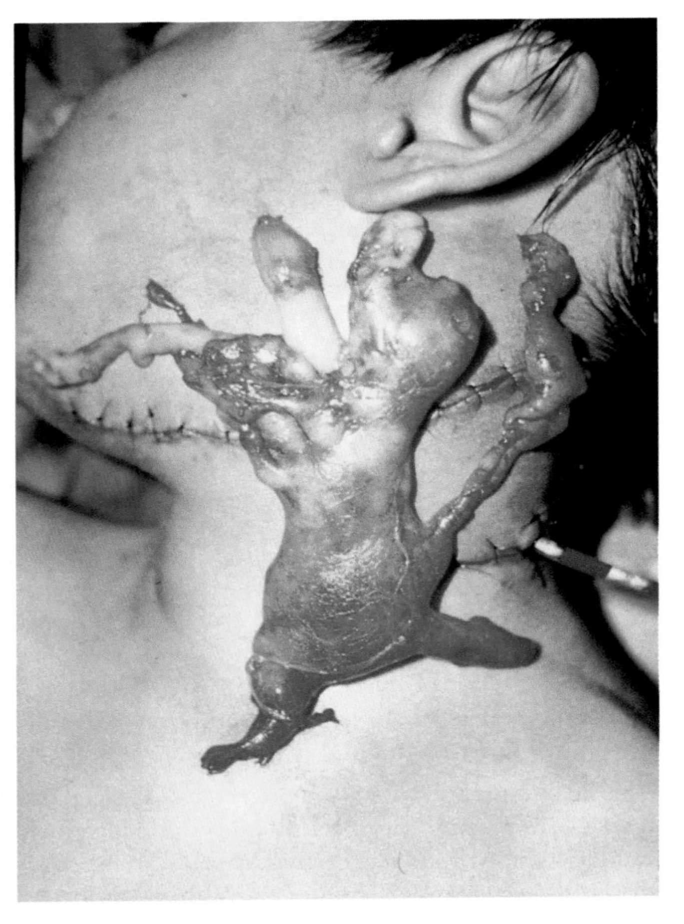

Fig.45.3 Large neurilemmoma with multiple branches reaching up to chin, occiput, posterior triangle and mediastinum, removed intact through a submandibular incision

- 'Intramuscular' injection of a drug into the radial nerve. Wrist drop results, with inability to extend the fingers. Anesthesia is found over the ball of the thumb.

Median nerve

This nerve may be injured at the *elbow* due to fracture at the lower end of the humerus. The index finger cannot be flexed--*the pointing index*--but the other fingers can be flexed by the portion of flexor digitorum profundus which is supplied by the ulnar nerve (Fig.45.4). The thenar muscles are wasted. Sensation is lost over the lateral three and a half digits in front. Trophic changes occur, specially in the index finger.

Injuries at the *wrist* are common due to cuts etc. The thenar muscles are paralysed and wasted. No part of the hand is completely anesthetic.

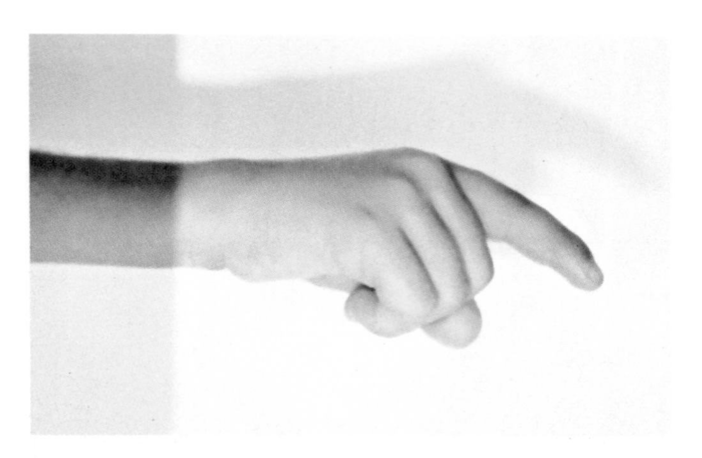

Fig.45.4 Pointing index finger' due to division of median nerve.

Ulnar nerve

This nerve may be injured at the *elbow* from:

- Fracture of the medial condyle.
- Being stretched due to cubitus valgus from old injury of the humerus with increase of the carrying angle.

The small muscles of the hand are paralysed, except the thenar muscles and lateral two lumbricals. The patient cannot abduct or adduct the fingers, and cannot grip a piece of paper between the fingers. Wasting is obvious in the interosseous spaces and along the inner border of the hand. Sensations are lost over the medial one and a half fingers.

Injury at the *wrist* occurs due to cuts. Paralysis and wasting of the small muscles of the hand occurs. Sensation is lost only over the front of the medial one and a half fingers.

Transposition of the ulnar nerve

This procedure is indicated if due to stretching of the nerve there is pain or wasting in the distribution of the nerve. The nerve is mobilized and brought in front of the medial epicondyle, shortening its course and relaxing it.

NERVES OF THE LOWER LIMB

Injury to the *ilioinguinal nerve* may occur on the right side during appendicectomy, and on the left side during iliac colostomy. The conjoint tendon becomes weak, predisposing to an inguinal hernia.

Sciatic nerve

This nerve is injured by wounds, fractures or intramuscular injections. The flexors of the knee are paralysed, but some flexion is possible due to the action of the sartorius and gracilis muscles. There is complete sensory loss below the knee, except for a strip along the inner side of the leg and foot supplied by the saphenous nerve. Trophic ulcers form on the sole of the foot.

Lateral popliteal nerve

This nerve is injured by fractures of, or during excision of, the upper end of the fibula, and by pressure from plasters or splints. There is complete paralysis of the extensors and peroneal muscles, with talipes equinovarus and sensory loss over the outer side of the leg and dorsal aspects of the toes. Trophic changes also occur in this area.

Medial popliteal nerve

This nerve is not injured very often.

Intramuscular injections

To close this discussion of injuries to peripheral nerves, mention may be made of the preferred sites for intramuscular injections. Most such injections are made in the deltoid, triceps and the gluteus maximus. Now, each of these sites contains a major nerve: circumflex, radial and sciatic respectively, which can be damaged by the injection.

It should be remembered that the ideal site for intramuscular injections is the lateral aspect of the thigh with its huge vastus lateralis muscle and no recognized nerves or vessels. If multiple injections have to be given, the site can also be changed each time.

Chapter

46 FACE AND MOUTH

The face develops from five processes around the primitive mouth. At the cephalic side lies the frontonasal process, and on each side a maxillary and mandibular process. Mesoderm grows medially from each maxillary process to join in the midline and form the palate. Anteriorly, the two maxillary processes join with the frontonasal process to form the upper lip.

CLEFT LIP AND PALATE

Failure of fusion between the above-mentioned development processes results in a cleft involving the following structures:

- Lip alone.
- Lip and alveolus.
- Lip, alveolus and palate.
- Palate alone.

During the first two months of pregnancy exposure to x-rays, vitamin deficiency and certain virus infections, e.g. rubella, is associated with an increased incidence of these abnormalities. The overall incidence of cleft lip and palate deformities in Pakistan is 1.91 per 1000 live births. In 12% of cases the condition is familial.

Effects

Cleft lip

A cleft lip can ruin the symmetry and appearance of an otherwise beautiful face (Fig.46.1). Cleft lip also impairs all functions of the lip, including speech, sucking and facial expressions. The cleft may be unilateral or bilateral, with the left unilateral cleft twice as common as the right. The cleft may be a notch in the lip (incomplete), or may extend all the way to the nose (complete).

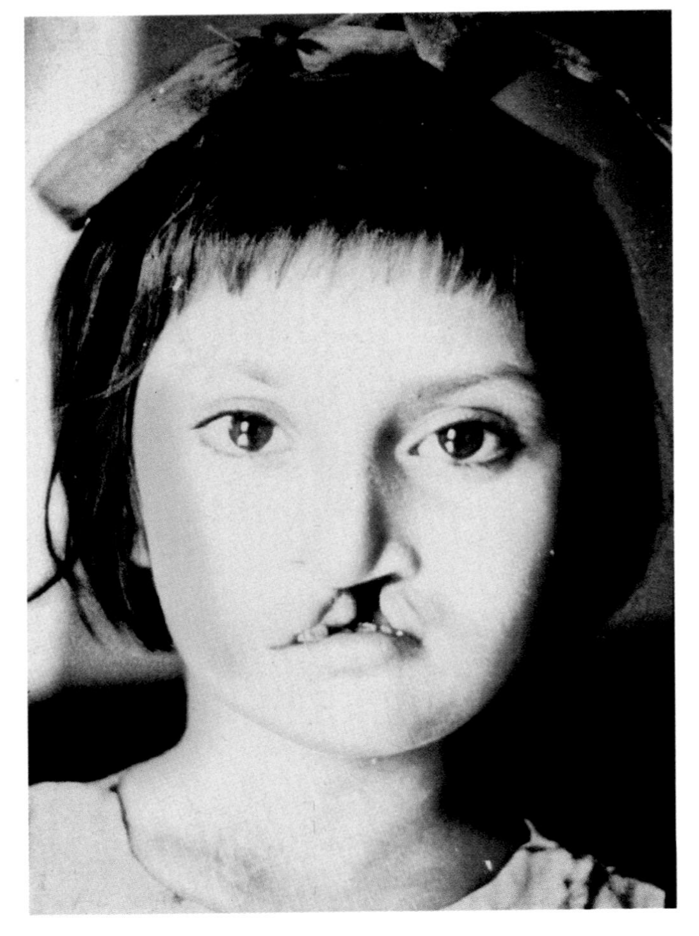

Fig.46.1 Cleft lip in a young girl, destroying the symmetry of an otherwise beautiful face

Cleft palate

This interferes with numerous important functions:

Sucking

With cleft palate the infant may be unable to suck, as negative pressure cannot be established in the oral cavity. Most cases can be dealt with by enlarging the hole in the teat; for this purpose a red hot sewing needle may be passed through the hole.

Speech

Because air escapes into the nose the patient with cleft palate cannot make consonants (e.g. B, D and T), and has a nasal speech.

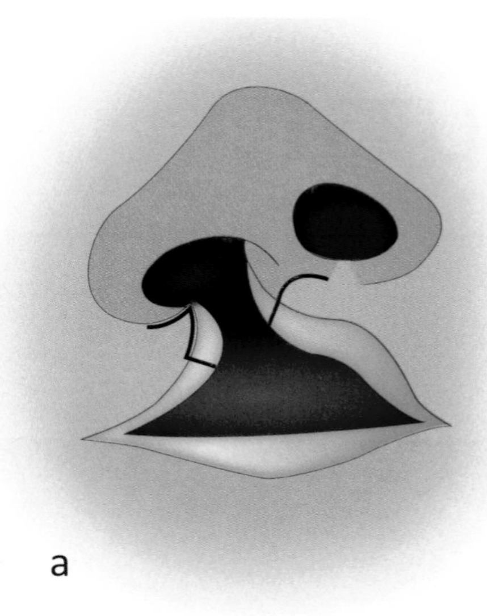

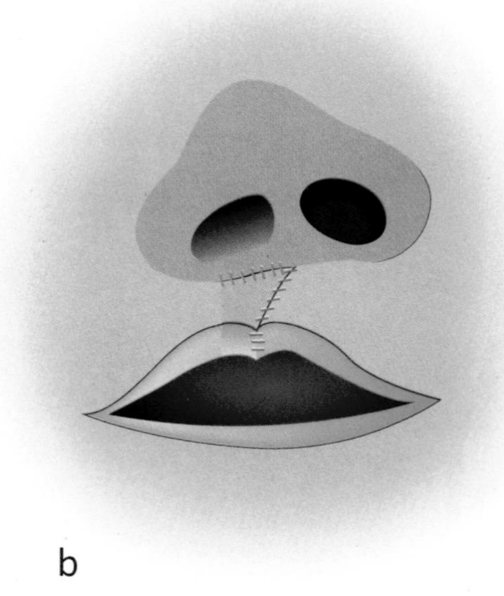

Fig.46.2 a, b Millard operation for unilateral cleft lip a. Flaps outlined b. Incisions made

Hearing

There is a slight loss of hearing because regurgitated food causes inflammation of the pharynx and eustachian tubes. At the same time, middle ear infections are more common in cases of cleft palate, the reason being as follows: in the normal person, acting from below, the tensors and levators palati open out the inner ends of the eustachian tubes during swallowing, allowing air to enter and equalize the pressure inside and outside the tympanic membrane. In cleft palate, as these muscles are severed in the midline they are put out of action. The middle ear remains closed, air gets absorbed, the tympanic membrane caves in and may rupture. Early closure of the cleft palate removes this source of ear infections.

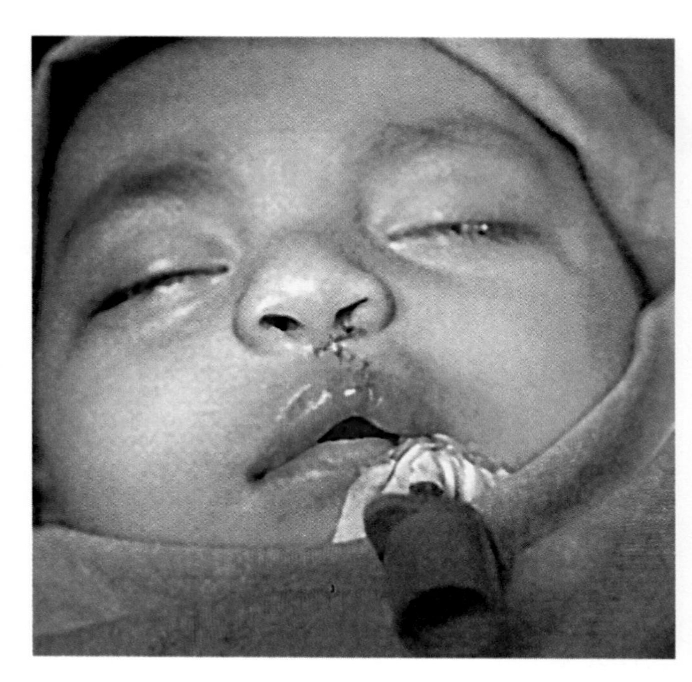

Fig.46.3 Unilateral cleft lip repaired with Millard's operation

Teeth

The teeth are out of line and require orthodontic management.

Treatment

Cleft lip

The aim is to improve the appearance. Operation is performed at the age of about three months, when the baby is putting on weight. The most popular operation is by Millard [1], in which the deficiency of tissue on the medial side of the defect is made good by an advancement flap from the lateral side, which lies in the position of, and looks like, the missing philtrum column, producing a very good result (Figs. 2 and 3). Fine sutures of monofilament polypropylene (size 7/0) result in a scar without stitch marks (Fig.46.4).

1 Le Meurier published his operation for cleft lip in 1949. The article consisted of just one paragraph with before-and-after drawings, yet it held the world's centre-stage for a quarter century. Then in 1975 Millard showed his procedure in a world congress, where he got only 2 ½ minutes for the presentation. Yet it has been the most popular operation since that date. This shows that the popularity of a presentation depends not on its length but its quality.

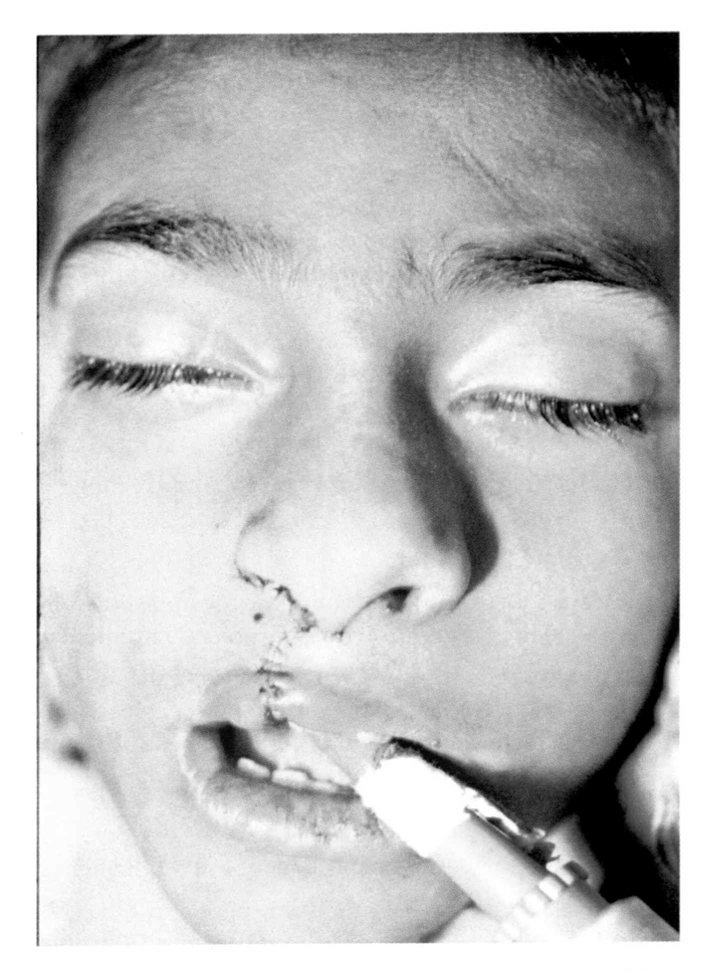

Fig.46.4 Ulilaterl cleft lip repaired with sutures of fine polypropylene

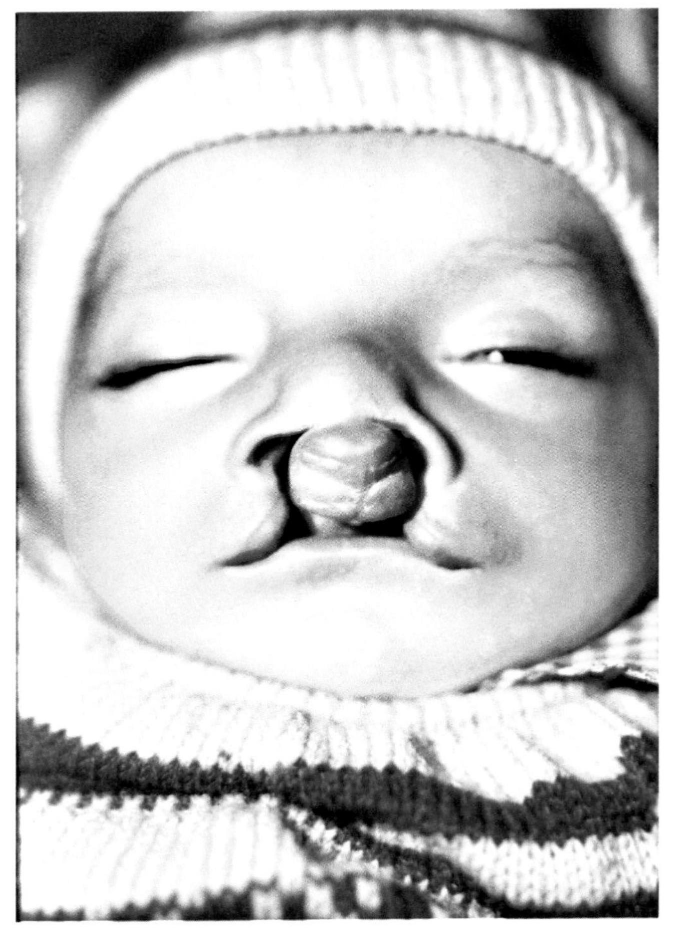

Fig.46.5 Bilateral complete cleft lip with protruding premaxilla

When there is a *bilateral* cleft lip with unfused premaxilla (Fig.46.5), both sides are operated upon together, the better to repair the orbicularis oris across the midline. The constant pull exerted by the reconstructed orbicularis oris ensures that the protruding premaxilla moves back to its normal position. The short columella results in a depressed tip of the nose, which generally requires correction later.

Cleft palate

The aim is adequate speech and dentition, swallowing without nasal regurgitation, and no loss of hearing. Operation is undertaken at the age of 12 to 18 months. The mucosa of the palate is mobilized in the form of flaps. The mucosa on the nasal aspect of the palate is also mobilized. Both layers are sutured. The muscle of the soft palate is stitched carefully.

Before operation the parents must be told that in a small number of cases the cleft palate repair can break down, due to the fact that it is a thin, moist membrane, which is subject to very high pressures during the act of swallowing. The care of an infant with cleft palate should be the responsibility of a team effort between a surgeon, an orthodontist, an otorhino-laryngologist, and a speech therapist.

Pharyngoplasty

Even after operation, a gap may remain behind the repaired palate due to its shortness, allowing some air to escape via the nose and interfering with proper speech. Cineradiography in the lateral position helps clarify the situation. If speech therapy fails to deal with the matter, a flap from the posterior wall of the pharynx may have to be raised and its free edge attached to the posterior margin of the soft palate, to remedy the situation ('pharyngoplasty').

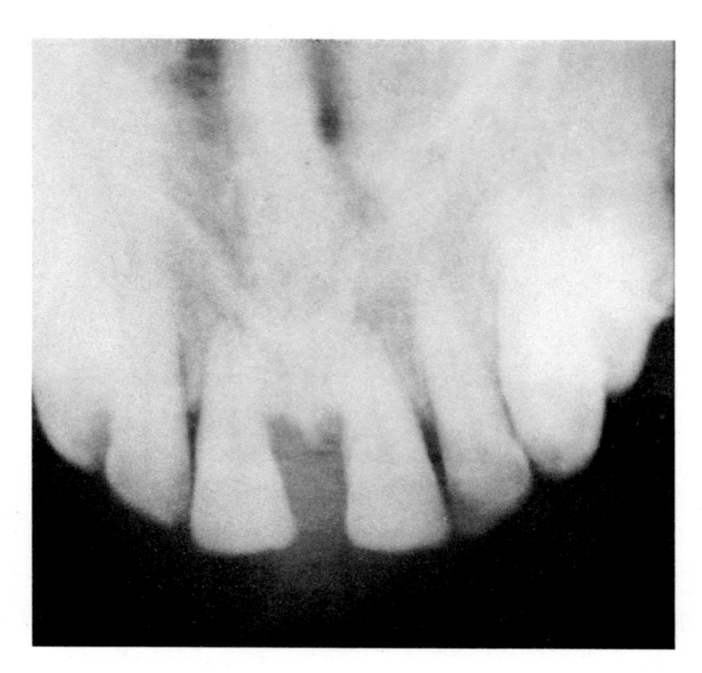

Fig.46.6 Diastema (gap between central incisors)

Micrognathia

In this condition the horizontal ramus of the mandible is poorly developed and short. Usually a cleft palate is also present, when the condition is called *Pierre Robin syndrome*. The pharyngeal airway is narrow, resulting in attacks of dyspnoea and cyanosis.

The baby should be nursed in the prone position so that the tongue cannot fall back and obstruct the pharynx. If this is done, there is no need of the 'tongue stitch' of the past. To hold the chin off the bed in the prone position, a 'cap' of tubinette gauze is worn, which is suspended from an overhead frame.

In about six weeks the mandible grows sufficiently, so that symptoms of respiratory difficulty disappear. In adult life the ramus can be lengthened by bone-grafting or, preferably, distraction osteogenesis[1]. However, in many cases, the ramus grows adequately so that recourse to such a procedure is not required.

Preauricular sinus

Six tubercles join to form the external ear. Imperfect fusion results in a preauricular sinus, the opening of which lies in front of the tragus. If the opening closes, a cyst may form. If it becomes infected and bursts an ulcer may result. The only curative treatment is complete excision of the sinus.

1 In later childhood the ramus can be lengthened by ***distraction osteogenesis***. The rami of both sides of the mandible are divided by osteotomy. An external distractor is placed in position, and opened at 1mm a day for about a month until the ramus is lengthened to the desired extent. New bone forms in the gap created.

Prominent maxillary frenum

If the midline mucosal fold in the upper vestibule of the mouth (maxillary 'frenum') is thickened, a gap between the medial incisors (diastema) may result, which is cosmetically unattractive (Fig.46.6).

Causes of diastema

These include:

- Prominent labial frenum, hereditary.
- Habits (e.g. sucking on a pencil, or keeping a matchstick there).
- Unerupted supernumerary tooth in midline.

If the cause is a prominent frenum, the mucosal fold should be incised transversely and sutured longitudinally.

It should be remembered that sometimes the medial incisors come together in spite of the presence between them of a thick, fleshy frenum. This suggests that the frenum may not always stand in their way.

Swellings on the palate

A swelling on the palate may be one of the following:

- A tumor of the palatal mucosa or bone.
- An ectopic salivary tumor.
- A carcinoma of the maxillary antrum.
- An alveolar abscess.

External angular dermoid

Each half of the face develops from a frontonasal, a maxillary and a mandibular process. Between the former two processes, at the external angle of the eye, some skin gets buried and produces a hemispherical fluctuant swelling (Fig.46.7). The treatment is excision.

NEOPLASMS OF THE LIPS

Lymphangioma and cavernous hemangioma occur from time to time.

Carcinoma of the lip

This tumor is common in men between sixty and seventy years of age, specially fair-skinned individuals who have followed an outdoor occupation, as excessive exposure to sunlight predisposes to this condition. Thus the condition is very common in Australia. The lower lip is affected in 95 percent cases. It is a squamous-celled carcinoma, and presents as a non-healing ulcer, usually with the typical everted edge. Any ulcer on the lip which does not heal readily should be viewed with suspicion and biopsied.

Treatment

Carcinomas of the lip are usually slow-growing and surgery and external beam radiotherapy are effective therapies, the 5 year survival rate being above 80%.

- *Early* (T1) tumors can be managed by wedge resection, including at least 0.5cm of normal tissue.
- *More advanced* lesions require combined surgery and radiotherapy.
- If a tumor is advanced or recurs after radiotherapy, surgical excision leaves behind a large defect, which has to be repaired by rotating a local flap, commonly from the nasolabial area, or by a forearm flap.

Involvement of submental or deep cervical nodes occurs late. If they are mobile, a neck dissection is performed. The tendency is to remove the lymph nodes only in the supraomohyoid region of the neck. If the nodes are fixed or the patient is elderly or weak, radiotherapy is used instead. Careful follow-up of all cases is essential.

FACIAL INJURIES

In a bilateral fracture of the mandible the airway may be obstructed by blood, or by the tongue falling back. The patient should be placed on his side or semi-prone. A complete examination can be carried out in the operation theatre under anesthesia. The blood supply to the face is good, so wounds in this area heal well. They can be treated by primary suture even if 24 hours have elapsed since the injury. Dirt and pieces of glass must be removed. Sutures on the facial skin are removed in 2 to 4 days to avoid stitch marks.

Fractures of the face

The nasal bones

The injury may be lateral, causing impaction of one nasal bone under the other; or frontal, which compresses the nasal structures backwards, at times resulting in a naso-ethmoidal fracture. Under general anesthesia the bones are gripped in special forceps, disimpacted and manipulated into position. They are protected by a fibre-glass cast, malleable metallic or plaster of paris cast.

The malar bone

The malar bone may be fractured and depressed by a direct blow. There may be diplopia and inability to open the mouth, subconjunctival ecchymosis and numbness of the infraoribital region.. A notch, or step-defect can be palpated on the infraorbital margin.

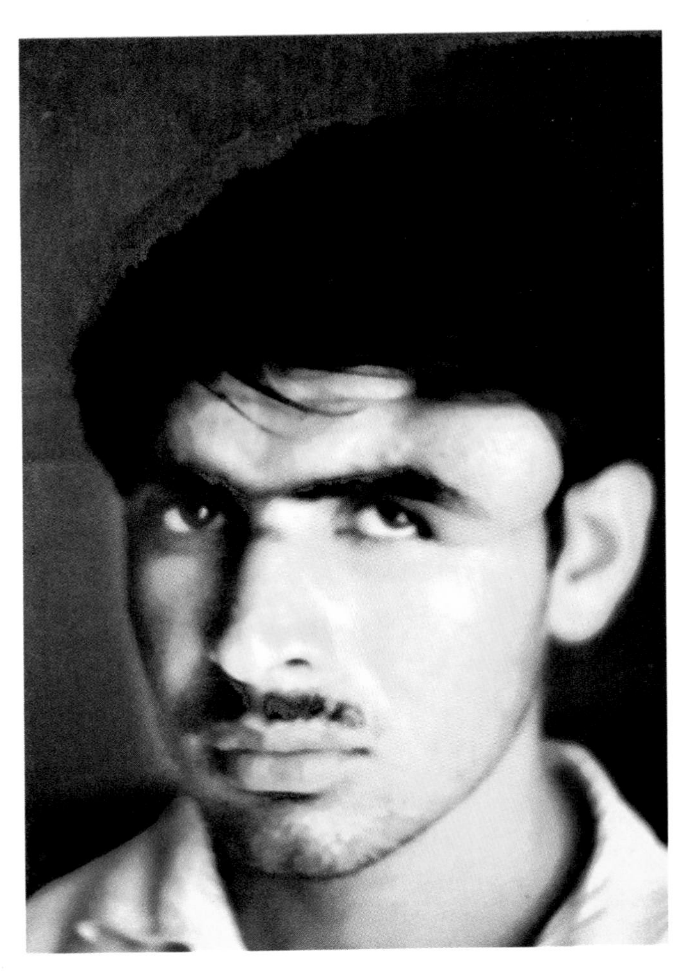

Fig.46.7 External angular dermoid. Hemi-spherical fluctuant mass above outer canthus

The bone is elevated by a bone lever introduced through an incision in the temple behind the hair margin (Gillie's approach). It is fixed by wiring or plating it to the frontal bone and maxilla.

The maxilla

These fractures are classified according to Le Fort (Fig.46.8):

- In *Le Fort I* fracture the alveolus is separated from the maxilla.
- In *Le Fort II* the maxilla is separated from the rest of the skull.
- In *Le Fort III* the maxilla, malar bones, nasal bones, ethmoids and palatal bones are separated from the base of the skull. The fracture is frequently comminuted The patient may be unable to close the jaws.

In Le Fort II and III there may be diplopia due to displacement of the floor of the orbit. In Le Fort III the cribriform plate may be injured and cerebrospinal fluid rhinorrhoea may result.

Treatment

A tracheostomy may be necessary. The displaced maxilla is freed by rocking with bone forceps, restored to its normal position, and held in place by one of the following methods:

- By internal *wire sutures* or *mini-plates* between maxilla, malar and frontal bones.
- By wiring a pliable *metal bar* to the teeth and fixing this by a system of extra-oral rods to a steel frame around the skull.

At the same time the upper and lower jaws may be wired together; the procedure is called *inter-maxillary fixation.*.

The mandible

The mandible may be fractured at the following sites:

- *Neck of the condyle.* The neck is pulled forwards by the external pterygoid muscle. These fractures are most common and result in malocclusion (upper and lower teeth do not meet properly). A short period of immobilization needs to be followed by active mobilization to prevent ankylosis of the temporomandibular joints.
- *Ascending ramus*, usually near the angle of the jaw; little displacement occurs. The only symptom is persistent pain.
- *Angle of the mandible.* These are commonly closed fractures resulting in malocclusion. Impacted wisdom teeth near the angle weaken this portion and predispose to fractures.
- *Body of the jaw* is fractured frequently, usually by a direct blow. The fracture commonly occurs at the site of the canine tooth, the long root of which weakens the bone. If the fracture is bilateral the central portion of the jaw is displaced downwards by the anterior bellies of the digastric muscles etc. The fracture is nearly always open due to the firm attachment of the mucoperiosteum to the bone.

Diagnosis

This is obvious, as speech and swallowing are impaired. Blood-stained saliva trickles from the mouth. The line of the teeth is irregular, and there is malocclusion, where the upper and lower teeth do not align when the patient closes the jaws.

Favourable and unfavourable fractures

Fractures of the body of the mandible are rated as favourable or unfavourable according to the direction of the fracture line:

- Fractures that run downwards and forwards are favourable. The posterior fragment is pulled upwards by the masseter, the anterior fragment downwards by the mylohyoid and digastric; thus the fragments are brought together, which helps in reduction and immobilization.
- The reverse is true if the fracture line runs downwards and backwards.

Treatment

- *Compression plates* or mini-plates produce maximum contact and stabilization of the fractures; the need for temporarily fixing the jaws together (intermaxillary fixation) is eliminated, so that motion at the temporomandibular joint is allowed; this prevents stiffness at the joint.
- If plating systems are not available, open exposure of the fracture and *direct wiring with intermaxillary fixation* for 4–6 weeks is required, fluids being taken through a tube.

Warm antiseptic mouthwashes reduce the chances of infection in this compound fracture. Antibiotic cover is required.

Complications include:

- Necrosis of bone.
- Delayed union.
- Aspiration pneumonia.
- Temporomandibular joint ankylosis.

Boils on the face

Boils in the 'mask' area of the face should never be squeezed, as the infection can reach the cavernous sinus by venous connections and cause cavernous sinus thrombosis.

SWELLINGS OF THE JAWS

The portion of each jaw bearing the sockets ('alveoli') for the teeth is called the alveolar process of that jaw. Because of the teeth contained inside the alveolus, the swellings arising here are different from those arising elsewhere in the jaws.

Swellings on the alveolar process

These include the epulides and the odontomes.

Epulides

Epulide literally means 'on the gum'. An epulide is any lump situated on the fixed mucosa of the gum or the movable mucosa over the alveolar process. There are four varieties of epulides:

- ***Granulomatous epulis,*** i.e. a mass of granulation tissue, usually around a carious tooth. The tooth should be extracted and the granulations scraped.
- ***Fibrous epulis,*** i.e. a fibroma arising from the periodontal membrane. The adjacent tooth and a wedge of bone (including the portion of the gum containing the growth) must be removed.
- ***Giant cell epulis***, i.e. osteoclastoma. Ulceration and hemorrhage can occur. X-rays show bone destruction. Small tumors are curetted, large ones radically excised.
- ***Vascular epulis,*** i.e. hemangioma, clinically referred to frequently as a pyogenic granuloma or pregnancy epulis. Excision, along with scaling of the involved teeth is required.
- ***Carcinomatous epulis,*** *i.e.* an epithelioma of the gum, which can ulcerate, invade the bone and spread to the cervical lymph nodes.

Odontomes

These are cysts, tooth malformations or tumors arising from the epithelial or mesothelial elements of the teeth. Only epithelial odontomes are important, namely dental cyst, dentigerous cyst and adamantinoma.

Dental cyst

This occurs at the root of a normally erupted but chronically infected pulpless (non-vital) tooth. Epithelial cells from the enamel organ form the lining. Usually the fluid is clear and uninfected and the condition is painless.

Dentigerous cyst

This cyst contains an unerupted permanent tooth, usually a third molar.

Treatment of both the above-mentioned cysts is excision of the whole epithelial lining of the cyst.

Adamantinoma

An adamantinoma is an epithelial tumor probably arising from enamel-forming cells (ameloblasts). It looks histologically and behaves like a basal cell carcinoma, being locally invasive. It is solid, but with areas of cystic degeneration. An x-ray shows large and small loculi.

Treatment

The tumor recurs after enucleation, so the treatment is resection of the affected portion of the jaw with a margin

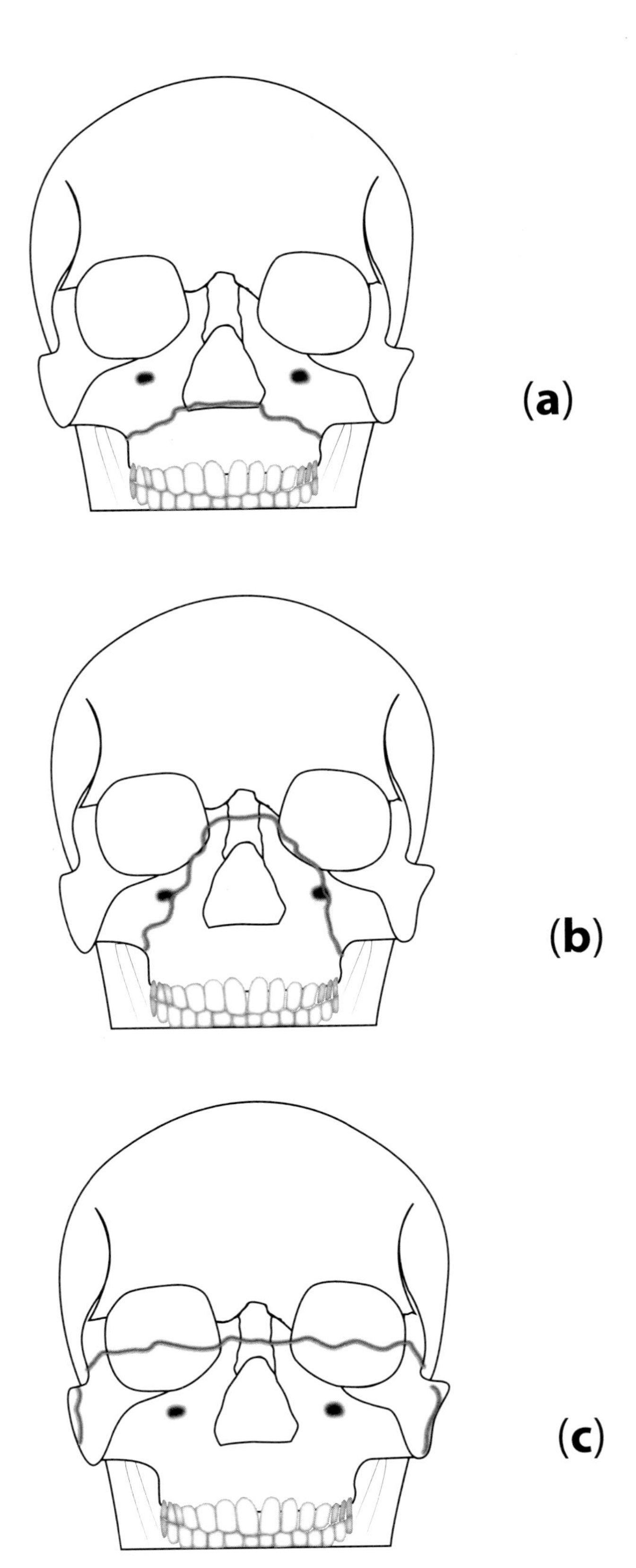

Fig.46.8 Fractures of the face: (a) Lefort (I), (b) Lefort (II), (c) Lefort (III).

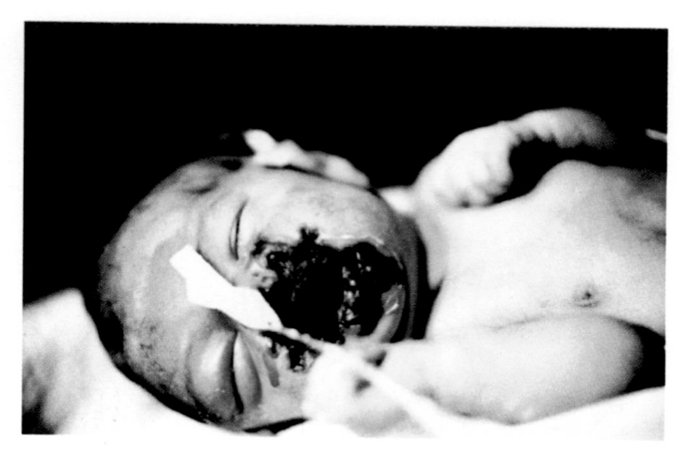

Fig.46.9 Cancrum oris

of healthy tissue. The defect in the jaw is bridged by a bone graft.

Swellings elsewhere on the jaws

These may be benign swellings or tumors.

Benign swellings

Fibro-osseous group

These are probably disorders of ossification in membrane bones. They contain fibrous tissue and bone. Examples are ivory osteomas and fibrous dysplasias.

Giant-celled reparative granuloma

This probably results from a hemorrhage within the jaw. It occurs between 10 and 25 years of age, i.e. at an earlier age than osteoclastoma. Its treatment is by thorough curettage.

Tumors

Osteoclastomas occur from time to time in both mandible and maxilla.

Mandible

A primary or secondary cancer is rare in the mandible. However, the mandible may be involved by the spread of a carcinoma of the lip, tongue or floor of mouth. Irradiation causes bone necrosis; therefore, the affected area of mandible must be resected.

Maxilla

Osteogenic sarcoma and squamous-cell carcinoma from the hard palate or gum are seen occasionally.

Colummar-celled carcinoma from the *maxillary antrum* produces a foul blood-stained discharge from the nose. It may grow:

- Medially to cause nasal obstruction.
- Upwards to produce diplopia.
- Forwards to produce a facial swelling.
- Downwards to bulge out from the palate.

High-voltage irradiation is given. If lymph nodes are palpable a neck dissection is performed.

All nasal polyps should be biopsied to avoid missing a malignancy; fragments of the tumor may be washed out by antral lavage and examined microscopically.

THE MOUTH

Stomatitis

This is a general term applied to inflammatory, erosive and ulcerative conditions affecting the oral mucosa. *Gingivitis* refers to similar conditions confined to the gums. If they spread to other parts of the oral mucosa the term gingivostomatitis is used.

Infecting organisms

The mouth contains many organisms. Most of them are harmless under normal circumstances. Their ability to cause damage is reduced by:

- Regular desquamation of surface cells.
- Constant washing of the mouth by saliva.
- Integrity of the epithelium.

Types of pathogens

Some organisms produce specific infections (*true pathogens*). Others take advantage of any weakness in the defences of the oral mucosa to produce an infection (*facultative pathogens*).

An oral ulcer is soon colonized by facultative pathogens e.g. streptococci, staphylococci and Vincent's organisms. A non-specific acute inflammation results. This secondary infection can be treated by 0.2% solution of chlorhexidine as a mouthwash.

Predisposing factors

The following factors predispose to the development of stomatitis:

- Deficiency of iron, vitamin B_{12}, folic acid and other B vitamins causes atrophy of the epithelium. The patient may present with a red, burning tongue and angular cheilitis due to secondary infection by Candida albicans.
- Severe protein deficiency produces a similar condition.
- Chronic lead poisoning leads to a blue line at the gum margin.

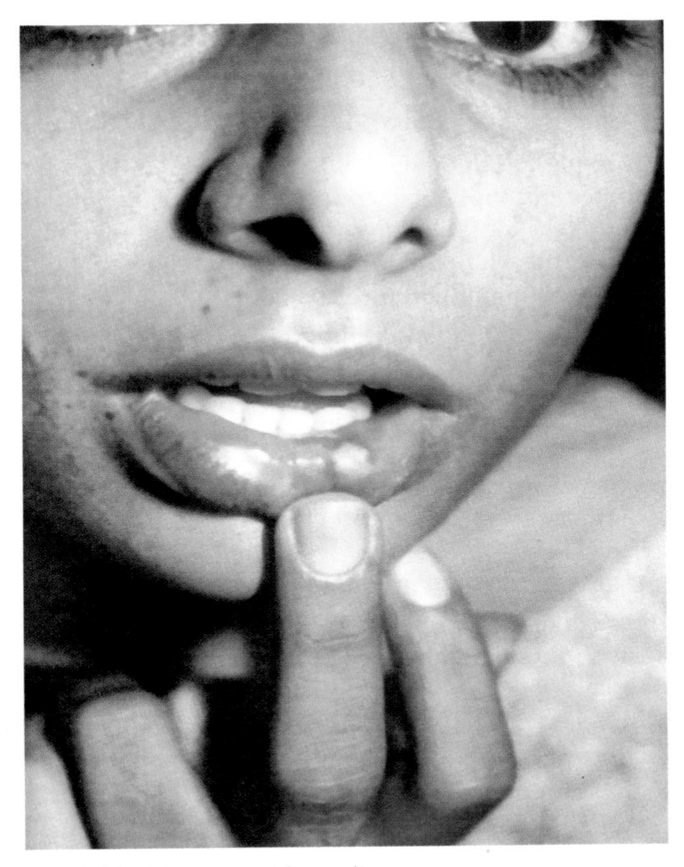

Fig.46.10 Mucous cyst lower lip

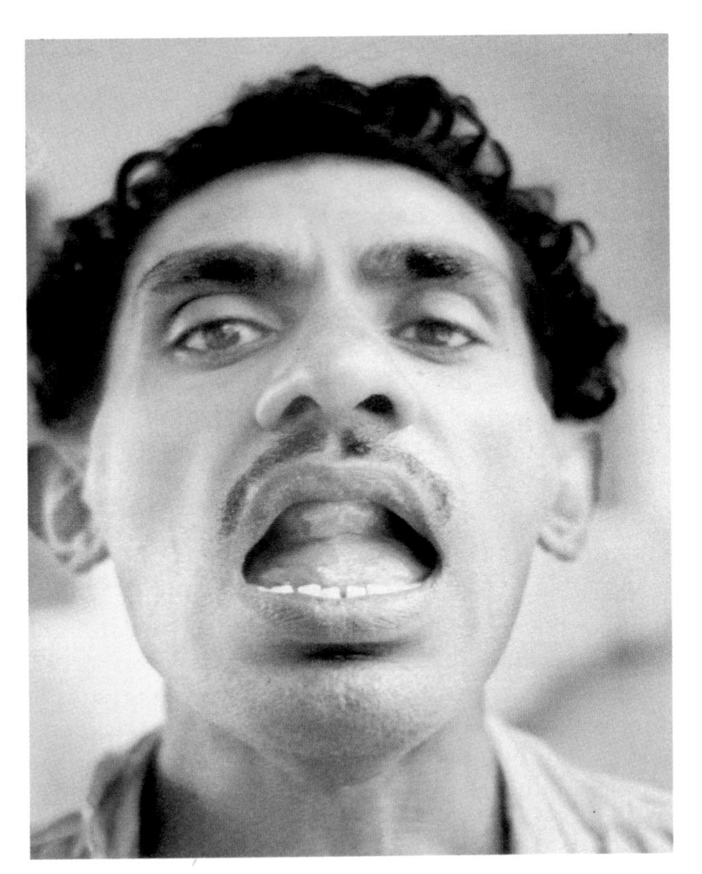

a

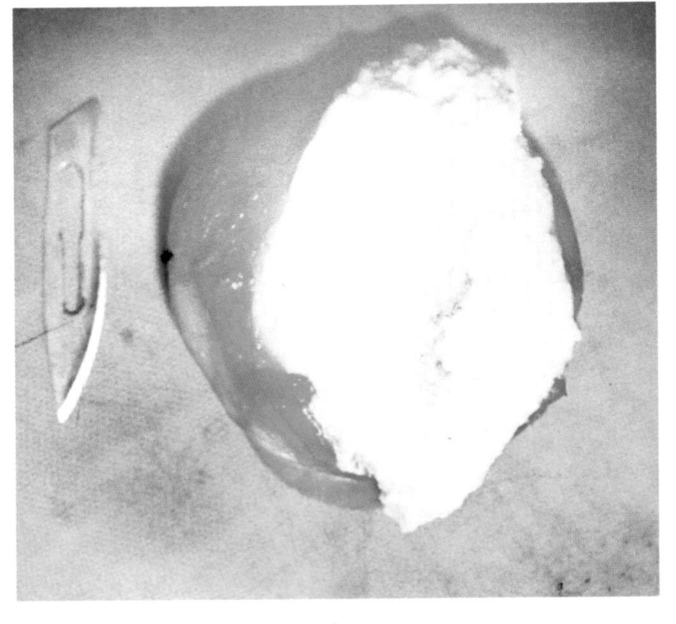

b

Fig.46.11 Sublingual dermoid. a. In situ. b. Cut open to show white keratin paste

- Excessive intake of iodides results in a sore mouth and salivation.
- Cytotoxic drugs, agranulocytosis, aplastic anemia and hypogammaglobulinaemia reduce the ability to deal with secondary infection.

Aphthous stomatitis

(Greek. *Aphtha:* small ulcer). *Minor* aphthae appear in crops on a cyclical basis. The ulcers are 5–10mm across, with a yellow base and red margin, and are painful. They heal within a fortnight.

Major aphthae are larger and deeper, and heal with scarring. A mouthwash of 0.2% chlorhexidine or tetracycline helps healing.

Herpes simplex infections

Herpes simplex is caused by a virus from the *Herpesviridae* genus. The infection may be subclinical or may result in stomatitis. Vesicles appear and break down to form small (<5mm across) ulcers that coalesce. There is fever and lymphadenitis. An analgesic elixir and 0.2% chlorhexidine mouthwash are prescribed. Healing takes place in 10 to 14 days.

Herpes labialis

This consists of a reactivation of the herpes virus on exposure to cold winds, bright sunlight etc. It is infectious, so doctors and nurses should take due precautions.

Vincent's gingivostomatitis

This occurs due to symbiosis between *Borrelia vincenti* and *Fusiformis fusiformis*, both anaerobic and gram negative organisms. It produces a deep ulcer crater covered with greenish grey necrotic tissue, which bleeds readily, and has a characteristic smell. There is fever, ache in the part and salivation. Both organisms are sensitive to penicillin and metronidazole. However, local factors also need treatment by a dentist.

Cancrum oris

This is a severe form of stomatitis affecting poorly nourished children as a complication of measles etc. During states of toxemia and dehydration, thrombosis of branches of the facial arteries develops, and results in necrosis of the tissues. Ulceration starts from the gums and spreads into the jaws. It also spreads to the lips and cheeks producing full-thickness tissue loss (Fig.46.9). Treatment should be prompt, with systemic penicillin and metronidazole, local irrigation and a high-protein, vitamin-rich diet through a nasogastric tube. Defects of the lips can be filled by nasolabial flaps. More extensive cheek defects may require repair by tubed pedicle flaps.

Monilial stomatitis

Candida albicans infection occurs in the form of thrush. This affects debilitated infants and persons with diminished resistance, e.g. the chronically ill, the elderly, and during treatment with steroids and cytotoxic agents. Small soft white plaques form, looking like milk curds. When these are wiped off, bleeding erosions are revealed. Acute candidiasis also occurs after treatment with broad spectrum antibiotics. The lateral part of the tongue is smooth and red with a burning sensation. 1% aqueous gentian violet is used in infants, and amphotericin B lozenges in older patients.

Angular stomatitis

This condition is seen in infants who suck a thumb, and in the elderly, due to leakage of saliva. There are moist cracks at the angles of the mouth, with infection by candida and staphylococci. Treatment is by nystatin cream and fucidate ointment.

The single oral ulcer

The most common cause of this condition is acute or chronic trauma, e.g. from a toothbrush or a denture. If an ulcer persists for weeks or months the possibility of malignancy must be ruled out by biopsy.

Mucous cysts (Mucocele)

These may occur on the lips and cheeks. They arise due to retention in, or extravasation from, minor salivary glands. They are small soft round blue-purple swellings (Fig.46.10). The treatment is excision along with the underlying minor salivary gland.

Ranula

This arises due to extravasation of saliva from a sublingual gland. A translucent swelling forms in the floor of the mouth. There is a delicate fibrous capsule lined by a layer of macrophages. The entire mass of gland and extravasation should be removed by gentle dissection.

Sublingual dermoid

This condition arises due to inclusion of skin during fusion in the ventral midline. This produces an opaque swelling. It is lined by stratified squamous epithelium and filled with paste-like keratin. It commonly presents in the midline of the floor of the mouth (Fig.46.11).

Carcinoma of the cheek

Most of these are squamous cell carcinomas. The incidence is increased by smoking, drinking alcohol and chewing betel leaf.

Radiotherapy is the treatment of choice, using external beams. Surgery is required for residual or recurrent tumor, or if radiotherapy is not available. If a full-thickness defect results, this is repaired by tubed pedicle flaps from the deltopectoral area. Enlarged neck nodes are treated by neck dissection.

TONGUE

Tongue-tie

Tongue-tie and ankyloglossia are terms applied to a short lingual frenum (Fig.46.12). Attempts to protrude the tongue result in heaping up of the mid-portion of the tongue. The condition can result in considerable speech impediment.

It is not commonly realized that stretch on the short frenum can irritate the neighbouring opening of the duct of the submandibular salivary gland, and occasionally result in excessive salivation. Characteristically, the patient complains that when he wakes up in the morning his mouth is full of saliva. It is only after he has spat it out that he can talk to anyone. The short frenum should be divided across. The wound takes on a linear shape in the vertical direction, and should be closed with fine absorbable sutures.

Lingual thyroid

The thyroid descends from the foramen cecum to its final position in the neck. If it does not do so, it may be seen as a midline swelling at the junction of the middle and posterior thirds of the tongue, i.e. at the foramen cecum. If large, it may cause difficulty in breathing and swallowing. However, before it is removed, *a radioiodine uptake scan should be carried out, to ensure that there is some thyroid tissue at its normal site* in the neck; if it is not, the removed lingual thyroid should be sliced, and some of the slices implanted among the muscles of the neck.

CARCINOMA OF THE TONGUE

Carcinomas of the tongue constitute about half of all oral cancers. 97 percent are squamous cell in type, the remainder being salivary and connective tissue tumors. Squamous cell carcinoma predominantly occurs in older men. However, it has also been seen in younger individuals and should therefore not be overlooked in this population. Poor oral hygiene and the use of tobacco and alcohol are considered to be important in its causation. When tobacco and alcohol are used together over a period of time, the risk is greatly increased. Tumors arising from the ventral surface of the tongue extend directly to the floor of the mouth, and it is difficult to distinguish them from tumors arising primarily at this site.

Clinical features

Symptoms

Anterior two-thirds

Tumors of the anterior two-thirds of the tongue present most often as painful ulcers (Fig.46.13) or visible swellings. Dysphagia, or the presence of a lump in the neck, are uncommon features.

Posterior third

Carcinomas of the *posterior third* of the tongue are very different from those of the anterior two thirds; they behave like tumors of the oropharynx, many of them being non-Hodgkin lymphomas. They commonly present either with local pain or dysphagia. A lump of lymph nodes in the neck is also a fairly frequent occurrence.

If there is any fixation of the tongue, difficulty will be experienced in propelling food backwards from the mouth into the pharynx. A lesion near the alveolus may result in toothache or in difficulty in wearing dentures. If a tooth is extracted, its socket may not heal. Generally speaking, the more anterior the lesion the earlier the patient seeks advice.

Extensive lesions of the tongue may extend posteriorly to involve the *larynx*. Even if the larynx is not infiltrated, involvement or resection of the base of the tongue may predispose the patient to aspiration pneumonia.

Signs

Inspection will show whether the lesion is ulcerative or exophytic. The patient should be asked to move the tongue from side to side; this allows the degree of fixation to be assessed.

Palpation is an essential part of the examination of any lesion in the oral cavity. Tongue ulcers are like icebergs; while a small part of the tumor may be visible, there may be many times the volume in the deeper tissues of the tongue. This can be assessed only by palpation.

Staging is based on size and this should be recorded. The extent of induration is also included in this estimate of *size*.

Nerve involvement is difficult to assess:

- Anesthesia indicates infiltration of the lingual nerve, and since this lies deep, its involvement means extensive spread of the tumor.
- In the hard palate anesthesia signifies infiltration of the greater palatine nerve, and such patients are incurable.

Mandibular involvement is best assessed on x-ray, but any fixation to bone must be noted clinically.

Metastases

Finally, the neck should be palpated for metastatic nodes. These usually lie in the submandibular area or the deep jugular chain, but the tongue also has direct drainage to the jugulo-omohyoid node in the lower part of the neck. Lesions in the posterior part of the tongue may spread to the retropharyngeal nodes, and pressure from these on the sympathetic chain may result in Horner's syndrome.

Lymph node metastases constitute the most important factor in prognosis. In their absence as many as 80 percent patients survive for five years or more; in their presence only 40 percent. This shows the importance of early diagnosis.

Investigations

X-rays

If spread to the mandible is suspected, x-rays should be taken. They also show the state of the teeth and the presence of any root abscesses; these facts have an important bearing on the use of radiotherapy, which

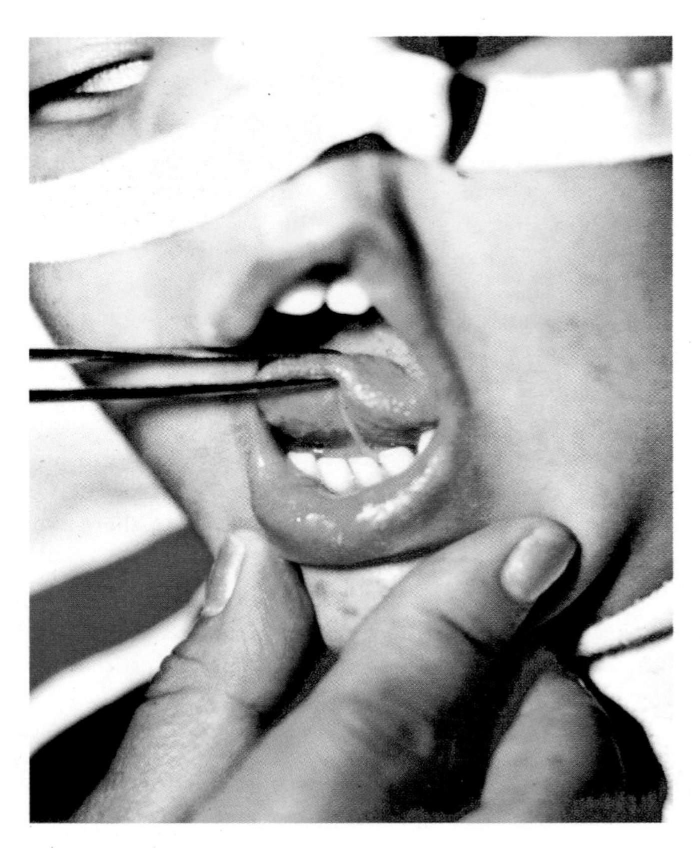

Fig.46.12 Tongue-tie

should be postponed until these infections have been dealt with.

CT scan

If spread to the retropharyngeal area is suspected, CT scan is useful.

Biopsy

This should be carried out under general anesthesia; local anesthesia causes a rise in the tissue pressure, which may result in spread of the tumor. A representative part of the tumor should be chosen for biopsy, not the necrotic centre. General anesthesia also allows examination of the oro-pharynx for a concurrent second primary, present in up to 10% cases.

Treatment

Anterior two-thirds of the tongue

Radiotherapy

Carcinomas of the anterior two-thirds of the tongue can be treated by radiotherapy, either using an external beam or by interstitial implantation of tubes into which radium needles or iridium 192 can be placed. External radiation in doses of 6500 rads is useful, but interstitial radiation can deliver doses over 10,000 rads over a small area with greater effect.

Surgery

In general, surgical treatment is required for tumors that:

- are large,
- involve the mandible,
- have recurred after radiotherapy, and
- are accompanied by palpable neck nodes.

Surgical therapy consists of resection of the tumor with a margin of normal tissue and block dissection of the regional lymph nodes. Hemiglossectomy is generally carried out for any lesion of the lateral tongue. Due to uncertainty about the ability to obtain clear margins, surgery is often followed by adjuvant radiotherapy.

Posterior one-third of the tongue

Radiotherapy

Carcinomas of the posterior one-third of the tongue are more radiosensitive, so that 2-year local control rates of 75% for T1 lesions and 67% for T2 lesions are obtained.

Surgery

Advanced disease at the primary site or disease with cervical metastases requires surgery. If the lesion is lateral enough, partial glossectomy may suffice, otherwise total glossectomy with or without laryngectomy is required. The 3-year survival rate after total glossectomy is around 50 percent, and 90% of patients can maintain adequate nutrition by the oral route. If the larynx is preserved, 80% have intelligible speech.

Neck nodes

If *neck lymph nodes* are palpable a neck dissection should be carried out. Fixed nodes are not necessarily a contraindication to radical neck dissection, as the structure to which they are fixed can often be removed.

Preoperative radiotherapy and surgery

If preoperative radiotherapy is employed followed by surgery, the cure rate is increased but complications like infection, wound breakdown and bone necrosis are also more frequent. If a tumor recurs after surgery, radiotherapy seldom rescues the patient; on the other hand where radiotherapy has failed, surgery succeeds in about one-third of the cases.

Post-irradiation care

Radiotherapy tends to cause periodontal disease and xerostomia, which results in rampant radiation caries.

Thus if a patient with intact teeth is irradiated he should undergo a *6 monthly dental check-up* for the rest of his life. If he fails to do this and caries starts, pulpitis and apical abscess formation quickly follow, and in the irradiated case the mandible may be lost due to osteoradionecrosis.

It is therefore wiser to extract all infected and diseased teeth and those which may cause future problems before radiating an oral cavity. This usually does not meet with any resistance, because patients with a carcinoma of the tongue often have badly diseased teeth. Modern sets of artificial teeth are a lot better than diseased and irradiated teeth.

Reconstruction

Resection of cancers of the tongue or floor of the mouth can leave large defects in the latter. If more than half the tongue is removed or less than 1cm of the floor of the mouth remains, replacement of soft tissues by a flap is required.

Pectoralis major myocutaneous flap

This is a very useful flap. It consists of a pedicle of pectoralis major muscle carrying the pectoral branch of the acromiothoracic artery on its deep surface and an ellipse of skin on its superficial aspect. It is elevated upto the clavicle, tunnelled underneath the skin of the neck and passed through the defect in the floor of the mouth. It is sutured in such a manner that the skin island lies in the mouth and the muscle pedicle lies over and protects the carotid sheath.

Free jejunal graft

In cases where laryngectomy is also required, the resulting gap between the pharynx and the trachea is bridged by a free graft of the jejunum. For blood supply, the supplying artery of the graft is anastomosed to the superior thyroid artery, the vein (end-to-side) to the internal jugular vein, using microvascular techniques.

A number of carcinomas of the tongue are incurable on presentation due to:

- Distant metastases.
- Very advanced local disease.
- Bilateral neck glands.
- Poor general condition.

SALIVARY GLANDS

Investigations

Sialography

A radiopaque liquid such as sodium diatrizoate is injected into the parotid duct using a fine catheter, and antero-posterior and lateral x-rays taken. They outline

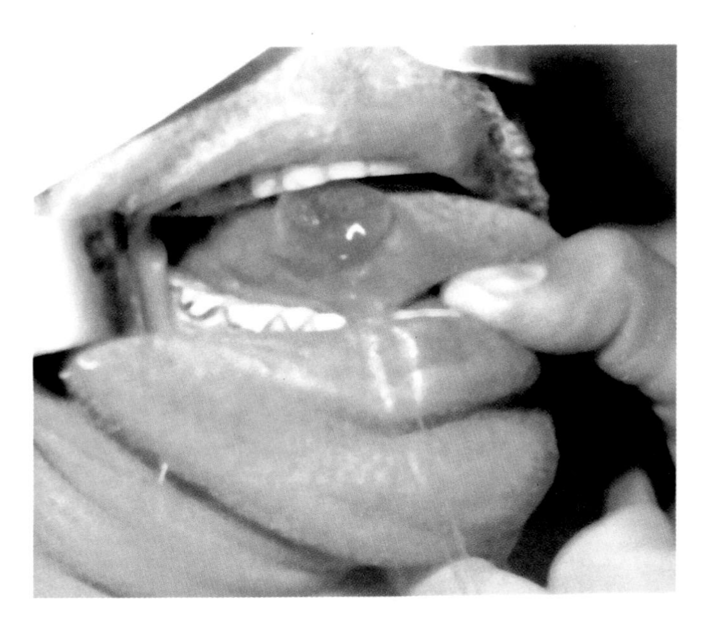

Fig.46.13 Carcinoma of the tongue presenting as an ulcer with raised edges

dilatations or constrictions of the duct, as well as any displacements of the ducts due to an expanding lesion.

Immunological studies and analysis of *blood chemistry* are valuable in the evaluation of patients whose salivary problems are related to underlying conditions such as Sjogren's syndrome, lymphoma, arthritis or other collagen or autoimmune diseases.

Inflammations

Acute parotitis

The two common causes of acute parotitis are mumps and postoperative suppurative parotitis.

Mumps

Mumps arises due to infection by a virus. High fever is accompanied by painful swelling of both parotid glands, often along with acute orchitis; this is occasionally followed by atrophy of the testes.

Suppurative parotitis

Suppurative parotitis is commonly seen in patients who are severely toxaemic, and where marked dehydration occurs in the postoperative period. *Staphylococcus aureus* is the usual infecting organism. A hard, tender and painful swelling is seen in the parotid region. An abscess often forms, and requires drainage.

Prevention

For prevention of acute suppurative parotitis, adequate hydration must be ensured during the postoperative period. Regular mouthwashes help maintain a proper standard of oral hygiene, so that bacteria cannot multiply.

Treatment

Antibiotics and analgesics are administered. The patient's state of hydration and his general condition are improved. Oral hygiene should be attended to, including the use of toothpaste applied with a soft toothbrush. If the general condition does not improve and an abscess forms, it should be incised and drained.

Chronic sialadenitis

The most common cause of recurrent or chronic sialadenitis is obstruction of the duct of the gland due to a calculus.

Salivary calculus

The secretion of the *submandibular gland* is thick in consistency, and the duct has a tortuous course. Therefore, salivary calculi are seen most commonly in these glands. A submandibular salivary calculus can be felt in the floor of the mouth by bi-manual palpation. It is shown up by x-rays because it is radiopaque due to its calcium content. For its removal, an incision is made in the floor of the mouth over the duct under local anesthesia.

TUMORS OF THE SALIVARY GLANDS

Benign tumors

Pleomorphic adenoma

Also called a mixed salivary tumor, this is by far the most common neoplasm of the salivary glands. The sex distribution is equal and the peak age incidence is in the fifth decade. It is a very slow-growing tumor, and forms a smooth, firm lump, usually over the lower pole of the parotid. When the tumor attains a large size it becomes lobulated (Fig.46.14). It is usually symptomless, apart from the lump. Pain and facial paralysis should raise the suspicion of malignancy.

On *microscopic examination* the tumor shows a mixed appearance. Epithelial cells appear in strands, while others take on a duct-like arrangement. In parts of the tumor a mucoid material is produced between the cells, resulting in an appearance resembling cartilage. The tumor is classified as benign, but strands of tumor cells penetrate the capsule of the gland. Therefore *simple enucleation is not advised*, as it can leave behind residual tumor and lead to a recurrence. Occasionally, a long-standing pleomorphic adenoma may change to a carcinoma.

Investigations

In suspected neoplastic disease of the parotid, *MRI or CT* scanning should be carried out.

Fine needle aspiration biopsy should be used routinely in the assessment of suspected neoplastic disease of the salivary glands.

Open incisional or excisional biopsies may be required if a granulomatous or autoimmune condition is suspected. However, such biopsies should be undertaken only after careful consideration, since they carry the risk of dissemination of mixed tumors or malignancy.

Treatment

The superficial lobe of the *parotid* gland containing the tumor should be removed, with preservation of the branches of the facial nerve. The main trunk of the nerve is identified outside the stylomastoid foramen, and each branch traced forwards.

In the case of the *submandibular* salivary gland, the entire gland is removed through a submandibular incision, avoiding the mandibular branch of the facial nerve, which supplies muscles at the angle of the mouth.

Adenolymphoma (Warthin's tumor)

This tumor presents a slowly enlarging soft swelling. It is much more common in males, the peak age incidence being in the seventh decade. Bilateral tumors are sometimes encountered. Unlike other salivary tumors, an adenolymphoma produces a 'hot' spot in a ^{99}Tcm scan, so a firm preoperative diagnosis is possible without biopsy.

Malignant tumors

Carcinomas of the salivary glands

The histological types of carcinomas include adenocarcinoma, squamous cell carcinoma and undifferentiated carcinomas. The adenocarcinomas contain the various cell types found in the salivary glands. The epidermoid and undifferentiated carcinomas resemble those seen at other sites. All these neoplasms tend to produce signs of malignancy at an early stage; these include fixation, resorption of adjacent bone, pain, anesthesia, and paralysis of muscles.

An *adenoid cystic carcinoma* is the most common malignant tumor of the salivary glands. It is associated with a poor prognosis, because it infiltrates over long distances in the perineural tissues of adjacent nerves, and in the medullary cavity of neighbouring bones, before causing bone resorption. Thus, the tumor is always more extensive than the physical signs or radiological appearances suggest. The most common presenting feature is pain, and the growth may be present for some years before diagnosis. During this period the patient often consults different specialists for facial pain.

Treatment

Carcinoma of a salivary gland should be treated by radical excision of the gland:

- In the case of the *parotid*, the facial nerve should be resected if its preservation is likely to result in incomplete resection of the tumor. Restoration of continuity of the nerve will require primary nerve grafting.
- In the case of the *submandibular* gland radical excision with, if necessary, removal of the adjacent tongue, presents no difficulty.

In *mucoepidermoid* and *squamous cell* carcinoma of the parotid and submaxillary glands, metastases to regional lymph nodes occur in about 40 percent of the patients. Therefore in these cases regional node dissection should be carried out. If lymph nodes are palpable neck dissection should be carried out in all cases.

Surgery may be *contraindicated* if the disease is extensive or the patient severely debilitated; radiotherapy or chemotherapy can then be employed.

Postoperative radiotherapy is indicated if surgical margins are close or positive for tumor cells, and in high grade mucoepidermoid carcinoma that shows a propensity for early metastasis.

Survival

Five-year survival rates vary from 40 percent for high-grade tumors to 90 percent in low-grade neoplasms.

COMMON FEATURES OF HEAD AND NECK TUMORS

Most malignant tumors developing in the anatomic area above the clavicles are squamous cell carcinomas originating from the respiratory and stratified epithelium of the upper aerodigestive tract. The change from normal to malignant epithelium passes through the stages of hyperplasia and hyperkeratosis (grouped together as leukoplakia) and erythroplakia or red patch, the last-named of which is premalignant.

Leucoplakia

In the past, leukoplakia was considered a precursor of malignancy, and removal of all leukoplakic areas of mucosa was advised. However, recent thinking suggests that this change is not in itself premalignant but simply evidence of chronic irritation; therefore surveillance rather than removal is recommended.

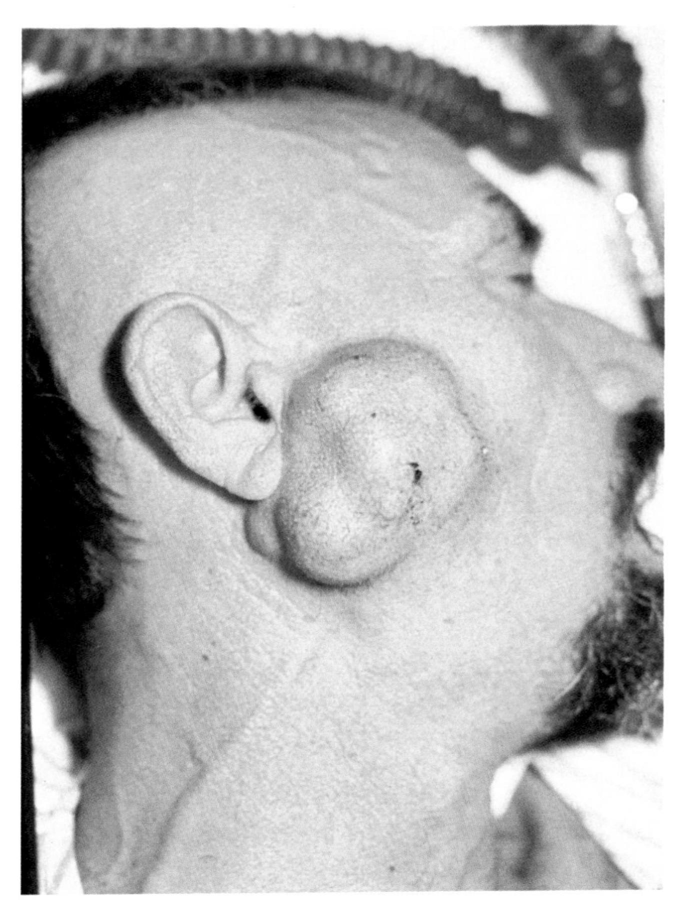

a

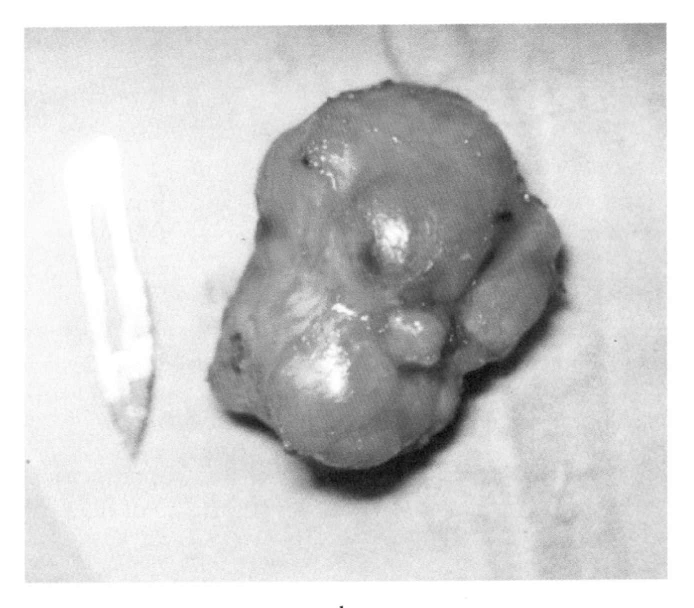

b

Fig.46.14 a: Mixed parotid tumor (pleomorphic adenoma) of many years' duration, so that it has become lobulated. b: The lobules perceptible on inspection are seen on the specimen.

Extent of dysfunction

Malignant tumors of the head and neck cause more disruption of local function than tumors at other sites. The two main vegetative functions of the human body---alimentation and respiration---are dependent on the harmonious function of the bone, muscle and mucosa-lined cavities that constitute the head and neck. Invasive carcinoma disrupts these functions with resultant malnutrition, upper airway obstruction and recurrent aspiration pneumonia.

Cause of death

Thus, whereas with tumors in other parts of the body death is usually caused by disseminated malignancy, 60% of patients dying with head and neck cancers have no distant metastases.

Prognosis

As with most solid tumors, the best *prognosticator* of head and neck cancer is the presence or absence of lymph node metastases. Again, extracapsular spread of tumor is a bad prognostic sign.

Flaps for repairing skin and soft tissue defects in the head and neck

While removing advanced cancers in the head and neck considerable areas of the skin and soft tissues have often to be removed. If a simple split-skin graft is used to resurface the area, a depressed and wrinkled area of skin may remain. For this reason a variety of skin flaps are employed:

Random flaps

These include advancement, transposition, and rotation flaps, and Z-plasties as explained and illustrated in chapter 4 on burns and grafts.

Axial flaps

An axial flap is based on an artery running down its long axis. Therefore it can be a good deal longer than broad, i.e. it can be designed without regard to the length to width ratio. Some examples follow:

- *Median forehead flap* based on the supratrochlear vessels, for replacement of loss of the tip of the nose or an ala.
- *Scalping flap* based on the superficial temporal artery, for loss of the whole nose.
- *Deltopectoral flap* from the upper chest is supplied by the perforating branches of the internal mammary artery. It may be used to supply skin cover, as well as lining in the mouth.

Myocutanous flaps

This type of flap is required where skin as well as underlying soft tissue has been lost. It consists of a large-sized muscle vascularized by a defined artery and vein. The skin covering the muscle, usually in the shape of an ellipse, is left attached to its surface. The muscle is detached from its origin or insertion, or from both. It is tunnelled under the skin lying between the donor and recipient sites. At its destination the skin is sutured into the epithelial defect, while the muscle fills any soft tissue gap, besides acting as a vascularized pedicle for the skin patch.

Pectoralis major myocutaneous flap

Resection of cancer of the floor of the mouth may leave a defect in place of the excised portions of the tongue, the floor of the mouth, and the mandible. A suitable flap for reconstruction is the pectoralis major myocutaneous flap. The muscle is detached from its origin and insertion but is left attached to an overlying ellipse of skin and its supplying thoracoacromial vessels. It is tunnelled under the skin of the neck and into the mouth. It is a brilliantly designed flap:

- The patch of skin fills the mucosal and tongue defect.
- If a radical neck dissection has been done, the pectoralis major:
  - o Fills the hollow left by removal of the sternomastoid and restores the contour of the neck.
  - o Provides cover to the carotid arteries.

Free microvascular flaps

Unlike the above-mentioned flaps, a microvascular flap is completely divided from its donor site, i.e. it is a *free graft*. Its supplying artery is anastomosed to an equal-sized artery at the recipient site. As these arteries are small, microvascular techniques have to be employed, using an operating microscope and extremely fine instruments and sutures. The whole operation takes many hours, but can transfer composite grafts over long distances for a very good cosmetic effect, and provides a one-stage procedure for the resolution of a complex problem.

Chapter

47 NECK

Branchial cyst

In the fetus, on the side of the neck four bars appear; these are the branchial arches, which are separated by the branchial clefts. The first cleft persists as the external auditory meatus. The second arch grows over the third and fourth arches to fuse with the fifth. The enclosed epithelium disappears. If it persists, a branchial cyst results. If the second arch fails to fuse with the fifth, the opening persists as a branchial fistula.

A branchial cyst is lined by squamous epithelium and its contents are normally like white paste, containing keratinous cellular debris and cholesterol crystals. It lies under the anterior border of the upper third of the sternomastoid as a fluctuant swelling. If it is infected, it may be confused with lymphadenitis. It should be removed through an incision parallel to the skin creases of the neck.

Branchial fistula

A branchial fistula represents a persistent second branchial cleft. The external orifice of the fistula is located at the anterior border of the sternomastoid muscle, at the junction of its middle and lower thirds. The tract proceeds superiorly and passes inwards through the bifurcation of the carotid artery. The internal orifice lies close to the tonsil, or the track may end blindly outside the lateral pharyngeal wall. The discharge of the fistula consists of mucus or muco-pus.

Treatment

In order to get rid of the troublesome discharge of mucus as well as the possibility of repeated infections, branchial fistulae should be excised. Dissection of the tract is facilitated by passing a fine probe into the orifice and utilizing it as a guide for dissection. It is also useful to inject methylene blue dye into the opening. As the tract is followed up in the neck, a series of two or three small transverse incisions in a stepladder pattern are preferable to a long oblique incision, which is cosmetically undesirable.

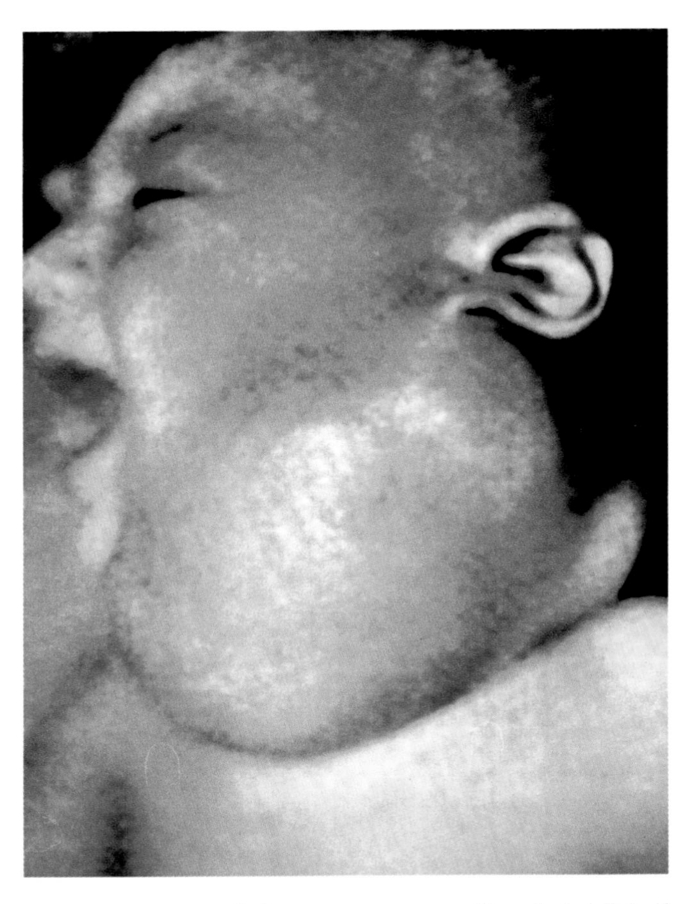

Fig.47.1 Huge cystic hygroma occupying the whole left half of the neck

Cystic hygroma

In the early embryo primitive lymph sacs develop, one on either side of the neck. Normally they disappear. However, if one of them becomes sequestrated and persists, a cystic hygroma results. It consists of a collection of cysts, like a mass of soap bubbles. A cystic hygroma is usually present at birth; it may occasionally be so large as to obstruct labour. Occasionally, if it is very large (Fig.47.1), it may compress the trachea and produce respiratory distress. It usually lies in the lower part of the posterior triangle of the neck. The swelling is soft and cystic. It is brilliantly transilluminant, and this characteristic distinguishes it from all other swellings in the neck.

Treatment

Excision of all the cysts at an early age is the treatment of choice; if left untreated, the hygroma can be subject to repeated infections in its cysts. However, radical ablative surgery is not advised in this benign lesion. Conservative unroofing of remaining cysts is advised, preserving all adjacent crucial structures. Postoperative wound drainage is desirable and is best accomplished by the suction technique.

INFLAMMATORY CONDITIONS

Ludwig's angina

In this condition there is an indurated, inflamed and swollen area in the submandibular region and the floor of the mouth. The cause is a virulent, usually streptococcal, infection of these parts. If the condition remains untreated, it may assume dangerous proportions. The swollen tongue is pushed towards the palate and forwards through the open mouth. Ludwig's angina is an infection of a closed space, and untreated the inflammation spreads to the submucosa of the glottis, so that the patient's life is in danger from edema of the glottis.

Treatment

If the condition is diagnosed very early, antibiotics may abort the infection. If the swelling does not subside with such treatment, a transverse curved incision is made below the jaw and the mylohyoid muscles divided. This decompresses the closed fascial space.

Cervical lymphadenitis

Nearly half the lymph nodes in the body lie in the neck; they guard the portals of entry into the respiratory and gastrointestinal tracts. Bacteria entering these tracts often pass through the mucosa of the throat and reach these nodes; therefore inflammation of the lymph nodes of the neck is very common, and occurs from the oral and nasal cavities, the ear, the scalp, and the face.

Acute lymphadenitis

The affected nodes are enlarged and tender, and there is usually a degree of pyrexia. If the patient comes early, antibiotics and fomentation may help in resolving the infection. If an abscess forms, incision and drainage is required.

Tuberculous lymphadenitis

This condition is described in detail in chapter 43 on lymphatics and lymph nodes. In the neck, usually the upper jugular chain of nodes is first affected. If widespread lymphadenitis is present, periadenitis often occurs, as shown by matting together of the nodes. If the patient's natural resistance is good, or he receives appropriate treatment, fibrosis or calcification may occur. If not, the caseating material liquefies and a cold abscess forms.

Collar-stud abscess

If the pus erodes the overlying deep fascia and flows into the subcutaneous tissues of the neck, it is called a collar-stud abscess. If left untreated, the skin over it becomes reddened, and soon a discharging sinus forms, through which secondary infection can occur.

Chemodectoma (Carotid body tumor)

The carotid body, which lies at the bifurcation of the carotid artery, contains chemoreceptors sensitive to changes in the pH of the blood. Tumors arising in this structure are usually very slow-growing; only occasionally do they metastasize to the lymph nodes. This tumor is common in middle age. As it is attached to the carotid artery *it can be moved from side to side but not vertically*. Expansion of the tumor can lead to paresis of cranial nerves, usually the vagus and hypoglossal, with hoarseness, choking or dysphagia.

Diagnosis

The possibility of a carotid body tumor should be kept in mind in a patient who presents with a lump in the region of the carotid bifurcation. A misdiagnosis of lymph node enlargement with attempt at excision biopsy can result in excessive blood loss and a great deal of embarrassment.

Ultrasound pinpoints the diagnosis by:

- Confirming the relationship of the tumor with the carotid bifurcation with splaying of the carotid arteries.
- Showing up the internal vascularity of the neoplasm ('tumor blush').

MRI, specially with enhancement by gadolinium, provides greater soft tissue contrast. This allows the detection of tumors down to 5mm in diameter, as well as better assessment of the extent of invasion by a large tumor.

Because these tumors are vascular, preoperative biopsy is contraindicated.

Treatment

If the tumor is asymptomatic and growing slowly and the patient is elderly, removal is probably not required. However, it is easier and safer to remove the tumor before extensive local invasion, and so generally excision while the tumor is small is advocated. With tumors greater than 3cm in diameter it may be an advantage to shrink them preoperatively by embolization.

Operation

If excision is to be carried out, the surgeon must be prepared to replace the artery with a length of saphenous vein. During the grafting procedure the circulation to the brain should be continued by diverting the blood from the common to the internal carotid artery through a silicone tubing. This shunt also devascularizes the tumor by excluding the external carotid artery from the circulation.

Secondary carcinoma in the neck

Secondary carcinoma is quite commonly seen in the lymph nodes of the neck. In such a case a search must be made for the primary, by examining the possible sites in the region, including the thyroid, the tongue, the larynx, the pharynx, the jaws, the paranasal sinuses, as well as distant sites, such as the breast, the bronchus, the stomach and the testis.

Management

This varies with the situation:

- If the primary tumor is being treated by surgery and the cervical nodes are palpable, they may be excised en bloc with the primary.
- If lymph nodes become palpable some time after successful treatment of the primary, a neck dissection should be carried out.
- If radiotherapy results in resolution of the primary but the metastatic nodes persist, they can be dealt with by a neck dissection.

Neck dissection

For over a century now, cervical lymph nodes have been removed in cases of head and neck malignancies in order to eradicate disease in the primary lymphatic field. However, the extent of dissection recommended has undergone a reduction with the passage of time:

- In the *classical radical neck dissection* carried out by Crile in 1906, the cervical lymph nodes were removed en bloc along with those structures intimately associated with them, i.e. the internal jugular vein, the sternomastoid muscle, and the accessory nerve.
- *Preservation of accessory nerve.* A major factor in the morbidity of classical neck dissection is paralysis of the trapezius muscle by resection of the accessory nerve, and preservation of this nerve was recommended many years ago.
- *Prophylactic (elective) neck dissection.* Other surgeons have demonstrated techniques where the jugular vein and sternomastoid can also be left intact. These methods are particularly useful in prophylactic (elective) neck dissections where the lymph nodes are not enlarged.
- *Selective neck dissection.* Finally, it has been suggested that only those lymph nodes at risk should be resected. The concept of *selective* neck dissection, customized to the site of the primary disease, has gained support. Thus, for example:
    - For carcinoma of the lip, anterior tongue and floor of the mouth, *supraomohyoid* neck dissection might be used.
    - In thyroid disease an *anterior compartment* neck dissection may be appropriate.
    - For a nasopharyngeal lesion a *posterolateral* neck dissection may be employed.

Chapter

48 THYROID GLAND

Anatomy

Arterial blood is supplied to the thyroid through the superior thyroid artery at the upper pole, and the inferior thyroid artery at the lower pole. During thyroidectomy care should be taken when these vessels are ligated:

- The superior pedicle should be ligated close to the gland to prevent damaging the superior laryngeal nerve which runs along the artery.
- The inferior pedicle should be ligated a little away from the gland to prevent injury to the recurrent laryngeal nerve.

The parathyroid glands are located on the posterior side of the lobes of both sides.

INVESTIGATIONS

Laboratory

Thyroid function tests

Of all the tests the most commonly used test is the estimation of serum levels of T3, T4 and TSH.

Serum thyroid stimulating hormone (0.5–5 μU/mL)

Nowadays the ultrasensitive TSH assay is largely used as the most sensitive and specific test for diagnosing hypo- or hyperthyroidism. It is also utilized to optimize T4 therapy.

In euthyroid patients having thyroid nodules, TSH is the only test necessary. The reason is this: the secretion of TSH is secondary to the serum level of free T4, there being an inverse relationship between the free T4 level and TSH concentration. With a change in free T4 there is a shift in TSH levels in the opposite direction.

For screening purposes estimation of total T4 and T3 along with TSH are a routine protocol.

Total T4 (55–150 nmol/L) and T3 (1.5–3.5 nmol/L)

Serum total T4 and T3 are measured by radioimmunoassay. This includes both the free and bound fractions of the hormones.

T3. Estimation of T3 level is a better indicator of metabolism and generally not suited for screening purposes.

T4. Different conditions affect the levels of T4:

Increase in levels. The levels of serum total T4 are increased in hyperthyroidism, but also in:

- Pregnancy.
- Oral contraceptive use.
- Certain congenital diseases.

Decrease in levels. Decreased total T4 levels indicate hypothyroidism. They are also seen in:

- Protein-losing disorders like nephrotic syndrome.
- Use of anabolic steroids.

Individuals with these latter disorders may be euthyroid if their free T4 levels are normal.

In clinically hyperthyroid patients with normal T4 levels, measurement of total T3 levels is important, because they may have T3 thyrotoxicosis.

Free T4 (12–28 pmol/L) and Free T3 (3–9 pmol/L)

As already mentioned free T4 and free T3 fractions of the thyroid hormones are the biologically active forms. These radioassays are not routinely performed and are only done on demand whenever thyroid disease (early hyperthyroidism) is suspected.

Thyrotropin-releasing hormone

Thyrotropin-releasing hormone (TRH) is a hormone of hypothalamic–pituitary–thyroid axis and its determination helps to assess the secretory function of the pituitary gland. The anterior pituitary when stimulated by TRH responds by secreting TSH. While performing this test about 500 μg of TRH is administered intravenously and serum TSH levels are documented after one hour. Normally, TSH levels increase by 6μ IU/mL from the baseline. It is helpful in cases of borderline hyperthyroidism.

Antibodies

These antibodies include:

- Antithyroglobulin (anti-Tg) antibody.
- Antimicrosomal antibody.
- Thyroid-stimulating immunoglobulin.

The disorders associated with antibodies include:

- Hashimoto's thyroiditis.
- Graves' disease.
- Multinodular goitres.
- Occasionally thyroid neoplasms.

Serum calcitonin

This hormone is secreted by the parafollicular C cells and works to decrease the levels of serum calcium. The normal level is 0–4 pg/mL. It is a sensitive marker of medullary thyroid carcinoma.

Imaging

Radionuclide imaging

Isotope scanning provides graphic information about the size and shape of the thyroid and the distribution of functional activity in the gland. Thus it is used to screen and treat patients with differentiated thyroid cancers for metastatic disease. The ^{123}I or 99mTC (technetium pertechnetate) employed today have a short half-life and result in a lower dose of irradiation to the thyroid:

- The areas which trap less radioactivity are termed *cold*.
- Those that demonstrate increased activity are termed *hot*.
- Sometimes uptake of the isotope by the nodule is similar to the rest of the gland; these lesions are referred to as *warm* nodules.

Risk of malignancy

This is higher in "cold" lesions (20%) compared to "hot" or "warm" lesions (<5%):

- Most carcinomas are 'cold', while an autonomous toxic nodule is 'hot'.
- The scintillation scan may be of value in determining the presence of abnormally positioned thyroid tissue, such as substernal or lingual thyroid.
- After total thyroidectomy, whole body scanning after a tracer dose of radioisotope can demonstrate metastases. For this purpose ^{99}mTC is particularly sensitive.

However, if the thyroidectomy was partial the metastases are not shown up because they cannot compete with the remaining normal thyroid tissue in the uptake of iodine. This is an important reason why total thyroidectomy is preferred in the treatment of thyroid malignancies.

Ultrasound

Ultrasound is a noninvasive tool for assessing thyroid disorders. It helps to evaluate the size and multicentricity of thyroid nodules and whether the lesions are solid or cystic. Ultrasound can also guide the ultrasonographer when performing fine-needle aspiration biopsy (FNAB).

CT and MRI

Computed tomography and magnetic resonance imaging are also very helpful for imaging the thyroid gland. They can assess the size and extent of the lesions and their fixity to the underlying structures.

Biopsy

Biopsy of the thyroid is particularly helpful in two situations: in establishing a diagnosis of thyroiditis, and in differentiating between benign and malignant thyroid nodules. A core biopsy may be obtained with a Trucut needle, but the incidence of complications is high; with advancements in cytology it is not much used nowadays.

Fine needle aspiration cytology

In this test the aspirate of a nodule obtained by a 25-gauge needle on a 10ml syringe is evaluated. Interpretation should be made only by a trained cytologist. In the case of follicular lesions the technique cannot distinguish between benign and malignant lesions since no information is available about capsular and vascular invasion.

CONGENITAL ANOMALIES

The thyroid arises as a bud from the foramen cecum and descends to its final position in the neck. Some residual thyroid tissue may be found along the course of the thyroglossal tract. Very rarely the whole gland is ectopic.

Lingual thyroid

Most or all of the thyroid may be located at the back of the tongue at the foramen cecum, where it forms a swelling which may cause dysphagia, impairment of speech, respiratory obstruction or hemorrhage. It may be treated medically by L-thyroxine to keep the TSH

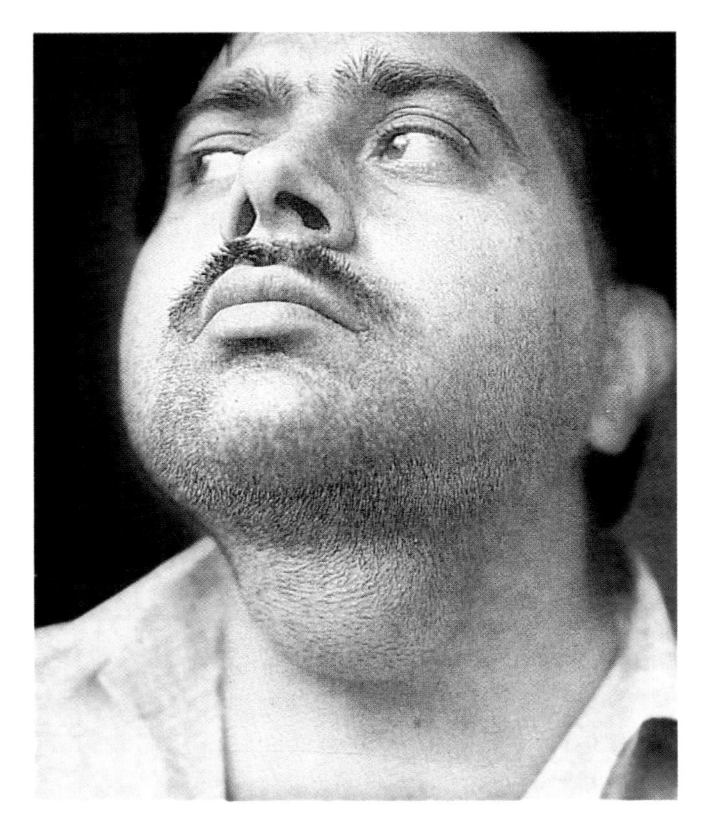

Fig.48.1 Thyroglossal cyst, located just below hyoid bone

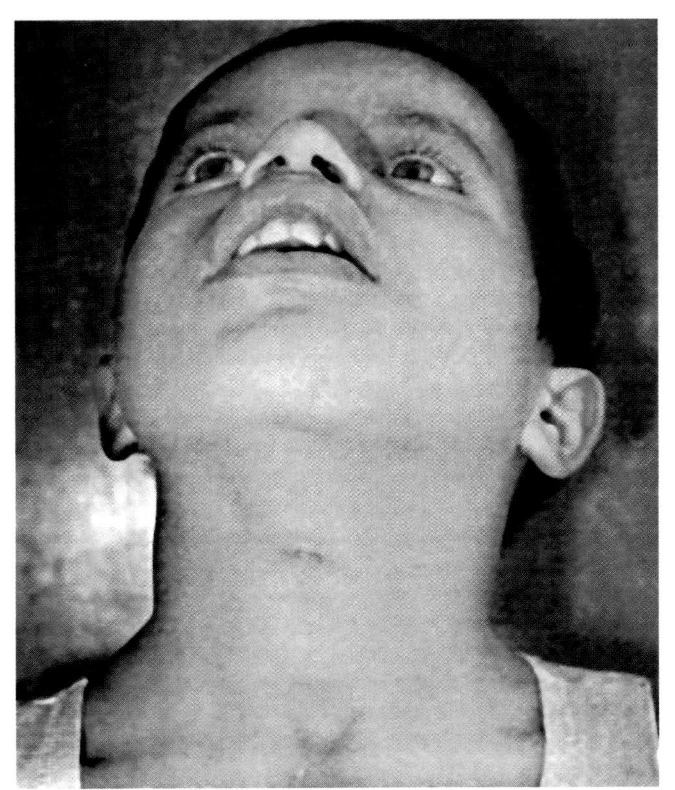

Fig.48.2 Thyroglossal fistula. The upper margin is crescentic, indicating the upward direction of the fistula.

suppressed when it usually becomes smaller. If it does not, it may have to be removed.

Before embarking upon surgery, radioactive iodine uptake scan of the neck must be done to determine the presence of normal thyroid tissue, which in 70% of cases may not be present at the normal site. In such a case removal of the lingual thyroid will result in hypothyroidism. The removed thyroid is sliced, and some of the slices implanted into the muscles of the neck, in view of the rich blood supply of muscular tissue.

Thyroglossal cyst

Thyroglossal cysts constitute the most commonly encountered congenital thyroid anomaly. The lumen of the thyroglossal duct begins to obliterate during the fifth week of gestation and the duct disappears by the eighth week. Sometimes the duct may persist and present as a central cystic neck swelling anywhere along the path of the thyroid; it is then called a thyroglossal cyst. It is commonly located just below the hyoid bone (Fig.48.1). Because it is attached to the foramen cecum of the tongue *it moves upwards not only on swallowing but also on protrusion of the tongue*. These cysts are usually asymptomatic but occasionally become infected by oral bacteria.

Treatment

A thyroglossal cyst should be treated by excision (Sistrunk operation). If the chances of recurrence are to be minimized, the central portion of the body of the hyoid must be removed with the cyst, as the tract is intimately related to the hyoid. Further, the dissection must be carried upwards to the base of the tongue. An infected cyst may be mistaken for a simple abscess and incised, in which case a thyroglossal fistula often results.

Before removing what appears to be a thyroglossal cyst, the surgeon must make sure by isotope scanning that thyroid tissue is present at the normal site. Sometimes the mass is an ectopically placed thyroid instead of a thyroglossal cyst, and the child may be rendered athyreotic by its removal.

Thyroglossal fistula

A thyroglossal fistula arises when a thyroglossal cyst becomes infected and bursts, or is inadequately removed. As the track proceeds upwards, characteristically its upper margin is sharp and crescentic, indicating the upward direction of the track (Fig.48.2). It discharges mucus and becomes repeatedly inflamed. The body of the hyoid must be removed along with the fistula, in order to avoid a recurrence.

Lateral aberrant thyroid

In the past, if thyroid tissue was found in the lateral part of the neck it was either considered to be an ectopically placed (or 'aberrant') thyroid or a remnant of the lateral anlage that had failed to fuse with the main thyroid. We now know that these represent thyroid cancers metastasizing to the lymph nodes. The carcinoma of the thyroid in such cases may be too small to be palpable.

'HYPOTHYROIDISM'

Hypothyroidism is defined as a condition in which there is a deficiency of circulating levels of thyroid hormone. There is failure of the thyroid gland to maintain an adequate plasma level of thyroid hormone. In adults it is called hypothyroidism while in neonates it is referred to as cretinism, which is characterized by neurologic impairment and mental retardation. Hypothyroidism also may occur in Pendred's syndrome (associated with deafness) and Turner's syndrome.

Importance for the surgeon

Hypothyroidism is important for the surgeon due to the following reasons:

- Removal of most of the thyroid, or putting it out of action by radioactive iodine, is an important cause of hypothyroidism.
- The clinical features of hypothyroidism may mimic different surgical illnesses.
- It is important to recognize the hypothyroid state in the pre-operative patient, because major surgery in a grossly hypothyroid patient is associated with an increased mortality rate.

Etiology

Hypothyroidism may result from one of the following:

- Aplasia of the thyroid.
- Replacement of the gland by a non-functional goitre or autoimmune thyroiditis.
- Hypopituitarism.
- Total or subtotal thyroidectomy.
- Radioactive iodine therapy for hyperthyroidism.

Clinical features

In newborns and infants

Functional failure of the thyroid in the newborn is termed *cretinism*. This is not seen at birth, because during pregnancy the mother's thyroid hormones reach the fetus across the placenta. The condition becomes manifest later in infancy. The infant is markedly retarded mentally, and shows a poor growth pattern. The remaining features are similar to those in adults, as described below.

In adults

Spontaneous hypothyroidism in adults commonly follows lymphocytic thyroiditis, most patients being female. Whether hypothyroidism is spontaneous or follows an ablative procedure on the thyroid, the clinical features come on gradually. Its manifestations affect most systems:

- In mild cases only *tiredness* and an increase in weight may be present.
- In severe cases there is increasing fatigue and *apathy*.
- *Mental* and *physical processes* are slowed, and speech may be impaired.
- These patients commonly complain of *shortness of breath*.
- Congestive *heart failure* may be present.
- The *bowel* moves sluggishly, so that constipation and abdominal distension are commonly seen.
- There is decreased *libido* in both men and women and the females may suffer from menorrhagia.

Investigations

Hypothyroidism is associated with low circulating levels of T4 and T3 in the blood.

TSH

- If TSH levels are raised primary thyroid failure should be suspected.
- In secondary hypothyroidism serum TSH levels are decreased along with thyroid hormones. This decrease in TSH is nonresponsive to TRH stimulation.

In patients with autoimmune disease (Hashimoto's thyroiditis, Graves' disease) the *autoantibodies* may be raised.

ECG

This shows sinus bradycardia, diminished voltage and inverted or flattened T waves.

Blood tests

These usually reveal the presence of anemia. Serum cholesterol is commonly raised above 300mg/dl.

Treatment

Thyroxine

The treatment of adult hypothyroidism is very effective, and aims at producing a normal metabolic state. Standard treatment is T4 (L-thyroxine) administered in a dose varying between 50 to 200μg/per day, depending upon the patient's levels of thyroid hormones. The treatment is usually begun in doses of 100 μg of T4 daily. In elderly patients, especially those having co-morbid heart disease or profound hypothyroidism, even lower doses like 25 to 50 μg daily should be given at the start.

These patients are likely to be suffering from hypercholesterolemia and atherosclerosis. The dose can be slowly titrated over weeks to months until a euthyroid state is achieved. The level of the drug is determined by quantitative chemical analysis to avoid cardiac problems arising due to a sudden increased metabolic demand on the myocardium.

Most of the time the maintenance dose is 2–3 tablets/day.

HYPERTHYROIDISM

Hyperthyroidism refers to a spectrum of clinical manifestations which are due to excessive production and secretion of thyroid hormone. Many conditions are associated with hyperthyroidism, including:

- Graves' disease (toxic diffuse goitre).
- Toxic multinodular goitre.
- Toxic adenoma.

Pathology

Graves' disease

Graves' disease is the most common cause of hyperthyroidism worldwide and accounts for about 60 to 80% of cases. This is an autoimmune disease with a strong familial predisposition. The peak incidence is between the ages of 40 to 60 years, with a definite female preponderance (5:1).

Generally Graves' disease is a disorder regarded as a systemic autoimmune disease *characterized* by:

- Hyperthyroidism.
- Exophthalmos.
- A dermopathy called pretibial myxoedema, with or without a diffuse goitre.

Certain other manifestations that may sometimes be associated but are not characteristic for the disease, include:

- Thyroid acropachy (clubbing of fingers and toes due to new bone formation).
- Gynecomastia.

It is believed that TSH receptor antibodies are produced that bind the receptor and stimulate thyroid cells to grow and synthesize excess thyroid hormone. Evidence supporting its recognition as an autoimmune process includes:

- Presence of IgG, IgM and IgE in the thyroid.
- Lymphocytic infiltration of the gland.
- Generalized lymphadenopathy often seen in Graves' disease.

The thyroid of the patient with Graves' disease is moderately and diffusely enlarged, the surface being characteristically smooth. Microscopically the thyroid is hyperplastic, the epithelium is columnar and only a minimal amount of colloid is present. The nuclei may exhibit mitoses and the hyperplastic epithelium is thrown into papillary projections. There may be aggregates of lymphoid tissue, and the vascularity is greatly increased.

Toxic multinodular goitre

In this condition toxicity is usually superimposed on a multinodular goitre. Grossly, the gland contains multiple nodules, many of which contain aggregates of irregular large cells and a scant amount of colloid. These areas basically are the autonomous functioning nodules. The severity of hyperthyroidism is normally less than that associated with Graves' disease.

Solitary toxic adenoma

This is a benign tumor. Like the multinodular toxic goitre it is capable of functioning independently of TSH, and the administration of exogenous thyroid fails to suppress the secretion of T3 and T4.

Clinical features

The *age* of onset is different in the three main pathological processes:

- Graves' disease most commonly becomes clinically apparent in young patients.
- Toxic adenoma occurs during the thirties or forties.
- A toxic multinodular goitre becomes manifest after the age of fifty except in endemic areas.

The patient *feels warmer* than other people in the same environment and becomes intolerant to heat. The excess heat resulting from the hypermetabolic state has to be dissipated; for this purpose there is increased *sweating*, which in turn results in increased *thirst* due to the fluid loss.

As the body furnace is burning at a higher than normal rate, there is *loss of weight* despite increased appetite and food intake; this feature is more marked in patients with toxic multinodular goitre and toxic adenoma.

The *cardiovascular manifestations* of thyrotoxicosis are more prominent in the older patients with toxic multinodular goitres or toxic adenomas. They include tachycardia, frequent atrial fibrillation and congestive heart failure. Hyperthyroidism increases the force and rate of the heart beat, probably because of sensitization to adrenergic stimuli. Sleeping pulse rate is over 80 per minute. Palpitations are common. Due to peripheral vasodilatation the pulse pressure is increased. Atrial fibrillation may occur, especially among older patients.

The patient is *excitable*, restless, and emotionally unstable, often with insomnia. The emotional and neurogenic signs are more marked in Graves' disease.

Muscle wasting and *fatigue* are common. The extended and abducted fingers show a fine *tremor*. The *skin* is warm and moist with facial flushing and perspiration. The *hair* is fine and readily falls off with combing. *Menstrual periods* are scanty.

Graves' disease

In Graves' disease goitre, thyrotoxicosis and exophthalmos occur together. A bruit is heard over the gland due to the extreme vascularity.

Eye signs

A number of eye signs are a distinctive feature of thyrotoxicosis. These include

- Lid lag (von Graefe's sign).
- Spasm of the upper eyelid (lid retraction) revealing the sclera above the corneoscleral limbus (Dalrymple's sign).
- A prominent stare, due to catecholamine excess.
- True infiltrative eye disease results in:
    - Periorbital edema.
    - Conjunctival swelling and congestion (chemosis).
    - Proptosis.
    - Keratitis.
    - Even blindness, due to optic nerve involvement.

The eye signs vary from minimal to severe.

Proptosis

It should be remembered that proptosis means protrusion of the eyeball and the term exophthalmos is generally referred to as proptosis due to thyrotoxicosis:

- To *detect* proptosis the examiner stands behind the seated patient and asks him to look forwards. The upper eyelid is drawn upwards and the cornea appears to be bulging forwards.
- When *measuring* proptosis the examiner sits on one side of the patient. He places a transparent ruler against the lateral orbital margin and reads the distance the cornea is bulging out of the orbital margin. He then repeats the same procedure on the opposite side and records the measurements.

Toxic multinodular goitre

In this condition the thyroid contains many nodules, which have been present for a long time. Pressure effects on the trachea or esophagus are more common than in Graves' disease but exophthalmos and other extrathyroidal manifestations are rare.

Toxic adenoma

Hyperthyroidism from a single hyperfunctioning nodule usually occurs in the younger age group. There is a slowly growing mass in the neck. Very rapid growth may be due to central necrosis and hemorrhage, when because of necrosis the signs of thyrotoxicity may show spontaneous remission. Radioimmunoassay scanning shows a "hot" nodule with suppression of the rest of the thyroid gland. Exophthalmos is absent.

Investigations

In thyrotoxicosis T3 and/or T4 levels are elevated. The thyroidal radioiodine uptake is markedly elevated in Graves' disease, less markedly so in toxic multinodular goitre and toxic adenoma.

In toxic adenoma the isotope scan demonstrates uptake of tracer in the area of the nodule, while the rest of the normal gland is not visualized. If exogenous TSH is now given, the remaining part of the gland will take up the isotope.

Anti-thyroglobulin is elevated in upto 75% of patients, but is not specific.

Elevated TSH receptor or thyroid-stimulating immunoglobulins (TSAb) are diagnostic of Graves' disease and are increased in about 90% of patients. Graves'ophthalmopathy can be evaluated by MRI scans of the orbits.

Treatment

Hyperthyroidism can be treated by antithyroid drugs, radioactive iodine, or surgical excision of thyroid tissue. The method chosen depends upon the pathological process involved and the patient's age and general health.

Antithyroid drugs

Most antithyroid drugs interfere with the organic binding of iodine in the thyroid and inhibit the coupling of iodotyrosines. They have no effect on the underlying cause of the disease. It takes these drugs about six weeks to restore a euthyroid state. The treatment is monitored by clinical observation and by noting the patient's pulse and weight.

Most patients with Graves' disease are treated with antithyroid drugs in the hope that a natural remission will occur after the patient is rendered euthyroid. If treatment is continued for 6 months and then the drugs are stopped, only about 40 percent patients have long-lasting remissions. Side-effects include skin rash, fever and peripheral neuritis, serious complications being agranulocytosis and aplastic anemia. If the white blood cell count falls significantly the drug must be stopped.

The commonly used drug is carbimazole in the form of 5mg tablets. This is given initially in a dose of 10 to 30mg daily in three divided doses, then once daily. Curative treatment for Graves' disease is reserved for patients with:

- Goiters which are small (< 40 g) and nontoxic.
- Goitres with mild elevation of thyroid hormone.
- Goitres that decrease rapidly in size after medication with antithyroid drugs.

The sympathetic response due to thyrotoxicosis is dealt with by beta-blockers, which also decrease the peripheral conversion of T4 to T3. The beta blocker commonly used is propranolol given in a dose of 20 to 40mg four times daily.

Radioactive iodine

In some centres radioactive iodine is considered as the treatment of choice for Graves' disease. The average dose is 8 to 10 mC of ^{131}I, which delivers approximately 6,000 rads. The advantage of radioiodine therapy lies in the avoidance of a surgical procedure with its attendant complications of recurrent laryngeal nerve paralysis or hypoparathyroidism. The disadvantages include:

- The time required to control the disease.
- The incidence of permanent myxoedema.
- The development of nodules.

80 to 98% patients show remission. Unfortunately, in the long term more than half the patients develop hypothyroidism due to overdosage.

The incidence of thyroid cancer or leukemia is not increased by the use of radioiodine. At the same time the possibility of genetic abnormalities following radioiodine treatment is very remote. Most centres limit the use of radioiodine to women thirty-five years of age or older, who have relapsed after medical or surgical therapy and those in whom antithyroid drugs or surgery are contraindicated.

Radioiodine should never be given to *pregnant or lactating women* because it crosses the placenta, is excreted in milk, and could destroy the fetal thyroid.

Surgical treatment

Surgery is indicated in cases where the patient:

- Has confirmed cancer or suspicious thyroid nodules.
- Is young.
- Is pregnant or has the desire to conceive soon after treatment.
- Has had severe reactions to antithyroid medications.
- Has a large goitre causing compressive symptoms.
- Is reluctant to undergo radioimmunoassay therapy.

Preoperative preparation

Operation on a patient with hyperthyroidism cannot be carried out straightaway. First the patient must be rendered euthyroid:

- Commonly, antithyroid drugs are used for this purpose.
- Iodine is then added to this regimen 8 to 10 days prior to the operation to decrease the vascularity of the gland.
- Some surgeons add thyroxine to the regimen to prevent hypothyroidism and to decrease the size of the gland.
- The beta-adrenergic blocker, propranolol, has added safety to the operation for hyperthyroid patients. It reduces the pulse rate and the finger tremors, and is also helpful in preventing thyroid storm, although the patient remains thyrotoxic. Some use propranolol alone for 5 to 7 days. But it is probably better to use antithyroid drugs along with propranolol.

Results of operation

Subtotal thyroidectomy provides rapid correction of the thyrotoxic state in over 95% of cases.

The *advantages* of surgical therapy include:

- Prompt control of the disease.
- A lowered incidence of myxoedema as compared with radioiodine therapy.

The disadvantages of thyroidectomy include the following:

- Possibility of recurrent laryngeal nerve paralysis.
- Possible damage to the parathyroid glands resulting in tetany.
- In a few patients permanent hypothyroidism develops; in others hyperthyroidism recurs.

Selection of therapy

Graves' disease

In young patients with Graves' disease antithyroid drugs are used initially. If prolonged drug therapy is required, or if recurrence of thyrotoxicosis follows the discontinuation of the drugs, thyroidectomy is used. Antithyroid drugs cross the placenta and may cause hypothyroidism and goitre in the fetus, so they cannot be used in pregnancy. If during pregnancy thyrotoxicosis is severe and cardiac symptoms herald cardiac failure later in pregnancy, subtotal thyroidectomy should be undertaken in the middle trimester, which is safe and effective. These drugs can be used in lactating mothers as their excretion into milk is at a level too low to cause hypothyroidism in the infant.

Toxic multinodular goitre

The preferred treatment for this condition is surgical excision. A subtotal thyroidectomy, leaving a 4-to 7-g remnant, is recommended for patients suffering from a toxic multinodular goitre. Remnants less then 3 grams are recommended for children.

Hyperfunctioning adenoma

Similarly, surgical resection of the hyperactive part of the thyroid gland in a case of *hyperfunctioning adenoma* is so straightforward that the other methods of treatment need not be seriously considered unless the patient is medically unfit for surgery. The preferred treatment for such cases is surgery (lobectomy and isthmectomy).

Treatment of exophthalmos

The treatment of hyperthyroidism does not always improve the situation in respect of exophthalmos. Treatment is essentially symptomatic:

- The eyes should be protected against wind and sun.
- The patient should sleep in a sitting position to reduce venous congestion.
- If the edema is severe the eyelids may be opposed by suturing them together (tarsorraphy) to prevent corneal ulceration.
- Steroid eye drops may help.
- If the intraorbital pressure threatens vision, the lateral bony wall of the orbit may be removed by operation to allow the orbital contents to expand (orbital decompression).

THYROIDITIS

Inflammatory processes of the thyroid may be acute, subacute or chronic. Chronic thyroiditis includes Hashimoto's disease and Riedel's thyroiditis.

Acute suppurative thyroiditis

This is a rare condition. It is essentially an abscess of the thyroid, which nearly always follows upon an acute upper respiratory tract infection. Other causes include direct spread via thyroglossal duct cysts or fistulae, or trauma. There is sudden severe pain with dysphagia, fever and chills. The diagnosis can be achieved by leukocytosis and aspiration for Gram's stain, culture, and cytology. CT scan is used to delineate the extent of infection. Treatment consists of incision and drainage.

Subacute thyroiditis (de Quervain's disease)

This condition occurs at almost any age, being more common in women. Although the disease is considered to be of viral origin, the exact cause is yet to be established. The gland is adherent to the surrounding structures, but can be dissected free. There is infiltration by mononuclear cells, lymphocytes and neutrophils. Epithelioid type of giant cells are present. There is swelling and pain, with fever and malaise.

Treatment

Needle biopsy helps establish the diagnosis. The acute pain can be alleviated by aspirin and a beta-blocker. If this fails, 20 to 30mg of prednisolone daily for one month usually provides relief. Thyroxine may be required if hypothyroidism develops. Surgery is only required if the diagnosis is uncertain on fine-needle cytology.

Hashimoto's disease (lymphadenoid goitre)

Hashimoto's disease, or chronic lymphocytic thyroiditis, is the most common form of chronic thyroiditis. It is an autoimmune process in which the thyroid gland becomes sensitized to its own thyroglobulin and cell constituents. The serum contains antithyroid antibodies, which are either antimicrosomal or antithyroglobulin. The disease sometimes runs in a family where there is an increased incidence of Hashimoto's disease, goitre, spontaneous hypothyroidism and thyrotoxicosis.

Pathology

There is usually a symmetrical enlargement of the thyroid which is firm and pale on gross examination. Microscopically, the gland is diffusely infiltrated with small lymphocytes, plasma cells and occasionally shows well-developed germinal centers. Thyroid follicles are small with reduced amounts of colloid and increased interstitial connective tissue. The follicles contain Hurthle or Askanazy cells, having abundant eosinophilic, granular cytoplasm. The epithelial cells are disrupted and the basement membrane fragmented. Gradually, the thyroid tissue may degenerate or be replaced by fibrous tissue.

Clinical features

Most patients are middle-aged women. The neck is enlarged with pain and tenderness in the region of the thyroid. There may be dyspnoea and dysphagia. Most patients are euthyroid or hypothyroid. Other autoimmune disorders, e.g. rheumatoid arthritis, hemolytic anemia, may coexist with Hashimoto's disease.

Investigations

Early in the course of the disease thyroid function tests may occasionally indicate hyperfunction. Later, T4 and T3 are often abnormal. Diagnosis is confirmed by demonstrating high titres of thyroid antibodies in the serum. If the glandular enlargement is nodular or asymmetrical, large needle biopsy or needle aspiration with cytology may be necessary to rule out the diagnosis of carcinoma.

Treatment.

If the thyroid is symmetrical and non-nodular, and if there are no symptoms of compression, the patient should be managed by suppressive doses of thyroxin if there is evidence of a goitre. Symptoms of pressure on the trachea and esophagus are common and may be relieved by prednisolone 20mg/day.

If there is no goitre and the patient is euthyroid, *no treatment* is required.

Surgical treatment, i.e. subtotal thyroidectomy, is required only if:

- There are marked compression symptoms e.g. dysphagia.
- A cancer is suspected.
- For cosmetic reasons as in the case of a very large gland.

Suppressive therapy with thyroid hormone should be continued postoperatively.

Riedel's thyroiditis

Riedel's thyroiditis is a rare chronic inflammatory disorder of the thyroid, often extending to the surrounding structures like fascia, muscles, trachea etc. The disease mostly affects middle-aged persons, specially women. Some workers regard it as a terminal stage of Hashimoto's disease. Microscopically, a few small follicles are seen, surrounded by dense fibrous tissue, which may constrict and narrow the trachea. When the lesion is only on one side, it is difficult to distinguish it from carcinoma. Tests may indicate the presence of hypothyroidism.

Treatment consists of the administration of thyroid hormones. If symptoms of tracheal or esophageal obstruction are present surgical intervention is required for their relief.

GOITRE

Goitre is defined as any enlargement of the thyroid gland. However, in common usage the term is employed for benign enlargements of the gland. Toxic and inflammatory goitres have already been described. What remains to be discussed is the condition called simple goitre.

Simple goitre

Etiology

Simple goitre arises as follows: either due to a deficiency of iodine in the diet or a defect of synthesis of the thyroid hormones, the level of the circulating thyroid hormones falls. This results in increased secretion of thyroid stimulating hormone (TSH) by the anterior pituitary. TSH stimulates the thyroid gland which enlarges in size, and a goitre results.

Iodine deficiency

In certain areas both food and water have a very low content of iodine. Usually these are mountainous regions, where rain water washes away the iodides from the soil. In the advanced countries iodine is added to table salt to remedy any possible deficiency of iodine in the diet, and this simple step has greatly reduced the incidence of deficiency goitre in many regions where it used to be endemic.

Defects of synthesis of thyroid hormones

These may arise due to one of the following causes:

- *Inherited defects of synthesis.* Sometimes many members of a family are seen to be suffering from goitre. Those coming from a non-endemic area are thought to be suffering from an inherited defect of thyroid hormone synthesis. The metabolic defect may impair iodine accumulation, organification or coupling of iodotyrosine; or it may be related to a disorder affecting the serum iodoprotein. As the thyroid hormones are not synthesized in sufficient amounts, the inhibitory action of these hormones on the secretion of TSH is reduced. Increased secretion of TSH stimulates the thyroid so that a goitre results.

- *Goitrogens*. Certain chemicals block one or the other step in the synthesis of the thyroid hormones, and thus act as goitrogens. These include drugs such as para-aminosalicylic acid and the antithyroid drugs.

Evolution of a simple goitre

- ***Diffuse hyperplastic goitre***. Due to iodine deficiency or a defect of synthesis of thyroid hormones persistent TSH stimulation occurs, and causes diffuse hyperplasia. All lobules are composed of active follicles, and iodine uptake is uniform. This is a diffuse hyperplastic goitre which may persist for a long time but is reversible if TSH stimulation ceases. Diffuse hyperplasia represents the first stages of the natural history of a simple goitre.
- ***Puberty goitre***. Such a goitre usually appears at puberty when the accelerated metabolism results in an increased demand for iodine which outstrips the supply (puberty goitre). If TSH stimulation ceases the goitre may regress, but can recur later at a time of stress. The goitre is soft and diffuse.
- ***Colloid goitre.*** A colloid goitre is a late stage of diffuse goitre, when many follicles are inactive and full of colloid; it is firm in consistency and has a smooth saface (Fig.48.3).
- ***Multinodular goitre.*** Persistent but fluctuating TSH stimulation leads to progressive nodule formation. The nodules may be cellular or colloid, but cystic degeneration, hemorrhage, and even calcification may be seen. The diagnosis is easily made on finding multiple smooth, firm nodules in a patient who is euthyroid (Fig.48.4). The goitre is painless and moves freely on swallowing. If a nodule appears suddenly and enlarges rapidly it may raise the suspicion of carcinoma; however, this is more often due to hemorrhage into a simple nodule.

Investigations

Thyroid function tests should be performed to evaluate the functional status of the goitre.

Estimation of *thyroid antibody titres* helps exclude Hashimoto's goitre.

Plain *x-ray* of the neck should be taken to show up any tracheal deviation or compression, and any calcification in the thyroid.

Complications

The important complications to which a simple goitre is prone are the following:

- *Pressure effects*. The trachea may be obstructed due to gross lateral deviation or compression. Hemorrhage into a nodule may produce acute respiratory obstruction.
- A small number of patients with nodular goitres develop *hyperthyroidism*.
- *Carcinomas*, commonly of the follicular type, also arises in a few cases.

Treatment

Adding one part of potassium iodide to 10,000 parts of table salt provides virtually complete *prophylaxis* against the development of simple goitre, and is universally employed in the advanced countries.

In its *early* stages a *diffuse* hyperplastic goitre can be made to regress if thyroxine is given in maximum doses, i.e. 0.2mg per day for several months. If regression does not occur thyroidectomy may be indicated for cosmetic reasons or pressure effects.

On the other hand the pathological changes in a *nodular goitre* are irreversible. It should be treated by subtotal thyroidectomy because it is unsightly and uncomfortable; besides, it is prone to the complications of pressure effects, toxic change and malignancy. Resection aims at leaving about 8gm of thyroid tissue on each side.

Prevention of recurrence

The causative factors often persist after operation, and therefore a *recurrence* is quite likely unless further TSH stimulation is prevented. For this purpose 0.1mg of thyroxine is given daily till after the menopause, or even better, for the rest of the patient's life.

The clinically solitary nodule

A frequent and important clinical problem is seen when the thyroid is the seat of a single nodule. Such a nodule can be an adenoma, a carcinoma, or a colloid nodule in a multinodular goitre in which the other nodules are too small in size to be palpable. Sudden painful enlargement of a solitary nodule can indicate hemorrhage into the nodule (Fig.48.5).

Clinical features

A colloid nodule (Fig.48.6) is usually firm in consistency. If it has degenerated into a cyst the consistency may be soft; however, if the cyst contains fluid under a good deal of tension the nodule may be tense. An adenoma is firm, whereas a carcinoma is usually hard to the feel. The remainder of the thyroid should be carefully palpated for the presence of other smaller nodules, which would show that this is really a multinodular goitre. The presence of fixity of the nodule, hoarseness of the voice, or enlarged hard lymph nodes in the lateral neck tends to label a nodule as malignant.

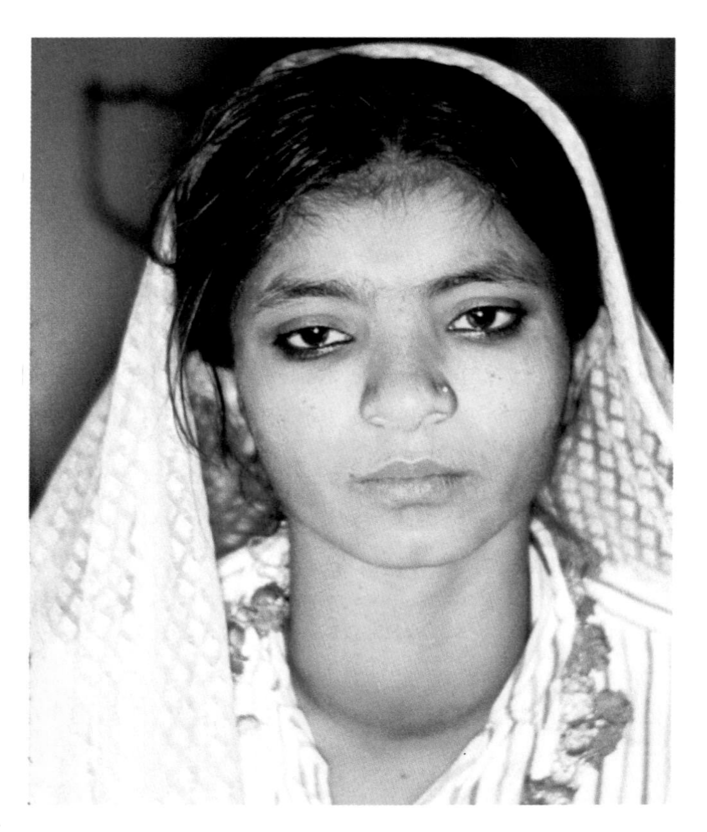

Fig.48.3 Colloid goitre in young woman

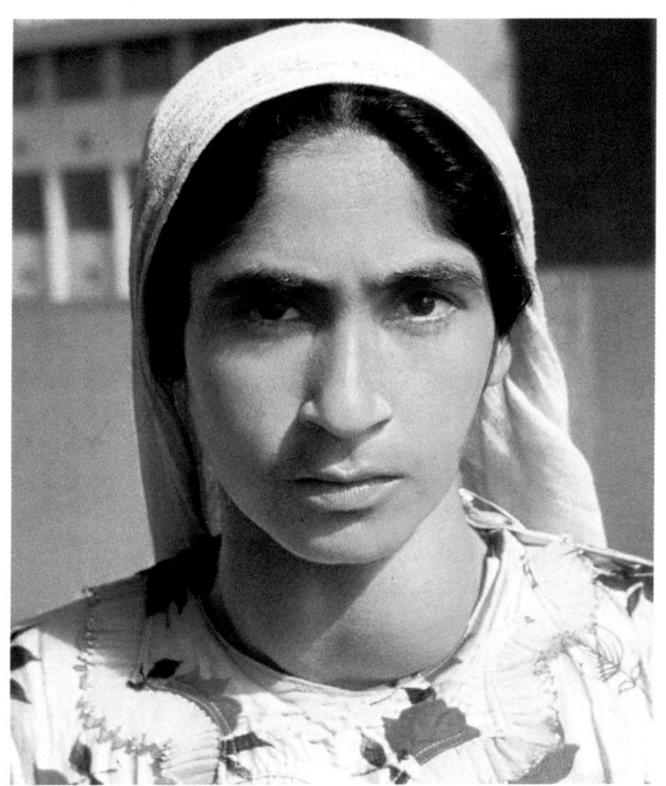

Fig.48.4 Multinodular goitre at a rather young age

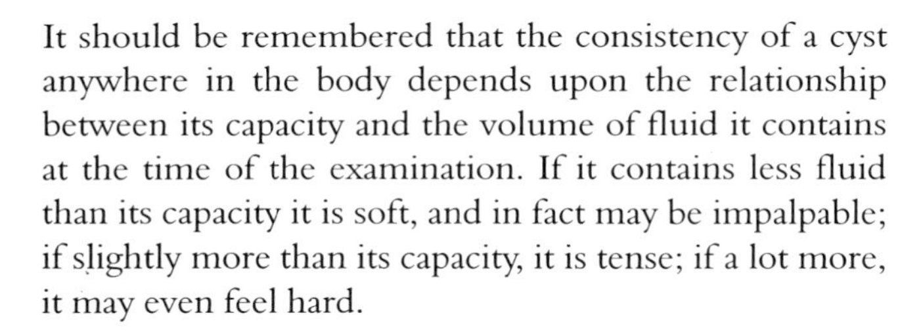

It should be remembered that the consistency of a cyst anywhere in the body depends upon the relationship between its capacity and the volume of fluid it contains at the time of the examination. If it contains less fluid than its capacity it is soft, and in fact may be impalpable; if slightly more than its capacity, it is tense; if a lot more, it may even feel hard.

Investigations

Radio-isotope scanning

On isotope scanning:

- A colloid nodule and a carcinoma are usually 'cold', i.e. they do not take up radioiodine.
- An adenoma is often 'warm', i.e. both the nodule and the surrounding thyroid take up the isotope.
- A toxic adenoma is 'hot'; not only does the adenoma take up the isotope, but the surrounding thyroid tissue does not. Here the normal thyroid tissue is inactive because the nodule is producing such high levels of thyroid hormone that TSH secretion is suppressed.

Ultrasound

An ultrasound examination can distinguish between a swelling which is solid and one which contains fluid, i.e. is cystic. When it is remembered that most cystic nodules in the thyroid are benign and most solid nodules neoplastic, it will become obvious that ultrasound examination has a role to play in the differential diagnosis of a solitary nodule. At the same time, ultrasound examination helps demonstrate the presence of additional small nodules if any such are present, which shows that the case is one of a multinodular goitre. In that case the possibility of a malignancy becomes quite remote.

A CT scan can provide the same information as an ultrasound.

Fine-needle aspiration cytology (FNAC)

This method is simple and quick to perform in the outpatients department, and has a high diagnostic accuracy. It can distinguish between colloid nodules, thyroiditis, papillary, medullary and anaplastic carcinoma, and lymphoma.

Treatment

A *solitary toxic nodule* is never malignant, it is a toxic adenoma; it is best treated by surgical excision and histopatholgy.

A *euthyroid warm* nodule is either a functioning adenoma or a simple nodule. Rarely, it may be a well-differentiated carcinoma; therefore it should be excised and examined by a histopathologist.

A *euthyroid cold nodule* can be a carcinoma; therefore it should be excised by total lobectomy. Incisional biopsy should never be carried out as it could result in seeding of malignant cells.

NEOPLASMS OF THE THYROID

Benign tumors

The common benign tumor of the thyroid is a *follicular* neoplasm, which presents as a slowly growing nodule. When solitary nodules removed at operation are examined microscopically, 80 percent of the specimens prove to be benign, while 20 percent are malignant.

On the other hand when a tumor has a *papillary* structure it is nearly always malignant, even though of a very low grade; a pure papillary adenoma probably does not exist.

Treatment

When a solitary nodule of the thyroid shows up on ultrasound examination as a solid lesion, it is highly likely to be a neoplasm, whether benign or malignant. In such a case the best treatment is lobectomy. Ideally, the lobectomy specimen should be examined by frozen section while the patient is still under anesthesia. If it proves to be an adenoma nothing further needs to be done.

MALIGNANT TUMORS

The common malignant tumors of the thyroid are all carcinomas. Papillary, follicullar and anaplastic carcinomas arise from the follicular cells, while medullary carcinoma is derived from parafollicular cells. In addition, lymphomas and metastatic carcinomas are seen from time to time.

Papillary carcinoma

Papillary and follicular carcinomas are referred to as the differentiated thyroid cancers. Papillary carcinoma is the most common thyroid malignancy, accounting for two-thirds of all thyroid carcinomas. The peak age incidence occurs in the third and fourth decades of life, three-fourths of the patients being women.

Pathology

Papillary carcinoma contains columnar epithelium arranged in papillary projections and characteristic pale, empty nuclei called *Orphan Annie nuclei*. The tumor may contain localized deposits of calcium arranged in concentric layers (psammoma bodies). Papillary carcinoma is the most slowly growing of thyroid cancers, but has a tendency to become more malignant with advancing age. The tumor is very frequently multicentric in origin, and there is some evidence that its growth is dependent on TSH stimulation.

Some of these tumors contain both papillary and follicular elements. However, if any papillary structure is present the tumor behaves as a papillary carcinoma.

Clinical features

The lesion usually presents as an asymptomatic mass in the thyroid or as a solid swelling in a lymph node draining the thyroid. Fixation of the thyroid, signs of pressure on adjacent structures, and metastases are all evidence of advanced disease.

Investigations

An *x-ray* of the neck may show calcium flecks suggesting psammoma bodies [Greek. *Psammos*=sand].

Isotope scan demonstrates a lack of iodine uptake. An *ultrasound* scan shows a solid lesion. *Fine-needle aspiration* cytology is usually diagnostic.

Treatment

The treatment of choice for a papillary carcinoma of the thyroid is surgery. While considering surgical treatment, papillary carcinomas are best divided into two groups:

- *Minimal or occult papillary carcinoma.* This term refers to a small papillary tumor, *less than 1cm* in diameter and without invasion through the thyroid capsule or lymph node metastases, and usually found in the specimen in a young person when thyroidectomy has been done for another benign condition. In such a case lobectomy is sufficient.
- *Standard treatment.* For tumors *larger than 1cm* in diameter, a near-total or total thyroidectomy should be carried out. Usually the best course to follow is to excise the mass completely by lobectomy, and submit the excised lobe to frozen section examination. If the lesion is reported to be benign, or smaller than 1cm with no capsular invasion, nothing more needs to be done; otherwise a near-total or total thyroidectomy is carried out.

Decision between lobectomy and total thyroidectomy can be arrived at by a scoring system devised to identify low-and high-risk patients based on four variables: age, grade, extent, and size (AGES); a higher score on each indicates a poorer prognosis and the need for more radical surgery.

The *advantages* of carrying out a total thyroidectomy are the following:

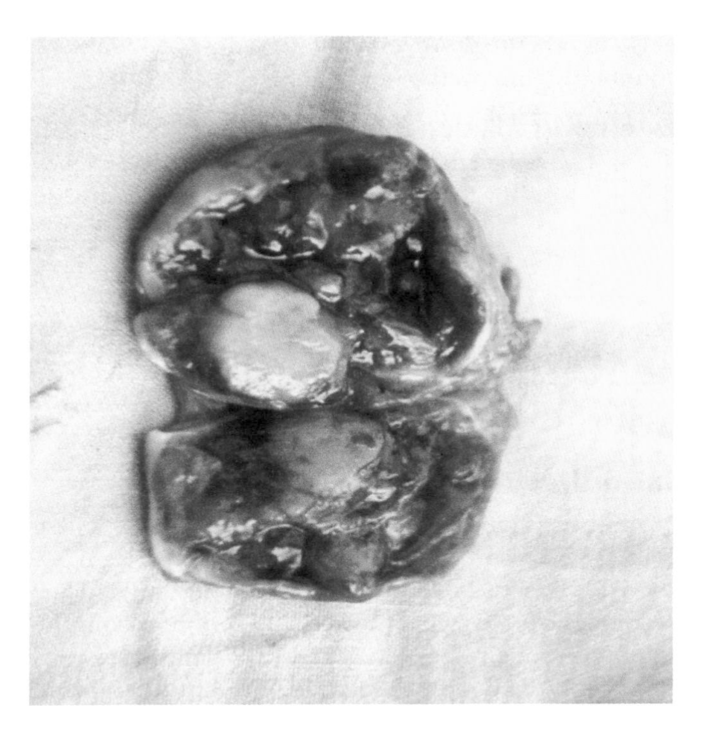

Fig.48.5 Solitary nodule slit open to show large area of hemorrhage

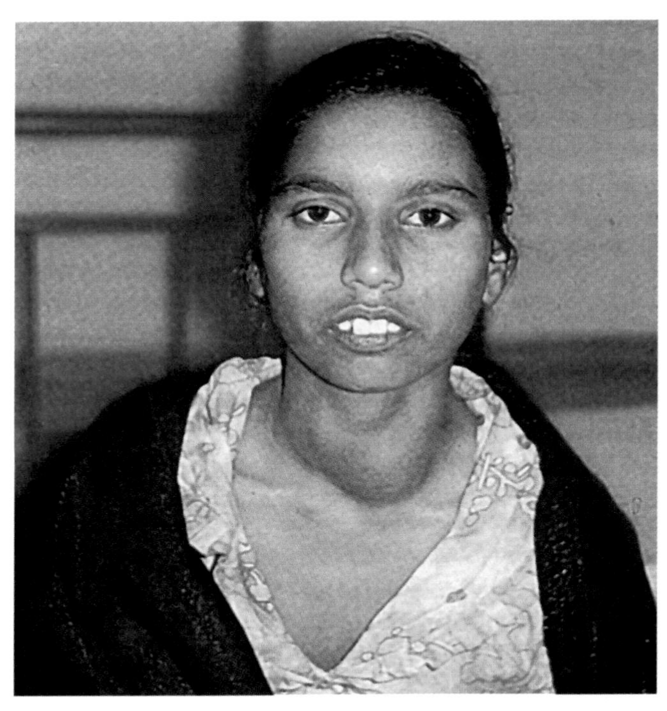

Fig.48.6 Colloid nodule in left lobe thyroid in young woman

- Papillary carcinoma is very often multicentric; therefore the likelihood of eradicating the disease is much greater after total thyroidectomy.
- The best method of follow-up for metastases is by repeated isotope scans. If some functioning thyroid tissue is present, metastases do not show up. Therefore total thyroidectomy facilitates follow-up for metastases, and their treatment by radioiodine.
- If after total thyroidectomy a measureable amount of thyroglobulin is detected in the serum it means that metastatic disease is present, and requires localization by isotope scanning and treatment by radioiodine.

About the lymph nodes

Any abnormal lymph nodes in the tracheo-esophageal groove should be removed. A neck dissection should be carried out only if the lateral neck nodes are involved with tumor. To determine this, a lymph node from the jugular chain should be removed for biopsy using the frozen section technique.

Follow-up

- After operations for differentiated thyroid cancers, it is standard practice to place all patients *on thyroid hormone for life* to suppress serum TSH levels, and to follow them up at regular intervals. T3 in a daily dose of 80 microgram is usually appropriate. T3 is preferred over T4 because it need be stopped for only 1 week before scanning. T4 has to be discontinued for 1 month and during this time mild hypothyroidism may occur.
- The measurement of *serum thyroglobulin* is of value in the follow-up for detecting metastatic disease after surgery for differentiated thyroid cancer. It is a good example of a 'tumor marker'. A sensitive radioimmunoassay for thyroglobulin is available. It provides a more convenient means of follow-up than scanning with radioiodine, as thyroid suppression therapy does not have to be stopped. However, if a rise in the level occurs a scan should be carried out to confirm and localize the metastatic disease for needful.
- Radiotherapy and chemotherapy are described along with follicular carcinoma.

Prognosis

If the disease is limited to the thyroid and regional lymph nodes, it carries one of the most favourable prognoses of all forms of cancer, with 5-year survivals of 90%, scarcely reduced at 10 years. Patients with extrathyroidal disease i.e. extending to the trachea or esophagus, do not fare so well.

Follicular carcinoma

Follicular carcinoma of the thyroid occurs at a somewhat later age, with a peak incidence in the fifth decade, again being three times more common in women.

Pathology

Grossly, the tumor appears encapsulated. The follicles are crowded with cells, there being hardly any colloid. Capsular and vascular invasion are prominent features. The tumor is much less often multicentric than papillary carcinoma; however its malignant potential exceeds that of the latter tumor. Spread to the regional lymph nodes occurs in only a few cases, while hematogenous spread to distant sites such as bone, lung and liver predominates and occurs early.

Clinical features

The common presentation is as a solitary nodule in the thyroid, though sometimes there is a long history of goitre with recent change in the gland. Although carrying a better prognosis than most cancers, it is more aggressive and dangerous than papillary carcinoma. Regional lymph nodes are seldom enlarged, but distant metastases are frequent. The metastases usually possess the ability to concentrate iodine.

Treatment

For the treatment of a follicular carcinoma of the thyroid, some favour hemithyroidectomy with removal of the isthmus but others, including the author, favour total or near-total thyroidectomy, not because of multicentricity, but rather to facilitate later scanning of the body with radioiodine and treatment with ^{123}I if metastases are found. The usual method is to withhold thyroxine after thyroidectomy for 3 to 6 weeks so that the patient becomes hypothyroid. The increased TSH secretion makes the secondaries hungry for iodine and therefore more likely to be identified by a radioisotope scan.

Since lymph node metastases are uncommon, neck dissection is rarely required. Overall, the survival rate of follicular tumors is about 70%, being about 45% if invasiveness is present, and as high as 85% if the tumor is not invasive.

Other methods of treatment for differentiated tumors

Radioiodine therapy

After thyroidectomy for a differentiated carcinoma a total body scan should be carried out to locate any metastases. If 30 millicuries (mC) of radioiodine are now given, this will ablate most small remnants of normal thyroid in the neck. In order to destroy metastases a dose of 150 mC is commonly employed.

External irradiation therapy

This is used when thyroid cancer has invaded the trachea or esophagus, or for the treatment of metastatic disease that no longer takes up radioiodine.

Chemotherapy

Widely metastatic lesions that no longer take up radioiodine can be treated with moderate success with systemic chemotherapy. Adriamycin has been the single most successful agent.

Medullary carcinoma

Medullary carcinoma is composed of C cells. These cells are derived from the neural crest, and are part of the APUD series of polypeptide-secreting cells. They secrete calcitonin, which lowers the serum calcium by inhibiting bone resorption. The tumor sometimes runs in a family, being inherited as an autosomal dominant. It spreads both via the lymphatics and through the bloodstream.

Clinical features

Patients present with a single nodule or with multiple nodules. In addition, these tumors may present with very distinct symptoms. Diarrhea is a very common complaint. It may be due to 5-hydroxytryptamine or prostaglandin produced by the tumor.

Combinations with other tumors

- Medullary carcinoma can occur in combination with phaeochromocytoma and hyper-parathyroidism in the syndrome known as multiple endocrine neoplasia *(MEN type IIa)*.
- If the tumor occurs with neuromas involving the lips and tongue the syndrome is called *MEN type IIb*.

Calcitonin

As would be expected these tumors are not hormone-dependent and do not take up radioiodine. Calcitonin is a good marker for this tumor; therefore close relatives of the patient should be screened by determining their serum calcitonin levels. At the same time, the progress of the tumor can be monitored after surgery by serial estimations of serum calcitonin.

Treatment

Total thyroidectomy is the procedure of choice in view of the high incidence of multicentric lesions in both familial and sporadic disease. The upper poles and the lymph nodes in the primary lymphatic area should be completely resected. Lymph nodes in the secondary drainage areas should be sampled, and if positive removed by neck dissection.

Before operation, a coexisting phaeochromocytoma or parathyroid tumor should be excluded, as failure to attend to these tumors first may be catastrophic.

Anaplastic carcinoma

In these tumors local infiltration is an early feature, with spread both by the lymphatics and the blood stream. They affect predominantly the older age groups. Anaplastic thyroid tumors are very lethal, and survival beyond four years is unusual. There is rapid progressive swelling with voice changes due to involvement of the recurrent laryngeal nerves and stridor from tracheal compression. Whenever possible an attempt should be made to decompress the trachea by surgery to relieve respiratory obstruction. External radiotherapy is normally used in addition although the tumor is rarely very sensitive. Chemotherapy has little place in treatment.

SURGERY OF THE THYROID

Anatomy

(Fig.48.7) shows, in a cross section of the neck, the structures relevant in operations on the thyroid. The common operations carried out on the thyroid include subtotal or total lobectomy on one or both sides.

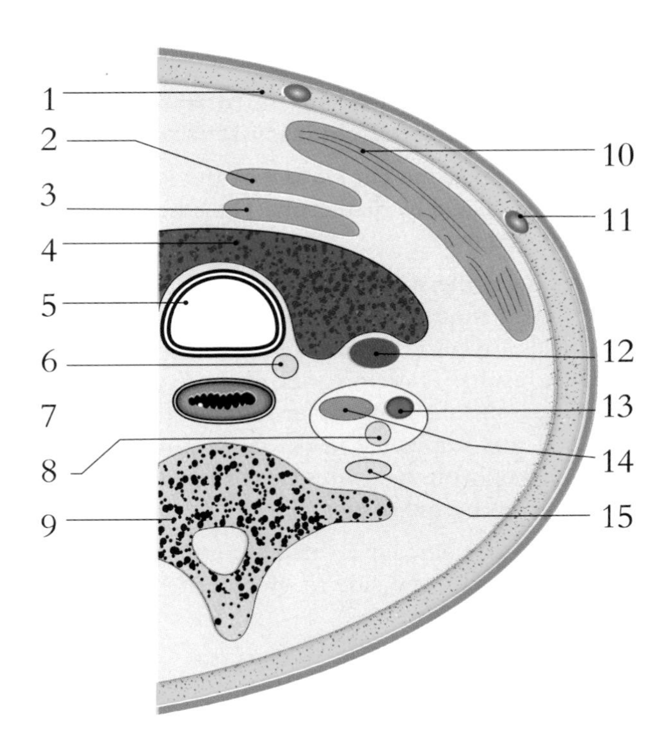

Fig.48.7. Transverse section through neck at level of thyroid isthmus 1. anterior jugular vein 2. sternohyoid mastoid muscle 3. sternothyroid muscle 4. thyroid isthmus 5. trachea, 6, recurrent laryngeal nerve 7. esophagus 8. vagus nerve 9. vertebral body 10. sternomastoid muscle 11. external jugular vein 12. parathyroid gland 13. common carotid artery 14. internal jugular vein 15. sympathetic trunk

Exposure

Most operations on the thyroid are carried out through a transverse collar incision. If a skin crease is present at approximately this site, the incision should be made through it. If a nodule is to be removed from only one side, the skin incision should still be extended equally on either side, otherwise the asymmetrical scar is more noticeable. The platysma muscle is divided with the skin. The upper flap is now dissected upwards to the thyroid cartilage and the lower one downwards to the suprasternal notch. The deep fascia is divided vertically in the midline, separating the strap muscles. If more exposure is required, the strap muscles can be divided; in such a case the anterior jugular veins also require ligation.

Control of blood supply

Each lobe in turn is now delivered outside, and the blood vessels supplying it ligated. At the upper pole of the lobe the superior thyroid artery is ligated and divided. In the proximal part of its course this artery is accompanied by the external branch of the superior laryngeal nerve; therefore it is ligated low down, close to the thyroid, to avoid injury to the nerve, which results in loss of the characteristic quality (timbre) of the voice. At the middle of the outer border of the lobe, the middle thyroid vein enters the internal jugular vein. It is next ligated and divided, and allows a more complete delivery of the lobe. The inferior thyroid artery is now located, running across from behind the carotid sheath to the thyroid lobe. When it is traced towards the thyroid the recurrent laryngeal nerve comes into view, which runs upwards either through or behind the branches of the artery. The artery is ligated in continuity to reduce the blood supply to the lobe. If, instead, branches of the artery are ligated after they have given off supply to the parathyroid glands, postoperative parathyroid deficiency is prevented. Finally, the inferior thyroid veins are ligated and divided at the lower pole of the thyroid.

Resection

The blood supply having been controlled, the desired amount of the lobe is now removed, being sectioned off with a knife or scissors. In a subtotal lobectomy three to six grams of thyroid tissue is left behind on either side. This confers two incidental benefits:

- It protects the recurrent laryngeal nerve from injury.
- This part of the lobe contains the parathyroid glands, so they are protected from inadvertent removal.

Bleeding points on the cut surface of the lobe are next ligated or coagulated by diathermy. The cut surface may now be sutured over.

In *total lobectomy* the whole lobe is removed, care being taken to avoid injury to the recurrent laryngeal nerve. If both lobes are being removed completely, tetany very commonly results. Therefore, one or more parathyroids are dissected out of the posterior border of the thyroid lobe, sliced, and implanted in the neck muscles, whose rich blood supply often ensures survival and function of the grafted parathyroid tissue.

In a *near-total thyroidectomy* a small amount of thyroid is left on the contralateral side to protect the parathyroid glands and recurrent nerve.

Postoperative complications

Thyroidectomy can be followed by serious complications:

- *Hemorrhage* A ligature on the superior thyroid artery may slip; alternatively, bleeding may take place from a thyroid remnant or a thyroid vein. If the blood has already compressed the trachea and produced dyspnoea the sutures should be removed in the ward to relieve the pressure, before taking the patient to the theatre for evacuation of the hematoma, followed by visualization and control of the bleeding point.
- *Respiratory obstruction* The most common cause of respiratory obstruction is laryngeal edema, which itself may be due either to a hematoma or trauma to the larynx by anesthetic intubation. If evacuation of the hematoma does not immediately relieve the obstruction, an endotracheal tube should be passed at once and may require to be left in place for a few days.
- *Recurrent laryngeal nerve paralysis* This may be transient or permanent. In unilateral injury the voice is husky. Bilateral injury is much more serious because both cords can assume a medial position and cause airway obstruction. Often tracheostomy is required.
- *Thyroid insufficiency* This can develop after a subtotal or total thyroidectomy. It comes on imperceptibly and may be difficult to recognize.
- *Parathyroid insufficiency* This is rarely the result of removal of all the parathyroid glands, but more commonly due to disruption of their blood supply. It can be minimized by ligating the branches of the inferior thyroid artery on the thyroid capsule distal to their supply of the parathyroid glands. Symptoms include circumoral numbness and tingling in the fingers and toes. The serum calcium level should be measured daily for a few days. In patients with symptoms 1g (10ml of 10%) calcium gluconate should be given i.v. over 10 minutes, followed by several grams in each liter of i.v. solution. Oral calcium should also be started (2 to 4 g calcium carbonate daily).
- *Thyroid Storm.* This is a condition mostly associated with surgery in an inadequately prepared patient. It is accompanied by fever, central nervous system agitation or depression and cardiovascular dysfunction. It is due to release of the thyroid hormone into the circulation during surgery. In the past thyroid storm had a high mortality rate.

Treatment. The condition needs to be managed in an intensive care unit setting:

- Corticosteroids are given intravenously and constitute the main stay of therapy. They are helpful in preventing adrenal exhaustion and blocking hepatic thyroid hormone conversion.
- An intravenous beta blocker (propranolol 40mg 6 hourly) is given to reduce peripheral T4 to T3 conversion and decrease the hyperthyroid symptoms.
- Carbamizole 15mg blocks the formation of new thyroid hormone and reduces peripheral conversion of T4 to T3.
- To decrease iodine uptake and thyroid hormone secretion, intravenous sodium iodate or Lugol's iodine are administered.
- The patient is given supplemental oxygen and intravenous hemodynamic support.
- Non-aspirin compounds can be used to treat pyrexia.
- Digoxin is given for uncontrolled atrial fibrillation.
- Sedation is also an essential part of therapy.

Chapter

49 PARATHYROIDS AND ADRENALS

Parathyroids

Anatomy

Generally there are four parathyroid glands present in the body, two being located along the posterior border of each lobe. These are the superior parathyroid glands (dorsal to the recurrent laryngeal nerve) and the inferior glands (ventral to the nerve). Normally they are light brown in color. each measuring around 7mm. They are present in loose tissue or fat, therefore during surgery it is difficult to distinguish them from the surrounding fat.

Location

The position of the superior parathyroid glands is relatively constant, 80% being present near the posterior aspect of the upper and middle thyroid lobes. The commonest site of the inferior glands is within 1cm from a point centered where the inferior thyroid artery and recurrent laryngeal nerve cross. Approximately 15% of inferior glands are found in the thymus, or the chest.

HYPOPARATHYROIDISM

Hypoparathyroidism is defined as a condition caused by greatly reduced or absent function of the parathyroid gland. A wide variety of conditions may lead to this problem:

- The commonest cause of hypoparathyroidism is total thyroidectomy.
- Temporary hypocalcemia following thyroid procedures is usually due to ischemia of the parathyroid glands.
- Sometimes hypoparathyroidism is a result of subtotal resection or total parathyroidectomy.
- Tetany in the first few days of life may be seen in an infant born of a mother suffering from undiagnosed hypoparathyroidism.

Clinical features

Symptoms

Post-hypoparathyroidism hypocalcemia causes a decrease in ionized calcium and the patients exhibit increased neuromuscular excitability. Initially they suffer from tingling and numbness around the mouth and fingertips. There may be anxiety, confusion, and depression. In extreme cases cramps in the hands and feet are very painful.

Symptoms usually appear on the second or third postoperative day, and often clear up in a few days or weeks. Such events should be anticipated; if the patient is not managed appropriately the condition may prove fatal.

Signs

On examination Trousseau's sign and Chvostek's sign are positive. Tonic-clonic seizures, carpopedal spasm, and laryngeal stridor are suggestive of tetany induced by hypoparathyroidism.

Carpopedal spasm

The extended fingers are flexed at their metacarpophalangeal joints, with the thumb strongly adducted. The toes are plantar flexed and the ankle joints extended. Tonic and clonic convulsions of the respiratory muscles and laryngeal stridor cause great distress, and may prove fatal. In chronic hypoparathyroidism cataracts and mental changes may occur.

In mild cases of hypocalcemia, tetany may be precipitated by one of the following tests:

- ***Trousseau's sign.*** A sphygmomanometer cuff applied to the arm and inflated above the systolic pressure for about two minutes produces carpo-pedal spasm.
- ***Chvostek's sign.*** Tapping over the branches of the facial nerve at the angle of the jaw produces twitching of the corners of the mouth, the alae of the nose, and the eyelids.

Treatment

Management of these patients includes oral calcium and vitamin D supplements; IV calcium infusion is rarely required except in patients with preoperative osteitis fibrosa cystica.

Acute cases

In these cases the slow intravenous injection of 10 to 20ml of a 10% solution of calcium gluconate rapidly relieves the symptoms. This should be repeated until the patient's serum calcium level becomes stabilized.

Long-term management

For long-term management the absorption of calcium is enhanced by oral administration of the most active metabolite of vitamin-D, namely dihydoxycholecalciferol. This substance accelerates the active absorption of calcium and phosphorus, raising the calcium level to normal in a few days.

HYPERPARATHYROIDISM

Hyperparathyroidism, or excessive secretion of parathyroid hormone, occurs in three different forms:

Primary hyperparathyroidism

The cause of this condition is:

- Commonly a parathyroid adenoma.
- Sometimes hyperplasia of the parathyroids.
- Rarely a parathyroid carcinoma.

Unlike secondary hyperparathyroidism, the excessive parathyroid secretion here is not a response to a lowered serum calcium concentration; it is an unstimulated and inappropriately high level of parathormone due to an autonomous tumor or hyperplasia.

Secondary hyperparathyroidism

In this condition the excessive secretion of the parathyroid occurs in response to a low serum calcium concentration; this in turn may be due to:

- Insufficient absorption of calcium from the gut.
- One of the malabsorption syndromes.
- Excessive urinary excretion of calcium in chronic renal failure.

All four parathyroid glands are involved.

Tertiary hyperparathyroidism

This is a further stage of reactive hyperplasia, where the parathyroids become autonomous, as they no longer respond to physiological stimuli. It mostly occurs in cases of renal transplantation.

PRIMARY HYPERPARATHYROIDISM

Primary hyperparathyroidism is a disorder involving autonomous parathyroid hormone secretion which is independent of the negative feedback regulation by serum calcium. Increased parathormone causes reduced renal calcium clearance, increased intestinal absorption of calcium, and increased production of vitamin D3, and the patient eventually presents clinically with hypercalcemia or the sequelae of longstanding hypercalcemia. The condition occurs twice as often in women as in men, and its incidence peaks in the sixth decade.

Clinical features

The mode of presentation varies a great deal from asymptomatic to the classical features of stones, bones, tones, abdominal groans and pschiatric moans:

- There may be *no symptoms*; in the advanced countries the most common presentation is the detection of unsuspected hypercalcemia by routine biochemical scanning employing multichannel chemical analyzers.
- There may be *non-specific symptoms*, e.g. polyuria, thirst, anorexia, weight loss, and muscle weakness. If such symptoms cannot be explained, the serum calcium level should be determined.
- There may be *generalized decalcification of bones* along with cysts (the 'osteitis fibrosa cystica' of the past). Early radiographic changes appear in the phalanges, consisting of subperiosteal erosions and osteoporosis. Therefore, if the condition is suspected the phalanges are x-rayed.
- *Kidney stones* may be present. Hyperparathyroidism must be considered in every case of renal calculus, especially in the case of recurrent stones.
- *Dyspepsia* may be present, due to a peptic ulcer or pancreatitis. These two conditions are commonly seen along with hyperparathyroidism, although the association has not been explained. For surgeons it is important because these patients have an increased incidence of cholelithiasis, probably due to an increase in biliary calcium leading to the formation of calcium bilirubinate stones.
- *Psychiatric cases* may have hyperparathyroidism as the underlying cause. If hypercalcemia is severe the patient may suffer from psychosis, obtundation, or coma, while in milder cases there may be tiredness, listlessness, depression, anxiety and other personality changes. The clinician should remain on his guard, in order not to miss the correct diagnosis.

On *physical examination* nothing abnormal may be found, except for any pathological fractures or bony swellings.

Differential diagnosis

Hypercalcemia is caused by a variety of conditions. Hyperparathyroidism along with malignancy is responsible for over 90% of cases of hypercalcemia. Malignancies associated with hyperparathyroidism include bone metastases and soft tissue tumors (lung, breast, kidney, head and neck, and ovary).

It is easy to differentiate hyperparathyroidism from other causes clinically and with appropriate investigations.

Investigations

Biochemical assays

Increased serum calcium with intact parathormone or two-site parathormone levels and reduced urinary calcium levels are almost diagnostic of primary hyperparathyroidism.

- ***Calcium.*** *The plasma calcium is estimated* (normal 2.35–2.55mmol/l) Calcium is mainly bound to albumin so its levels in the serum are directly related to plasma albumin levels. It is therefore mandatory to estimate the plasma albumin (normal 35–50g/l) in conjunction with serum calcium. Any alterations in the albumin level have to be taken into account and the plasma calcium corrected accordingly.
- ***Phosphorus.*** The plasma phosphorus is estimated (normal 1.0–1.5mmol/l). Parathormone inhibits renal tubular reabsorption of phosphorus, thus promoting urinary excretion of phosphorus and leading to hypophosphotaemia..
- ***Serum alkaline phosphatase.*** 10% of patients may show increased levels which indicates high bone turnover.

Immunoradiometric assay (IRMA)

This test is carried out for parathyroid hormone (PTH) (normal 0.9–5.4 pmol/l).

X-rays

Abdominal x-rays may show renal calculi or nephrocalcinosis. *High*-definition x-rays of the hand may show subperiosteal erosions in the middle or terminal phalanges.

Hydrocortisone suppression test

If steroids (hydrocortisone 40mg thrice daily) are given for 10 days, normally the plasma calcium level is suppressed, but not so in hyperparathyroidism.

Ruling out 2ndary hyperparathyroidism

The following tests are next carried out to rule out different causes of secondary hyperparathyroidism:

- *Plasma electrophoresis.* This is carried out to exclude myeloma.
- *Serum TSH and T3* levels are determined to exclude thyrotoxicosis.
- Biopsy is performed to rule out sarcoidosis.

Localization tests

Localization is generally not required if parathyroid surgery is not planned but once it is decided to perform resection a battery of tests can be used to facilitate surgery. The advantages of localization include:

- Lower morbidity rates (hypoparathyroidism and recurrent laryngeal injury).
- Decreased operative times.
- Reduced duration of hospital stay.
- Improved cosmetic outcomes.
- Better cost effectiveness.

Localization by imaging and blood tests

The following imaging tests help in localization of the adenoma:

- *CT scan.* Very high resolution is required.
- *MRI.* This may prove more sensitive.
- *Radioactive subtraction scan.* This method of isotope scanning is quite interesting. Technetium is taken up by the thyroid, while thallium is taken up both by the thyroid and the parathyroids. Technetium 99m is first given and a scan carried out to outline the thyroid. Next, thallium 201 is administered which is taken up by both thyroid and parathyroids, and another scan is performed. A computer now subtracts the digital figures representing the thyroid image from the those of the thyroid plus parathyroids. The enlarged parathyroid remains as a 'hot spot'.
- *Barium swallow.* This may show indentation of the esophagus by an adenoma.
- *Catheterization of the parathyroid veins* to measure parathormone. This is usually reserved for cases where previous operation has failed to localize the adenoma.

Tests before re-exploration

If *re-exploration* is required, the following tests may be carried out:

- High frequency neck ultrasound identifies three quarters of enlarged glands.
- Technetium-99m labeled sestamibi (MIBI) also detects a similar number of abnormal glands; further, it discovers glands in the mediastinum which ultrasound cannot.

- Single photon emission computed tomography (SPECT) gives a 3-D image which is useful for orientation before surgery.

A combination of ultrasound and MIBI allows accurate localization.

These tests are not indicated for first-time neck exploration.

Treatment

The only curative treatment is surgical removal of the overactive gland or glands.

In *mild* hyperparathyroidism the following are helpful:

- A low calcium diet.
- Avoidance of diuretics and lithium which aggravate dehydration and hypercalcemia.
- Calcium reducing agents e.g. biphosphonates.

Hypercalcemic crisis

If the serum calcium level rises above 16mg/dl, confusion, nausea and abdominal pain can occur, with cardiac arrhythmias, hypotension and acute renal failure, followed by severe vomiting, dehydration, oliguria, and finally coma. This is sometimes called acute hyperparathyroidism or parathyroid crisis, but since it occurs during hypercalcemia from any cause (for example in advanced breast cancer), it is better referred to as hypercalcemic crisis.

Treatment should be with intravenous saline and biphosphonate therapy (pamidronate), to correct the dehydration and hypercalcemia, in an intensive care unit. Patients whose hypercalcemia is not due to hyperparathyroidism should be treated by a medical regimen to lower the serum calcium concentration.

Indications for parathyroidectomy

The indications for parathyroidectomy in primary hyperparathyroidism include:

- Kidney stones.
- Reduced bone density.
- Deteriorating kidney function.
- High serum calcium.
- Symptoms of hypercalcemia.

In symptomatic patients the indication for operation is clear cut. However, patients in whom hypercalcemia has been discovered incidentally, e.g. during routine screening, are often asymptomatic and the decision to proceed with operation is more difficult.

There is a general consensus that with renal disease or bone involvement, surgery is indicated, as there is no medical treatment. Apart from this:

- Those patients who are *asymptomatic* should receive careful follow-up; if renal, bony or other symptoms appear, surgical treatment should be undertaken.
- If the plasma calcium is mildly raised, most researchers feel that if even *mild symptoms* of hypercalcemia, are present, parathyroidectomy should be carried out.
- Since the advent of minimal access techniques, clinicians are more inclined to recommend parathyroidectomy because of lower operative morbidity.

Surgery

Adenomas, either single or multiple, are removed. If all four glands are hyperplastic, three and a half glands are removed, leaving half a gland with intact blood supply. If it is desired to avoid repeated potentially difficult explorations of the neck, parathyroid tissue can be successfully autotransplanted into the muscles of the forearm in the form of eight to ten fragments of 1 cu mm each. Parathyroid surgery should be performed only by surgeons with both proper training and experience.

Prognosis

With successful surgery, bones recalcify and pseudotumors resolve. Kidney stones do not disappear, but the incidence of recurrence after surgical removal is reduced and deterioration in renal function prevented. Psychiatric patients often show a remarkable recovery.

Adrenal Glands

Anatomy

There are two adrenal glands located one on top of each kidney. Each gland consists of a cortex and a medulla. The glands are supplied by the superior, middle and inferior adrenal arteries which are branches of the inferior phrenic artery, aorta and the renal arteries respectively. These vessels form a rich plexus beneath the capsule and during adrenalectomy need to be dissected out carefully before ligation and division. The venous drainage of each gland is by a single adrenal vein. The right adrenal vein is short and drains directly into the inferior vena cava, so care is required while ligating it.

ADRENAL CORTEX

Hypocorticism

Adrenocortical insufficiency may be acute or chronic.

Acute hypocorticism

Acute adrenocortical insufficiency arises due to bilateral adrenal infarction. The common situations in which it occurs include the following:

- In the newborn, after a long and difficult labour.
- In cases of fulminating sepsis, commonly meningococcal, but occasionally streptococcal, staphylococcal or pneumococcal; this is called the Waterhouse-Friderichsen syndrome.
- After major and extensive surgery, especially in cases suffering from intra-abdominal sepsis, pneumonia, coagulation defects and cancer.

Clinical features

The blood pressure falls precipitously, and the patient goes into a severe state of shock. Other evidence of acute adrenal failure is seen in the form of vomiting, diarrhea and mental confusion. In cases of septicemia, hyperpyrexia and rigors may be seen, along with petechial hemorrhages and purpuric patches. Eosinophilia is very suggestive, but the most useful laboratory finding is a low plasma cortisol.

Treatment

Treatment consists of the intravenous administration of hydrocortisone hemisuccinate. 100mg is first given very rapidly in 500ml of isotonic saline, and is repeated in about an hour. If there is a response, it should be continued in a dose of 50mg every 6 hours. When the patient's condition is stabilized, treatment with a synthetic oral steroid should be substituted. In cases with sepsis, appropriate antibiotic therapy must be immediately started by the intravenous route.

Chronic hypocorticism (Addison's disease)

This condition occurs due to adrenocortical deficiency from progressive destruction of first the cortex and then the medulla of the adrenal glands. The most common cause is supposed to be an autoimmune disease, other causes being tuberculosis, metastatic carcinoma and amyloidosis.

Clinical features

Addison's disease is most often seen in young adults. The leading features are muscular weakness and a low blood pressure. Increased pigmentation is seen at points of pressure and at the flexion creases. The mucous membrane of the mouth becomes pigmented. Episodes of acute adrenal insufficiency occur from time to time.

Treatment

The treatment is medical. Most patients need 20 to 30mg of cortisone daily in divided doses, along with 0.05mg fludrocortisone as mineralocorticoid replacement. If an excess of the drugs is given there is hypertension, hyperkalaemia and edema; if enough is not given there is fatigue and hypotension. By the use of cortisone, the patient's life expectancy is greatly increased.

Hypercorticism

Cushing syndrome

Etiology

Cushing syndrome consists of a set of symptoms and signs which is caused by excessive hydrocortisone concentrations. The causes of the syndrome include the following conditions:

- Most often, Cushing syndrome results from the *long-term administration of corticosteroids*, in the treatment of different illnesses specially rheumatoid arthritis, and in patients receiving transplants, where steroids are given to suppress the rejection of the transplant.
- The next most common cause of the syndrome is *Cushing disease*, which is produced as follows: a basophil adenoma of the anterior pituitary secretes an excess of adrenocorticotrophic hormone (ACTH). This leads to hyperplasia of the adrenal cortex and hypersecretion of hydrocortisone (cortisol) resulting in the signs and symptoms of Cushing syndrome.
- Rarely, certain *non-adrenal neoplasms may secrete* ACTH leading to Cushing syndrome. Sometimes it may be part of MEN-I (multiple endocrine neoplasia-I) where the symptoms may be the result of:
    - o ACTH-secreting primary adrenal neoplasms.
    - o Ectopic ACTH-secreting carcinoid tumors.
    - o Pituitary tumors.
- Cushing syndrome can be caused by an adrenocortical adenoma or carcinoma, which secretes hydrocortisone independently of ACTH control.

Causes of cushing syndrome

ACTH-dependent:

- Pituitary adenoma.
- Ectopic ACTH production.
- Ectopic Corticotrophin Releasing Hormone (CRH) production.

ACTH-independent:

- Adrenal hyperplasia (micronodular or macronodular).
- Adrenal adenoma.
- Adrenal carcinoma.

Other:

- Pseudo-Cushing syndrome.
- Iatrogenic: exogenous administration of steroids.

Clinical features

Cushing syndrome is most often seen in young females, in whom there is an excessive deposition of fat in certain unusual situations. The face becomes rounded like a full moon, the abdomen becomes protuberant, the neck is thick, and the supraclavicular fossae are obliterated. The arms and legs are thin, and the patient complains of increasing weakness. As the corticosteroids inhibit fibrous tissue, the skin becomes inelastic and feels like tissue-paper. Purple striae are seen on the abdomen, and the patient bruises easily. There is increased growth of hair, and acne is common. Amenorrhoea is frequent and in the male, impotence.

Due to a negative calcium balance severe osteoporosis occurs, and pathological fractures commonly result. Mild glycosuria is often seen and hypertension is frequent, often resulting in congestive cardiac failure. In more than half the cases a psychosis eventually supervenes. Cushing syndrome is rare in children; when it occurs, an adrenal tumor is usually the cause.

To sum up, the clinical features of Cushing syndrome include:

Weight gain.

Supraclavicular pads of fat.

Hypertension.

Hirsutism, purple striae, acne.

Emotional lability, psychosis, depression.

Generalized weakness, osteopenia.

Diabetes, hyperlipidemia.

Decreased libido, menstrual irregularities.

Adrenogenital syndrome

A condition similar to Cushing syndrome is the adrenogenital syndrome, which is caused by an excessive secretion of adrenal androgens, and commences in females shortly after puberty. The onset of amenorrhoea is followed by excessive growth of hair on the face, acne, atrophy of the breasts and muscular development, with deepening of the voice and enlargement of the clitoris.

Investigations

In Cushing syndrome:

- Cortisol levels in the plasma in the morning and at midnight are raised.
- 24-hour urinary cortisol excretion is not suppressed by administration of dexamethasone.
- ACTH-dependent and ACTH-independent disease are distinguished from each other by serum ACTH levels.

In 80–90% of cases raised ACTH levels indicate a pituitary tumor, necessitating an MRI of the pituitary. If this is negative, the abdomen and chest should be examined by a CT scan to detect an ectopic ACTH-producing neoplasm.

Treatment

ACTH-producing tumors

- ACTH-producing pituitary tumors are treated by resection through the trans-sphenoidal route or by radiotherapy.
- An ectopic ACTH-producing tumor will require resection.

Adrenal tumors and hyperplasia

- A unilateral adenoma requires adrenalectomy.
- A carcinoma necessitates radical resection. Postoperative radiotherapy and cytotoxic chemotherapy improve survival.
- Bilateral adrenal hyperplasia is treated by bilateral adrenalectomy.

ADRENAL MEDULLA

Tumors

Tumors of the adrenal medulla include:

- Tumors of the sympathetic neurones:
    - o Ganglioneuroma.
    - o Neuroblastoma.
- Tumor of chromaffin cells, namely phaeochromocytoma.

Ganglioneuroma

Ganglioneuroma is a tumor of the sympathetic neurons and arises from the neural crest cells. This tumor can occur at any age below 60 years. It is symptomless, and can slowly grow to a large size. Only a small percentage occur in the adrenal medulla, the remainder arise anywhere along the sympathetic chain. Pathologically, ganglioneuromas are solid, firm tumors that typically are white when seen with the naked eye. Most often they are found incidentally by CT or MRI performed for another condition.

Treatment is by surgical excision. If this tumor is removed early, a cure can be expected.

Neuroblastoma

A neuroblastoma of the adrenal medulla arises in infants and children. It is a reddish-grey tumor that is highly malignant. It grows rapidly to a large size, filling nearly the whole abdomen, and although arising on one side, extends across the midline. At this stage it can be confused with a Wilms' tumor (nephroblastoma), which is the other common large-sized abdominal tumor of infancy. The nodular feel of the neuroblastoma may help the distinction, because the Wilms' tumor has a smooth surface.

Unusual biological behavior

- Occasionally, a neuroblastoma exhibits rather curious behaviour. Sometimes a baby is brought when his tumor is so advanced that only a piece is removed for biopsy. However, the tumor undergoes spontaneous remission, so much so that even the secondaries disappear.
- Again, if the case is borderline between ganglioneuroma and neuroblastoma, and large doses of folic acid are given, the tumor sometimes becomes converted into a ganglioneuroma and the prognosis is improved.

Investigations

Imaging

Ultrasonography

This distinguishes neuroblastoma (solid and extrarenal) from cystic lesions and renal tumors.

X-ray

X-ray detection of calcification in the tumor suggests neuroblastoma. *Skeletal survey* and *chest x-ray* are essential to detect possible metastases.

Table 49.1 Staging of neuroblastoma

Stage I
Confined to organ of origin and totally excised
Stage II
Extends beyond organ but not across midline
Stage III
Extends across midline
Stage IV
Distant metastases
Stage IVs
Primary tumor localized; disseminated only to liver, skin or marrow

CT scan

This gives good anatomical data about the tumor.

MRI

This provides the same, as well as evidence of vascular involvement and extension into the spinal cord.

Laboratory tests

MIBG (*m-iodobenzyl guanidine)* resembles adrenaline, and is specifically taken up by neurectodermal tumors. Labelled with ^{123}I it is used for localizing the primary tumor as well as for detecting residual and metastatic disease.

Monoclonal antibodies to neuroblastoma are available and can be radiolabelled for similar purposes.

Neuroblastomas produce high levels of *catecholamines* and their metabolites:

- A vanilmandelic acid spot test is used for screening.
- The metabolites can be quantified by analysis of a 24-hour urine collection. The higher the ratio of vanilmandelic acid to homovanilic acid the better the prognosis.

Staging

A staging system for neuroblastoma is presented in Table 49.1.

Treatment

The recommended treatment regimes for neuroblastoma in the different stages are given in Table 49.2.

Prognosis

This depends upon the factors presented in Table 49.3.

Patients with early, intermediate and late tumors have

Table 49.2 Treatment regimens for neuroblastoma in the different stages

Stage	Treatment
Stage I:	Total excision alone
Stage II:	Total excision +-chemo and/or radiotherapy
Stage III:	Resectable tumors: excision + chemo + radiotherapy Unresectable tumors: cyto-reduction with chemo and radiotherapy, followed by excision of shrunken tumor
Stage IV:	Combination chemotherapy. If response, excise residual tumor
Stage IVs:	Excision of primary tumor

Note: A rapidly enlarging liver may embarrass respiration. It should be treated as follows:

- o By low dose irradiation, or.
- o By enlarging the abdominal cavity temporarily by putting a silastic patch in the abdominal wall.

Table 49.3 Prognostic factors in neuroblastoma

Factors	Good prognosis	Poor prognosis
-Age	< 1 year	> 1 year
-Stage	I and II (all ages) III (if >1 year)	III and IVs(if<1 Year) IV (all ages)
-DNA content	Euploidy	Hyperploidy
-Histology	Differentiated	Undifferentiated
-Urinary catecholamine metabolites	Low HVA:VM	High HVA:VM

3-year survival rates of 90, 80 and 30 % respectively, showing the importance of early diagnosis.

Pheochromocytoma

Pheochromocytomas are tumors of the adrenal medulla and related chromaffin tissues elsewhere in the body that release epinephrine, norepinephrine, or both, resulting in episodic or intermittent hypertension, and other symptoms of catecholamine secretion. They occur in two forms:

- Sporadically as isolated tumors in patients with no other disease.
- As part of a multiple endocrine neoplasia syndrome (MEN-II), in which the other neoplasms include:
  - o Medullary carcinoma of the thyroid.
  - o Neurofibromas.
  - o Ganglioneuromas.
  - o Hyperparathyroidism.

Pathology

Pheochromocytomas are reddish-brown vascular tumors. They feel firm but may be multicystic, and necrotic areas are common. Although the tumor is benign, the veins and the capsule may be invaded.

Clinical features

The clinical features in cases of pheochromocytoma are very variable. Therefore it is recommended that every new case of hypertension should be investigated to exclude pheochromocytoma as the cause. In actual fact, however, this tumor makes up only 0.5% of all the cases of hypertension.

The classic *symptoms* are those one would expect from an injection of epinephrine. They include:

- Episodic hypertension.
- Pallor followed by flushing.
- Palpitations.
- Headache.
- Excessive perspiration.
- Nervousness and anxiety.

In about half the cases, phaeochromocytomas cause *sustained* hypertension with or without evidence of excessive catecholamine secretion.

The usual *signs* include:

- Tachycardia.
- Retinopathy.
- Emotional lability.
- Weight loss.

The clinical findings may mimic hyperthyroidism. Excessive secretion of epinephrine raises the blood glucose level and therefore may be confused with diabetes mellitus.

Investigations

Biochemical tests

- Levels of the products of breakdown of adrenaline and noradrenaline, namely metanephrine and normetanephrine, are determined in a 24-hour urine collection, and levels upto 30 times greater than the normal will be found in patients suffering from the condition.

- Plasma-free levels of metanephrine and normetanephrine are also raised.

Localization of the tumor

MRI is preferable, because the agent used for a CT scan with contrast may cause seizures in this condition. Single-photon emission tomography (SPECT) detects both tumors and metastases.

Differential diagnosis

The differential diagnosis of phaeochromocytoma includes:

- Different causes of hypertension.
- Hyperthyroidism.
- Acute attacks of anxiety.
- Carcinoid syndrome.

Complications

The complications of phaeochromocytoma are usually the sequelae of hypertension i.e.:

- Stroke.
- Renal failure.
- Myocardial infarction.
- Cardiac decompensation.

Treatment

Medical

Once the biochemical diagnosis is established, treatment with an *alpha-blocker* should be started. The aim of treatment is to control the blood pressure and protect the patient from the danger of a severe hypertensive attack with its potential complications. Phenoxybenzamine is the usual drug employed for this purpose. Propranolol, a *beta-blocker*, is useful when cardiac arrhythmias are present, but should only be given after the patient has received an alpha-blocker, otherwise a hypertensive crisis may occur.

Inspite of the above measures abrupt changes in pulse rate and blood pressure may occur and require sudden administration of *pressors* or *vasodilators*.

Surgical

The definitive treatment of phaeochromocytoma is *excision*. Tumors up to 8cm in diameter can be removed laparoscopically, those above this size need an open operation. An arterial catheter and continuous ECG should be employed, for constant monitoring of the arterial pressure and heart action.

Phentolamine or nitroprusside and propranolol should be immediately available to treat sudden hypertension or cardiac arrhythmias that often occur when the tumor is manipulated. The surgeon should ligate the adrenal veins early in the procedure to avoid these crises. The results of surgery for the usual benign tumors are very gratifying. Although some hypertension commonly persists, it is easily treated with drugs.

Chapter

50 SKIN

Naevi

Definition

A naevus is a circumscribed stable malformation of the skin which is not due to external causes and is therefore presumed to be of hereditary origin. It is a hamartomatous malformation of the skin. (A hamartoma is a benign tumor-like nodule composed of an overgrowth of mature cells that normally occur in the part, but with one element predominating).

Naevi may be composed of epidermal or dermal elements.

Epidermal naevi are wart-like papules which may form linear plaques. They are asymptomatic and have little effect on the general health.

Connective tissue naevi are firm, flesh-coloured papules. They are harmless and are excised for cosmetic reasons.

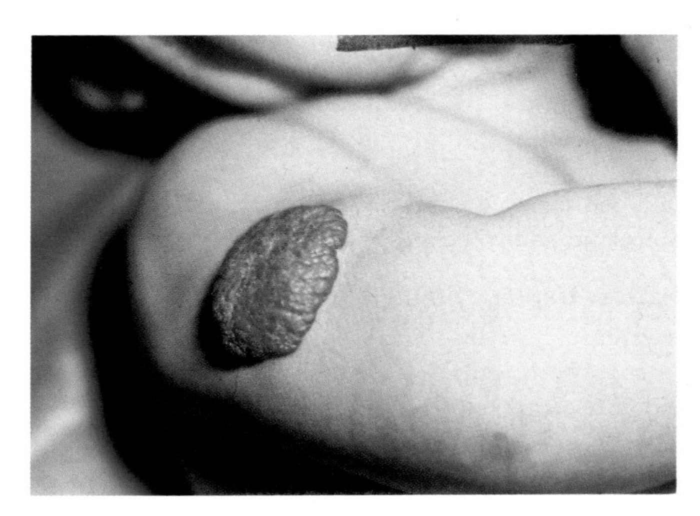

Fig.50.1 Strawberry hemangioma upper arm in a young child

Hemangiomas

Hemangiomas are proliferations of vascular elements. Their endothelium-lined vascular spaces are commonly capillary-sized, but large 'cavernous' spaces are also found. The most common types of hemangiomas include strawberry and cavernous hemangiomas:

Strawberry hemangiomas

These may be present at birth, but more commonly appear during the first few weeks of life (Fig.50.1). They are lobular, bright red nodules with a spongy consistency, so that blood can be compressed out of them. The surface is studded with small capillary tufts so that the lesion resembles a strawberry.

Treatment

These lesions seldom require treatment, because the vast majority involute spontaneously by the age of about 6 years. However:

- Treatment may be required for lesions situated on the eyelids, nose or lips, where they cause functional impairment.
- Rapidly growing strawberry hemangiomas are usually first treated by corticosteroids, which may stimulate gradual involution.

Cavernous hemangiomas

These also may present at birth and grow rapidly during the first few months of life, after which they involute spontaneously. They are situated just beneath the skin and appear as soft, bluish masses. A typical strawberry hemangioma may form the cutaneous component of a cavernous hemangioma.

Emptying sign

In infants, in the case of every soft swelling, the possiblity of hemangioma should be excluded by testing the swelling for the 'emptying' sign, which is a hallmark of a hemangioma. Firm, continuous pressure should be applied to see if the swelling empties. The importance of carrying out the test is this: most hemangiomas in infants, after enlarging for some time, regress spontaneously over a period of months. Therefore, specially if they are located in the vicinity of important structures which

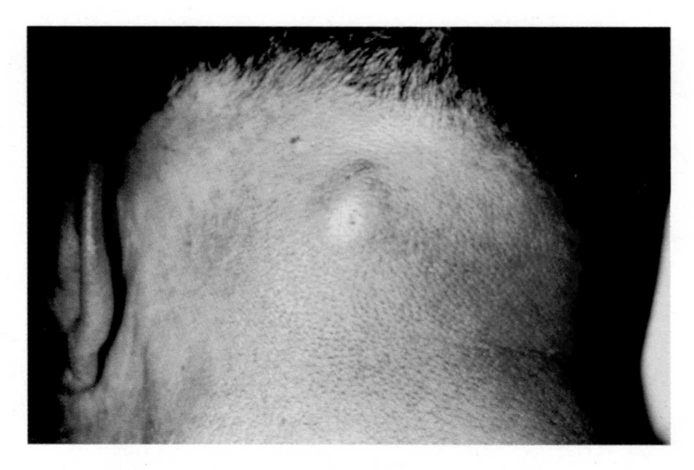

Fig.50.2 Sebaceous cyst back of neck showing punctum.

could be damaged by the dissection, they should be left well alone, and will regress with time.

Platelet-trapping hemangioma

A problem can arise if a hemangioma is very large, because the blood flows through its spaces sluggishly, and platelets get trapped in the mass. When this happens on a massive scale, the thrombocytopenia results in a bleeding tendency. When this bleeding takes place in the hemangioma itself, the mass continues to enlarge, and specially if located in the vicinity of the trachea, may produce respiratory obstruction. Such a condition is called a platelet-trapping hemangioma.

Cysts

Epidermal (sebaceous) cysts

These cysts, which are commonly known as sebaceous cysts, are the most common cysts of the skin. The most frequent sites are the scalp, face and back. They may be solitary or multiple, and present as 0.5 to 3cm spherical, slightly compressible intradermal masses. A follicular orifice, the 'punctum', usually connects the cyst to the skin surface at the dome of the cyst (Fig.50.2). The wall consists of stratified squamous epithelium. Desquamated keratin cells are shed into the cavity of the cyst, forming a cheesy white material. Infection can lead to fibrosis of the surrounding dermis and make the cyst difficult to dissect.

Treatment

If the cyst is infected, it should be incised and drained, and later removed about two months after the infection has subsided. It must be removed *in toto* to avoid recurrence.

Pigmented lesions

Benign

These include benign and dysplastic naevi.

Benign naevi

These include junctional, compound and blue naevi. They differ from dysplastic naevi as follows:

- They are usually less than 6mm in diameter.
- They have a uniform colour throughout.
- They possess a sharp, clear-cut border.

Dysplastic naevi

These contain increased numbers of abnormal melanocytes in the epidermis. Around 7 percent of them become melanomas. They:

- are larger in size than benign naevi,
- contain a mixture of light brown and black within the same naevus, and
- have irregular borders.

Dysplastic naevi are markers of increased risk for, or even precursors to, cutaneous melanoma. They should be excised with a good margin.

Neurofibromatosis

This is an inherited disorder which is transmitted as an autosomal dominant. Two types are seen.

- Neurofibromatosis Type 1 occurs approximately once in every 4,000 births. Its common manifestations include multiple cutaneous neurofibromas (Fig.50.3), cafe au lait spots[1], freckles in the axillae and groins, and nodules of the iris.
- Neurofibromatosis Type 2 is less common (one in 100,000 births). It is manifested by multiple intracranial and spinal tumors, specially bilateral acoustic neuromas.

TUMORS

Premalignant

Keratoacanthoma

These tumors appear suddenly and grow rapidly, achieving a diameter of several centimeters within a few weeks. They are benign and typically regress spontaneously within one year. However, the behaviour of large keratoacanthomas is more like that of squamous

1 *Café au lait* (Fr.) coffee with milk. Café au lait spots: pigmented macules of a light brown colour, as in neurofibromatosis and Albright's syndrome

cell carcinomas, with locally destructive growth and the potential for invasion.

The tumor is domed with a central crater containing a keratin plug. Histologically it resembles a squamous cell carcinoma, and differentiation between the two may be difficult. However, unlike the latter tumor its base is flat and it does not show invasion of the deeper dermis. Therefore, the biopsy should extend into the subcutaneous fat so as to include this deeper portion of the tumor. The treatment of choice is surgical excision.

Malignant

Basal cell carcinoma

Basal cell carcinomas contain cells that resemble the basal cell layers of the epidermis. They are locally destructive but rarely metastasize. They are common in males over the age of 40 years and occur mostly on the upper and central parts of the face.The tumor is much commoner in white-skinned persons

Starting as a translucent papule the tumor may assume one of several forms:

- The noduloulcerative type is the most common. When a large ulcer has formed, such a lesion is often called a 'rodent ulcer'.
- Pigmented basal cell carcinomas need to be distinguished by biopsy from melanoma.
- Superficial basal cell cancers form red, scaly lesions difficult to distinguish from other skin conditions.

Basal cell carcinomas are slow growing, and patients often neglect these lesions for years. Metastasis and death are extremely rare, but the tumors cause extensive local destruction.

Treatment

The preferred treatment is surgical excision with a margin of 4–6mm of normal tissue. Histological confirmation that the margins do not contain tumor is required.

Moh's surgery

Around the eyes, nose and ears one may wish to allow less wider margins. In that case Mohs' micrographic surgery has to be employed. The dermatological surgeon carries out the excision, examines the frozen section slides for residual tumor, and removes more skin as required, because the recurrence rate depends entirely on the adequacy of the margins. Mohs' surgery can also be used for cases of squamous cell carcinoma[1].

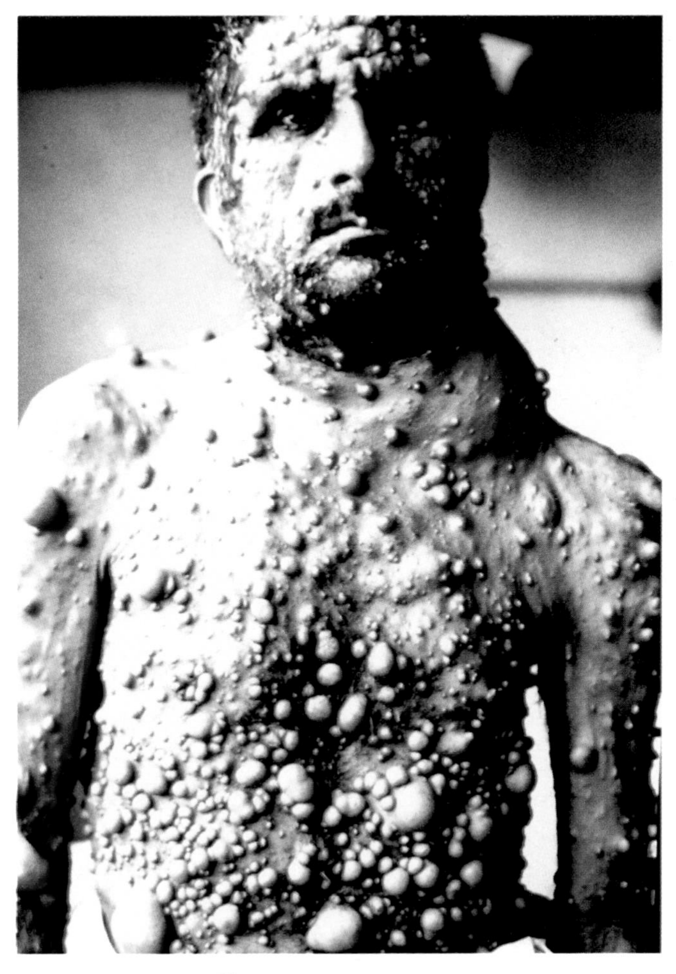

Fig.50.4 Neurofibromatosis

In elderly and frail patients radiation may be employed with recurrence rates similar to surgery.

Squamous cell carcinoma

This tumor arises in the keratinizing cells of the epidermis, and after basal cell carcinoma is the most common malignant tumor of the skin.

Etiology

In white-skinned people it arises most often due to chronic damage by sunlight, most patients being elderly.

It also develops:

- At mucocutaneous interfaces as a result of the use of tobacco or papilloma virus infection.
- At sites treated with radiation.
- In the scars of burns.
- In chronic ulcers of the skin.

1 Interestingly, Mohs' technique was developed as far back as 1938 by Frederic Mohs, a general surgeon.

Table 50.1 Risk factors for cutaneous melanoma (in decreasing order of importance)

Risk factor
Mole exhibiting persistent changes
Dysplastic naevus in patient with family history of melanoma
Family history of melanoma
Dysplastic naevus, no family history
Personal history of melanoma
Caucasian patient
Immunocompromised individual
Excess exposure to sunlight

Tumors caused by sunlight rarely metastasize and usually require only local excision; those due to other factors are aggressive and metastasize frequently. These tumors occur more often in immunosuppressed patients, specially following organ transplantation.

The tumor presents as a nodule or plaque, which may ulcerate. In white-skinned patients the lesions are typically pink or flesh-coloured; in those with darker complexions they may be hypopigmented or hyperpigmented.

Broder's histological grading divides the tumor into grades according to the ratio of de-differentiated and normal cells.

Treatment

Squamous cell carcinomas should be *treated* by excision with a 1cm margin if possible, and the fact that the margins are not involved by tumor confirmed by histological examination. As far as the regional lymph nodes are concerned:

- They should be excised only if clinically palpable (therapeutic lymph node dissection).
- However, lesions arising in chronic wounds behave more aggressively and are more likely to spread to regional lymph nodes. In these cases lymph nodes should be excised even if not palpable (prophylactic lymph node dissection).

Alternatives to surgical therapy include radiation and topical applications of 5-fluorouracil; these should be employed in patients unfit or unwilling for surgery. Distant metastases indicate a poor prognosis.

Cutaneous melanoma

Cutaneous melanoma is malignancy of the pigment producing cell, the melanocyte, which is normally located in the basal layer of the epidermis. It is common in light-skinned Caucasians. Patients used to present late and die rapidly of the disease. However, since the early signs of the disease have been widely publicized, the 5 year survival rates have more than doubled. The most frequent site for cutaneous melanoma is the upper back in men and the lower leg as well as upper back in women. (Table 50.1) lists the risk factors in decreasing order of importance; the highest risk is associated with a persistently changing mole. Increase in size and change in colour are the two most common characteristics of early cutaneous melanoma.

Biopsy

Total excisional biopsy with narrow margins is the procedure of choice for the diagnosis of cutaneous melanoma; this provides the entire specimen for histopathological examination and also provides definitive therapy for benign lesions. Where total excisional biopsy is not easily accomplished, removal of a partial biopsy specimen is a reasonable course of action. Either punch (trephine) or incisional biopsy can be used. When a partial biopsy is performed, biopsy from the most raised portion is usually sufficient for diagnosis. In flat lesions biopsy of the darkest portion produces a representative specimen.

Prognosis

The *thickness of the primary tumor* in millimetres is the single most important prognostic factor in patients with no clinical evidence of disease elsewhere.

Apart from this, the following are associated with a poor prognosis:

- Increased numbers of mitoses.
- The presence of an ulcer.
- The presence of microscopic satellites.

Thus, early recognition followed by prompt surgery offers the best chance of cure.

Treatment. Classical treatment consisted of excision of the tumor with 5cm surgical margins. It has recently been shown that in the case of tumors 1mm or less in thickness 1cm margins are adequate, while in thicker tumors 3cm margins are required; these latter usually require a graft or a flap to resurface the wound.

Lymph node dissection.

- Tumors thinner than 1mm rarely have nodal metastases, so that elective nodal dissection is not considered necessary.

- Tumors thicker than 4mm have systemic metastases, hence node dissection does not improve their prognosis.

Studies are being conducted to determine whether or not melanomas of a thickness of 1.5 to 4mm benefit from lymph node dissection. Until the results are available, elective nodal dissection in these patients should be carried out at the discretion of the surgeon, after discussion with the patient.

Limb perfusion. At specialized centres perfusion of the affected extremity with phenylalanine mustard at elevated temperatures has produced good control of in-transit lesions and satellite lesions. This is accepted as a palliative measure. However, its benefit as an adjuvant in the treatment of primary extremity melanomas has not been established.

In the presence of *disseminated disease* a systemic approach is appropriate, the response to chemotherapy being greatest in the case of tumors in the skin, lymph nodes and lungs.

INDEX

B

C

D

E

F

G

H

I

J

K

L

M

N

O

P

R

S

T

U

V

W

Z